D1560979

BRONCHOSCOPY

BRONCHOSCOPY

Editor

Udaya B. S. Prakash, MD, FRCP(C), FACP, FCCP

Professor of Medicine
Mayo Medical School and
Mayo Graduate School of Medicine
and
Consultant in Thoracic Diseases and Internal Medicine
Director of Bronchoscopy
Mayo Clinic and Mayo Medical Center
Rochester, Minnesota
and
President, *American Association for Bronchology*
Editor-in-Chief, *Journal of Bronchology*
Editor-in-Chief, *Mayo Clinic Proceedings*
Editor, Bronchoscopy Section, *Chest*

Raven Press New York

Raven Press, Ltd., 1185 Avenue of the Americas, New York, New York 10036

Made in the United States of America

Library of Congress Cataloging-in-Publication Data

Bronchoscopy / [edited by] Udaya B. S. Prakash.
p. cm.
Includes bibliographical references and index.
ISBN 0-7817-0095-7
1. Bronchoscopy. 2. Bronchoscopy—Atlases. I. Prakash, Udaya B. S.
[DNLM: 1. Bronchoscopy—atlases. WF 17 B869 1992]
RC734.B7B77 1993
616.2'307545—dc20
DNLM/DLC
for Library of Congress 93-7652
CIP

The material contained in this volume was submitted as previously unpublished material, except in the instances in which some of the illustrative material was derived.

Great care has been taken to maintain the accuracy of the information contained in the volume. However, neither Raven Press nor the editors can be held responsible for errors or for any consequences arising from the use of the information contained herein.

Materials appearing in this book prepared by individuals as part of their official duties as U.S. Government employees are not covered by the above-mentioned copyright.

9 8 7 6 5 4 3 2 1

To
Pushpa
and
Apurva, Anna, and Amita
for their
love, patience, and encouragement

Contents

Contributors

W. Mark Brutinel, M.D. *Assistant Professor of Medicine, Mayo Medical School and Mayo Graduate School of Medicine; Consultant, Thoracic Diseases and Internal Medicine, Mayo Clinic and Mayo Medical Center, 200 First Street, S.W., Rochester, Minnesota 55905*

Sergio Cavaliere, M.D. *Director, Center for Respiratory Endoscopy and Laser Therapy, Pulmonary Division, Spedali Civili, I-25125 Brescia, Italy*

Henri G. Colt, M.D. *Assistant Clinical Professor of Medicine, Division of Pulmonary and Critical Care Medicine, University of California at San Diego, 225 Dickinson Street, San Diego, California 92103*

Denis A. Cortese, M.D. *Professor of Medicine, Mayo Medical School and Mayo Graduate School of Medicine; Consultant, Thoracic Diseases and Internal Medicine, Mayo Clinic Jacksonville, 4500 San Pablo Road, Jacksonville, Florida 32224*

José P. Díaz-Jiménez, M.D. *Head, Endoscopy Laser Unit, Hospital Principes da España, Feixa Llarga s/n, 08907 Hospitalet, Barcelona, Spain*

Jean-François Dumon, M.D. *Hopitaux SUD Sainte Marguerite, 270 Boulevard de Sainte-Marguerite, B.P. 29, 13274 Marseille CEDEX 09, France*

Eric S. Edell, M.D. *Assistant Professor of Medicine, Mayo Medical School and Mayo Graduate School of Medicine; Consultant, Thoracic Diseases and Internal Medicine, Mayo Clinic and Mayo Medical Center, 200 First Street, S.W., Rochester, Minnesota 55905*

Mark H. Ereth, M.D. *Assistant Professor of Anesthesiology, Mayo Medical School and Mayo Graduate School of Medicine; Senior Associate Consultant, Anesthesiology, Mayo Clinic and Mayo Medical School, 200 First Street S.W., Rochester, Minnesota 55905*

Lutz Freitag, M.D. *Assistant Medical Director, Department of Bronchology, Center for Chest Medicine and Thoracic Surgery, Ruhrlandklinik, 43 Essen 16, Germany*

Richard A. Helmers, M.D. *Assistant Professor of Medicine, Mayo Medical School and Mayo Graduate School of Medicine; Consultant, Thoracic Diseases and Internal Medicine, Mayo Clinic Scottsdale, 13400 East Shea Boulevard, Scottsdale, Arizona 85259*

Lauren D. Holinger, M.D. *Professor and Head, Pediatric Otorhinolaryngology, Head Section of Bronchoesophagology, Children's Memorial Hospital, Northwestern University, Box 25, 2300 Children's Plaza, Chicago, Illinois 60614*

Harubumi Kato, M.D., Ph.D. *Professor and Chairman, Department of Surgery, Tokyo Medical College, Vice-President; Tokyo Medical College Hospital, 6-7-1 Nishishinjuku Shinjuku-Ku, Tokyo 160, Japan*

Willane S. Krell, M.D. *Assistant Professor of Medicine, Wayne State University, Harper Hospital, 3990 John R, Detroit, Michigan 48201*

Marsha J. Kulas, R.N. *Charge Nurse, Bronchoscopy, Mayo Medical Center and Rochester Methodist Hospital, 201 W. Center Street, Rochester, Minnesota 55905*

Paul A. Kvale, M.D. *Senior Staff Physician, Pulmonary Division, Henry Ford Hospital, 2799 West Grand Boulevard, Detroit, Michigan 48202*

Robert L. Lennon, D.O. *Associate Professor of Anesthesiology, Mayo Medical School and Mayo Graduate School of Medicine; Consultant, Anesthesiology, Mayo Clinic and Mayo Medical Center, 200 First Street, S.W., Rochester, Minnesota 55905*

John C. McDougall, M.D. *Assistant Professor of Medicine, Mayo Medical School and Mayo Graduate School of Medicine; Consultant, Thoracic Diseases and Internal Medicine, Mayo Clinic and Mayo Medical Center, 200 First Street, S.W., Rochester, Minnesota 55905*

Atul C. Mehta, M.D. *Head, Section of Bronchology, Department of Pulmonary and Critical Care Medicine, Pulmonary Diseases, The Cleveland Clinic Foundation, One Clinic Center, 9500 Euclid Avenue, Cleveland, Ohio 44195*

Jeffrey L. Myers, M.D. *Associate Professor of Pathology, Mayo Medical School and Mayo Graduate School of Medicine; Consultant, Surgical Pathology, Mayo Clinic and Mayo Medical Center, 200 First Street, S.W., Rochester, Minnesota 55905*

David E. Midthun, M.D. *Assistant Professor of Medicine, Mayo Medical School and Mayo Graduate School of Medicine; Senior Associate Consultant, Thoracic Diseases and Internal Medicine, Mayo Clinic and Mayo Medical Center, 200 First Street, S.W., Rochester, Minnesota 55905*

Peter C. Pairolero, M.D. *Professor of Surgery, Mayo Medical School and Mayo Graduate School of Medicine; Consultant, Thoracic and Cardiovascular Surgery; Chairman, Section of Thoracic Surgery, Mayo Clinic and Mayo Medical Center, 200 First Street, S.W., Rochester, Minnesota 55905*

Richard J. Pisani, M.D. *Assistant Professor of Medicine, Mayo Medical School and Mayo Graduate School of Medicine; Consultant, Thoracic Diseases and Internal Medicine, Mayo Clinic and Mayo Medical Center, 200 First Street, S.W., Rochester, Minnesota 55905*

Udaya B. S. Prakash, M.D. *Professor of Medicine, Mayo Medical School and Mayo Graduate School of Medicine; Consultant, Thoracic Diseases and Internal Medicine; Director of Bronchoscopy, Mayo Clinic and Mayo Medical Center, 200 First Street, S.W., Rochester, Minnesota 55905*

David R. Sanderson, M.D. *Professor of Medicine, Mayo Medical School and Mayo Graduate School of Medicine; Chairman, Department of Internal Medicine, Consultant, Thoracic Diseases and Internal Medicine, Mayo Clinic Scottsdale, 13400 East Shea Boulevard, Scottsdale, Arizona 85259*

Stanley M. Shapshay, M.D. *Professor of Otorhinolaryngology, Lahey Medical Center, 41 Mall Road, Burlington, Massachusetts 01805*

Edward G. Shaw, M.D. *Assistant Professor of Oncology, Mayo Medical School and Mayo Graduate School of Medicine; Consultant, Radiation Oncology, Mayo Clinic and Mayo Medical Center, 200 First Street, S.W., Rochester, Minnesota 55905*

Mickie J. Stelck, C.S.T. *Surgical Technician, Bronchoscopy, Mayo Medical Center and St. Mary's Hospital, 200 First Street, S.W., Rochester, Minnesota 55905*

Samuel E. Stubbs, M.D. *Assistant Professor of Medicine, Mayo Medical School and Mayo Graduate School of Medicine; Consultant, Thoracic Diseases and Internal Medicine, Mayo Clinic and Mayo Medical Center, 200 First Street, S.W., Rochester, Minnesota 55905*

Robert E. Wood, M.D., Ph.D. *Professor of Pediatrics, Chief, Pediatric Pulmonary Medicine, University of North Carolina, 635 Burnett-Womack Building, Chapel Hill, North Carolina 27599*

James P. Utz, M.D. *Assistant Professor of Medicine, Mayo Medical School and Mayo Graduate School of Medicine; Senior Associate Consultant Thoracic Diseases and Internal Medicine, Mayo Clinic and Mayo Medical Center, 200 First Street, S.W., Rochester, Minnesota 55905*

Preface

Bronchoscopy had its origins during the waning years of the nineteenth century. The next century witnessed tremendous advances in the application of bronchoscopy in clinical practice. The improvements in the design of the rigid bronchoscope, the advent of flexible fiberoptic bronchoscope, and the greatly increased safety of anesthesia and anesthetic agents further enhanced the application of this important clinical procedure. Recent years have seen newer clinical applications, techniques, and instruments as they relate to bronchoscopy practice. As the twenty-first century approaches, bronchoscopy has become perhaps the most commonly employed invasive procedure in the practice of pulmonary medicine. Instead of being a simple technical procedure, bronchoscopy now requires extensive knowledge and training in all aspects of pulmonary diseases. Thus, in spite of many excellent color atlases available on the market, there is a need for a comprehensive text that can provide detailed information on bronchoscopy.

My coauthors and I are truly pleased to present this volume as the mark of our cooperative objective to pen a comprehensive text for the apprentice as well as the expert bronchoscopist. We have attempted to provide detailed information on the various instruments, techniques, indications, complications, bronchoscopy training, and analysis of optimal bronchoscopy practices in both pediatric and adult bronchoscopy. Individual chapters are devoted not only to common and established topics (i.e., hemoptysis, tracheobronchial foreign bodies, etc) but also to newer areas (tracheobronchial prosthesis, brachytherapy, etc). We hope that this book will become the standard reference on bronchoscopy and continually provide detailed discussions based on the authors' thorough review of the literature as well as extensive personal experience gathered from numerous medical centers around the world.

My co-authors and I eagerly look forward to the reactions and comments from the readers.

Udaya B. S. Prakash

Acknowledgments

I am greatly indebted to my co-authors for their painstaking attenion to detail and hard labor in bringing forth this project. Their letting me impose on them my convictions regarding the contents and formats of the chapters speaks highly of their trustworthy nature. My special thanks go to Edward C. Rosenow, III, M.D., for his wholehearted support for this project. Encouragement and suggestions by Arthur M. Olsen,M.D.,were invaluable.One of the major driving forces, always firm yet gentle and encouraging, has been Kathey Alexander of Raven Press, the publishers of this book. I am personally indebted to Ms. Alexander for accepting this project and bringing it to fruition. Thanks are also given to Nicholas Radhuber, the production editor who guided this rather complex manuscript into its final format, and to Diana Andrews and James Garrity for the cover design. My co-authors and I are grateful to the following for their splendid contribution to the book: Joan M. Beck (design and illustration), John Desley and Lisa Shoemaker (illustration), and Anthony Nelson, Anne M. Johnson, Mary Lou Broz, and Laura Ledsworth (typesetting, paste-up, and production), and M. Alice McKinney for coordinating the art work. Special thanks to Monica J. Farrell for the superb secretarial assistance.

Bronchoscopy,
edited by U. B. S. Prakash.
Mayo Foundation © 1994.
Published by Raven Press, Ltd., New York.

Introduction

Udaya B. S. Prakash

The title of each chapter is self-explanatory as to its subject matter. Because of some overlap in the topics covered, some redundancy is inevitable. Several bronchoscopic images appear more than once to stress an entirely different and unrelated clinical point. To avoid confusion and to simplify the text, all chapters, photographs, and figures use the following terminologies and pictorial orientation.

NOMENCLATURE

The term ***rigid bronchoscope*** is used instead of "open tube bronchoscope," "ventilating bronchoscope," "straight bronchoscope," "stiff bronchoscope," "laserscope," "laser bronchoscope," or "traditional bronchoscope." The term ***flexible bronchoscope*** is employed instead of "flexible fiberoptic bronchoscope," "fiberoptic bronchoscope," "fiberbronchoscope," "fibrebronchoscope," or "bronchofiberscope."

The terms "transbronchoscopic," and "transbronchial" are used interchangeably in clinical practice as well as publications to denote special procedures, such as lung biopsy or needle aspiration, performed through the bronchoscope. Semantically analyzed, the prefix "trans" means "across" rather than "through." Therefore, a percutaneous transthoracic lung aspiration or biopsy can also be "transbronchial" because the needle may inadvertently pierce a bronchus during its transthoracic sojourn. Furthermore, many bronchoscopists wrongly describe the submucosal needle aspiration of a bronchial lesion as transbronchial needle aspiration. Despite the risk of becoming accused of historic revisionism, the text will use the terms ***bronchoscopic lung biopsy*** and ***bronchoscopic needle aspiration*** or ***biopsy,*** avoiding "trans" as much as possible.

U. B. S. Prakash: Division of Thoracic Diseases and Internal Medicine, Mayo Clinic, Rochester, Minnesota 55905.

The chapter on anatomy for the bronchoscopist (Chapter 2) introduces the reader to the classification of the tracheobronchial tree. The descriptions of bronchi in the text and the labels of the figures use the numbering system (e.g. "Fig. 1") to indicate the location of the abnormality. For example, the terms RB-3 and LB-9 are used to describe respectively the bronchus to the anterior segment of right upper lobe and the bronchus leading to the lateral segment of left lower lobe.

ORIENTATION OF FIGURES AND DRAWINGS

Bronchoscopists vary in their method of introducing the flexible bronchoscope into the tracheobronchial tree; some introduce it nasally or orally facing the patient whereas others insert it by standing behind the head of the supine patient. Depending on the bronchoscopist's position, the anatomy of the tracheobronchial tree is mentally pictured as shown in Fig. 1 or 2. However, all rigid bronchoscopic procedures are performed with the anatomic orientation as depicted in Fig. 2. The majority of the authors of this textbook also perform the procedure with the mental conceptualization of the tracheobronchial tree as shown in Fig. 2. The traditional orientation of the tracheobronchial tree in almost all publications on bronchoscopy has also used the upside-down format. Further, the recent resurgence of rigid bronchoscopy for laser procedures and stent placements necessitates maintenance of the traditional format. For these reasons, the line drawings of the tracheobronchial tree adjacent to many of the bronchoscopic images are arranged with the trachea at the bottom of the figure and the distal bronchi at the top (Fig. 3). To commiserate with the orientation of the upside-down tracheobronchial tree, the bronchoscopic images and circular line drawings are also appropriately rotated (see below).

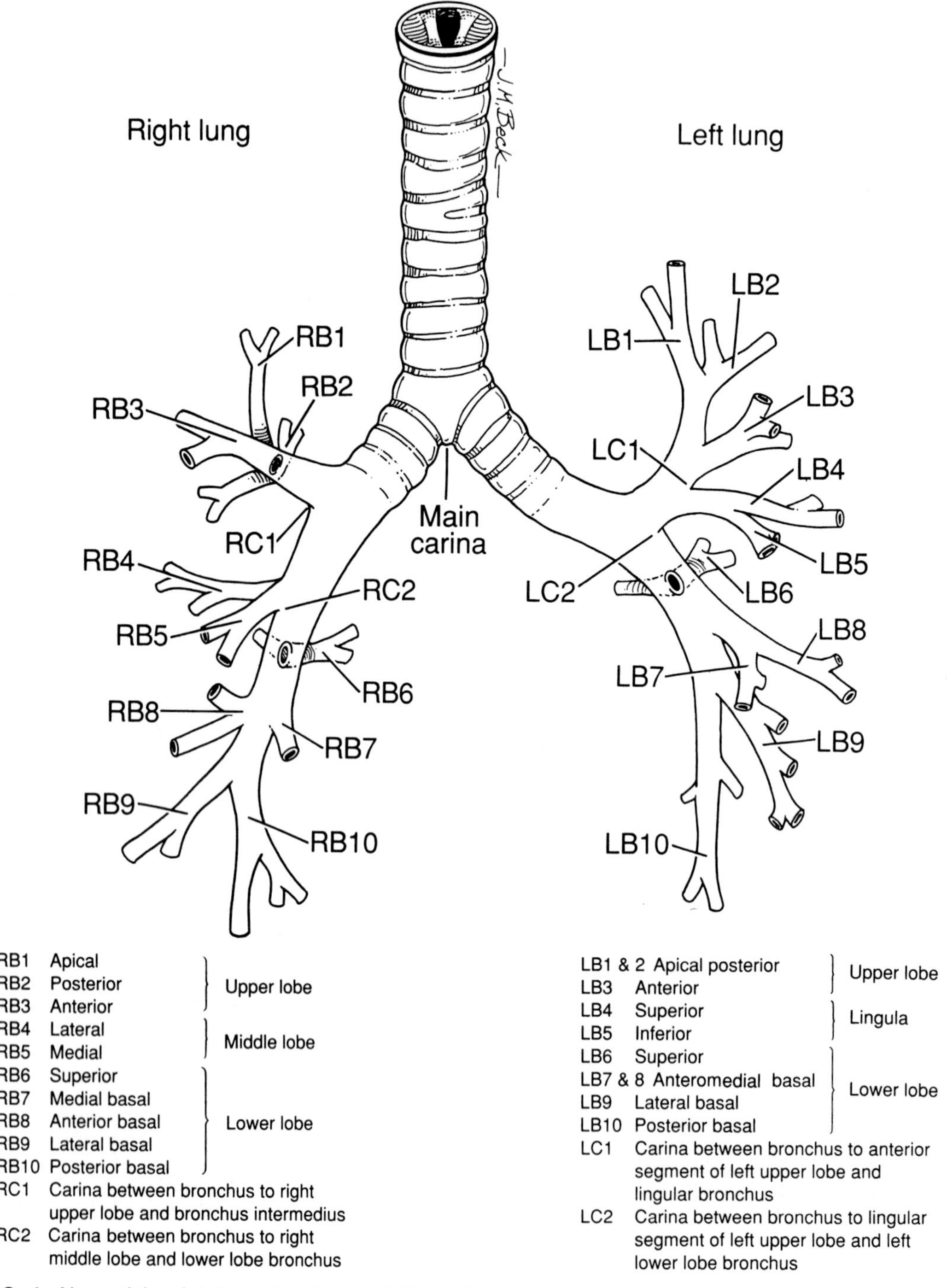
J.M. Beck
Right lung
Left lung
RB1
RB2
RB3
RC1
Main carina
RB4
RC2
RB5
RB6
RB8
RB7
RB9
RB10
LB1
LB2
LB3
LC1
LB4
LB5
LC2
LB6
LB8
LB7
LB9
LB10
RB1 Apical
RB2 Posterior
RB3 Anterior
Upper lobe
RB4 Lateral
RB5 Medial
Middle lobe
RB6 Superior
RB7 Medial basal
RB8 Anterior basal
RB9 Lateral basal
RB10 Posterior basal
Lower lobe
RC1 Carina between bronchus to right upper lobe and bronchus intermedius
RC2 Carina between bronchus to right middle lobe and lower lobe bronchus
LB1 & 2 Apical posterior
LB3 Anterior
Upper lobe
LB4 Superior
LB5 Inferior
Lingula
LB6 Superior
LB7 & 8 Anteromedial basal
LB9 Lateral basal
LB10 Posterior basal
Lower lobe
LC1 Carina between bronchus to anterior segment of left upper lobe and lingular bronchus
LC2 Carina between bronchus to lingular segment of left upper lobe and left lower lobe bronchus

FIG. 1. Normal (upright) anatomic orientation of the tracheobronchial tree in an adult human.

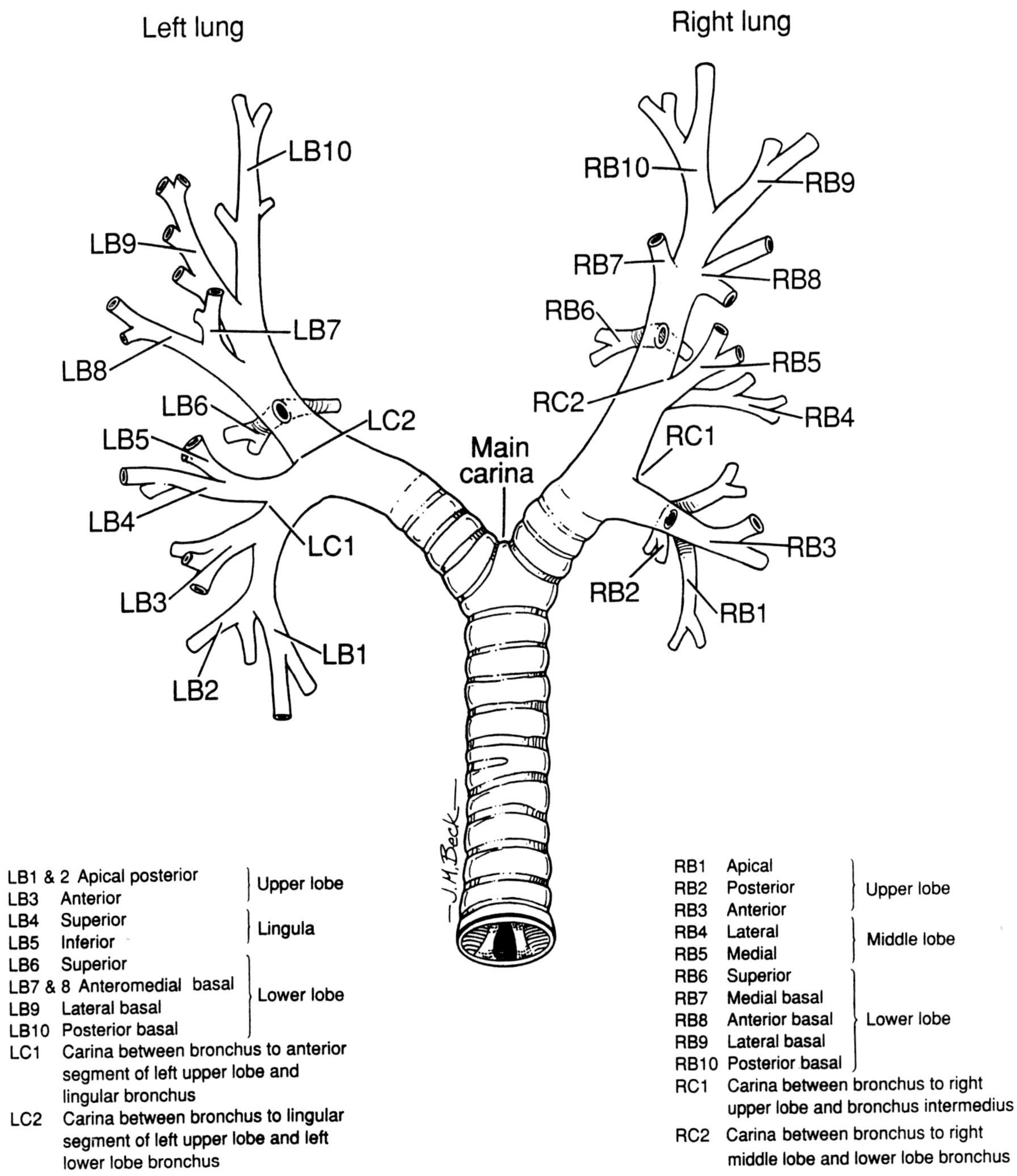

FIG. 2. Traditional (upside down) orientation of the tracheobronchial tree for bronchoscopy.

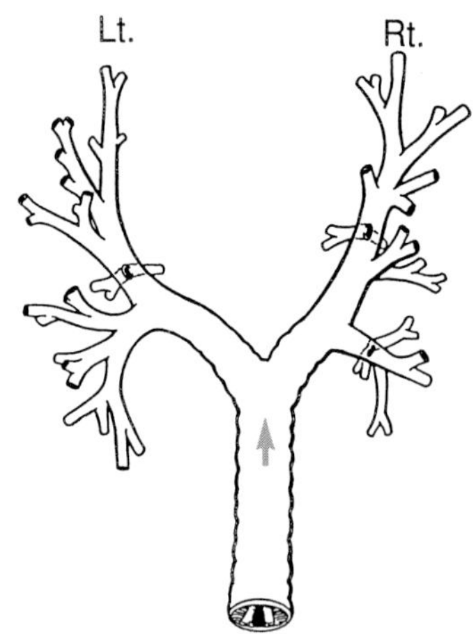

FIG. 3. An upside-down line drawing of the tracheobronchial tree utilized in this book.

An explanation of the figures that portray the bronchoscopic findings is in order. In the atlases and books on bronchoscopy, it is a common practice to always show the pointer at the 12 o'clock position in the bronchoscopically obtained photographs (Fig. 4). The outcome is the loss of anatomic orientation unless the figure is properly labeled. In this textbook, the bronchoscopically obtained photographs are arranged so that the top (12 o'clock position) of the photograph always represents the patient's anterior and the bottom (6 o'clock position) the posterior, irrespective of the location of the pointer (Fig. 5). Therefore, the reader should ignore the location of the pointer in the photographs. Nevertheless, the circular line drawings depicting the adjacent bronchoscopic photographs further clarify the location of the anatomic region illustrated (Fig. 6). A sagittal view of the neck is drawn to orient the reader to the lesions in the upper trachea (Fig. 7). The colored arrow inside the line drawing of the tracheobronchial tree marks the location of the tip of the bronchoscope in the tracheobronchial tree from where the photograph was taken and the direction of bronchoscopic visualization (Fig. 6).

PHOTOGRAPHY

Unless specified, all bronchoscopic images in this book were photographed by the members of the section of bronchoscopy, Division of Thoracic Diseases, at Mayo Medical Center and Mayo Medical School, Rochester, Minnesota. The contributions of bronchoscopic photographs and figures by others is gratefully acknowledged here and in the figure legends.

There are several special bronchoscopic images accompanied by line drawing of the tracheobronchial tree

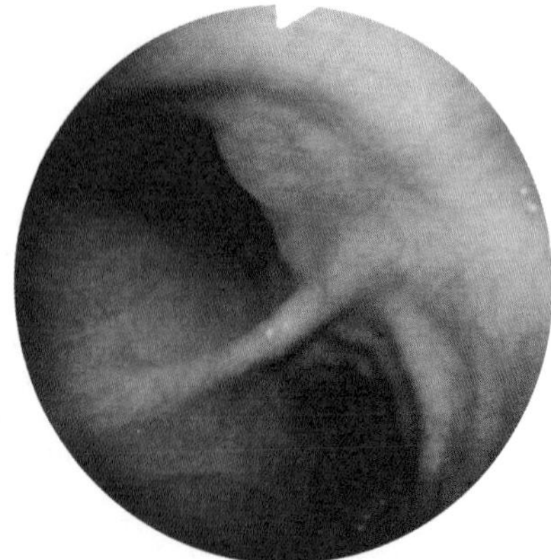

FIG. 4. The bronchoscopic pointer at the 12 o'clock position. The patient's true anterior (indicated by the anterior aspect of main carina) is at 2 o'clock and the true posterior (posterior aspect of main carina) is directed toward 8 o'clock.

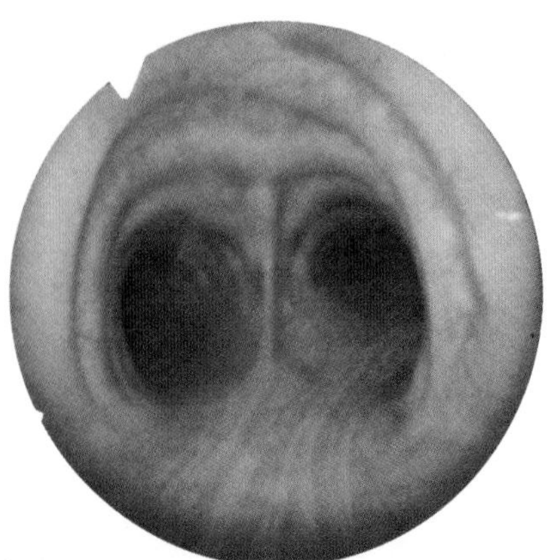

FIG. 5. The bronchoscopic pointer is not at the 12 o'clock position but the image is rotated so that anatomic orientation of distal trachea and main bronchi is depicted properly to show anterior portion of main carina at the 12 o'clock position, in contrast to the alignment in Figure 4.

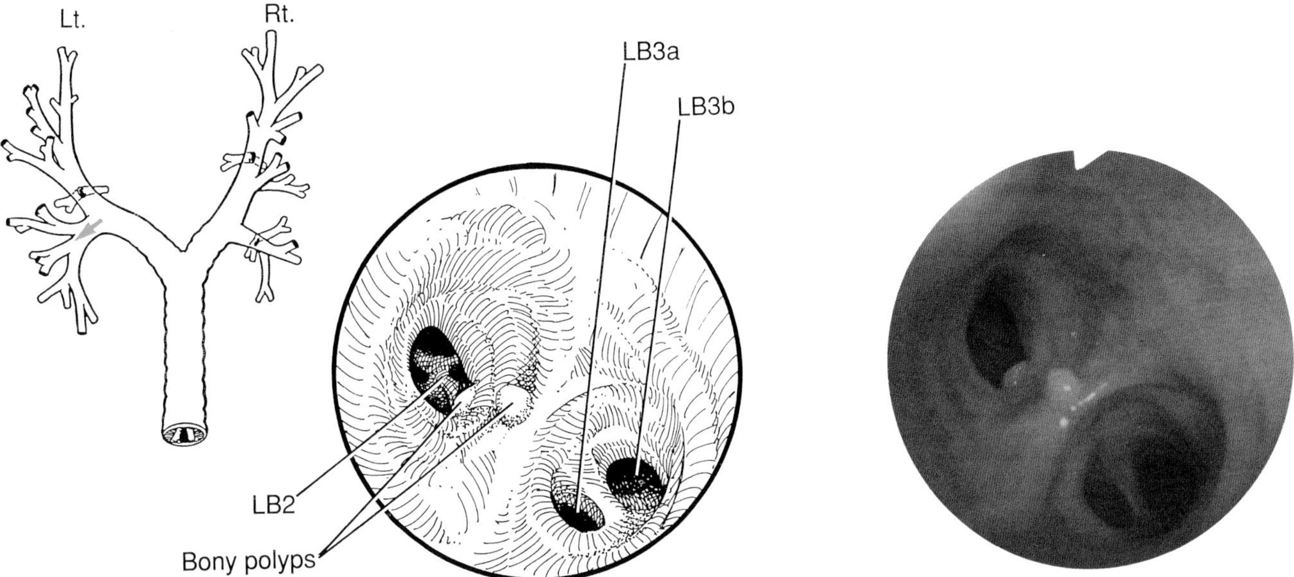

FIG. 6. Line drawings of an upside down tracheobronchial tree, labeled circular drawing mimicking the bronchoscopic image, and the actual photographic image. The arrows inside the line drawing of the tracheobronchial tree mark the location of the tip of the bronchoscope in the bronchial tree from where the photograph was taken and the direction of bronchoscopic visualization.

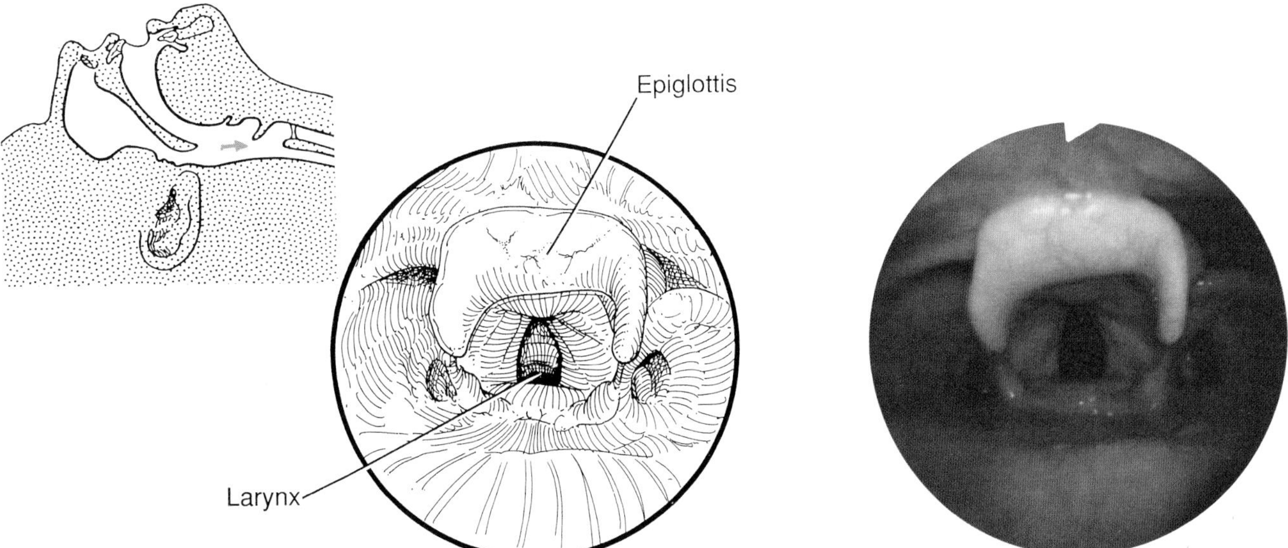

FIG. 7. A sagittal view of the neck and upper airway to orient the reader to the anatomic location of the abnormality depicted in the bronchoscopic image and circular drawings.

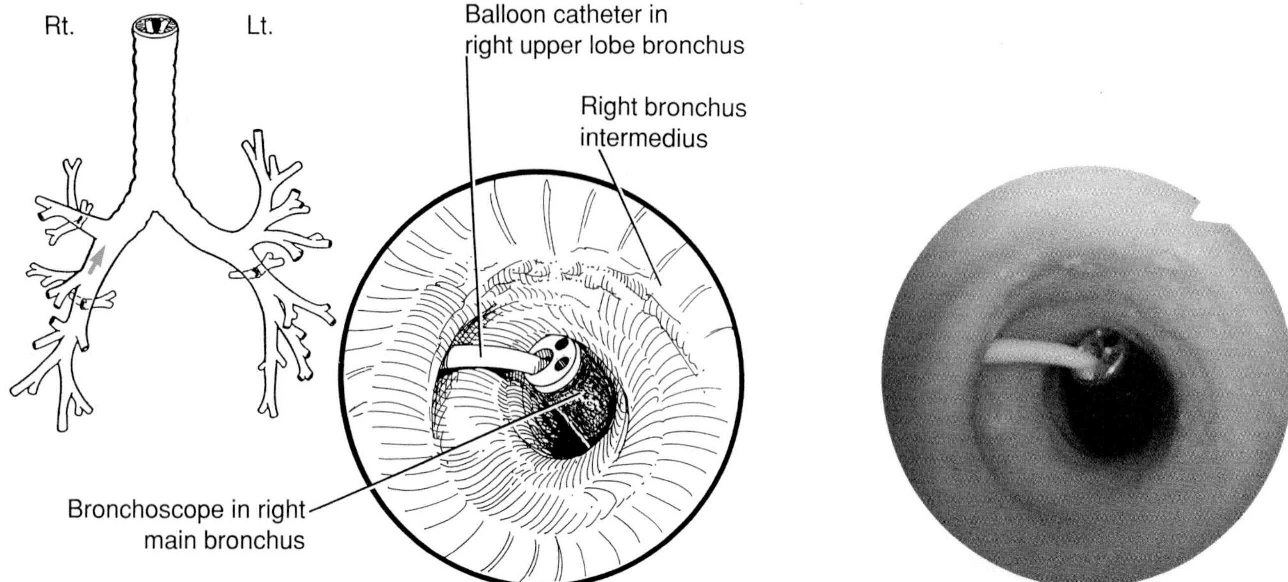

FIG. 8. Line drawings of an upright tracheobronchial tree, labeled circular drawing mimicking the bronchoscopic image, and the actual photographic image of the "reverse" or cephalad view show a distally located bronchoscope viewing another bronchoscope in action in the proximal bronchial tree.

in an upright mode (Fig. 8). These images provide a "reverse" or cephalad view from the distal bronchial tree. To wit, if one bronchoscopist were to introduce a bronchoscope into a distal bronchus from the outside (transthoracic route) and advance it proximally (toward the larynx), he or she would see these images of another bronchoscopist's instrument (introduced into the airway in the traditional manner) in action within the tracheobronchial tree. These special images were bronchoscopically photographed by the editor of this textbook using modified models of the tracheobronchial tree.

Bronchoscopy,
edited by U. B. S. Prakash.
Mayo Foundation © 1994.
Published by Raven Press, Ltd., New York.

CHAPTER 1

History of Bronchoscopy

Eric S. Edell and David R. Sanderson

Examination of internal body cavities has been of scientific interest for centuries. The ruins of Pompeii have produced speculi that were likely used by some of the earliest healers (1). Inspection of the airway was probably first accomplished by highly polished metal mirrors, although history does not document by whom the first instrument was used. History does tell us that in 1743 Monsieur Leuret developed a speculum through which he could remove polyps from the nose and throat (1). This instrument was a polished mirror plate that utilized the reflection of external sunlight for inspection. In 1807, Bozini, of Frankfurt, Germany, illuminated the interior of various canals using a small metal tube (2). His paper, entitled "The Light Conductor, or a Description of a Simple Apparatus for the Illumination of Internal Cavities and Spaces in the Human Body," was immediately dubbed as quackery. This invention was termed the "magic lantern in the human body." Bozzini's "magic" proved to be of little value, but it did stimulate subsequent investigators to develop various tools for examination of the upper part of the larynx.

Endoscopic examination of the larynx was first thought feasible in 1828 when Horace Green noted that the larynx could tolerate the presence of a foreign body (2,3). A probang of whalebone was used to introduce a piece of sponge soaked in silver nitrate solution. Using this technique, Green eventually became proficient at catheterizing the larynx and trachea. A gum elastic catheter was inserted through the larynx and passed into the lower bronchi. Silver nitrate solution was then introduced with a syringe. Green presented this technique and results of his work at the Surgical Society of New York in 1847. The technique was condemned as "an anatomical impossibility and an unwarranted innovation in practical medicine." Green was subsequently asked to resign from membership of the society. The next several decades resulted in further developments and Green's claims were universally conceded.

Stenosis of the larynx was a severe complication of diphtheria. After several years of work, Joseph O'Dwyer perfected an intubation tube in 1885 that he used to relieve such strictures. O'Dwyer was also given credit for noting the severe complications of retained foreign bodies in a bronchus (4). He constructed a thin-walled tube to facilitate expulsion of foreign bodies from the trachea or bronchus. The work of Green and O'Dwyer established the principles of bronchoscopy used today, namely, the ability of the larynx to tolerate the initial and continued presence of a foreign body.

THE RIGID BRONCHOSCOPE

Kirstein examined the interior of a patient's larynx directly with O'Dwyer's tube in 1895. He also confirmed Rosenheim's discovery that it was possible to get a straight tube into the trachea, but did not pursue this further. In fact, Kirstein warned against entering the lower trachea as a dangerous practice (5). It was in 1897 that Gustav Killian, known as the "father of bronchoscopy," reportedly investigated the lower trachea and main stem bronchi using a Kirstein laryngoscope (5). It is believed that Killian convinced a retired hospital janitor in Freiburg, Germany, to submit to an examination for small amounts of money. It was originally believed that the bronchus was too rigid for close inspection; however, reporting at the Society for Medical Doctors in Freiburg, Killian reported that "there is no bleeding afterwards."

Later in the same year, a 63-year-old farmer from the Black Forest was referred to Dr. Killian after apparently swallowing a piece of pork bone. Symptoms

E. S. Edell: Division of Thoracic Diseases and Internal Medicine, Mayo Clinic, Rochester, Minnesota 55905.

D. R. Sanderson: Division of Thoracic Diseases and Internal Medicine, Mayo Clinic, Scottsdale, Arizona 85259.

of severe cough, dyspnea, and hemoptysis prompted this referral. Using a Kirstein laryngoscope, Killian was able to identify a solid object that resided in the right main stem bronchus. Killian's first reaction was to provide the patient with tracheostomy; however, not being a surgeon he was not permitted to do this operation. At that time, Geheimrat Kraske was the laryngologist allowed to do the tracheostomy. After consultation, it was decided against surgery, and Killian was given permission to attempt removal of the foreign body using a Mikulicz–Rosenheim esophagoscope. Under local cocaine anesthesia, the foreign body was removed. In 1898, in the Congress of Southwest German Laryngologists in Heidelberg, Killian reported three cases of foreign body extractions from the tracheobronchial tree (5). He called the method "direct bronchoscopy" and subsequently demonstrated the necessity for side openings in the lower end of the bronchoscope to enable ventilation of the healthy lung while the bronchoscope occluded the bronchus during extraction of the foreign body. Thus began the era of bronchoscopic examination (Fig. 1).

The first bronchoscopy done in the United States was by Algernon Coolidge, Jr., on May 11, 1898 (6). Using an open urethroscope, a head mirror, and reflected sunlight, Dr. Coolidge removed a portion of hard, rubber tracheotomy cannula from the right bronchus of a 22-year-old man. In 1890, Dr. Chevalier Jackson developed an esophagoscope with which he removed a denture from an adult and, using a smaller version, a coin from a child. It was a natural extension of his interest in the esophagus and larynx to begin bronchoscopy in 1899. Jackson practiced his techniques sequentially in mannequins, cadavers, and dogs, designing and building many of the special instruments himself. In 1890, Jackson was appointed to the Chair of Laryngology at the Western Pennsylvania Medical College, later to become part of the University of Pittsburgh, and he drew increasing referrals as his reputation grew.

In 1916, Jackson was invited to Philadelphia to become Professor of Laryngology at Jefferson Medical College. The next two decades might be called the golden age of open tube bronchoscopy and Philadelphia was its focal point. There Jackson had the singular honor, probably unique in medical education, of simultaneously holding academic appointments in all five medical colleges of Philadelphia. In each institution he developed strong training programs and disciples to train others. Doctor Louis Clerf at Jefferson continued the tradition. Among Clerf's students was Dr. Jo Ono, who introduced peroral endoscopy to Japan. Doctor Gabriel Tucker, Sr., became chairman at the University of Pennsylvania and Dr. C. L. Jackson succeeded his father at Temple University. It was in 1904 that Chevalier Jackson developed a bronchoscope with a small light at the distal end. About the same time, Dr. Jackson also developed an instrument with an auxiliary tube for lighting and an additional tube for draining.

By 1912 the bronchoscope had become an accepted instrument for inspection of the trachea and main stem bronchi. Its use was limited almost exclusively to the removal of foreign bodies. Surgical removal of foreign bodies of the main stem bronchi had such a high mortality that bronchoscopy was a welcomed addition to the surgeon's armamentarium. In those early days, bronchoscopy also had an appreciable mortality, but subsequent perfection of the technique and the elimination for the need for general anesthesia reduced the mortality significantly. Through the work of various endoscopists, but primarily that of Dr. Chevalier Jackson, instruments were developed that improved the ease

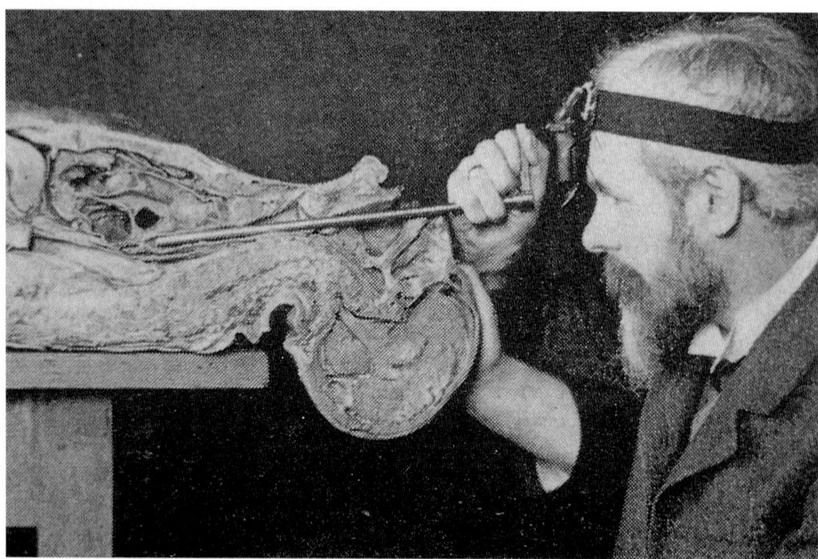

FIG. 1. Gustav Killian demonstrating the bronchoscope on a cadaver in 1898. From *Arch Otolaryngol* 1965; 82:656, with permission.

with which foreign bodies were removed (Fig. 2). The mortality from foreign body removal was subsequently lowered to approximately 1%. The demand rose for a magnified field of vision providing better inspection of the distal bronchi. This resulted in the development of two accessories. One was a telescope that could be inserted into the rigid tube for magnification. Another Jackson protege, Dr. Edwin N. Broyles, developed the optical telescope with forward and angle viewing, which permitted inspections of the upper as well as the lower lobes of the lung. Jackson's skill as an artist provided many of the early illustrations used for teaching. Photography of the remote reaches of the bronchial tree was difficult and it was Dr. Paul H. Holinger who developed many of the techniques and instrumentation for recording on film the visual images seen with the endoscope.

Although primarily used as an instrument for foreign body removal, the continued development of the rigid bronchoscope led to its use in other pulmonary diseases. Many interesting and vitally important discoveries were made once objective examination of the interior of the tracheobronchial tree had been perfected. In his address to the Boston Surgical Society in 1928, Chevalier Jackson commented on several such discoveries (6). These include its use in the treatment of atelectasis, posttonsillectomy pulmonary suppuration, spirochetosis, vegetable bronchitis, asthma, and pneumonia.

The rigid bronchoscope remained the primary tool for diagnosis and, under certain circumstances, treatment of disorders of the trachea and major bronchi. Little change occurred over the next several decades. One major advance was the report by H. A. Andersen, in 1965, where biopsy material was obtained from patients with diffuse lung disease (7). A subsequent report of 450 cases in 1972 documented the safety of transbronchoscopic lung biopsy using a rigid bronchoscopy (8). Another major development was the solid rod lens by H. H. Hopkins, which greatly improved the optical quality. Despite these advancements in technology, the rigid bronchoscope had limitations, particularly in patients with peripheral lesions of the upper lobes. The development of fiberoptic systems led to the next phase of bronchoscopy.

FLEXIBLE BRONCHOSCOPE

In 1870, John Tyndall described the optical properties of glass fibers created when a glass rod was heated and rapidly pulled apart. It was not until 1927 and 1930 that J. L. Baird and C. W. Hansell put forth a proposal that this property could be utilized. In 1930, H. Lamb,

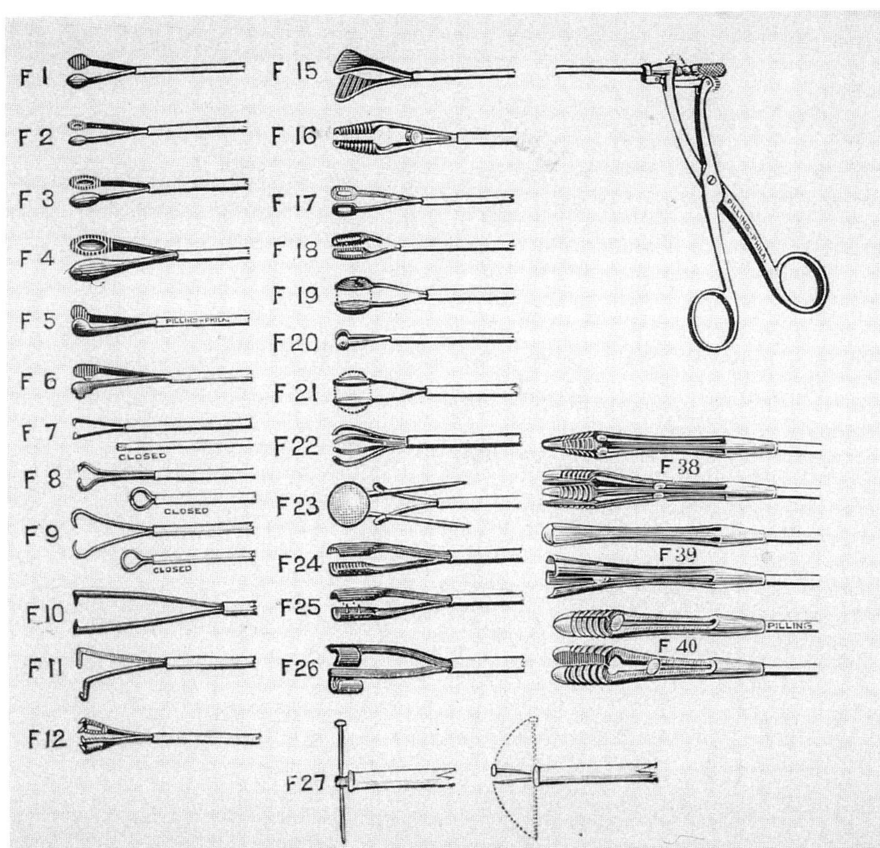

FIG. 2. Bronchoscopic and esophagoscopic forceps with the most frequently used forms of jaws that were available to Dr. Chevalier Jackson. From Jackson C, Jackson CL: *Diseases of the air and food passages of foreign body origin.* Philadelphia: WB Saunders; 1936:294, with permission.

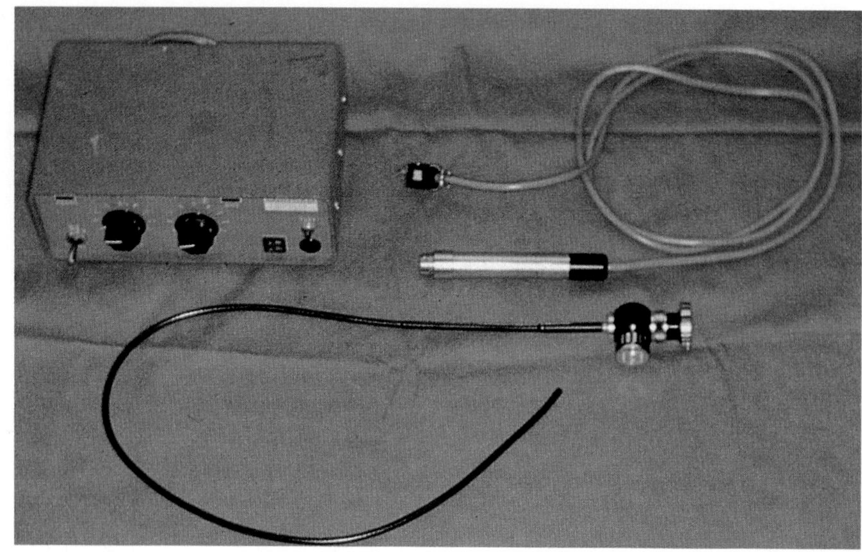

FIG. 3. Prototype of the first flexible bronchoscope by Machida.

a German, advocated the application of the glass fibers to a flexible gastroscope. Real progress was not made on research into the optical properties of this glass fiber until the 1950s (9). When bundles of fibers are used, the exterior of each light-transmitting fiber requires coating with a glass of lower refractive index than the core fiber. This process, called cladding, is an invention by V. Heel and B. O'Brien (10). H. H. Hopkins and N. S. Kapany invented a means for arranging these fiber bundles and named it the fiberscope (11). A flexible bundle is comprised of a large number of optic fibers gathered together with both ends tightly fixed. When arranged this way, an image entering one end of the bundle is transmitted to the other. For accurate image transmission, the fibers must be arranged identically at both ends. The smaller the fiber, the better the

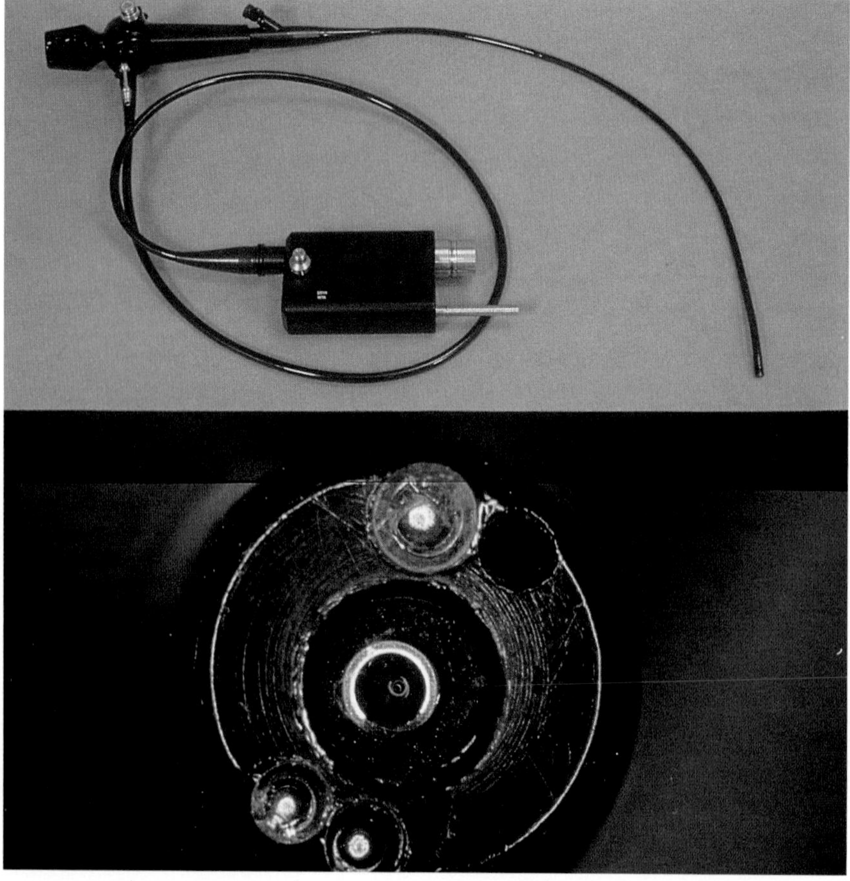

FIG. 4. Prototype of the first video bronchoscope using a charge-coupled device by Pentax Corp.

optical resolution. If a fiber is too thin, it loses both its mechanical strength and its light transmission capacity. Five micrometers has been quoted as the lowest practical limit.

Hopkins and Kapany brought the first fiberscope to the United States, where further investigations were carried out at the University of Rochester, in association with Bausch and Laumb Optical Technology Inc. In 1957 Basil Hirschowitz worked separately on the gastrofiberscope at the University of Michigan. Hirschowitz presented the first clinical fiberscope at the Gastroscopic Society of America (12).

Doctor Shigeto Ikeda established standards for the first flexible bronchoscope in 1964 (Fig. 3). Doctor Ikeda's interest in early diagnosis of lung cancer stimulated him to design an instrument that could enter subsegmental bronchi and directly visualize lesions and obtain specimens for tissue and cytological diagnosis. Prototypes of the bronchofiberscope were completed by Machida Endoscopic Company Ltd. and Olympus Optical Company Ltd. in 1966. Doctor Ikeda performed a series of clinical trials and perfected the first commercially available bronchofiberscope in July 1967 (13).

In April 1970, Doctor Ikeda presented his instrument and early experience to the annual meeting of the American Bronchoesophagology Association (14). Its introduction led to a second era in the exploration and documentation of the anatomy of the tracheobronchial tree. The flexible bronchoscope has become the standard tool for this inspection. Endoscopic examination of the tracheobronchial tree has progressed from the rigid technique originally described by Killian to flexible fiberoptics applied by Dr. Ikeda. Current standard equipment utilizes state-of-the-art fiberoptic systems that have allowed accurate anatomic and pathological documentation. Diagnosis of various disorders of the tracheobronchial tree have resulted from the application of these flexible fiberoptic systems. The current flexible bronchoscopes have image resolution of exceedingly good quality. Unfortunately, the fiber bundle is prone to damage and repair is quite expensive. Also image quality is limited by the presence of the fiber bundle.

In an attempt to improve image quality, Dr. Ikeda has again been the forerunner in the development of the most recent bronchoscope. In February 1987 he introduced a prototype videobronchoscope (15). This system eliminated the optical fiber bundle and replaced it with a charge-coupled device (CCD) image sensor that transmits the image to a video processor for display on a television monitor (Fig. 4). The advantages of the videobronchoscope are its improved image resolution and the ability to manipulate a digitized signal on various recording medias. The videobronchoscope offers the potential to become the next-generation instrument for visualizing the tracheobronchial tree.

REFERENCES

1. Tyson EB. Development of the bronchoscope. *J Med Soc NJ* 1957;54:26–30.
2. Patterson EJ. History of bronchoscopy and esophagoscopy for foreign body. *Laryngoscopy* 1926;36:157–75.
3. Donaldson F. The laryngology of Trousseau and Horace Green. An historical review. *Proc Am Laryngol Assoc* 1891:10.
4. Birkett HS. Transatlantic development of rhinolarngology. *Laryngoscope* March 1923;609–611.
5. von Eiken C. The clinical application of the method of direct examination of the respiratory passes and the upper alimentary tract. *Arch Laryngol Rhinol* Nov. 1904;15.
6. Jackson C. Bronchoscopy: past, present and future. *N Engl J Med* 1928;199:758.
7. Andersen HA, Fontana RS, Harrison EG, Jr. Transbronchoscopic lung biopsy in diffuse pulmonary disease. *Dis Chest* 1965; 48:187–192.
8. Andersen HA, Fontana RS: Transbronchoscopic lung biopsy for diffuse pulmonary diseases: technique and results in 450 cases. *Chest* 1972;62:125–128.
9. Ikeda S. *Atlas of flexible bronchofiberoscopy*. Tokyo: Igaku Shoin Ltd; 1974:6–10.
10. Van Heel ACS. A new method of transporting optical images without aberrations. *Nature* 1954;173:39.
11. Hopkins HH, Kapany NS. A flexible fiberscope using static scanning. *Nature* 1954;173:39–41.
12. Hirschowitz BL, Curtiss LE, Peters CW, Pollard HM. Demonstration of a new gastroscope, the "fiberscope." *Gastroenterology* 1958;35:50–53.
13. Ikeda S, Yanai N, Ishikawa S. Flexible bronchofiberscope. *Keio J Med* 1968;17:1.
14. Ikeda S. Flexible bronchofiberoscope. *Ann Otol* 1970;79:916.
15. Ikeda S. The development and progress of endoscopes in the field of bronchoesophagology. *J Jap Bronchoesophagol Soc* 1988;39:85–96.

Bronchoscopy,
edited by U. B. S. Prakash.
Mayo Foundation © 1994.
Published by Raven Press, Ltd., New York.

CHAPTER 2

Anatomy for the Bronchoscopist

Denis A. Cortese and Udaya B. S. Prakash

During the bronchoscopy training, every bronchoscopist should acquire a solid fund of knowledge in the tracheobronchial anatomy. Particular attention should be extended to variations in normal anatomy, differences in adult and pediatric populations, and the relationship of the tracheobronchial tree to its adjacent structures. Knowledge of pulmonary vascular anatomy and its relation to the tracheobronchial tree is essential to the performance of optimal laser bronchoscopy and transtracheal/bronchial needle aspiration or biopsy. Further, the bronchoscopist should possess knowledge of chest roentgenologic interpretation and indications for other imaging procedures that may provide additional information on the anatomy of the lung and tracheobronchial tree as it applies to the practice of bronchoscopy. These studies will lead to a three-dimensional conceptualization of the tracheobronchial tree that in turn will make it easier to apply bronchoscopic skills to patient management. In this chapter, we provide brief discussion on the developmental aspects of the tracheobronchial tree. The normal anatomy of the tracheobronchial tree as viewed by the bronchoscope is dealt with in more detail and the discussion is specifically oriented to the bronchoscopy procedures.

DEVELOPMENT OF THE TRACHEOBRONCHIAL TREE

The tracheobronchial tree and lungs develop in a progressive fashion beginning with the large airways, smaller airways, acini, vessels, and alveoli as the fetus approaches full term. The lung matures from the original simple tube that branches from the foregut early in the fourth week of gestation, and it becomes surrounded by mesenchyme and a vascular network as it develops. This process has been studied extensively by Boyden who categorized them into stages (1–6). The stages have been modified by Langston into the following phases: embryonic, pseudoglandular, canalicular, saccular, alveolar (7).

Embryonic Phase

The major airways develop between the fourth and sixth weeks. The lung bud appears during the fourth week, branching from the anterior surface of the foregut. The bud extends and elongates caudally and divides into right and left branches. With further elongation of the main bronchi, early "lung sacs" develop with shallow external creases indicating lobes and segments. Variations in segmental and subsegmental bronchi may appear at this time and are due to atypical origins of primary or secondary subpulmonary buds as they form. The embryonic bronchopulmonary tree becomes ensheathed in an arterial plexus. Abnormal or aberrant vascular patterns may emerge from this plexus explaining the varied arterial patterns found during life.

Pseudoglandular Phase

This phase, between the seventh and the sixteenth weeks of gestation, is characterized by the formation of all conducting airways and the development of acini. The name for this period derives from the fact that with continuous elongation and growth there are multiple dichotomous divisions of the airways that are lined by cuboidal epithelium. The lung has the histological appearance of a gland. Cartilage begins to appear in some of the larger airways. As growth continues, there is additional branching and ingrowth of mesenchyma that will eventually become capillaries. Additional airways

D. A. Cortese: Division of Thoracic Diseases and Internal Medicine, Mayo Clinic, Jacksonville, Florida 32224.
U. B. S. Prakash: Division of Thoracic Diseases and Internal Medicine, Mayo Clinic, Rochester, Minnesota 55905.

continue generating until, by the end of the sixteenth week, all conducting airways of the lung, including the terminal bronchioles, have been formed. Complete development of the bronchial tree by the sixteenth week of gestation has been described as Reid's first law of lung development (8).

Canalicular Phase

This occurs between the 16th and 28th weeks of gestation and is characterized by the development of acini and progressive vascularization. This is a critical period in which the essential components of the acinus and the respiratory unit can be identified. These components include a terminal bronchiole, two to four respiratory bronchioles, and six to seven generations of buds destined to become the saccules of the terminal sac. Capillaries appear over the periphery of these sacs. Respiratory bronchioles are lined partly by columnar epithelium similar to the epithelium of the distal airways and partly by cuboidal epithelium that is destined to eventually form alveoli.

Saccular Phase

This phase occurs between the 29th and 36th weeks of gestation. It is characterized by a decrease in interstitial tissue, further differentiation of saccules, and the development of surfactant. Saccule walls are progressively thin so that there is less interstitial tissue and the sacs have a deeper, sac-like appearance. Some of the sacs subdivide into smaller units called subsaccules, which are the immediate precursors of alveoli. The capillary network around the saccules and subsaccules continues to develop. The most important feature of this period is the production of surfactant by maturing type 2 pneumocytes at approximately 30 weeks of gestation.

Alveolar Phase

True alveoli form between the 37th week and birth, as saccules differentiate. Langston et al. defined alveoli as "a thin-walled, flask-shaped or multifaceted polygonal structure with a single capillary network" (7). The rate of alveolar development in this phase appears variable, but a mean of 50 million alveoli is reported.

Pulmonary Vessels

During the embryonic phase, the fourth week of intrauterine life, the pulmonary artery begins to form from the right and left sixth aortic arches. The right sixth arch soon disappears leaving the left sixth aortic arch to form the main trunk, right and left pulmonary arteries. The remnant of the left sixth aortic arch remains attached to the dorsal aorta and becomes the ductus arteriosus. The developing pulmonary arteries grow into and with the developing lungs and bronchial trees, eventually fusing with vascular channels developing from the mesenchyma and capillaries. The terminal bronchioles and acinar structures at birth are accompanied by nonmuscular arteries. After birth, muscular and partly muscular arteries appear in association with respiratory bronchioles. After 2 years of age, the muscular arteries progressively extend adjacent to alveolar ducts. During the second decade of life muscular and partly muscular arteries develop adjacent to alveoli, which is the final development of the adult pulmonary arteries.

Coinciding with the development of the pulmonary arteries, the pulmonary veins begin to form as outgrowths from the dorsal aspects of the common cardiac atrium. This common chamber eventually branches into the four main pulmonary veins, which are subsequently incorporated into the left atrium. The developing large veins are in continuity with the vascular plexus within the mesenchyma that covers the developing lung buds. It is from this mesenchymal vascular plexus that the small intrapulmonary veins arise and complete the development of the pulmonary venous structures.

Lung After Birth

The number of alveoli greatly increase in early childhood; there are approximately 127 million alveoli by the first year and 280 million by the eighth year of life. Additional alveoli develop beyond the sixteenth generation of airways distal to the last cartilage-containing airways. Diverticula perforate the subepithelial mucosal layer surrounding these bronchioles and develop into thinned-walled spherical sacs that are subsequently invaded by capillaries and finally converted to alveoli. These alveoli develop at sporadic intervals and do not result in the reduction in the number of airways but merely add to the number of alveoli in the terminal bronchioles. Reid's second law of lung development states that "alveoli develop after birth, increasing in number until the age of eight years and in size until growth of the chest wall finishes with adulthood" (8). The canals of Lambert arise in the distal portions of the bronchiolar tree particularly in the preterminal bronchioles. These are tubular structures lined by cuboidal epithelium and communicate with surrounding alveoli. Alveolar pores of Kohn are openings in the alveolar wall that permit intraalveolar collateral ventilation. It is not known when these structures develop.

BRONCHOSCOPIC ANATOMY

Upper Airway

The bronchoscope can be inserted into the human airways via the nasal passages, oral route, or through a tracheostomy stoma. Therefore, it is essential that the bronchoscopist possess a knowledge of upper airway anatomy (Fig. 1). An important landmark in the oropharynx is the base of the tongue. In this location, the glandular mucosal surface of the tongue meets and joins the anterior surface of the epiglottis and forms the medial and lateral glossoepiglottic folds or vallecula. Approximately opposite and superior to this location is the uvula in the midline (Fig. 2). Lateral to the lateral glossoepiglottic folds are the pyriform sinuses of the pharynx. While inserting the bronchoscope, it is possible to enter these blind pouches and become disoriented (Fig. 3).

In order to see the anatomic structures of the larynx, it is important to first recognize the epiglottis (Fig. 4), then pass posterior to the tip of the epiglottis as the bronchoscope is advanced caudally (Fig. 5).

The flexible bronchoscope can also be introduced through the nose and directed to the posterior pharynx before entering the larynx. The bronchoscope is introduced through the nasal vestibule along the floor of the nose, passing between the inferior turbinate, which is lateral, and the nasal septum, which is medial, through the posterior choana into the upper oropharynx just beyond the soft palate. The epiglottis is then easily visualized and the bronchoscope can be advanced to the larynx.

The larynx begins at the opening bounded anteriorly by the free border of the epiglottis, laterally by the aryepiglottic folds, and posteriorly by the corniculate tubercles of the arytenoid cartilages (Fig. 6). A membrane covers the epiglottis and continues around poste-

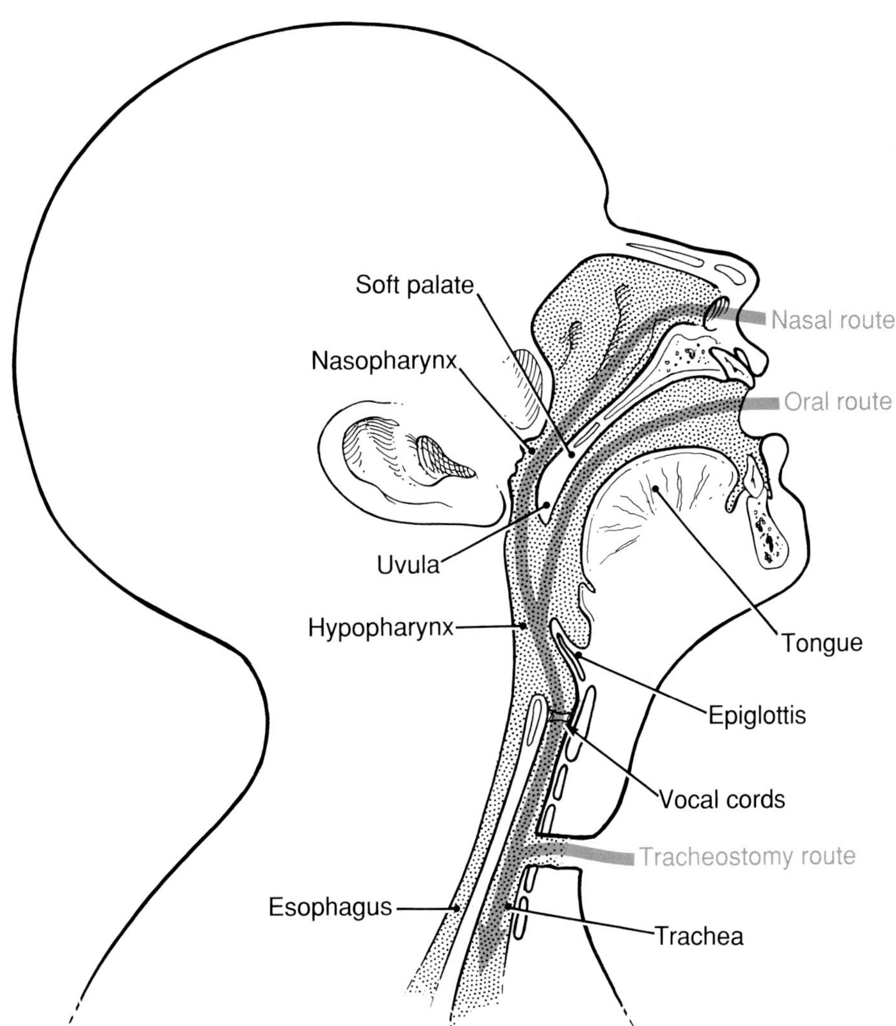

FIG. 1. Upper airway anatomy as it pertains to routes of insertion of flexible bronchoscope. Rigid bronchoscope can be inserted by oral or tracheostomy route.

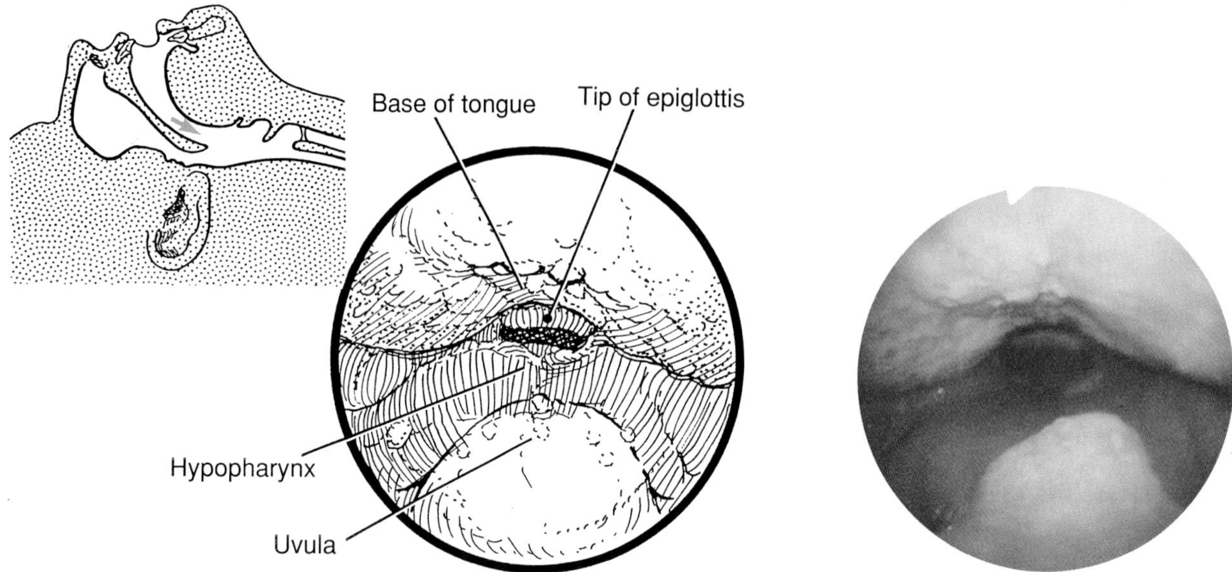

FIG. 2. Important anatomic landmarks in the upper airway include the base of the tongue and the uvula.

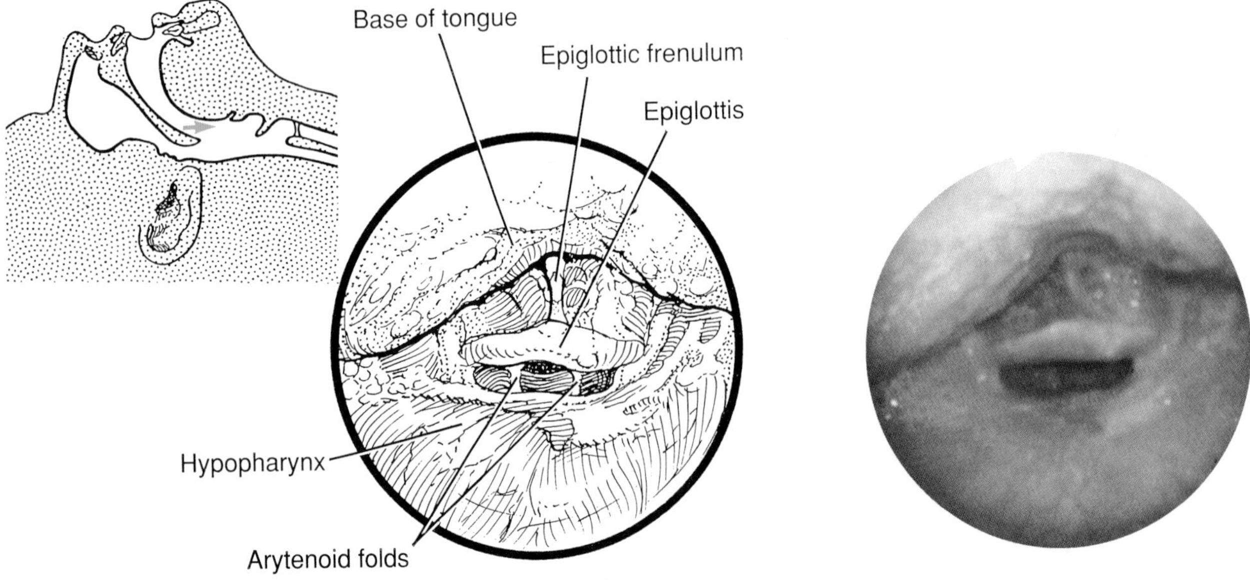

FIG. 3. Important anatomic structures located beyond the base of the tongue.

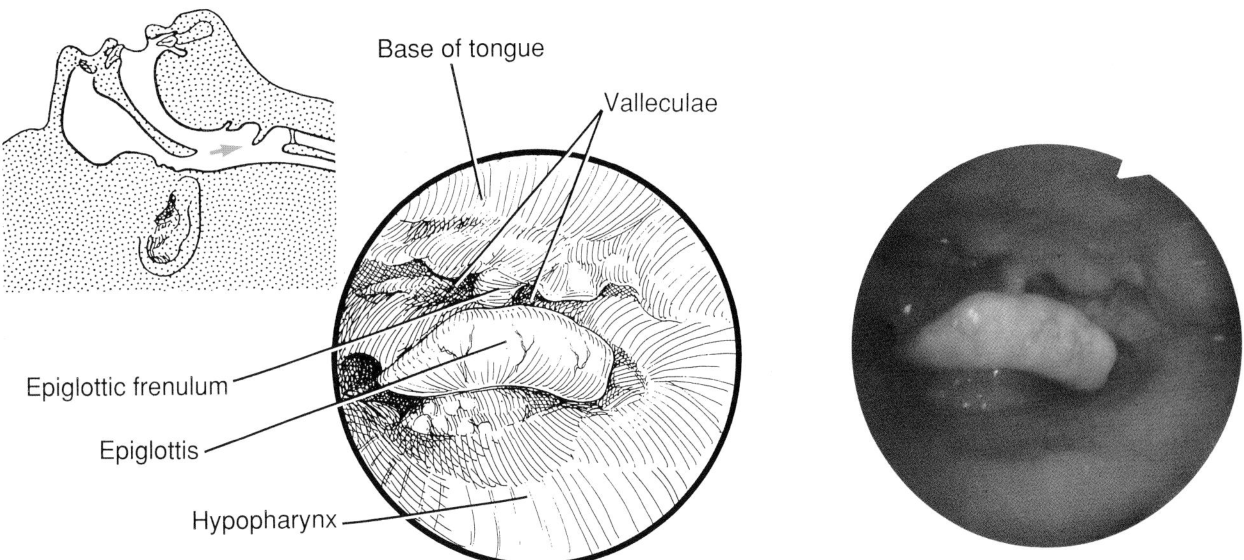

FIG. 4. Supraepiglottic area depicts certain anatomic landmarks that may disorient the bronchoscopist if the bronchoscope is inadvertently introduced to these areas.

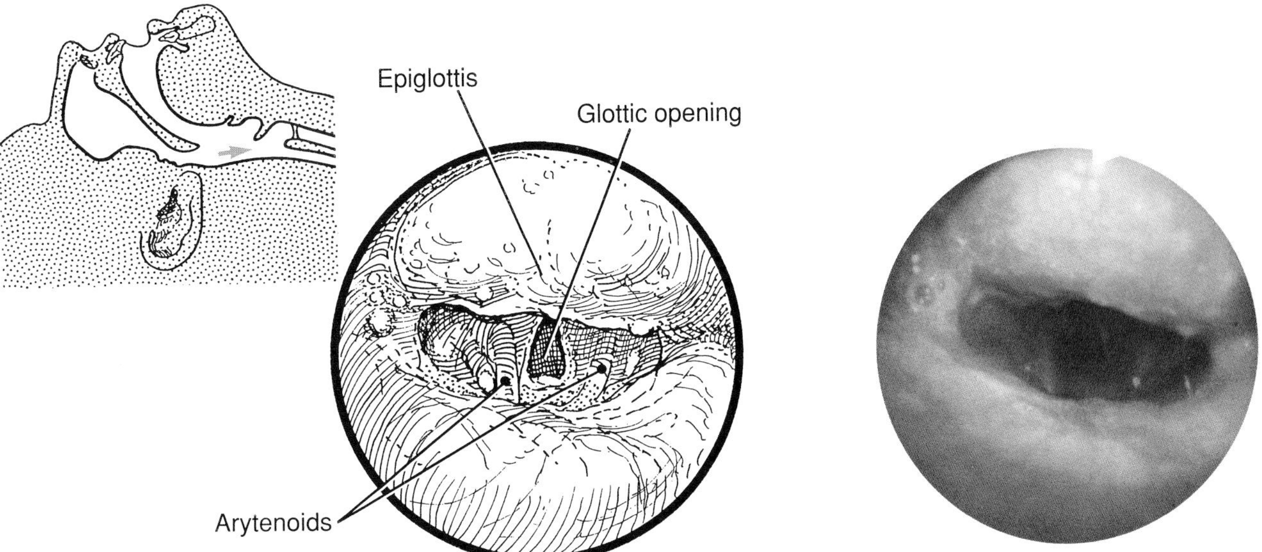

FIG. 5. Bronchoscopic view from just beyond the tip of the epiglottis.

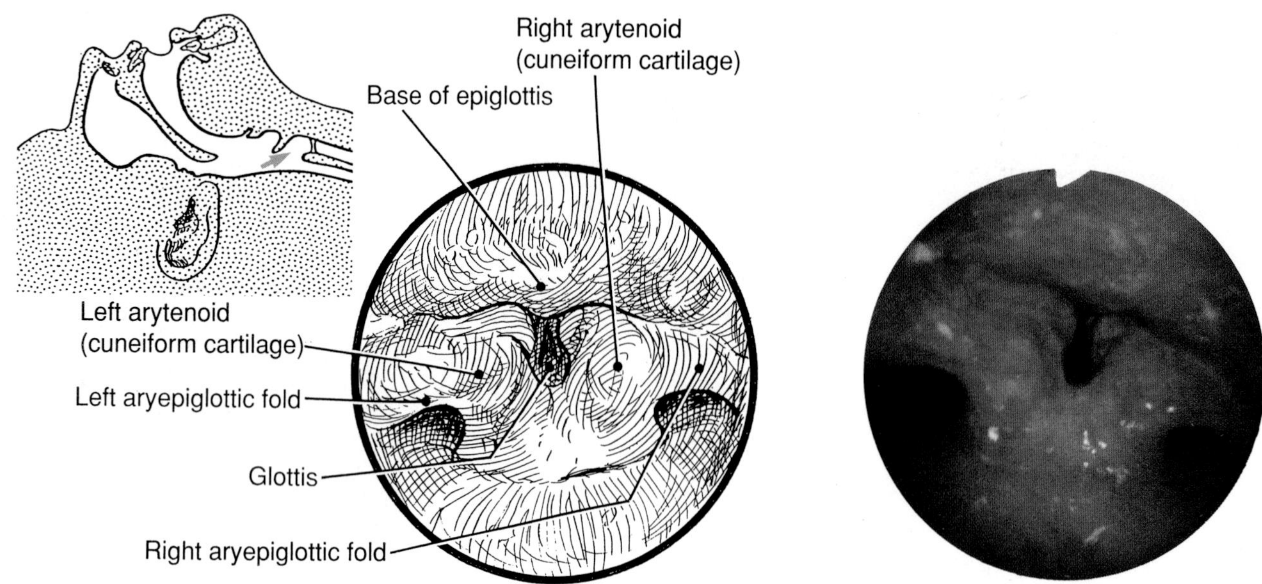

FIG. 6. Close-up view of the laryngeal structures.

riorly to envelope the crescents of the arytenoid cartilages forming the aryepiglottic folds. Just beyond these structures, the ventricular folds may be seen (false vocal cords), which are tissue folds lateral, parallel, and superior to the true vocal cords (Fig. 7). Immediately below the false vocal cords, the true vocal cords are formed by tough fibroelastic bands that extend forward from the anterior surface of the arytenoid cartilages to the midline of the thyroid cartilage. The two vocal cords form an opening into the trachea which is the glottis. When open, the vocal cords form an isosceles triangle with the apex anteriorly along the thyroid cartilage beneath the epiglottis (Fig. 8). The cricoid cartilage is suspended from the inferior aspect of the thyroid cartilage. This forms a complete ring at the inferior aspect of the larynx and is fixed to the tracheal rings.

The innervation of the larynx is predominantly by the vagus nerve. The internal branch of the superior laryngeal branch of the vagus nerve is sensory to the mucosa of the larynx and the epiglottis. This branch passes below the mucosa covering the pyriform sinuses lateral to the larynx. Motor innervation of the vocal cords is via the recurrent laryngeal branches of the

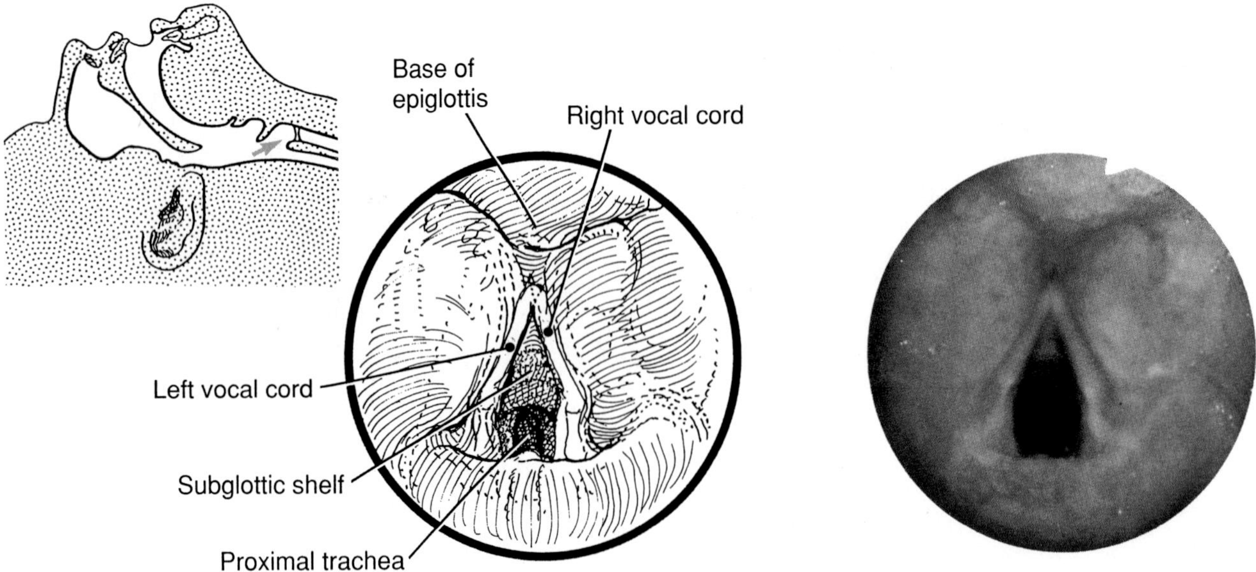

FIG. 7. Bronchoscopic view of the vocal apparatus. The bulging folds just proximal to vocal cords are the false cords.

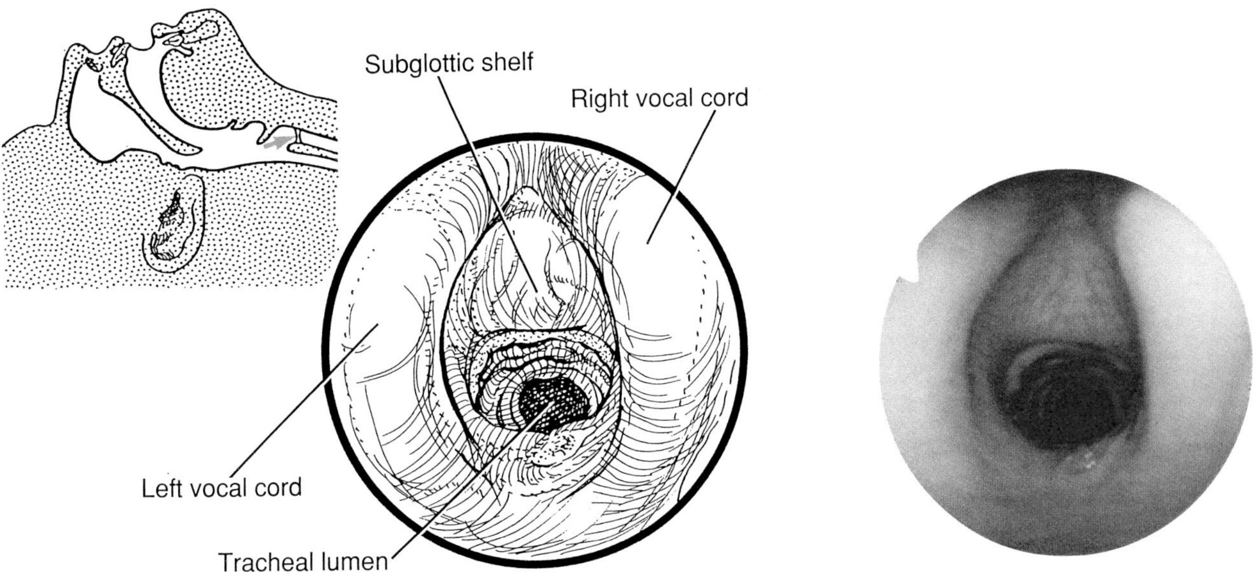

FIG. 8. Close-up view of vocal cords, subglottic space, and proximal trachea.

vagus nerve. On the left side, the recurrent laryngeal nerve loops around the aortic arch from anterior to posterior and it ascends in the mediastinum to the larynx. On the right side, it takes a similar course around the right subclavian artery before entering the larynx. Both nerves ascend in the laryngotracheal grooves and supply motor fibers to the intrinsic muscles of the larynx and sensory fibers to the mucosa below the vocal cords.

Trachea

The length and diameter of the trachea and angle of branching of the main stem bronchi vary from infant to adult (Fig. 9). Even the intra- and extrathoracic components of trachea change from infancy to old age (Fig. 10). The trachea is entered after passing through the cricoid cartilage and ends at the division into the right and left main stem bronchi at the carina. The carina

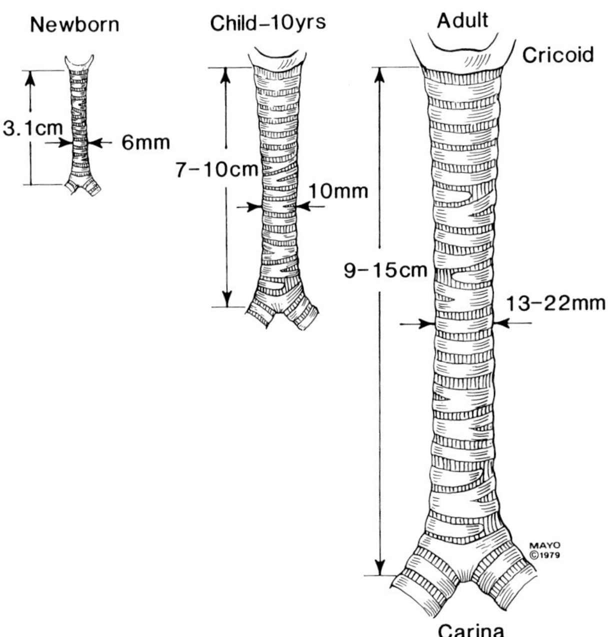

FIG. 9. The length and external diameter of trachea in the newborn, a 10-year-old child, and an adult.

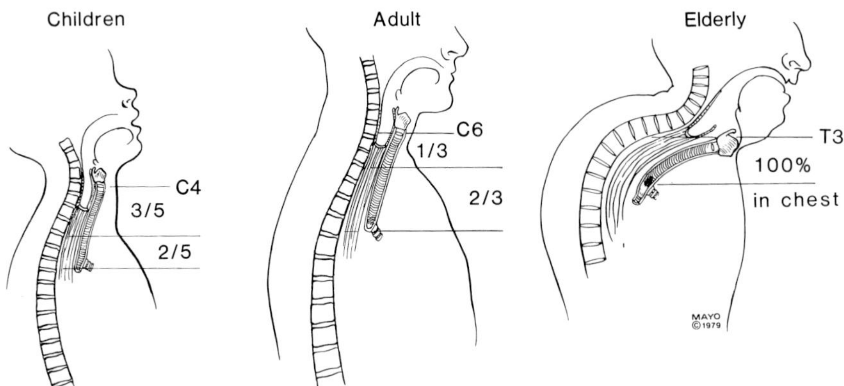

FIG. 10. The intrathoracic extension of trachea increases as the person gets older. C4 and C6 represent fourth and sixth cervical vertebrae, respectively, and T3 is the third thoracic vertebral body. The fractions indicate the extent of intra- and extrathoracic trachea.

usually appears as a sharp, keel-like structure and is usually oriented in the vertical position. Variations can occur, and the angle of the carina may vary as much as 45° from the vertical in either direction. The angle between the longitudinal axis of the trachea and the bifurcation of the main bronchi may range from 30° to 105° (Fig. 11). The angle of the right main bronchus is usually 10–15° less than that of the left main bronchus. The normal internal diameter of the trachea ranges from 1.2 to 1.5 cm (Fig. 9). The tracheal caliber varies at different levels (Fig. 11) and may also vary with respiration particularly along the posterior membrane, which may move anteriorly during expiration (Figs. 12 and 13).

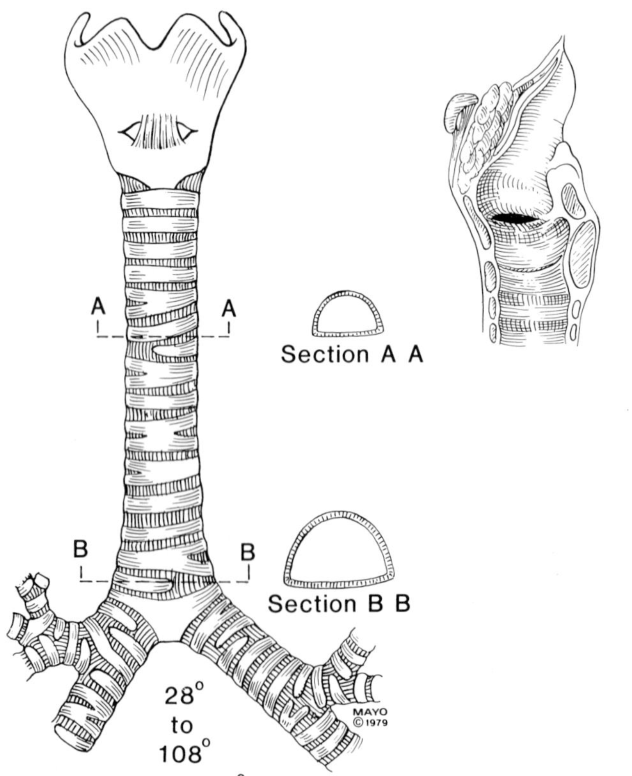

Main Carina

As the name implies, the main carina is keel-shaped and oriented in an anteroposterior plain (Fig. 14). It is a very important landmark and signifies the branching of the trachea into right and left main stem bronchi. It is normally sharp and its anteroposterior dimensions increase during inspiration and decrease during expiration. In infants and children, the main carina is not as sharp and is in fact quite blunt. Widened main carina in adults may indicate subcarinal lymphadenopathy.

Right Bronchial Tree

The right main stem bronchus is approximately 1.5 cm in length and its normal internal diameter is 1.0–1.2 cm (Fig. 15). The right upper lobe bronchus is the first branch off of the right main stem. It branches laterally from the right main stem bronchus of an angle of approximately 100°. Accessory bronchus to the right upper lobe is a commonly encountered anatomic variation (Fig. 16). The right upper lobe bronchus itself may have a length of 1 cm and quickly gives rise to three segmental bronchi. Beyond the origin of the right upper lobe bronchus, the right main stem bronchus continues as the bronchus intermedius (Fig. 17). This bronchus may extend for 2.0–2.5 cm at which point it gives rise to the middle lobe bronchus anteriorly, the superior segment of the right lower lobe posteriorly, which is frequently directly across from the middle lobe orifice, and the right lower lobe bronchus. The right middle lobe bronchus diameter is usually 0.8 cm, and the length may range from 1.0 to 1.2 cm terminating in two segmental bronchi. At the point of origin of the right middle lobe, there may be an area of sudden narrowing,

FIG. 11. Angle of bifurcation of trachea and cross-section of trachea at different levels.

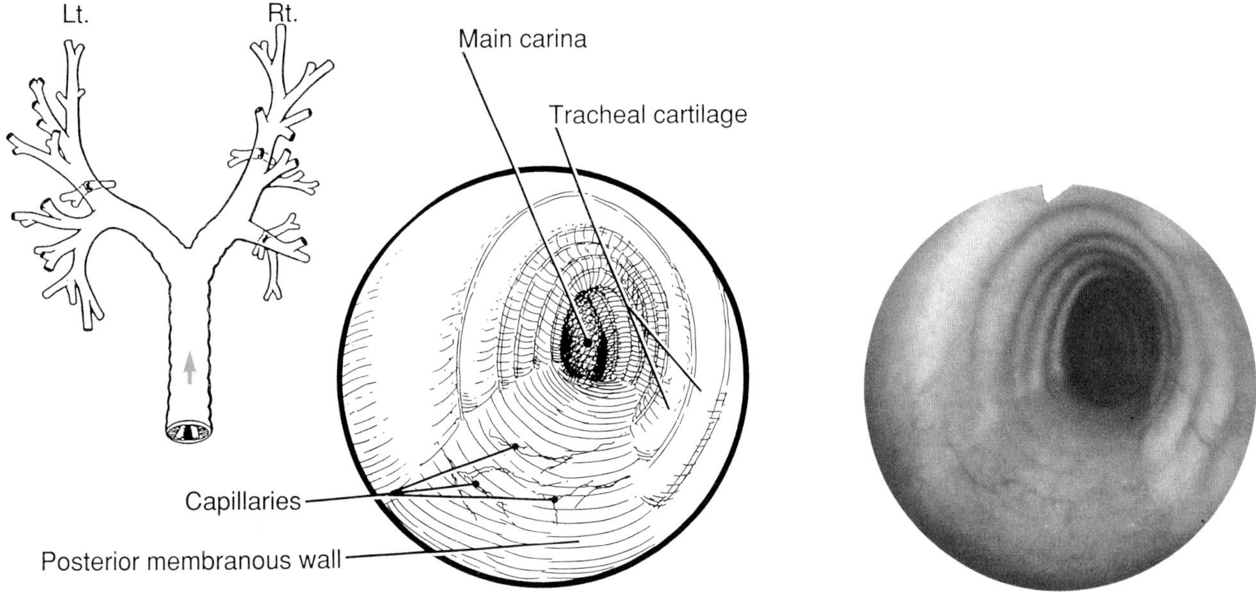

FIG. 12. Normal trachea during inspiration shows posterior displacement of the posterior membranous wall of the trachea.

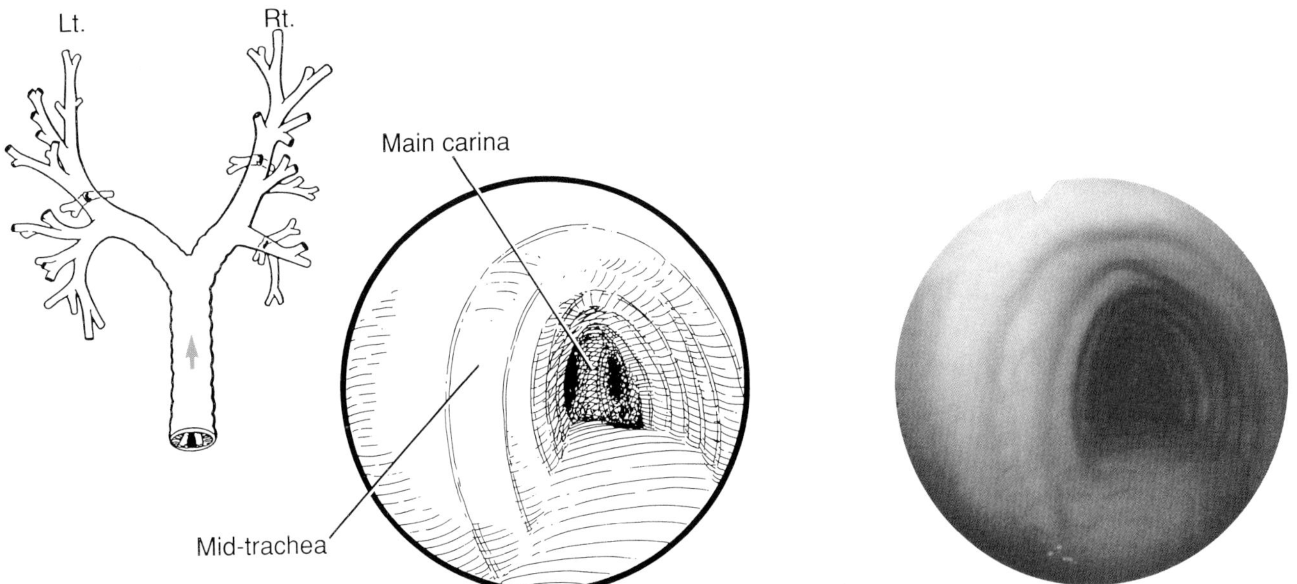

FIG. 13. Normal trachea during expiration shows mild anterior bulging and displacement of the posterior membranous wall of the trachea.

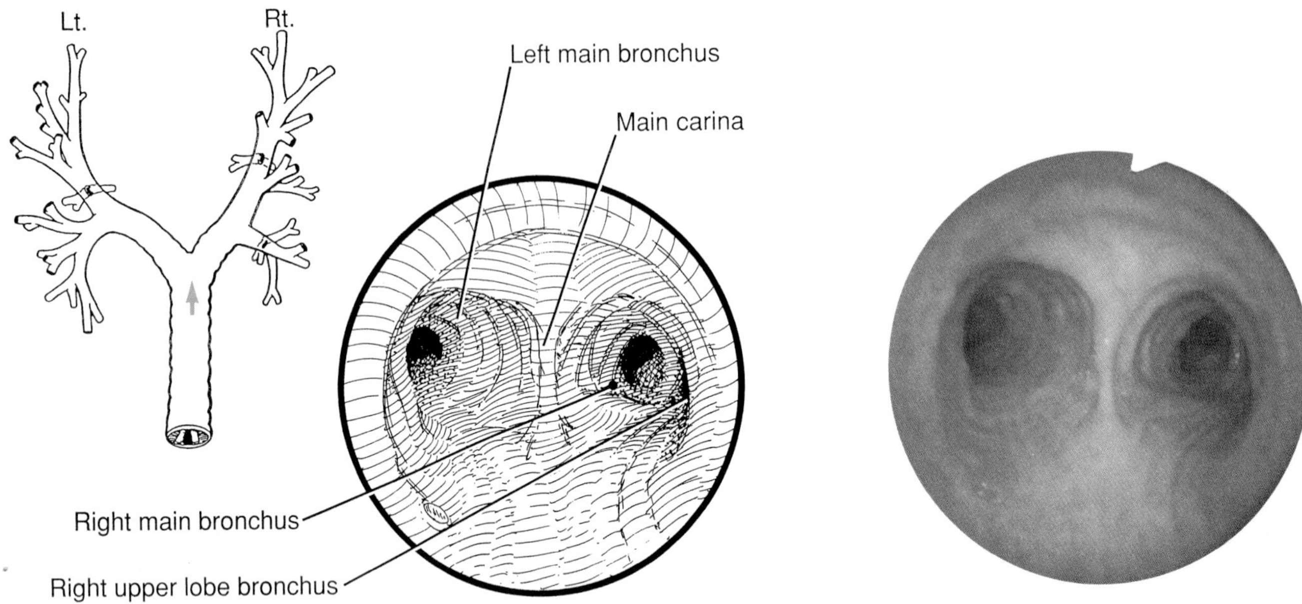

FIG. 14. Normal main carina. Note the sharp keel-like appearance.

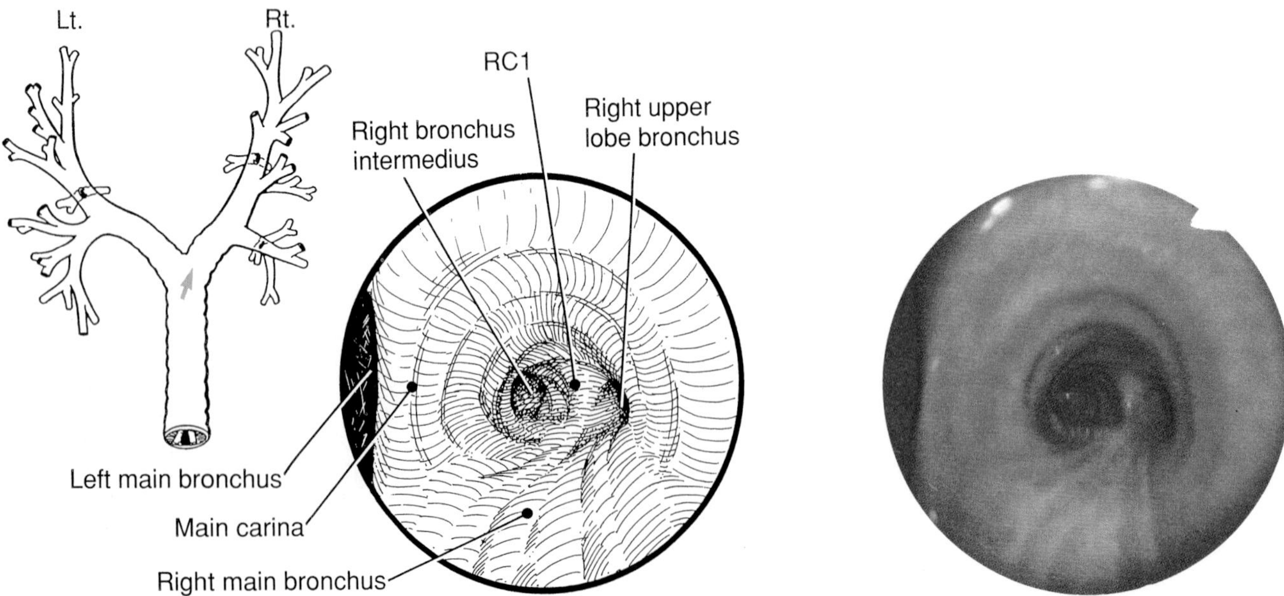

FIG. 15. The right main stem bronchus and distal branching.

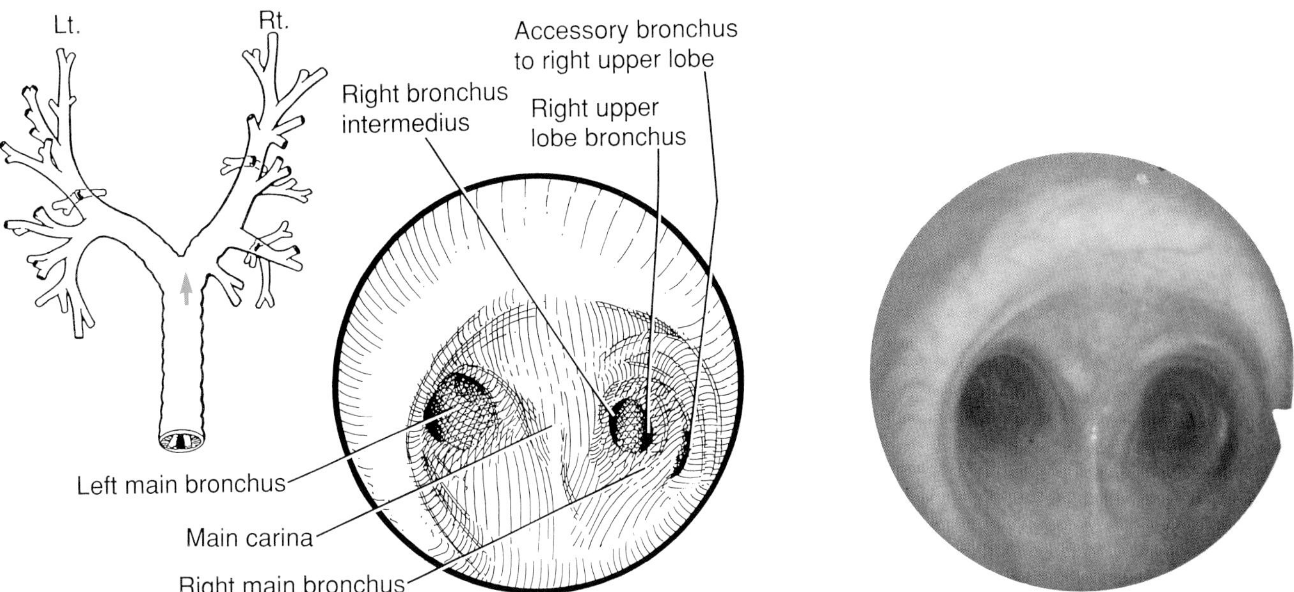

FIG. 16. Main carina, main stem bronchi, bronchus intermedius, right upper lobe bronchus, and an accessory bronchus to right upper lobe.

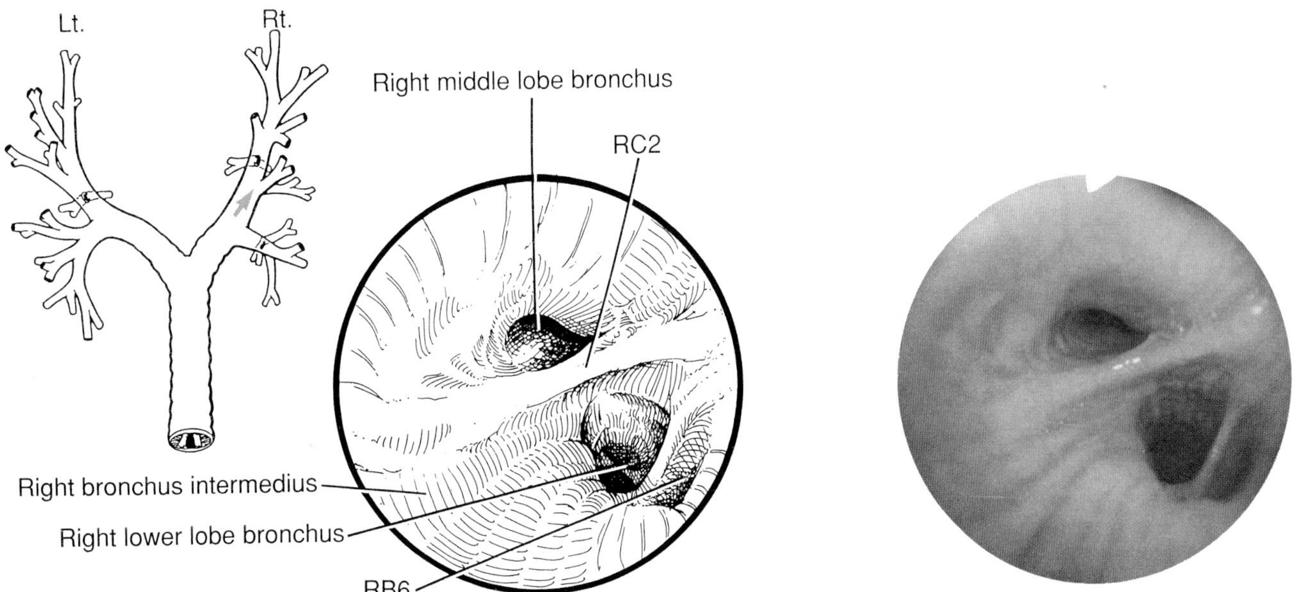

FIG. 17. Distal bronchus intermedius, RC2, and bronchi to right middle and lower lobes.

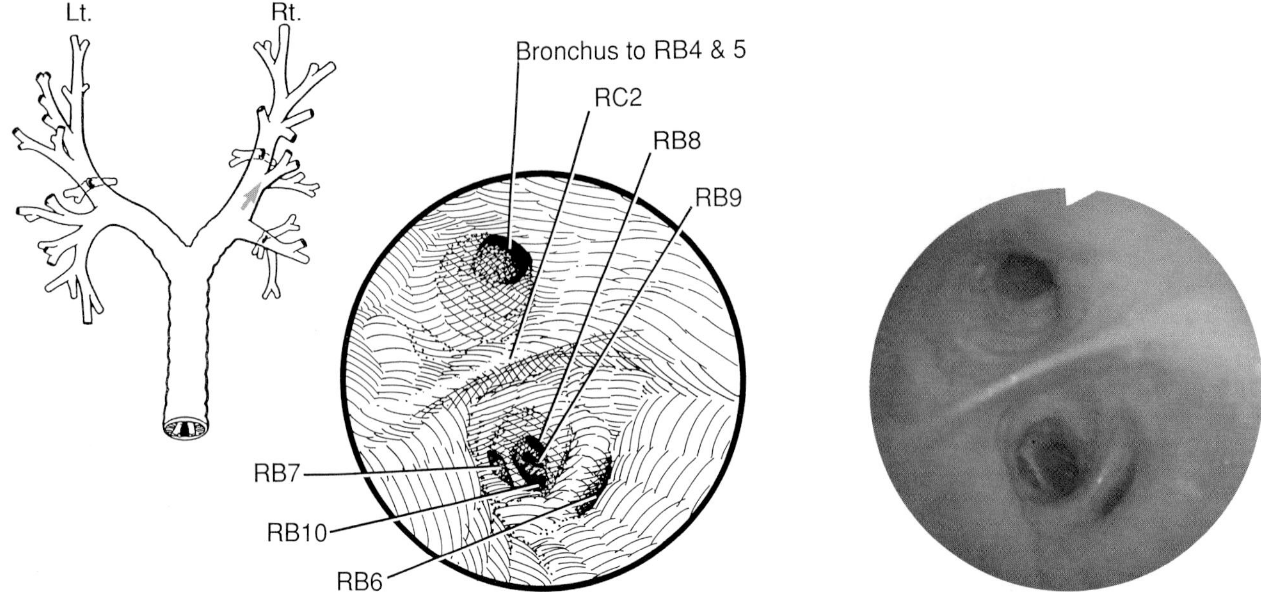

FIG. 18. Bronchi to right middle and lower lobes.

which is a normal finding and not related to an extrinsic process. Beyond the origin of the superior segment of the right lower lobe, the branches to the other lower lobe segmental bronchi are usually found (Fig. 18).

Left Bronchial Tree

The left main stem bronchus makes more of an angle with the trachea than the right main stem (Fig. 19). It descends further into the lung before dividing; its usual length is 4.0–4.5 cm and tends to progress posteriorly, inferiorly, as well as laterally. The left main stem bronchus terminates in a bifurcation into the left upper lobe and lower lobe bronchi (Fig. 20). The left upper lobe bronchus is generally 0.8–1.0 cm in diameter and approximately 1 cm in length. As the bronchus ascends superiorly, the lingular bronchus arises and extends slightly downward in an inferior-lateral direction. The upper division bronchus of the left upper lobe passes beyond the orifice of the lingula. Its length may vary from a few mm to 1.0 mm. It frequently gives rise to a common bronchus serving the apical and posterior segments of the left upper lobe and an independent bronchus serving the anterior segment of the left upper lobe (Fig. 21). The lingular division of the left upper

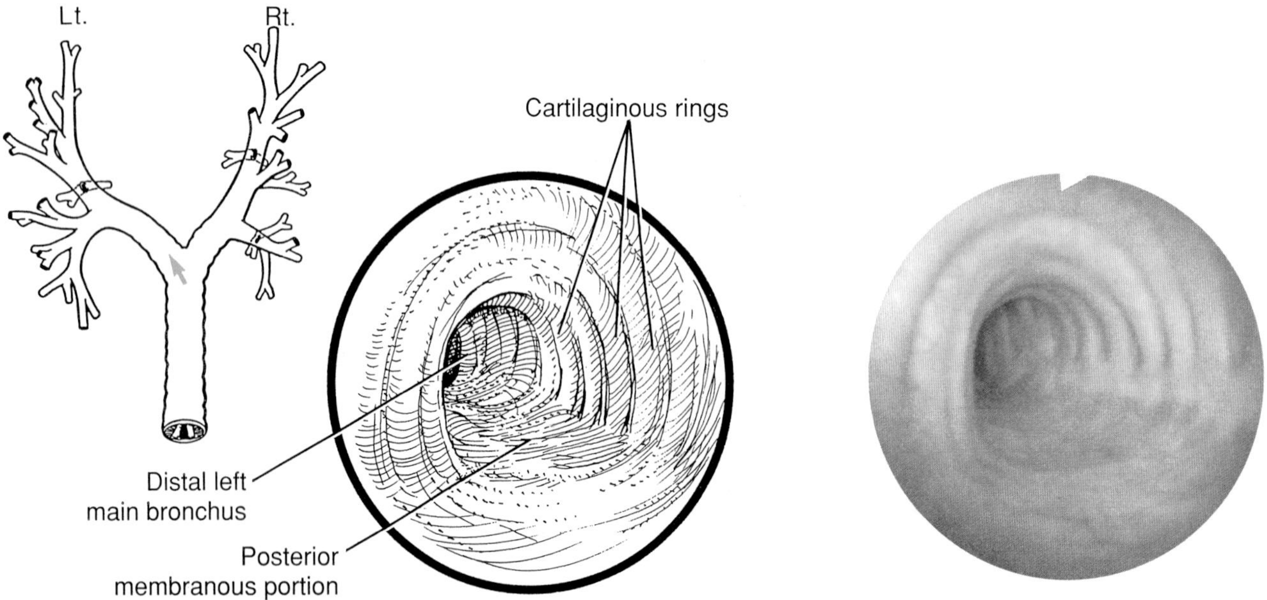

FIG. 19. Left main stem bronchus, proximal half.

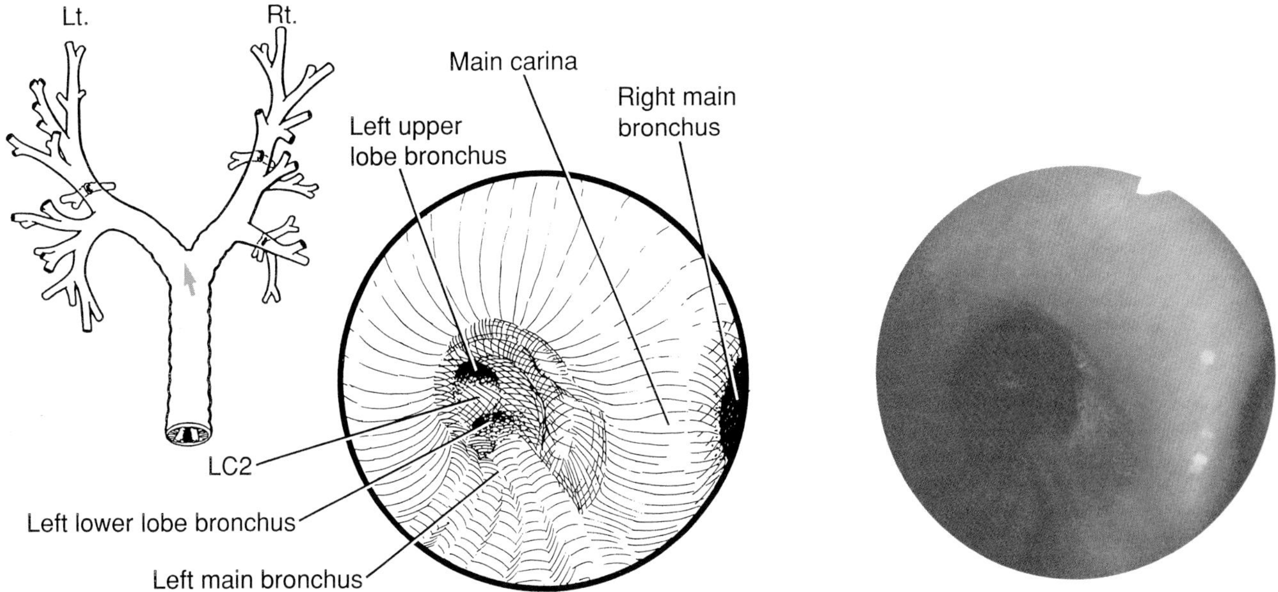

FIG. 20. Left main stem bronchus and origins of bronchi to left upper and lower lobes.

lobe is approximately 1 cm in length before giving rise to segmental bronchi. The left lower lobe bronchus is usually slightly larger than the right lower lobe bronchus. Immediately on entering the left lower lobe bronchus, the superior segment of the left lower lobe bronchus arises and descends posteriorly (Fig. 21). The left lower lobe bronchus beyond the origin of the superior segment is usually 1 cm in length before giving rise to the basilar bronchi.

NOMENCLATURE OF THE TRACHEOBRONCHIAL TREE

Bronchial Tree

The above discussions have focused on the normal anatomy of the tracheobronchial tree. However, the bronchoscopist's approach to the tracheobronchial

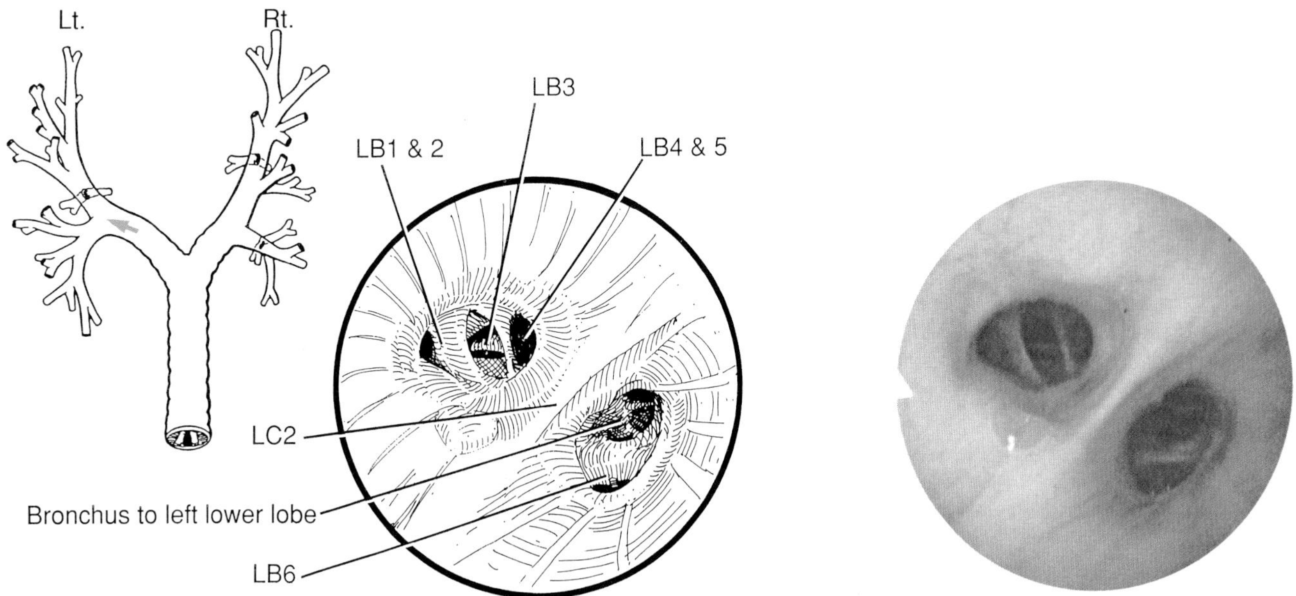

FIG. 21. View from distal left main stem bronchus shows segmental bronchi to left upper and lower lobes.

tree is somewhat different for several reasons. As noted in the introductory chapter on the interpretation of figures in this textbook, some bronchoscopists insert the instrument facing the patient, whereas others insert the bronchoscope by standing at the head of the patient. The mental orientation of the tracheobronchial tree is reversed in these two approaches (see Figs. 1 and 2 in the introductory chapter). Nevertheless, the classification of the tracheobronchial tree remains unchanged. Therefore, it is important to become familiar with the classification of the tracheobronchial tree. The use of appropriate terminologies to describe the bronchi in the recordings of the bronchoscopic findings will aid in the optimal communication among physicians. It is unfortunate that there are some variations in the bronchial nomenclature between the British and the commonly used system. The following description is primarily based on the needs of the bronchoscopist.

The present system of bronchial nomenclature is based on the pioneer studies in the 1940s by Jackson and Huber (9), Boyden and associates (10–16), and Shinoi (17). More detailed classifications of subsegmental bronchi have been described by Nagaishi (18) and Ikeda (Figs. 22–24) (19). Ikeda further classified the distal bronchial tree (Fig. 25). While such classification is needed for the detailed anatomic study of the tracheobronchial tree, its clinical application in the current practice of bronchoscopy is limited. Until the identification of cancer in its earliest stages in the distal bronchial tree is achieved and its treatment without sacrificing a lobe or a lung discovered, the routine naming of sub-subsegmental bronchi in clinical bronchoscopic recordings should be avoided. This does not imply that the bronchoscopist should limit the visual examination to segmental bronchi. The commonly accepted and clinically (and bronchoscopically) used classification of the tracheobronchial tree is depicted in Fig. 26). In the majority of cases, the proper identification of segmental bronchi is sufficient in terms of the presence of an abnormality.

We highly recommend that the term "apical" bronchus or segment be reserved for the apical segments of upper lobes, and the term "superior" bronchus or segment be reserved for the superior segment (sometimes called the apical segment) of lower lobes. Worldwide uniformity in describing the bronchi and carinae will help avoid confusion in the interpretation of bronchoscopic findings.

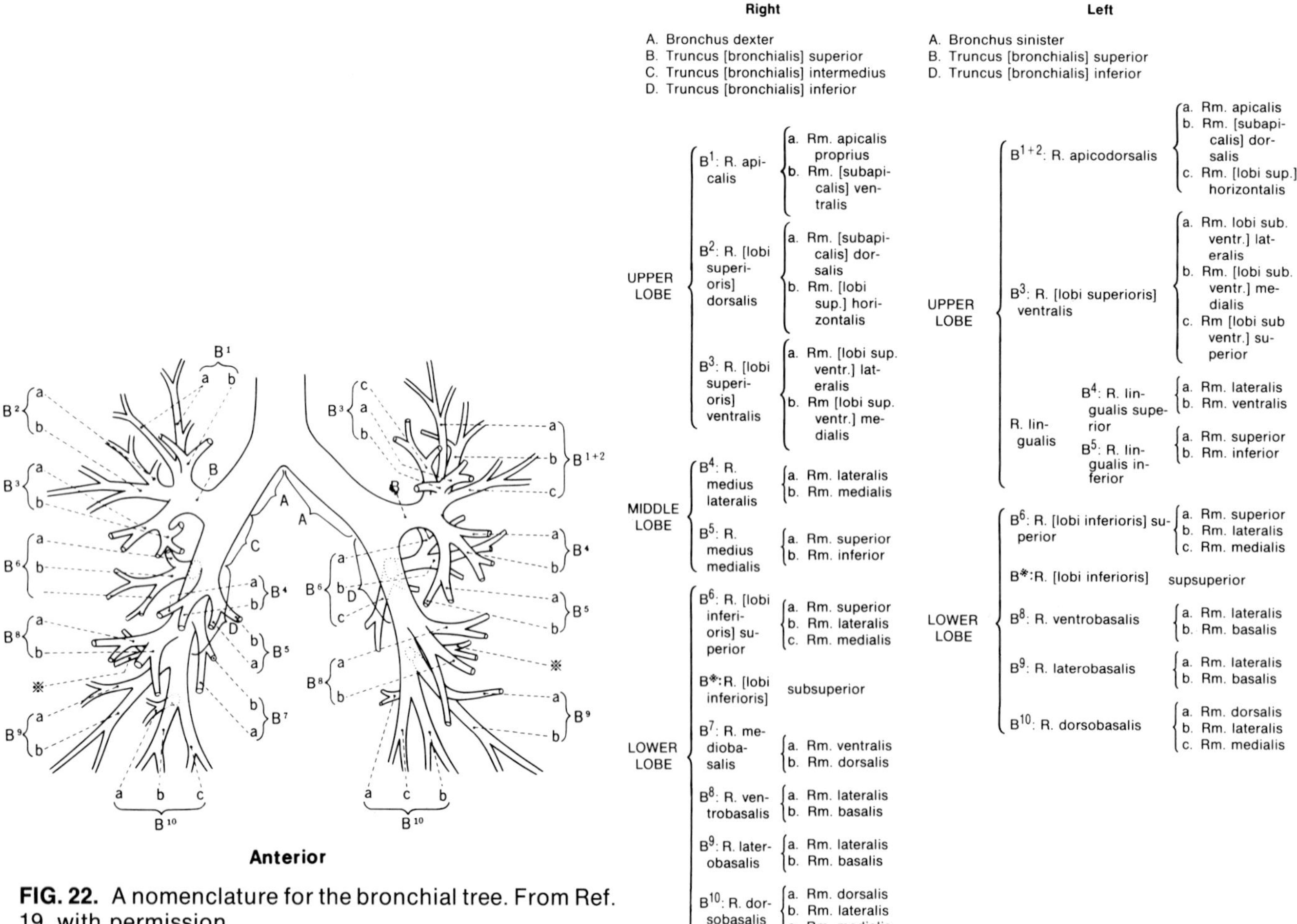

FIG. 22. A nomenclature for the bronchial tree. From Ref. 19, with permission.

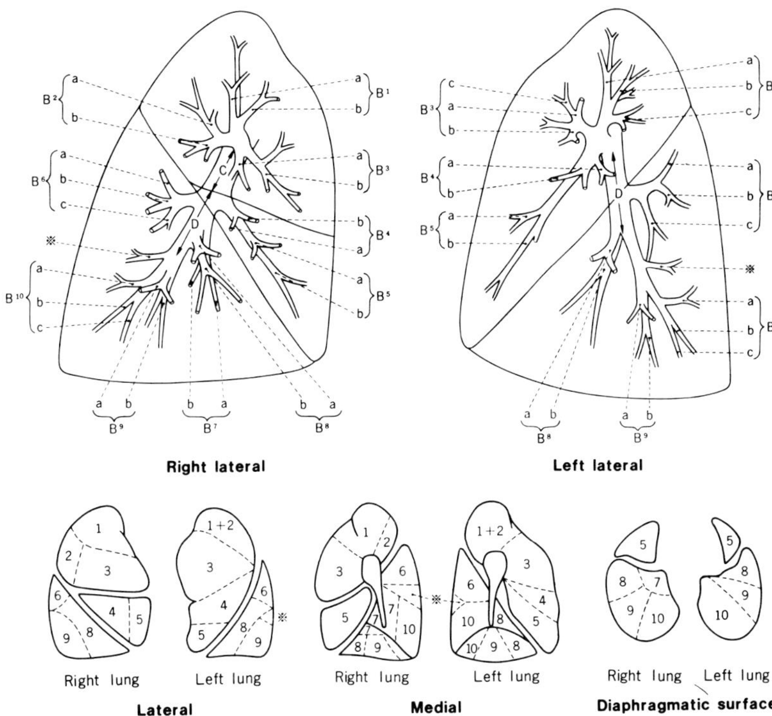

FIG. 23. A nomenclature for the bronchial tree (top) and lung segments (bottom). See Fig. 22 for description of abbreviations. Note that this classification does not differentiate LB7 from LB8. Instead they are together named LB8-b and LB8-a, respectively. From Ref. 19, with permission.

Distal Carinae

The carinae, including the main carina, are sometimes described as "spur," "wedge," "branching angle," or "bifurcating point of bronchi." We suggest that the term *carina* be used consistently to describe these structures. The main carina is part of the trachea and because its involvement by the neoplastic process usually denotes unresectability, the bronchoscopist should record such finding. Prakash and Fontana (20)

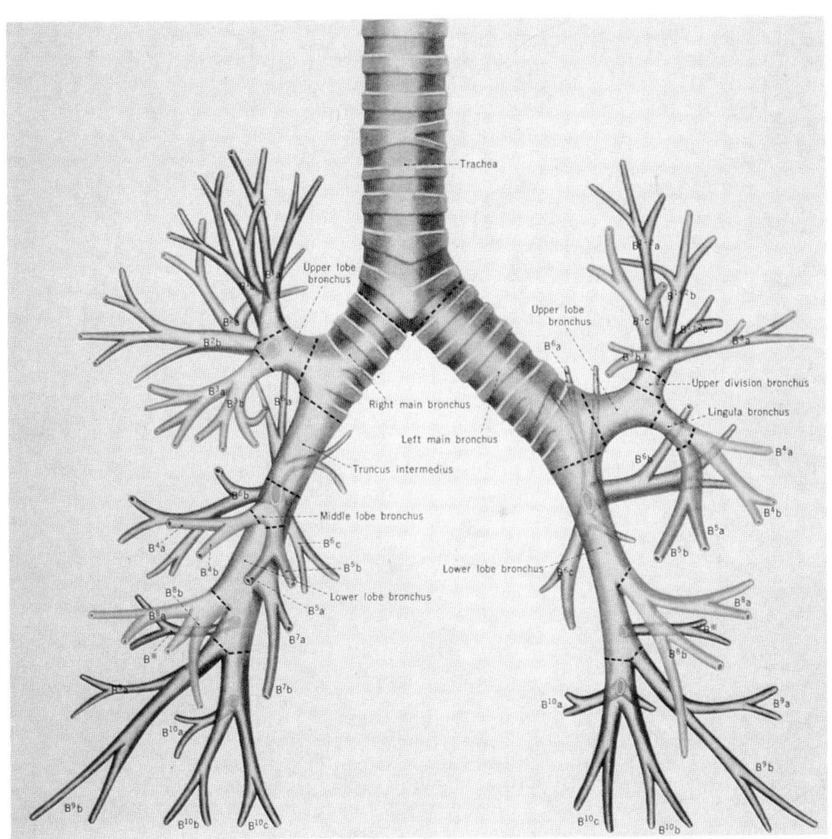

FIG. 24. The tracheobronchial tree. See Fig. 22 for the nomenclature. From Ref. 19, with permission.

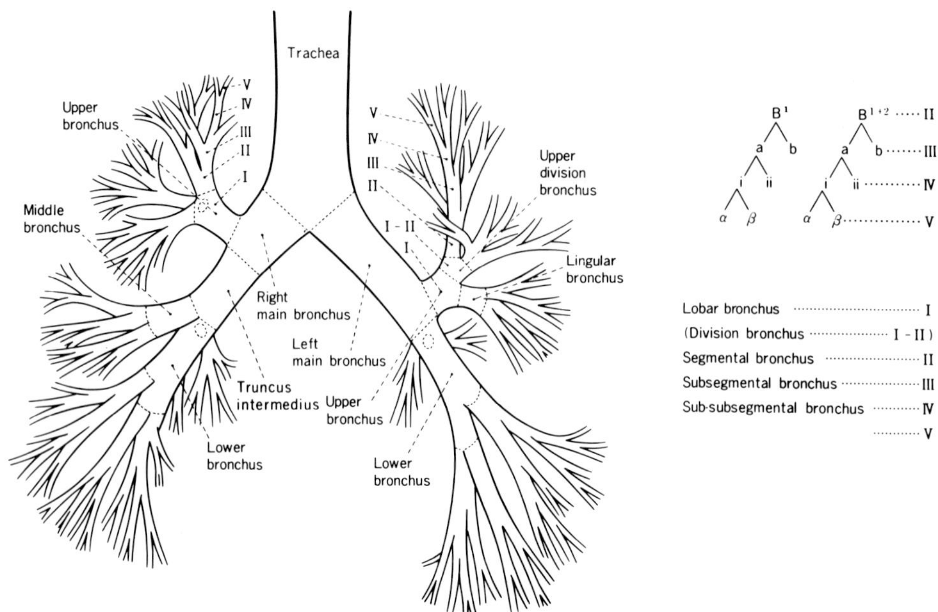

FIG. 25. Classification of bronchi to sub-subsegmental level and beyond. Conventionally, the letters a, i, and α are used to name a bronchus that is posterior or lateral or inferior, and b, ii, and β are used to designate a bronchus that is anterior or medial or superior. From Ref. 19, with permission.

described a classification and a method to name the bronchial carinae (Figs. 1 and 2 in the introductory chapter). Their classification is an attempt to provide further information regarding the extent of neoplastic involvement of the bronchial tree so that appropriate surgical treatment can be planned.

The carina dividing the bronchus to the right upper lobe and right bronchus intermedius is termed right

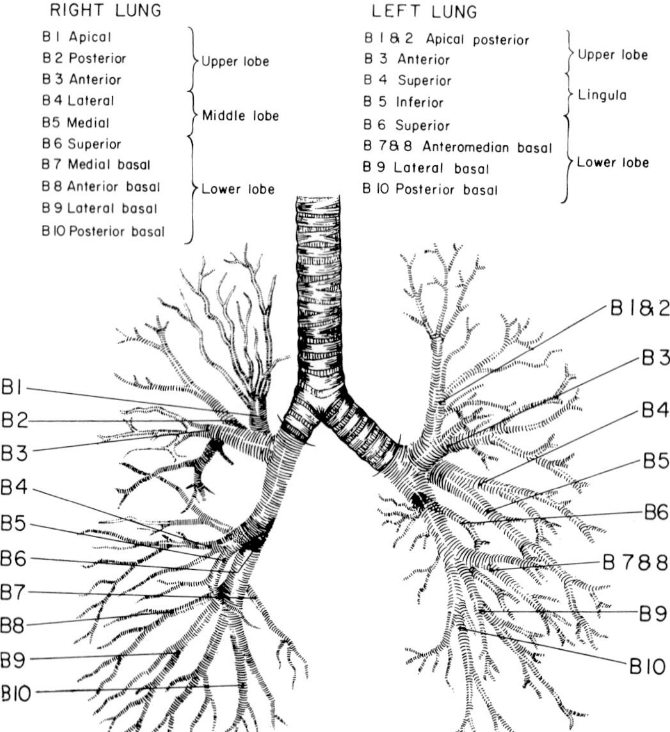

FIG. 26. Standard bronchial nomenclature used in current practice of bronchoscopy.

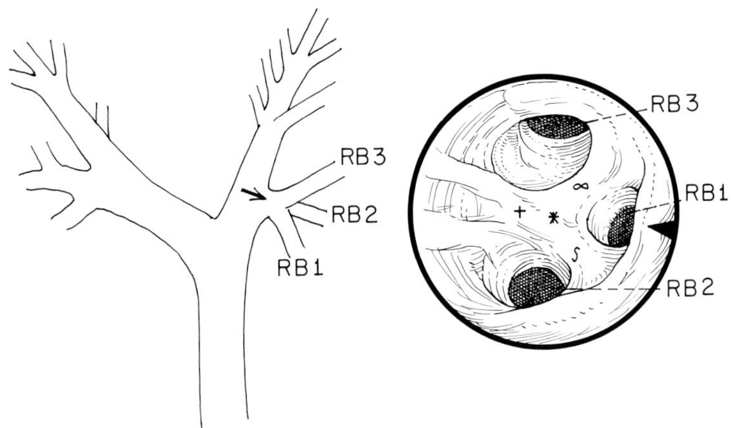

FIG. 27. Example of description of segmental carinae. Common anatomic arrangement of three minor carinae in right upper lobe. Carina at + is termed "carina RB2–3," and likewise, carinae at *s* and ∞ are named "carina RB1–2" and "carina RB1–3," respectively. Similarly, associated minor carinae can be described by noting relationship between bronchi and each carina formed by bronchial branching. From Ref. 20, with permission.

carina 1 or RC-1, and the carina between the right middle lobe bronchus and the bronchus to the right lower lobe is termed right carina 2 or RC-2. Similarly LC-1 (left carina 1) describes the carina between the bronchus to the anterior segment of left upper lobe and bronchus leading to the lingular segments. LC-2 (left carina 2) is the carina that separates bronchus to lingular segment of left upper lobe and left lower lobar bronchus. Distal carinae can be similarly described (Fig. 27).

The reasoning behind the above nomenclature is related to clinical application, particularly in assessing the extent of neoplastic involvement and the surgical resection required. For instance, the involvement of LC-2 automatically denotes that the patient will require pneumonectomy unless a tailored bronchoplasty is planned.

PULMONARY LOBES AND SEGMENTS

An understanding of the lobar and segmental anatomy of the lungs is particularly helpful in interpreting the appearance of the plain chest roentgenograph in the posteroanterior and lateral projections. We believe that the bronchoscopist should acquire sufficient expertise in the interpretation of chest roentgenograms as well as plain and computed tomograms of the thorax. Such knowledge not only provides confidence in approaching difficult problems but also increases the diagnostic and therapeutic yield from bronchoscopy.

Right Lung

The right lung is composed of three lobes: upper, middle, and lower. There are ten bronchopulmonary

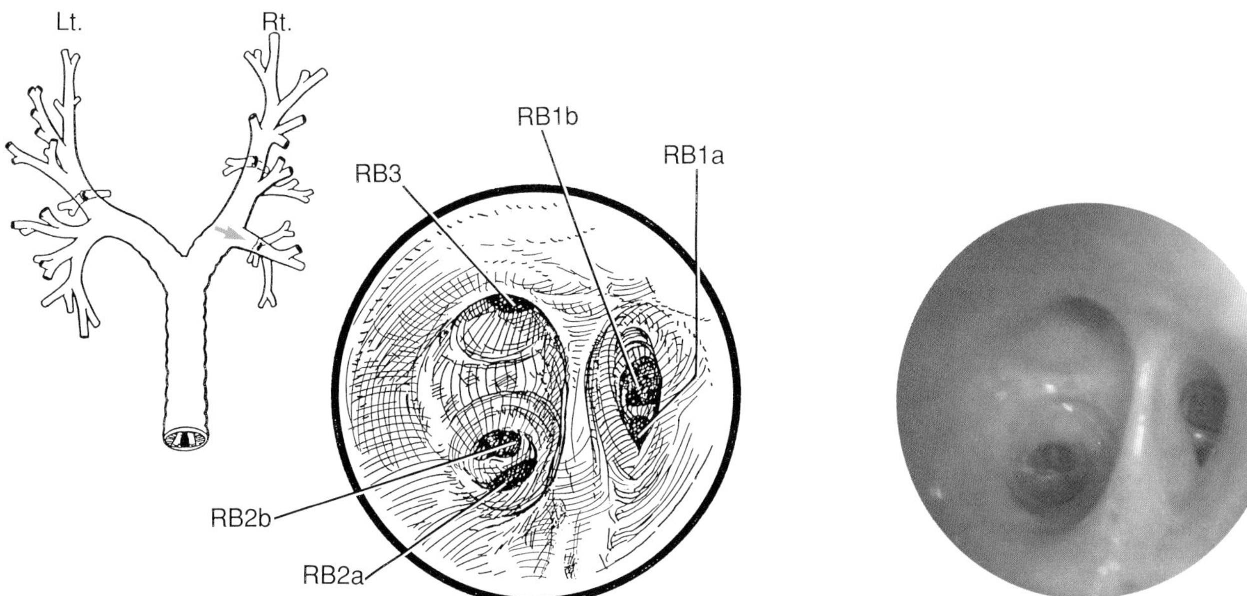

FIG. 28. A bronchoscopic view of segmental bronchi to right upper lobe.

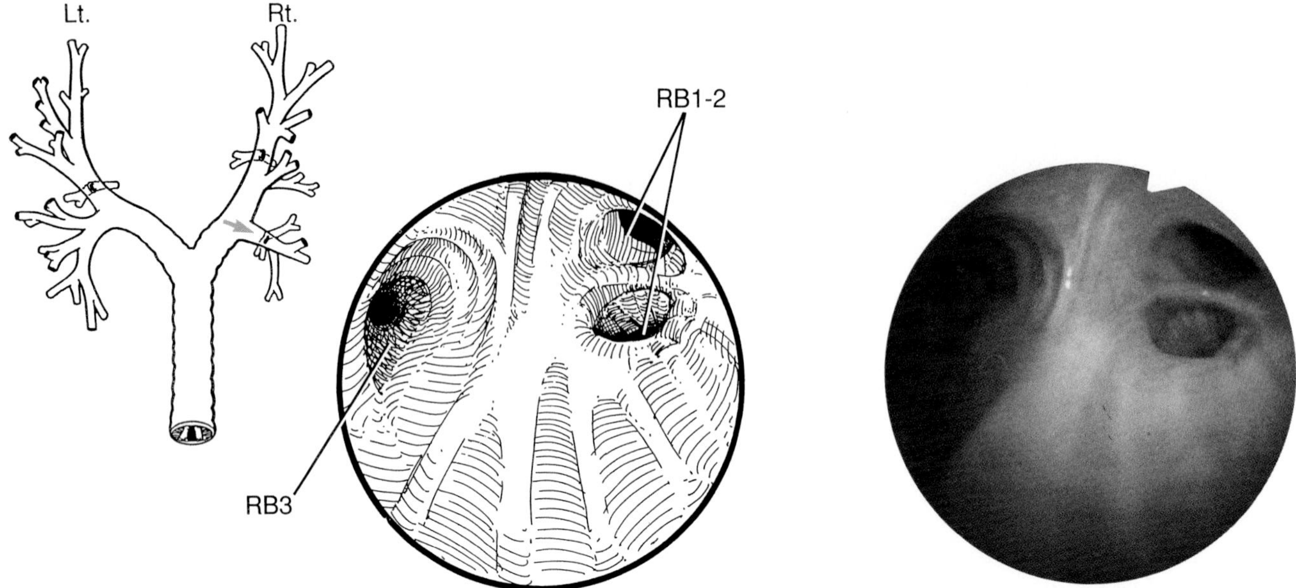

FIG. 29. Bifurcation (instead of usual trifurcation) of segmental bronchi to right upper lobe.

segments distributed throughout these three lobes. The right upper lobe contains three segments (Fig. 28). The apical segment of the right upper lobe, RB1, composes the apex of the lung. The posterior segment of the right upper lobe, RB2, composes the posterior portion of the right upper lobe, abuts the major fissure, and is contiguous with the superior segment of the right lower lobe. The anterior segment of the right upper lobe, RB3, comprises the anterior portion of the right upper lobe, abuts the chest wall anteriorly and the minor fissure inferiorly, and therefore is contiguous with the middle lobe. Not infrequently, only two branches are seen in the right upper lobe, similar to the normal arrangement in the left upper lobe (Fig. 29).

The minor fissure of the right lung is located between the right upper lobe and the right middle lobe. On the posteroanterior roentgenogram, this fissure is occasionally visible as a faint line. It is this fissure that produces the linear shadow seen with right upper lobe collapse. The minor fissure posteriorly abuts the major fissure in the midportion of the lung and passes anteriorly to the anterior chest wall. As it passes from the posterior to anterior direction, it has a slight slant inferiorly. This structure is less than 1 mm in thickness and

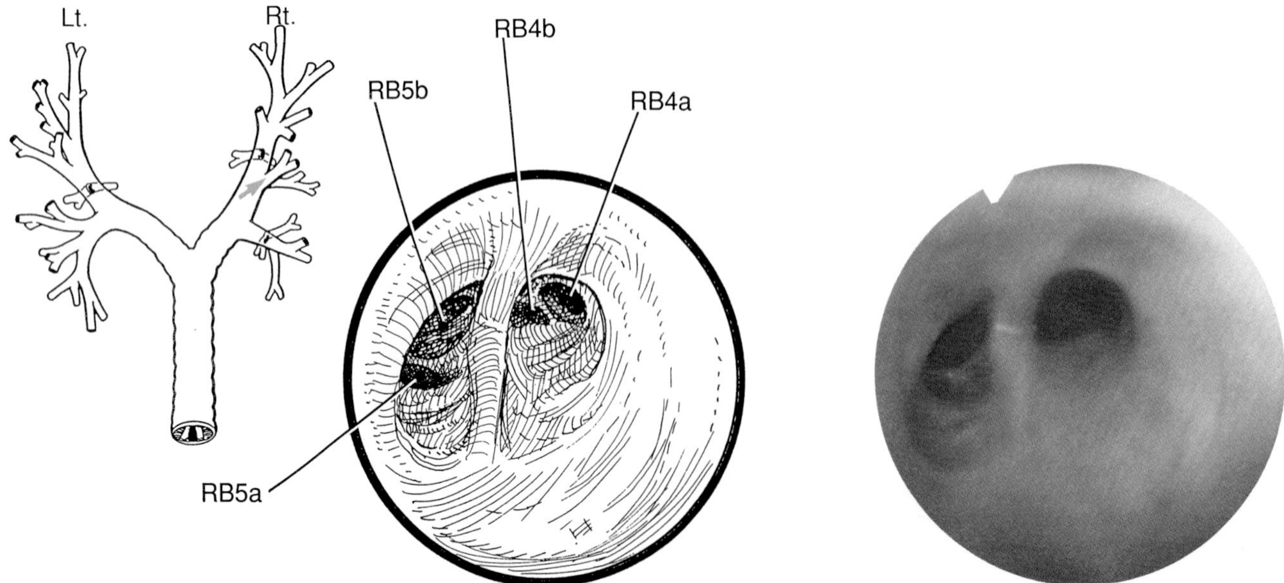

FIG. 30. Bronchi to right middle lobe segments.

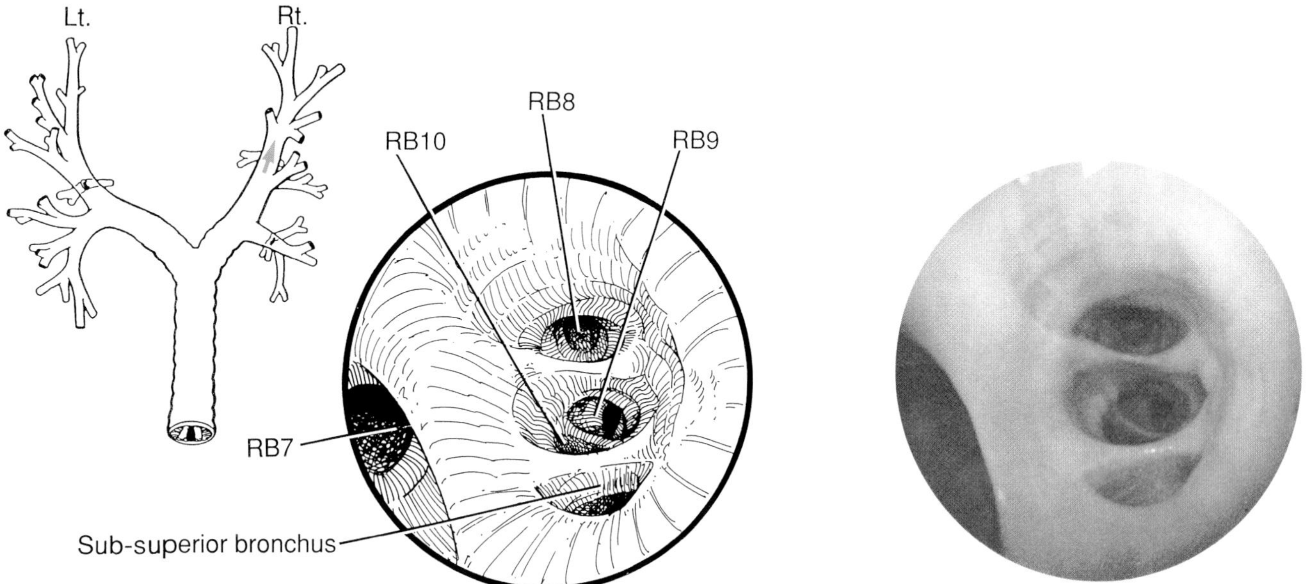

FIG. 31. Bronchi to right lower lobe segments. A subsuperior segment is shown. Superior segment (RB6) is proximal to this view and hence not seen.

therefore may be difficult to see on a posteroanterior roentgenogram because of its slight downward deflection on this view.

The right middle lobe is divided into a lateral segment, RB4, and a medial segment, RB5 (Fig. 30). The medial segment of the right middle lobe abuts the right atrium on the posteroanterior projection. On the lateral projection, the right middle lobe segments reach the inferior aspect of the lung shadow abutting the anterior costophrenic angle.

The right lower lobe consists of the superior segment, RB6; the medial basal segment, RB7; an anterior basal segment, RB8; a lateral basal segment, RB9; and a posterior basal segment, RB10 (Fig. 31). Superior segment (RB6) usually trifurcates (Fig. 32). Occasionally, a subsuperior segment between RB6 and RB10 is also evident (Fig. 31). On the lateral projection, the right lower lobe constitutes the lung shadow that borders the diaphragm, along the posterior chest wall, and reaches superiorly to the fifth–sixth vertebral body.

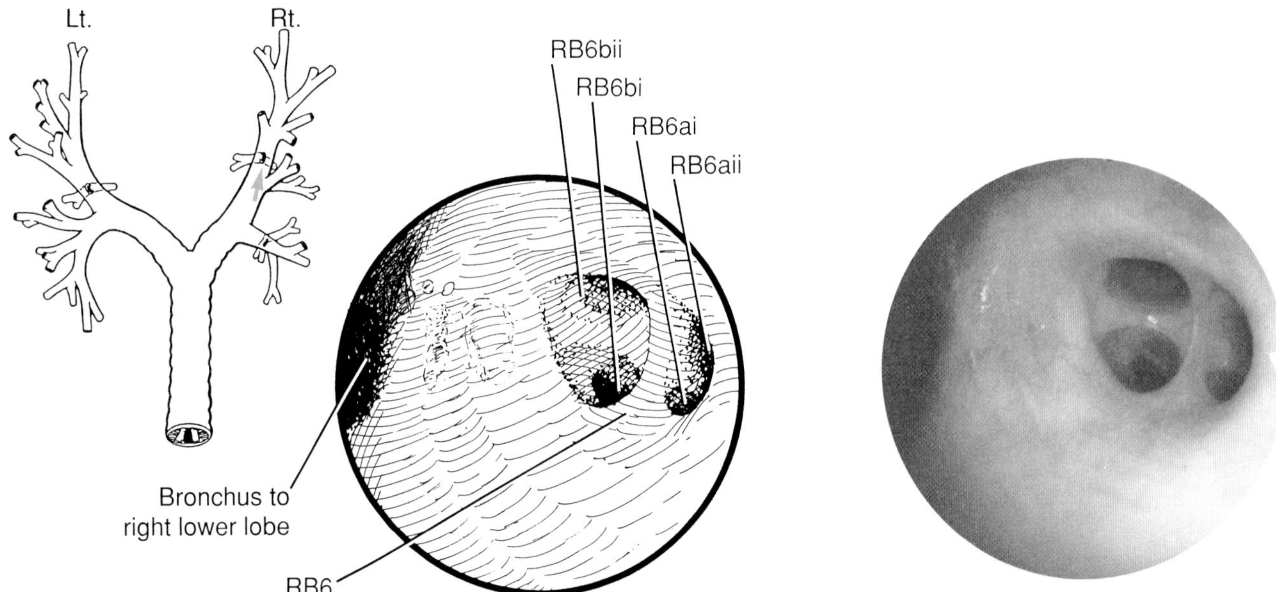

FIG. 32. Bronchus to superior segment of right lower lobe (RB6). Trifurcation is normal for this bronchus.

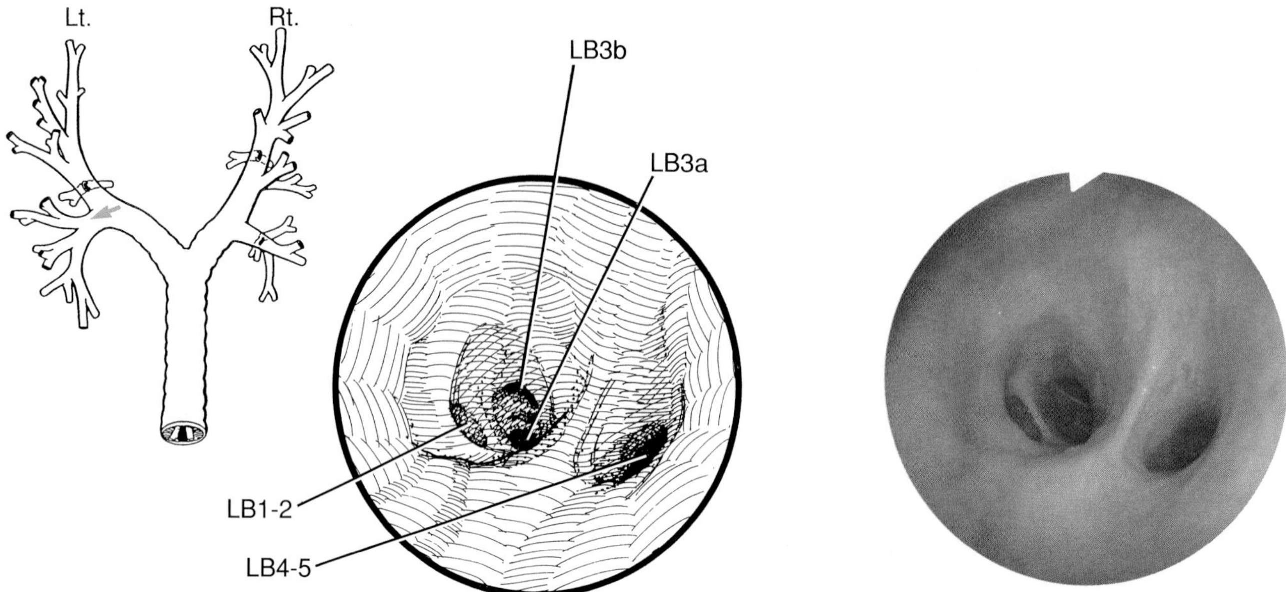

FIG. 33. Bronchi to left upper lobe segments, including lingula.

The major fissure passes obliquely from posterior to the anterior direction as it descends caudally from the level of the fifth–sixth vertebral body. It separates the right lower lobe from the right upper and middle lobes. There is variability in the distribution of the anterior, lateral, and posterior basal segments of the right lower lobe; and it is not always possible to name these orifices with certainty. However, bronchoscopically, the relationship of these orifices is rather clear and their names correspond with the appropriate direction of the bronchus as it passes into the periphery.

Left Lung

On the left side, there are two lobes—the left upper lobe and the left lower lobe—and ten bronchopulmonary segments. On the lateral projection, the left major fissure passes between the left upper and the left lower lobes. This fissure arises slightly higher on the left than on the right at approximately the fourth or fifth vertebral body and passes obliquely anteriorly as it proceeds from superior to inferior aspect.

The left upper lobe consists of an upper division that

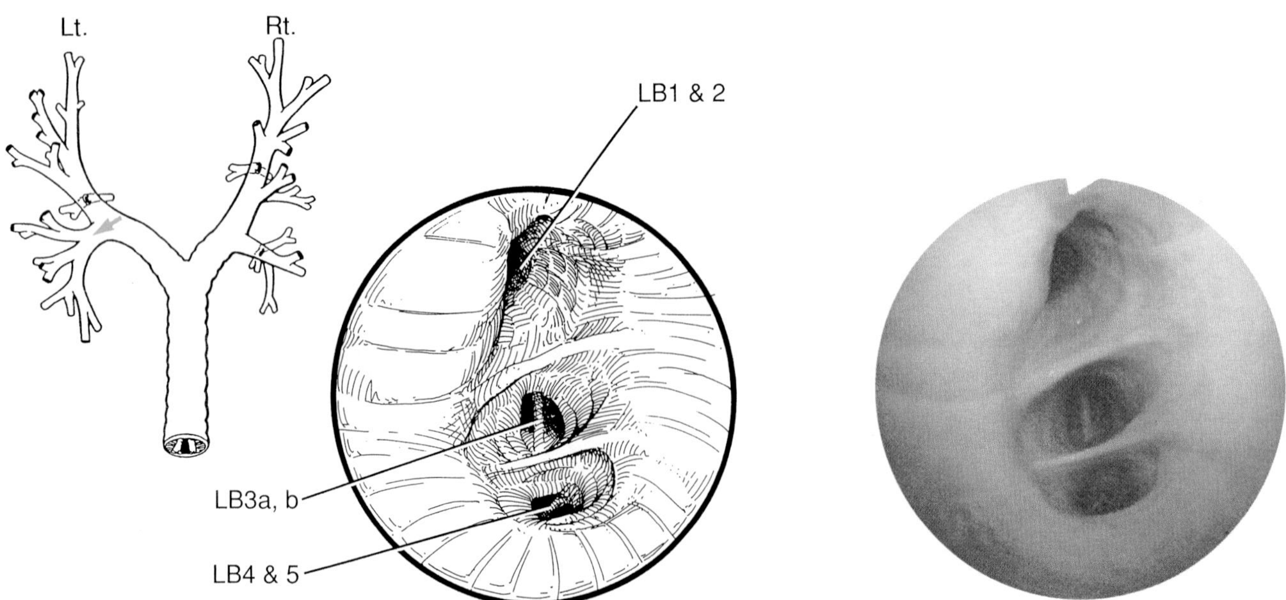

FIG. 34. Closer view of bronchi to LB1&2, LB3, and LB4&5.

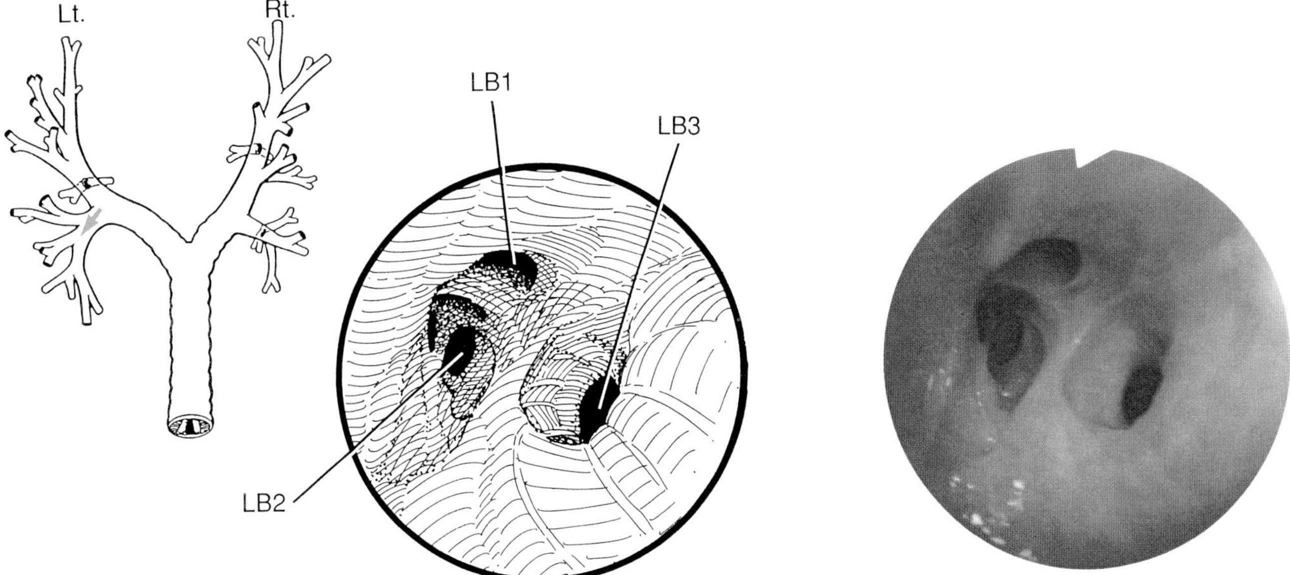

FIG. 35. Left upper lobe bronchial branching as the mirror image of right upper lobe bronchial branching.

corresponds to the right upper lobe and a lingular division that corresponds to the right middle lobe (Figs. 33 and 34). The upper division of the left upper lobe gives rise to a common apical posterior segment of the left upper lobe, LB1 + 2, which occupies the apex and the posterior areas of the lung. The anterior segment of the left upper lobe, LB3, is located along the anterior aspect of the lobe. There is variability in the appearance of the left upper lobe bronchus and occasionally there will be three bronchi arising simultaneously and presenting as a mirror image of the right side with independent segments leading to the apical, posterior, and anterior segments of the left upper lobe (Fig. 35). The lingular division of the left upper lobe gives rise to the superior segment, LB4, and the inferior segment, LB5, which composes the inferior portion of the left upper lobe (Fig. 36). The lingula abuts the anterior chest wall and the left heart border.

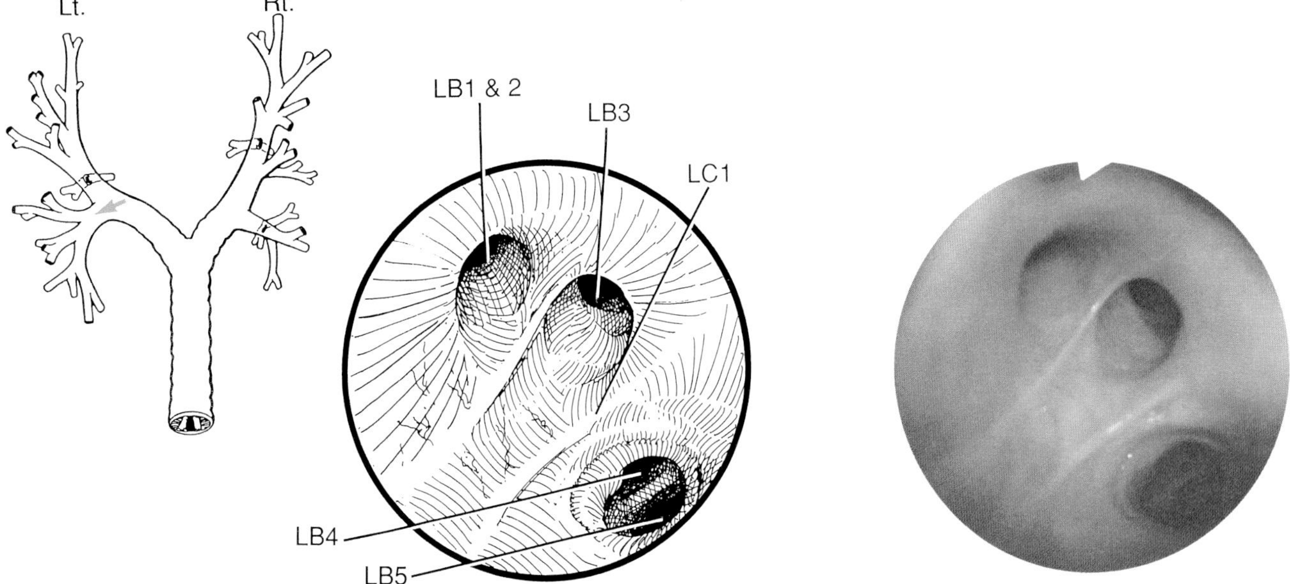

FIG. 36. Branching of lingula (LB4&5), LB1&2, and LB3. This is the most common anatomic arrangement of left upper lobe bronchial branching.

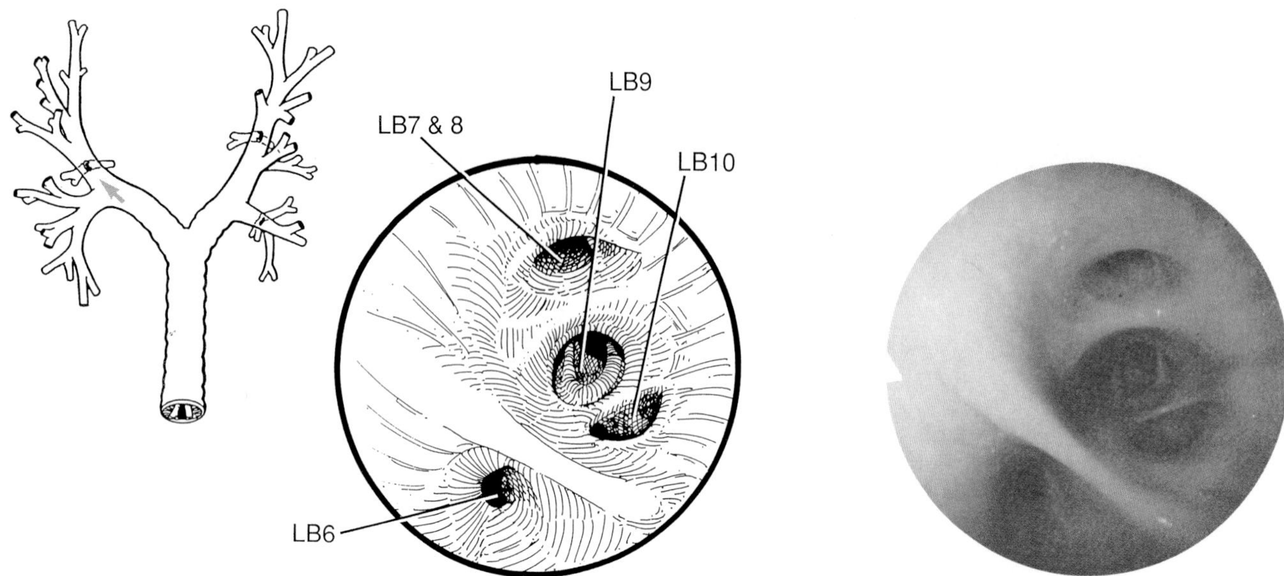

FIG. 37. Typical division of bronchi to segments of left lower lobe.

The left lower lobe is composed of a superior segment, LB6; usually a common anteromedial basal segment, LB7–8; a lateral basal segment, LB9; and a posterior basal segment, LB10 (Fig. 37). Occasionally, there is also a subsuperior segment between LB6 and LB10 as may be found on the right side (Fig. 38).

Mediastinum

We will concentrate on the anatomy of the mediastinum as it pertains to the bronchoscopist with particular emphasis on vascular structures and lymph node anatomy. Thorough knowledge of the mediastinal anatomy is required before performing procedures relating to treatment and staging of lung cancer that involve the use of laser bronchoscopy as well as transtracheal and transbronchial needle aspirations and biopsies. The American Joint Committee for Cancer Staging and End Results Reporting classifies mediastinal lymph nodes into superior mediastinal nodes, aortic nodes, and inferior mediastinal nodes (21).

The superior mediastinal nodes are subcategorized into the highest mediastinal nodes, upper paratracheal

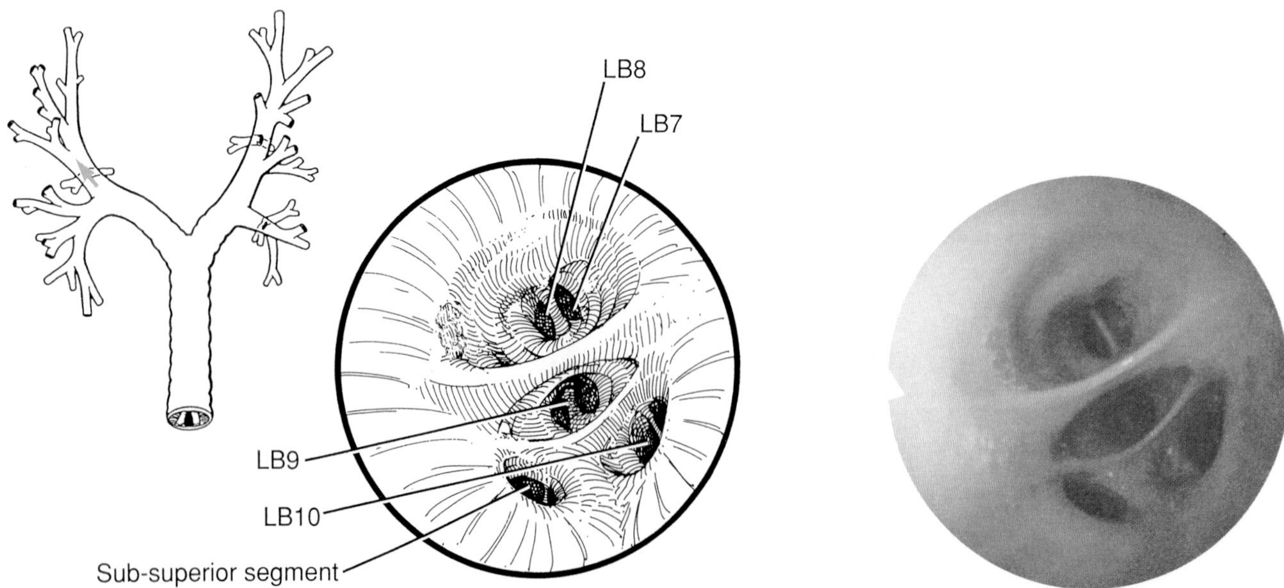

FIG. 38. Closer view of bronchi to segments of left lower lobe. Note the bronchus to subsuperior segment.

nodes, pre- and retrotracheal lymph nodes, and lower paratracheal lymph nodes. The aortic lymph nodes are located along the course of the aorta on its lateral aspect. There are groups of subaortic, aortic window, and paraaortic lymph nodes (ascending aorta or phrenic). The inferior mediastinal lymph nodes are grouped into the subcarinal nodes, the paraesophageal nodes, and the pulmonary ligament nodes. If any of the mediastinal nodes are involved with tumor, they are classified in the N2 or N3 category of the TNM classification as recommended by the American Joint Committee on Cancer (AJCC) and the Union Internationale Contre Cancer (UICC) and described by Mountain (22). N2 means metastases to ipsilateral mediastinal lymph nodes and subcarinal lymph nodes. N3 means metastases to contralateral mediastinal lymph nodes, contralateral hilar lymph nodes, and ipsilateral or contralateral scalene or supraclavicular lymph nodes. N1 lymph nodes include those that are not within the mediastinum. The groups include hilar lymph nodes, interlobar lymph nodes, lobar lymph nodes, and segmental lymph nodes. According to the TNM classification, N1 implies metastases to lymph nodes in the peribronchial or ipsilateral hilar region, or both, including direct extension.

Relationship of the Vascular Structures to the Tracheobronchial Tree

Bronchoscopists who plan on practicing laser bronchoscopy and bronchoscopic needle aspiration/biopsy should be particularly familiar with the vascular structures that surround the tracheobronchial tree. The following is description of the essential vascular anatomy for the bronchoscopist.

The thyroid gland lies along the thyroid cartilage in the cervical trachea. Along the lower edge of the thyroid gland, there are veins that drain away from the trachea into the left innominate vein, usually immediately behind the manubrium sternum and not in immediate contact with the trachea. However, there are arterial structures in close proximity to the trachea below the thyroid gland. The course of the brachycephalic artery passes from left to right immediately in front of the trachea. This vessel is the first large vessel to arise from the arch of the aorta and passes across the trachea, frequently bifurcating in close proximity to the trachea at the base of the neck. The right common carotid may run obliquely across the front of the cervical trachea while the right subclavian passes laterally. Both common carotid arteries are in contact with the sides of the trachea at their origins and move laterally away from the trachea as they ascend into the neck. The left innominate vein passes anteriorly to the aortic arch in a horizontal direction. As it enters the mediastinum, it joins the right innominate vein slightly to the right of the trachea and their junction forms the superior vena cava (Figs. 39 and 40).

The superior vena cava descends vertically in front and slightly to the right of the trachea. As the superior vena cava passes inferiorly, and just prior to joining the right atrium, it receives the large azygos vein posteriorly. The azygos vein passes through the posterior mediastinum just lateral to the airway where the trachea and the right main stem bronchus join. It courses over the lateral right side of the bottom of the trachea and joins the superior vena cava (Fig. 41).

The aortic arch passes obliquely from anterior to posterior and from right to left across the left anterior aspect of the trachea. Bronchoscopically, an indenta-

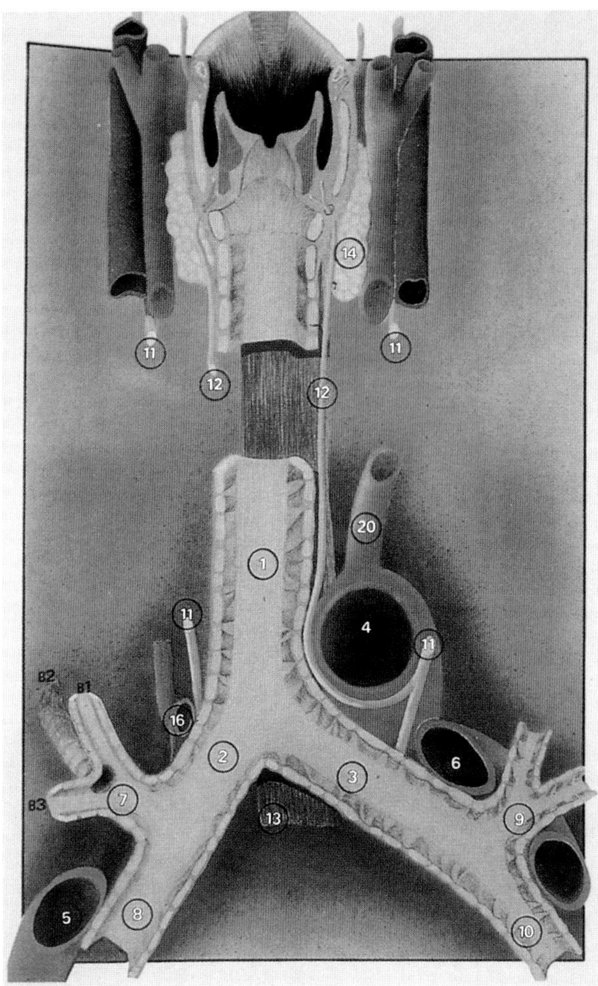

FIG. 39. Cross section of the tracheobronchial tree: anterior view. 1, Trachea; 2, right main stem bronchus; 3, left main stem bronchus; 4, aorta; 5, right pulmonary artery; 6, left pulmonary artery; 7, right upper lobe bronchus; 8, bronchus intermedius; 9, left upper lobe bronchus; 10, left lower lobe bronchus; 11, vagus nerve; 12, recurrent laryngeal nerve; 13, esophagus; 14, thyroid gland; 16, azygos vein. Figs. 39–49 use identical numbering system to identify various structures. (Courtesy of J.-F. Dumon, M.D.)

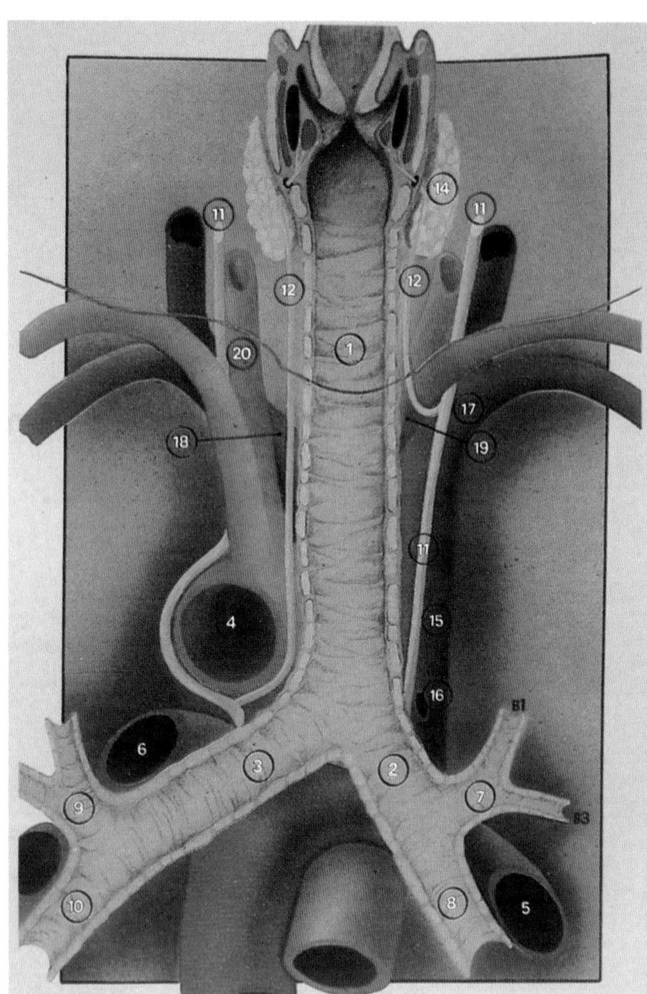

FIG. 40. Cross-section of the tracheobronchial tree: posterior view. 1, trachea; 2, right main stem bronchus; 3, left main stem bronchus; 4, aorta; 5, right pulmonary artery; 6, left pulmonary artery; 7, right upper lobe bronchus; 8, bronchus intermedius; 9, left upper lobe bronchus; 10, left lower lobe bronchus; 11, vagus nerve; 12, recurrent nerve; 14, thyroid gland; 15, superior vena cava; 16, azygos vein; 17, right innominate vein; 18, left innominate vein; 19, innominate artery; 20, left carotid artery. (Courtesy of J.-F. Dumon, M.D.)

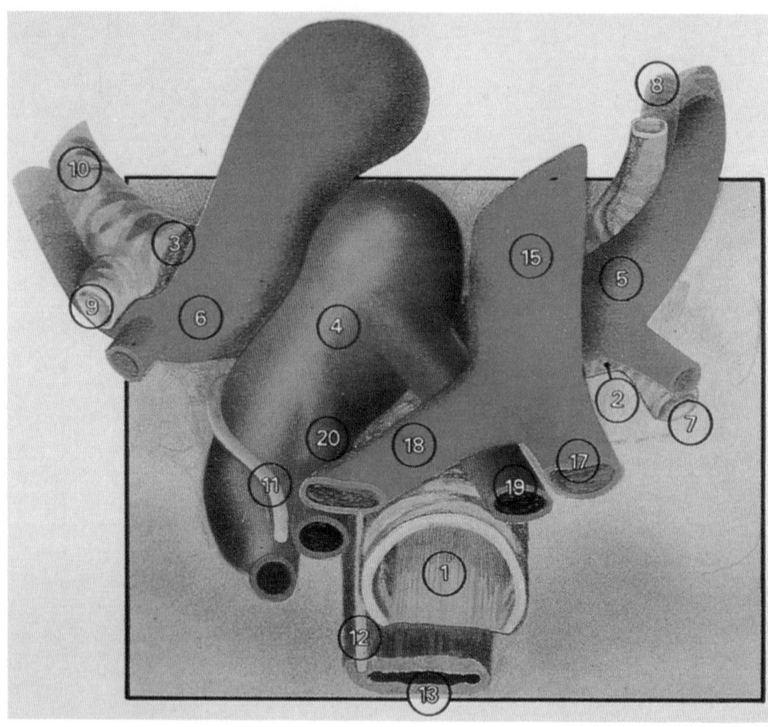

FIG. 41. Above the aortic arch. 1, trachea; 2, right main stem bronchus; 3, left main stem bronchus; 4, aorta; 5, right pulmonary artery; 6, left pulmonary artery; 7, right upper lobe bronchus; 8, bronchus intermedius; 9, left upper lobe bronchus; 10, left lower lobe bronchus; 11, vagus nerve; 12, recurrent nerve; 13, esophagus; 15, superior vena cava; 17, right innominate vein; 18, left innominate vein; 19, innominate artery; 20, left carotid artery. (Courtesy of J.-F. Dumon, M.D.)

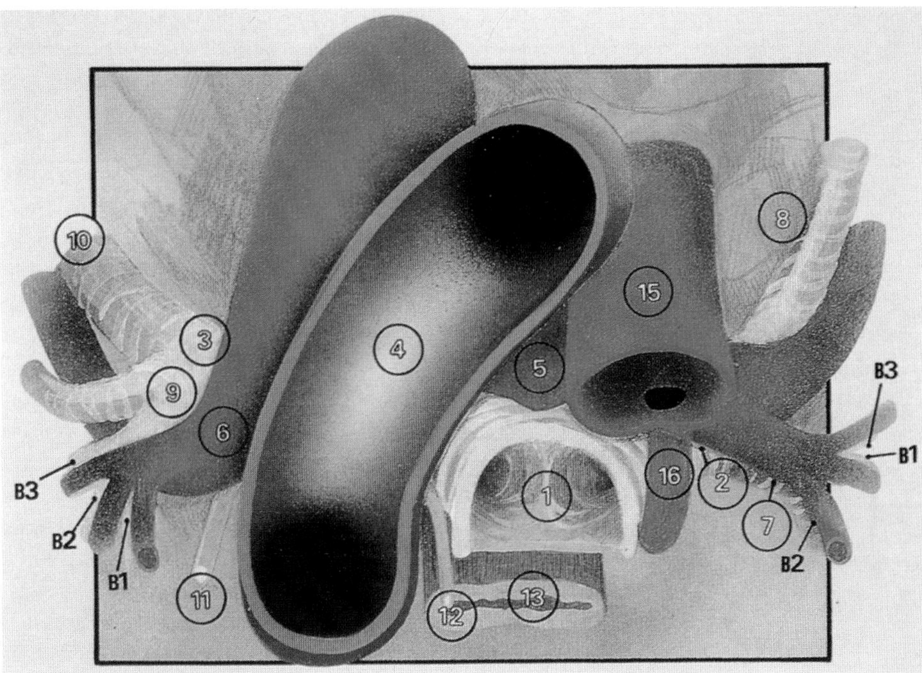

FIG. 42. At the aortic arch level. 1, trachea; 2, right main stem bronchus; 3, left main stem bronchus; 4, aorta; 5, right pulmonary artery; 6, left pulmonary artery; 7, right upper lobe bronchus; 8, bronchus intermedius; 9, left upper lobe bronchus; 10, left lower lobe bronchus; 11, vagus nerve; 12, recurrent nerve; 13, esophagus; 15, superior vena cava; 16, azygos vein. (Courtesy of J.-F. Dumon, M.D.)

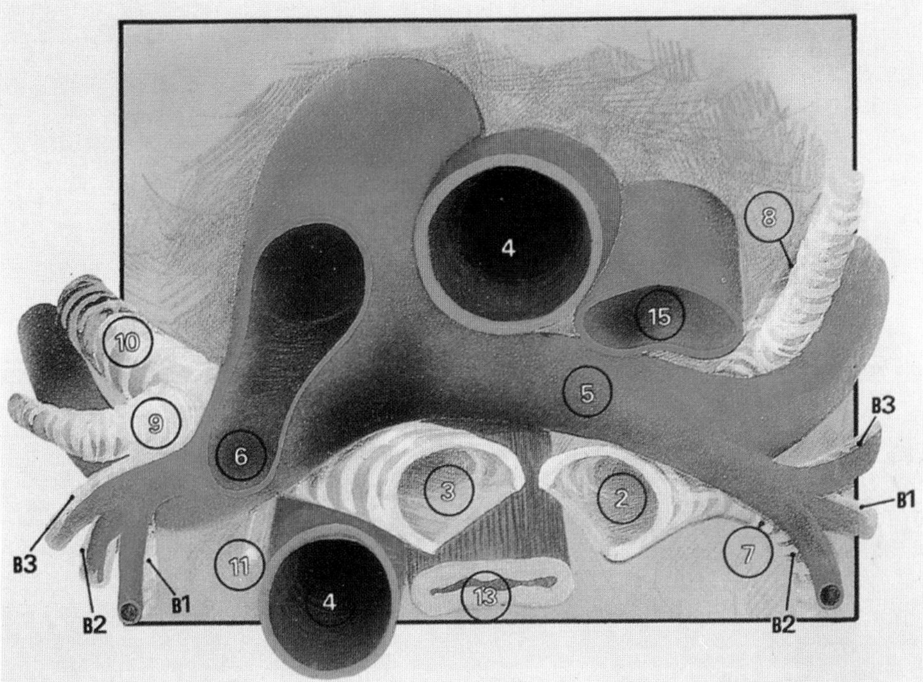

FIG. 43. Below the carina. 2, right main stem bronchus; 3, left main stem bronchus; 4, aorta; 5, right pulmonary artery; 6, left pulmonary artery; 7, right upper lobe bronchus; 8, bronchus intermedius; 9, left upper lobe bronchus; 10, left lower lobe bronchus; 11, vagus nerve; 13, esophagus; 15, superior vena cava. (Courtesy of J.-F. Dumon, M.D.)

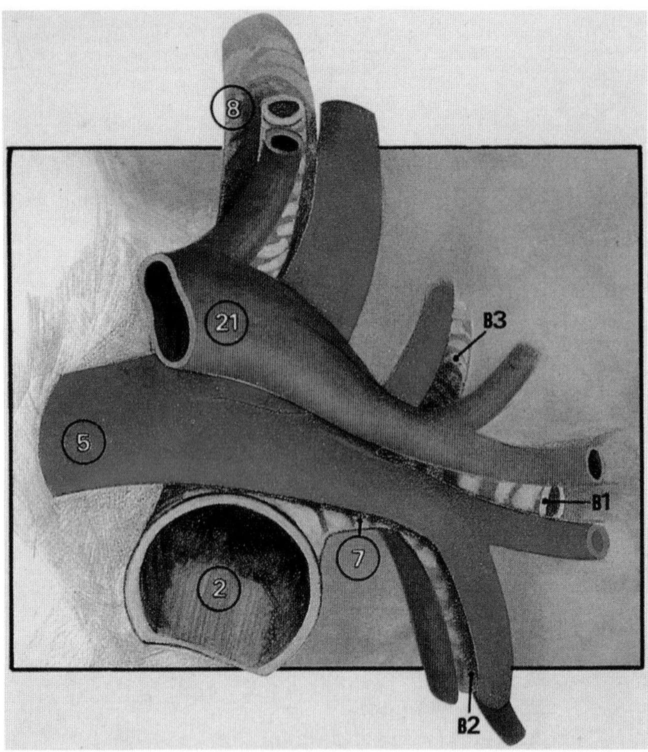

FIG. 44. Right main stem bronchus. 2, right main stem bronchus; 5, right pulmonary artery; 7, right upper lobe bronchus; 8, bronchus intermedius; 21, right upper pulmonary vein. (Courtesy of J.-F. Dumon, M.D.)

tion can be seen along the left anterior lateral wall of distal trachea where the aortic arch abuts the trachea. The aortic arch winds over the left main stem bronchus and descends against the vertebral column. The level of the arch of the aorta gives rise to the right brachycephalic artery (innominate artery) just in front of the trachea. This artery ascends to the right side of the trachea and at the base of the neck divides into the right subclavian artery and the right common carotid artery. The left common carotid artery arises further back and against the left side of the trachea. It passes laterally away from the trachea as it ascends into the neck. The left subclavian artery arises at some distance lateral to the trachea, courses obliquely forward and laterally, and is not in direct contact with the trachea (Fig. 42).

At the tracheal bifurcation, there are several important relationships. The bifurcation of the main trunk of the pulmonary artery is located slightly below, anterior, and to the left of the bifurcation of the trachea. The right pulmonary artery passes in front of the main carina and along the anterior portion of the right main stem bronchus. The aortic arch is situated to the left of the trachea directly at the tracheal bifurcation. The esophagus comes in immediate contact with the posterior wall of the proximal left main stem bronchus as this bronchus arises from the carina. The right pulmonary artery is in close proximity to the anterior wall of the

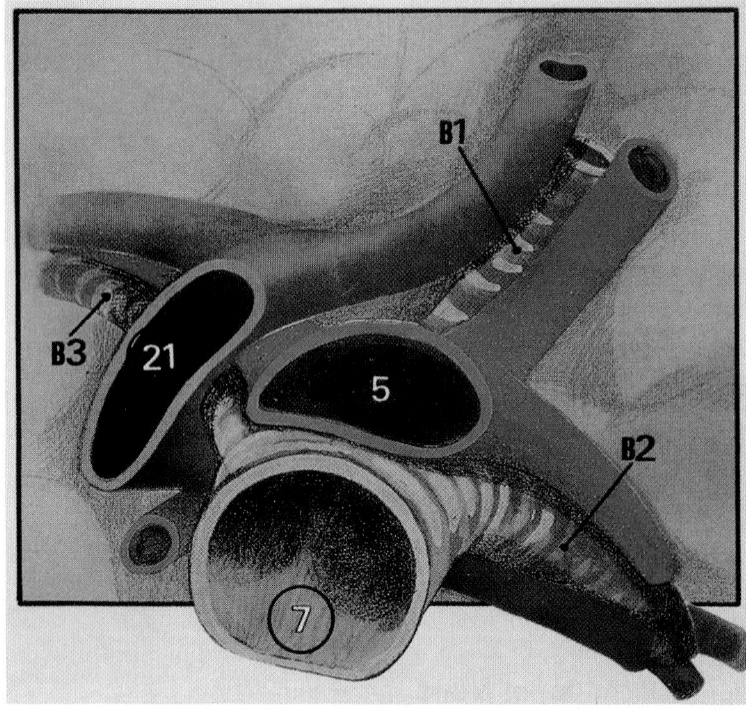

FIG. 45. Right upper lobe bronchus. 5, right pulmonary artery; 7, right upper lobe bronchus; 21, right upper pulmonary vein. (Courtesy of J.-F. Dumon, M.D.)

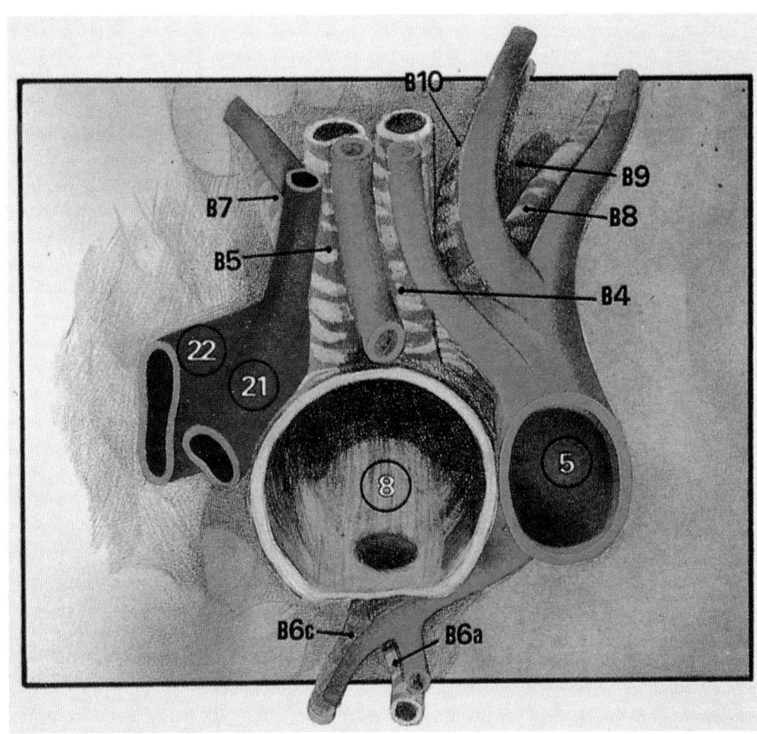

FIG. 46. Middle lobe and right lower lobe bronchi. 5, right pulmonary artery; 8, bronchus intermedius; 21, right upper pulmonary vein; 22, right lower pulmonary vein. (Courtesy of J.-F. Dumon, M.D.)

right main stem bronchus as this vessel passes laterally into the hilum (Fig. 43).

The right upper lobe bronchus is joined by the right upper lobe artery, which lies along the superior and anterior aspects of the bronchus. The pulmonary vein is lower and not in contact with the bronchus. The right middle lobe bronchus is usually joined by the middle lobe artery along the lateral side of the bronchus while the right middle lobe veins are usually along the medial wall of this bronchus (Figs. 44–46).

The left main stem bronchus is surrounded by several structures. The aortic arch is in contact with the superior and posterior aspects of the proximal left main stem bronchus. The esophagus is adherent to the first 2 cm of the posterior portion of the left main stem bronchus. Anterior to the proximal left main stem bronchus

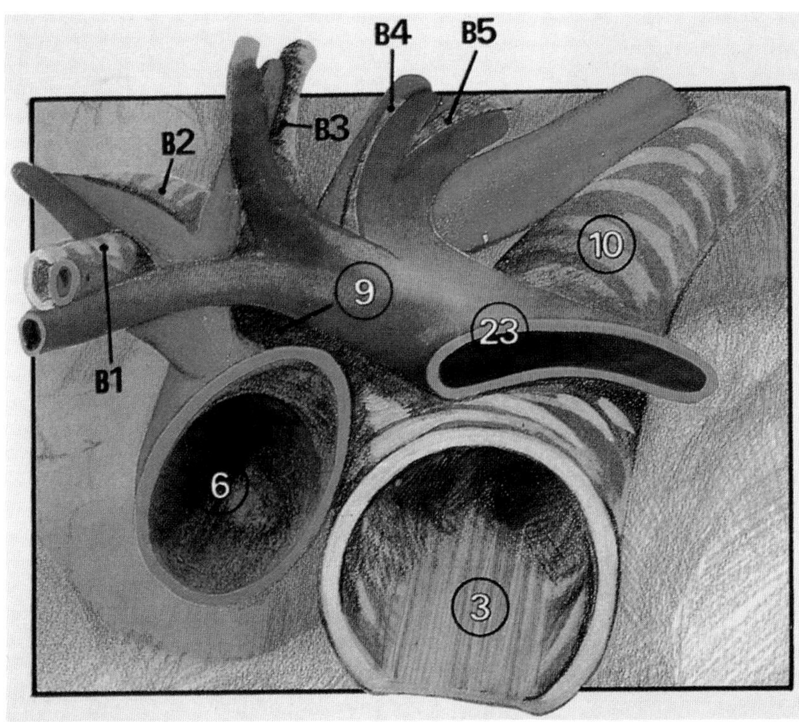

FIG. 47. Left main stem bronchus. 3, left main bronchus; 6, left pulmonary artery; 9, left upper lobe bronchus; 10, left lower lobe bronchus; 23, left upper pulmonary vein. (Courtesy of J.-F. Dumon, M.D.)

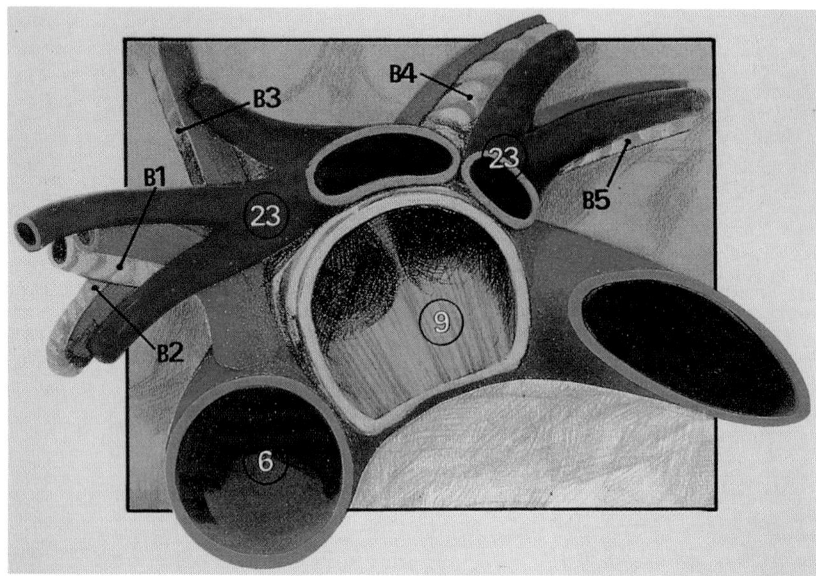

FIG. 48. Left upper lobe bronchus. 6, left pulmonary artery; 9, left upper lobe bronchus; 23, left upper pulmonary vein. (Courtesy of J.-F. Dumon, M.D.)

is the trunk of the right pulmonary artery separating the aorta from the left main stem bronchus. The left pulmonary artery is short and passes immediately anterior to the middle portion of the left main stem bronchus as the artery ascends to the left upper lobe bronchus. The pulmonary veins on the left side are anterior to the main stem bronchus and pass lateral and inferior to the pulmonary artery. At the origin of the left upper lobe bronchus, the left pulmonary veins are in contact with the anterior, inferior wall of the distal left main bronchus as they enter the left atrium (Fig. 47).

The left upper lobe bronchus is short, rapidly dividing into the upper division and lingular bronchi. The pulmonary artery is in significant relationship to these bronchi. The pulmonary artery is in contact with the superior and the posterior aspects of the distal left main bronchus as the artery ascends, passes around, and then descends behind the left upper lobe bronchus. As this artery ascends, it gives rise to branches of the anterior segment of the left upper lobe and the lingula (Fig. 48). The pulmonary artery then descends behind the left upper lobe bronchus supplying branches to the left

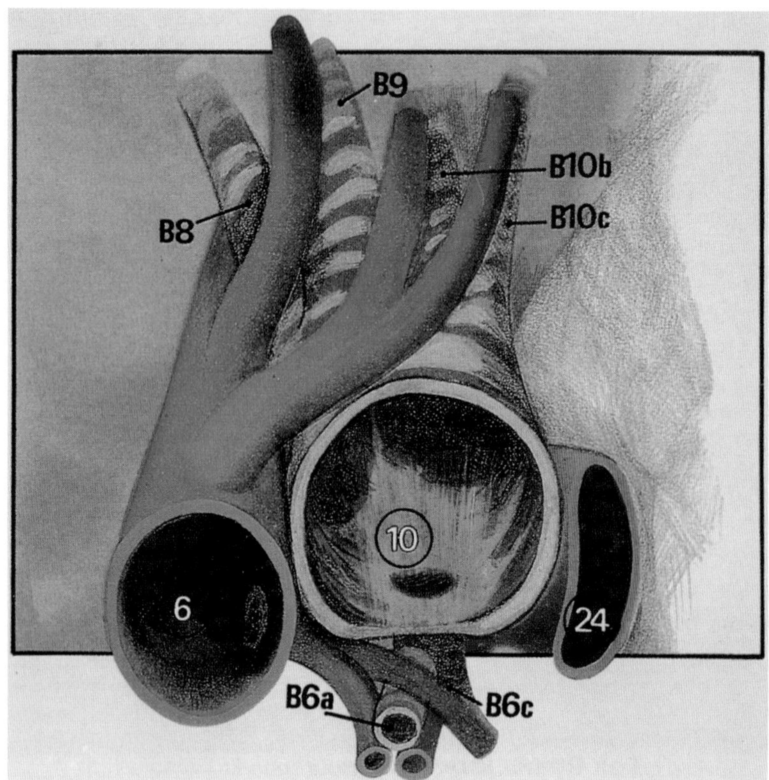

FIG. 49. Left lower lobe bronchus. 6, left pulmonary artery; 10, left lower lobe bronchus; 24, left lower pulmonary vein. (Courtesy of J.-F. Dumon, M.D.)

lower lobe. The left lower lobe bronchus is surrounded by the left lower lobe pulmonary artery on its lateral aspect and the left lower lobe pulmonary veins posteriorly and medially (Fig. 49).

The right pulmonary artery passes in front of the carina and along the anterior portion of the right main stem bronchus. The right pulmonary artery is in close proximity to the anterior wall of the right main stem bronchus as this vessel passes laterally into the hilum. The right upper lobe bronchus is joined by the right upper lobe artery, which lies along the superior and anterior aspects of the bronchus. The pulmonary vein is lower and not in contact with the bronchus. The right middle lobe bronchus is usually joined by the middle lobe artery along the lateral side of the bronchus while the right middle lobe veins are usually along the medial wall of this bronchus.

GETTING TO KNOW THE TRACHEOBRONCHIAL TREE

Before beginning to apply specialized bronchoscopic techniques in clinical practice, the apprentice bronchoscopist must understand the normal anatomy and the variations of normalcy. Once the bronchoscope is introduced into the tracheobronchial tree, the bronchoscopist should be able to acknowledge the anatomic location of the tip of the bronchoscope and how it got there. To quote Straddling, "one's position in the peripheral bronchial tree can only be appreciated by knowing how one got there" (23). The first step toward mastering tracheobronchial anatomy is to study the topic in a textbook. To gain proficiency in the handling of the bronchoscope, models of tracheobronchial tree specially designed for bronchoscopy training should be used to identify various bronchi and to maneuver comfortably within the tracheobronchial tree. Bronchoscopy practice on live animal models will further instruct the student in movement of the tracheobronchial tree in relation to respiratory motion and cough. Further details regarding bronchoscopy training and teaching are discussed in Chapter 29 of this volume.

Once the bronchoscope has entered the tracheobronchial tree, the bronchoscopist should imagine that he or she is actually within the airways. The bronchoscopist should then "walk down" the trachea and bronchi, and then enter the lobar, segmental, and subsegmental bronchi. It is extremely important for the bronchoscopist to be reminded of the relationship between the bronchoscope's location and the true anterior of the patient's body. It is very easy to become disoriented, even for an expert, and to get lost in the distant depths of the bronchial tree, if the bronchoscopist does not keep track of where the bronchoscope is and how it got there. When one gets lost in the distal bronchial tree, the best recourse is to withdraw the tip of the bronchoscope proximal to the main carina and start all over. The main carina is the only dependable landmark (Fig. 50). Major carinae (RC1, RC2, LC1, and LC2) as well as distant carinae and bronchi can be misleading landmarks (Fig. 51).

The small peripheral triangular pointer in the flexible bronchoscope is extremely helpful in orienting the bronchoscopist and the observer or student looking through the lecturescope (teaching arm). The pointer is located in the same position as the suction outlet. The student or observer using the lecturescope can

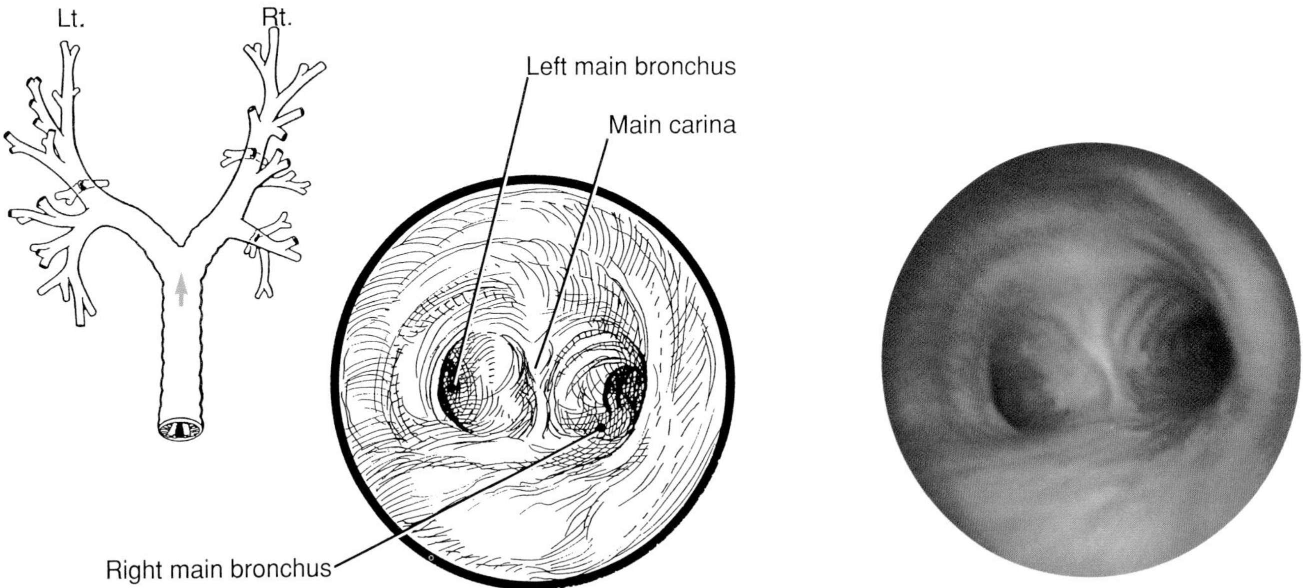

FIG. 50. The main carina is the major landmark for the bronchoscopist.

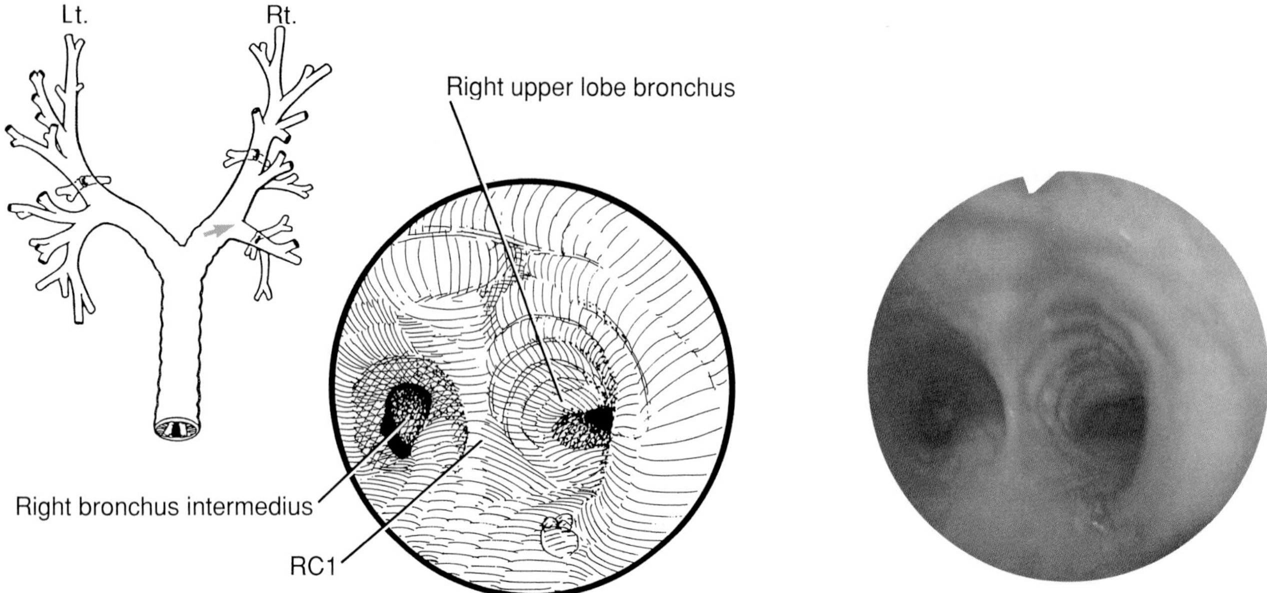

FIG. 51. Right bronchus intermedius and large right upper lobe bronchus can easily mimic left and right main stem bronchi, respectively, and RC1 can be mistaken for the main carina, unless the bronchoscope is withdrawn proximally and the main carina identified.

turn the head of the lecturescope in the same direction as the suction outlet on the bronchoscope to become oriented "inside" the bronchial tree.

REFERENCES

1. Boyden EA, Tompsett DH. The changing patterns of the developing lungs of infants. *Acta Anat* 1965;61:164–192.
2. Boyden EA. The terminal air sacs and their blood supply in a 37-day infant lung. *Am J Anat* 1965;116:413–428.
3. Boyden EA. Notes on the development of the lung in infancy and early childhood. *Am J Anat* 1967;121:749–762.
4. Boyden EA. The structure of the pulmonary acinous in a child of six years and eight months. *Am J Anat* 1971;132:275–300.
5. O'Rahilly R, Boyden EA. The timing and sequence of events in the development of the human respiratory system during the embryonic period proper. *Z Anat Entwicklungsgesh* 1973; 141:237–250.
6. Boyden EA. Development and growth of the airways. In: *Development of the lung*. Hodson WA, ed. New York: Marcel Dekker; 1977;3–35.
7. Langston C, Kida K, Reed M, Thurlbeck WM. Human lung growth in late gestation and in the neonate. *Am Rev Resp Dis* 1984;129:607–613.
8. Hislop A, Reed L. Growth and development of the respiratory system. In: Davis JA, Dopping J, eds. *Scientific foundations of pediatrics*. London: Heineman; 1974;214–254.
9. Jackson CL, Huber JF. Correlated applied anatomy of the bronchial tree and lungs with a system of nomenclature. *Dis Chest* 1943;9:319–326.
10. Boyden EA, Hartmann JF. An analysis of variations in the bronchopulmonary segments of the left upper lobes of 50 lungs. *Am J Anat* 1946;79:321–360.
11. Boyden EA, Scannel JG. An analysis of variations in the bronchovascular pattern of the right upper lobes of 50 lungs. *Am J Anat* 1948;82:27–74.
12. Boyden EA, Hamre CJ. An analysis of variations in the bronchovascular pattern of the middle lobe in 50 dissected and 20 uninjected lungs. *J Thorac Surg* 1951;21:172–188.
13. Boyden EA. *Segmental anatomy of the lungs: a study of the patterns of the segmental bronchi and related pulmonary vessels*. New York: McGraw-Hill; 1955.
14. Berg RM, Boyden EA, Smith FR. An analysis of variations of the segmental bronchi of the left lower lobe of 50 dissected, and ten injected lungs. *J Thorac Surg* 1948;18:216–236.
15. Scannel JG. A study of variations of the bronchopulmonary segments in the left upper lobe. *J Thorac Surg* 1947;16:530–537.
16. Scannel JG, Boyden EA. A study of variations of the bronchopulmonary segments of the right upper lobe (in 13 injected specimens). *J Thorac Surg* 1948;17:232–237.
17. Shinoi K. A proposal on bronchial nomenclature. *Jap J Thorac Surg* 1948;1:118–125.
18. Nagaishi C. *Functional anatomy and histology of the lung*. Baltimore: University Park Press; 1972.
19. Ikeda S. *Atlas of flexible bronchofiberscopy*. Tokyo: Igaku-Shoin; 1974.
20. Prakash UBS, Fontana RS. Functional classification of the bronchial carinae. *Chest* 1984;770–772.
21. *American Joint Committee on Cancer, Task Force on Lung: Staging of Lung Cancer, 1979*. Chicago: American Joint Committee on Cancer; 1979.
22. Mountain CF. Staging of lung cancer: the new international system. *Lung Cancer* 1987;3:4–11.
23. Stradling P, Stradling JR. *Diagnostic bronchoscopy: a teaching manual*. Edinburgh: Churchill Livingstone; 1991.

Bronchoscopy,
edited by U. B. S. Prakash.
Mayo Foundation © 1994.
Published by Raven Press, Ltd., New York.

CHAPTER 3

The Bronchoscopy Suite, Equipment, and Personnel

Udaya B. S. Prakash, Mickie J. Stelck, and Marsha J. Kulas

At the very outset, we underscore the fact that a surgical suite totally dedicated to bronchoscopy is not only unnecessary but unrealistic at all medical centers practicing bronchoscopy and related procedures. The need for such a suite, however, will depend on the number of bronchoscopies and special bronchoscopy-related procedures, such as laser therapy, stent placement, pediatric bronchoscopy, and complicated rigid bronchoscopy. While it is convenient to have a dedicated operating room or other facility, bronchoscopy can be performed safely in other areas, provided trained personnel and equipment are available to deal with any complications that may develop (1).

The results of a mail survey of 871 bronchoscopists in the United States and Canada by the American College of Chest Physicians revealed that many performed bronchoscopy in several locations: the operating room (49.5%), patient's room (55.6%), physician's office (11.0%), bronchoscopy suite/laboratory or pulmonary function test laboratory (17.2%), and intensive care unit (2.5%) (2). Outpatient bronchoscopy (in the hospital) was practiced by 62.8% of physicians (2). The safety of outpatient bronchoscopy, including transbronchoscopic lung biopsy, has been well documented (3–6). Several factors contribute to the choice of location for the procedure and choice of assistants such as personal preference, convenience, available facilities, and availability of personnel or paramedical training programs.

Before the introduction of the flexible bronchoscope into clinical practice, evaluation of the tracheobronchial tree of infants required transportation to the operating room for rigid bronchoscopy. Presently, however, the availability of the small-diameter (ultrathin) flexible bronchoscope allows safe performance of bronchoscopy in the neonatal intensive care unit (7,8). Nevertheless, rigid bronchoscopy can also be performed in the neonatal intensive care unit, as noted in a report on five cases (9).

U. B. S. Prakash, M. J. Stelck, and M. J. Kulas: Division of Thoracic Diseases and Internal Medicine, Mayo Clinic, Rochester, Minnesota 55905.

THE BRONCHOSCOPY SUITE

An ideal bronchoscopy suite should have adequate space for the following: storage of bronchoscopy-related equipment, prebronchoscopy preparation of the patient, performance of the procedure, and post-bronchoscopy observation of the patient. The size of the suite may depend on the case load of each bronchoscopist and medical center. The major advantages of a dedicated bronchoscopy suite are the availability of any type of instrument and the facility to perform all types of bronchoscopy-related procedures. At medical centers that perform a significant number of complicated bronchoscopic procedures such as laser bronchoscopy, stent placement, pediatric bronchoscopy, and complicated rigid bronchoscopy, it may be convenient to locate the bronchoscopy suite adjacent to surgical operating rooms so that the expertise of thoracic surgeons and anesthesiologists is readily available. Irrespective of where the bronchoscopy is performed, personnel and equipment to provide resuscitation should be readily available.

Patient Preparation Area

Prior to bronchoscopy, administration of premedications and instillation of topical anesthesia may be accomplished in a separate area or in the location where bronchoscopy is performed. The bronchoscopist and the bronchoscopy team should assemble the equipment required to prepare the patient. A method to deliver supplemental oxygen and resuscitation measures should be handy in the preparation area. The bronchoscopist should be able to prepare the patient single-handedly unless the patient is too sick to adequately cooperate and requires additional help from a nurse or another physician.

The Procedure Area

Depending on the bronchoscopist's preference, the procedure can be performed on an operating table, on patient's bed, in a regular chair, or in a chair similar to that used by dentists. The facility to place the patient in reverse Trendelenburg position should be available in case of severe bronchoscopy-induced bleeding or hypotension. There should be adequate room around the patient to handle various equipment and deal with an emergency, should it arise. It is equally important that the bronchoscopist and the assisting personnel also have sufficient space, particularly around the patient's head. The instruments used should be immediately accessible to the bronchoscopist. In our practice, all bronchoscopy-related implements are stored in the bronchoscopy suite as well as in the mobile bronchoscopy cart.

The major advantages of performing bronchoscopy in the patient's room include the fact that the procedure is performed in familiar surroundings and the patient does not have to be moved to another area. The disadvantages are that all necessary equipment, such as a fluoroscopy or laser system, cannot be readily brought to the patient's room. Almost all rigid bronchoscopies and bronchoscopies requiring general anesthesia cannot be provided in the patient's room.

The Postbronchoscopy Area

Most patients require a period of observation to ensure that there are no complications from the pharmaceutical agents used during the procedure or the procedure itself. Depending on the setup at each medical center, this area may include the bronchoscopy suite itself, the postsurgical recovery suite, a room adjacent to the bronchoscopy suite, a waiting room, or the patient's room if bedside bronchoscopy is performed. The important point is that the personnel engaged to observe the patient following bronchoscopy are trained to recognize the potential complications and have the resuscitative equipment at their disposal. In the survey of North American bronchoscopists, 56.5% reported using an area adjacent to bronchoscopy suite as the postbronchoscopy recovery area, whereas 42.6% used a separate area such as an outpatient waiting area, the procedure room, or the emergency room for this purpose (2). Postbronchoscopy observation should be undertaken by the bronchoscopist, another physician, or a nurse trained to recognize postbronchoscopy complications.

THE MOBILE OR PORTABLE BRONCHOSCOPY UNIT

Not all bronchoscopists perform the procedure in dedicated bronchoscopy suites or operating rooms. In fact, 55% of the bronchoscopists in the North American survey reported that they did bronchoscopy at the bedside in the patient's room (2). The bronchoscopists who prefer to provide the bronchoscopy service in the patient's room should develop and maintain a mobile bronchoscopy unit to facilitate the optimal performance of the procedure. The major disadvantages and advantages of doing bronchoscopy in patient's room are discussed above. In our practice, although two ded-

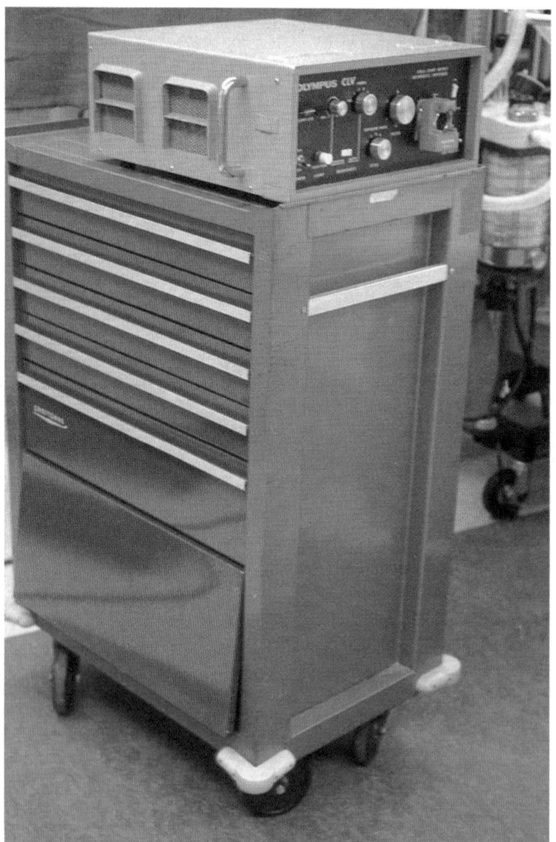

FIG. 1. Mobile bronchoscopy cart contains most of the equipment necessary to perform standard diagnostic bronchoscopic procedures and essential instruments for therapeutic bronchoscopy in critical care units. It is also equipped with emergency and resuscitation equipment.

icated suites for bronchoscopy are available 24 hours a day, we utilize a mobile cart (Fig. 1) to perform a majority of the procedures. These carts are stocked with all necessary equipment for both diagnostic and therapeutic flexible bronchoscopy and can be taken instantly to any area within the hospital.

Critical care units at our institution are also equipped with mobile bronchoscopy carts and respiratory therapists trained in the care and setup of the equipment because many patients admitted to the critical care unit frequently require diagnostic and therapeutic bronchoscopy. However, patients admitted to the intensive or critical care unit may require transportation to another area for certain bronchoscopic procedures such as laser therapy and bronchoscopic lung biopsy.

BRONCHOSCOPY EQUIPMENT

While there are many varieties of bronchoscopes and related equipment, not all are required to provide optimal bronchoscopy service. Depending on the needs and the type of bronchoscopy practice, each bronchoscopist should plan her or his own setup. The bare minimum required for performing flexible bronchoscopy to obtain biopsies of the lesions in the tracheobronchial tree and therapeutic bronchoscopy in adults includes an adult-size flexible bronchoscope, a light source, several cytology brushes and biopsy forceps, specimen containers, suction apparatus, and supplemental oxygen and equipment for resuscitation. Some of the equipment required for basic or standard flexible and rigid bronchoscopic procedures are shown in Figs. 2 and 3. Even in the absence of a large-volume bronchoscopy practice, the bronchoscopist is well advised to have an extra bronchoscope and several biopsy forceps in case of equipment breakdown. Any other bronchoscopic procedure will require additional implements. The following is a brief description of various instruments available. The instruments not described here are discussed in other chapters. The care of the bronchoscopes and other bronchoscopy-related instruments, photographic equipment, lasers, and other equipments are discussed elsewhere in this book.

Bronchoscopes

The bronchoscopes are manufactured by various firms and the details of the specifications of the flexible bronchoscopes and rigid bronchoscopes are discussed in Chapters 4 and 5 of this volume, respectively. The number and types of bronchoscopes required will depend on the needs of each individual bronchoscopist. The bare minimum required is described above. The novice bronchoscopist in the process of organizing a

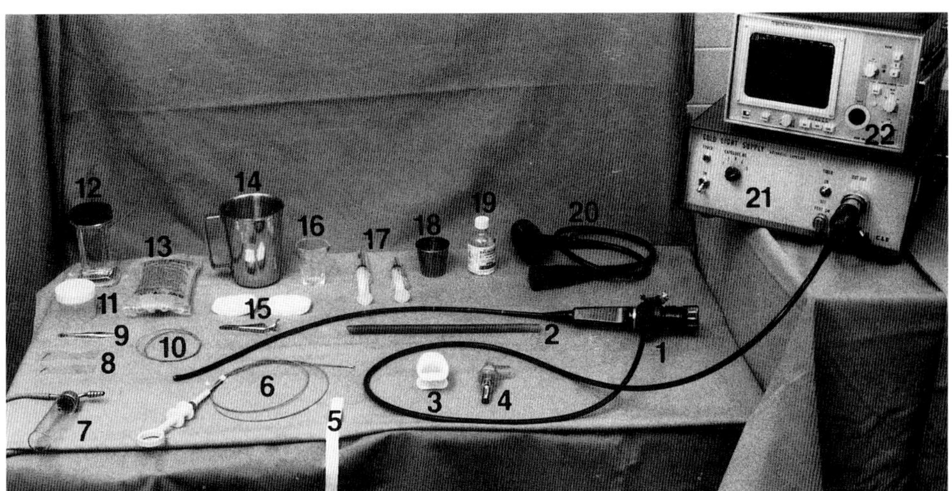

FIG. 2. Essential instruments required for standard flexible bronchoscopy. Instrument setup for flexible bronchoscopy: (1) flexible bronchoscope; (2) soft, uncuffed, and noncollapsible endotracheal (ET) tube; (3) bite-block (mouthpiece); (4) ET tube adapter for supplemental oxygen delivery; (5) 20-cm-long adhesive tape to fasten ET tube; (6) flexible biopsy forceps; (7) sterile glass container to collect bronchial lavage; (8) glass slides for cytological smears; (9) pickup forceps to remove biopsy specimens from biopsy forceps; (10) bronchial brush; (11) specimen jar with formaldehyde; (12) slide container with 95% alcohol; (13) lactated Ringer's solution for bronchial lavage; (14) metal container with warm water to defog and clean the bronchoscope tip; (15) eye pads and towel clip; (16) medicine jar with lactated Ringer's solution; (17) syringes—one with lactated Ringer's solution and the other containing 4% lidocaine; (18) metal cup containing 4% lidocaine; (19) 4% lidocaine; (20) lecturescope; (21) cold-light source; and (22) electrocardiographic monitor. Not shown in the figure are a tube of lubricating jelly and gauze pads. (From *Semin Resp Med* 1981;3:19, with permission.)

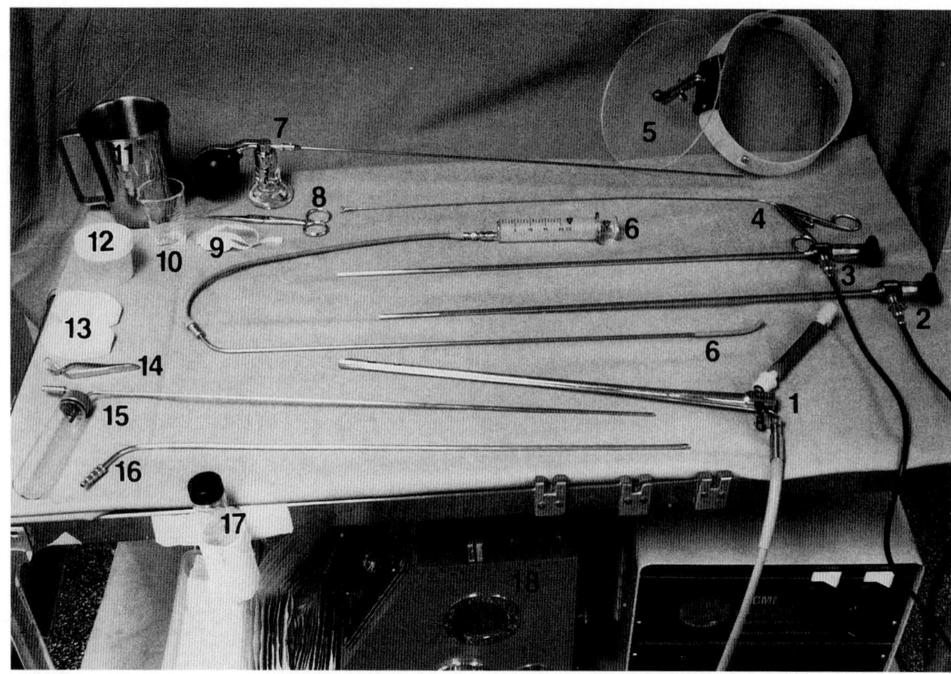

FIG. 3. Essential instruments required for standard rigid bronchoscopy. Instrument setup for rigid bronchoscopy: (1) rigid bronchoscope with light supply cord below and oxygen delivery tube above; (2) straight-view telescope; (3) 90° view telescope; (4) biopsy forceps; (5) eye shield; (6) syringe and long rubber-tipped metal tube for bronchial lavage through rigid bronchoscope; (7) atomizer containing 4% lidocaine—for topical anesthetic application through rigid bronchoscope to anesthetize bronchial mucosa; (8) pair of scissors; (9) "umbilical tape" to pack severely hemorrhaging bronchus; (10) medicine cup containing lavage fluid; (11) container with warm water to clean biopsy forceps, telescope tips, etc.; (12) specimen jar with formaldehyde; (13) eye pads; (14) towel clip; (15) container to collect bronchial lavage fluid; (16) long suction cannula; (17) bronchial lavage container; and (18) light source.) (From *Semin Resp Med* 1981;3:19, with permission.)

bronchoscopy unit should recognize that instruments made by one manufacturer may not be compatible with those made by a different manufacturer. Therefore, it is better to purchase the bronchoscope and related equipment made by the same manufacturer. It is also essential to ascertain that repair service is prompt and excellent. A bronchoscopist or the medical center involved in all aspects of bronchoscopy may require flexible and rigid bronchoscopes of various sizes to accommodate adult as well as pediatric patients. Several types of both flexible and rigid bronchoscopes may be needed if laser bronchoscopy, stent placement, and removal of foreign bodies are to be undertaken. Pediatric bronchoscopy will require ultrathin flexible bronchoscopes and rigid bronchoscopes of smaller diameters (Chapters 23 and 24 of this volume).

Light Source

Light sources are different for the flexible and rigid bronchoscopes. Properly functioning light sources should be available for use in the mobile cart and for still photography as well as for videobronchoscopy. The proper maintenance of the light sources is mandatory. Extra bulbs and fuses should be available for an uninterrupted functioning of the light source.

Endotracheal Tubes

Endotracheal tubes are used by many bronchoscopists to facilitate flexible bronchoscopic examination. For most adult flexible bronchoscopies, the minimum inner diameter of the endotracheal tube required is 7.5 mm. While any type of endotracheal tube can be used, soft latex wire-spiral tubes without cuff are easier to use over a flexible bronchoscope and better tolerated by patients (10). As the ultrathin flexible bronchoscopes used in pediatric practice have varying diameters (1.8 to 32 mm), endotracheal tubes of different diameters should be available.

Cytology Brushes for the Flexible Bronchoscope

Both disposable and reusable cytology brushes are available. Brushes can be sheathed or unsheathed and

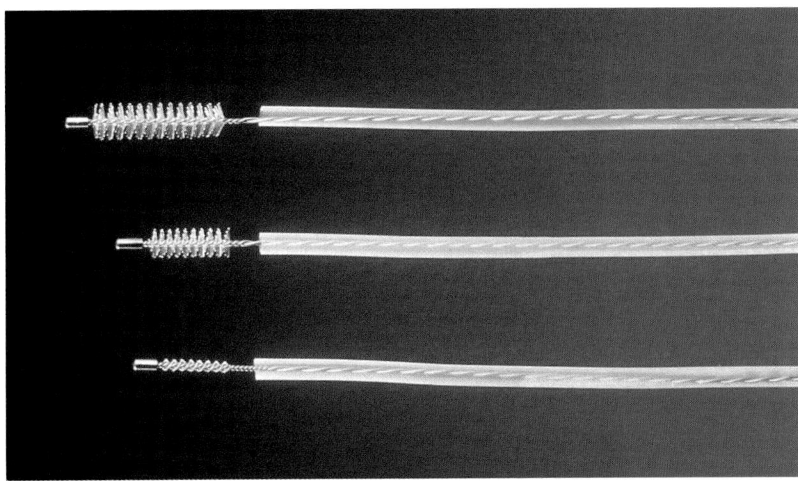

FIG. 4. Cytology brushes of various bristle lengths.

lined with bristles that have varying degrees of stiffness or flexibility (Fig. 4). The efficacy of various cytology brushes has been studied. One study examined the cellular yield expressed as the number of cells recovered with two different types of sheathed cytology brushes, one with slightly longer and wider bristles. The latter provided greater yield in total number of cells recovered per brush (11). On the other hand, another study using sheathed brushes of 1.00, 1.73, and 3.0 mm diameter showed no significant difference in cell recovery among the three brushes (12). It is important to recognize that the techniques of brushing and preparing cytology smears are far more significant than the type of brush used (13).

Biopsy Forceps for the Flexible Bronchoscope

Biopsy forceps also come in many varieties and shapes. The standard adult flexible bronchoscopes have working channels that range from 2.0 to 2.8 mm in diameter. There are no forceps that can traverse the working channel of pediatric (ultrathin) flexible bronchoscopes. Therefore, the bronchoscopist should make sure that the biopsy forceps can easily traverse the working channels of the flexible bronchoscope. The three basic types include those with serrated edge (alligator), smooth edge with fenestrated or unfenestrated cups, and "spiked" (impaler needle between the cups) (Fig. 3–5). Some forceps are manufactured with longer blades. The latter type of forceps is helpful in obtaining a biopsy from mucosal abnormalities along the tracheal wall or from lesions from which the regular forceps easily slip or slide.

The choice of biopsy forceps depends on the individual bronchoscopist and the performance of the forceps. Wang and associates studied the efficacy of three different types of forceps to obtain a transbronchoscopic lung biopsy and reported that larger forceps and serrated forceps provided larger specimens, but the size of the biopsy specimen itself did not significantly alter the diagnosis (14). The nondisposable forceps have a finite life and a study observed that biopsy forceps be-

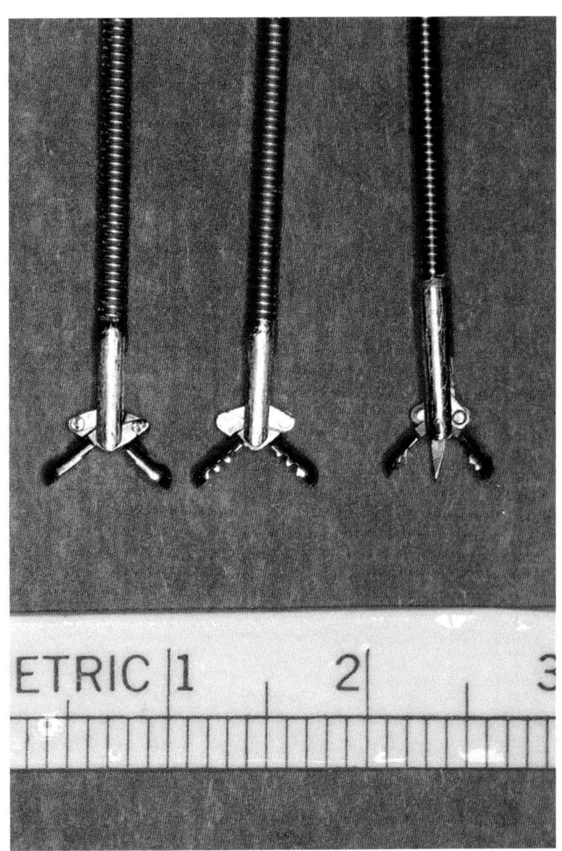

FIG. 5. Bronchoscopic biopsy forceps; cup forceps **(left)**, toothed forceps **(middle)**, and forceps with an impaler needle **(right)**.

come dull after 20 or 25 applications (15). Dull forceps tend to produce artifact by crushing the tissue.

Biopsy Forceps for the Rigid Bronchoscope

The types of forceps available for use with the rigid bronchoscope are many and are aimed at handling almost all types of problems within the airways. Even a bronchoscopic lung biopsy can be obtained with special forceps (16). Specialized forceps are available for the removal of various types of foreign bodies. In design the forceps are usually much larger than those used with the flexible bronchoscope, slightly rigid in performance, and stronger. The forceps for use with the pediatric rigid bronchoscope are identical in structural details but smaller.

Bronchoscopy Needles

In recent years, bronchoscopic needle aspiration and biopsy have been used to sample paratracheal, hilar, and subcarinal lymph nodes. The majority of the needles available are disposable and in our experience each needle can be used only once. Two sizes (19 and 21 gauge) are available and the larger needle is used to obtain tissue biopsy whereas the smaller needle is designed for obtaining cytology aspiration. Retractable and nonretractable needles as well as metallic and plastic needles are available. Many manufacturers have discontinued the sale of nonretractable needles because of the high risk of injury to the inner lining of the flexible bronchoscope.

Baskets and Claws

The presently available baskets and claws, mainly for the removal of tracheobronchial foreign bodies, are rather flimsy and not as effective as instruments available for the removal of foreign bodies with a rigid bronchoscope. However, the basket and claws have been used for the recovery of tracheobronchial foreign bodies and for the removal of thick mucous plugs with a flexible bronchoscope.

Protected Catheters

The protected catheter brushes are used for obtaining respiratory specimens for bacterial culture (17–19). Various types are available and all are meant for single use. The preference for these catheters depends on the individual bronchoscopist and the performance of the catheter. We once again stress that appropriate technique of use of the catheters is far more important than the type of brush.

Specimen Traps

Specimen traps to collect bronchial washings and bronchoalveolar lavage effluent and special containers to hold cytology slides and biopsy specimens are commercially available. Many bronchoscopists improvise their own system with spare parts. Major medical centers may have these manufactured to their specifications. The bronchoscopist is well advised to discuss her or his needs with the personnel in pathology and microbiology laboratories so that mutually acceptable equipment can be designed and procured.

Fluoroscopy

Biplane fluoroscopy equipment is essential for accurate localization to obtain a bronchoscopic lung biopsy. By demonstrating the location of the biopsy forceps relative to a lesion or pleura, fluoroscopy helps to minimize the risk of pneumothorax, particularly following bronchoscopic lung biopsy. Even though bronchoscopic lung biopsy can be performed without fluoroscopic guidance, the incidence of pneumothorax associated following bronchoscopic lung biopsy is less than 1.8% when fluoroscopy is used and the incidence significantly increases to 2.9% without fluoroscopy (20).

The fluoroscopy machines are either fixed or mobile (portable). If the latter is not available, the patient who requires fluoroscopy-guided bronchoscopic lung biopsy will have to be transported to the location of the fluoroscopy unit, generally in the chest roentgenology suite. The portable units are quite handy for the performance of bronchoscopic lung biopsies in patient rooms and other areas. The fluoroscopy machines are expensive and therefore a fluoroscopy unit dedicated only to bronchoscopy is not feasible for most bronchoscopists. The mail survey of 871 bronchoscopists in North America noted that a fluoroscopy facility dedicated to bronchoscopy was reported by 20.9% of the respondents and fluoroscopy was shared with nonbronchoscopists by 74.1%. Several participants complained that their roentgenology departments did not allow them to use fluoroscopy machines (2). In many institutions, the fluoroscopy machines are managed by roentgenology departments and the bronchoscopists may have to use the equipment with the approval of roentgenologists.

Monitoring Equipment

Noninvasive measures such as sphygmomanometry, electrocardiographic monitoring, and pulse oximetry provide the necessary information during the bronchoscopy and should therefore be utilized in the majority of patients. Pulse oximetry is useful to assess the adequacy of oxygenation whether or not supplemental oxygen is given (21–23). In the mail survey mentioned above (2), routine use of pulse or other oximetry was practiced by 84.2% of the respondents and electrocardiographic monitoring by 74.6%. Supplemental oxygen should always be available.

Other Equipment

Suction apparatus, extra tubings, cleaning materials, and commonly used pharmaceutical agents are among the miscellaneous equipment necessary for the optimal practice of bronchoscopy. All equipment and medications necessary for cardiopulmonary resuscitation should be readily available at the bronchoscopy location.

The Storage Area

The size of the storage for the bronchoscopy equipment area depends on the diversity of bronchoscopy practice. If a bronchoscopist is limited to simple bronchoscopy (only flexible bronchoscopy and no pediatric bronchoscopy or other special procedures), then all the bronchoscopy equipment can be stored in a mobile cart in a corner of a storage room in the hospital or office. Bronchoscopists specializing in laser bronchoscopy, rigid bronchoscopy, and other complex procedures will require more spacious areas to store their equipment.

The flexible bronchoscope is a delicate instrument and requires proper handling and storage (Fig. 6).

THE BRONCHOSCOPY PERSONNEL

We strongly recommend that the procedure be performed by physicians who are skilled and appropriately trained in the procedure. It is also important that the training of the future bronchoscopists should encompass assisting the bronchoscopist during bronchoscopy and related procedures (see Chapter 29).

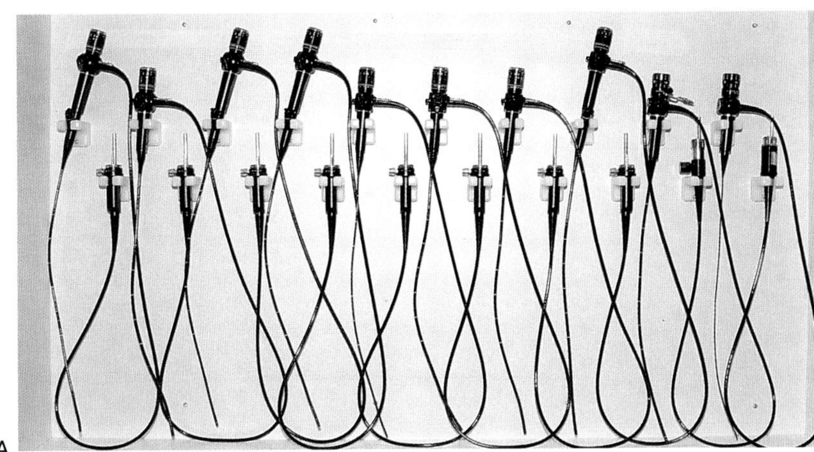

A

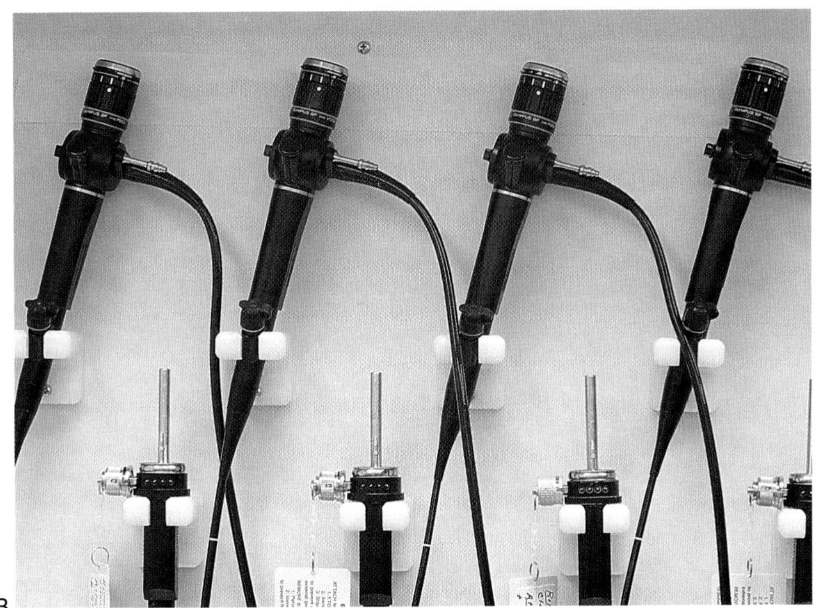

B

FIG. 6. Special storage cupboard for flexible bronchoscopes **(A)**; and a close-up view **(B)**. Hanging them as shown prevents development of curves in the shaft of the instrument.

The mail survey described above reported that nurses alone assisted 39.0% of the bronchoscopists during the procedure whereas 26.2% of the bronchoscopists utilized nurses and other assistants; respiratory therapists were the sole assistants to 14.7% of bronchoscopists, and 7.6% of physicians utilized respiratory therapists and others (nurses, laboratory technicians, residents, etc.). Pulmonary function technicians and other paramedical personnel assisted 12.4% of the bronchoscopists. Physicians were mentioned as bronchoscopy assistants by 15.3% (2). Since many bronchoscopy suites are adjacent to or part of a pulmonary function testing laboratory or respiratory therapy department, many institutions train the technicians in these areas to assist in bronchoscopy. As in any surgical procedure, the team concept is vital to the performance of bronchoscopy.

Training of Paramedical Personnel

The training of the paramedical personnel to provide assistance to the bronchoscopist should include the education needed to understand bronchoscopy and related procedures, a period of observation of the procedure and assistance provided to the bronchoscopist, opportunities to assist the trained bronchoscopy nurse/surgical technician, and personal performance of required duties.

First, the trainee should be provided with didactic teaching in the basic anatomy of the tracheobronchial tree, the reasoning behind the procedures, and a working knowledge of the equipment, indications and contraindications, potential complications, and administrative policies and procedural details pertaining to the institution.

Second, the trainee should be encouraged to observe all aspects of bronchoscopy and related procedures, beginning with the preparation of the patient and ending with the care of the patient in the postbronchoscopy and final dismissal. The period of observation should also include maintenance and cleaning of bronchoscopy equipment.

The third phase of the training consists of active participation of the trainee in assisting the bronchoscopy nurse/technician. The responsibilities are gradually increased with the trainee is able to comfortably assist the charge nurse/technician in complex procedures. During this period, the bronchoscopist and the charge nurse/technician should correct any deficiencies and provide remedial training if necessary.

The final phase consists of the fully trained nurse/technician being in charge of the organization of the bronchoscopy procedures and in ascertaining that each procedure is smoothly organized and completed. Periodic didactic sessions in continuing education in the procedure and new developments should be encouraged to maintain competence.

The Anesthesiologist and the Nurse Anesthetist

The majority of flexible bronchoscopies in adults can be performed without general anesthesia. Assistance from the anesthesiologist or the nurse-anesthetist is rarely required for routine flexible bronchoscopy procedures. Technically difficult procedures, most rigid bronchoscopies, most time-consuming laser bronchoscopies, and extreme patient apprehension are circumstances that merit consideration of using general anesthesia. The performance of rigid bronchoscopy, particularly in children, will require general anesthesia and hence the assistance from the anesthesiologist and/or nurse-anesthetist. It is of interest that nearly 8% of the participants in the mail survey routinely used assistance from the anesthesiologist/anesthetist during bronchoscopy and 16.5% used general anesthesia for bronchoscopy (2). A mail survey of the British bronchoscopists reported that general anesthesia was used by 12% (20). In our practice, we utilize nurse-anesthetists for monitoring of patients during bronchoscopy.

REFERENCES

1. Prakash UBS, Stubbs SE. The bronchoscopy survey: some reflections. *Chest* 1991;100:1660–1667.
2. Prakash UBS, Offord KP, Stubbs SE. Bronchoscopy in North America: the ACCP survey. *Chest* 1991;100:1668–1675.
3. De Fenoyl O, Capron F, Lebeau B, Rochmaure J. Transbronchial lung biopsy: a five year experience in outpatients. *Thorax* 1989;44:956–959.
4. Ahmad M, Livingston DR, Golish JA, Mehta AC, Wiedemann HP. The safety of outpatient transbronchial lung biopsy. *Chest* 1986;90:403–405.
5. Ackart RS, Foreman DR, Klayton RJ, Donlan CJ, Munzel TL, Schuler MA. Fiberoptic bronchoscopy in outpatient facilities. *Arch Intern Med* 1983;143:30–31.
6. Aelony Y. Outpatient fiberoptic bronchoscopies (letter). *Arch Intern Med* 1983;143:1837.
7. Myer CM, Thompson RF. Flexible fiberoptic bronchoscopy interest neonatal intensive care unit. *Int J Pediatr Otorhinolaryngol* 1988;15:143–147.
8. Fan LL, Sparks LM, Dulinski JP. Applications of an ultrathin flexible bronchoscope for neonatal and pediatric airway problems. *Chest* 1986;89:673–676.
9. Muntz HR. Therapeutic rigid bronchoscopy in the neonatal intensive care unit. *Ann Otol Rhinol Laryngol* 1985;94:462–465.
10. Hodgkin JE, Rosenow EC III, Stubbs SE: Oral introduction of the flexible bronchoscope. *Chest* 1975;68:88–90.
11. Michaelson ED, Serafini SM. Quantitative differences in the cellular yield of two bronchial brushes. *Am Rev Resp Dis* 1975;112:267–268.
12. Hanson FN, Wesselius LJ: Effect of bronchial brush size on cell recovery. *Am Rev Resp Dis* 1987;136:1450–1452.
13. Parker RL, Haesart SP, Kovnat DM, Bachus B, Snider GL. Bronchial brushing in bronchogenic carcinoma. Factors influencing cellular yield and diagnostic accuracy. *Chest* 1977;71:341–345.

14. Wang KP, Wise RA, Terry PB, et al. Comparison of standard and enlarged forceps for transbronchial lung biopsy in the diagnosis of lung infiltrates. *Endoscopy* 1980;12:151–154.
15. Saltzstein SL, Harrell JH II, Cameron T. Brushings, washings, or biopsy? Obtaining maximum value from flexible fiberoptic bronchoscopy in the diagnosis of cancer. *Chest* 1977; 71:630–632.
16. Andersen HA, Fontana RS. Transbronchoscopic lung biopsy for diffuse pulmonary diseases: technique and results in 450 cases. *Chest* 1972;62:125–128.
17. Bartlett JG, Alexander J, Mayhew J, Sullivan-Sigler N, Gorbach SL. Should fiberoptic bronchoscopy aspirates be cultured? *Am Rev Resp Dis* 1976;114:73–78.
18. Wimberley NW, Bass JB Jr, Boyd BW, Kirkpatrick MB, Serio RA, Pollock HM. Use of bronchoscopic protected catheter brush for the diagnosis of pulmonary infections. *Chest* 1982; 81:556–562.
19. Faling LJ. A tale of two brushes. *Chest* 1981;79:155–156.
20. Simpson FG, Arnold AG, Purvis A, Belfield PW, Muers MF, Cooke NJ. Postal survey of bronchoscopic practice by physicians in the United Kingdom. *Thorax* 1986;41:311–317.
21. Eichhorn JH, Cooper JB, Cullen DJ, Maier WR, Philip JH, Seeman RG. Standards for patient monitoring during anesthesia at Harvard Medical School. *JAMA* 1986;256:1017–1020.
22. Tyler IL, Tantisira B, Winter PM, Motoyama EK. Continuous monitoring of arterial oxygen saturation with pulse oximetry during transfer to the recovery room. *Anesth Analg* 1985; 64:1108–1112.
23. Temper KK, Barker SJ. Pulse oximetry. *Anesthesiology* 1989; 70:98–108.

Bronchoscopy,
edited by U. B. S. Prakash.
Mayo Foundation © 1994.
Published by Raven Press, Ltd., New York.

CHAPTER 4

The Rigid Bronchoscope

Udaya B. S. Prakash and José P. Díaz-Jiménez

The science of bronchoscopy was born at the end of the nineteenth century when Gustav Killian examined the trachea with a laryngoscope. Later, Killian used an esophagoscope to extract a foreign body from the trachea and labeled the technique "direct bronchoscopy" (1). The historical details of the development of the rigid bronchoscope are described in the initial chapter of this textbook. During the early days of bronchoscopy, the rigid esophagoscope doubled as a bronchoscope. Successive structural modifications were introduced until the rigid bronchoscope became a well-established surgical instrument. Chevalier Jackson popularized the technique (2). The majority of the rigid bronchoscopies, however, were for the extraction of tracheobronchial foreign bodies. Development of the Hopkins light rod telescope system for use through the rigid bronchoscope further enhanced its diagnostic capabilities.

Traditionally, the rigid bronchoscope has been employed by surgeons. A survey from the United Kingdom (3) reported that although only 2% of the 39,564 bronchoscopies performed between 1974 and 1986 employed the rigid bronchoscope, more than 90% of the rigid bronchoscopies were done by surgeons. In another mail survey, conducted by the American College of Chest Physicians (4), only 8% of the 871 respondents, almost all pulmonary physicians, used the rigid bronchoscope. The reasons for the diminished frequency of use of the rigid bronchoscope in the current bronchoscopy practice include the demonstrated versatility of the flexible bronchoscope, the decreasing number of cases in which the rigid bronchoscopy is indicated, and the increasing frequency with which the surgeons, who traditionally used the rigid bronchoscope, now utilize the flexible bronchoscope. These factors are also responsible for the rapidly diminishing number of experts available to provide the training in rigid bronchoscopy.

The advent of the flexible bronchoscope in the early 1970s revolutionized the diagnostic and therapeutic approach to diseases of the airways and lungs. The flexible bronchoscope has made relentless strides and at present is the most commonly used instrument in bronchoscopy. Nevertheless, the more recent developments in bronchoscopic therapy of airway problems has demonstrated the resurgence of rigid bronchoscopes. The superiority of rigid bronchoscopy for the management of massive hemoptysis (5,6), laser procedures (7–10), removal of tracheobronchial foreign bodies (11–14), dilatation of tracheobronchial strictures, and placement of airway stents (15–19) is well established.

THE INSTRUMENT

The rigid bronchoscope is also described as "open tube bronchoscope," "ventilating bronchoscope," "stiff bronchoscope," or "straight bronchoscope." We will use the term *rigid bronchoscope* in this chapter. As the name implies, the rigid bronchoscope is a rigid, straight, and hollow metallic tube (Fig. 1). The thickness of the wall varies from 2 to 3 mm and the length varies from a very short instrument for use in small babies to a longer tube for use in adults. The external diameter varies from 2 to 9 mm.

The earlier rigid bronchoscopes had larger luminal diameters proximally and tapered toward the distal end. The more recent rigid bronchoscopes, designed for laser bronchoscopy, have a uniform diameter throughout the length of the instrument. The luminal shape is more or less circular in contrast to the antero-

U. B. S. Prakash: Division of Thoracic Diseases and Internal Medicine, Mayo Clinic, Rochester, Minnesota 55905.

J. P. Díaz-Jiménez: Endoscopy Laser Unit, Hospital Durán y Reynals, Ciudad Sanitaria y Universitaria de Bellevitge, Barcelona, Spain.

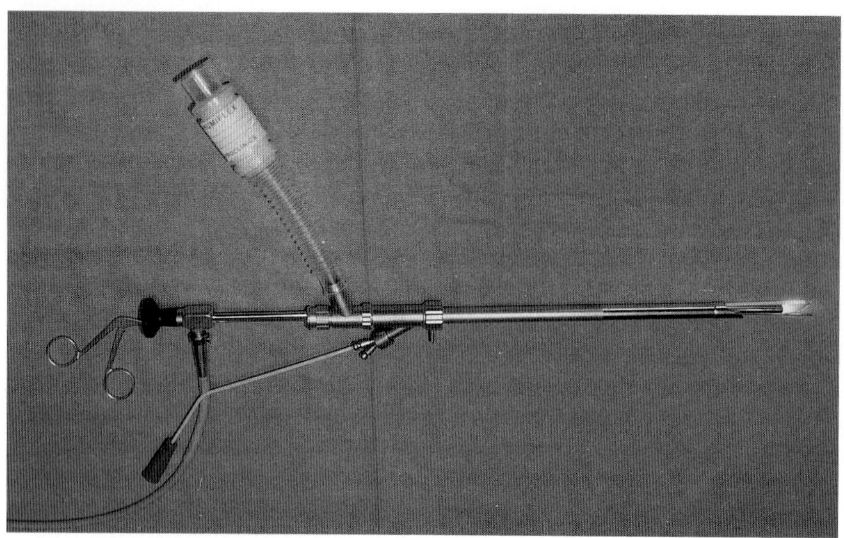

FIG. 1. Rigid bronchoscope with telescopically guided biopsy forceps, semirigid suction catheter, and a ventilating unit (top) to provide oxygenation and gaseous anesthesia.

posteriorly flattened diameter of the rigid esophagoscope. The proximal end of the instrument has special attachments to accommodate passage of a light-carrying wand, a side ventilation port, and in certain models special attachments can be used during laser bronchoscopy and stent placement. A proximal detachable glass cover prevents leakage of anesthetic gases. Rigid telescopes, made of glass fibers, of various lengths and diameters can be passed through the proximal opening of the rigid bronchoscope. The distal end of the rigid bronchoscope is beveled to facilitate insertion of the instrument through the larynx. In the earlier versions of the rigid bronchoscopes, the light is carried by a straight rigid wand with a detachable light bulb distally. A lumen within the wall of the bronchoscope facilitates the passage of the light wand. The newer rigid bronchoscopes have modifications that allow laser bronchoscopy, placement of tracheobronchial stents, and dilatation of tracheobronchial stenosis.

The newer rigid bronchoscopes provide the following additional advantages: the use of 11–12 interchangeable tubes with increasing diameters as well as two lengths (Fig. 2). The short tubes, without lateral holes to avoid loss of ventilation at the pharynx, are well suited for tracheoscopy and the longer tubes for examination of the bronchial tree. The latter have lateral windows to ventilate the contralateral bronchial tree. A principal entry tube, 14 mm in diameter, can adapt different sizes of tubes within it as well as allow the simultaneous passage of ancillary instruments such as telescope, forceps, and suction catheter. The larger diameter of the tracheoscope permits introduction of a flexible bronchoscope either to aspirate blood and secretions or to reach areas inaccessible to the rigid

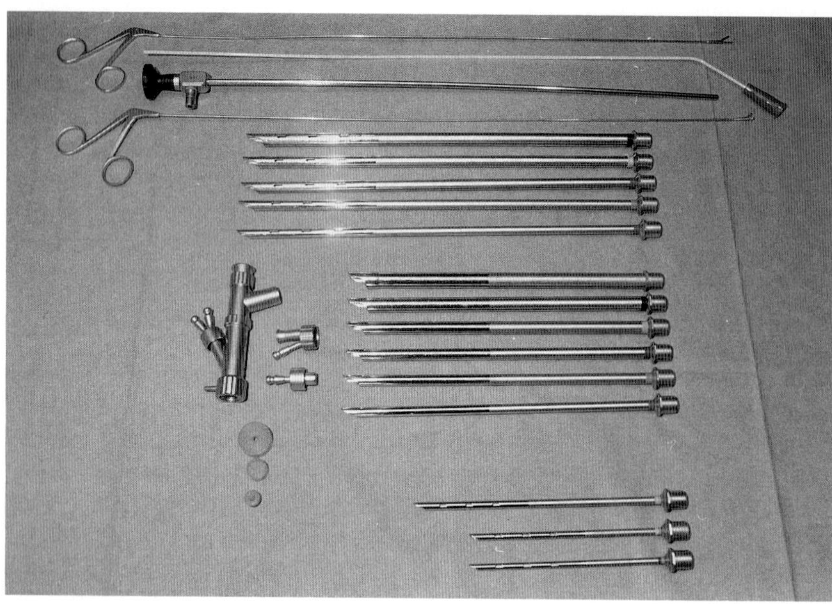

FIG. 2. The newer rigid bronchoscopes are available in several lengths and diameters.

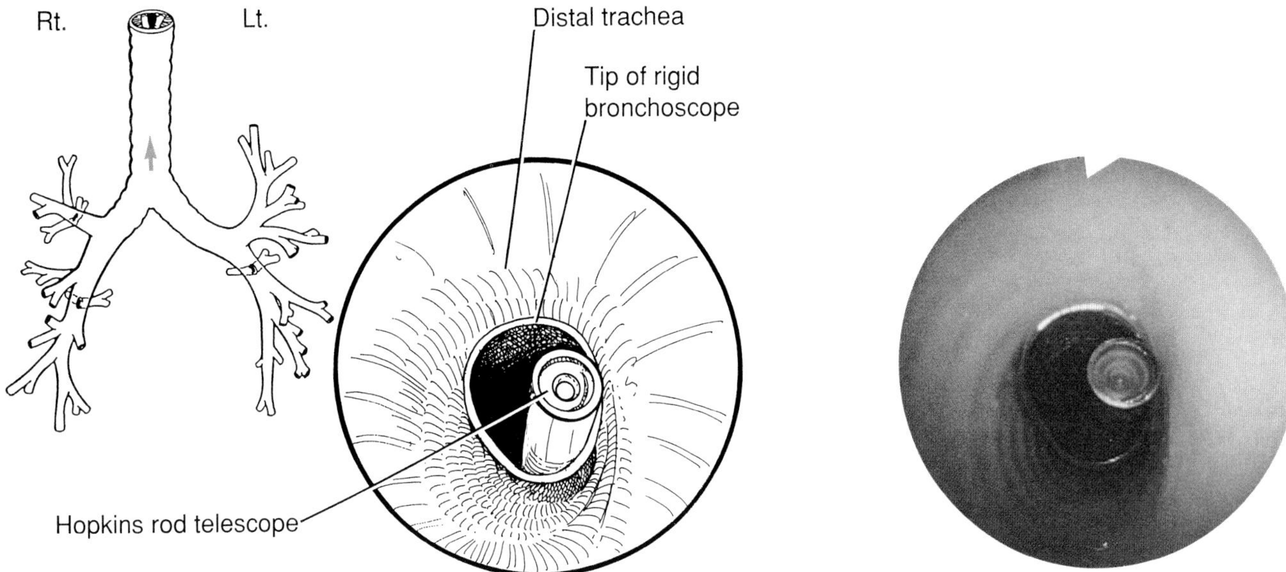

FIG. 3. Cephalad view of the tip of a rigid bronchoscope in the distal trachea of a tracheobronchial tree model. The tip of the telescope is shown. There is ample room for ventilation around the telescope. Photograph obtained by a flexible bronchoscope in the distal trachea.

bronchoscope. The proximal end of this instrument is equipped with side entrances for the separate introduction of suction catheter and laser fiber.

Telescopes

The clarity of the visual images seen through the rigid bronchoscopy telescopes far surpasses that obtained with any of the flexible bronchoscopes. The advent of the Hopkins rod lens system has made it possible to obtain a larger viewing angle, which facilitates excellent orientation in the airways. Hopkins rod telescopes, available in various lengths and diameters, can provide superb visualization of the tracheobronchial tree (Figs. 3 and 4). Telescopes with objective lens located at 90, 135, and 180° enable visualization of upper lobe bronchi and bronchi leading to the superior segments of the lower lobes. However, the flexible bronchoscope has greatly extended the range of visualization possible. This fact can be used advantageously by simultaneously utilizing both the rigid and flexible bronchoscopes. If the distal bronchial tree is to be visualized, the flexible bronchoscope can be easily passed through the rigid instrument.

The past two decades have seen the introduction of new optic systems and lens systems for rigid bronchoscopy. The increasing use of videobronchoscopy equipment for use with the flexible bronchoscope has encouraged the development of similar systems for the rigid bronchoscope. Using high-refraction lens and prisms, it is possible to increase the field of vision to 110°. These improvements provide a panoramic view through the rigid bronchoscope.

Light Sources

The light emitted by the lamp in the light source must be well localized so that light is not lost in the conductor cable. This is usually accomplished by using a cold-light reflector that allows the passage of light. Between the optical system and the light conductor cable, a thermal filter filters the infrared light.

Ancillary Instruments

Besides a straight telescope, the lumen of the rigid bronchoscope accommodates various biopsy forceps, laser fibers, and suction tubing. The introduction of the optical biopsy forceps (forceps and telescope used

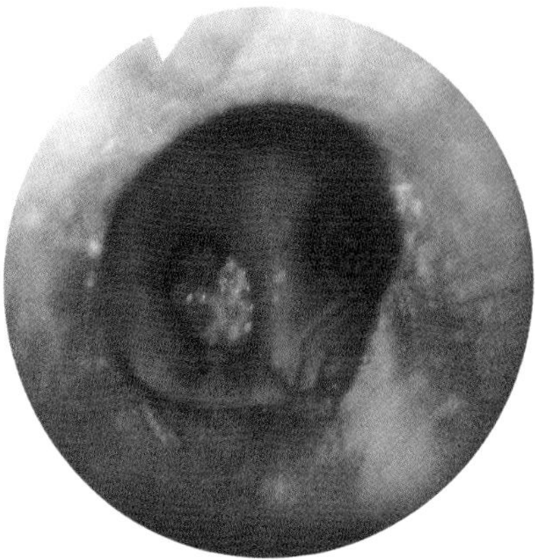

FIG. 4. View of the distal trachea and main stem bronchi through the Hopkins rod telescope. Inner aspect of the distal tip of the rigid bronchoscope is also seen.

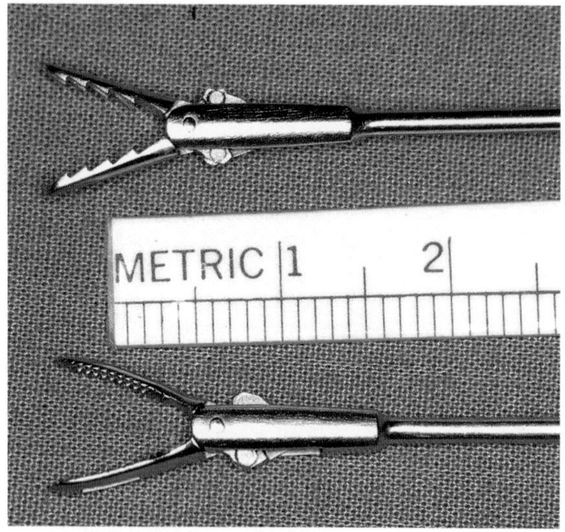

FIG. 5. Toothed (top) and nontoothed curved biopsy forceps (bottom) in open position.

as a single unit) permits more accurate tissue sampling. Likewise, the optical foreign body forceps is of great help in fast and precise manipulations (20). The increased light transmission produces a brighter image and easier perception.

The forceps used through the rigid bronchoscope permit biopsy of larger samples of mucosa and submucosal tissue. Removal of tracheobronchial foreign body, as well as placement and removal of airway stents, is also easier with these forceps (Fig. 5). One disadvantage of the optical biopsy forceps, particularly during laser bronchoscopy, is that they occupy a significant space in the bronchoscope (Fig. 6). Cleaning of obstructing film of mucous or blood is also more time consuming. In general, it is important to remember that the diameter of the optical biopsy unit must be small enough to permit easy manipulation in the bronchial tree.

A semirigid or rigid suction catheter is necessary in rigid bronchoscopy. Traditionally, the rigid suction catheters have been made of steel. Recently, semirigid plastic catheters have come into use with increasing frequency during laser bronchoscopy (Fig. 6). In addition to the removal of secretions, clots, and debris from the tracheobronchial tree, the suction catheters are also useful in the instillation of topical anesthetics and irrigating solution. The diameter of this catheter is normally 3 mm.

Other ancillary equipment available includes flexible and deflectable brush and biopsy forceps.

ADVANTAGES AND DISADVANTAGES

Advantages

The major advantages of the rigid over the flexible bronchoscope include the complete control of the airway, the ability to deliver and maintain adequate oxygenation, the capability of obtaining large biopsies and controlling massive bleeding from the tracheobronchial tree, and the ease with which laser bronchoscopy, removal of foreign bodies, and dilatation of tracheobronchial stenosis can be carried out. The disadvantages include the inability to visualize beyond the subsegmental bronchi and biopsy of lesions in the upper lobes. It may also be somewhat difficult to biopsy localized peripheral lesions. Bronchoscopic lung biopsy was indeed first performed through a rigid bronchoscope (21). It can still be accomplished if one wishes. It should be pointed out that most of the flexible bronchoscopes can be easily passed through the rigid bronchoscope, if necessary (Fig. 7). The large internal diameter of the rigid bronchoscope permits adequate oxygenation and excellent control of the airway, whether general anesthesia or topical anesthesia is used. The telescope system provides a superb bronchoscopic view and magnification. The wide variety of ancillary instruments such as forceps, baskets, and various grasping devices enable the bronchoscopist to easily extract tracheobronchial foreign bodies. The

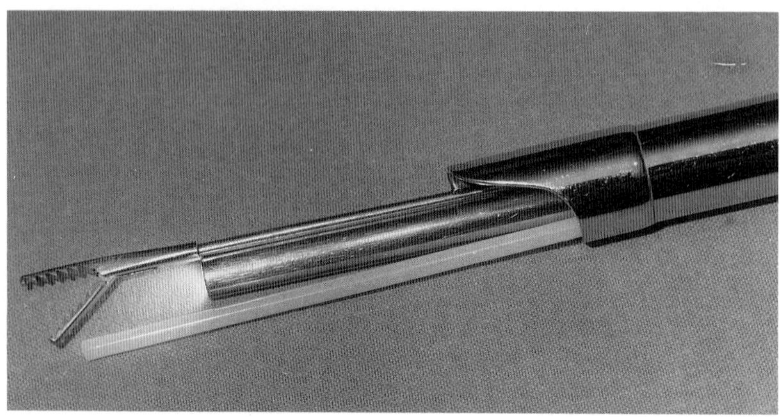

FIG. 6. Telescopically guided forceps and semirigid suction catheter shown exiting the distal end of a rigid bronchoscope. These ancillary devices can occupy significant space in the bronchoscope.

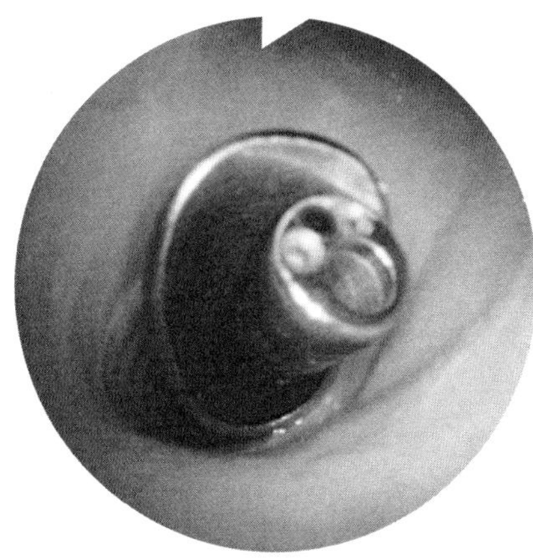

FIG. 7. Cephalad view of the distal tip of a rigid bronchoscope in the distal trachea. A flexible bronchoscope has been passed through the rigid bronchoscope. Note the ample space for ventilation around the flexible bronchoscope.

rigid bronchoscope is better for laser application, tracheobronchial stent therapy, and management of massive bleeding in the airways. In fact, almost anything that can be done with a flexible bronchoscope can be done with a rigid instrument.

Disadvantages

The majority of rigid bronchoscopy procedures require general anesthesia or deep intravenous sedation. Therefore, the procedure requires an operating room and extra personnel. Bedside bronchoscopy employing a rigid bronchoscope is almost impossible. Ankylosis of the cervical vertebrae as well as the patient's inability to extend the neck or open the jaw generally precludes rigid bronchoscopy. Bronchoscopic examination of the distal airways is more difficult even when special telescopes are used. The risk of trauma to airways and oropharyngeal structures is higher than with the flexible bronchoscope. Rigid bronchoscopy is more difficult to learn and therefore requires special training.

INDICATIONS

The rigid bronchoscope can be used for almost all the diagnostic and therapeutic indications outlined in Chapter 6 and Tables 1 and 2 of that chapter. One indication for which the rigid bronchoscope cannot be used is the assessment of endotracheal tube placement. In spite of the recent revival of and interest in rigid bronchoscopic applications and techniques, there are some who have questioned its usefulness (22–26). The latter viewpoint may indicate a want of training in rigid bronchoscopy and therefore a lack of awareness of the utility of the instrument. Granted that general anesthesia or deep intravenous sedation is required in most cases, rigid bronchoscopy is as safe as flexible bronchoscopy in trained hands. The negative commentaries in the literature on the role of rigid bronchoscopy seem unjustified without supporting evidence and are reminiscent of comparable disapproval of the flexible bronchoscope when it was first instituted in clinical practice more than two decades ago (27–29). In fact, recently the documentation of the importance of rigid bronchoscopy in the current clinical practice has proven wrong the earlier pronouncements that the flexible bronchoscope would ultimately displace the rigid bronchoscope (30,31). The flexible bronchoscope and the rigid bronchoscope should complement rather than compete with each other (32).

The rigid bronchoscope is notable for its exceptional ability to extract tracheobronchial foreign body, dilatation of tracheobronchial stricture and stenosis, placement of tracheobronchial stents, control of massive hemoptysis, laser bronchoscopy, removal of tenacious mucous plugs and blood clots, removal of necrotic tracheobronchial mucosa, and intraoperative assistance during resection and anastomosis of trachea or main bronchi. It has been also used in bronchoscopic electrocautery and cryotherapy. The role of the rigid bronchoscope in several of these situations is discussed below.

Unusual clinical situations may not permit the passage of the flexible bronchoscope. For example, extreme rigidity of the trachea, as in tracheopathia osteoplastica, may not only prevent the passage of the flexible bronchoscope but also damage it (Fig. 8).

Airway Malignancy

The rigid bronchoscope was used in the mid-1930s to treat airway malignancy. In 1935, Kramer and Som (64,65) published the first results of bronchoscopic resection in 23 patients with bronchial carcinoid and observed 15 years later that of the 14 cases that they had considered adequately treated, 50% were cured or free of symptoms. Even though laser bronchoscopy has become more popular for the treatment of unresectable tracheobronchial malignant lesions, simple rigid bronchoscopic biopsy forceps removal of obstructing neoplastic tissue may open up an occluded airway. In patients who present with progressive respiratory distress due to obstructing tracheobronchial neoplasms, palliation of symptoms and establishment of an airway in acute obstruction is the goal. The rigid bronchoscope can be used to "core out" obstructing tracheobronchial neoplastic tissue (Fig. 9). Mathisen and Grillo (33) used this technique in 56 patients to relieve obstruction from airway neoplasms. A single

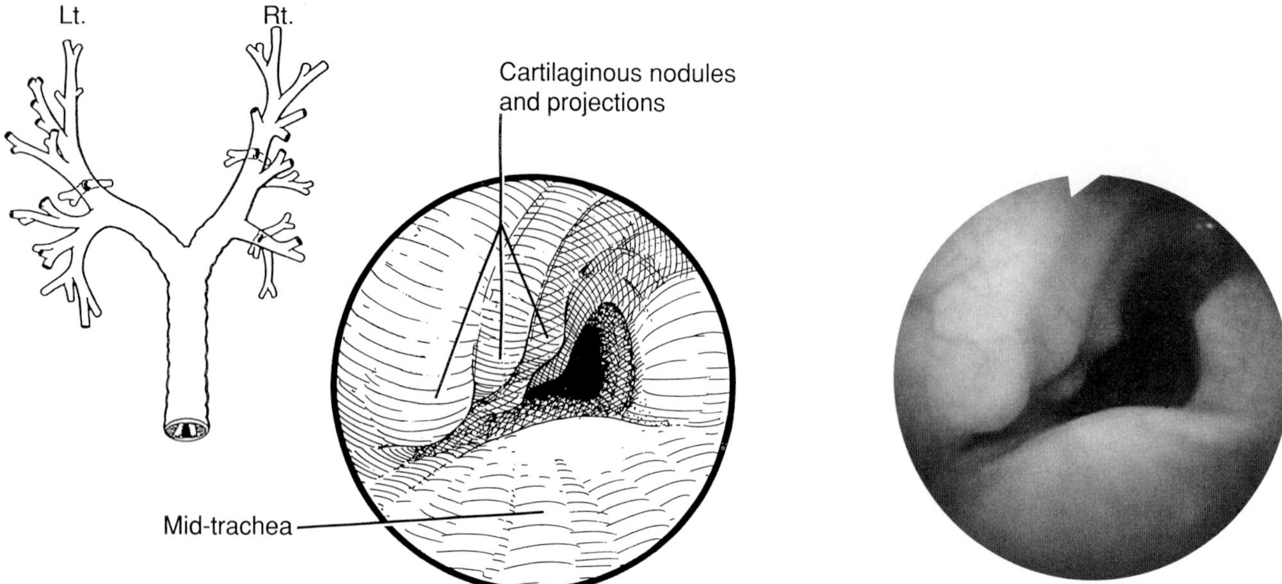

FIG. 8. Extremely rigid trachea in a patient with tracheopathia osteoplastica. The passage of a flexible bronchoscope through this was almost impossible because the bony polyps gripped the instrument and did not permit entrance to the distal tracheobronchial tree. A small caliber rigid bronchoscope was able to traverse the tracheobronchial tree easily.

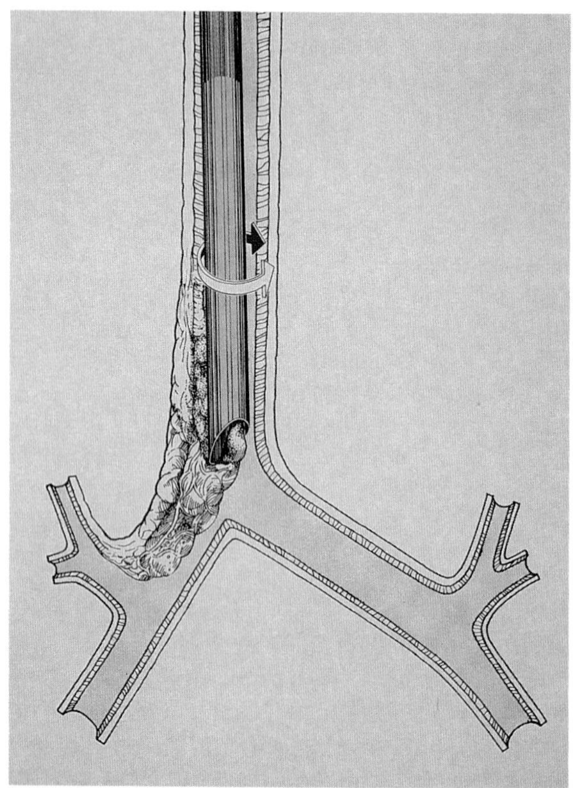

FIG. 9. The sharp tip of the rigid bronchoscope itself can be used to "core out" the tracheal neoplasm by rotating and simultaneously advancing the instrument. (Courtesy of J.-F. Dumon, M.D. and J. P. Díaz-Jiménez, M.D.)

bronchoscopy was sufficient in 96% and improvement in the airway was accomplished in 90% of patients. The location of the obstruction was trachea in 16 patients, carina in 24, main bronchi in 8, and distal airway in 8. The authors concluded that the coring technique was superior to laser therapy. Benign neoplasms can be completely resected through the rigid bronchoscope. Sahin and colleagues (34) successfully removed an endobronchial hamartoma of the right lower lobe bronchus in a 60-year-old patient.

Laser Bronchoscopy

The introduction of laser treatment of airway malignancy was mainly responsible for the resurrection of rigid bronchoscopy. Rigid bronchoscopy is the preferred technique for the administration of carbon dioxide laser therapy (35–37). In a report from a hospital in Toronto (35), rigid bronchoscopy with Venturi ventilation was used in 24 patients, with the CO_2 laser therapy directed down the open end of the bronchoscope; the complication rate was minimal. Diaz-Jimenez and associates (38) performed over 400 YAG:Nd procedures in 252 patients using rigid bronchoscopy under general anesthesia and experienced no significant complications. Cavaliere et al. (39) reported their experience with 1,000 patients who underwent Nd:YAG laser therapy; 92% of treatments utilized rigid bronchoscopy under general anesthesia. At the Mayo Clinic, the bronchoscopists have been employing the rigid bronchoscope as the main instrument in all the Nd:YAG laser bronchoscopies and have concluded that rigid bronchoscopy is far superior to flexible bronchoscopy (32). Bronchoscopists with considerable experience in rigid bronchoscopy have discerned that the "laser ablation" of large-airway tumors is, to a vast degree, smoothly accomplished via the rigid bronchoscope with extraction of large portions of obstructing tissue by a biopsy forceps and the use of the rigid bronchoscope itself as a coring instrument (Fig. 9). Most of the tumor mass is indeed removed this way, while the laser is used to coagulate and cauterize vascular lesions and vascular stalks of pedunculated tumors.

Furthermore, the rigid bronchoscope itself serves as a dilator of the narrowed airway. The rigid instrument can achieve the opening of an occluded airway in a much shorter time than the flexible bronchoscope. There is a notable and statistically significant difference in the number of laser sessions required by flexible bronchoscopy and rigid bronchoscope. The rigid bronchoscopy requires only one session and the flexible bronchoscopy requires a mean of two sessions to treat the airway occlusion (9,40). In fact, bronchoscopists who use only the flexible bronchoscope for laser resection of large-airway lesions require several sessions because of the long duration involved in removing large tumors with the laser via the flexible bronchoscope.

The reasoning that flexible bronchoscopy is better suited for laser therapy of distal or peripheral airway lesions is rather unconvincing because such cases are uncommon and the indication for palliative therapy debatable (32). Even in those infrequent situations, we feel that the rigid bronchoscope is the instrument of choice because a flexible bronchoscope can be passed, if required, through the rigid bronchoscope to apply laser therapy (Fig. 10) (41). This strategy combines the safety of the rigid bronchoscope with the maneuverability of the flexible bronchoscope (9).

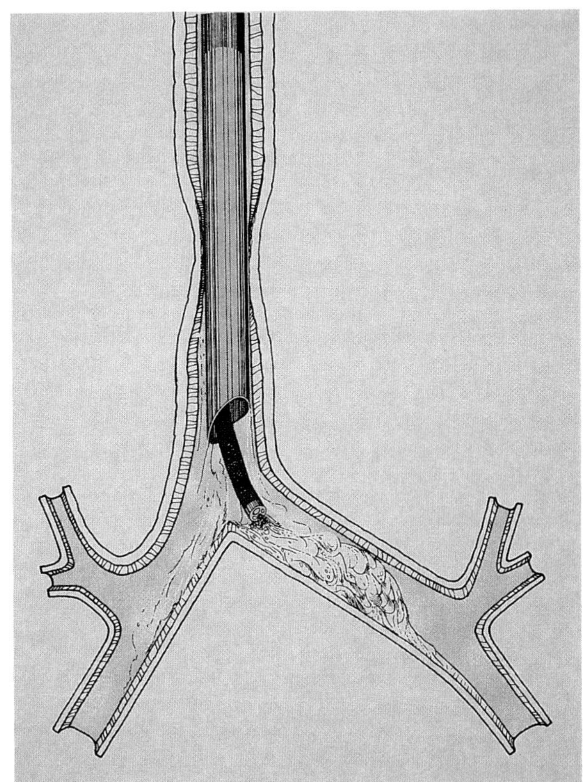

FIG. 10. Flexible bronchoscope can be passed through the rigid bronchoscope to deliver laser therapy to lesions not accessible to rigid bronchoscope. (Courtesy of J.-F. Dumon, M.D. and J. P. Díaz-Jiménez, M.D.)

Foreign Body

The rigid bronchoscope is the instrument of choice for removal of foreign bodies from pediatric airways. Rigid bronchoscopy in children suspected to have aspirated a tracheobronchial foreign body is a safe, effective, and sometimes life-saving procedure (42). The vast array of ancillary instruments such as forceps, baskets, and other instruments available for use with the rigid bronchoscope is incomparable; almost any type of tracheobronchial foreign body can be extracted. Many bronchoscopists have championed the use of flexible bronchoscopy for the removal of tracheobronchial foreign bodies in adults. One retrospective study of 60 adults with tracheobronchial foreign bodies observed that the flexible bronchoscope was successful in 61% of patients whereas the rigid instrument accomplished the extraction of foreign body in 96% (13). While small foreign bodies in the tracheobronchial tree can be extracted with a flexible bronchoscope, larger ones will require the rigid bronchoscope.

The formation of granuloma secondary to chronic retention of a tracheobronchial foreign body may require rigid bronchoscopy for the application of laser therapy to remove the obstructing tissue before attempting the extraction of the underlying foreign body.

Massive Hemorrhage

Massive hemorrhage in the tracheobronchial tree is a daunting problem to encounter with the flexible bronchoscope. The limiting factor with the flexible instrument is its inability to aspirate large quantities of blood or blood clot. Stradling and Stradling (43) are of the opinion that if significant hemoptysis is already occurring, rigid bronchoscopy should be the first choice. The rigid bronchoscope will not only permit aspiration of large volumes of blood or clots, but will also enable the bronchoscopist to effectively control the bleeding (Chapter 17 of this volume).

Airway Dilatation

In the treatment of strictures and stenoses of the tracheobronchial tree, the rigid bronchoscope is valuable as a mechanical dilator. The instrument itself is gently pushed through the narrowed airway to effect dilatation (44). If this is not possible, a balloon catheter or bougie can be used through the rigid bronchoscope to dilate the stenosis. The bronchoscopist who wishes to perform dilatation procedures should possess a thorough knowledge of the tracheobronchial anatomy and its relationship to the great vessels and the esophagus.

Airway Stents

Although the flexible bronchoscope has been used in the placement of wire-mesh stents to treat tracheobronchial stenosis, the majority of bronchoscopists use the rigid bronchoscope for insertion of various types of stents in the tracheobronchial tree. A rigid bronchoscope permits easy insertion, manipulation, and removal of airway stents (45,46). There are several modifications of the rigid bronchoscope to facilitate this procedure and these are discussed elsewhere in this book.

The insertion technique of the stents will depend on the location and the prothesis model used. The length and diameter of the stenotic area is first measured. For silicone stents (Dumon stents) two methods can be used. One is to place the stent in the distal lumen of the rigid bronchoscope and push the stent with the telescope. The other method consists of folding the stent and loading it into the specially made stent introducer. The prothesis is then pushed into place through the bronchoscope. Special stent introducers are available for placement of stents of different sizes in different locations in the tracheobronchial tree (Fig. 11). Stainless steel wire stents (Gianturco) are placed using either rigid or flexible bronchoscopy. The sheath is pushed in place using a special delivery catheter.

Mucous Plugs

Tenacious or thick mucus plugs are occasionally difficult to aspirate or remove with the flexible bronchoscope. This is particularly true in pediatric patients with cystic fibrosis, asthma, and postoperative atelectasis. Rigid bronchoscopic removal is much easier and more rapidly accomplished.

Pediatric Bronchoscopy

As discussed in Chapter 23 of this volume, the rigid bronchoscope continues to be as important as the flexible bronchoscope in pediatric patients with airway problems. The role of the rigid bronchoscope for the extraction of foreign bodies from the pediatric tracheobronchial tree is discussed above and in Chapter 18 of this volume. The ability to control the pediatric airway with the rigid bronchoscope is a major advantage.

Cryotherapy

Airway narrowing due to obstructing tissue growing into the tracheal or bronchial lumen may cause progressive dyspnea and hypoxemia. Rigid bronchoscopic cryotherapy is an alternative method to remove the obstructing lesions (66). The tissue is exposed to extremely low temperatures by means of a super-cooled liquid that is circulated through a tube introduced via the bronchoscope so as to apply cryotherapy to the abnormal tissue. The cryoprobes used in bronchial cry-

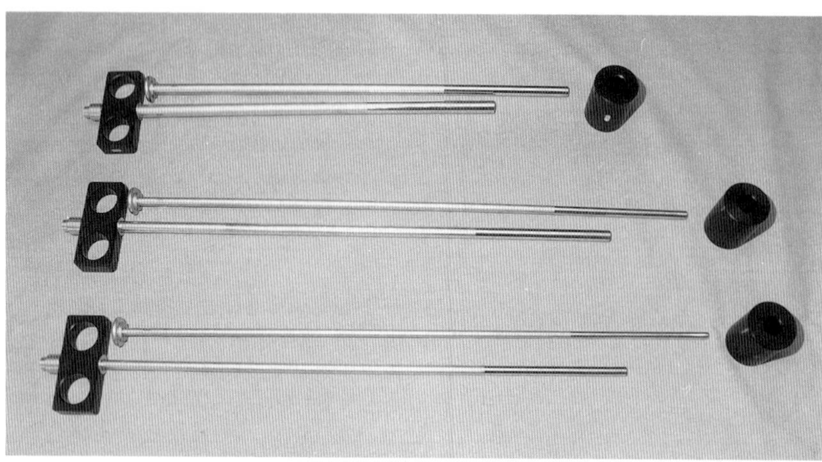

FIG. 11. Stent introducer system for rigid bronchoscope.

otherapy employ nitrous oxide cryoprobes. There are two kinds of cryoprobes: rigid cryoprobes of 3 mm diameter, for use through the rigid bronchoscopes, and flexible cryoprobes of 2–3 mm diameter for use through flexible bronchoscopes.

Other Indications

Rigid bronchoscopes have been used during the resection and anastomosis of tracheal strictures. With the distal tip of a rigid bronchoscope in the trachea distal to the surgical site, the patient's ventilation can be easily maintained while the surgeon proceeds with the resection and anastomosis. Further discussion on this aspect is discussed in Chapter 22 of this volume. The rigid bronchoscope can be a life-saving instrument in clinical situations besides tracheobronchial foreign body aspiration and massive hemoptysis. A report described two pediatric patients with acute airway compromise due to benign tracheal mucocele both of whom developed acute respiratory distress following upper airway infection. The mucoceles were "unroofed" and drained through rigid bronchoscopes (47).

During the past decade, transtracheal and bronchoscopic needle aspiration and biopsy of lymph nodes adjacent to the airways have been used to diagnose benign and malignant disease as well as to stage lung cancer. Even though most bronchoscopists now use the flexible bronchoscope for this purpose, this technique was originally accomplished through the rigid bronchoscope (48–51). Pauli and associates (52) performed rigid bronchoscopy and bronchoscopic needle aspiration/biopsy of lymph node biopsies and forceps bronchial biopsies in 258 patients with suspected sarcoidosis and noted the presence of noncaseating granulomas in 66.3% of patients. When bronchoscopic needle aspiration biopsies were combined with forceps bronchial biopsies, the positive rate increased to 77.7%. No major complication occurred during bronchoscopic needle aspiration.

In difficult endotracheal intubations, a flexible bronchoscope can be used to guide the endotracheal tube into the trachea. Occasionally, when even this technique fails, the rigid bronchoscope itself can be used as an endotracheal tube (53).

CONTRAINDICATIONS

The contraindications to both flexible and rigid bronchoscopy are discussed in Chapter 6 of this volume. There are very few absolute contraindications to bronchoscopy. Some clinical situations, however, should be considered as relative contraindications to rigid bronchoscopy. An unstable neck that precludes excessive motion of the neck during bronchoscopy, microstomia, and technical difficulties due to cervical ankylosis and severe kyphoscoliosis are among the major contraindications. Absolute contraindications to bronchoscopy include an unstable cardiovascular status, life-threatening cardiac arrhythmias, extremely severe hypoxemia that is likely to worsen during bronchoscopy, and an inadequately trained bronchoscopist and/or bronchoscopy team.

THE TECHNIQUE

Preparation of the Patient

The preparation of the patient for bronchoscopy is discussed in Chapter 8 of this volume. Even when general anesthesia is used for rigid bronchoscopy, application of topical anesthesia to vocal cords, oropharynx, inner lips, and gums is important. Clinical studies have shown that patients who received lidocaine for rigid bronchoscopy under general anesthesia had no significant rise in blood pressure and heart rate from baseline following the introduction of the rigid bronchoscope (54). Whether general anesthesia or deep intravenous anesthesia is used, it is preferable to maintain spontaneous breathing so that the risk of hypoventilation is minimized. However, it may be necessary to induce total muscle relaxation if the initial attempts to insert the bronchoscope are unsuccessful. General anesthesia is remarkably safe for rigid bronchoscopy. It is difficult to acquiesce with some reports that maintain that rigid bronchoscopy under general anesthesia is fraught with significant complications (55). To minimize the risks, it is imperative that the bronchoscopist discuss the procedural plans with the anesthesiologist and maintain communication with the anesthesiologist before and during the procedure.

Once the patient is anesthetized, the teeth, lips, gums, and eyes should be protected by use of wet gauze or commercially available guards for teeth and eyes. Dentures should be removed before submitting the patient to anesthesia. Nonremovable dental appliances should be protected from damage. Certain steps are necessary to facilitate easy visualization of the laryngeal structures so that the rigid bronchoscope can be inserted swiftly and effortlessly. To achieve this, a roll of blanket or towel is placed between the shoulder blades so that the upper trachea is thrust forward and the cervical spine extended. Another option is to have the patient's head suspended over the edge of the operating table while an assistant holds it carefully and moves it up or down depending on the bronchoscopist's instructions. If this technique is used, the bronchoscopist places her or his foot on a stool so that the patient's head can be supported by the bronchosco-

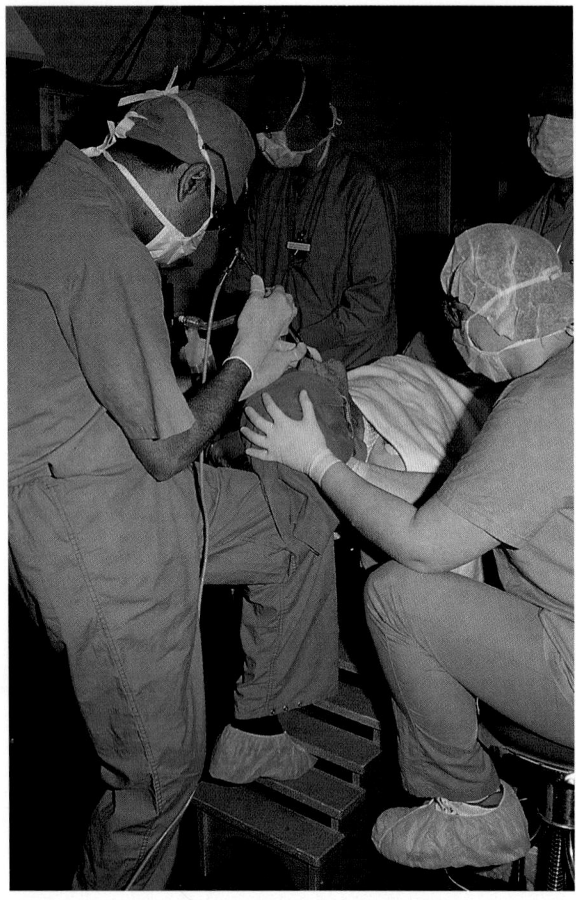

FIG. 12. Bronchoscopist introduces the instrument while supporting the patient's head on his knee while an assistant also supports the patient's head. Note the specially made stool with steps at different levels to allow proper positioning of the bronchoscopist's foot.

pist's bent knee (Fig. 12). The standard method is to place the patient's head on a firm pillow and extend the head on it so that the chin points vertically upward, i.e., the position usually assumed when shaving the chin (Fig. 13) (43).

Methods of Insertion

As there are several methods of insertion of the rigid bronchoscope, the details of the particular technique to be used should be discussed with the anesthesiologist and the bronchoscopy team before general anesthesia is administered. The different methods of insertion of the rigid bronchoscope are briefly described below. In each of these, the beveled tip (the long axis) of the bronchoscope is usually maintained in an anterior orientation in relation to patient's body. Both hands of the bronchoscopist are used. The hand (generally the right hand) holding the proximal end of the instrument aids in moving the distal tip up or down, rotating the instrument on its long (luminal) axis, and moving it from side to side. The forefinger and thumb of the other hand (usually the left hand if the bronchoscopist is right-handed) hold the bronchoscope, where the instrument crosses the upper teeth, and protect the teeth, lips, and gums (Fig. 14). The left thumb should function as the fulcrum to lift or lower the distal tip of the bronchoscope. The upper teeth or gum should never be used as the fulcrum. The movement of the patient's head is controlled by inserting the third, fourth, and fifth fingers of the left hand inside the mouth so that the left side of the hard palate is in contact with the fingers and the left palm is in contact with the skin over the left cheek. This "hold" on the patient's head permits the bronchoscopist to move the patient's head and bronchoscope en masse. This system is ideal for the standard insertion of the rigid bronchoscope. Other methods of insertion do not necessarily require this maneuver.

It is important to maintain the bronchoscope in the midline during the insertion so that laryngeal structures are quickly exposed and the bronchoscope is introduced into the trachea. The bronchoscope can be introduced while the bronchoscopist visualizes the anatomic landmarks through the bronchoscope's lumen or by using the telescope through the bronchoscope's lumen (Fig. 15). If the telescope is used through the bronchoscope, the distal tip of the instrument should be maintained within the lumen of the bronchoscope so that mucous films do not cover the telescopic lens. If excessive secretions are a problem, they should be thoroughly aspirated before attempting bronchoscopy. A small amount of lubricant should be applied to the outer aspect of the distal few centimeters of the instrument; an alternate lubricating agent is warm saline. Care should be taken to ensure that the upper lip is separated from the upper teeth by the use of gauze or towel because the upper lip or the tongue can easily get caught between the rigid bronchoscope and the upper teeth and sustain significant trauma.

Direct Insertion

Once the patient's neck is maintained in the extended position, the bronchoscope is inserted almost vertically into the oral cavity. Ideally, the patient's chin, tip of nose, and the long axis of the bronchoscope should be in a straight line. This path will invariably lead to the larynx. If the patient's tongue pushes the bronchoscope or if the teeth do not permit midline insertion, then the bronchoscope should be inserted on the side of tongue while pushing it out of the way, and the tip of the instrument moved over to midline. Occasionally, the movement of the tongue is stimulated by the bronchoscope. An effort should be made

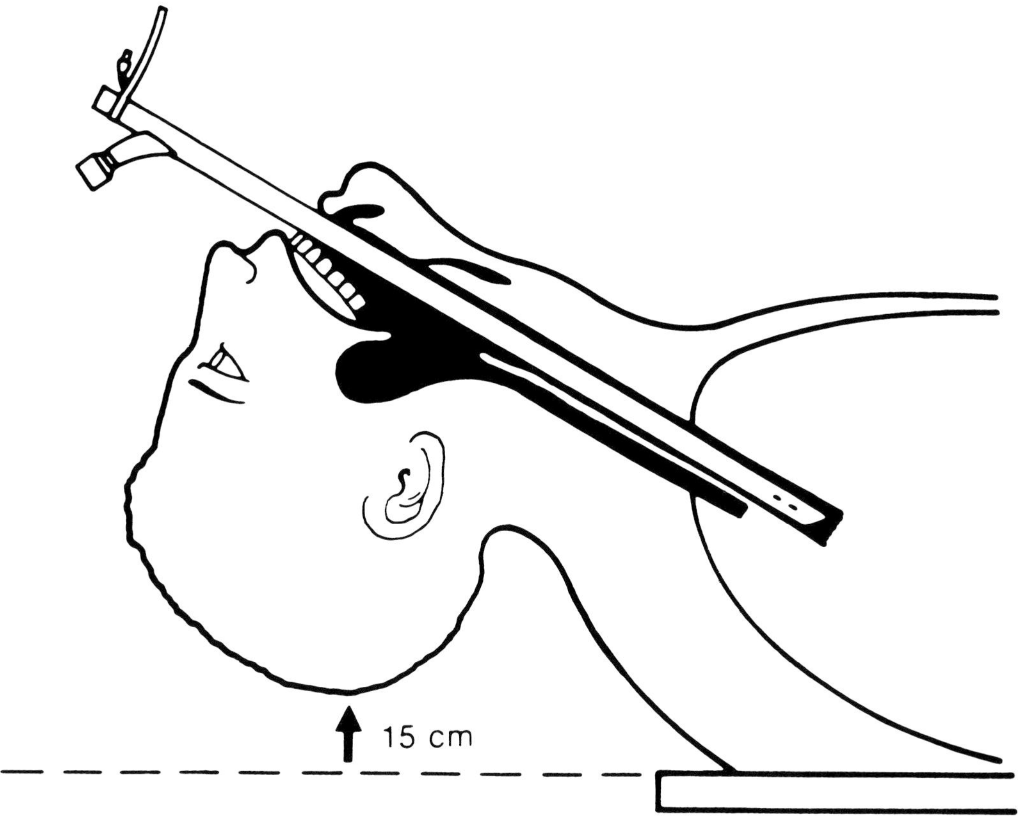

FIG. 13. The chin of the patient is the highest part of the body during introduction of the rigid bronchoscope. (From Ref. 62, with permission.)

to avoid any contact with the tongue. This can be accomplished by gently sliding the distal tip of the bronchoscope along the roof of the mouth until the uvula is passed. Interference by the tongue is generally not a problem in an anesthetized patient. When the distal tip of the instrument is close to the uvula, the left thumb gently pushes the bronchoscope upward while at the same time the right hand moves the proximal end of the instrument inferiorly, until the tip of the epiglottis comes into view. The epiglottis is an important landmark during the insertion of rigid as well as flexible bronchoscopes. Excessive anterior positioning of the bronchoscope will lead it to the blind valleculae (space between epiglottis and tongue), whereas an extreme

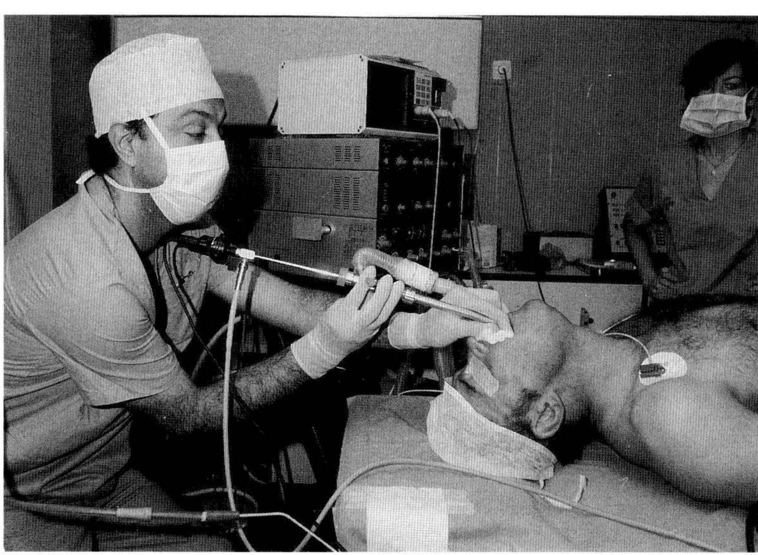

FIG. 14. The bronchoscopist protects the patient's teeth, gum, and tongue with the left hand while the right hand advances and manipulates the rigid bronchoscope.

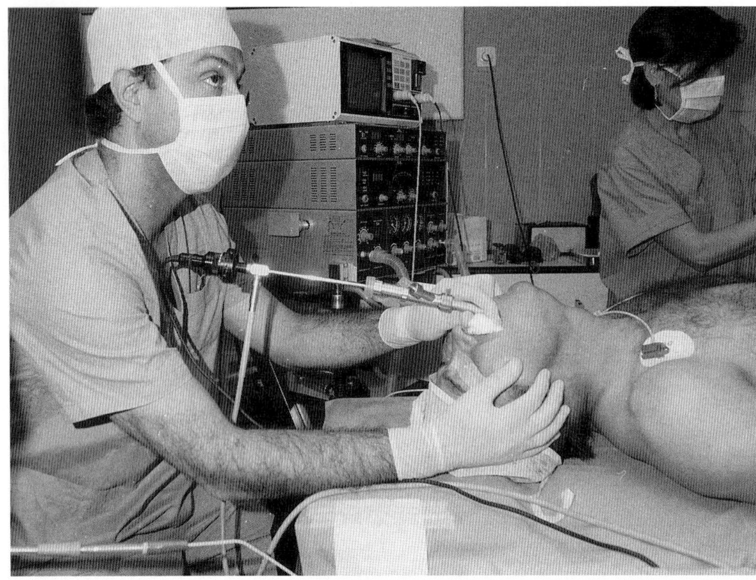

FIG. 15. The bronchoscopist views the video monitor to assess progress of the rigid bronchoscope in the tracheobronchial tree. A video adapter is attached to the proximal end of the telescope.

posterior approach will guide the instrument into the pharynx and esophagus. If the epiglottis is missed, the bronchoscope should be withdrawn proximally and reoriented to identify the epiglottis.

As soon as the epiglottis is lifted up with the tip of the bronchoscope, the tip of the bronchoscope is directed anteriorly until the larynx is visualized (Fig. 16). The crucial part of this maneuver is to not lose sight of the vocal cords as the instrument is advanced further. The bronchoscope is advanced until it is just about to traverse the glottic opening. Then the bronchoscope is rotated clockwise 90° on its long axis such that the bevel is parallel to the glottic chink. Once the trachea is entered, the instrument is again rotated 90° clockwise to maintain the long axis along the posterior wall of the trachea. However, the bronchoscope can be rotated in the trachea to provide best visualization.

It is possible to insert the rigid bronchoscope into the trachea without the use of the telescope. To realize this technique, the bronchoscopist should develop monocular vision by practicing through the lumen of the bronchoscope without telescope. Another requirement is that a light-carrying rod be incorporated into the instrument. When the telescope is used, its distal tip should be maintained within the lumen of the bronchoscope, usually at a distance of 1.5 cm from the tip of the bronchoscope. During insertion, there is an involuntary tendency for the bronchoscopist's forehead or glasses to push the telescope tip out of the bronchoscope. If mucous film or secretions block the vision, the oropharynx should be suctioned with a straight suction rod and the distal tip of the telescope treated with an antifog agent. If the bronchoscope cannot be advanced into the trachea by gentle manipulation, force should not be used. Instead, a bronchoscope with a smaller diameter should be tried.

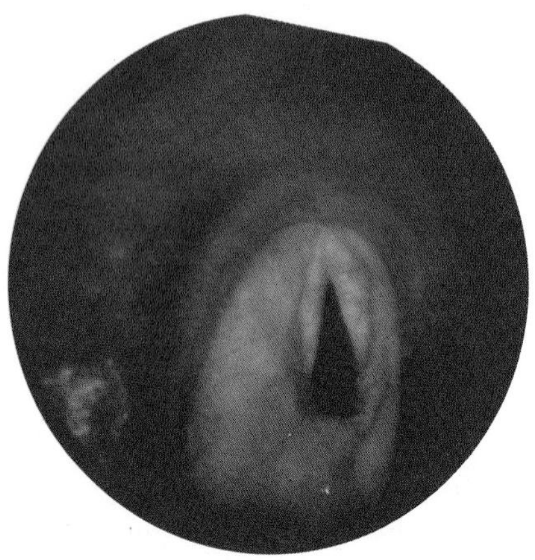

FIG. 16. Rigid bronchoscopic view of larynx.

Insertion Guided by Endotracheal Tube

If an endotracheal tube is placed prior to the insertion of the rigid bronchoscope, the endotracheal tube can be used as a guide to insert the bronchoscope. A major advantage is that excellent ventilation can be maintained through the endotracheal tube until just before the rigid bronchoscope replaces it. In this technique, the rigid bronchoscope is inserted into the oral cavity and gently slid along the anterior wall of the endotracheal tube until the vocal cords are reached. At this point, the distal progression of the instrument is halted and the distal tip of the bronchoscope held close to the vocal cords without losing site of the glottic opening. The bronchoscopist should instruct the anesthesiologist or an assistant to gradually remove the endotracheal tube while the bronchoscopist constantly visualizes the vocal apparatus. As soon as the tip of the endotracheal tube comes out of the larynx, the rigid bronchoscope is quickly introduced into the trachea by the technique for direct insertion described above.

The bronchoscope can also be slid along the posterior wall of the endotracheal tube, but this requires extra effort to lift the rigid bronchoscope anteriorly and the bronchoscope tends to slide off to one side or the other. Excessive lubricant applied to the bronchoscope or the endotracheal tube also tends to produce slippage of the bronchoscope over the endotracheal tube. To avoid the slippage, the bronchoscopist must ascertain that the bronchoscope is held firmly to maintain constant visualization of the airway lumen.

Laryngoscopic Insertion

Either a straight or curved laryngoscope is used to lift the epiglottis and expose to laryngeal opening. The rigid bronchoscope is then introduced into the trachea in a manner similar to that of endotracheal intubation. This method may entail a tangential approach to the glottic opening because the laryngoscope occupies the midline space, and the bronchoscopist should make sure that the laryngeal apparatus is not damaged during the insertion. This technique is more useful in pediatric patients.

Insertion via Laryngeal Suspension

This method provides the bronchoscopist an easy access to the tracheobronchial tree using the rigid bronchoscope. The bronchoscope can be removed and reinserted at will. One disadvantage is that side-to-side movement of the patient's head is somewhat limited. After general anesthesia is established, the laryngoscope is used to lift the glottis and, with the use of special equipment, laryngeal suspension is established.

Insertion Through Tracheostomy Stoma

The tracheostomy cannula should be removed before attempting rigid bronchoscopy. The degree of discomfort is tolerable and general anesthesia is not necessary. Topical anesthesia should be applied to the stoma and the airways. The chin and mandibular margins prevent midline insertion of the bronchoscope. The bronchoscopist should approach the stoma from the left or right side of the patient's neck or flex the patient's neck in the opposite direction. Hyperextension of the patient's head by letting it dangle over the edge of the bed permits midline insertion.

Using the Flexible Bronchoscope as a Guide

This technique is not recommended for routine use because of the high risk of damage to the delicate flexible bronchoscope. We have used this method in a small number of patients. This method is easier to use when a shorter rigid bronchoscope (sometimes called a tracheoscope) has to be inserted. The rigid bronchoscope is threaded over a well-lubricated flexible bronchoscope. After the trachea is entered with the flexible bronchoscope, the bronchoscopist helps an assistant to gently slide the rigid bronchoscope over the flexible bronchoscope. The patient's head should be maintained as described above for other modes of insertion. The major complication is the high risk of damage to the outer lining of the flexible bronchoscope by the relatively sharp and hard bevel of the rigid instrument. We do not recommend this method on a routine basis .

Manipulation Within the Tracheobronchial Tree

As soon as the distal tip of the rigid bronchoscope is inserted into the trachea, appropriate attachments are connected to the vents in the bronchoscope to provide oxygen and anesthesia gases. Gum protectors made of plastic or rubber should be positioned properly. The bronchoscopist should assume the normal operating posture and by looking the through the bronchoscope lumen adjust the position of patient's head, operating table, or the sitting height of the bronchoscopist's chair to obtain maximal view of the trachea. The distal movement of the instrument should be gentle and not forced. Excessive movement of the proximal portion of the bronchoscope tends to traumatize the laryngeal structures and may cause edema and bleeding. If cough is a problem, topical anesthetic can be applied via a long metal cannula inserted through the lumen of the bronchoscope. The space around the patient's head should be free so that the bronchoscopist can easily change her or his position around the head. If the bronchoscopist wishes to sit down to perform the procedure, a chair with wheels permits easy movement around the patient's head.

Once the teeth, lips, and gums are protected, the bronchoscope can be relatively fixed by packing the oropharynx around the bronchoscope with wet gauze. This will prevent undue movement of the instrument as well as the escape of anesthetic gases from the patient's tracheobronchial tree. Commercially available equipment can be used to fix the bronchoscope so that the bronchoscopist's hands are free to manipulate ancillary instruments. This is particularly useful in performing prolonged procedures such as laser bronchoscopy. An alternative is to have an assistant hold and stabilize the bronchoscope while the bronchoscopist carries out manipulations within the airway.

The left bronchial tree is harder to examine because of the more horizontal as well as lengthy course of this airway. To enter the left bronchial tree, the patient's head is turned and flexed slightly to the left and the proximal portion of the bronchoscope moved toward the right angle of the mouth. Slight lateral pressure (to the right) at the angle of the mouth may be necessary to align the bronchoscope with the lumen of left main stem bronchus. The right bronchial tree is easier to examine and may not require positioning of the patient's head or movement of the bronchoscope to the extreme left corner of the mouth. The distance to which the tip of the bronchoscope is introduced depends on the size of the bronchoscope and the diameter of the bronchi. If the bronchoscope cannot enter the distal bronchi, then the telescope should be used to examine the distal bronchi. A special angled telescope should be employed to examine the upper lobe bronchi and other inaccessible bronchi (superior segments, etc.). Use of the angled telescope requires some practice. Another option available is the use of a flexible bronchoscope through the rigid instrument to examine the distal bronchial tree.

Use of Ancillary Equipment

Aspiration of secretions is accomplished by inserting a long metal cannula through the lumen of the instrument. The tip of the suction cannula should be able to protrude out of the distal end of the bronchoscope for a distance of at least 1.5 cm. Excessive suction of mucosa should be avoided. The proper use of ancillary instruments such as biopsy forceps and foreign body removal equipment requires some practice. Depending on the rigid bronchoscope model used, the ancillary instruments can be used in conjunction with a telescope to provide direct visualization of the tracheobronchial tree. If the telescope and the biopsy forceps cannot be inserted simultaneously, the bronchoscopist should first visualize the lesion and fix the bronchoscope so that the distal lumen of the bronchoscope does not move in relation to the object in question. Then a biopsy forceps, without telescopic visualization, is used to obtain specimens in a somewhat blind fashion. With practice, good results can be expected with this method. The newer models of rigid bronchoscope have separate channels for the insertion of suction catheter and laser fiber. The better approach to biopsy of endobronchial lesion is to employ telescopically guided forceps (Figs. 6 and 17).

The techniques of rigid bronchoscopic control of tracheobronchial hemorrhage, foreign body removal, laser bronchoscopy, dilatation of tracheobronchial stenosis, and stent placement are discussed elsewhere.

The newer tracheoscopes permit maintenance of airway using the large-caliber tracheoscopes through which rigid bronchoscopes of various calibers can be introduced to place stents and dilatations (Figs. 18).

Removal of the Bronchoscope

The steps adopted for removal of the rigid bronchoscope after the examination is completed are the reverse of insertion. The removal should be done visually to make sure that mucosal trauma is avoided. The larynx should be examined for any trauma related to procedure and to make sure that the function of vocal cords is unchanged. The teeth, gums, lips, and dentures should be protected during instrument withdrawal. The laryngeal area should be suctioned thor-

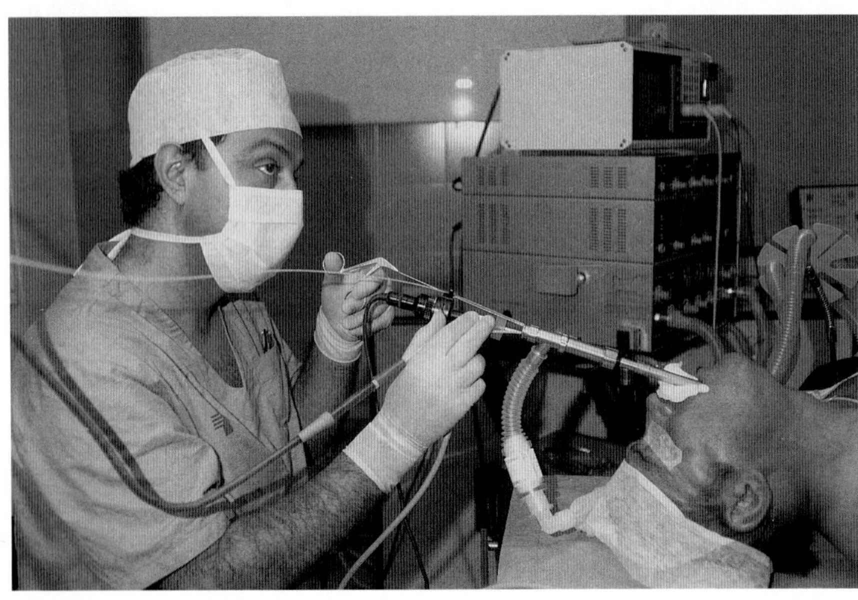

FIG. 17. The bronchoscopist uses video guidance to obtain a biopsy through the rigid bronchoscope.

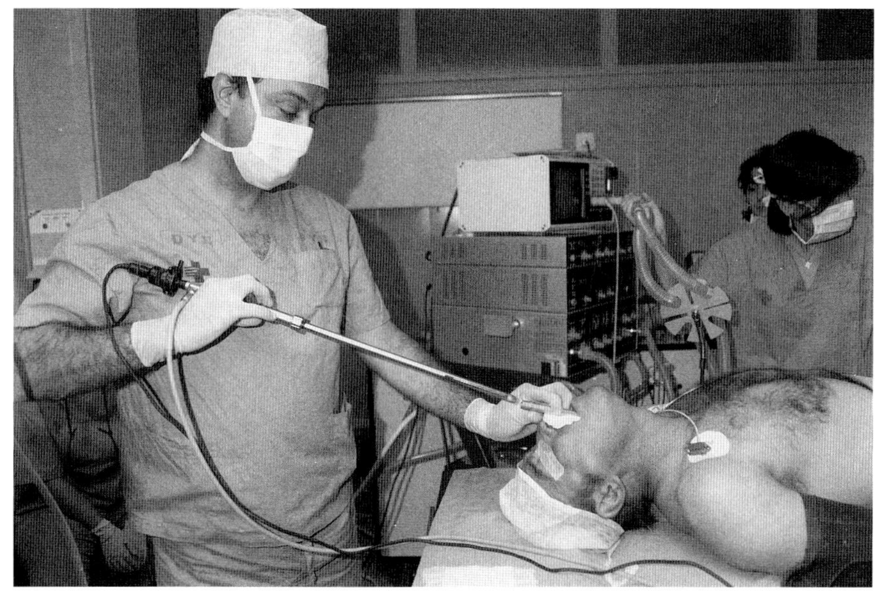

FIG. 18. With the tracheoscope in place, the bronchoscopist is about to introduce a longer bronchoscope through the tracheoscope.

oughly before removing the instrument from the patient's mouth.

COMPLICATIONS

Complications of bronchoscopy are discussed in Chapter 25 of this volume. Complications peculiar to rigid bronchoscopy include trauma to teeth, lips, gums, or throat. Mild laryngeal edema is not uncommon but it seldom causes clinical problems. Sore throat and neck stiffness last for 24–36 hr.

An uncommon complication of bronchoscopy is the disruption of the posterior tracheal wall. One report described six children with posterior tracheal wall disruptions; three were associated with tracheotomy, one with bronchoscopy, and another with endotracheal intubation (56). Appropriate training and techniques in bronchoscopy should prevent such complications.

Mathisen and Grillo (33) used the rigid bronchoscope to core out obstructing malignant airway lesions in 56 patients and observed 19 complications occurring in 11 patients: pneumonia in 5, bleeding in 3, pneumothorax in 2, hypoxia and or hypercarbia in 2, arrhythmia in 6, and laryngeal edema in 1. There were 4 deaths, within 2 weeks of core-out, related to respiratory failure.

It may intuitively appear that insertion of a telescope through the rigid bronchoscope will increase resistance to ventilation and result in derangements in oxygenation. Clinical studies in anesthetized patients have shown that the presence of telescope in the bronchoscope does not impair ventilation and oxygenation (57). In a study of 100 patients who underwent rigid bronchoscopy under intravenous general anesthesia with oxygen Venturi ventilation, no major complications were observed. Another study measuring serial arterial blood gases in ten patients showed carbon dioxide retention in nine patients even though ventilation was adequate in all (58).

Rapid changes in oxygenation and ventilation can occur during Nd:YAG laser procedures. Lennon and associates (59) showed that pulse oximetry is clinically useful during Nd:YAG laser resection of tracheobronchial tumors through the rigid bronchoscope. In a study of 14 patients, they found that transcutaneous oxygen and carbon dioxide monitors responded slowly to these changes and frequently provided misleading values.

One of the disadvantages of rigid bronchoscopy under general anesthesia, if inhalational anesthetic is used, is leakage of the anesthetic gas from the patient's airway and contamination of the bronchoscopist's breathing zone. In a study (60), the leakage of nitrous oxide during bronchoscopy in 14 adult patients was 11.4 ± 3.2 L/m and the median value of the nitrous oxide concentration in the breathing zone of the bronchoscopist was greater than 300 ppm. Experimental studies have indicated that halothane anesthesia for bronchoscopy administered by conventional techniques is a source of air pollution in the operating room and exposes the bronchoscopist to subanesthetic levels of halothane that may affect psychomotor functioning (61). The use of the gas-scavenging system can lower the concentrations of halothane and nitrous oxide in the bronchoscopist's breathing zone. We believe these problems can be minimized by packing the oropharynx around the bronchoscope and proper communication with the anesthesiologist during the procedure. One scavenging system described consists of a vacuum pump applied to the open ventilating rigid bronchoscope sidearm connection during intratracheal administration of a nitrous oxide, oxygen, and halothane gas mixture (61).

TRAINING IN RIGID BRONCHOSCOPY

Several aspects of training in bronchoscopy are discussed in Chapter 29 of this volume. Rigid bronchoscopy is more difficult to master. Repeated laryngoscopy and tracheal intubation prior to surgical procedures will provide good basic training in the manipulation of the upper airway. We have provided bronchoscopic training using properly anesthesized dogs and cats. The upper airway anatomy in the cat mimics to a large extent the pediatric oropharyngolaryngeal anatomy. Mannequins provide additional help in understanding the tracheobronchial anatomy. Needless to say that repeated performance of rigid bronchoscopic procedures are necessary to maintain proficiency in the procedure. Every opportunity to insert a rigid bronchoscope should be utilized by the novice rigid bronchoscopist. Special training courses are provided by various medical centers in laser bronchoscopy and other rigid bronchoscopic techniques.

SHOULD ALL BRONCHOSCOPISTS BE PROFICIENT IN RIGID BRONCHOSCOPY?

We believe that an ideal bronchoscopist should be proficient in both rigid and flexible bronchoscopy in adult as well as pediatric patients. Stradling (43) stated that "ideally, all aspiring bronchoscopists should be trained to use both rigid and flexible apparatus under operating room conditions and thus be equipped for all eventualities." However, the current trends in training and the increasing use and versatility of the flexible bronchoscope has made it difficult to attain this goal. Some authorities have indicated that the rigid bronchoscope is not needed in bronchoscopy practice (24). Zavala (62) concluded that expertise in both techniques is theoretically sound and ideally desirable, but in practice may not be absolutely necessary. It is important, in his view, for the flexible bronchoscopist to become familiar with rigid bronchoscopy, so that he or she may have a better understanding of its uses and limitations. Zavala further stated that "it is wise to have a rigid bronchoscope available to handle the unusual event of massive hemorrhage from forceps biopsy or an outpouring of thick material from a ruptured abscess" (62). If one does not know how to use the rigid bronchoscope, there is very little to gain by having a rigid bronchoscope handy. The readers should note that Zavala's comments were made before the advent of laser bronchoscopy, tracheobronchial stents, and other newer bronchoscopic procedures. In the earlier paragraphs of this chapter, we have discussed the superiority of the rigid bronchoscope in certain applications.

Those bronchoscopists who wish to develop expertise in these newer bronchoscopic techniques will be better off learning rigid bronchoscopy. Guidelines for laser bronchoscopy training have been outlined (63). Those who wish to limit their bronchoscopy practice to standard procedures may not require training in rigid bronchoscopy. Some in the latter group will invariably encounter situations such as massive hemoptysis, flexible bronchoscopy–induced massive bleeding, large foreign body in the tracheobronchial tree, or tenacious mucus plug that may require rigid bronchoscopic intervention. If rigid bronchoscopy cannot be performed in these circumstances, then the flexible bronchoscopist should have at her or his disposal alternate means to deal with these problems.

REFERENCES

1. von Eiken C. The clinical application of the method of direct examination of the respiratory passes and the upper alimentary tract. *Arch Laryngol Rhinol Nov 1904*;15.
2. Jackson C. *Bronchoscopy and esophagoscopy: a manual of peroral endoscopy and laryngeal surgery*. Philadelphia: WB Saunders; 1927.
3. Simpson FG, Arnold AG, Purvis A, Belfield PW, Muers MF, Cooke NJ. Postal survey of bronchoscopic practice by physicians in the United Kingdom. *Thorax* 1986;41:311–317.
4. Prakash UBS, Offord KP, Stubbs SE. Bronchoscopy in North America: the ACCP survey. *Chest* 1991;100:1668–1675.
5. Wedzicha JA, Pearson MC. Management of massive hemoptysis. *Resp Med* 1990;84:9–12.
6. Editorial. Life-threatening hemoptysis. *Lancet* 1987; 1:1354–1356.
7. Dumon J-F, Shapshay S, Bourcerau J, Cavaliere S, Meric B, Garbi N, et al. Principles for safety in application of neodymium-YAG laser in bronchology. *Chest* 1984;86:163–168.
8. Beamis JF Jr, Shapshay S. More about the YAG. *Chest* 1985; 87:27–28.
9. Hetzel MR, Smith SGT. Endoscopic palliation of tracheobronchial malignancies. *Thorax* 1991;46:325–333.
10. Chan AL, Tharratt RS, Siefkin AD, Albertson TE, Volz WG, Allen RP. Nd:YAG laser bronchoscopy. Rigid or fiberoptic mode? *Chest* 1990;98:271–275.
11. Nunez H, Rodriguez EP, Alvarado C, Vergara C, Golpe A, Reboiras SD, Zapatero J. Foreign body aspiration extraction (letter). *Chest* 1989;96:697.
12. Weissberg D, Schwartz I. Foreign bodies in the tracheobronchial tree. *Chest* 1987;91:730–733.
13. Limper AH, Prakash UBS. Tracheobronchial foreign bodies in adults. *Ann Intern Med* 1990;112:604–609.
14. Holinger PH, Holinger LD. Use of the open tube bronchoscope in the extraction of foreign bodies. *Chest* 1978;73:721–724.
15. Cooper JD, Pearson FG, Patterson GA, Todd TRJ, Ginsberg RJ, Goldberg M, Waters P. Use of silicone stents in the management of airway problems. *Ann Thorac Surg* 1989;47:371–378.
16. Dumon J-F. A dedicated tracheobronchial stent. *Chest* 1990; 97:328–332.
17. Freitag L, Firusian N, Stamatis G, Greschuchna D. The role of bronchoscopy in pulmonary complications due to mustard gas inhalation. *Chest* 1991;100:1436–1441.
18. Prakash UBS. Chemical warfare and bronchoscopy. *Chest* 1991; 100:1486–1487.
19. Wallace MJ, Charnsangavej C, Ogawa K, Carrasco H, Wright KC, McKenna R, et. al. Tracheobronchial tree: expandable metallic stents used in experimental and clinical applications. *Radiology* 1986;158:309–311.
20. Berci G. Chevalier Jackson Lecture. Analysis of new optical systems in bronchoesophagology. *Ann Otol Rhinol Laryngol* 1978;87:451–460.

21. Andersen HA, Fontana RS. Transbronchoscopic lung biopsy for diffuse pulmonary diseases: technique and results in 450 cases. *Chest* 1972;62:125–128.
22. Dedhia HV, Lapp NL. Nd:YAG laser bronchoscopy: rigid or fiberoptic mode? *Chest* 1991;100:587–588.
23. Whitlock WL, Brown CR, Young MB. Tracheobronchial foreign bodies (letter). *Ann Intern Med* 1990;113:482.
24. Oho K, Amemiya R. *Practical fiberoptic bronchoscopy*. Tokyo; Igaku-Shoin; 1984.
25. de Castro FR, Lopez L, Varel A, Freixinet J. Tracheobronchial stents and fiberoptic bronchoscopy (letter). *Chest* 1991;99:792.
26. Lan RS, Lee CH, Chiang YC, Wang WJ. Use of fiberoptic bronchoscopy to retrieve bronchial foreign bodies in adults. *Am Rev Resp Dis* 1989;140:1734–1737.
27. Tucker GF, Olsen AM, Andrews AH Jr, Pool JL. The flexible fiberscope in bronchoscopic perspective. *Chest* 1973; 64:149–150.
28. Grant IWB. Safety and fibreoptic bronchoscopy. *Br Med J* 1974; 4:464.
29. Stradling P, Poole G. Safety and fibreoptic bronchoscopy. *Br Med J* 1974;4:717–718.
30. Elliott RC, Smiddy JF. The "territorial domain" of hemoptysis. *Chest* 1964;65:703.
31. Wilson JAS. The flexible fiberoptic bronchoscope. *Ann Thorac Surg* 1972;14:686–688.
32. Prakash UBS, Stubbs SE. The bronchoscopy survey: some reflections. *Chest* 1991;100:1660–1667.
33. Mathisen DJ, Grillo HC. Endoscopic relief of malignant airway obstruction [see comments]. *Ann Thorac Surg* 1989;48:469–473; discussion 473–5.
34. Sahin AA, Aydiner A, Kalyoncu F, Tokgozoglu L, Baris YI. Endobronchial hamartoma removed by rigid bronchoscope. *Eur Resp J* 1989;2(5):479–480.
35. Goldberg M, Ginsberg RJ, Basiuk JP. Endobronchial carbon-dioxide laser therapy. *Can J Surg* 1986;29(3):180–182.
36. McElvein RB, Zorn GL Jr. Carbon dioxide laser therapy. *Clin Chest Med* 1985;6(2):291–295.
37. McElvein RB, Zorn GL Jr. Indications, results, and complications of bronchoscopic carbon dioxide laser therapy. *Ann Surg* 1984;199(5):522–525.
38. Diaz-Jimenez JP, Canela-Cardona M, Maestre-Alcacer J, Balust-Vidal M, Fontanals-Tortra J, Balust-Vidal J. Treatment of obstructive tracheobronchial disease with the Yag-Nd laser: 400 procedures in a 4-year experience. *Med Clin (Barc)* 1989; 93:244–248.
39. Cavaliere S, Foccoli P, Farina PL. Nd:YAG laser bronchoscopy. A five-year experience with 1,396 applications in 1,000 patients. *Chest* 1988;94(1):15–21.
40. George PJM, Garrett CPO, Nixon C, Netzel MR, Nanason EM, Millard FJC. Laser treatment for tracheobronchial tumours: local or general anesthesia? *Thorax* 1987;42:656–660.
41. Brutinel WM, Cortese DA, Edell ES, McDougall JC, Prakash UBS. Complications of Nd:YAG laser therapy. Editorial. *Chest* 1988;94:902–903.
42. Vane DW, Pritchard J, Colville CW, West KW, Eigen H, Grosfeld JL. Bronchoscopy for aspirated foreign bodies in children. Experience in 131 cases. *Arch Surg* 1988;123(7):885–888.
43. Stradling P, Stradling JR. *Diagnostic bronchoscopy: a teaching manual*. Edinburgh: Churchill Livingstone; 1991:23.
44. Iles PB. Multiple bronchial stenoses: treatment by mechanical dilatation. *Thorax* 1981;36:784–786.
45. Colt HG, Janssen JP, Dumon JF, Noirclerc MJ. Endoscopic management of bronchial stenosis after double lung transplantation. *Chest* 1992;102:10–16.
46. Tsang V, Williams AM, Goldstraw P. Sequential silastic and expandable metal stenting for tracheobronchial strictures. *Ann Thorac Surg* 1992;53:856–860.
47. Redmond FA, Rogers CS. Acute airway compromise due to tracheal mucocele. *Ann Emerg Med* 1987;16(4):445–446.
48. Wang KP, Terry P, Marsh B. Bronchoscopic needle aspiration biopsy of paratracheal tumors. *Am Rev Resp Dis* 1978; 118(1):17–21.
49. Wang KP, Britt EJ, Haponik EF, Fishman EK, Siegelman SS, Erozan YS. Rigid transbronchial needle aspiration biopsy for histological specimens. *Ann Otol Rhinol Laryngol* 1985;94(4 Pt 1):382–385.
50. Schieppati E. Mediastinal lymph node puncture through the trachea carina. *Surg Gynecol Obstet* 1958;107:243–246.
51. Lemer J, Malberger E, Konig-Nativ R. Transbronchial fine needle aspiration. *Thorax* 1982;37:270–274.
52. Pauli G, Pelletier A, Bohner C, Roeslin N, Warter A, Roegel E. Transbronchial needle aspiration in the diagnosis of sarcoidosis. *Chest* 1984;85(4):482–484.
53. Rigg D, Dwyer B. The use of the rigid bronchoscope for difficult intubations. *Anaesth Intensive Care* 1985;13(4):431–433.
54. Gaumann DM, Tassonyi E, Fathi F, Griessen M. Effects of topical laryngeal lidocaine on sympathetic response to rigid panendoscopy under general anesthesia. *J Otorhinolaryngol* 1992; 54:49–53.
55. Lukomsky GI, Ovchinnikov AA, Bilal A. Complications of bronchoscopy: comparison of rigid bronchoscopy under general anesthesia and flexible fiberoptic bronchoscopy under topical anesthesia. *Chest* 1981;79:316–321.
56. Crysdale WS, Forte V. Posterior tracheal wall disruption: a rare complication of pediatric tracheotomy and bronchoscopy. *Laryngoscope* 1986;96:1279–1282.
57. Saarnivaara L, Tarkkanen J. The effect of instrumentation with a telescope during bronchoscopy on arterial oxygen tension and acid-base balance. *Acta Anaesthesiol Scand* 1983;27:242–244.
58. Godden DJ, Willey RF, Fergusson RJ, Wright DJ, Crompton GK, Grant IW. Rigid bronchoscopy under intravenous general anaesthesia with oxygen Venturi ventilation. *Thorax* 1982; 37:532–534.
59. Lennon RL, Hosking MP, Warner MA, Cortese DA, McDougall JC, Brutinel WM, Leonard PF. Monitoring and analysis of oxygenation and ventilation during rigid bronchoscopic neodymium-YAG laser resection of airway tumors. *Mayo Clin Proc* 1987; 62(7):584–588.
60. Sorensen BH, Thomsen A. Bronchoscopy and nitrous oxide pollution. *Eur J Anaesthesiol* 1987;4(4):281–285.
61. Ostfeld E, Blonder J, Szeinberg A, Dagan J. Gas scavenging during bronchoscopy under general anesthesia. *Ann Otol Rhinol Laryngol* 1984;93(2 Pt 1):146–149.
62. Zavala DC. *Flexible fiberoptic bronchoscopy: a training handbook*. University Iowa Press; 1978:6–7.
63. Kvale PA. Training in laser bronchoscopy and proposals for credentialing. *Chest* 1990;97:983–989.
64. Kramer M, Som M. Further study of adenoma of the bronchus. *Ann Otol Rhinol Laryngol* 1935;44:861–878.
65. Som ML. Adenoma of the bronchus. Endoscopic treatment in select cases. *J Thorac Surg* 1949;18:464–478.
66. Vergnon JM, Guichenez P, Fournel P, Emonot A. Efficiency of cryotherapy in bronchial tumors) *Am Rev Resp Dis* 1990; 141:402.

Bronchoscopy,
edited by U. B. S. Prakash.
Mayo Foundation © 1994.
Published by Raven Press, Ltd., New York.

CHAPTER 5

The Flexible Bronchoscope

Udaya B. S. Prakash and Harubumi Kato

The advances in the understanding of optical properties of glass fibers in the mid-1950s eventually led to the development of the fiberscope during the next decade (1–3). Ikeda and colleagues (3–6) established standards for the first flexible fiberoptic bronchoscope in the mid-1960s and introduced the instrument into clinical practice during the early 1970s. The flexible bronchoscope has since undergone several modifications and presently flexible bronchoscopes are available for application even in neonates. In current practice, the flexible instrument is employed in the majority of bronchoscopic procedures. At the Mayo Medical Center, for instance, in excess of 2,000 adult and pediatric bronchoscopies are performed each year and an analysis reveals that the flexible bronchoscope is used in 94% of procedures; the rigid bronchoscope is used for almost all laser bronchoscopies, placement of tracheobronchial stents, removal of tracheobronchial foreign bodies, and other complicated bronchoscopic procedures. At Tokyo Medical College Hospital, an equivalent number of procedures are performed, but the flexible bronchoscope is used exclusively. Oho and Amemiya (7) reported finding no indication for rigid bronchoscopy in over 15,000 bronchoscopy cases. Thoracic surgeons have traditionally used the rigid bronchoscope, have universally accepted the flexible instrument after initially wondering whether the flexible instrument was a "diagnostic tool or medical toy" (8).

A mail survey of 871 bronchoscopists (98.2% were pulmonary physicians) in North America, conducted by the American College of Chest Physicians (9), revealed that 91.6% of bronchoscopists did not utilize the rigid bronchoscope; only 8.4% indicated that they used the rigid bronchoscope in their practice. Only 0.6% of respondents did not do flexible bronchoscopy. An earlier mail survey of British bronchoscopists (10) reported that although only 2% of 39,564 bronchoscopies performed between 1974 and 1986 involved the rigid bronchoscope, more than 90% of the rigid bronchoscopies were done by surgeons. That report also noted that the flexible bronchoscopy was used by 81% of bronchoscopists, both flexible and rigid instruments by 9%, and flexible bronchoscope through the rigid instrument by 8%.

THE INSTRUMENT

Physical Properties

The flexible fiberoptic bronchoscope, as the name implies, is flexible and is made up of bundles of optical fibers, a longitudinal channel to facilitate suction and biopsy, a mechanism to flex the distal tip of the bronchoscope with a proximal control lever, and an objective lens at the distal tip (Figs. 1–3). The proximal control section contains the eyepiece with diopter adjustment and the proximal end of the inner channel where suction can be applied, anesthetic or saline instilled, or cytology brushes and biopsy forceps, catheters, etc., introduced (Fig. 4). The entire length of the insertion cord (also known as shaft or tube) is covered by a specially treated flexible vinyl tube. The external diameter of currently available flexible bronchoscopes range from 1.8 mm (ultrathin) to 6.4 mm (most adult instruments average 6.0 mm), and the length (usable length) of the insertion cord varies from 400 to 600 mm (most measure 550–600 mm). The diameter of the working channel measures from 0.6 to 3.2 mm (the majority have diameters of 2.0–2.2 mm). The upward or superior deflection ranges from 120° to 180° (most instruments have 160–180°), whereas the downward or

U. B. S. Prakash: Division of Thoracic Diseases and Internal Medicine, Mayo Clinic, Rochester, Minnesota 55905.
H. Kato: Department of Surgery, Tokyo Medical College, Tokyo, Japan.

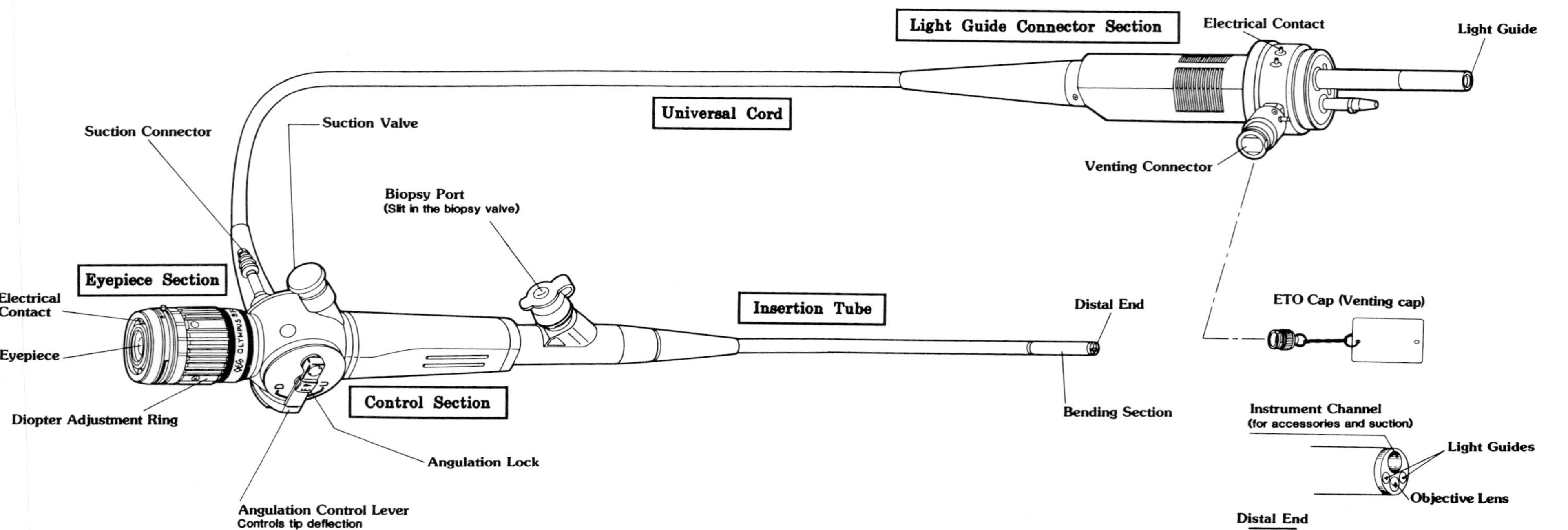

FIG. 1. Components of a flexible bronchoscope (a model manufactured by Olympus Corp.).

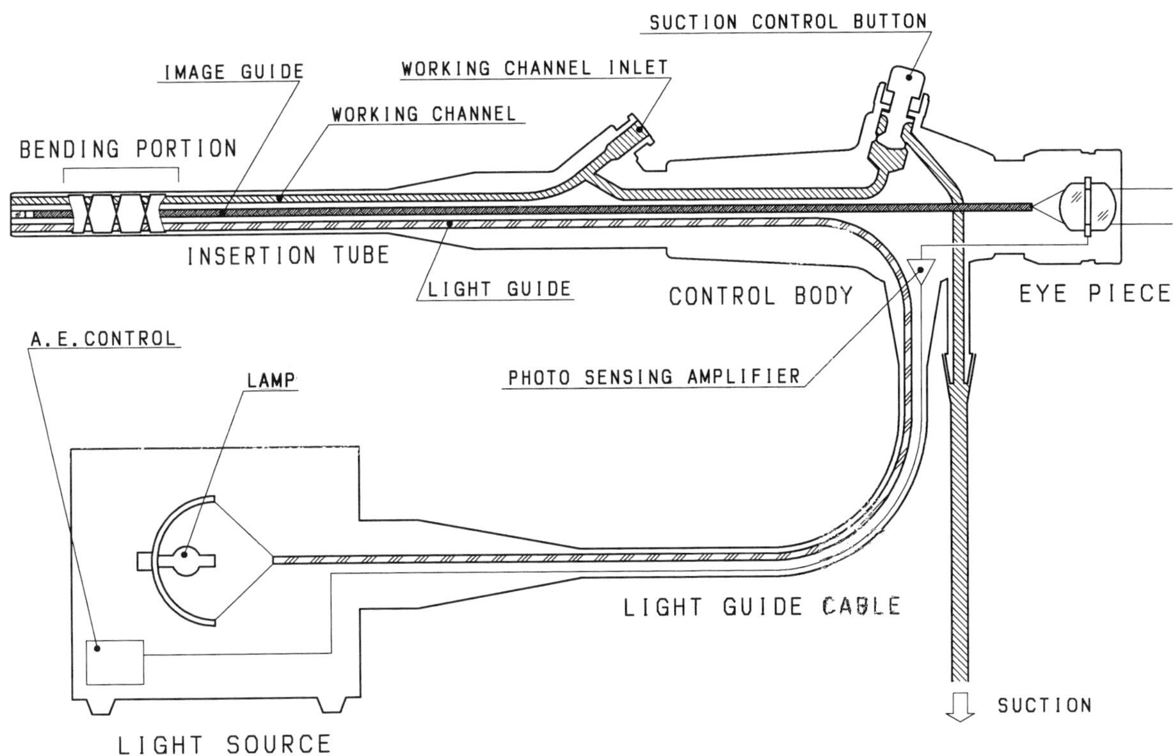

FIG. 2. Components of a flexible bronchoscope (a model manufactured by Pentax Corp.).

inferior deflection varies from 60° to 130° (most bronchoscopes deflect 100–130°). The field of view ranges from 60° to 120°.

The fiberoptic apparatus consists of a number of optical fibers bundled together with both ends tightly fixed. An optical image enters one end of the bundle and is transmitted to the other end (11). In order to reproduce a precise image, the fibers are arranged identically at both ends, the so-called coherent bundle. Each fiber in the bundle is coated (cladding) with a layer of another type of glass to achieve complete optical isolation. Even though smaller fibers provide better optical resolution, extremely thin fibers (less than 8 μm) lose illumination. Another bundle (light guide) of optic fibers conducts light from an external light source to the distal end of the bronchoscope so that the tracheobronchial tree can be illuminated. All flexible bronchoscopes are "frontal view" instruments, i.e., the objective lens is perpendicular to the longitudinal axis of the instrument. The insertion cord (shaft) of the

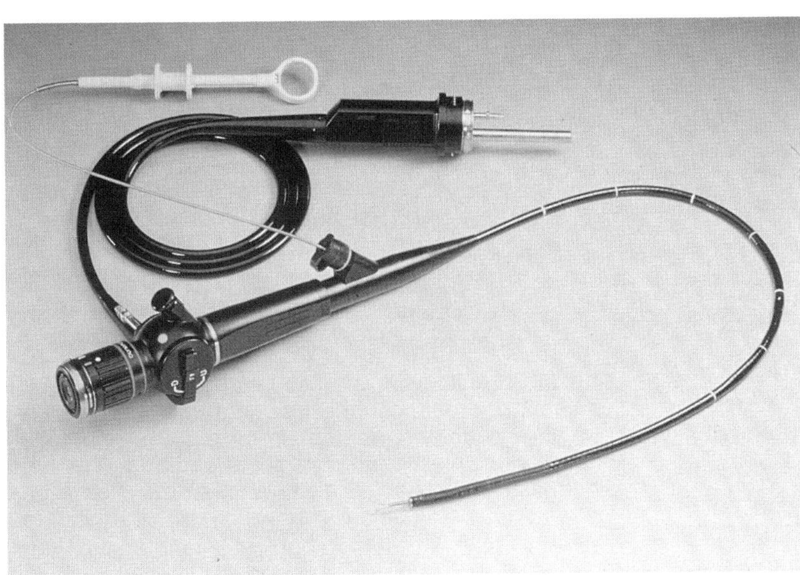

FIG. 3. A flexible bronchoscope with a biopsy forceps through its working channel (a model manufactured by Olympus Corp.).

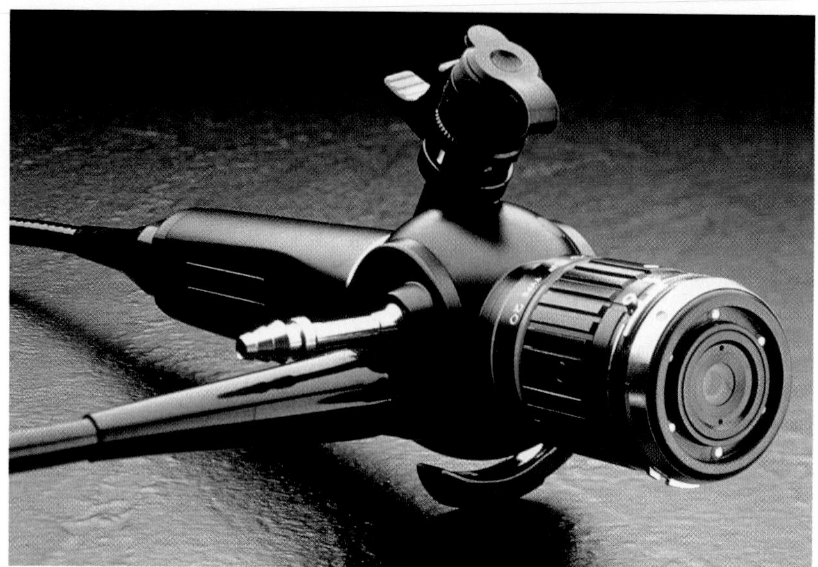

FIG. 4. Proximal end of a flexible bronchoscope (a model manufactured by Olympus Corp.).

flexible bronchoscope is "torque-free," meaning that the tip remains at the same angle to which it is adjusted. Any inadvertent twisting motion of the shaft on itself will break the fiberglass bundles and irreparably damage the instrument. Exposure to excessive radiation during fluoroscopy has been shown to discolor the fiberoptic bundles (12).

The handle of the flexible bronchoscope is designed to be held in the left hand. The cord carrying the fiberoptic bundle from the external light source is meant to be caught between the thumb and forefinger of the left hand in case of an accidental slippage of the instrument from the hand. The lever or knob for controlling the distal tip is normally held away from the patient and operated by the left thumb. The intrinsic mechanism of the lever includes two separate wires that traverse from the lever to the hinge mechanism in the distal tip of the instrument. Bending the lever down moves the distal tip superiorly or anteriorly, whereas pushing the lever up will orient the distal tip inferiorly or posteriorly. Long-term use of the lever invariably results in a gradual loss of full flexion capability. The working channel (for suction, biopsy, etc.) is located toward the patient and the suction control button is designed to be operated by the left forefinger. Most flexible bronchoscopes have a tip-locking lever to lock the distal bending tip at the desired position, but it is rarely used during routine bronchoscopy.

The insertion cord or shaft of the flexible bronchoscope is the part of the instrument that is inserted in the tracheobronchial tree. The insertion cord is flexible and contains the light guide, image transmission bundle, working channel, and two control wires to bend the distal tip. The distal tip is made more flexible by a series of metal rings joined by hinges along the two sides. The hinges are regulated by two wires connected to the control lever in the handle (Fig. 5). To allow more flexibility, the distal tip is coated with rubber. Heavy use and improper storage of the instrument results in the gradual development of torque in the insertion tube.

The focusing of the image is done by rotating the diopter ring on the handle. The flexible bronchoscope

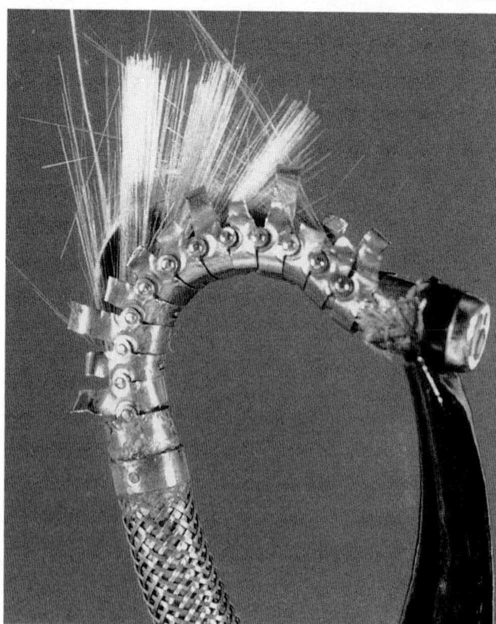

FIG. 5. Glass fibers at the distal end of the insertion cord of a flexible bronchoscope. Each light-carrying (incoherent) and image-carrying (coherent) glass fiber bundle is enclosed in a plastic tube and separated from the others. The plastic tube is opened to expose the glass fibers. Dissected bending section shows cut metal rings joined by hinges to metal wires to provide maximum bending at the distal tip. (From ref. 13, with permission.)

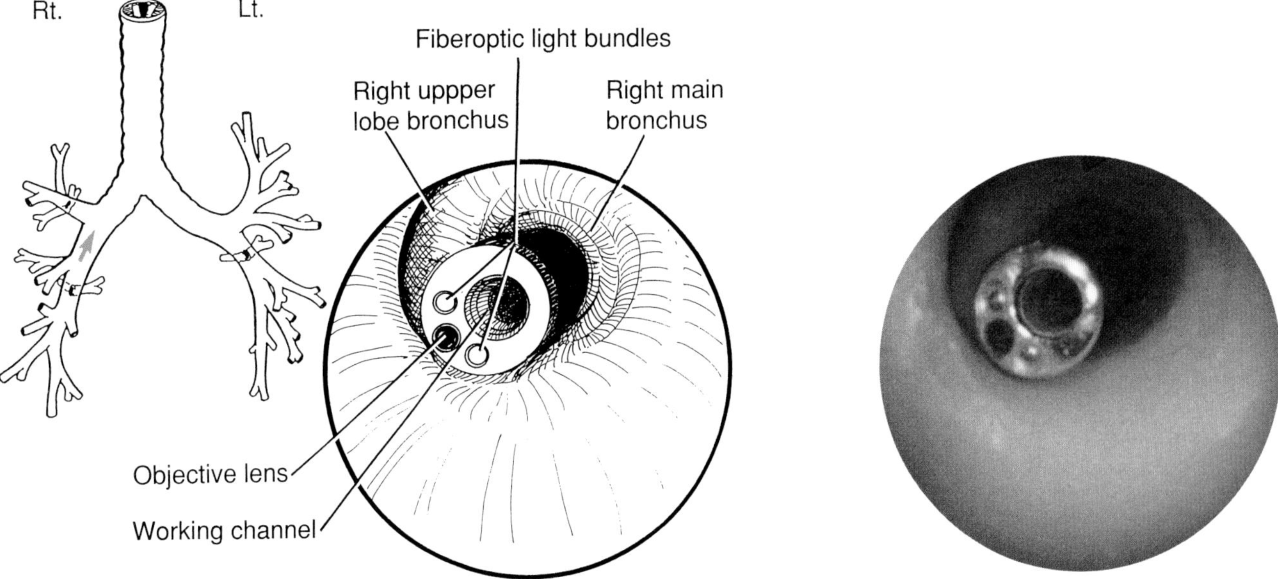

FIG. 6. A cephalad view of the right main stem bronchus into which the tip of the flexible bronchoscope has entered. The bronchoscopic image was obtained with another flexible bronchoscope placed in the distal right bronchus intermedius of a model of tracheobronchial tree.

has a fixed focus at the distal end (Fig. 6); the light reflected from the object is focused by the objective lens onto the distal end of the image transmission bundle (object face). This image is then transmitted to the proximal end of the image transmission bundle to the face near the eyepiece (image face) (13). The range of the flexible bronchoscope continues to expand, with the newer models providing wider and clearer views of the tracheobronchial tree. The field of view is regulated by the number of fibers and the amount of field allotted to each fiber.

The working channel for most flexible bronchoscopes is around 2 mm in diameter. The ultrathin flexible bronchoscopes have no working channel and some larger bronchoscopes have wider channels. Some manufacturers have put in two channels for specialized procedures. The insertion of most biopsy forceps will require a channel diameter of at least 2 mm.

Types

The flexible bronchoscopes are produced by several manufacturers most of whom provide worldwide sales and service. Continuous modifications have been occurring at a rapid pace and therefore it is impossible to evaluate the equipment made by different manufacturers. The following are our recommendations to novice bronchoscopists. Each bronchoscopist should assess personal needs and decide on the type and number

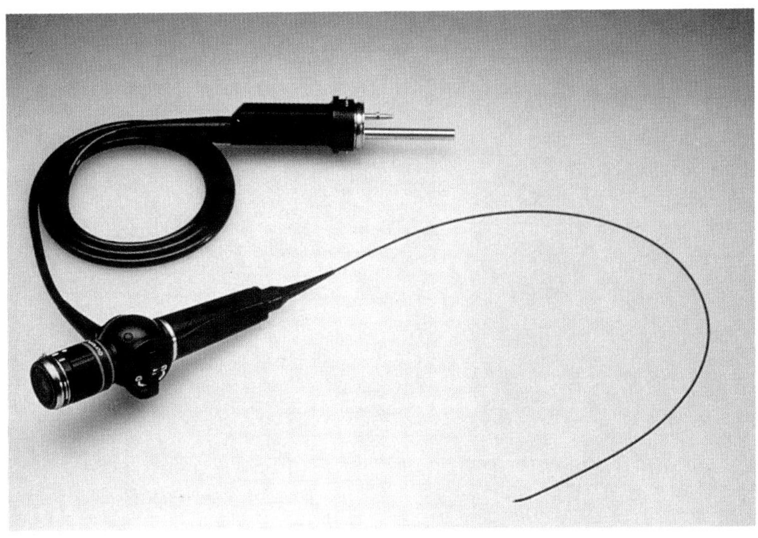

FIG. 7. An ultrathin flexible bronchoscope is useful for pediatric bronchoscopy (a model manufactured by Olympus Corp.).

of flexible bronchoscopes and accessories. A busy bronchoscopy practice will obviously require more than one bronchoscope, and even a very light bronchoscopy practice may warrant a spare bronchoscope in case of damage to the frequently used instrument. A purely pediatric bronchoscopy practice demands ultrathin instruments (Fig. 7) (14,15). The ultrathin bronchoscopes have been used in adults to reach bronchi not reached with standard flexible bronchoscopes (16,17). Interestingly, a disposable flexible bronchoscope has been described for use in pediatric patients (18). Those who wish to perform specialized procedures such as laser bronchoscopy, bronchoscopic dilatation, stent placement, and other procedures will need specific equipment.

Once the decision is made regarding the type and number of flexible bronchoscopes, the prospective buyer should evaluate instruments from several manufacturers to learn about the long-term service, turnaround time for repairs, update of newer developments, and the financial aspects of purchasing the implements. Most manufacturers permit use of their bronchoscopes on a trial basis. It behooves the bronchoscopist to know that the bronchoscopes fabricated by one manufacturer may not be compatible with the accessory equipment made by another. Totally submersible bronchoscopes are preferable to older models as the disinfecting and sterilization procedures are easier and more efficient with the former.

ANCILLARY EQUIPMENT

The accessory equipment used in flexible bronchoscopy includes the light source, cytology and microbiology brushes, curettes, biopsy forceps, protected brush and balloon catheters, and catheters for brachytherapy, balloon dilatation, application of fibrin glue, Fogarty type balloon catheter, and laser therapy (Fig. 8). Needles for transtracheal or transbronchial aspiration and biopsy, baskets and claws for extraction of tracheobronchial foreign bodies, and supplies for specimen collection are the other implements. Specialized ancillary instruments include gadgets for stent placement, laser bronchoscopy, cryotherapy, and electrocautery, as well as cameras for still photography, videocameras, video playback equipment, and the teaching attachment (lecturescope). These are discussed in Chapter 3 and in the chapters dealing with the respective topics.

ADVANTAGES AND DISADVANTAGES

Advantages

The advantages of the flexible bronchoscope are obvious. The versatility of the flexible bronchoscope carries with it many advantages. It can be employed in almost all the situations indicated in Chapter 6 (Tables 1 and 2).

Disadvantages

Flexible bronchoscopic extraction of moderate to large tracheobronchial foreign bodies is decidedly not as efficient as the rigid bronchoscopic extraction. This is particularly true in pediatric patients. Even in adults with tracheobronchial foreign bodies, the rigid bronchoscope is far superior to the flexible instrument. In a report from the Mayo Clinic (19), 60 adults with tracheobronchial foreign bodies underwent bronchoscopic removal. The rigid bronchoscopy was successful in 94% and the flexible instrument in 61%. The currently available forceps, claws, and baskets for use with the flexible bronchoscope are less robust and sometimes do not permit a good grasp of the foreign body.

Significant or massive hemorrhage in the tracheobronchial tree is difficult to control with the flexible bronchoscope. The factors responsible for this limitation include the narrow suction channel and obscura-

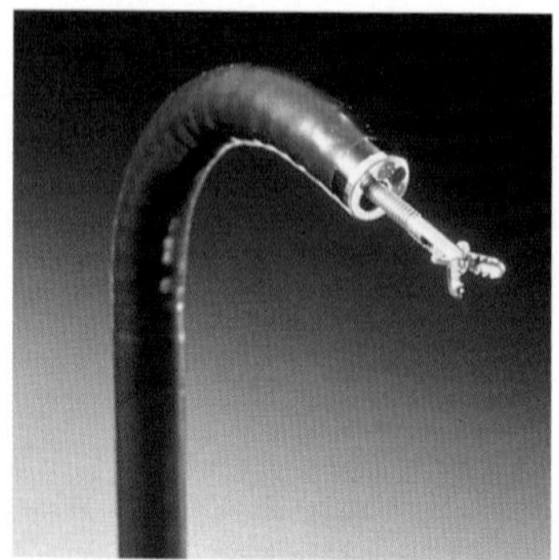
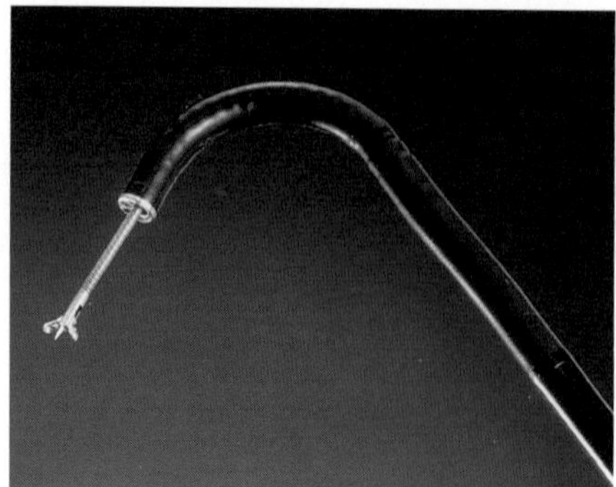
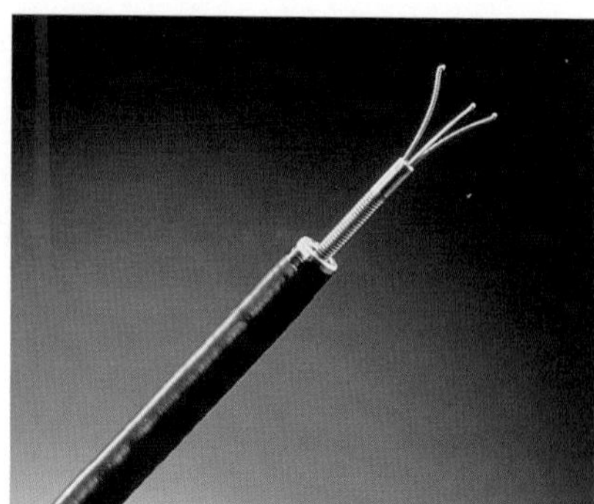

FIG. 8. A toothed biopsy forceps **(left)**, biopsy forceps with an impaler needle **(middle)**, and a claw **(right)** can easily traverse the working channel of a standard flexible bronchoscope. Courtesy of Olympus Corp.

tion of the bronchoscopic view by blood. The flexible bronchoscopes with larger or double channels are better equipped to handle massive hemorrhage. However, in the presence of active significant bleeding, the rigid bronchoscope is still the instrument of choice (20).

The flexible bronchoscope, although employed by many bronchoscopists for laser bronchoscopy, placement of stent, and tracheobronchial dilatation, is not as functional as the rigid bronchoscope. The rigid bronchoscope is mandatory for carbon dioxide laser therapy.

The quality of the bronchoscopic image and photographs obtained through the flexible instrument are not as vivid as those captured through the rigid bronchoscope. The newer models of flexible bronchoscopes, specially manufactured for the purposes of photography, may circumvent this problem.

In patients with significant tracheal strictures, the flexible bronchoscope can compromise the air passage and precipitate acute respiratory distress. On the other hand, the rigid bronchoscope will not only dilate the narrowed airway but also provide a wider channel for adequate ventilation.

INDICATIONS, CONTRAINDICATIONS, AND COMPLICATIONS

The flexible bronchoscope can be used in the majority of the conditions listed in Chapter 6 and Tables 1 and 2 of that chapter. The situations where the rigid bronchoscope is more applicable are discussed above under "disadvantages." The reader is referred to Chapter 6 regarding contraindications. The complications from flexible bronchoscopy are discussed in Chapter 25.

TECHNIQUE

Preparation of the Patient

The details of this aspect and premedication are outlined in Chapters 7 and 8. The most important and essential consideration is the careful and simple explanation to the patient of the procedure and what it entails. Demonstration of the bronchoscope and its function will go a long way toward allaying the apprehension.

Positioning the Patient

The patient's body position to undergo bronchoscopy depends on the route of insertion, location of bronchoscopy, and the clinical situation. If a nasal insertion is planned, it is more convenient to have the patient assume a supine, semirecumbent, or sitting position facing the bronchoscopist. Before inserting the instrument, the patient should be asked whether the position selected is comfortable. Obviously, a totally supine posture is most comfortable for the patient. A semirecumbent position in a bed or couch is somewhat awkward as it allows the patient to slide down during the procedure. If an oral route is used, the bronchoscopist can either face the patient or stand behind the patient's head, with the patient in a supine position. In carrying out bronchoscopy in intensive care units or at bedside, the bronchoscopist has to improvise and adapt appropriately so that the position is comfortable for the patient. The most important goal to accomplish is for the patient to be comfortable and the patient's position convenient for the bronchoscopist.

The novice as well as the experienced bronchoscopist should remember the reversal of spatial orientation of the tracheobronchial anatomy when the bronchoscopist's operating position changes in relation to the patient.

Methods of Insertion

The flexible bronchoscope can be inserted nasally, orally, through a nasotracheal or orotracheal tube, through a tracheostomy stoma, or through a rigid bronchoscope (4,21–26). Each has its advantage and every bronchoscopist should be proficient in all modes of insertion.

Nasal Insertion

After assuring optimal topical anesthesia of the larger of the two nasal passages, the well-lubricated tip of the flexible bronchoscope is gently inserted into the nostril and advanced along the floor of the nose, in the manner akin to the insertion of a nasogastric tube. If resistance is encountered, visual guidance through the bronchoscope can be used to direct the tip. Maintaining the insertion cord (shaft) of the bronchoscope as straight as possible provides good control of the instrument. The general direction of the advancing tip is caudad. Once the nasopharynx is reached, the bronchoscope tip is further deflected caudally and advanced until the base of the tongue and epiglottis are identified. By pursuing a course posterior to the epiglottis, the instrument is passed through the larynx into the trachea. The major advantages of the nasal route are the absence of tongue movements, which can displace the bronchoscope, and the avoidance of teeth, which can harm the delicate fiberoptic mechanism.

Oral Insertion

A bite block or similar appliance is necessary to prevent damage to the flexible instrument from teeth or gums. A disadvantage of inserting the bite block initially is the loss of the bronchoscopist's ability to control the movement of patient's tongue, which can easily push the bronchoscope from side to side. An alternate method is to have an assistant wrap the tip of the tongue with a dry gauze and pull it out of the mouth as far as possible. Allowing the patient to do this is not recommended as the patient may not be able to follow the instructions because of premedication, sedation, and anxiety. If the tongue is held outside the mouth, the bite block should be threaded over the bronchoscope before the instrument is inserted into the mouth and as soon as the bronchoscope enters the trachea the bite block is threaded down and placed in position, and only then is the tongue let go. Letting go of the tongue before placing the bite block involves the danger of the patient biting and damaging the flexible instrument. Another problem that should be taken care of before insertion of the bite block is the accumulated secretions in the back of the mouth and oropharynx. The patient should be instructed to swallow the secretions or the secretions should be removed by a suction catheter.

The flexible bronchoscope is held straight without any curves or loops in its insertion cord and is inserted through the lumen of the bite block with the tip advanced past the uvula and as far as the back of the tongue and then deflected caudally. Maintaining a route along the midline is important to identify prominent landmarks such as the uvula, back of the tongue, and epiglottis. The bronchoscopist should try as far as possible to avoid contact with the mucosa and glottic apparatus to minimize gagging and deglutition reflexes in order that the anatomy and function of the vocal cords and surrounding areas can be examined properly. If cough interferes with the procedure, topical anesthetic should be instilled through the channel of the bronchoscope. After the completion of the laryngeal examination, the bronchoscope is inserted in the trachea.

Insertion Through an Endotracheal Tube

If a decision is made to insert the bronchoscope through an endotracheal tube, the bronchoscopist must make sure that the diameter of the endotracheal tube will permit easy passage of the flexible bronchoscope through it. The majority of standard (adult) flexible bronchoscopes available in the market will pass through an endotracheal tube with an inner diameter of 7.5 mm or larger. The longer the endotracheal tube, the more difficult it is to pass the flexible instrument. Adequate but not excessive lubrication will facilitate this process. It is a good practice to routinely check the passage of the flexible instrument through the intended endotracheal tube before either is introduced into the patient's tracheobronchial tree. One may pass a nasotracheal or an orotracheal tube before insertion of the flexible bronchoscope using indirect laryngoscopy and an endotracheal tube with a stylet. Alternately, the bronchoscope is threaded through the endotracheal tube before insertion into the patient and intubation accomplished readily by initially intubating the trachea with the flexible bronchoscope and passing the endotracheal tube over the flexible bronchoscope through the vocal cords into the trachea. This technique is applicable to oral as well as nasal endotracheal intubation.

For nasotracheal intubation, the above steps can be applied or modified as follows: The nasotracheal tube is inserted into the nostril until its tip reaches the nasopharynx. This initial step will permit easy rotation and manipulation of the nasotracheal tube during its sojourn through the nasal passage. Once the tip of the nasotracheal tube reaches the nasopharynx, the flexible bronchoscope is inserted into the nasotracheal tube and passed through the tube into the trachea. Then the nasotracheal tube is advanced into the trachea using the bronchoscope itself as a guide.

Several types of endotracheal tubes are available for bronchoscopic intubation. In general, they are the same tubes used for induction of general anesthesia. The stiffer endotracheal tubes tend to catch at the vocal cords or subglottic shelf. A rotational maneuver to allow the beveled tip to enter the glottic chink will facilitate entrance into the trachea. Softer wire-spiral noncuffed latex tubes are slightly easier to insert. If the endotracheal tube fails to pass the vocal cords, the patient's neck should be slightly extended or flexed. Instructing the patient to cough will permit posttussive inspiration to abduct the vocal cords at which point the tube should be inserted.

Insertion of the endotracheal tube into the trachea should be confirmed by bronchoscopic visualization and the tip of the tube should be located at a distance of approximately 2 cm proximal to the main carina. The tube is then secured with a piece of tape, and an adaptor to provide supplemental oxygen may be attached. The patient is now ready for the examination.

Insertion Through Tracheostomy

The inner cannula of the tracheostomy apparatus is removed before bronchoscopy. If a mature stoma is present, the bronchoscope can be passed through it. Before the insertion of the bronchoscope, topical anesthetic agent is trickled down the wall of the trachea. An endotracheal tube can be inserted into the trachea if necessary. To avoid forceful expulsion of respiratory secretions out of the stoma, a thin gauze is placed over the stoma, ensuring that ventilation is not affected, and the bronchoscope is passed through a small hole in the gauze.

Insertion Through a Rigid Bronchoscope

Most newer models of rigid bronchoscopes for adults allow easy passage of the flexible bronchoscope through the lumen. The flexible bronchoscope can be passed through the rigid instrument to examine the distal bronchial tree after completion of laser therapy. Occasionally, laser-resected pieces of tumor become lodged in the distal bronchial tree and may not be visible to the rigid bronchoscope. Flexible bronchoscopic identification can be followed by either rigid or flexible bronchoscopic removal of the loose tissue. The blood that collects in the distal bronchial tree after completion of laser bronchoscopy is easily removed by bronchial washing through the flexible instrument.

Tracheobronchial foreign bodies can be multiple. Occasionally, during an attempt to extract a single tracheobronchial foreign body, the foreign body may break off and the smaller fragments may migrate distally. If the rigid bronchoscope is used as the primary instrument, the smaller pieces lodged in the distal bronchial tree may not be visible. This is another clinical example of a situation where the passage of the flexible bronchoscope through the rigid device will permit identification of foreign bodies in the distal bronchial tree. One of us (UBSP) uses this technique almost routinely in pediatric patients with a suspected or documented tracheobronchial foreign body.

The proximal opening of the rigid instrument can be fitted with a slit diaphragm that will permit the passage of the flexible bronchoscope without allowing the anesthetic gases to escape.

Other Routes of Insertion

In intubated and mechanically ventilated patients, the bronchoscopist is well advised to ascertain the diameter of the endotracheal tube before attempting flexible bronchoscopy. It may be necessary to replace the existing tube with a larger one. The multiple mechanical gadgets attached to the proximal end of the endotracheal tubes in these patients often hinders the easy insertion of the flexible bronchoscope. As many of such fixtures as possible should be removed before bronchoscopy. If the patient is receiving positive pressure ventilation, a special diaphragm to cover the proximal end of the endotracheal tube is required. This too can hinder the easy insertion of the bronchoscope.

When the trachea is transected during tracheoplasty procedures, the flexible bronchoscope has been used to guide insertion of smaller endotracheal tubes into distal tracheal segments or the main stem bronchus. This, however, is better accomplished with a rigid bronchoscope that can be used to ventilate the lung.

On rare occasions, the flexible bronchoscope has been used to examine the tracheobronchial tree via bronchopleurocutaneous fistulas or esophagotracheal fistulas by introducing the flexible instrument through the cutaneous tract or the esophagus, respectively (27). The flexible bronchoscope has been used in the past to perform thoracoscopy (28,29). Currently, however, dedicated thoracoscopes are widely available.

Manipulation Within the Tracheobronchial Tree

The previous chapter mentioned that rigid bronchoscopy is difficult to master. It does not mean that flexible bronchoscopy is easier to learn. Adequate training is essential to obtain maximum benefit from the procedure (Chapter 29 of this volume). The bronchoscopist should develop excellent hand–eye coordination and techniques of flexion and rotation of the bronchoscope as well as hands, wrists, and elbows. Although the flexible bronchoscope has been designed to be held in the left hand, the bronchoscopist should develop ambidexterity so that maximum efficiency can be extracted from the instrument. The ability to perform bronchoscopy with either hand is invaluable when the bronchoscopist is faced with severe anatomic distortions of the tracheobronchial tree or has to operate in difficult surroundings such as the cramped space in the intensive care unit, the patient's room, or during thoracic surgery when the patient is placed in the lateral decubitus position (Chapter 22).

The use of ancillary equipment such as brushes, curettes, and biopsy forceps also requires training and experience. There are many nuances and problems associated with the performance of various flexible bronchoscopic procedures. Many of these are addressed in Chapter 9 of this volume.

Training

Teaching and training techniques in flexible bronchoscopy are discussed in detail in Chapter 29 of this volume.

Electronic Videobronchoscopy

With reductions in the size of charge-coupled devices, which are essentially miniature video cameras at the tips of endoscopes, it has become possible to produce video endoscopes that are small enough in diameter to be employed for bronchoscopy. The slimmest instrument available at present is the Pentax EB-1830, which has an outer diameter of 6.3 mm and a working channel of 2.0 mm. The insertion cord is 6.0 mm in diameter.

The video endoscope electronically transmits the digitalized image to a monitor screen that can be viewed by more than one person at the same time and the images can be stored in a variety of video formats, 35 mm, floppy disks, and laser disks. The electronic videobronchoscope is opening up a new era in bronchoscopy as it makes possible the use of a wide variety of image-processing techniques and automation-assisted diagnostic techniques (30).

REFERENCES

1. Van Heel ACS. A new method of transporting optical images without aberrations. *Nature* 1954;173:39.
2. Hopkins HH, Kapany NS. A flexible fiberscope using static scanning. *Nature* 1954;173:39–41.
3. Hirschowitz BL, Curtiss LE, Peters CW, Pollard HM. Demonstration of a new gastroscope, the "fiberscope." *Gastroenterology* 1958;35:50–53.
4. Ikeda S, Yanai N, Ishikawa S. Flexible bronchofiberscope. *Keio J Med* 1968;17:1.
5. Ikeda S. Flexible bronchofiberoscope. *Ann Otol* 1970;79:916.
6. Ikeda S. *Atlas of flexible bronchofiberoscopy*. Tokyo: Igaku Shoin, 1974:6–10.
7. Oho K, Amemiya R. *Practical fiberoptic bronchoscopy*. Tokyo: Igaku-Shoin; 1984.
8. Taylor FH, Evangelist FA, Barham BF. The flexible fiberoptic bronchoscope: diagnostic tool or medical toy? *Ann Thorac Surg* 1980;29:546–550.
9. Prakash UBS, Offord KP, Stubbs SE. Bronchoscopy in North America: the ACCP survey. *Chest* 1991;100:1668–1675.
10. Simpson FG, Arnold AG, Purvis A, Belfield PW, Muers MF, Cooke NJ. Postal survey of bronchoscopic practice by physicians in the United Kingdom. *Thorax* 1986;41:311–317.
11. Epstein M. Fiber optics in medicine. *Crit Rev Biomed Eng* 1982; 7:79–120.
12. Kato H, Suzuki T, Ito A, Tanaka M, Urahashi S. Changes in optic glass-fibers due to X-ray irradiation. *Chest* 1979; 76:672–677.
13. Ovassapian A. *Fiberoptic airway endoscopy in anesthesia and critical care*. New York: Raven Press; 1990.
14. Kleeman PP, Jantzen JP, Bonfils P. The ultra-thin bronchoscope in management of the difficult paediatric airway. *Can J Anaesth*. 1987;34:606–608.
15. Fan LL, Sparks LM, Dulinski JP. Applications of an ultrathin flexible bronchoscope for neonatal and pediatric airway problems. *Chest* 1986;89:673–676.
16. Prakash UBS. The use of the pediatric fiberoptic bronchoscope in adults. *Am Rev Resp Dis* 1985;132:715–717.
17. Tanaka M, Satoh M, Kawanami O, Aihara K. A new bronchofiberscope for the study of diseases of very peripheral airways. *Chest* 1984;85:590–594.
18. Finkelhor BK, Healy GB. Disposable flexible fiberoptic minibronchoscope for evaluating the pediatric airway. *Otolaryngol-Head-Neck-Surg* 1989;101:511–512.
19. Limper AH, Prakash UBS. Tracheobronchial foreign bodies in adults. *Ann Intern Med* 1990;112:604–609.
20. Stradling P, Stradling JR. *Diagnostic bronchoscopy. A teaching manual*. Edinburgh: Churchill Livingstone; 1991:23.
21. Wanner A, Amikam B, Sackner MA. *Chest* 1972;61:287–288.
22. Sackner MA. State of the art: bronchofiberscopy. *Am Rev Resp Dis* 1975;111:62–88.
23. Harrell JH II. Transnasal approach for fiberoptic bronchoscopy. *Chest* 1978(Suppl);73:704–706.
24. Hodgkin JE, Rosenow EC III, Stubbs SE. Diagnostic and therapeutic techniques in thoracic medicine. *Chest* 1975;68:88–90.
25. Stubbs SE, Rosenow EC III. Flexible fiberoptic bronchoscopy. *Minn Med* 1973;56:831–835.
26. Sanderson DR, McDougall JC. Transoral bronchofiberoscopy. *Chest* 1978;73(Suppl):701–703.
27. Chowdhury JK. Percutaneous use of fiberoptic bronchoscope to investigate bronchopleurocutaneous fistula. *Chest* 1979; 75:203–204.
28. Ratliff JL, Johnson N, Clever JA. Pleuroscopy and cautery control of intrathoracic hemorrhage with a flexible fiberoptic bronchoscope. *Chest* 1977;71:216–217.
29. Ben-Isaac FE, Simmons DH. Flexible fiberoptic pleuroscopy: pleural and lung biopsy. *Chest* 1975;67:573–576.
30. Kato H, Barron JP: *Electronic videobronchoscopy*. Chur, Switzerland: Harwood Academic, 1993.

Bronchoscopy,
edited by U. B. S. Prakash.
Mayo Foundation © 1994.
Published by Raven Press, Ltd., New York.

CHAPTER 6

Indications for and Contraindications to Bronchoscopy

James P. Utz and Udaya B. S. Prakash

The bronchoscope was first used by Killian in 1889 to extract a tracheal foreign body (1). Modifications of the rigid bronchoscope and the introduction of the flexible bronchoscope have greatly increased the diagnostic utility of bronchoscopy. Presently, bronchoscopes are utilized in several clinical situations. The indications for bronchoscopy can be broadly classified into diagnostic and therapeutic. It is not uncommon to observe that in many patients both therapeutic and diagnostic bronchoscopy are performed simultaneously. In this chapter, we discuss the indications for and contraindications to bronchoscopy. Further discussion of this topic relating to pediatric patients is included in Chapters 23 and 24 of this volume. In this chapter, Tables 1 and 2 list the indications for both diagnostic and therapeutic bronchoscopy and indicate the chapters in which many of these are discussed.

The increasing use of the bronchoscope for laser therapy of tracheobronchial lesions, dilation of tracheobronchial strictures, and stent placement to treat stenoses of the tracheobronchial tree has made therapeutic bronchoscopy increasingly important. Of the 871 bronchoscopists in North America who participated in the survey on bronchoscopy by the American College of Chest Physicians, 56% indicated that therapeutic bronchoscopy for lobar and segmental atelectasis was one of the five most common indications for bronchoscopy (2). Among patients in critical care units, 47% to nearly 75% of bronchoscopies have been performed for therapeutic purposes (3–5). The indications for therapeutic bronchoscopy are listed in Table 2. In clinical practice it is common to perform bronchoscopy for both diagnostic and therapeutic purposes simultaneously. For example, a single bronchoscopic procedure may demonstrate a mucoid impaction causing lobar collapse that can be aspirated during the same procedure, thereby providing diagnostic and therapeutic utility. The two most important determinants of the need for bronchoscopy are clinical parameters and chest roentgenographic abnormalities. The discussions that follow pertain to indications not discussed elsewhere in the text.

J. P. Utz and U. B. S. Prakash: Division of Thoracic Diseases and Internal Medicine, Mayo Clinic, Rochester, Minnesota 55905.

INDICATIONS FOR DIAGNOSTIC BRONCHOSCOPY

Cough

Cough is one of the most common indications for diagnostic bronchoscopy. In the absence of any abnormality on the chest roentgenograph, the diagnostic role of bronchoscopy is rather limited in patients with chronic cough (6–10). Nevertheless, in the survey of 871 bronchoscopists conducted by the American College of Chest Physicians, nearly 25% of bronchoscopists listed cough as one of the five most common indications for bronchoscopy in their practice (2). The aim of bronchoscopy is to exclude a tracheobronchial etiology for chronic cough. It is our bias that bronchoscopy is overused in this group of patients. However, in carefully selected patients with chronic cough, bronchoscopy can be of use. Sen and Walsh retrospectively reviewed their experience with bronchoscopy in patients with chronic cough and nonlocalizing chest roentgenograms in whom diagnostic efforts had failed and empiric bronchodilator or antitussive therapy had failed (11). Under these conditions, bronchoscopy appeared to be a useful diagnostic procedure. Seven of 25 patients (28%) had diagnostic findings on bronchoscopy,

TABLE 1. *Indications for diagnostic bronchoscopy*

Cough
Wheeze and stridor
Abnormal chest roentgenogram
Persistent pneumothorax
Diaphragmatic paralysis
Vocal cord paralysis and hoarseness
Chemical and thermal burns of tracheobronchial tree
Refractory lung abscess
Thoracic trauma
Bronchography
Hemoptysis (Chapter 17)
Abnormal or atypical sputum cytology (Chapter 15)
Diagnostic bronchoalveolar lavage (Chapters 13 and 14)
Suspected pulmonary infections (Chapters 13 and 14)
Suspected tracheoesophageal or bronchoesophageal fistula (Chapters 16 and 22)
Follow-up of bronchogenic carcinoma (Chapter 15)
Carcinoma of the lung (Chapter 15)
Mediastinal neoplasm (Chapter 22)
Esophageal carcinoma (Chapter 22)
Suspected foreign body in the tracheobronchial tree (Chapter 18)
Obstructing neoplasms (Chapters 19–21)
Tracheobronchial strictures and stenoses (Chapter 21)
Bronchopleural fistula (Chapters 16 and 22)
Assessment of endotracheal tube placement (Chapter 16)
Assessment of potential endotracheal tube–related injury (Chapter 16)
Postoperative assessment of tracheal, tracheobronchial, or bronchial anastomosis (Chapter 22)
Research

including broncholithiasis (2), tracheopathia osteoplastica (2), tuberculous bronchostenosis (1), laryngeal dyskinesia (1), and an arytenoid polyp (1).

Unless postobstructive atelectasis or localized wheezing is present, the clinician may not consider tracheobronchial malignancy in the differential diagnosis of cough, though malignant neoplasms of the tracheobronchial tree may present with cough and an initially normal chest roentgenogram. Shure reported that chest roentgenograms may be negative in patients with complete endobronchial obstruction demonstrated at bronchoscopy (12). Patients with obstruction of segmental bronchi were more likely to have a negative chest roentgenogram than patients with obstruction of more proximal airways.

It would therefore seem reasonable to consider diagnostic bronchoscopy in selected patients with chronic cough. Cough that suggests an airway lesion or cough that is associated with hemoptysis, localized wheeze, or an abnormal chest roentgenogram provides a more compelling indication for bronchoscopy than chronic cough alone. In patients without these findings, bronchoscopy may be useful in selected cases. Patients with prolonged refractory cough (arbitrarily 6 months or longer) and nonlocalizing chest roentgenograms should be considered for bronchoscopy if empiric medical therapy has failed and if other evaluations such as methacholine challenge, otorhinolaryngological examination, and barium esophagram (and/or esophageal pH study) are nondiagnostic.

Wheeze and Stridor

Auscultation of the chest in patients with established asthma and suspected asthma may reveal bilateral polyphonic inspiratory and expiratory wheezes. Nonasthmatic etiologies for chronic intermittent or persistent wheezing are listed in Table 3. At times asthmatic wheezes may be difficult to differentiate from wheezes caused by localized narrowing of a bronchus. Localized tracheobronchial lesions may produce wheezing or stridor that may be misinterpreted as asthma. Localized wheezing that is produced by a change in body position may indicate a partially obstructing bronchial lesion. In a patient with wheezing, pulmonary function tests may show a reduction in maximum voluntary ventilation and abnormal flow volume curves in cases of large airway lesions. Bronchoscopy is indicated under these conditions to rule out an upper airway lesion. Localized wheezing, refractory "asthma" despite aggressive therapy, and "asthma" associated with a roentgenologic abnormality should alert the physician to the possibility of a nonasthmatic cause of wheezing and bronchoscopy is often helpful in the evaluation of such a condition.

Partial obstruction of the trachea may produce a wheeze of varying pitch and intensity. Stridor suggests

TABLE 2. *Indications for therapeutic bronchoscopy*

Retained secretions, mucous plugs, clots
Necrotic tracheobronchial mucosa
Foreign bodies in the tracheobronchial tree (Chapter 18)
Hemoptysis (Chapter 17)
Obstructing neoplasms (Chapters 15, 19, 20, and 21)
Strictures and stenoses (Chapter 21)
Pneumothorax
Bronchopleural fistula (Chapters 16 and 22)
Lung abscess
Bronchogenic cysts
Mediastinal lesions
Intralesional injection
Endotracheal tube placement
Cystic fibrosis
Asthma
Thoracic trauma (also Chapter 22)
Therapeutic bronchoalveolar lavage (pulmonary alveolar proteinosis)
Brachytherapy (Chapter 20)
Laser bronchoscopy (Chapter 19)
Photodynamic therapy (Chapter 19)
Electrocautery (Chapter 16)
Cryotherapy (Chapter 16)

Unless specified in parentheses, see Chapter 16 for all other indications for therapeutic bronchoscopy.

TABLE 3. *Nonasthmatic causes of wheezing*

Tracheobronchial neoplasm (benign or malignant)
Broncholithiasis
Tracheobronchial stricture or stenosis
Tracheobronchial foreign body
Extrinsic compression of the tracheobronchial tree
Bronchopleural fistula
Acute aspiration pneumonia
Acute pulmonary embolism
Toxic inhalation
Drug-induced bronchospasm
Congestive cardiac failure (nocturnal cardiac asthma)
Paradoxic vocal cord dysfunction
Carcinoid syndrome
Mastocytosis

a serious narrowing of the upper airway or trachea. When the diagnosis of stridor is made, emergent laryngoscopy and bronchoscopy are often required to evaluate these patients. In the pediatric patient with stridor, the most common diagnoses include epiglottitis, croup, rapidly progressive laryngomalacia, laryngeal papillomata, and tracheal foreign body. In adults, the onset of acute stridor is not as commonly encountered. Causes of acute stridor in adults include acute bilateral vocal cord paralysis, rapidly growing tracheal lesions, and extrinsic compression of the trachea by mediastinal and esophageal lesions. In situations where emergent diagnostic bronchoscopy is indicated for evaluation of life-threatening stridor, the bronchoscopist is well advised to have at her or his disposal the services of an anesthesiologist and a laryngologist so that, if needed, emergency tracheostomy can be performed to secure an optimal airway and adequate ventilation. In fact, in cases where glottic and subglottic lesions may be responsible for the stridor, an emergent tracheostomy may be needed before proceeding with bronchoscopy. If acute or life-threatening tracheal obstruction is secondary to an obstructing neoplasm or stricture, the bronchoscopist should be prepared to proceed with both a simultaneous diagnostic and therapeutic bronchoscopy. Under these conditions, the rigid bronchoscope is well suited for dilatation of the airway, for forceps biopsy debulking of tumor with or without laser therapy, and, more recently, for endobronchial stenting procedures.

The unusual occurrence of acute tracheal obstruction has been noted in patients with large anterior mediastinal masses who are subjected to general anesthesia (13). Several reports have described acute obstruction of the major airways during general anesthesia, some with fatal outcomes (14–17). Flexible bronchoscopy in such cases has demonstrated near-total obstruction of the distal half of the trachea secondary to an extrinsic compression. This acute tracheal obstruction is more common in children than adults. Potential factors responsible for the tracheal obstruction include the following: the effect of anesthesia on pulmonary mechanics, the supine body position, the elimination of glottic regulation of airflow through the endotracheal tube, changes related to the surgical manipulation of the tumor itself, size and location of the mediastinal mass, the young age of the patient, and preexisting airway disease (13). Measures to prevent tracheobronchial compression during general anesthesia in patients with anterior mediastinal masses should include the following: the use of topical anesthesia and intubation with a flexible bronchoscope, the advancement of an endotracheal tube distally close to the main carina as soon as intubation is carried out, the periodic bronchoscopic assessment of airway patency and its dependence on body position and depth of anesthesia, the avoidance of muscle relaxants, and, at least initially, the maintenance of spontaneous respiration as long as possible. If airway compromise is observed in spite of these precautions, the anesthesiologist should change the patient to the lateral decubitus, prone, or sitting position and pay attention to the position of the neck. The efficacy of these interventions should be confirmed by bronchoscopy (13). The need for diagnostic bronchoscopy in these situations is clear.

Abnormal Chest Roentgenogram

Not all patients with abnormal chest roentgenograms require diagnostic bronchoscopy. Abnormal chest radiographic findings for which bronchoscopy is indicated are listed in Table 4. Most of the acute infectious

TABLE 4. *Abnormal roentgenologic findings for which diagnostic bronchoscopy may be indicated*[a]

A. Localized Abnormality
   1. Mass lesion (solid or cavitated)
   2. Recurring pulmonary infiltrates
   3. Unresolved pulmonary infiltrates
   4. Persistent atelectasis/collapse
      a. segmental
      b. lobar
      c. lung
   5. Unilateral hyperinflation or hyperlucency (? foreign body)
   6. Mediastinal and hilar abnormalities
   7. Pleural effusion
   8. Abnormalities of the tracheobronchial air bronchogram
   9. Paratracheal lymphadenopathy/mass

B. Diffuse Parenchymal Lung Disease[b]
   1. Immunocompetent host
   2. Nonimmunocompetent host

[a] This list does not exclude other chest roentgenologic abnormalities.

[b] Diffuse infiltrates can be asymmetric, patchy, or unilateral.

and other inflammatory processes that produce pneumonitis do not initially require a diagnostic bronchoscopy. Patients with rapidly progressive processes may require emergent bronchoscopy with diagnostic bronchoalveolar lavage to identify potential pathogenic organisms, particularly when patients are immunocompromised hosts. In an otherwise healthy individual who develops community-acquired pneumonia, routine bronchoscopy is generally not indicated.

Typical chest roentgenologic abnormalities that indicate a need for diagnostic bronchoscopy include atelectasis of a lung, lobe, or segment; enlarging or suspicious pulmonary parenchymal nodules; cavitated pulmonary lesions; mediastinal masses; diffuse parenchymal processes without an established diagnosis; rapidly progressive pulmonary infiltrates in immunosuppressed patients; and sudden disruption of tracheobronchial air shadows or air bronchograms.

Atelectasis may result from intraparenchymal etiologies such as resolving pneumonitis, bronchiectasis, pulmonary infarction, or adult respiratory distress syndrome. Bronchoscopy may be indicated to exclude intrabronchial obstructive lesions and extrinsic compression of bronchi. While atelectasis may result from postobstructive collapse of pulmonary parenchyma, an endobronchial obstructive lesion may produce a "ball-valve" type of obstruction. This results in the air entering the alveoli but not exiting with normal expiration. The chest roentgenograph in such cases may show hyperinflation and hyperlucency of the lung parenchyma rather than atelectasis and loss of volume. Pediatric patients with a foreign body in the main bronchi are more likely to demonstrate this phenomenon. Obtaining chest roentgenograms following full inspiration and expiration may show this and bronchoscopy may confirm the diagnosis of a foreign body (Chapter 18, this volume).

Pleural Effusion

The presence of pleural effusion on the plain chest roentgenograph has been used as an indication for diagnostic bronchoscopy (18). However, many studies have shown that in the absence of roentgenologic or clinical features suggesting an endobronchial lesion, bronchoscopy is unlikely to aid in the diagnosis of a lone pleural effusion (19–23). One study evaluated the role of bronchoscopy in 245 patients presenting with pleural effusion and reported that of the 46 patients who had bronchoscopy, a positive yield was obtained in 13, though in 5 of these a second pleural aspiration was also diagnostic (19). Bronchoscopy was more diagnostic in patients presenting with a cough (12/24) than in those with no cough (1/22), and in those whose chest roentgenograms revealed significant abnormalities such as hilar enlargement, lung mass, or persisting consolidation (12/29), as opposed to those without such changes (1/17). To our knowledge, only one publication has concluded that bronchoscopic examination is of value in the evaluation of patients with undiagnosed pleural effusions without roentgenographic evidence of mass lesion or atelectasis (18). Large pleural effusions may obscure underlying parenchymal lesions and a postthoracentesis chest roentgenograph or a computed tomography of the chest may be required to uncover the lesion. Nevertheless, the role for bronchoscopy in pleural effusion without other obvious chest roentgenologic abnormality is limited. When bronchoscopy is performed in patients with pleural effusion and no other obvious chest roentgenologic abnormalities, the endobronchial findings consist of slight narrowing and crowding of the bronchi that lead to the pulmonary segment or segments compressed by the pleural fluid. Occasionally, thin secretions may be seen exuding from the distal bronchial tree. In our judgment, routine bronchoscopy is not justified in the evaluation of pleural effusions. It is of interest to note that the bronchoscope (both flexible and rigid) itself has been used as a pleuroscope or thoracoscope to diagnose and treat pleural effusion (24).

Persistent Pneumothorax

Patients with persistent pneumothorax or continued air leak following placement of a chest tube may have a lesion of the bronchus as the underlying etiology. In our experience, however, such an occurrence is unusual unless the chest roentgenograph shows a suspicious abnormality in addition to the pneumothorax. Bronchoscopy is sometimes utilized in such cases to exclude an inapparent bronchial lesion. In our experience, bronchoscopy in these patients seldom reveals an endobronchial abnormality. The role of bronchoscopy in the treatment of air leaks is discussed elsewhere (Chapter 16, this volume).

Diaphragmatic Paralysis

Although unilateral diaphragmatic paralysis may indicate a neoplastic process or other lesion adjacent to the path of either phrenic nerve, most cases are of unknown etiology (25). Because of the common association of bronchogenic carcinoma and metastatic hilar lymphadenopathy, clinicians should consider pulmonary neoplasms in the differential diagnosis of diaphragmatic paralysis. Neoplasms that cause diaphragmatic paralysis are usually large enough to be visualized on a plain chest roentgenograph. However, subtle hilar lymphadenopathy can be easily overlooked on the plain chest roentgenograph. Computed tomography of the chest has assumed a major role in the evaluation of diaphragmatic paralysis (26). Bronchoscopy with transbronchial needle aspiration/biopsy of the perihilar lymph nodes is another diagnostic option (Chapter 12, this volume).

Vocal Cord Paralysis and Hoarseness

The anatomic course of the left recurrent laryngeal nerve takes it around the left pulmonary artery and hence it is in close proximity with the structures in the left hilum. Any significant pathological process that affects the left hilar structures, particularly the lymph nodes in the aortopulmonary window, can compress or destroy the nerve and cause paralysis of the left vocal cord. When patients present with vocal cord paralysis, the clinician should consider the possibility of a left hilar lesion as the etiological factor. Other causes of vocal cord paralysis should be excluded. Computed tomography of the chest may help in better delineation of the hilar structures. As in the patient with diaphragmatic paralysis, the presence of respiratory symptoms may indicate a need for a diagnostic bronchoscopy. Paralysis of the right vocal cord by an intrathoracic process is rare unless the pathological process extends toward the right side of the neck.

Hoarseness may result from vocal cord paralysis or other vocal cord pathology, including malignant tumor, polyps, and postintubation injury. Vocal cords are examined at the time of bronchoscopy and may disclose these problems. Laryngoscopy frequently is performed to evaluate isolated hoarseness in the absence of other complaints or abnormal findings.

Chemical and Thermal Burns of the Tracheobronchial Tree

The inhalation of certain chemicals, gases, and superheated air can produce acute, subacute, and chronic pulmonary complications. Victims exposed to these agents may develop acute inflammation of the larynx and tracheobronchial tree. Depending on the clinical status of the patient and the degree of respiratory impairment, emergent diagnostic bronchoscopy may be indicated. Thermal injury to the airway should be suspected when any of the following findings are present in a patient exposed to fire: facial burns, soot in the nares or sputum, singeing of the nasal hair, or hoarseness. In the acute stages of chemical burns and thermal injury, the tracheobronchial mucosa will demonstrate severe edema and erythema. If the mucosa is burned, areas of mucosal elevation with some suggestion of mucosal sloughing may be visible. It should be pointed out that the severely inflamed and edematous laryngeal area may make it difficult to visualize the vocal cords, and the bronchoscopic procedure itself may exacerbate the problem by aggravating the preexisting mucosal edema. Careful evaluation of the laryngeal structures is essential to assure that an urgent tracheostomy is not needed.

In those exposed to smoke, diffuse soot deposition may be visible in the tracheobronchial tree. Simple bronchial washing and suctioning using minimal amounts of normal saline will help remove the sooty material and enable the bronchoscopist to better visualize the mucosa. When victims of chemical and thermal burns become unconscious, the threat of pulmonary aspiration of orogastric contents rises. If a diagnostic bronchoscopy is performed under these conditions to assess the degree of mucosal burns, the bronchoscopist should exclude an aspirated foreign body in the tracheobronchial tree.

The respiratory complications are proportional to the quantity and concentration of chemicals inhaled and these complications can be divided into acute, subacute, and chronic phases (27). In the acute stage, upper airway obstruction from mucosal edema and respiratory failure from pulmonary edema and or hemorrhage are the main features. The subacute stage may last from hours to several days and is manifested by necrosis of the tracheobronchial mucosa, hemorrhagic tracheobronchitis, persistent pulmonary edema/hemorrhage, and secondary infection. Weeks to months later, the chronic stage may result, with development of scarring and stenoses of the tracheobronchial tree, bronchiectasis, formation of granulation tissue, recurrent infections, bronchiolitis obliterans, and progressive respiratory insufficiency.

Freitag and associates demonstrated the invaluable role of bronchoscopy in the diagnosis and treatment of this special group of patients (28). In the acute stage, bronchoscopy helps assess the extent of damage to the upper airway mucosa and may help facilitate tracheobronchial patency by removing charred and necrotic mucosa. It is unlikely that bronchoalveolar lavage (BAL) will benefit the patient during the acute stage. Bronchoscopy is useful to obtain materials for culture and to remove thick purulent secretions. Significant stenoses are common occurrences in the subacute and chronic stages. Several bronchoscopic examinations may be necessary to evaluate and treat the tracheobronchial complications.

While the progression and recurrence of tracheobronchial stenoses may be relentless, bronchoscopic dilatation, stent placement, and Nd:YAG laser therapy seem to lessen respiratory distress and prolong the life of these patients. Although balloon dilatation via the flexible bronchoscope has been employed in the management of tracheobronchial stenoses (28–30), it is important to stress that rigid bronchoscopy is far more versatile in managing the stenotic lesions of the airways, particularly when stent placement is contemplated (31–34). Repeated bronchoscopy has the potential to further irritate the already damaged tracheobronchial mucosa, but it is unlikely that carefully performed bronchoscopy promotes the formation of airway strictures or other pulmonary complications. Repeated bronchoscopic examinations should be avoided unless they contribute to the diagnosis and management of these patients.

Refractory Lung Abscess

In a patient with refractory lung abscess, an obstructing bronchial lesion complicated by postobstructive pneumonitis and secondary abscess formation should be considered. Bronchoscopy is occasionally indicated in these patients to exclude an endoscopically obvious lesion. Additionally, bronchoscopy is performed to obtain materials for culture from the abscess cavity. Bronchoscopic drainage of lung abscesses is discussed in Chapters 14 and 16 of this volume.

Thoracic Trauma

Diagnostic bronchoscopy has been recommended for all cases of major thoracic trauma (35–37). The main indication for bronchoscopy in patients with recent chest trauma is to rule out serious airway injury (38). These injuries may not lead to significant initial symptoms and one needs to maintain a high index of suspicion in cases of significant chest trauma. Bronchoscopy is also useful in the assessment and management of other problems encountered in acute trauma. Bronchoscopy for lung, lobar, or segmental collapse may reveal aspirated material or thick secretions and mucous plugging that can be removed at the time of bronchoscopy. Bronchoscopy for hemoptysis following chest trauma may reveal pulmonary contusion and hemorrhage.

The Mayo Clinic experience with 48 patients with blunt chest trauma over a 10-year period revealed that most were due to motor vehicle accidents, crush injuries, and falls (39). Physical and radiographic findings included pneumothorax, subcutaneous emphysema, hemothorax, pulmonary contusion, mediastinal emphysema, atelectasis, flail chest, and hemoptysis. Bronchoscopy was of diagnostic use in 55% of patients revealing a variety of findings including complete tracheal transection, tracheal laceration, complete bronchial transection, bronchial laceration, bronchial contusion, ongoing distal hemorrhage, pulmonary contusion, aspirated material, mucous plugging/thick secretions, and supraglottic lesions. Ongoing distal hemorrhage secondary to pulmonary contusion was found in 25% of the patients in the Mayo Clinic series. In two patients this prompted the insertion of a double-lumen endotracheal tube and in one the placement of a Fogarty balloon catheter for tamponade. Aspirated material was found in 11% and mucous plugging and thick secretions were found in 29%.

When there is suspicion of airway trauma, bronchoscopy has proven useful in the evaluation of airway injury (40–44). Ecker et al. reported on 24 patients admitted with traumatic tracheal or bronchial injuries, of whom 13 had immediate bronchoscopy. In each instance, the diagnosis was either established or confirmed bronchoscopically (40). In the 14 patients with major tracheal or bronchial injury evaluated by Grover and associates, bronchoscopy was diagnostic in all six patients on whom it was performed (41). Kelly and colleagues noted that in only 1 of 24 patients with combined injuries of the trachea and esophagus did bronchoscopy fail to identify the lesion (42). Jones and associates observed that bronchoscopy was diagnostic in 85% of patients with acute airway injury (43). Occasionally, bronchoscopy may fail to disclose signs of traumatic airway lesions (44). Because of the possibility that a lesion might be overlooked by initial bronchoscopy, repeat bronchoscopic examination should be performed if the clinical situation suggests that a lesion is present (39).

Examination of the cervical trachea, larynx, and supraglottic region should also be performed. It is important to perform bronchoscopy at the time of extubation in patients who have had blind intubation done in an acute trauma setting. In one series, 15% of patients had laryngeal injury discovered in this way (37).

Bronchography

In cases of suspected bronchiectasis, bronchography has often been used to confirm the diagnosis and to assist in planning medical or surgical management. The contrast material used during bronchography may be applied to the bronchial tree via a flexible bronchoscope. The advent of conventional and high-resolution computerized tomography scanning has greatly reduced the need for bronchography (45–47). Bronchography has been used to localize roentgenologically and bronchoscopically occult bronchogenic carcinoma (60). It is our opinion that the role of bronchography is limited in the diagnosis of bronchogenic carcinoma.

Bronchoscopy in Thoracic Malignancy

One of the major roles played by bronchoscopy is in the diagnosis and treatment of primary and metastatic intrathoracic malignancies. In patients with primary bronchogenic carcinoma, the authentication of small cell carcinoma by bronchoscopy will generally obviate more invasive diagnostic or therapeutic measures. Likewise, if the bronchoscopic specimens establish the presence of metastatic malignancy in the tracheobronchial tree or pulmonary parenchyma, further diagnostic procedures may be unnecessary. The bronchoscope has assumed an increasing role in the staging of lung cancer by its ability to allow the bronchoscopist to obtain needle aspiration and biopsy from lymph nodes adjacent to major airways. This is discussed in more detail in Chapter 12. As much of the decision on treatment of primary and metastatic malignancy in the thoracic cage depends on the tissue diagnosis, bronchoscopy has a vital role in the therapeutic decisions.

The type of surgical treatment for primary bronchogenic carcinoma (non–small cell type) is dependent on the stage of the cancer. While imaging procedures and other diagnostic procedures such as thoracentesis, mediastinoscopy, madiastinotomy, and thoracotomy are also used in the staging procedure, bronchoscopy is the first and most commonly used procedure for this purpose. The finding of cancer in the trachea or in the main stem bronchi within a distance of 2 cm from the main carina places the tumor in stage 3. The bronchoscopic finding of vocal cord paralysis indicates advanced stage.

The role of bronchoscopy in the early detection of cancer, occult bronchogenic cancer, and various bronchoscopic treatments is discussed elsewhere in this textbook.

Other Indications

There are many other important indications for diagnostic bronchoscopy. Suspected or confirmed tracheobronchial aspiration of gastric contents has been recommended as an indication for bronchoscopy (61). Depending on the pH and volume of the material aspirated into the tracheobronchial tree, various degrees of mucosal inflammation can be seen. In our opinion, unless the aspiration of large particulate matters results in lobar or segmental atelectasis, there is very little to be gained by performing bronchoscopy in all cases of aspiration.

Continuous monitoring of upper airway dynamics in patients with disordered sleep problems can be accomplished with bronchoscopy and video recording. For this, a smaller caliber flexible bronchoscope is introduced nasally and the distal tip of the instrument is stationed proximal to the larynx.

Other indications for diagnostic and therapeutic bronchoscopies are discussed in other chapters as indicated in Table 1.

INDICATIONS FOR THERAPEUTIC BRONCHOSCOPY

Table 2 lists the indications for therapeutic bronchoscopy. The majority of topics on therapeutic bronchoscopy are discussed in Chapter 16 of this volume. Other indications for therapeutic bronchoscopy are discussed at length in various chapters and the reader is referred to Table 2 for the chapter numbers.

CONTRAINDICATIONS TO BRONCHOSCOPY

There are very few absolute contraindications to either diagnostic or therapeutic bronchoscopy. The safety of bronchoscopy has been documented by several earlier multicenter studies (48–50). Even though many new bronchoscopic applications and wide variations in the techniques have evolved since these studies were published, the finding of very low rates of both minor and major complications among recently surveyed bronchoscopists has once again confirmed the safety of bronchoscopy (2). Bronchoscopy and bronchoalveolar lavage are safe even in severely thrombocytopenic patients and in those requiring mechanical ventilation (3–5,51,52). Even severe respiratory dysfunction in immunosuppressed patients with diffuse pulmonary infiltrates is only a relative contraindication to bronchoscopy (3,53). Nevertheless, the proven safety of bronchoscopy should not lead to complacency and indiscriminate use of the procedure. Life-threatening complications can be appalling experiences for both the patient and the bronchoscopist. These experiences should be rare, however, for competent and experienced bronchoscopists who consider the potential problems and risks that might be associated with bronchoscopy in an individual patient and who prepare to deal with them (53).

Absolute contraindications to bronchoscopy include an unstable cardiovascular status, life-threatening cardiac arrhythmias, extremely severe hypoxemia that is likely to worsen during bronchoscopy, and an inadequately trained bronchoscopist and bronchoscopy team. Contraindications to rigid bronchoscopy include an unstable neck, a severely ankylosed cervical spine, and severely restricted motion of the temporomandibular joints. Contrary to an earlier assertion (61), the presence of hepatitis B virus and untreated pulmonary tuberculosis should not be considered as absolute contraindications to bronchoscopy.

A hemorrhagic diathesis is not an absolute contraindication to bronchoscopy to inspect the tracheobronchial tree and to obtain bronchoalveolar lavage. Biopsies, needle aspirations, and laser resections should not be attempted without first correcting the coagulopathy. Although platelet dysfunction is common in patients with renal failure, the degree of platelet dysfunction and the risk of bleeding in these patients is unclear (54). A blood urea nitrogen level of >30 mg/dl is considered a contraindication to transbronchoscopic lung biopsy (55,56). Zavala stated that "any biopsy procedure is avoided, if at all possible, on a uremic patient because of hemorrhage" (55). In our practice, a serum creatinine level of >3 mg/dl is considered a relative contraindication to transbronchoscopic lung biopsy (53). Patients with platelet counts <50,000/dl should receive 6–10 units of platelets before transbronchoscopic lung biopsy (56,57).

No single test can predict bleeding following transbronchoscopic lung biopsy or other bronchoscopic procedures. Routine bleeding time screening is not indicated because of the failure of this test to accurately predict the risk of hemorrhage in individual patients (58,59). Similarly, routine measurement of prothrombin time and the activated partial thromboplastin time is not necessary to screen for potential bleeding problems unless clinical findings suggest an underlying disorder of coagulation.

REFERENCES

1. Killian von Eiken C. The clinical application of the method of direct examination of the respiratory passes and the upper alimentary tract. *Arch Laryngeal Rhinol* Nov 1904.
2. Prakash UBS, Offord KP, Stubbs SE. Bronchoscopy in North America: the ACCP survey. *Chest* 1991;100:1668–1675.
3. Olopade CO, Prakash UBS. Bronchoscopy in the intensive care critical care unit. *Mayo Clinic Proc* 1989;64:1255–1263.
4. Stevens RP, Lillington GA, Parsons GH. Fiberoptic bronchoscopy in the intensive care unit. *Heart and Lung* 1981; 10:1037–1045.
5. Lindholm CE, Ollman B, Snyder J, Millen E, Grenvik A. Flexible fiberoptic bronchoscopy in critical care medicine. Diagnosis, therapy, and complication. *Crit Care Med* 1974;2:250–261.
6. Irwin S, Curley FJ, French CL. Chronic cough. The spectrum and frequency of causes, key components of the diagnostic evaluation, and outcome of specific therapy. *Am Rev Resp Dis* 1990; 141:640–647.
7. Poe RH, Israel RH, Utell MJ, Hall WJ. Chronic cough: bronchoscopy or pulmonary function testing. *Am Rev Resp Dis* 1982; 126:160–162.
8. Poe RH, Harder RV, Israel RH, Kallay MC. Chronic persistent cough: experience in diagnosis and outcome using an anatomic diagnostic protocol. *Chest* 1989;95:723–728.
9. Irwin RS, Curley FJ. Is the anatomic, diagnostic work-up of chronic cough not all that it is hacked up to be? [editorial]. *Chest* 1989;95:711–713.
10. Irwin RS, Corrao WM, Pratter MR. Chronic persistent cough in the adult: the spectrum and frequency of causes and successful outcome of specific therapy. *Am Rev Resp Dis* 1981; 123:413–417.
11. Sen RP, Walsh TE. Fiberoptic bronchoscopy for refractory cough. *Chest* 1991;99:33–35.
12. Shure D. Radiologically occult endobronchial obstruction in bronchogenic carcinoma. *Am J Med* 1991;91(1):19–22.
13. Prakash UBS, Abel MA, Hubmayr RD. Mediastinal mass and tracheal obstruction during general anesthesia. *Mayo Clin Proc* 1988;63:1004–1011.
14. Neuman GG, Wiengarten AE, Abramowitz RM, Kushins LG, Abramson AL, Ladner W. The anesthetic management of the patient with an anterior mediastinal mass. *Anesthesiology* 1984; 60:144–147.
15. Keon TP. Death on induction of anesthesia for cervical node biopsy. *Anesthesiology* 1981;55:471–472.
16. Piro AH, Weiss DR, Hellman S. Mediastinal Hodgkin's disease: a possible danger for intubation anesthesia. *Int J Radiat Oncol Bio Physiologic* 1976;1:415–419.
17. Bittar D. Respiratory obstruction associated with induction of general anesthesia in a patient with mediastinal Hodgkin's disease. *Anesth Analg* 1975;54:399–403.
18. Williams T, Thomas P. The diagnosis of pleural effusions by fiberoptic bronchoscopy and pleuroscopy. *Chest* 1981; 80:566–569.
19. Upham JW, Mitchell CA, Armstrong JG, Kelly WT. Investigation of pleural effusion: the role of bronchoscopy. *Aust NZ J Med* 1992;22:41–43.
20. Kelly P, Fallouh M, OBrien A, Clancy L. Fibreoptic bronchoscopy in the management of lone pleural effusion: a negative study. *Eur Resp J* 1990;3:397–398.
21. Heaton RW, Roberts CM. The role of fiberoptic bronchoscopy in the investigation of pleural effusion. *Postgrad Med J* 1988; 64:581–582.
22. Chang SC, Perng RP. The role of fiberoptic bronchoscopy in evaluating the causes of pleural effusions. *Arch Intern Med* 1989; 149:855–857.
23. Feinsilver SH, Barrows AA, Braman SS. Fiberoptic bronchoscopy and pleural effusion of unknown origin. *Chest* 1986; 90:516–519.
24. Sarkar SK, Purohit SD, Sharma TN, Sharma VK, Ram M, Singh AP. Pleuroscopy in the diagnosis of pleural effusion using a fiberoptic bronchoscope. *Tubercle* 1985;66:141–144.
25. Piehler JM, Pairolero PC, Gracey DR, Bernatz PE. Unexplained diaphragmatic paralysis: a harbinger of malignant disease. *J Thorac Cardiovasc Surg* 1982;84:861–864.
26. Shin MS, Ho KJ. Computed tomographic evaluation of the pathologic lesion for the idiopathic diaphragmatic paralysis. *J Comput Tomogr* 1982;6:257–259.
27. Winternitz W. Chronic lesions of the respiratory tract initiated by inhalation of irritant gases. *JAMA* 1919;73:689–691.
28. Freitag L, Firusian N, Stamatis G, Greschuchna D. The role of bronchoscopy in pulmonary complications due to mustard gas inhalation. *Chest* 1991;100:1436–1441.
29. Cohen MD, Weber TR, Rao CC. Balloon dilatation of tracheal and bronchial stenosis. *Am J Roentgenol* 1984;142:477–478.
30. Carlin BW, Harrell JH, Moser KM. The treatment of endobronchial stenosis using balloon catheter dilatation. *Chest* 1988; 93:1148–1151.
31. Prakash UBS. Chemical warfare and bronchoscopy. Editorial. *Chest* 1991;100:1486–1487.
32. Cooper JD, Pearson FG, Patterson GA, Todd TRJ, Ginsberg RJ, Goldberg M, Waters P. Use of Silicone stents in the management of airway problems. *Ann Thorac Surg* 1989;47:371–378.
33. Dumon JF. A dedicated tracheobronchial stent. *Chest* 1990; 97:328–332.
34. Wallace MJ, Charnsangavej C, Ogawa K, Carrasco H, Wright KC, McKenna R, McMurtrey M, Gianturco C. Tracheobronchial tree: expandable metallic stents used in experimental and clinical applications. *Radiology* 1986;158:309–311.
35. Payne WS, DeRemee RA. Injuries of the trachea and major bronchi. *Postgrad Med* 1971;49:152–158.
36. Travis SPL, Layer GT. Traumatic transection of the thoracic trachea. *Ann R Coll Surg Engl* 1983;65:240–241.
37. Angood PB, Attia EL, Brown RA, Mulder DS. Extrinsic civilian trauma to the larynx and cervical trachea—important predictors of long-term morbidity. *J Trauma* 1986;26:869–273.
38. Kirsh MM, Orringer MB, Behrendt DM, Sloan H. Management of tracheobronchial disruption secondary to nonpenetrating trauma. *Ann Thorac Surg* 1976;22:93–101.
39. Hara K, Prakash UBS. Fiberoptic bronchoscopy in the evaluation of acute chest and upper airway trauma. *Chest* 1989; 96:627–630.
40. Ecker RR, Libertini RV, Rea WJ, Sugg WJ, Webb WR. Injuries of the trachea and bronchi. *Ann Thorac Surg* 1971;11:289–298.
41. Grover FL, Ellestad C, Arom KV, Root HD, Cruz AB, Trinkle JK. Diagnosis and management of major tracheobronchial injuries. *Ann Thorac Surg* 1979;28:384–391.
42. Kelly JP, Webb WR, Moulder PV, Moustouakas NM, Lirtzman M. Management of airway trauma II: Combined injuries of the trachea and esophagus. *Ann Surg* 1987;43:160–163.
43. Jones WS, Mavroudis C, Richardson JD, Gray LA, Howe WR. Management of tracheobronchial disruption resulting from blunt chest trauma. *Surgery* 1984;95:319–323.

44. Roxburgh JC. Rupture of the tracheobronchial tree. *Thorax* 1987;42:681–688.
45. Swenson SJ, Aughenbaugh GL, Brown LR. High-resolution computed tomography of the lung. *Mayo Clin Proc* 1989; 64:1284–1294.
46. Joharjy IA, Bashi SA, Adbullah AK. Value of medium-thickness CT in the diagnosis of bronchiectasis. *Am J Roentgenol* 1987; 149:1133–1137.
47. Grenier P, Marice F, Musset D, Menn Y, Nahum H. Bronchiectasis: assessment by thin-section CT. *Radiology* 1986; 161:95–99.
48. Pereira W Jr, Kovnat DM, Snider GL. A prospective cooperative study of complications following flexible fiberoptic bronchoscopy. *Chest* 1978;73:813–816.
49. Credle JF Jr, Smiddy JF, Elliot RC. Complications of fiberoptic bronchoscopy. *Am Rev Resp Dis* 1974;109:67–72.
50. Suratt PM, Smiddy JF, Bruber B. Deaths and complications associated with fiberoptic bronchoscopy. *Chest* 1976; 69:747–751.
51. Stover DE, Zaman MB, Hajdu SI, Lange M, Gold J, Armstrong D. Bronchoalveolar lavage in the diagnosis of diffuse pulmonary infiltrates in the immunosuppressed host. *Ann Intern Med* 1984; 101:1–7.
52. Chastre J, Viau F, Brun P, Pierre J, Dauge MC, Bouchama A, Akesbi A, Gilbert C. Prospective evaluation of the protected specimen brush for the diagnosis of pulmonary infections in ventilated patient. *Am Rev Resp Dis* 1984;130:924–929.
53. Prakash UBS, Stubbs SE. The bronchoscopy survey: some reflections. *Chest* 1991;100:1660–1067.
54. George JN, Shattil SJ. The clinical importance of acquired abnormalities of platelet function. *N Engl J Med* 1991;324:27–39.
55. Zavala DC. Transbronchial biopsy in diffuse lung disease. *Chest* 1978;73:727–733.
56. Cunningham JH, Zavala DC, Corry RJ, et al. Trephine air drill, bronchial brush, and fiberoptic transbronchial lung biopsies in immunosuppressed patients. *Am Rev Resp Dis* 1977; 115:213–220.
57. Zavala DC. Pulmonary hemorrhage in fiberoptic bronchoscopy. *Chest* 1976;70:584–588.
58. Rodgers RPC, Levin J. A critical appraisal of the bleeding time. *Semin Thromb Hemost* 1990;16:1–20.
59. Lind SE. The bleeding time does not predict surgical bleeding. *Blood* 1991;77:2547–2552.
60. Brown SD, Foster WL. Localization of occult bronchogenic carcinoma by bronchography. *Chest* 1991;100:1160–1162.
61. Zavala DC. *Flexible fiberoptic bronchoscopy: a training handbook*. University of Iowa Press; 1978:123.

Bronchoscopy,
edited by U. B. S. Prakash.
Mayo Foundation © 1994.
Published by Raven Press, Ltd., New York.

CHAPTER 7

Bronchoscopic Pharmacology and Anesthesia

Mark H. Ereth, Samuel E. Stubbs, and Robert L. Lennon

Provision of anesthesia or sedation for patients undergoing bronchoscopy is necessary to facilitate the examination, minimize untoward physiological responses to airway stimulation, diminish patient movement, and improve patient safety and comfort. Techniques commonly used include topical anesthesia of the airway, intravenous sedation, regional blockade of nerves innervating the airway, and general anesthesia. Patients presenting for bronchoscopy have known or suspected pulmonary disease, and frequently coexisting cardiovascular disease, placing them at increased risk for development of complications (1). Knowledge of the patient's preexisting medical condition, current medication, prior anesthetic experience, and a detailed understanding of the agents and techniques used for anesthesia and sedation during bronchoscopy are necessary. The bronchoscopist and/or anesthesiologist can then choose the appropriate technique and agents best suited for any given patient to maximize safety and minimize discomfort.

BRONCHOSCOPY TEAM PREPARATION

Bronchoscopy should be carried out by a team of individuals who are familiar with the procedure and its complications, and have the knowledge and resources available to respond in the event of an emergency. We believe this is ideally accomplished in a dedicated setting with the assistance of anesthesiology personnel as indicated and nurses or technicians trained to assist the bronchoscopists. These dedicated personnel allow the bronchoscopist to focus attention on the primary objective: completion of a thorough and safe procedure.

M. H. Ereth and R. L. Lennon: Department of Anesthesiology, Mayo Clinic, Rochester, Minnesota 55905.
S. E. Stubbs: Division of Thoracic Diseases and Internal Medicine, Mayo Clinic, Rochester, Minnesota 55905.

EQUIPMENT AND MONITORING

Utilization of an anesthesia machine provides for delivery of oxygen, anesthetic gases, and positive pressure ventilation. Upon arrival to the bronchoscopy suite, a free-flowing intravenous line or capped intravenous catheter should be established. Patients are monitored with an electrocardiogram (lead II in patients with dysrhythmia, lead V-5 in patients with coronary artery disease, who are at risk for myocardial ischemia), pulse oximeter, and an automated noninvasive blood pressure device.

Should complications arise or resuscitation become necessary, emergency equipment that was prechecked prior to the procedure must be readily available. This includes equipment for airway management and tracheal intubation, and pharmacological and electrical therapy for cardiovascular emergencies (Table 1). Provisions must be made for suction and adequate oxygenation in the event of emesis or regurgitation.

General anesthesia may be indicated for rigid bronchoscopy, laser or photodynamic therapy, pediatric patients, or uncooperative patients. When general anesthesia is indicated, additional equipment and monitoring is required. The rigid bronchoscope and cuffed endotracheal tube for flexible bronchoscopy are the most commonly used methods of ventilation when general anesthesia is indicated. Jet ventilation may be employed, but it is usually reserved for patients with high tracheal lesions. Apneic oxygenation with oxygen insufflation through a catheter can be used but only for short periods of time due to the risks of hypercarbia and hypoxemia. A capnograph to measure expired carbon dioxide, an inspired oxygen concentration monitor, and a patient temperature probe are required during the administration of general anesthesia. A peripheral nerve stimulator is needed to estimate the intensity of neuromuscular blockade, predict degree of recovery, and confirm pharmacological reversal.

TABLE 1. *Equipment for rapid tracheal intubation, airway management, and resuscitation*

Equipment	Pulse oximeter
	Capnograph
	Electrocardiogram monitor and leads
	Suction (wall outlet with attachment or portable)
	Compressed oxygen (wall outlet with adapter or E cylinder)
	Defibrillator
Airway management	Laryngoscope with assorted blades
	Ambu bag
	Anesthesia masks (small, medium, and large)
	Assorted endotracheal tubes and intubating stylets
	Nasal airways
	Suction catheters, tubing, and tonsil-tipped firm catheters
Medications	Sodium thiopental
	Propofol
	Succinylcholine
	Epinephrine
	Bretylium tosylate
	Calcium chloride
	Sodium bicarbonate
	Lidocaine
	Phenylephrine
	Atropine
	Glycopyrrolate
	Narcotics and benzodiazepines as needed

These monitors are recommended by the American Society of Anesthesiologists who determine the standard of care for conduction of and monitoring during general anesthesia (2).

PREOPERATIVE PREPARATION OF THE PATIENT

Adequate preoperative preparation of the patient is imperative. This includes an appropriate review of systems and physical examination, optimization of preoperative medical conditions, discussion of the procedure and sedation or anesthesia, and premedication when warranted. Patients should refrain from eating and drinking for 6 hr prior to the examination to reduce the risk of aspiration. A detailed discussion of preparation of the patient for bronchoscopy is presented in Chapter 8 of this volume.

PREMEDICATION

There is much debate over the need for sedation before or during this procedure (3–6). Five minutes of conversation with a physician who is calm and confident can be as effective an anxiolytic as 5 mg intravenous diazepam (7).

Unsedated patients may become apprehensive and uncooperative. Medications given prior to bronchoscopy typically include a sedative for anxiolysis and patient comfort, and an antisialagogue to limit oropharyngeal and bronchial secretions. Commonly used premedicants include midazolam, diazepam, codeine, morphine, and hydroxyzine (8). The pharmacological characteristics of these and other useful compounds are summarized in Table 2.

The use of atropine, glycopyrrolate, or scopolamine as a drying agent is an important aspect of premedication for bronchoscopy (Table 3). Limiting secretions with these medications promotes a clearer airway, greatly improves visibility, and eases conduction of the procedure. Atropine and glycopyrrolate are most commonly used (9). Glycopyrrolate, with a lower incidence and magnitude of tachycardia (10), is the preferred agent in patients with coronary artery disease. Its quaternary ammonium structure prevents it from crossing the blood–brain barrier, resulting in none of the sedation or delirium that may be seen with atropine and, especially, scopolamine. Scopolamine's unpredictable tendency toward disorientation and prolonged activity makes it less desirable. Premedication should be individualized to the patient, clinical setting, and physician's personal preference.

SEDATION

A lightly sedated, cooperative patient will facilitate the conduct of the procedure, whereas an overly sedated patient may hypoventilate and become uncooperative. The resulting hypoxemia and hypercarbia may lead to agitation, tachycardia, hypertension, or other cardiopulmonary complications.

We believe that incremental intravenous doses of carefully chosen sedatives in the appropriately monitored patient are safe, reliable, and facilitate conduct of the procedure. Sedated and cooperative patients facilitate the bronchoscopist's work. Most patients are very appreciative of anxiolysis and amnesia. A wide variety of agents may be used for sedation (Table 2).

We prefer using incremental doses of a benzodiazepine and narcotic, specifically midazolam and fentanyl. Both benzodiazepines and narcotics may cause varying degrees of respiratory and myocardial depression (11). When used together they may act synergistically, warranting caution and careful monitoring (12). As with any therapeutic agent, one must balance the risks and the benefits.

TABLE 2. *Pharmacologic agents used in bronchoscopy*

Sedative	Pharmacological actions	Dosage	Onset	Duration	Untoward reactions
Benzodiazepines	Sedation, anterograde amnesia, antiepileptic				
Midazolam		IV, IM = 5–7 mg (0.075 mg/kg)	IV = 1–3 min	IV, IM = 2 hr	Respiratory impairment in high doses
Diazepam		IV = 2–7 mg (0.03–0.1 mg/kg), IM = not recommended, PO = 3–11 mg (0.05–0.15 mg/kg)	IV = <3 min IM = 15–30 min PO = 30–60 min	IV = min-hr	Respiratory impairment in high doses, thrombophlebitis, IV and IM injections painful; potential for recurrent sedation ≤ 24 hr
Narcotics	Analgesia, sedation				
Meperidine		IV, IM = 20–100 mg		2–4 hr	Relatively little antitussive activity
Codeine		IV = not recommended, IM = 20–120 mg			Effective antitussive
Morphine		IV, IM, SC = 2–10 mg	IV = 5–10 min IM = 15–30 min SC = 30–90 min	1–6 hr	Respiratory depression, bronchospasm, bradycardia, vomiting, hypotension, biliary spasm
Fentanyl		IV, IM = 50–100 μg	IV = 2 min IM = 10–15 min	IV, IM-30–45 min	Similar to morphine, chest wall rigidity, bronchospasm, hypotension, and biliary spasm are less common
Alfentanil		IV, IM = 250–1000 μg	<Fentanyl	<Fentanyl	Similar to fentanyl
Sufentanil		IV, IM = 5–70 μg	<Fentanyl	<Fentanyl	Similar to fentanyl
Miscellaneous					
Propofol	Sedation	IV = 50 μg/kg/min	<1 min	8–10 min	Respiratory depression, hypotension, cough
Droperidol	Sedation, antiemetic, indifference, neuroleptanalgesic	IV, IM = 0.65–5.0 mg	IV, IM = 5–20 min	IV, IM = 6–12 hr	Dysphoria, extrapyramidal symptoms, mild α-adrenergic antagonist, prolongs emergence from anesthesia
Ketamine	Disassociation, analgesia	IV, IM = 0.2–0.5 mg	30–60 sec		↑ secretions, emergence delusion ↓ secretions, with benzodiazepines 5–30%
Antagonists					
Naloxone	Narcotic antagonist	IV = 1–4 μg/kg	<1 min	30 min	Tachycardia, hypertension, reversal of analgesia
Flumazenil	Benzodiazepine antagonist	IV = 0.4–1.0 mg	5 min	1–4 hr	Reversal of sedation

Modified from Ref. 32.
IV, intravenous; IM, intramuscular; PO, oral; SC, subcutaneous.

SEDATIVE AGENTS

Benzodiazepines

Midazolam is a water-soluble benzodiazepine that predictably induces anxiolysis. It has a number of advantages over diazepam including the absence of pain with intravenous injection, rapid onset of action, short duration, and reliable amnesia (13). Midazolam is more potent than diazepam and should be given in small incremental doses to closely monitored patients. Elderly patients may be particularly susceptible to respiratory depression (13).

Diazepam is effective orally or intravenously. It is not as quick in onset as midazolam and may also be painful on injection. While it predictably produces anxiolysis and amnesia, its prolonged duration of action limits its desirability. Lorazepam's even greater dura-

TABLE 3. *Pharmacological comparison of atropine, glycopyrrolate, and scopolamine*

Anticholinergic	Dosage (mg)	Antisialagogue	Sedation	Onset	Increase heart rate	Duration	Untoward reactions	Relax smooth muscles
Atropine	0.4–0.8 IV, IM SC, PO	+	+	IV rapid IM, SC, PO 1–2 hr	+ + +	IM, PO, SC 4 hr	Tachyarrhythmias, PVCs, urinary retention, decreased GI motility, hypothermia, and delirium	+ +
Glycopyrrolate	0.1–0.2 IV, IM	+ +	0	IV 1–4 min IM, SC 20–40 min PO 1 hr	+ +	IV 2–4 hr IM, SC 4–6 hr PO 6 hr	Tachyarrhythmias, PVCs, urinary retention, decreased GI motility	+ +
Scopolamine	0.3–0.6 IV, IM, SC	+ + +	+ + +	IV 1 min	+		Delirium, more excitement, tachyarrhythmias, hypothermia, amnesia, sedation	+

Modified from Ref. 32.
0, none; +, mild; + +, moderate; + + +, marked.
IV, intravenous; IM, intramuscular; PO, oral; SC, subcutaneous; PVC, premature ventricular contractions.

tion of action limits the usefulness of this benzodiazepine in bronchoscopy.

Narcotic Agents

Opioids are powerful analgesic agents that produce their effect by binding to opiate receptors distributed throughout the central nervous system (CNS). Their analgesia, cough suppression, and anxiolysis have to be balanced with their adverse effects of respiratory depression, nausea, and vomiting. We recommend the use of the potent shorter acting narcotic fentanyl, although codeine, morphine, and meperidine are effective. Alfentanil and sufentanil provide little benefit over fentanyl and are much more expensive. At the low doses necessary for sedation, chest wall rigidity in patients given fentanyl, sufentanil, or alfentanil is uncommon (14).

Fentanyl is a synthetic opioid related to the phenyl piperidines. Its analgesic potency is 60 times greater than that of morphine. It has a very rapid onset of action with a limited duration of action. Fentanyl, in doses of 0.5–2.0 μg/kg, is an excellent addition to midazolam for use during bronchoscopy. Vigorous coughing may be suppressed by 50–100 μg fentanyl.

Sufentanil is a potent fentanyl derivative with an analgesic potency five to ten times greater than that of fentanyl (15). Comparisons of equipotent doses of fentanyl and sufentanil have demonstrated more rapid recovery and less respiratory depression with sufentanil (16). Because of its extreme potency, it is recommended that sufentanil be diluted to 5 μg/ml to limit the possibility of overdose.

Alfentanil is a synthetic derivative of fentanyl that is six to eight times less potent than fentanyl. It has a rapid onset and brief duration of action. It may be used in doses of 10–30 μg/kg as an adjunct to benzodiazepine sedation.

Other Agents

Propofol is a recently introduced phenol derivative that may be used for sedation or for induction and maintenance of anesthesia. It is lipid-soluble and formulated in a white aqueous emulsion containing soy bean oil and purified egg phosphatide in glycerol. This drug has a large volume of distribution and is rapidly eliminated by hepatic and extrahepatic metabolism (17). Its extremely short duration of activity has made it very useful for outpatient general anesthesia. Given in smaller doses, it can provide excellent sedation (18). Hypotension as well as myocardial and respiratory depression may result. This is more commonly seen in patients who are receiving barbiturates, are hypovolemic, or are elderly. Some patients may become apneic. While it may not be the optimal sedative agent for bronchoscopy, it appears to be an excellent choice providing stable hemodynamics for the majority of patients (19). The intravenous injection of propofol can be painful and is attenuated by prior intravenous injection of 100 mg of lidocaine. This may require administration of lower doses of lidocaine for topical anesthesia to limit toxic plasma concentration.

Droperidol is a potent antiemetic and neuroleptic agent that exerts its effect via the chemoreceptor trigger zone. This butyrophenone dissociates the patients from their environment. Its onset is slower than the benzodiazepines and has a very long duration of action. Occasionally, some patients may exhibit unpleasant mental agitation or develop a dysphoric response. They may express feelings of doom or undirected fear, yet they may appear calm. These symptoms can be treated with small doses of an anticholinergic such as atropine or be relieved with an opiate or benzodiazepine. Glycopyrrolate is not effective because it does not cross the blood–brain barrier.

Ketamine was included in the table for completeness. This powerful dissociative agent has potent analgesic properties and may be useful in small doses for selected cases. Larger doses of ketamine may be associated with vomiting and aspiration. Its tendency to produce copious secretions and hallucinogenic responses limits its application for bronchoscopy.

While receptor-specific antagonists are not routinely used, the availability of naloxone to antagonize narcotic agents and flumazenil to antagonize benzodiazepines provides an additional margin of safety in the use of these medications (20,21). These agents abruptly reverse analgesia and sedation that may result in tachycardia or hypertension. These antagonists are used only as a resuscitative measure.

Naloxone is an opiate antagonist that effectively reverses the CNS effects of all opiates. In low doses (25- to 50-μg increments), naloxone reverses opioid-induced ventilatory depression without affecting pain relief (20). The administration of larger doses of naloxone will terminate analgesia and may precipitate dysrhythmias, hypertension, and pulmonary edema.

Flumazenil is a receptor-specific benzodiazepine antagonist. When administered intravenously in titrated doses (0.1–0.4 mg), it effectively reverses benzodiazepine-induced sedation within 2 min but does not reliably reverse benzodiazepine-induced respiratory depression (22). It has been tolerated well, even in high-risk cardiac patients with no significant changes in heart rate or blood pressure (23).

ANESTHESIA OF THE AIRWAY

A thorough knowledge of topographic anatomy and sensory innervation of the airway is necessary in order to provide appropriate anesthesia for bronchoscopy. Vigorous physiological responses may result if adequate airway anesthesia is not ensured. Bronchoscopy performed under successful airway anesthesia results in minimal increases in mean arterial blood pressure and heart rate (24).

The complex innervation of the upper and lower airway necessitates a systematic approach in order to achieve adequate blocking of sensory input. Table 4 summarizes sensory innervation of the upper and lower airways. Airway anatomy should be reviewed prior to performing transtracheal and superior laryngeal nerve blocks (Fig. 1). Sensation to the inferior surface of the epiglottis, the pharynx, and the posterior one third of the tongue may also be blocked by anesthetizing the glossopharyngeal nerve (IX). We do not commonly use this block for airway anesthesia but include it as an option.

Sensory innervation of the upper airway is supplied by the trigeminal and lingual nerves (V). The glossopharyngeal (IX) and vagus (X) nerves provide additional innervation of the upper and lower airways. The internal branch of the superior laryngeal nerve provides sensory innervation of the upper larynx, specifically from the inferior aspect of the epiglottis to the vocal cords (Fig. 1; Table 4). The external branch of the superior laryngeal nerve provides motor innervation to the cricothyroid muscle. The recurrent laryngeal nerve carries both motor and sensory fibers. It provides sensory innervation to the vocal cords and trachea. It in-

TABLE 4. *Sensory innervation of airway structures*

Structure	Sensory innervation	Motor function
Nose	Trigeminal nerve (V)	
Tongue		
Anterior	Lingual nerve (V)	
Posterior	Glossopharyngeal nerve (IX)	
Pharynx	Glossopharyngeal nerve (IX)	
Upper larynx	Superior laryngeal nerve (X)	
	Internal branch of the superior laryngeal (vagus nerve)	Sensory from the inferior aspect of the epiglottis to (but excluding) the vocal cords (upper larynx)
	External branch of the superior laryngeal (vagus nerve)	Motor to the cricothyroid muscle
Vocal cords	Recurrent laryngeal nerve (X)	
	Recurrent laryngeal (vagus nerve)	Sensory from the vocal cords to lower larynx and trachea Motor to all laryngeal muscles except the cricothyroid muscle
Trachea	Vagus nerve (X)	

Modified from Reed AP. *Chest* 1992;10:2248.

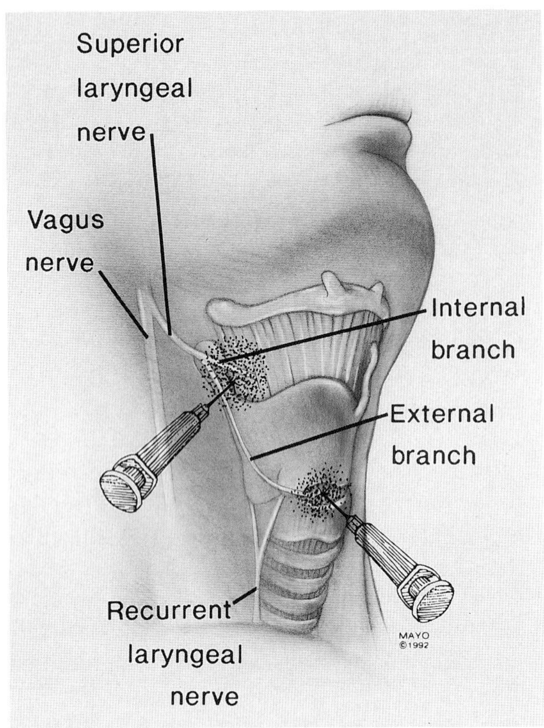

FIG. 1. Superior laryngeal nerve block and transtracheal block of the upper airway.

nervates all laryngeal muscles except the cricothyroid muscle.

Anesthetizing part or all of the airway may inhibit or obliterate protective airway reflexes. Patients may therefore be exposed to the risks of aspiration. Selected patients may benefit from the use of H_2 blocking agents to reduce the volume of gastric secretions and acidity in addition to limiting oral intake for 6 hr prior to the procedure.

TOPICAL ANESTHESIA

Direct placement of local anesthetics on the mucous membrane of the nose, mouth, and tracheobronchial tree produces topical anesthesia. The specific technique used for topical placement of local anesthetics is discussed in detail in Chapters 8 and 9 of this volume. Lidocaine (2–4%), tetracaine (2%), benzocaine (10–20%), and cocaine (4–10%) are effective agents. These agents inhibit ciliary activity and may impair secretion removal.

TRANSTRACHEAL BLOCK

Direct instillation of local anesthetics through the cricothyroid membrane into the trachea can provide excellent analgesia of the vocal cords and trachea. After palpating the midline depression between the thyroid and cricoid cartilages, a superficial skin wheal is made with local anesthetic. A 20-gauge or smaller, 3–5 cm, intravenous catheter over a needle is attached to a 3-cm^3 syringe and inserted through the skin wheal and advanced at 45° in a superior-to-inferior direction. Once the cricothyroid membrane has been pierced, aspiration of air confirms placement within the trachea. The needle and syringe are withdrawn, and the plastic catheter is held firmly in place. Four ml of 2–4% lidocaine is rapidly injected through the plastic catheter, usually resulting in abrupt, deep coughing. Immediately after injection, the catheter is fully withdrawn. In a cooperative patient who coughs vigorously, complete anesthesia of the lower and upper airway may be established.

SUPERIOR LARYNGEAL NERVE BLOCK

Bilateral superior laryngeal nerve blocks provide excellent anesthesia of the airway from the epiglottis to the vocal cords. With the patient's head extended, the hyoid bone is identified by its readily movable nature. After placing a subcutaneous wheal of local anesthetic, a 25-gauge, 2.5-cm needle is introduced laterally and directed at the greater corner of the hyoid bone. Immediately inferior to the greater corner of the hyoid, the needle is advanced 2–3 mm, piercing the thyrohyoid membrane. If aspiration for blood is negative, 3 cm^3 of 2–4% lidocaine may then be infiltrated. This procedure is repeated on the opposite side to ensure bilateral anesthesia.

LOCAL ANESTHETICS

Local anesthetics are used in bronchoscopy for topical anesthesia, to provide regional nerve blockade, and as intravenous adjuncts. Lidocaine has the widest margin of safety and is the most commonly used agent. Tetracaine, benzocaine, and cocaine can be equally effective, but have a narrow range of toxicity and other clinical limitations. Local anesthetics alter the permeability of nerve membranes to sodium ions, thus inhibiting transmission of nerve impulses (25). A pharmacological comparison of commonly used local anesthetics is presented in Table 5.

Lidocaine

This amide local anesthetic is the most widely used agent, in part because it is less toxic and shorter acting than tetracaine and cocaine. It is available in a wide variety of preparations and concentrations. Once absorbed, lidocaine is rapidly distributed into vessel-rich tissues and later redistributed into vessel-poor tissues

TABLE 5. *Pharmacological comparison of commonly used local anesthetics in bronchoscopy*

Anesthetic	Concentration (%)	Relative potency	Clinical use	Onset	Clinical duration (min)	Recommended maximum adult single dosage	Site of metabolism
Amides:							
Lidocaine	0.5–1	1	Infiltration	Fast	60–120	300 mg	Liver
	1–2		Nerve block	Fast	60–180	500 mg with epinephrine	
	2–4		Topical	Moderate	30–60	500 with epinephrine (7 mg/kg)	
Bupivacaine	0.25	4	Infiltration	Fast	2–4 hr	175 mg (2 mg/kg)	Liver
	0.25–0.50		Nerve block	Slow	4–12 hr	225 mg	
Esters:							
Benzocaine	10–20		Topical	Fast	15–30	200 mg	
Procaine	1.0	1	Infiltration	Fast	30–60	1000 mg	Plasma
	1–2.0		Nerve block	Slow	30–60	1000 mg	
Tetracaine	2.0	4	Topical	Slow	30–60	20 mg (0.2 mg/kg)	Plasma
Cocaine	4–10.0		Topical	Slow	30–60	150 mg (3 mg/kg)	Plasma and liver

Modified from Scott, DB, Cousins MJ. Clinical pharmacology of local anesthetic agents. In: Cousins MJ, Bridenbaugh PO, eds. *Neural blockade in clinical anesth and management of pain.* 1980: 88–89.

(26). The resulting serum concentration of lidocaine is directly related to total dose administered, regardless of solution concentration. Toxic symptoms may appear at plasma levels exceeding 5 μg/ml. It is metabolized by hepatic microsomes, and less than 10% is excreted in the urine. Patients with hepatic dysfunction may develop high plasma levels of lidocaine more rapidly (27).

Benzocaine

This commonly used, water-insoluble, ester-based local anesthetic is a derivative of *para*-aminobenzoic acid. It provides rapid onset of anesthesia within 15–30 sec when applied to mucous membranes. Its duration of action of 5–10 min is too short for many procedures, and it has a narrow margin of safety that limits its utility. Administration in the aerosolized form (benzocaine 20%) for more than 4 sec may exceed safe dosage limits. Methemoglobinemia may result following excessive topical administration of benzocaine and other local anesthetics (28,29).

Tetracaine

Tetracaine, another ester-type agent, is a potent local anesthetic with a longer duration of action than lidocaine or cocaine. Like cocaine, tetracaine is hydrolyzed by plasma cholinesterases, but at slower rates. Administered topically, tetracaine is much more toxic than cocaine and lidocaine. A topically applied dose of tetracaine should not exceed 40 mg (30). Unfortunately, the first sign of toxicity may be sudden death. We do not routinely use this drug for topical anesthesia in bronchoscopy because of its very narrow margin of safety. Tetracaine should not be used for infiltration due to its slow onset of anesthesia and its high potential for systemic toxicity.

Cocaine

Cocaine, a natural alkaloid, was the first local anesthetic to be discovered. It is the only one that produces both topical anesthesia and vasoconstriction when applied to mucous membranes. It is most commonly used in lower concentrations to limit toxicity. The metabolism of cocaine involves a plasma cholinesterase. Caution should be used in patients with a history of plasma cholinesterase deficiency, atypical cholinesterase, or in patients taking cholinesterase inhibitors such as echothiophate. It should be used with caution in patients who have coronary artery disease, hypertension, or who are taking monoamine oxidase inhibitors.

Toxic reactions appear to be more frequent when cocaine is applied to the tracheobronchial tree than to other mucous membranes (31). Tachycardia, hypertension, cardiac dysrhythmias, hyperthermia, tremors, and seizures may result from systemic absorption of cocaine in dosages greater than 1.5 mg/kg. α- and β-adrenergic antagonists may be used to blunt symptoms of excess sympathetic nervous system activity in overdoses of cocaine. Because of its possible toxicity, addictive nature, potential for abuse, required record keeping, and adequate alternatives, we do not commonly use cocaine for bronchoscopy.

Other Agents

Piperocaine, hexylcaine, dyclonine, and pramoxine are other local anesthetics that may be used as topical agents. However, they have clinical limitations and are not commonly used for topical anesthesia in bronchoscopy.

TOPICAL VASOCONSTRICTORS

The addition of epinephrine 1:200,000 (5 μg/cm^3) to a local anesthetic can approximately double the duration of infiltration anesthesia (32). Prolonging the duration of action by the addition of epinephrine is safer than increasing the dose of local anesthetic, which increases the chances of systemic toxicity (33,34). Systemic absorption of local anesthetics is reduced by one third with the addition of 1:200,000 epinephrine (35). Vasoconstriction may improve visualization by the shrinking of mucosal capillaries and may also limit nasopharyngeal bleeding.

Dilute epinephrine (e.g., 1:20,000) may be applied to tracheobronchial mucosa to control or prevent excessive bleeding due to brushing or biopsy. While very effective, the rapid uptake of this potent agent necessitates close observation of the patient's cardiac rhythm and hemodynamics.

Phenylephrine (0.125–0.5%) is often administered to the nasal mucosa and produces vasoconstriction, which limits systemic absorption and maintains drug concentration locally (Table 6). In vulnerable patients, systemic absorption of phenylephrine or epinephrine may accentuate hypertension and could result in further hemodynamic derangements. These potent agents should be administered with great care.

TABLE 6. *Recommended guidelines for phenylephrine dosage*

Weight (kg)	Concentration of solution (%)	Total amount administered (1 spray, 0.1 ml)[a]
0–15	0.125	2–3 sprays
16–30	0.125	4–6 sprays
31–40	0.125	4–6 sprays
41–60	0.25	4–8 sprays
61–100	0.5	4–8 sprays
101 and higher	0.5	8 sprays

Courtesy of ME Warner, MD and RA MacKenzie, DO.
[a] Utilizing atomizer.

TOXICITY OF LOCAL ANESTHETIC AGENTS

Systemic toxicity and allergic reactions are the primary side effects related to the use of local anesthetics. Clinically useful plasma concentrations of lidocaine may cause depression of the ventilatory response to hypoxia (36). In patients with chronic carbon dioxide retention whose resting ventilation is dependent on a hypoxic drive, the administration of lidocaine for treatment of ventricular dysrhythmias or for bronchoscopic procedures may result in further ventilatory depression. Systemic absorption of topically applied local anesthetics may produce plasma concentrations similar to those present following an intravenous injection. The rate of systemic absorption is dependent on dosage, injection site, vascularity, presence of vasoconstricting agents, and physical properties of the drug. The rate of drug absorption into the circulation, redistribution to inactive tissue sites, and metabolic clearance together determine the plasma concentrations of local anesthetics.

Excess plasma concentrations of these drugs lead to the signs of systemic toxicity. Toxic effects of local anesthetics are seen in the cardiovascular and central nervous systems. Individual variations between patients may significantly vary the threshold for toxicity. Following placement of tetracaine and lidocaine on the tracheobronchial mucosa, these high levels may cause CNS or cardiac toxicity (37).

Numbness of the tongue and circumoral tissues reflect delivery of low plasma concentrations of local anesthetics to these highly vascular areas. Profound hypotension due to relaxation of arterial vascular smooth muscle or myocardial depression may result when plasma concentrations of lidocaine reach 5–10 μg/ml. Local anesthetics also block sodium channels in the myocardium. In low concentrations, lidocaine is an antidysrhythmic, whereas excessive plasma concentrations block myocardial sodium channels, and automaticity and conduction are adversely depressed. Prolongation of the PR interval and QRS complex may be noted on the electrocardiogram.

At higher plasma concentrations, local anesthetics will produce a predictable pattern of CNS changes once they cross the blood–brain barrier. Initially patients may exhibit restlessness, tinnitus, vertigo, and difficulty with visual focusing. As concentrations in the CNS increase, slurred speech, drowsiness, and twitching of skeletal muscles may occur. The twitching is usually seen first in the face and extremities and is usually a premonition to the onset of tonic-clonic seizures. Classically, CNS depression follows a seizure, and concomitant hypotension and apnea may occur. Seizures are thought to result from a local anesthetic–induced inhibition of the release of neurotransmitters, especially γ-aminobutyric acid, or by depression of inhibitory corticoneurons. Because it may help detect nascent CNS toxicity, intermittent conversation with the patient is an excellent method to monitor for symptoms of toxicity.

Immediate treatment of local anesthetic–induced seizures includes support of ventilation and oxygenation and treatment of metabolic acidosis, which may occur rapidly during a generalized tonic-clonic seizure. Benzodiazepines such as midazolam and diazepam are the agents of choice to treat local anesthetic–induced seizures.

Intravenous injections of bupivacaine may result in precipitous hypotension, atrioventricular heart block, and other cardiac dysrhythmias. Bupivacaine is highly lipid-soluble and protein-bound. It dissociates very slowly from sodium channels, which accounts for its persistent myocardial depression and prolonged cardiac toxicity. As a result, resuscitative efforts in a patient who suffers a cardiac arrest secondary to bupivacaine toxicity should be prolonged. Bretylium tosylate, 20 mg/kg, reverses bupivacaine-induced cardiac depression and elevates the threshold for ventricular tachycardia (38). The less lipid-soluble lidocaine rapidly dissociates from cardiac sodium channels; its toxicity is thus short-lived. Because pregnancy increases sensitivity to local anesthetics, the cardiotoxic effects may also be accentuated and cardiopulmonary collapse may occur with smaller doses of bupivacaine in pregnant patients (39).

ALLERGY TO LOCAL ANESTHETIC AGENTS

True allergic reactions to local anesthetics are rare. It is likely that an allergic response to a local anesthetic is responsible for less than 1% of all adverse reactions attributed to local anesthetics (40). Manifestations of excess plasma concentrations of the local anesthetic or vasoconstricting agents (epinephrine and phenylephrine) are responsible for the majority of adverse responses that are often falsely labeled "allergic" in nature. Hypertension, syncope, or tachycardia in the presence of an epinephrine-containing local anesthetic solution is suggestive of accidental intravascular injection or systemic uptake.

The development of a rash, urticaria, laryngeal edema, or bronchospasm is highly suggestive of an allergic reaction. Documentation of allergy to the local anesthetic is based on the clinical history as well as intradermal testing (41). Even with the use of preservative-free agents, intradermal testing may not always provide an accurate result (42). True allergic reactions following the use of a local anesthetic may be due to methylparaben or similar substances that are used as preservatives. Many preservatives are structurally similar to the allergen *para*-aminobenzoic acid (PABA), and antibody production may be stimulated by the preservative and not the local anesthetic itself.

The metabolites of the ester class of local anesthetics are related to PABA, making them more likely to produce an allergic reaction than the amide class. The common metabolite PABA may result in cross-sensitivity between ester-type local anesthetics. However, this cross-sensitivity does not extend to the amide class of local anesthetics. In a patient with a documented allergy to an ester-type local anesthetic, an amide such as lidocaine in preservative-free solutions may be substituted without increased risk of experiencing an allergic reaction. In rare cases of a true lidocaine anaphylaxis or in an unsettled clinical situation, general anesthesia could be employed. If an allergy is doubted, one may elect to proceed, having full resuscitative equipment and medications immediately available.

AIRWAY MANAGEMENT

Consultation between the anesthesiologist and bronchoscopist prior to the procedure is imperative in special instances such as foreign body aspiration and major airway lesions. Prospective and coordinated cooperation provides a shared strategy for the shared airway. Contingencies for emergencies should be developed in advance. Consultation may also include discussion of the appropriate premedication. At the end of such cases, a true sense of accomplishment is felt by all team members confirming the spirit of the team approach.

EQUIPMENT

A documented, systematic, preparatory checklist is imperative. We recommend equipment as outlined in Table 1. Complete facilities for delivery of general anesthesia and airway management are required. Negative pressure suction as well as capabilities for positive pressure ventilation and resuscitation must be readily available. This includes a variety of masks, endotracheal tubes, and laryngoscope handles and the appropriately sized blades. Swivel adapters can be used to insufflate oxygen through a soft endotracheal tube. A tight-fitting sleeve for general anesthesia may be used. Double-lumen endotracheal tubes should be available in the event of the need to isolate one lung from the other. This may occur when acute hemorrhage results during laser surgery or when an empyema or nidus of infection needs to be isolated.

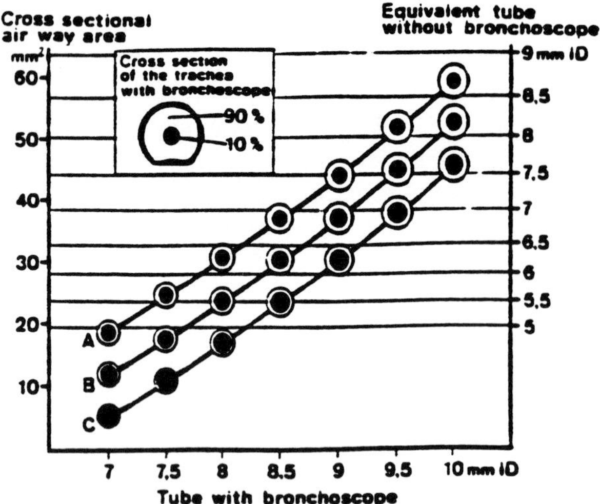

FIG. 2. Cross-section of different caliber tubes **(outer circle)** containing three different size bronchoscopes **(filled center)**: (A) 5-mm ED; (B) 5.7-mm ED. White area within the tubes shows available cross-sectional airway area. **Inserted**: Relation between available cross-sectional airway area of the trachea and the bronchofiberscope in nonintubated normal patients. From *Chest* 1978;74:4, with permission.

Resistance to air movement greatly increases with increased bronchoscope diameter (Fig. 2). Ideally, it is optimal to limit airway resistance as much as possible by using the largest endotracheal tube possible.

FLEXIBLE BRONCHOSCOPY

The most common procedure performed is flexible bronchoscopy. After local anesthetic is sprayed on the oropharynx, the larynx, and vocal cords, the patient is taken into the bronchoscopy room and administered oxygen. We pass a soft, lubricated oral endotracheal tube over the bronchoscope, through a bite block, with the bronchoscope acting as a stent. The patient insufflates oxygen supplied through a swivel adapter connected to the endotracheal tube. We prefer the oral approach for flexible bronchoscopy. It is easy to readily remove and reinsert the instrument to clean the lens and remove specimens or brushes. If the oral approach with an endotracheal tube is used and complications arise, control of the airway is ensured. We also use the nasal approach for brief bronchoscopic inspections. Nasal discomfort may persist for a few days after the bronchoscopy. Infrequently epistaxis occurs, and bacteremia may result. A full discussion on the preparation of the patient is presented in Chapter 8 of this volume.

RIGID BRONCHOSCOPY

The rigid bronchoscope may be employed with topical or general anesthesia. We formerly performed a mask induction with a volatile agent followed by passing the rigid bronchoscope. Because of the long delay in achieving adequate concentrations of volatile anesthetic, intravenous inductions are now used. After adequate and brief muscle relaxation, the trachea is intubated and the rigid bronchoscope passed alongside the endotracheal tube. As the vocal cords are approached, the endotracheal tube is withdrawn and the bronchoscope is passed through the cords.

Problems with the rigid bronchoscope include laryngeal or bronchial edema, laryngospasm, gastric distention, pneumothorax, and respiratory acidosis due to air trapping (43). Bronchoscope passage may be facilitated by intravenous lidocaine and/or small doses of muscle relaxant.

GENERAL ANESTHESIA

Anesthetic Induction

Anesthesia can be induced with spontaneous or controlled ventilation. There are specific reasons for choosing one over the other in many cases. Induction of general anesthesia is usually accomplished with sodium thiopental or propofol. The depolarizing muscle relaxant succinylcholine is used to facilitate tracheal intubation.

Anesthetic Gases

Volatile anesthetics such as halothane, enflurane, and isoflurane may all be used for varying reasons. They are diluted with oxygen and air combinations. Their use may result in some degree of myocardial and respiratory depression, which must be taken into consideration. Nitrous oxide may be used to facilitate anesthetic induction but is not used for maintenance because it requires 50–70% concentrations for clinical efficacy. The use of potent volatile anesthetics (1–2%) and a higher oxygen concentration increases the margin of safety.

Muscle Relaxants

We use the customary intubating bolus dose of succinylcholine (1–2 mg/kg). We do not give defacilitating doses of nondepolarizing agents because they have been shown to adversely affect the pulmonary dynamics and airway protection (44). They may also have lingering effects such as diplopia and weakness. Most of our patients are outpatients who are dismissed on the day of the procedure. We therefore avoid using long-acting agents. The short- and intermediate-acting nondepolarizing neuromuscular blocking agents mivacurium, atracurium, and vecuronium are well suited for those situations in which continued muscle relaxation is needed. We prefer not to administer neostigmine to reverse neuromuscular blockade because of potential pulmonary problems associated with anticholinergics.

LASER BRONCHOSCOPY

The neodymium-YAG (Nd:YAG) laser has a wavelength of 1064 nm. It is readily conducted through fiberoptics, is poorly absorbed by hemoglobin, and provides for good tissue penetration (45). In the initial 100 laser bronchoscopic procedures performed at the Mayo Clinic, we most commonly utilized the flexible bronchoscope. Thereafter, we have used the rigid bronchoscope as the primary instrument for these procedures and feel that it is far superior to the flexible bronchoscope.

The rigid bronchoscope provides for removal of large pieces of obstructing tumor by biopsy forceps and can itself be used as a coring instrument. In addition, the rigid bronchoscope may function as an airway dilator and can open an obstructed airway more rapidly than can the flexible bronchoscope. It is difficult to debulk a tumor through a flexible scope and retrieve large pieces of tissue. With the rigid bronchoscope, one can see more clearly, pass the forceps, and remove large amounts of charred tissue.

Anesthesia

Anesthesia may be induced with thiopental, midazolam, or propofol. The trachea is intubated after muscle relaxation is achieved with succinylcholine. We usually maintain anesthesia with fentanyl and isoflurane. A succinylcholine infusion or a nondepolarizing muscle relaxant is also given to ensure muscle relaxation. Ventilation is controlled with an FiO_2 of less than 0.5 in N_2 during the resection. Standard monitors including pulse oximetry and end-tidal carbon dioxide are used to gauge the level of oxygenation and ventilation (46). If any questions arise, arterial blood gasses are obtained. If desaturation is noted during prolonged periods of resection, laser therapy is interrupted and ventilation with high concentrations of oxygen is resumed until an adequate oxygen saturation is obtained. Apneic oxygenation can be provided with a continuous flow of oxygen through the rigid bronchoscope.

During laser resection of airway lesions, there are several potential anesthetic problems that may occur. As previously discussed, the bronchoscopist and the anesthesiologist must share the airway, and therefore ventilation and oxygenation may be compromised during prolonged tumor resections. Prolonged laser resection of airway lesions may require continued muscle relaxation with the attendant risk of residual neuromuscular blockade.

Many of the Nd:YAG laser procedures tend to be prolonged and may result in postoperative somnolence and respiratory depression. If significant, this may require continued intubation and ventilation. It is very important to monitor the patients in a postanesthesia care unit immediately adjacent to the operating (bronchoscopy) suite. Some patients may develop airway edema that may significantly compromise their ventilation within 24 hr postoperatively. Resection of tumors adjacent to vascular tissues may result in uncontrollable hemorrhage. If this occurs and one is unable to adequately clear the visual field, we utilize bronchial blockers or double-lumen endotracheal tubes to isolate the hemorrhage. Death due to exsanguination during use of the Nd:YAG laser can occur (47). Any patient who has had either a prolonged resection or removal of a large airway obstruction should be monitored carefully for 24 hr following surgery.

We choose to avoid nitrous oxide and maintain the FiO_2 at less than 0.5 to avoid supporting combustion (48,49). If the laser beam is delivered distal to the end of the endotracheal tube, the risk of endotracheal tube fires is not high. Red rubber endotracheal tubes can be wrapped with metal foil or metal endotracheal tubes can be used in laser surgery. Using copper or aluminum foil with a matte finish will limit reflection of the laser. It is important to remember that all endotracheal tubes are combustible.

In the event of a fire during laser surgery, a number of steps should be taken simultaneously. Oxygen flow should be discontinued, the endotracheal tube disconnected, the patient extubated. The fire is then extinguished with saline and the patient ventilated by a mask. The patient is reintubated with another endotracheal tube. Jet ventilation may be utilized for these procedures; however, we choose to use conventional controlled ventilation with volatile anesthetics.

PEDIATRIC BRONCHOSCOPY

Anesthesia

The goals in bronchoscopy for children include protecting the teeth, blunting laryngeal reflexes, having a well-relaxed jaw and glottis, having a cooperative patient, preventing arrhythmias, and providing for return of airway reflexes at the end of the procedure. Pediatric patients undergoing bronchoscopy require special attention. In addition to differing equipment needs, one must be readily prepared for possible emergencies. These patients will likely benefit from premedication to provide anxiolysis and limit oropharyngeal and bronchial secretions. Pediatric doses of

TABLE 7. *Pediatric doses of commonly used drugs for bronchoscopy*

Drug	Dosage
Fentanyl	1–2 μg/kg
Methohexital	15–25 mg/kg (rectal)
Ketamine	0.5–2 mg/kg (IV) 2–10 mg/kg (IM)
Sodium thiopental	2–7 mg/kg
Midazolam	0.05–0.3 mg/kg
Diazepam	0.02 mg/kg
Propofol	2.5–3.5 mg/kg
Atracurium	0.3–0.5 mg/kg, maint. 0.1 mg/kg
Succinylcholine	1.5–2.0 mg/kg (IV) 2–4 mg/kg (IM)
Vecuronium	0.1 mg/kg, maint. 0.04 mg/kg
Neostigmine	0.05 mg/kg
Glycopyrrolate	0.015 mg/kg
Naloxone	0.01–0.1 mg/kg
Aminophylline load	5–6 mg/kg, maint. 0.9 mg/kg/hr
Atropine	0.02–0.3 mg/kg
Sodium bicarbonate	1–2 meq/k
Dexamethasone	0.5–1.5 mg/kg
Racemic epinephrine 2%	<10 kg 0.25 ml in 2 ml NS >10 kg 0.25 ml
Lidocaine (topical)	Up to 4 mg/kg
Calcium chloride	5 mg/kg
Epinephrine	0.1–1 mg/kg/min
Lidocaine	1–1.5 mg/kg
Procainamide	3–6 mg/kg

commonly used sedatives and anesthetics as well as emergency medications are summarized in Table 7. Airway resistance is of particular importance in pediatric patients during partial occlusion of small endotracheal tubes with a bronchoscope (Fig. 2).

If a rigid bronchoscope is used, one must be immediately prepared to intubate with the appropriately sized endotracheal tube (Table 8). Airway anatomy in children is different from that in adults. The larynx is anterior and superior in relation to adults. The epiglottis is more round and less rigid (50).

In this special patient population, there are four options for the shared airway. Again, preoperative communication between the bronchoscopist and anesthesiologist is very important. One can use the rigid bronchoscope, a flexible fiberoptic bronchoscope with a side adapter for ventilation, a tracheostomy, or elect to not use an endotracheal tube and intermittently ventilate by mask or maintain spontaneous ventilation (51–52).

Insufflation pressures, irrespective of the technique, should be titrated to adequacy of chest wall excursion in 2–3 pounds per square inch (psi) increments. It is best to begin at 8 psi in infants or at 12–14 psi in primary school–aged children. Teenagers will usually tolerate beginning at 20 psi. Occasionally, apneic oxygenation can be utilized in which a small midtracheal catheter is placed and 0.2 L/kg/min oxygen is entrained. Adequate oxygenation can usually be maintained for up to 20 min; however, oxygen consumption and carbon dioxide production are quite high in pediatric and neonatal patients. As such, hypercarbia may rapidly develop, severely limiting the amount of time for apneic ventilation. If stridor or significant airway compromise develops postoperatively, it may be beneficial to reintubate those patients, evaluate neuromuscular function, and obtain a chest roentgenograph. If only minimal stridor occurs, it is helpful to administer a cool mist via close-fitting mask for an hour. Administration of nebulized racemic epinephrine, parental corticosteroids, and observation of the patient overnight may also be indicated.

TABLE 8. *Pediatric endotracheal tube size*

Age	Height (cm)	Weight (kg)		ETT size ID (mm)	Oral length (cm)	Nasal length (cm)
		Boys	Girls			
Neonate				3.0	9–10	12
3 mo	58	6	6	3.5	10–11	12
6 mo	66	8	8	4.0	11–12	14
9 mo	71	10	9	4.5	12–13	14
1 yr	76	11	10	4.5–5.0	13–14	16
2 yr	84	13	12	5.0	14–15	16
3 yr	96	15	15	5.0–5.5	15–16	18
4 yr	102	17	17	5.5	15–16	18
5 yr	109	19	19	5.5–6.0	16–17	19
6 yr	117	22	22	6.0	16–17	19
7 yr	122	25	25	6.0–6.5	17–18	20
8 yr	130	28	28	6.5	17–18	20
9 yr	134	31	31	6.5–7.0	18–19	21
10 yr	139	35	35	7.0	18–19	21
11 yr	146	38	40	7.0–7.5	19–20	22
12 yr	152	42	46	7.5	19–20	22

Modified from Steward DJ. *Manual of pediatric anesthesia*, 3rd ed. 66.
ETT, endotracheal tube; ID, internal diameter.

Foreign Bodies

Foreign bodies in the tracheobronchial tree offer unique challenges for airway management. Assessment of the patient's respiratory status to include severity of airway obstruction, respiratory distress, and level of consciousness must be ascertained prior to anesthetizing a child for foreign body removal. The nature and location of the foreign body, as well as a review of roentgenographs of chest and neck and inspiration-expiration films or fluoroscopy may be beneficial. Once these items have been reviewed and the oral intake status of the child is known, the anesthesiologist can determine the optimal anesthetic approach for the management of this emergency.

Removal of any foreign body is most safely performed in a lightly sedated or awake patient who is spontaneously ventilating with an intact cough mechanism. In infants and children, we usually administer a general anesthetic, maintaining spontaneous ventilation. In adults, we most commonly perform this procedure by topically applying local anesthetic in the customary manner.

EMERGENCIES

One should be prepared for emergencies during bronchoscopy such as airway obstruction, hemorrhage, hypoxemia, bronchospasm, and laryngospasm (1). Coordinated decisive action is needed by all members of the team in the presence of major airway emergencies. Of paramount importance is, again, recognition of the fact that the airway is shared by both the bronchoscopist and the anesthesiologist in this setting. A lost airway drill should be formulated and discussed in advance.

Complications from the use of double-lumen endotracheal tubes that are used in cases of uncontrollable hemorrhage may occur (53,54). A thorough knowledge of the working of the double-lumen tube and coordinated efforts by the team members is necessary when approaching this complex and life-threatening problem.

Cardiac irregularities and cardiopulmonary arrest are to be managed as recommended in the procedures of the advanced cardiac life support manual (55).

SUMMARY

Bronchoscopy can be safely completed with the appropriate use of premedication, sedation, topical or nerve block anesthesia, and general anesthesia. We believe it is best accomplished in a dedicated setting, carried out by well-prepared, coordinated team members. Carefully balancing the safety of the patient with the needs of the procedure is of paramount importance.

REFERENCES

1. Pereira W, Kovnat DM, Snider GL. A prospective cooperative study of complications following flexible fiberoptic bronchoscopy. *Chest* 1978;73:813.
2. Standards for basic intraoperative monitoring. American Society of Anesthesiologists. Approved 10/86, amended 10/90.
3. Colt HG, Morris JF. Fiberoptic bronchoscopy without premedication: a retrospective study. *Chest* 1990;98:1327.
4. Banerjee A, Banerjee SN, Nachiappan M. Premedication for fibreoptic bronchoscopy. *Indian J Chest Dis Allied Sci* 1986; 28:76.
5. Wisborg T. Rational bronchoscopy with the fibre bronchoscopy under local anesthesia. *Ugeskr Laeger* 1989;151:1740.
6. Mehta JB, Stubbs R. Fiberoptic bronchoscopy without premedication. *Chest* 1991;100:1179.
7. Egbert LD, Battit GE, Turndorf H, Beecher HK. The value of the preoperative visit by an anesthetist. A study of doctor-patient rapport. *JAMA* 1963;185:553.
8. Prakash UBS, Offord KP, Stubbs SE. Bronchoscopy in North America: the ACCP survey. *Chest* 1991;100:1668.
9. Mirakhur RK. Anticholinergic drugs. *Br J Anaesth* 1979;51:671.
10. Greenan J. Cardiac dysrhythmias and heart rate changes at induction of anaesthesia: a comparison of two intravenous anticholinergics. *Acta Anaesthesiol Scand* 1984;28:182.
11. Forster A, Gardaz J-P, Suter PM, Gemperle M. Respiratory depression by midazolam and diazepam. *Anesthesiology* 1980; 53:494.
12. Kanto J, Sjövall S, Vuori A. Effect of different kinds of premedication on the induction properties of midazolam. *Br J Anaesth* 1982;54:507.
13. Dundee JW, Halliday NJ, Harper KW, Brogden RN. Midazolam: a review of its pharmacological properties and therapeutic use. *Drugs* 1984;28:519.
14. Sokoll MD, Hoyt JL, Gergis SD: Studies in muscle rigidity, nitrous oxide, and narcotic analgesic agents. *Anesth Analg* 1972; 51:16.
15. Bovill JG, Sebel PS, Blackburn CL, Oei-Lim V, Heykants JJ. The pharmacokinetics of sufentanil in surgical patients. *Anesthesiology* 1984;61:502.
16. Monk JP, Beresford R, Ward A. Sufentanil: a review of its pharmacological properties and therapeutic use. *Drugs* 1988;36:286.
17. Adam HK, Briggs LP, Bahar M, et al. Pharmacokinetic evaluation of ICI 35 868 in man: single induction doses with different rates of injection. *Br J Anaesth* 1983;55:97.
18. Randell T. Sedation for bronchofiberoscopy: comparison between propofol infusion and intravenous boluses of fentanyl and diazepam. *Acta Anaesthesiol Scand* 1992;36:221–225.
19. Hill AJ, Feneck RO, Underwood SM, Davis ME, Marsh A, Bromley L. The haemodynamic effects of bronchoscopy. Comparison of propofol and thiopentone with and without alfentanil pretreatment. *Anaesthesia* 1991;46:266–270.
20. Evans JM, Hogg MIJ, Lunn JN, Rosen M. Degree and duration of reversal by naloxone of effects of morphine in conscious subjects. *Br Med J* 1974;2:589.
21. Klotz U, Ziegler G, Ludwig L, Reimann JW. Pharmacodynamic interaction between midazolam and a specific benzodiazepine antagonist in humans. *J Clin Pharmacol* 1985;25:400.
22. Baktai G, Szekely E, Marialigeti T, Kovacs L. Use of midazolam ("Dormicum") and flumazenil ("Anexate") in paediatric bronchology. *Curr Med Res Opin* 1992;12:552–559.
23. Geller E, Niv D, Nero Y, et al. Early clinical experience in reversing benzodiazepine sedation with flumazenil after short procedures. *Resuscitation* 1988;16:549.
24. Obassatian A, Yelick SJ, Dykes MHM, Brunner EE. Blood pressure and heart rate changes during awake fiberoptic nasal intubation. *Anesth Analg* 1983;62:951.
25. Ritchie JM, Greengard P. On the mode of action of local anesthetics. In: Elliott HW, ed. *Annual review of pharmacology*. Vol 6. Palo Alto: Annual Reviews Inc; 1966.
26. Boyes RN, Scott DB, Jebson PJ, et al. Pharmacokinetics of lidocaine in man. *Clin Pharmacol Ther* 1971;12:105.
27. Kirkpatrick MB. Lidocaine topical anesthesia for flexible bronchoscopy. *Chest* 1989;96:965.

28. Douglas WW, Fairbanks VF. Methemoglobinemia induced by a topical anesthetic spray (cetacaine). *Chest* 1977;71:587.
29. Collins JF. Methemoglobinemia as a complication of 20% benzocaine spray for endoscopy. *Gastroenterology* 1990;98:211.
30. Curran J, Hamilton C, Taylor T. Topical analgesia before tracheal intubation. *Anaesthesia* 1975;30:765.
31. Feehan HF, Mancusi-Ungaro A. The use of cocaine as a topical anesthetic in nasal surgery. *Plast Reconstr Surg* 1976;57:62.
32. Stoelting RK. Local anesthetics. In: *Pharmacology and physiology in anesthetic practice*. 2nd ed. Philadelphia: JB Lippincott; 1991.
33. Scott DB. Toxicity caused by local anaesthetic drugs (editorial). *Br J Anaesth* 1981;53:553.
34. Ueda W, Hirakawa M, Mae O. Appraisal of epinephrine administration to patients under halothane anesthesia for closure of cleft palate. *Anesthesiology* 1983;58:574.
35. Scott DB, Jebson PJR, Braid DP, et al. Factors affecting plasma levels of lignocaine and prilocaine. *Br J Anaesth* 1972;44:1040.
36. Gross JB, Caldwell CB, Shaw LM, Apfelbaum JL. The effect of lidocaine infusion on the ventilatory response to hypoxia. *Anesthesiology* 1984;61:662.
37. Viegas O, Stoelting RK. Lidocaine in arterial blood after laryngotracheal administration. *Anesthesiology* 1975;43:491.
38. Kasten GW, Martin ST. Bupivacaine cardiovascular toxicity: comparison of treatment with bretylium and lidocaine. *Anesth Analg* 1985;64:911.
39. Morishima HO, Pedersen H, Finster M, et al. Bupivacaine toxicity in pregnant and nonpregnant ewes. *Anesthesiology* 1985; 63:134.
40. Brown DT, Beamish D, Wildsmith JAW. Allergic reaction to an amide local anaesthetic. *Br J Anaesth* 1981;53:435.
41. Incaudo G, Schatz M, Patterson R, et al. Administration of local anesthetics to patients with a history of prior adverse reaction. *J Allerg Clin Immunol* 1978;61:339.
42. Fisher MM. Intradermal testing in the diagnosis of acute anaphylaxis during anaesthesia—results of five years experience. *Anaesth Intensive Care* 1979;7:58.
43. Lukomsky GI, Ovchinnikov AA, Bilal A. Complications of bronchoscopy: comparison of rigid bronchoscopy under general anesthesia and flexible fiberoptic bronchoscopy under topical anesthesia. *Chest* 1981;79:316.
44. Pavlin EG, Holle RH, Schoene RB. Recovery of airway protection compared with ventilation in humans after paralysis with curare. *Anesthesiology* 1989;70:381.
45. McDougal JC, Cortese DA. Neodymium-YAG laser therapy of malignant airway obstruction. *Mayo Clin Proc* 1983;58:35.
46. Lennon RL, Hosking MP, Warner MA, et al. Monitoring and analysis of oxygenation and ventilation during rigid bronchoscopic neodymium-YAG laser resection of airway tumors. *Mayo Clin Proc* 1987;62:584.
47. Warner ME, Warner MA, Leonard PF. Anesthesia for neodymium-YAG (Nd-YAG) laser resection of major airway obstructing tumors. *Anesthesiology* 1984;60:230.
48. Leonard PF. The lower limits of flammability of halothane, enflurane, and isoflurane. *Anesth Analg* 1975;54:238.
49. Vourc'h G, Tannieres ML, Toty L, Personne C. Anesthetic management of tracheal surgery using the neodymium-yttrium-aluminum garnet laser. *Br J Anaesth* 1980;52:993.
50. Eckenhoff JE. Some anatomic considerations of the infant larynx influencing endotracheal anesthesia. *Anesthesiology* 1951; 12:401.
51. Bailey AG, Valley RD, Azizkhan RG, Wood RE. Anaesthetic management of infants requiring endobronchial argon laser surgery. *Can J Anaesth* 1992;39:590–593.
52. Wood RE, Azizkhan RG, Lacey SR, Sidman J, Drake A. Surgical applications of ultrathin flexible bronchoscopes in infants. *Ann Otol Rhinol Laryngol* 1991;100:116–119.
53. Wagner DL, Gammage GW, Wong ML. Tracheal rupture following the insertion of a disposable double-lumen endotracheal tube. *Anesthesiology* 1985;63:698.
54. Clapham MC, Vaughan RS. Bronchial intubation. A comparison between polyvinyl chloride and red rubber double lumen tubes. *Anaesthesia* 1985;40:1111.
55. Albarran-Sotelo R, Atkins JM, Bloom RS, et al. *Textbook of Advanced Cardiac Life Support, Second Edition*. Dallas: American Heart Association; 1990.

Bronchoscopy,
edited by U. B. S. Prakash.
Mayo Foundation © 1994.
Published by Raven Press, Ltd., New York.

CHAPTER 8

Preparation of the Patient for Bronchoscopy

Samuel E. Stubbs and John C. McDougall

The indications and preparations for flexible bronchoscopy and rigid bronchoscopy are similar. Bronchoscopy today is largely flexible bronchoscopy (2), and when bronchoscopy is needed for patients on mechanical ventilators or for those with disease or trauma involving the skull, jaws, or cervical spine, the flexible bronchoscope is the instrument of choice. For massive hemoptysis, however, a rigid bronchoscope is the instrument of choice (3). Careful attention to the several steps involved in preparation of the patient for bronchoscopy can be rewarding for the patient and the examiner. Except where specifically indicated, the text will deal with the adult patient undergoing flexible bronchoscopy.

PREOPERATIVE CONSIDERATIONS

Although the indications for bronchoscopy are broad, one should use sound clinical judgment in determining its use in individual cases. The bronchoscopist should have a good appreciation of the patient's medical history, physical examination findings, and available laboratory data. Prior to bronchoscopy, one should go through a mental or written checklist regarding the risks of the procedure for the patient (2,4). Flexible bronchoscopy is a low-morbidity procedure; however, it is worthwhile for the bronchoscopist to consider situations in which the risk of bronchoscopy is increased. The increased risk situations, described by the American Thoracic Society's guidelines for flexible bronchoscopy in adults, are listed in Table 1 (3).

While any of the listed conditions may become contraindications or at least relative contraindications to bronchoscopy, the risk of the procedure must be weighed against the potential benefit for the patient. In certain situations, careful assessment and treatment in the hospital prior to examination may be necessary.

TABLE 1. *Clinical situations associated with increased risk from bronchoscopy*

1. Lack of patient cooperation
2. Recent myocardial infarction or unstable angina
3. Partial tracheal obstruction
4. Unstable bronchial asthma
5. Respiratory insufficiency associated with moderate to severe hypoxemia or any degree of hypercarbia
6. Uremia and pulmonary hypertension (possible serious hemorrhage after biopsy)
7. Lung abscess (danger of flooding the airway with purulent material)
8. Immunosuppression (danger of postbronchoscopy infection)
9. Obstruction of the superior vena cava (possibility of bleeding and laryngeal edema)
10. Debility, advanced age, and malnutrition
11. Unstable cardiac arrhythmia
12. Respiratory failure requiring mechanical ventilation
13. Disorders requiring laser therapy, biopsy of lesions obstructing large airways, or multiple transbronchial lung biopsies

From Ref. 3.

SPECIAL CIRCUMSTANCES

There are patients with conditions that require special consideration prior to bronchoscopy. Sound clinical judgment should be used in preparing the patient and in obtaining laboratory data prior to the procedure. Laboratory data obtained prior to examination should be individualized and based on the patient's medical history with consideration given to the cost and potential benefit to the patient.

S. E. Stubbs and J. C. McDougall: Division of Thoracic Diseases and Internal Medicine, Mayo Clinic, Rochester, Minnesota 55905.

Bacterial Endocarditis Prophylaxis

The American Heart Association currently recommends bacterial endocarditis prophylaxis for bronchoscopy with a rigid bronchoscope. Prophylaxis is recommended for patients with prosthetic cardiac valves, including bioprosthetic and homograft valves, previous bacterial endocarditis even in the absence of heart disease, most congenital cardiac malformations, rheumatic and other acquired valvular dysfunction even after valvular surgery, hypertrophic cardiomyopathy, and mitral valve prolapse with valvular regurgitation. Prophylaxis is not recommended for bronchoscopy with a flexible bronchoscope with or without biopsy. However, physicians may choose to administer prophylactic antibiotics even for flexible bronchoscopy in patients who have prosthetic heart valves, a previous history of endocarditis, or surgically constructed systemic-pulmonary shunts or conduits (5).

Bleeding Diatheses

Patients with bleeding diatheses require special attention, especially if biopsy is contemplated. A prothrombin time determination is indicated for patients taking oral anticoagulation. If biopsy is necessary, anticoagulation therapy should be discontinued allowing the prothrombin time to drift back to normal before proceeding. In cases where close anticoagulant control is desirable, temporary intravenous therapy with heparin may be useful. The heparin can be discontinued several hours prior to the planned procedure, and an activated partial thromboplastin time can be obtained prior to the examination. Thereafter, anticoagulation can be reestablished without excessive delay. It has been shown that patients with a blood urea nitrogen greater than 30 mg/dl have an increased incidence of bleeding complications leading to the recommendation that one should avoid, if possible, any biopsy procedure on uremic patients (6,7). It has been recommended that patients with platelet counts less than 50,000/mm^2 be given 6–10 units of platelets immediately prior to bronchoscopy if transbronchial lung biopsy is contemplated (7). In addition to chronic renal disease, platelet function may be adversely affected by drugs such as aspirin. After the ingestion of 650 mg of aspirin, an increase in the average bleeding time in normal subjects may persist for as long as 4 days. This increase in bleeding time is increased beyond the normal range in only half of normal subjects. The factors influencing the bleeding time are complex, but the forearm bleeding time can be useful in the diagnostic evaluation of platelet dysfunction (8).

Pulmonary Function Impairment

Depending on the patient's clinical status, preoperative assessment of patients may include some measure of pulmonary function including arterial blood gas determination. As with patients with acute arrhythmias, acute hypoxemia or acute hypercapnia should be corrected and the patient stabilized prior to proceeding with the examination (see Chapter 30, this volume, for further details).

Informed Consent

Once the indications and the potential risk for the patient have been considered, one should obtain informed consent from the patient or the patient's representative. Depending on the practice setting, informed consent should be documented in the patient's record or on a form designed for bronchoscopy to be kept with the patient's record. Using a review of the patient's medical status relative to potential complications as a baseline, a discussion with the patient, close relatives, or legal guardian, if necessary, should include not only the goals of the planned procedure but the possible risk and complications as well. One should remember to obtain informed consent before giving preoperative medication that includes sedatives. In some cases an interpreter may be necessary to adequately inform the patient. One may also use patient education materials effectively. Audiovisual material or pamphlets describing the planned procedure may provide reinforcement of the personal discussion with the patient. Specific instructions should be given regarding what is expected of the patient prior to the examination. Careful attention should be given to any questions or concerns the patient has about the planned procedure. Reassurance regarding unfounded fears will help establish rapport and the patient's full and relaxed cooperation.

If bronchoscopic lung biopsy is to be performed, the patient should be instructed in the importance of controlling cough and in reporting pleural pain if it occurs. A system of hand signals or other gestures facilitates communication during the performance of bronchoscopic lung biopsy (Chapter 11, this volume).

Fasting Instructions

We recommend that patients fast for 6 hr prior to the examination. This would require that the patient not eat or drink anything after midnight prior to the examination the following morning. If the examination is to be performed in the afternoon, one might permit the patient to have a small amount of clear liquid or black coffee and a piece of dry toast prior to 8:00 a.m. on the day of the examination. The patient may take oral medications with a small amount of water on the morning of the examination. The patient should be asked to remove materials such as chewing gum or removable dentures prior to the examination.

Premedication

The possibility of drug allergies should be considered in all patients prior to the administration of any drugs. Preoperative drugs to provide analgesia and sedation such as codeine, morphine, or meperidine may be combined with an antisialogogue such as atropine or glycopyrrolate and given intramuscularly 30–45 min prior to the examination (see Chapter 7, this volume). If additional sedation is anticipated, an intravenous line may be established for this purpose. This would also provide access to a vein should emergency drugs be needed in patients with increased risk for complication.

IN THE OPERATING ROOM

Topical Anesthesia

Certain basic equipment and appropriate drugs are required to facilitate application of topical anesthesia (Fig. 1). After the instrument and route of introduction are chosen, lidocaine is an effective topical anesthetic for an awake bronchoscopy. For flexible bronchoscopy using the transnasal approach, the nose should first be evaluated for structural deformities causing obstruction. An atomizer may be used to apply lidocaine in concentrations of 2–4% directly to the nasal mucosa preceded by the application of phenylephrine, 0.5% as a vasoconstrictor decongestant. Cotton-tipped applicators saturated with lidocaine, 2%, in carboxymethylcellulose may also be used effectively in the nose. For the oropharynx, glottis, and valleculae, one may choose to have the patient gargle a few milliliters of 2–4% lidocaine and expectorate the material. One can also use an atomizer of lidocaine or a multiple-dose canister of local anesthetic to initially anesthetize the oropharynx and adjacent structures. Facing the patient, one may now instill local anesthetic into the tracheobronchial tree using indirect laryngoscopy (Fig. 2). It is convenient to use a 10-ml ampule of lidocaine, 2%, containing a total of 200 mg. Five milliliters may be used for the initial preparation leaving 5 ml for subsequent use during the bronchoscopy if needed. After wrapping the patient's tongue with a piece of gauze, the patient is asked to hold the tongue while the glottis is viewed through the examining mirror. Aliquots of lidocaine may then be instilled using a syringe and

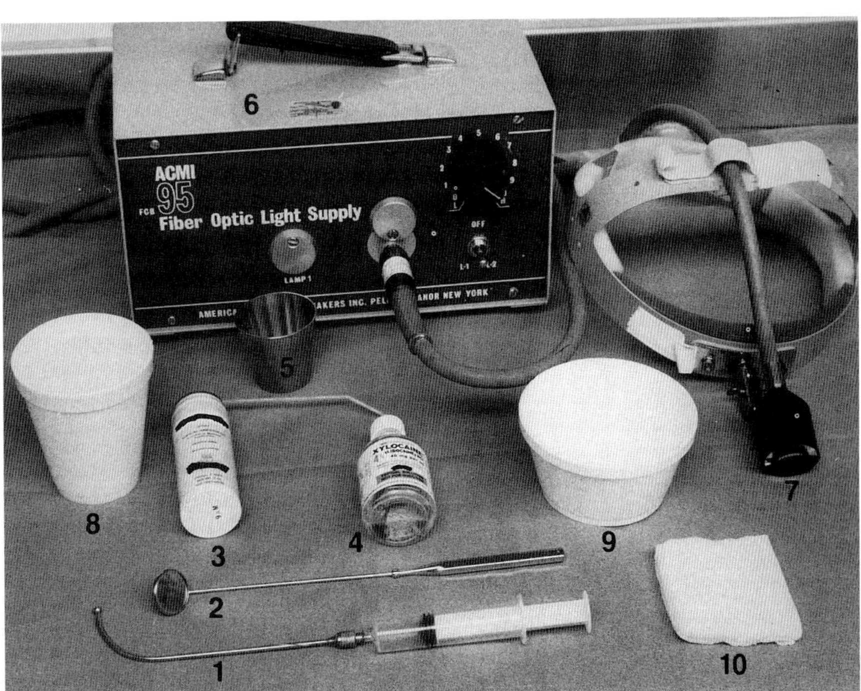

FIG. 1. Instrument setup for topical anesthetic application: (1) curved metal cannula attached to a syringe containing 3–4 ml of 4% lidocaine; (2) indirect laryngeal mirror to visualize vocal cords during application of topical anesthetic with curved metal cannula; (3) cannister containing aerosolizable topical anesthetic; (4) 4% lidocaine; (5) metal cup containing 4% lidocaine; (6) fiberoptic cold-light source; (7) headlight to visualize larynx during topical anesthetic application; (8) cup with warm water to defog laryngeal mirror; (9) emesis basin; and (10) gauze to secure and immobilize patient's tongue. (From Ref. 1, with permission.)

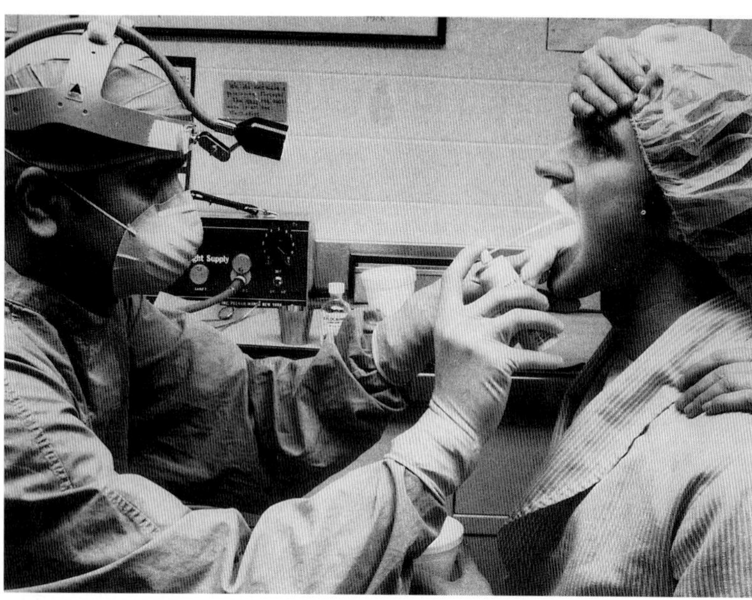

FIG. 2. Topical anesthetic application. With patient seated upright, the tongue is secured and immobilized. Aerosolized anesthetic is sprayed to the back of the throat. Then, using a laryngeal mirror and cannula with syringe, 4% lidocaine is trickled down onto the vocal cords and proximal trachea. (From Ref. 1, with permission.)

curved cannula, first onto the vocal cords and valleculae, and then through the cords into the trachea. Adequate time spent during this part of the procedure reaps significant rewards in patient comfort during the procedure (9). Topical anesthetic may also be administered through a tracheostomy tube or stoma if needed. An ultrasonic nebulizer has also been used effectively for the administration of topical anesthesia to the airways (10). Transtracheal instillation of a local anesthetic or local nerve block is a techique that has also been successfully used for bronchoscopy (Chapter 7, this volume) (11).

Modification of the technique of administering the topical anesthetic is necessary for patients who are ill and unable to sit upright. It may be necessary to administer the anesthetic while the patient is on a cart with the head of the cart elevated. The topical anesthetic may also be administered with the patient supine through the operating channel of the flexible bronchoscope. One-milliliter aliquots of topical anesthetic may be applied successively until the desired topical anesthesia is achieved. The application of topical anesthesia by an atomizer prior to use of this technique is helpful. Topical anesthesia is acceptable for the majority of patients. General anesthesia, however, may be desirable for patients who are very apprehensive, pediatric patients, and as part of special techniques such as laser work or stent placement in the major airways. Adapters with a close-fitting diaphragm attached to the endotracheal tube can be used effectively for flexible bronchoscopy under general anesthesia. Ventilating bronchoscopes are available for procedures requiring general anesthesia with rigid open tube instruments.

Positioning of the Patient for Examination

Flexible bronchoscopy can be performed with the patient seated or supine, in a bed, in the intensive care unit, or in the outpatient setting. Outpatient examinations should be performed in an operating room or in a procedure room dedicated for that purpose. Equipment and drugs should be readily available to deal with emergencies that may arise including cardiopulmonary resuscitation if necessary. The supine position is comfortable for the patient and ideal for monitoring of the blood pressure, electrocardiogram, and oximetry as indicated. At this point, one should consider giving additional sedation (see Chapter 7 of this volume), bronchodilators by inhalation, or nitroglycerin prophylactically if indicated. Other medications may be administered intravenously as needed or required. In the supine position, it is desirable to cover the eyes with protective pads that may be secured with a towel wrapped around the eyes and secured with a towel clip. At this point, a bite block should be inserted into the mouth, primarily to protect the flexible bronchoscope. If rigid bronchoscopy is planned, an assistant may be asked to hold the patient's head appropriately during the procedure.

Beginning the Examination

The flexible bronchoscope can be inserted through a rigid bronchoscope (12), transnasally (13–15), through the mouth without or with an endotracheal tube (16), or by tracheostomy (17). Supplemental oxygen may be administered through the ventilating rigid open tube bronchoscope if desired. Nasal prongs or a mask can provide supplemental oxygen for the transnasal approach. An adapter attached to an oxygen supply works well for providing supplemental oxygen if an endotracheal or nasotracheal tube is used. A tight-fitting diaphragm or inflated cuff is not necessary if the patient is awake and breathing normally. The need for or the success of oxygen supplementation during flexible bronchoscopy can be readily monitored with pulse oximetry. Once the bite block is in place, a brief inspection of the airways might also be accomplished without the use of an endotracheal tube. One may pass an endotracheal tube before insertion of the flexible bronchoscope using indirect laryngoscopy and an endotracheal tube with a stylet (12). In our experience, endotracheal intubation may be readily accomplished by initially intubating the trachea with the flexible bronchoscope and passing the endotracheal tube over the flexible bronchoscope through the vocal cords into the trachea (Fig. 3) (1,16). Once the endotracheal tube is in place, it may be secured with a piece of tape, and an adapter for providing supplemental oxygen may be attached. The patient is now ready for the examination.

Preparation and care of the patient before, during, and after bronchoscopy is a team effort. A nurse or trained paramedic may be the first person to review the planned procedure and provide support and relief from apprehension that may be experienced. All personnel directly involved with patients undergoing bronchoscopy should be familiar with the procedure, its risk, and its complications. The personnel responsible for giving the preoperative medication should be

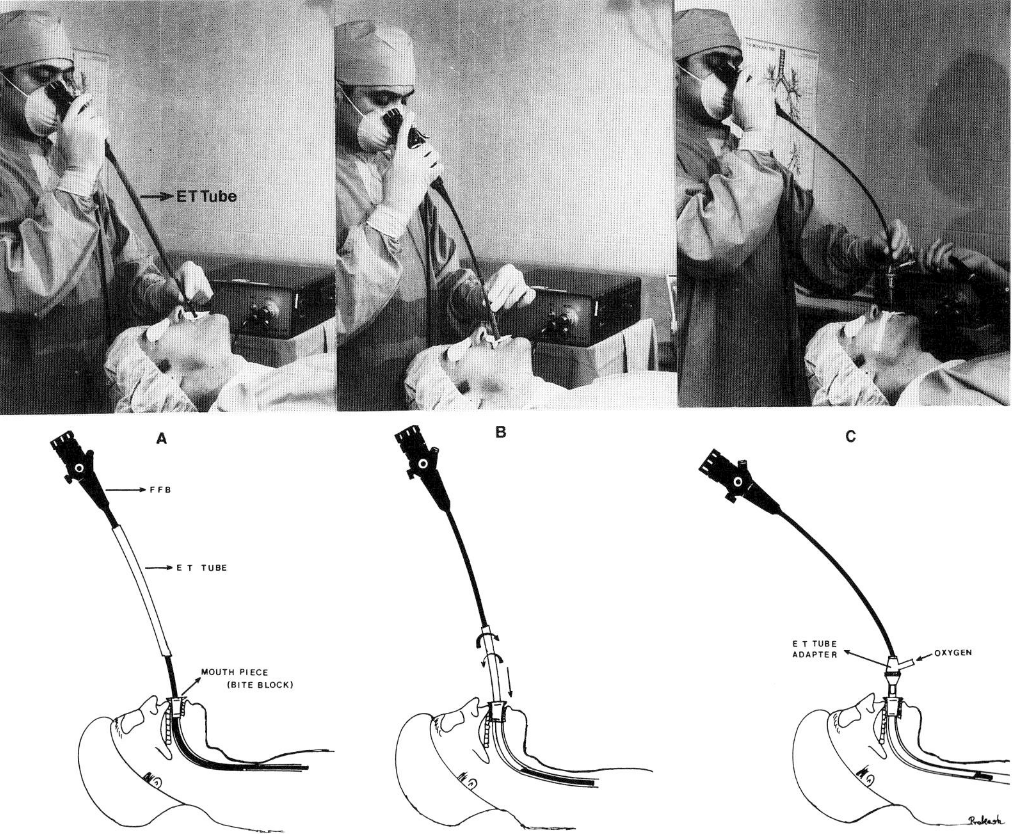

FIG. 3. Technique of orotracheal intubation using flexible bronchoscope (FB). **(A)**, After the oropharynx and larynx are anesthetized, the patient is placed on the operating table and the eyes are covered with soft eye pads. A plastic bite block is placed between the teeth to protect the FB. A soft, uncuffed latex endotracheal (ET) tube is threaded over the FB. The distal tip of the FB is then inserted through the bite block and larynx and held steady in the distal trachea. **(B)**, The ET tube is slid downward over FB in a circular motion until the distal tip of the ET tube reaches the junction of the mid and lower thirds of trachea. FB is then withdrawn from the ET tube. **(C)**, Proximal part of ET tube is fastened by means of tape to the patient's facial skin. ET tube adapter is inserted into the proximal portion of ET tube and supplemental oxygen tube attached to the side vent. Examination of tracheobronchial tree is then begun by passing the FB through the ET tube adapter and ET tube. (From Ref. 1, with permission.)

especially aware of the importance of documenting allergies, the patient's fasting status, and the use of medications that might suggest the presence of a condition involving increased risk for the patient. Thus, conscientious, well-trained personnel may prevent an oversight from resulting in a potentially serious complication. Continuing medical education programs (see Chapters 29 and 30) can be very helpful in maintaining the skills and knowledge of the medical and paramedical personnel involved with bronchoscopy. The work of each member of the team is important if bronchoscopy is to be performed in a manner that is effective and provides the patient with acceptable comfort and safety.

AFTER BRONCHOSCOPY

Following bronchoscopy, a period of observation in an area dedicated to and equipped for this purpose is appropriate. The intensity and duration of observation should be based on sound clinical judgment influenced by the patient's general medical status. A young, healthy adult who has only a brief inspection of the airways should require a shorter period of observation than a patient with severe obstructive lung disease with abnormal arterial blood gases (18). Close observation in the postbronchoscopy period for patients known to have significant increased risk for complications is imperative; some patients will require hospitalization for overnight observation after the procedure. After bronchoscopy, patients should be instructed to be alert for the development of signs or symptoms suggesting late complications. The sudden development of chest pain or worsening dyspnea may be associated with pneumothorax. Significant bleeding should be reported. If narcotic or sedative premedication is administered, the patient should not drive an automobile or work with potentially dangerous equipment for the remainder of the day of the examination.

Discussion with the patient of the bronchoscopic findings and recommendations based on those findings should be reserved until sedative and narcotic effects have resolved.

REFERENCES

1. Prakash, UBS, Stubbs, SE. Bronchoscopy: indications and techniques. *Semin Resp Med* 1981;3:42–53.
2. Prakash UBS, Stubbs SE. Bronchoscopy: indications and technique. *Semin Resp Med* 1981;3:17–24.
3. American Thoracic Society. Guidelines for fiberoptic bronchoscopy in adults. *Am Rev Resp Dis* 1987;136:1066.
4. Zavala DC. *Flexible fiberoptic bronchoscopy: a training handbook.* Iowa City: University of Iowa; 1978.
5. Dajani AS, Bisno AL, Chung KJ, et al. Prevention of bacterial endocarditis: recommendations by the American Heart Association. *JAMA* 1990;264:2919–2922.
6. Cunningham AJ, Zavala DC, Corry RJ, Keim LW. Trephine air drill, bronchial brush, and fiberoptic transbronchial lung biopsies in immunosuppressed patients. *Am Rev Resp Dis* 1977; 115:213–220.
7. Zavala DC. Transbronchial biopsy in diffuse lung disease. *Chest* 1978(Suppl);73:727–733.
8. George JN, Shattil SJ. The clinical importance of acquired abnormalities of platelet function (review article). *N Engl J Med* 1991;324:27–39.
9. Stradling P, Stradling JR. *Diagnostic bronchoscopy: a teaching manual*, 5th ed. London: Churchill Livingstone; 1986.
10. Christoforidis AJ, Tomashefski JF, Mitchell RI. Use of an ultrasonic nebulizer for the apploication of oropharyngeal, laryngeal, and tracheobronchial anesthesia. *Chest* 1971;59:629–633.
11. Fry WA. Techniques of topical anesthesia for bronchoscopy. *Chest* 1978(Suppl);73:694–696.
12. Ikeda S, Yanai N, Ishikawa S. Flexible bronchofiberscope. *Keio J Med* 1968;17:1–18.
13. Wanner A, Amikam B, Sackner MA. *Chest* 1972;61:287–288.
14. Sackner MA. State of the art: bronchofiberscopy. *Am Rev Resp Dis* 1975;111:62–88.
15. Harrell JH II. Transnasal approach for fiberoptic bronchoscopy. *Chest* 1978(Suppl);73:704–706.
16. Hodgkin JE, Rosenow EC III, Stubbs SE. Diagnostic and therapeutic techniques in thoracic medicine. *Chest* 1975;68:88–90.
17. Stubbs SE, Rosenow EC III. Flexible fiberoptic bronchoscopy. *Minn Med* 1973;56:831–835.
18. Albertini RI, Harrell JH II, Kurihara N, Moser KM. Arterial hypoxemia induced by fiberoptic bronchoscopy. *JAMA* 1974; 230:1666–1667.

Bronchoscopy,
edited by U. B. S. Prakash.
Mayo Foundation © 1994.
Published by Raven Press, Ltd., New York.

CHAPTER 9

Technical Solutions to Common Problems in Bronchoscopy

Udaya B. S. Prakash, Denis A. Cortese, and Samuel E. Stubbs

There are no specific standards established for any of the bronchoscopic techniques or procedures. The training of new pulmonary physicians in bronchoscopic techniques has to a great degree depended on their own teachers' training in the procedure and postgraduate courses. This has led to wide variations in the application of the bronchoscopic techniques in clinical practice (1). As with any surgical technique, bronchoscopic procedures also pose difficulties for the novice. With experience, each bronchoscopist develops personal preferences and expertise so as to obtain maximum diagnostic and therapeutic efficacy from the procedure. Several publications have described certain technical procedures used in bronchoscopy, but the coverage of problems and nuances associated with various techniques has been minimal (2–10).

Many of the specialized techniques employed in bronchoscopy practice are discussed in other chapters in this book. In this chapter, we discuss certain generally used techniques and provide practical solutions to commonly encountered problems in bronchoscopy practice. Much of the discussion here is based on our personal experiences. We recognize that there may be other solutions to the problems discussed below.

PREBRONCHOSCOPY CONSIDERATIONS

Preparation of the Patient

Anticipation and preparedness are two important factors that minimize complications and help improve the efficacy of bronchoscopy. The preparation of the patient for bronchoscopy was discussed in the previous chapter. Before the patient is subjected to bronchoscopy, it is important for the bronchoscopist and her or his team to go through a mental or a written checklist (Table 1) so that bronchoscopy is performed smoothly and the potential complications are anticipated and prevented (4,11,12). Depending on the results of the questions in the checklist, the bronchoscopist must modify plans for the procedure as indicated.

TABLE 1. *Prebronchoscopy checklist*

1. Is there an appropriate indication for bronchoscopy?
2. Has there been a previous bronchoscopy?
3. If the answer to the above question is yes, were there any problems or complications?
4. Does the patient [and close relative(s) if patient is unable to communicate] fully understand the goals, risks, and complications of bronchoscopy?
5. Does the patient's past medical history (allergy to medications and topical anesthesia) and present clinical condition pose special problems or predispose to complications?
6. Are all the appropriate tests completed and the results available?
7. Are the premedications appropriate and the dosages correct?
8. Does the patient require special consideration before (e.g., corticosteroid for asthma, insulin for diabetes mellitus, or prophylaxis against bacterial endocarditis) or during (supplemental oxygen, extra sedation) bronchoscopy?
9. Is the plan for post-bronchoscopy care appropriate?
10. Are all the appropriate instruments and personnel available to assist during the procedure and to handle the potential complications?

U. B. S. Prakash and S. E. Stubbs: Division of Thoracic Diseases and Internal Medicine, Mayo Clinic, Rochester, Minnesota 55905.

D. A. Cortese: Division of Thoracic Diseases and Internal Medicine, Mayo Clinic, Jacksonville, Forida 32224.

Premedications and Sedatives

The use of appropriate premedications and intravenous sedation (Chapter 7, this volume) will help one smoothly and speedily complete the bronchoscopy. If a patient is allergic to any of the medications scheduled to be used before or during bronchoscopy, then an alternative medication should be considered. A sound understanding of the basic pharmacological aspects of the commonly used medications in bronchoscopic practice is essential. Some authors have reported that bronchoscopy can be carried out with no premedication (13), but we believe that avoidance of premedication and sedation in all patients on a routine basis is unjustified. Routine use of an anticholinergic drug such as atropine or glycopyrrolate is generally recommended to reduce secretions and to prevent bradycardia (14–18). In addition to an anticholinergic, a drug capable of producing sedation or anxiolysis (e.g., codeine, meperidine, morphine, or barbiturate) should be administered approximately 30–45 min before the procedure. In the event that one cannot use a topical anesthetic, the bronchoscopist has to consider deep intravenous sedation or general anesthesia. Intravenous fentanyl has both sedative and anesthetic effects that can expedite the procedure.

Topical Anesthesia

If general anesthesia or deep intravenous sedation is not used or contraindicated, topical anesthesia is an absolute necessity in most adult and pediatric patients. The commonly used topical anesthetic agents include lidocaine, benzocaine, bupivacaine, procaine, tetracaine, and cocaine. There are several methods of administration of topical anesthesia, depending on whether the nasal or the oral route is used for insertion of the bronchoscope. Intravenous fentanyl has both sedative and anesthetic effects that can expedite the procedure.

Nasal Anesthesia

Most bronchoscopists use lidocaine (2%), spray or viscous form, to anesthetize the nasal passages. Some use vasoconstrictor agents such as phenylephrine or cocaine to effect decongestion of the nasal mucosa and thereby increase the cross-section of the nasal passage. The patient's head is hyperextended and the viscous or liquid lidocaine is dripped into the nasal passage. Then the opposite nasal passage is closed with finger and the patient is asked to sniff the anesthetic deep into the nasopharynx. Another alternative is to dip a cotton swab in the topical anesthetic, insert it into the nasal passage, and allow the medications to anesthetize the mucosa. Once the proximal nasal passage is anesthetized, the bronchoscope itself can be used as an anesthetizing instrument to anesthetize the distal nasal passage and the supraglottic areas by instilling the liquid lidocaine through the working channel of the bronchoscope as the instrument is gradually inserted into distal areas of the upper airways.

Oropharyngeal Anesthesia

In our practice, after the administration of premedication, the patient is asked to sit in a chair for both nasal and oral preparation while the bronchoscopist sits opposite the patient. The patient is given a cup in which to expectorate oral secretions. With the help of a tongue depressor, either benzocaine or lidocaine is sprayed to coat the oropharynx including the uvula and base of the tongue. The purpose of this initial anesthetic spray is to decrease the patient's tendency to gag during bronchoscopy and for the application of topical anesthetic to the remaining airways.

The dosages of topical anesthetics used in the supraglottic areas should be closely monitored. Excessive use of tetracaine, cetacaine, and other topical anesthetics has resulted in severe methemoglobinemia (19–21). The presence of candidiasis involving the oropharynx or the nasopharynx is reported to enhance absorption of local anesthetic from the affected mucosa and hence predispose to methemoglobinemia (22). To prevent this complication, we recommend that these topical anesthetics be sprayed in the supraglottic area for no more than 5–7 sec and each spraying maneuver should last for 0.5–2 sec. The patient should be allowed to catch her or his breath and clear the throat in between sprays. Timing the initial sprays to avoid inspiration may reduce the likelihood of inducing laryngospasm.

Laryngeal Anesthesia

After the oropharynx and the epiglottis are anesthetized, the patient is asked to stick her or his tongue as far out of the mouth as possible. The tongue is then wrapped in a thin gauze and held outside the mouth by either the patient or an assistant. Using a laryngoscopy mirror in one hand and the syringe with lidocaine in the other, the glottic structures are identified and lidocaine is dripped drop by drop onto the laryngeal structures including the epiglottis, arytenoid folds, false and true vocal cords, and subglottic mucosa. At this point, it is not important to anesthetize the trachea. Another method is to aerosolize the topical anesthetic agent by means of an ultrasonic nebulizer system (23). We find that this process is time consuming and may not concentrate the anesthetic agent in vital areas. Many patients who are not familiar with the use of ultrasonic nebulizers tend to swallow the anesthetic agent and therefore the airway does not get properly anesthetized. When performed correctly, the nebulizer technique can be very effective.

As in the preparation of the nasal passage, after the oropharynx is optimally anesthetized, the bronchoscope itself can be used to anesthetize the laryngeal and subglottic structures. This is also known as the spray-as-you-go technique and a vast majority of bronchoscopists employ it (15). Another effective method to produce excellent topical anesthesia is the use of laryngeal nerve blockade (24). The procedural details of transtracheal or cricoid block and superior laryngeal block are outlined in Chapter 7 of this volume. In a British survey of 231 bronchoscopists, it was reported that 29% of the bronchoscopists used the cricoid puncture (15).

Tracheobronchial Anesthesia

The bronchoscope is the best instrument to apply topical anesthesia to the tracheobronchial mucosa. Using the working channel of the instrument, small aliquots (0.5–1.0 ml) of lidocaine should be forcefully injected through a syringe. Since the working channel of a standard flexible bronchoscope has a volume of 3.5–6 ml, it is essential that the instillation of the topical anesthetic be forceful in order to eject the liquid out of the bronchoscope and be followed by injection of 5–8 ml of air soon after. To be effective, the working channel of the bronchoscope should be cleared of mucus and blood before instilling the topical anesthetic. Another practical point is that the topical anesthetic be allowed to stay on the mucosa for at least 10 sec and not be suctioned back into the bronchoscope as soon as it is injected through the instrument.

The blood concentration after topical application of lidocaine may be 30–50% of that obtained by rapid intravenous administration (25). Lidocaine is safer than tetracaine, with a more predictable sequence of toxicity (25–27). A total dose of lidocaine below 300 mg is well tolerated in a normal adult, with little risk of clinical toxicity or toxic blood levels (19,28). The dosage should be adjusted for the patient's weight, and also if the patient has had lidocaine for some other reason. Some individuals, particularly heavy smokers, may require higher doses. Higher doses, if necessary, should be administered with caution to patients with cardiac or hepatic disorders and to those with mucosal candidiasis. Many bronchoscopists routinely mix lidocaine with epinephrine before attempting a mucosal or bronchoscopic lung biopsy. The rationale and the usefulness of this is discussed in Chapter 17 of this volume.

Control of Gag Reflex

An urge to gag is a reflex phenomenon exhibited by many patients during the application of topical anesthesia and initial insertion of the bronchoscope. The intensity of gagging varies from patient to patient and the route of insertion of the bronchoscope. Gagging is more likely if bronchoscope is inserted orally. Indeed, the initial topical anesthetic is aimed at controlling the gagging reflex. If this is not possible, there are certain measures that can be undertaken to abolish or minimize this problem. The patient should be instructed to breathe in a slow but nonstop panting manner and to concentrate on this breathing pattern. The bronchoscopist should avoid pressure on or contact with the patient's tongue as much as possible. Before beginning the application of topical anesthetic, the patient should be made to gargle and swish (in the oropharynx) 2–3 ml of liquid lidocaine. Proper aerosolization of topical anesthetic by ultrasonic nebulizer may avoid the contact with the tongue and other sensitive oropharyngeal areas. Another means to avoid the sensitive structures is to insert the bronchoscope nasally. Deep intravenous sedation may also abolish gagging. In extreme situations, general anesthesia may be the only suitable alternative to the above techniques.

Control of Excessive Coughing

Excessive coughing by the patient is the main adversary of the bronchoscopist. Many a bronchoscopy procedure has been terminated because of excessive coughing. Not infrequently, certain procedures such as bronchoscopic lung biopsy cannot be performed safely if the patient coughs excessively. Cough is more likely to occur in those with chronic bronchitis secondary to tobacco abuse. Prebronchoscopy discussion with the patient regarding this and reassurance, as well as gentle censure, during the procedure are important. Antitussive medications may help some patients but in our experience there is no place for the use of these prior to bronchoscopy. Avoidance of excessive pressure on or contact with tongue and oropharyngeal structures during the insertion of the bronchoscope may help to some extent. Slow panting type of breathing as described above may also control excessive coughing. Excessive contact with and unnecessary instrumentation of tracheobronchial mucosa should be avoided by a conscious effort and meticulous technique to stay within the airway lumen. Quickness in completing the bronchoscopic examination is another approach to minimizing cough. The longer the time taken for the examination, the more likely that the effect of topical anesthetic will wear off. Excessive amounts of topical anesthetics may be needed in some

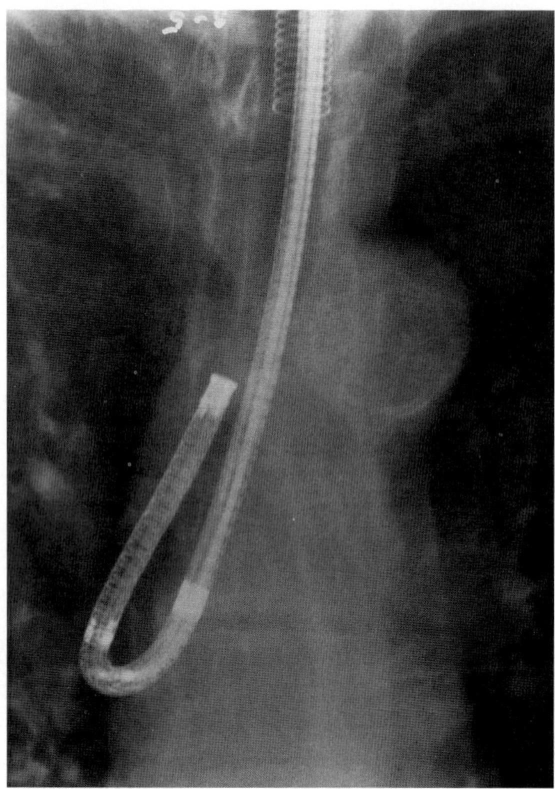

FIG. 1. An unusually rare example of excessive hard coughing resulting in acute "turnaround" of a flexible bronchoscope in the trachea. The hard coughing by the patient bent the tip of the instrument and further coughing moved the tip more proximally. The bronchoscope was gently removed with some difficulty.

instances to control excessive cough. An unusually rare complication of excessive and hard cough is shown in Fig. 1).

Deep intravenous sedation may control excessive coughing. However, it is important to recognize that when intravenous sedation is administered, the patient's ability to voluntarily control the cough is abolished and therefore coughing may worsen. If the excessive cough precludes any type of bronchoscopic procedure, than general anesthesia should be considered.

If, during an attempt at biopsy of a mucosal lesion, excessive coughing interferes with the procedure, then the patient should be instructed to hold her or his breath as long as possible. This usually results in the temporary abolition of cough and the bronchoscopist should quickly obtain the biopsy. Excessive suctioning of the mucosa also leads to coughing and should be avoided.

Endotracheal Tube

Most bronchoscopists who use the nasal passage for bronchoscopy do not insert a nasotracheal tube prior to bronchoscopy. For the insertion of a standard flexible bronchoscope, the minimal inner diameter of the nasotracheal tube should be 7.5 mm. The longer length of nasotracheal tube also produces increased resistance to passage of the bronchoscope. In patients who are already nasally intubated with a large-diameter tube, for the purposes of mechanical ventilation, for instance, bronchoscopy through the existing tube can be easily carried out. If the tube diameter does not allow passage of the bronchoscope, then the patient may have to be intubated with a larger nasotracheal tube.

The mail survey of 871 bronchoscopists in North America conducted by the American College of Chest Physicians observed that only 7% of the bronchoscopists "routinely" (in more than 85% of cases) used the endotracheal tube to facilitate bronchoscopy, whereas 14% used it "sometimes" (in 6–84% of cases), and 78% "rarely" (in less than 5% of cases) intubated their patients (1). Many of the respondents in the survey commented that they used the endotracheal tube in the following clinical settings: bronchoscopic lung biopsy, high-risk patients, respiratory failure, intensive care unit, laser bronchoscopy, serious hemorrhage, and hypoxemic patients.

We believe that soft endotracheal tubes, particularly for oral introduction of the bronchoscope, provide many advantages. First, the endotracheal tube provides an excellent control of the airway. Second, it allows administration of supplemental oxygen by a side port. Third, the frequent removal and reinsertion of the bronchoscope for cleaning the lens is facilitated. Fourth, if significant bleeding is associated with biopsy procedures, the bronchoscopist can advance the tube distally and selectively intubate the nonbleeding side so that flooding of that side by blood can be minimized and the patient can be well oxygenated. Fifth, if large biopsies are obtained, then the bronchoscope, with the biopsy forceps and biopsy specimen at the distal tip, can be removed without shearing off biopsy specimen. The same techniques can be used for obtaining specimens by brushes. Sixth, if the bleeding cannot be controlled with the flexible bronchoscope, the endotracheal tube can be used to insert suction catheters with larger lumen to suction the blood. The technique of inserting the endotracheal tube over the flexible bronchoscope is described in Chapter 8 of this volume.

SOLUTIONS TO PROBLEMS IN BRONCHOSCOPY

Inability to Bronchoscope Nasally

The larger of the two nasal passages should be utilized for passage of the flexible bronchoscope. Use of a mucosal decongestant or vasoconstrictor may facilitate entry of the bronchoscope and may reduce the chance of traumatic bleeding. Adequate lubrication is another solution to this problem. If the instrument cannot be passed through one nostril, then the opposite side should be tried. If a standard size bronchoscope cannot be inserted, a smaller (ultrathin) bronchoscope should be used. However, the smaller instruments either have very small working channels or no channels at all. Therefore, bronchoscopic biopsy may not be possible. Oral insertion of the bronchoscope is the ultimate answer to this problem.

Inability to See Laryngeal Structures

During the initial oral insertion of the bronchoscope, the oropharyngeal and laryngeal structures may not be optimally visible. This can result from excessive secretions in the oropharynx, blockage of objective lens by the mucous, or displacement of the tip of the bronchoscope by the patient's tongue and swallowing maneuvers. A small amount of liquid soap or lens-cleaning material applied to the objective lens of the flexible bronchoscope will improve the bronchoscopic image. If excessive secretions are the problem, then the bronchoscope should be removed from the oropharynx and the patient asked to swallow the oropharyngeal contents. Another solution to this problem is to suction the oropharyngeal secretions using the bronchoscope itself or a suction catheter. The tongue should be immobilized by instructing an assistant to wrap the distal tip of the tongue in gauze and pulling it out of the mouth to a distance of 2–3 cm. If none of these methods allow the passage of the bronchoscope, then deep intravenous sedation, general anesthesia, or nasal insertion of the bronchoscope should be considered.

Inability to Intubate the Larynx

In some patients, the passage of soft endotracheal tube, using the flexible bronchoscope as a guide, through the larynx into the trachea is difficult. The bronchoscopist should first ascertain that the laryngeal anatomy is normal and the endotracheal tube is not excessively large to traverse the larynx. If laryngospasm or closure of the larynx is observed, then extra application of topical anesthetic may relax the larynx. Adequate lubrication of the inner and outer lining of endotracheal tube and the exterior of the bronchoscope should be secured. A rotatory motion of the endotracheal tube may let the beveled tip of the tube enter the glottic chink and help to advance the rest of the endotracheal tube. The patient should be instructed to breathe in deeply, and during this motion the vocal cords abduct and the endotracheal tube should be quickly but gently inserted. Another method to accomplish this is to instruct the patient to cough hard. Invariably, the vocal cords abduct widely during the posttussive inspiration and this moment should be used to insert the endotracheal tube. Excessive flexion or extension of the patient's cervical spine occasionally precludes easy intubation. Another reason for the hangup of the tip of the endotracheal tube is the prominent subglottic shelf (Fig. 2). Gentle flexion and extension of patient's neck accompanied by an anterior jaw thrust may facilitate insertion of the endotracheal tube. If

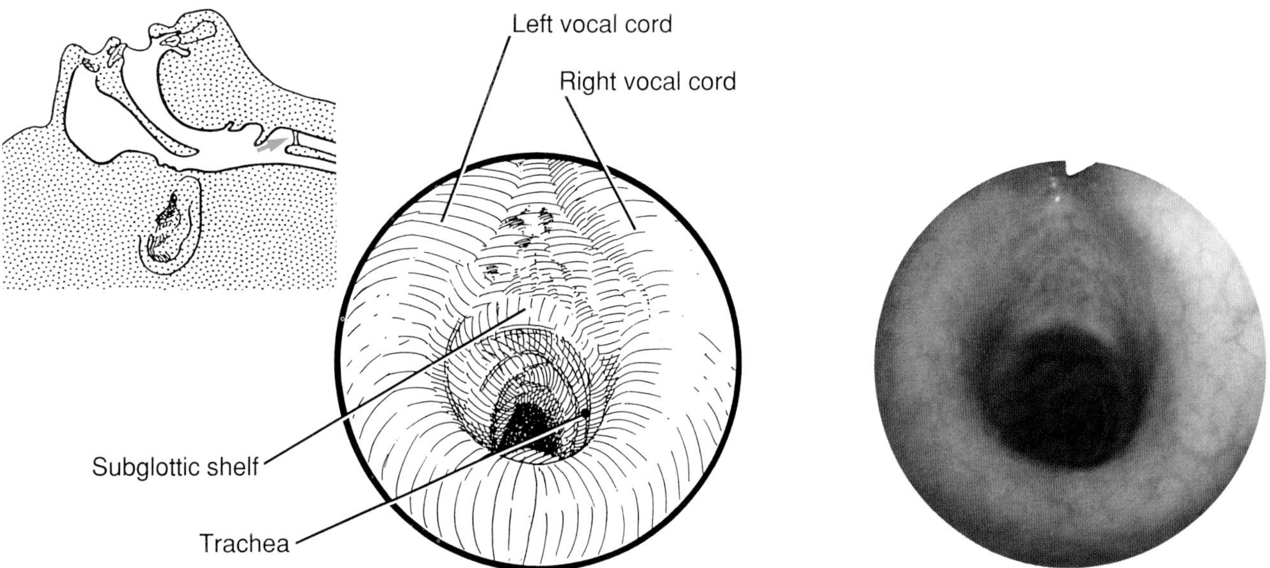

FIG. 2. Accentuation of normal subglottic shelf by hyperflexion or hyperextension of neck may make it difficult to insert an endotracheal tube.

none of these measures work, then bronchoscopy may need to be performed without an endotracheal tube. If endotracheal intubation is mandatory, intravenous sedation or general anesthesia should be used to accommodate laryngoscopy-guided insertion of the endotracheal tube.

Difficulty in Advancing the Bronchoscope

Occasionally, after passing through the larynx and subglottic trachea, it is difficult to advance the bronchoscope to the distal airways. To the bronchoscopist, it will feel as if the bronchoscope is firmly fixed to the endotracheal tube or the tracheal wall. When this happens, the bronchoscopist reassesses the size of the endotracheal tube used and replaces it with a larger tube if necessary. If a bite block or mouthpiece is not used to protect the bronchoscope, the patient's teeth or gums may be biting down on the bronchoscope and thus preventing its distal movement (Fig. 3). The use of a mouthpiece or bite block not only allows easy passage for the bronchoscope but also protects damage to the delicate instrument from patient's teeth. The bronchoscopy assistant, in an effort to secure the endotracheal tube or to protect the bronchoscope, may tightly pinch the endotracheal tube and/or the bronchoscope. This will prevent the bronchoscope from moving up or down.

Despite proper lubrication of the exterior of bronchoscope and the inner lining of the endotracheal tube, the distal progress of the bronchoscope is sometimes difficult or almost impossible. There are several problems associated with the lubricant. If the lubricant is applied long before the procedure, the dried lubricant in fact will function as an "antilubricant." Excessive lubricant use will also permit greater drying of the lubricant. Repeated application of the lubricant, in layer after layer, has a similar effect. When it becomes difficult to advance the bronchoscope, it should be removed from the trachea and the exterior cleaned with a gauze soaked in normal saline. Then a fresh thin film of lubricant should be used before reinserting the bronchoscope. A water-based lubricating agent is preferable to petroleum-based jelly because the latter damages the vinyl cover of the flexible bronchoscope. If, during the procedure, it becomes difficult to move the bronchoscope up or down, a few drops of saline deposited through the channel of the tube along the outer wall of the bronchoscope will provide excellent lubrication. We find that the normal saline is an excellent lubricant for the bronchoscope.

Bronchoscopic Suction

Many apprentice bronchoscopists, in our experience, use the suction apparatus of the flexible bronchoscope improperly. For some, it becomes a habit to apply continuous suction even when there is no mucous secretion or blood to aspirate. Continuous and excessive suction precipitates mucosal trauma and bleeding (Fig. 4), excessive coughing, and aspirates large amounts of inspired oxygen and anesthetic gases. Smaller bronchi are prone to suction trauma and bleeding, and therefore gentle suctioning is recommended. Mucous strands need not be suctioned unless they obstruct the view; instead, the bronchoscope should be passed next to them (Fig. 5). If small amounts of mucus or blood are encountered, brief and intermittent suction maneuvers should be used. One disadvantage of

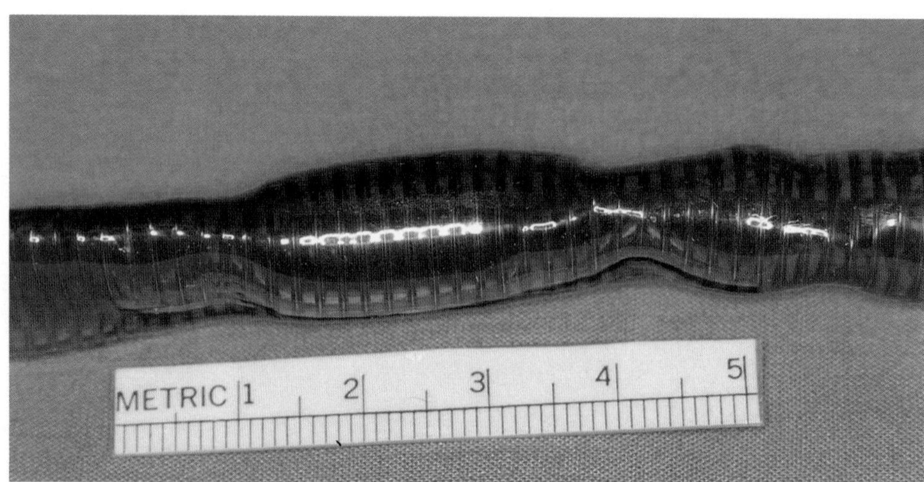

FIG. 3. Without a bite block (tooth guard) to protect the bronchoscope, the oral passage of a flexible bronchoscope can be difficult. A wire-spiral endotracheal tube crushed by a patient's teeth is shown. The bronchoscope was also severely damaged.

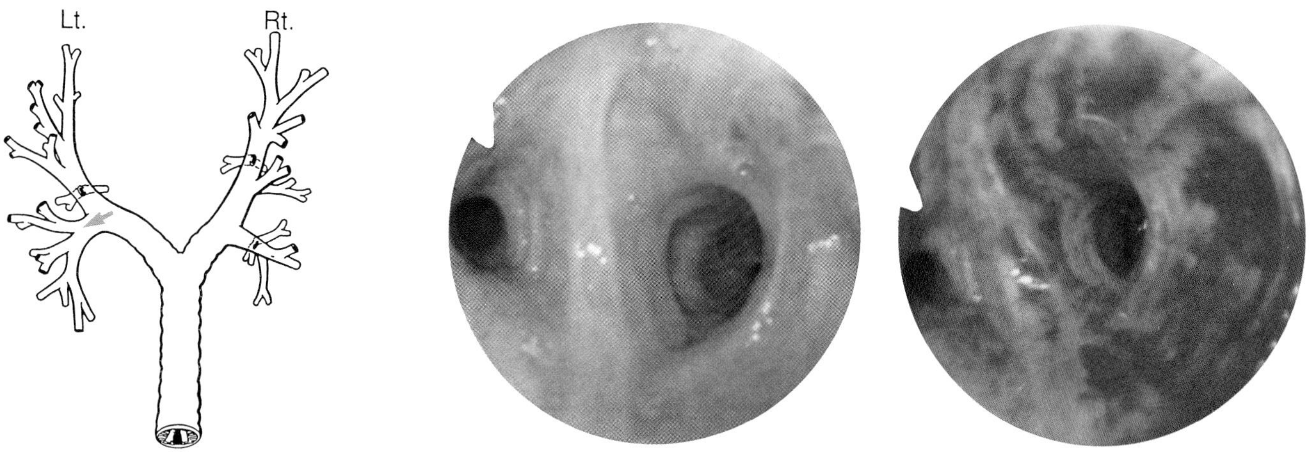

FIG. 4. Normal bronchi in the left upper lobe before bronchoscopic suction **(middle)** and same bronchi after excessive bronchoscopic suction **(right)**.

this technique is that the mucus and blood will fill the working channel (with a volume of 3.5–6 ml) of the bronchoscope, and when cytology brush or biopsy forceps is introduced, the secretions in the working channel are pushed in front of the brush or forceps and will be ejected out of the distal end of the bronchoscope to cover the objective lens and hinder the brushing and biopsy procedures. To avoid this problem, the bronchoscopists should first gently suction the secretions from the bronchi into the bronchoscope, then withdraw the instrument proximally into a larger bronchus, and then apply continuous suction for several seconds to clear the working channel. Another maneuver is to move the bronchoscope up and down rapidly, along the long axis of bronchus, with continuous suction applied to remove large amounts of secretions. This method works well especially when the patient is coughing hard and propelling the secretions proximally.

Thick secretions, mucous plugs, and blood can clog up even the larger bronchoscopes, especially when an intermittent "tap-tap" type of suctioning is applied. When this happens, the suctioning maneuver does not work. The bronchoscope should be completely removed from the tracheobronchial tree and normal saline, 5–10 ml, should be forcefully injected through the

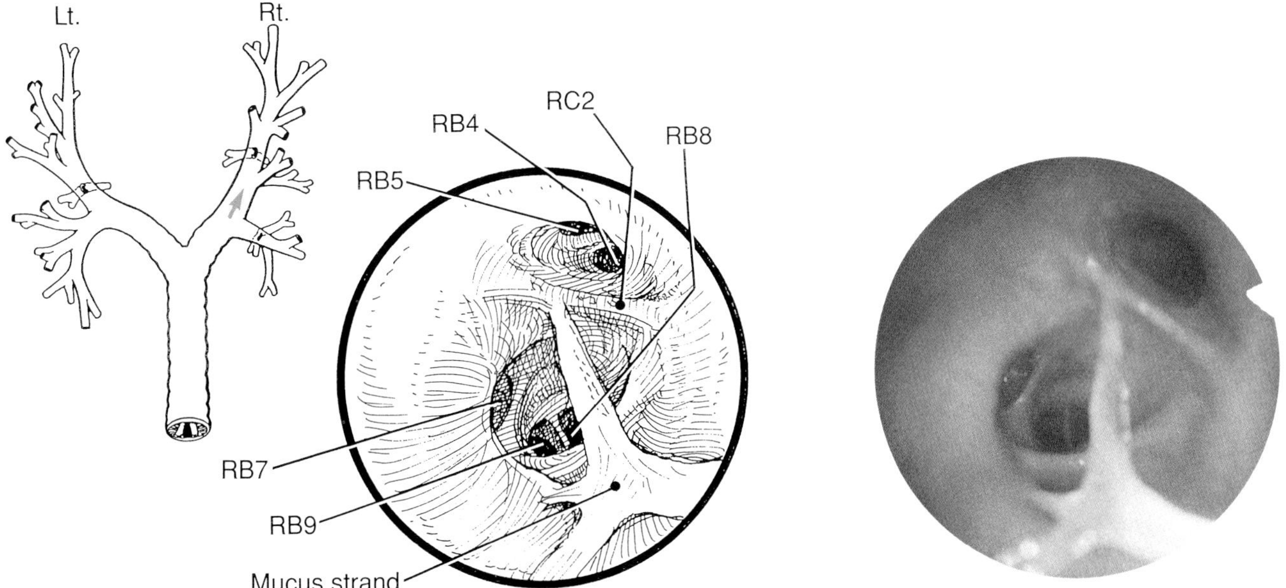

FIG. 5. Small strands of mucus in the bronchial tree need not be suctioned unless the bronchoscopic visualization is blocked.

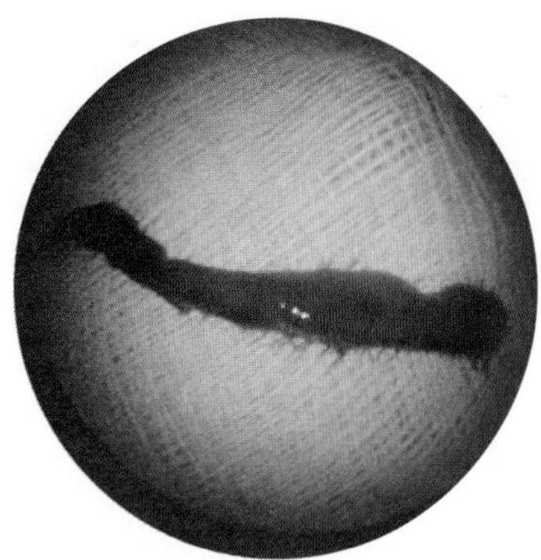

FIG. 6. A blood clot blocking the suction channel of a flexible bronchoscope ejected by forceful of saline instillation (*in vitro*) through the suction channel. The clot on a gauze pad was photographed through the bronchoscope.

proximal suction port to expel the thick secretions and blood clots out of the distal end of the bronchoscope (Fig. 6). If tracheobronchial bleeding is severe and unremitting, then continuous suctioning should be applied. If clot formation after an initial episode of bleeding is noted in a segmental bronchus, leaving the clot alone (without suctioning) is advisable (Fig. 7). The clot will eventually break up and be expectorated. Flexible bronchoscopes with smaller working channels are inefficient in suctioning even thin secretions. After suctioning smaller amounts, the bronchoscope should be removed from the tracheobronchial tree to clean the channel. Some methods for removing mucous plugs and blood clots are described in Chapter 16 of this volume.

Bronchoalveolar Lavage

The quantity of effluent collected after bronchoalveolar lavage amounts to approximately 60% of fluid instilled and it greatly varies from patient to patient. Poor returns are common. Most bronchoscopists use five aliquots of 20 ml each and apply suction after each aliquot is injected. Normally, the first return is poor, with only 3–5 ml of return. Increasing amounts are aspirated after the successive instillations. To improve the quality and quantity of the bronchoalveolar lavage effluent, the most abnormal lung segment, determined by chest roentgenography or computed tomography of chest, should be selected. The bronchoscope should be accurately wedged into the segmental bronchus. Excessive suction pressure will impede the return of bronchoalveolar lavage effluent by collapsing the airways. It is helpful if the bronchoscopist can see the bronchus through which the lavage solution is injected. The ability to see the distal bronchial segment through the lavage solution will aid in adjusting the suction pressure. Suction pressure below 100 cm H_2O is ideal. However, the suction pressure should be adjusted for each patient, depending on the lavage return and the collapsibility of distal bronchial segment. The patient should be instructed to breathe normally during the initial period of lavage return. When the lavage return decreases or stops, then the patient should be instructed to breath in deeply and hold the breath as long as possible. This attempt, if repeated 2–3 times at the end of each lavage aspiration, will greatly increase the quality and quantity of the lavage effluent.

When bronchoalveolar lavage is attempted from a dependent area of the lung, such as the posterior or superior segments of lower lobes, with the patient in

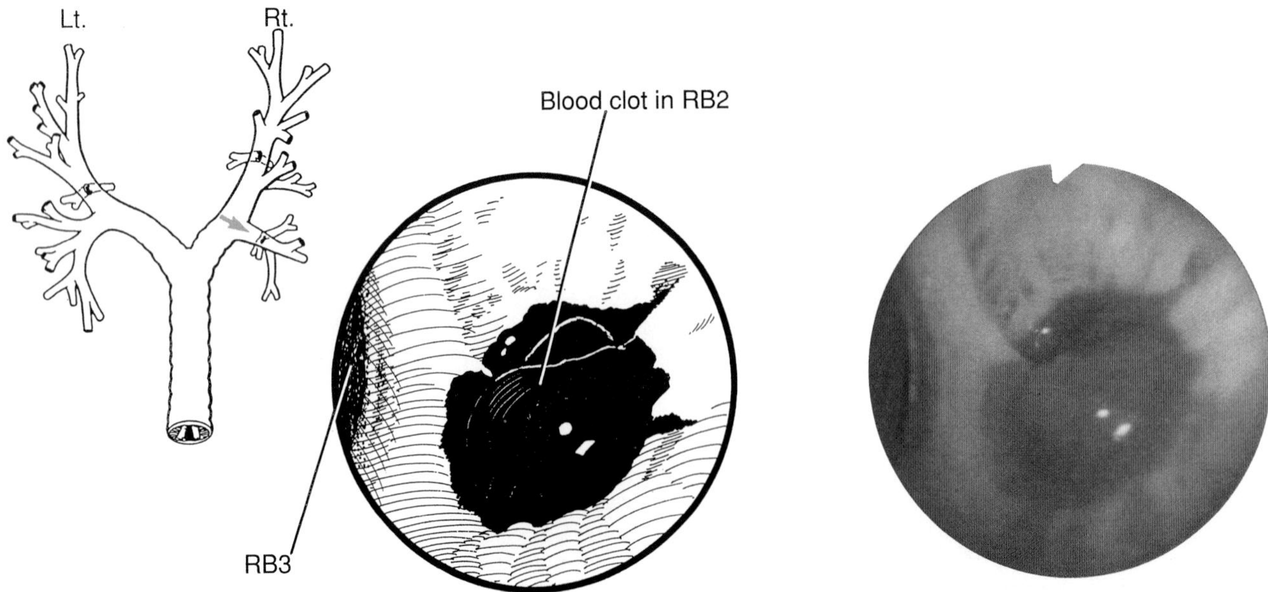

FIG. 7. A freshly formed blood clot in RB2 is left alone without suction or attempts to remove it.

supine position, the return tends to be low. If possible, the patient should be instructed to turn her or his body to one side so that the area to be lavaged is nondependent. In some patients the lavage return remains low in spite of the above maneuvers because of excessive collapsibility of distal bronchial segments. In this situation, a modified bronchoalveolar lavage technique should be considered. The bronchoscope is wedged as described above and each aliquot of lavage solution is instilled. As soon as the last part of each aliquot is injected, the bronchoscope is quickly withdrawn proximally so that the tip of the instrument is located at the entrance to the bronchus. This will prevent collapse of the airway and yet allow suctioning of the lavage effluent. Other technical details on bronchoalveolar lavage are described in Chapter 13 of this volume.

Inaccessible Bronchi

The newer flexible bronchoscopes allow the operator to reach almost all bronchi without much difficulty. However, the wide variation in individual bronchial anatomy makes it difficult to introduce the bronchoscope into the bronchi to the apical segments of upper lobes and superior segments of lower lobes. Even with total flexion of the bronchoscope, it is at times impossible to enter these bronchi. To facilitate the examination of these inaccessible bronchi, the bronchoscopist can try several maneuvers. If, for example, it is hard to enter the apical segment of the left upper lobe (B1 of LB1 + 2), flexion of the patient's neck to the opposite side (right) will enable the bronchoscope to enter the apical segment. Occasionally, only a part of the bronchus is seen in spite of flexing the bronchoscope in all directions. In this situation, the tip of the bronchoscope should be gradually slid along the wall of the bronchus to enter the bronchial lumen. If the bronchoscopist cannot fully flex her or his wrist, then moving around the patient's head, instead of firmly standing at the top of the table, will also help (Fig. 8). Using both hands to maneuver the bronchoscope is another technique that may accomplish the task. If the bronchus is small, the patient should be instructed to breathe in deeply. This method sometimes straightens the bronchus and enlarges the luminal diameter so that the bronchoscope can be advanced.

It is not uncommon for the bronchoscopists to be able to visualize the bronchus from a distance but unable to advance the bronchoscope into the bronchus. If such is the case, the bronchoscope should be maintained at a distance so as to visualize the bronchus, and a cytology brush should be introduced through the working channel into the inaccessible bronchus. Using the brush as a guide wire, the bronchoscope should be advanced distally. This method is very efficient.

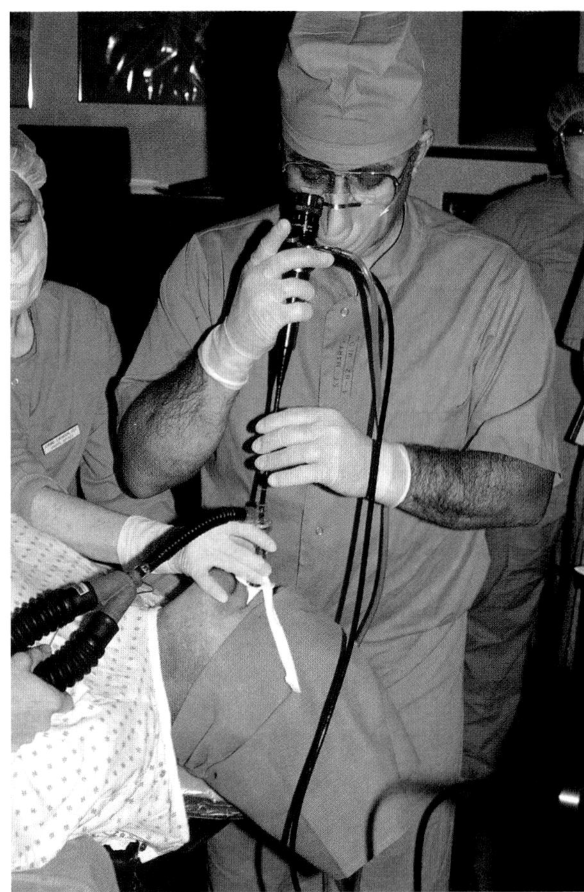

FIG. 8. In an effort to enter difficult-to-reach bronchi, the bronchoscopist should move around the patient's head if necessary to obtain optimal visualization and sampling of the bronchial tree.

Another technique that allows the entry of the bronchoscope into inaccessible bronchi relies on the flexible segment of the bronchoscope. As shown in Fig. 9, when the flexed segment of the bronchoscope assumes an angle suggested by the letter V, the distal tip of the instrument tends to move more laterally. By pushing

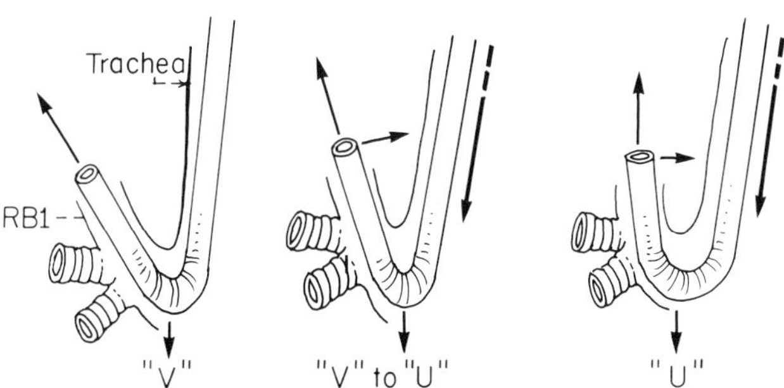

FIG. 9. Changing a V bend at the bending tip of flexible bronchoscope to a U bend by flexing the tip and simultaneously advancing the proximal portion of the instrument in an effort to reach an apical segment.

the bronchoscope "down" from above, the V can be changed to U. This allows the distal tip of the bronchoscope to move more medially to enter the B1 bronchus. If none of these methods work, then an ultrathin bronchoscope may be needed to examine the inaccessible bronchi.

Narrow or Collapsed Bronchus

It is common to encounter narrowed or collapsed bronchi, even though this finding is clinically unsuspected and there is no pathological reason for it. Etiologies for the narrowed and collapsed bronchi include congenital disorders, individual anatomic variations, the angulation of branching, pathological process in adjacent areas, extrinsic compression, antecedent pathology, and previous surgical resection. However, even a normal bronchus (without extrinsic or intrinsic airway pathology) may assume a "fish-mouth" appearance or be concentrically narrowed. The right middle lobe bronchus (RB4,5) commonly demonstrates the former. Gentle nudging of the bronchial opening and advancement of the bronchoscope may succeed in entry and proper examination of the distal airways. A slow and deep inspiration by the patient will occasionally open the apparently collapsed bronchus (Figs. 10 and 11). If these measures do not work, a cytology brush or biopsy forceps can be introduced into the collapsed bronchus to open it (Fig. 11). If the bronchial opening

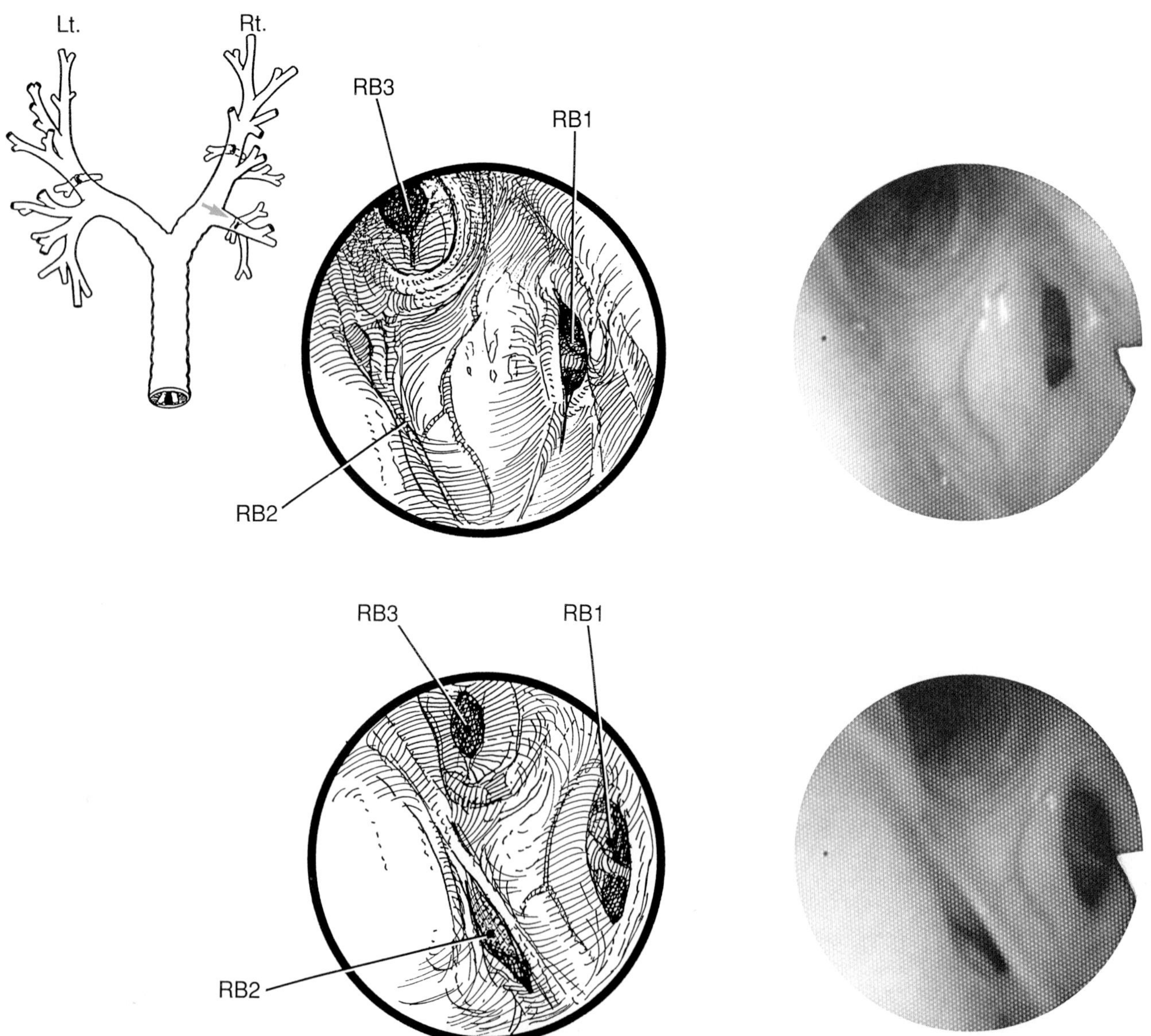

FIG. 10. An apparently collapsed RB2 during expiratory phase of breathing **(Top)** opens up during deep inspiration **(Bottom)**. There was no pathological process associated with this abnormality.

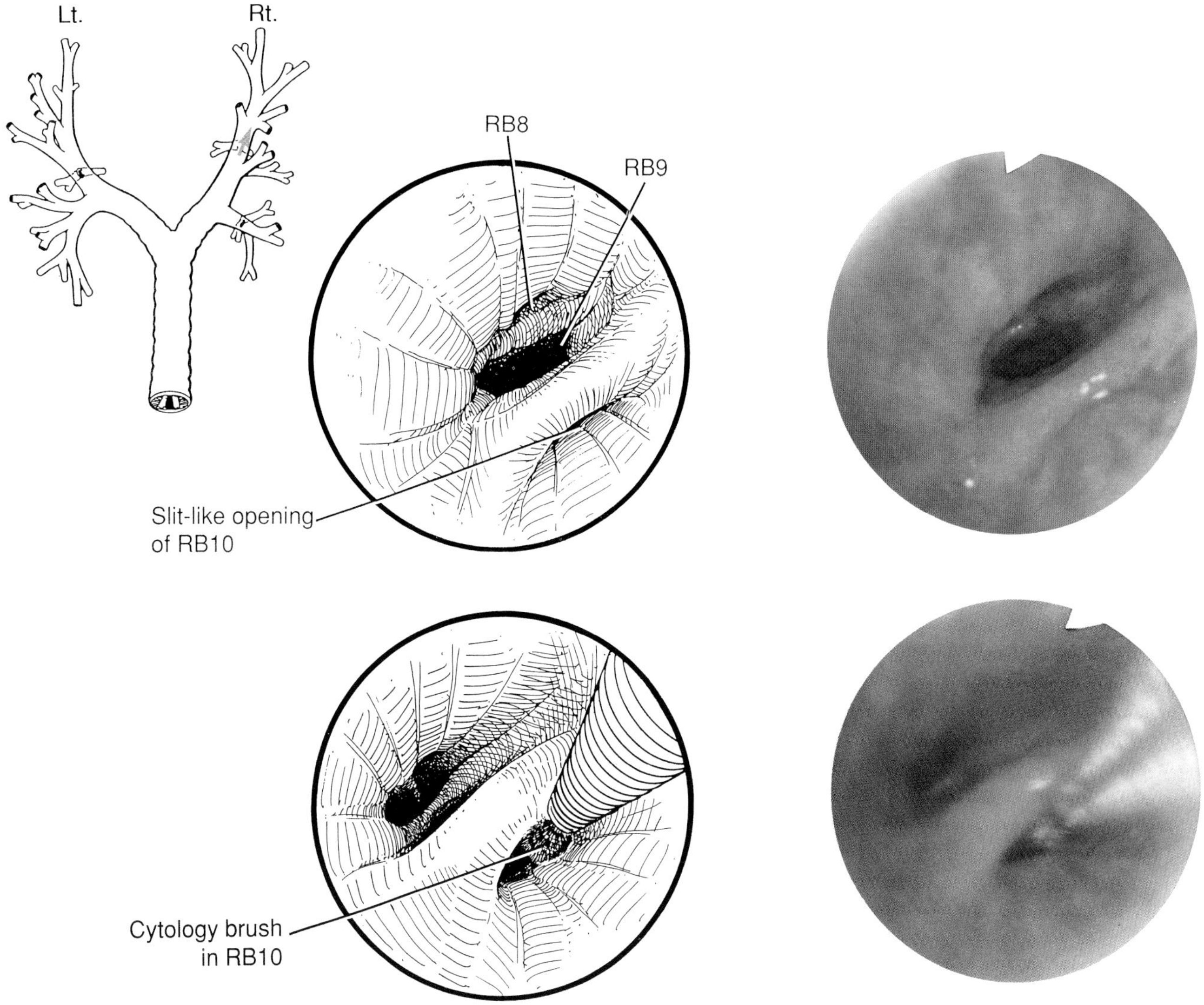

Lt. Rt.

RB8

RB9

Slit-like opening of RB10

Cytology brush in RB10

FIG. 11. Without an obvious etiology, bronchus to RB10 segment remained collapsed during both deep inspiration and expiration **(Top)**. However, a gentle nudging by cytology brush opened the bronchus and allowed examination of the distal bronchial tree **(Bottom)**.

is concentrically narrowed and looks like a stricture, it is unlikely that the bronchoscope can be advanced distally. A certain amount of force can be attempted but it may be better to try visualization using a bronchoscope with a smaller diameter.

One technique we have used successfully is saline dilatation of the bronchus. This is executed by first wedging the tip of the bronchoscope as close to the bronchial opening as possible (Fig. 12). Second, the suction is temporarily cut off so that there is no suctioning of the just-instilled saline. Third, 5–10 ml of normal saline is gently and continuously injected through the working channel while the bronchoscopist continues to observe the effect. Since the saline has no other place to go (except distally slowly), it dilates the bronchus (Fig. 13). The bronchoscopist can clearly

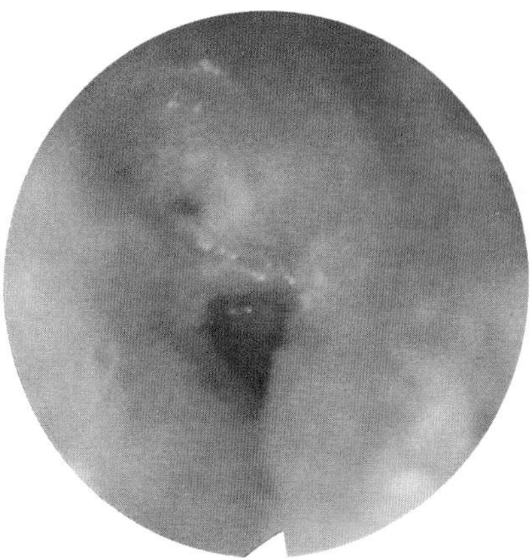

FIG. 12. The bronchus to right middle lobe is narrow and did not open on deep inspiration.

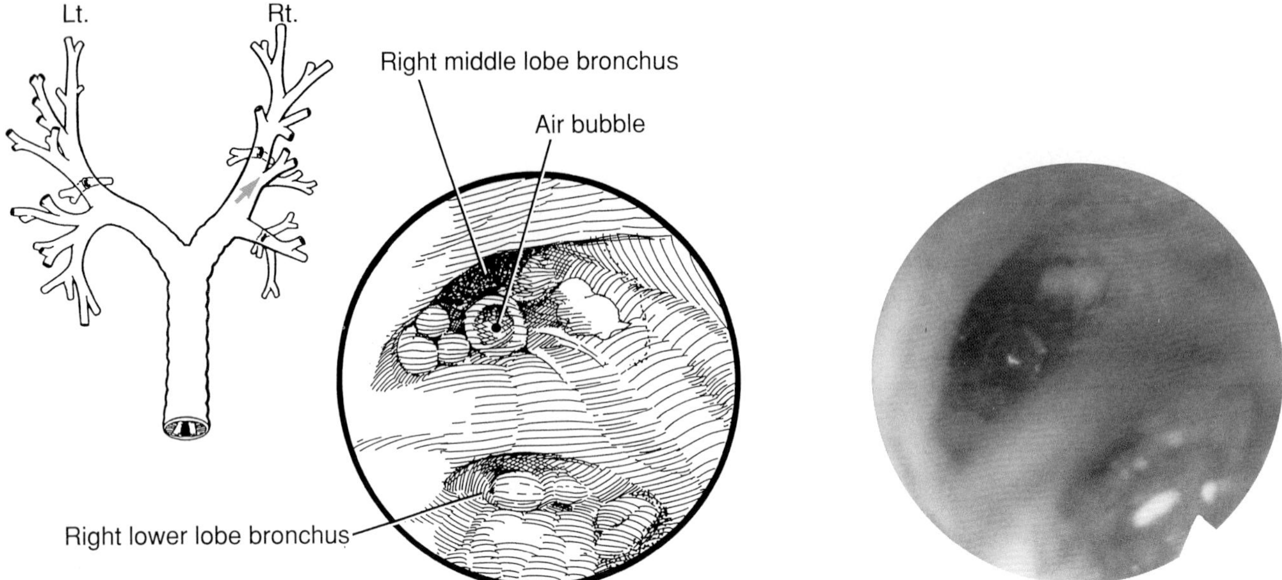

FIG. 13. Samé case as in Fig. 12. After the tip of a flexible bronchoscope was wedged into proximal opening of the right middle lobe bronchus, a forceful saline instillation dilated the bronchus. Without suctioning the instilled saline, an endobronchial examination (and photography) was successfully performed *through* the saline. No obvious pathology was noted distally.

visualize the distal bronchial tree through the saline and may attempt to advance the bronchoscope. More importantly, unexpected endobronchial abnormalities can be uncovered by this technique (Fig. 14). After the visualization is completed, the suction apparatus should be reattached to suction the saline.

Poor Visibility During Brush and Biopsy

Excessive secretions in the respiratory tract cause difficulty in brushing and obtaining a biopsy of mucosal lesions. Before attempting brushing or biopsy, the

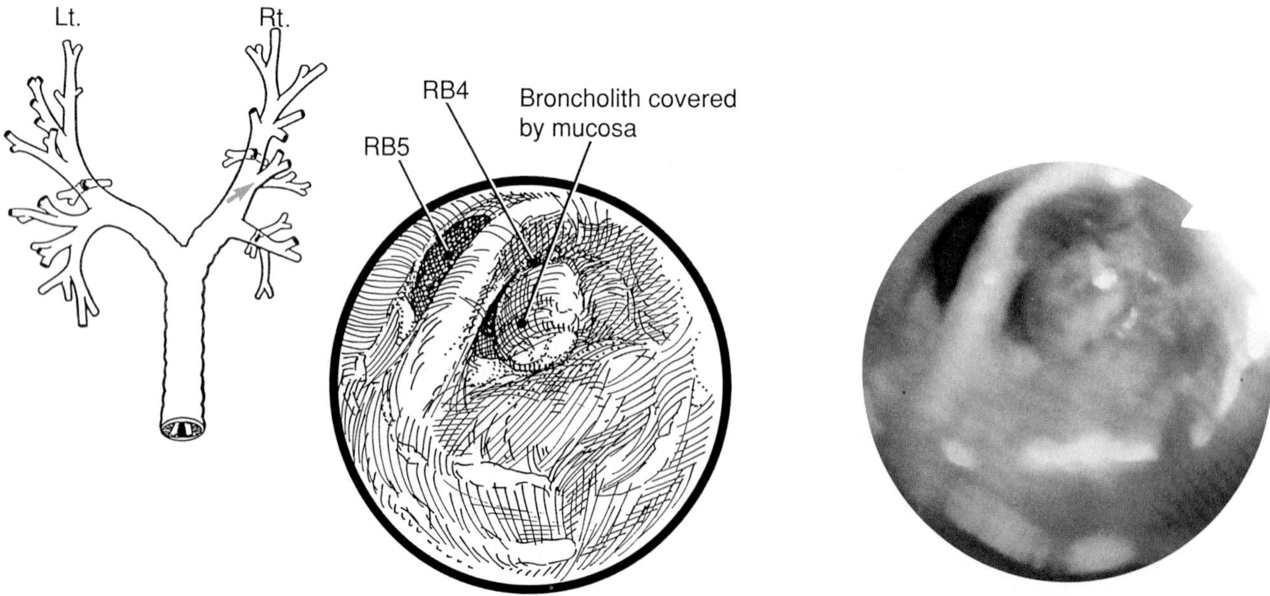

FIG. 14. Bronchoscopic saline dilatation of a collapsed bronchus to RB4 segment revealed a broncholith after the mucosa covering it was bronchoscopically removed. Bronchoscopic image obtained *through* saline.

bronchoscopist should take the precautions, as outlined above, to obtain proper visualization. The objective lens should be cleaned and a small amount of "antifog" material (diluted soap solution) applied to the lens. The focus should be checked and adjusted. If a thin film of mucus covers the objective lens and hinders the view, it is not necessary to remove the bronchoscope from the tracheobronchial tree. Instead, the tip of the bronchoscope should be flexed toward the nearest bronchial wall and gently rubbed against it to dislodge the mucous film. Injecting a few drops of normal saline will also dislodge the mucous film. The most important technical aspect is to keep the working channel free of mucus and blood by continuous suction before inserting the brush or biopsy forceps. If the buildup of mucous film cannot be avoided, then the bronchoscopist should consider "preloading" of the brush or biopsy forceps (Fig. 15). Before inserting the bronchoscope into the trachea, the brush or biopsy forceps should be inserted into the bronchoscope so that 3–4 mm of the brush or biopsy forceps is projecting out of the tip of the bronchoscope. This will keep the mucus away from the objective lens. If none of these methods provides excellent visualization of the lesion, the alternative is to get as good a visualization as possible and then "freeze" the bronchoscope tip aimed at the lesion and proceed with brush or biopsy. This somewhat blind method may have to be repeated to assure that appropriate samples are obtained.

Excessive Motion of Visible Lesions During Attempts to Biopsy

Visible lesions of the tracheobronchial mucosa vary in size from 2 mm to more than 2.5 cm. The larger lesions are easier to brush and biopsy. Poor cooperation on the part of the patient, excessive motion of the patient's body, coughing by the patient, movement of the tracheobronchial tree due to the patient's respiratory motions, and the vertical movement (along the long axis of the instrument) of the bronchoscope itself due to the patient's respiratory motions as well as the bronchoscopist's excessive manipulation of the instrument will make it more difficult to brush or biopsy smaller visible mucosal lesions of the tracheobronchial mucosa. The patient may require additional amounts of sedative so that excessive body motion can be controlled. To expedite optimal brushing and biopsy, the area surrounding the abnormality should be cleared of secretions and blood. The area to be brushed or biopsied should be centered in the field of vision and the tip of the bronchoscope maintained at an appropriate distance from the lesion. The bronchoscopist should immobilize the distal tip of the bronchoscope by freezing the motion of the elbow, wrist, and thumb controlling the bronchoscope and its distal tip. The assistant should be instructed to hold the bronchoscope where it enters the nostril or mouth so that vertical motion by the bronchoscope can be halted. Then the patient

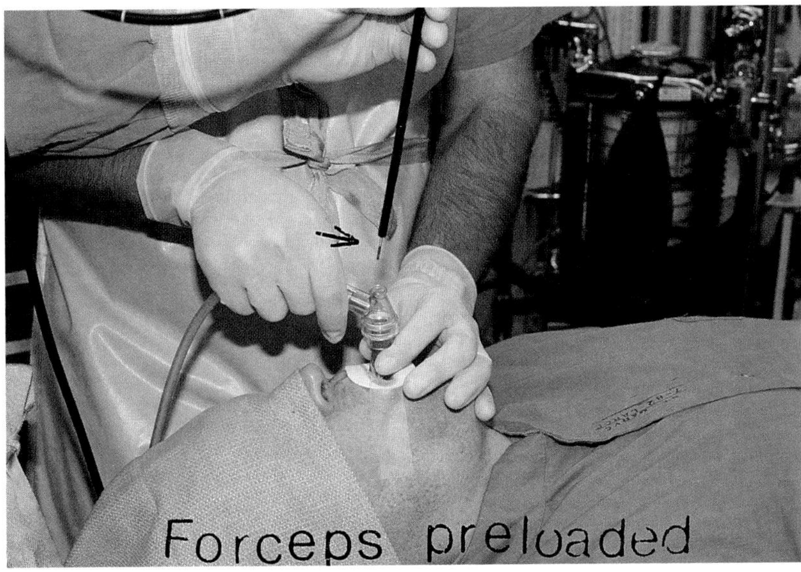

FIG. 15. "Preloading" the flexible bronchoscope with a biopsy forceps to avoid mucus (or blood) filling the suction channel and covering the objective lens of bronchoscope.

should be instructed to take in a breath and hold it as long as possible, for approximately 30 sec. This allows ample time for the bronchoscopist to obtain an optimal specimen. The bronchoscope can be held in the same position and the biopsy forceps alone removed for collection of the specimen. The entire sequence should be repeated if more biopsies are needed.

Problems with Biopsy Forceps

The new and unused as well as the old and overused biopsy forceps tend to be slow in the opening and closing operations, even outside the bronchoscope. This sluggish reaction becomes more pronounced when the forceps is inside the bronchoscope or in the airway. The time between the proximal part of the forceps is opened (or closed) to the time the distal cups open (or close) varies from 4 to 8 sec. The bronchoscopist and bronchoscopy team should check the forceps to assure that it works properly and that all parts are properly maintained and lubricated. Before insertion of the forceps through the flexible bronchoscope, the cups should be opened and closed several times. If the forceps does not open after traversing the working channel of the bronchoscope, the proximal end of the forceps should be maintained in the open position while the bronchoscopist quickly jiggles the entire forceps back and forth several times. It is important to visually ascertain that the forceps has closed, after the biopsy is obtained, prior to withdrawing it from the bronchoscope. If, after two or three tries, the forceps does not work to the bronchoscopist's satisfaction, then a new forceps should be tried.

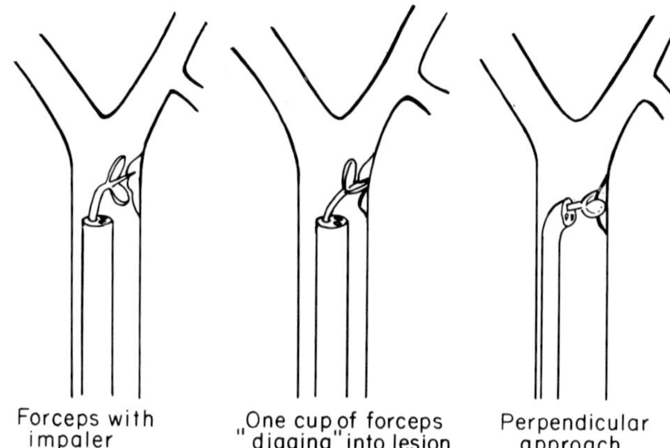

FIG. 16. Bronchoscopic biopsy techniques to obtain biopsy from tracheal wall. See text for details.

Keeping the biopsy forceps in proper functioning order is an important aspect of preventing dysfunction. Reusable forceps may require periodic lubrication of the hinge apparatus. Thorough drying after each use will prevent rust buildup and malfunction.

Biopsy of Lesions on Tracheobronchial Walls

Protruding or polypoid mucosal lesions of the trachea and main bronchi are easy to biopsy. On the other hand, if the lesions are flush with the mucosa, submucosal, or small, the forceps may slide off the wall without obtaining good biopsy specimens. Vigorous use of the cytology brush will produce a certain degree of

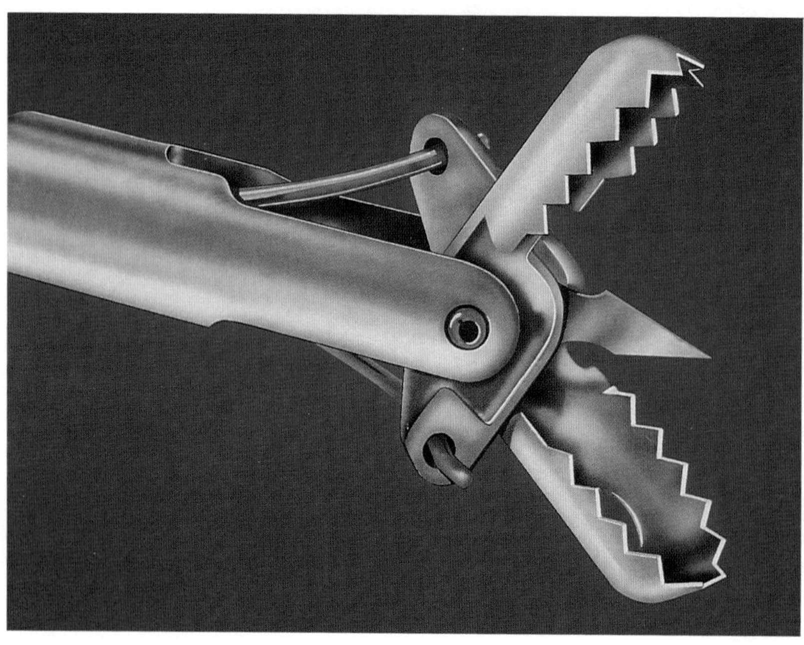

FIG. 17. A toothed (alligator) biopsy forceps with an impaler needle provides good grasp of lesions along tracheal wall. Figure courtesy of Microvasive Corp.

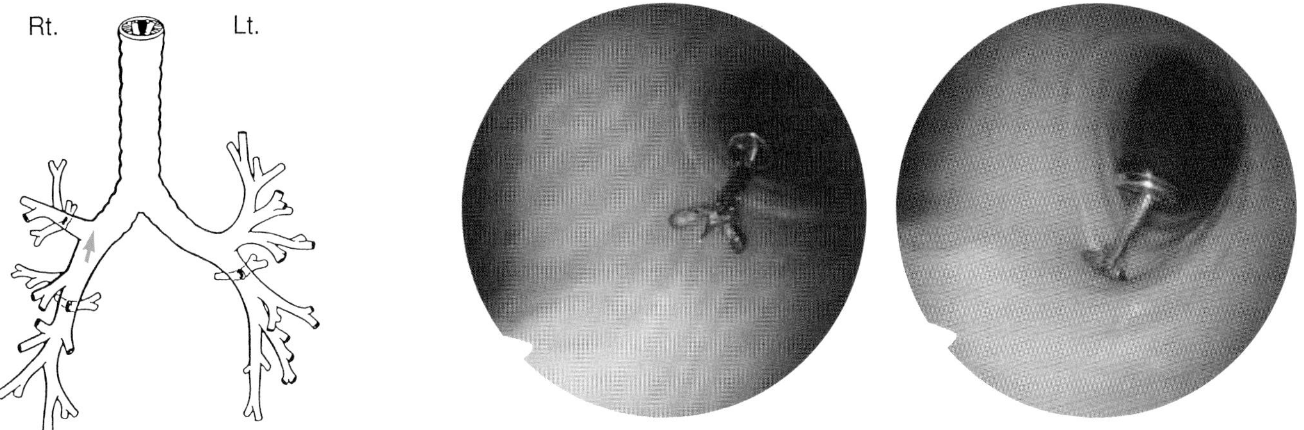

FIG. 18. Cephalad view of a model of the tracheobronchial tree shows simulated bronchial biopsy using forceps with an impaler needle **(Middle)**. Even in hard-to-biopsy locations (the superior aspect of right upper lobe take off shown here), the impaler needle secures a firm hold on the mucosa and permits biopsy of the lesion **(Right)**.

mucosal roughness and this may provide a slip-free surface for the forceps in addition to obtaining good cytological smears. If slippage of the forceps becomes a problem, several techniques can be tried to overcome this problem (Fig. 16). The use of biopsy forceps with an impaler needle should be contemplated (Figs. 16, 17, and 18). The needle will impale the abnormal mucosa so that the forceps cups can be closed around it (Fig. 16). Another method is to open the biopsy cups and use one cup to dig into the abnormality and then close the free cup to obtain a biopsy (Fig. 16). In the trachea, if the lumen is large, the bronchoscope and forceps can be bent to approach the lesion at an angle closer to perpendicular so that slipping of the forceps will not occur (Fig. 16). If the lesion is located within the shelf formed by tracheobronchial cartilages, then the biopsy forceps should be inserted into the shelf so that the forceps will not slide. Using a toothed (alligator) forceps (Fig. 19) instead of a toothless (regular cup) forceps will provide a firmer grip on the mucosal abnormality. Instructing the patient to hold his or her breath will also help in minimizing the slippage.

When attempting to biopsy lesions located on any carina, the open biopsy forceps may approach the carina in such a way that the cups may slip off the carina (Fig. 20). To avoid this problem, it is better to rotate

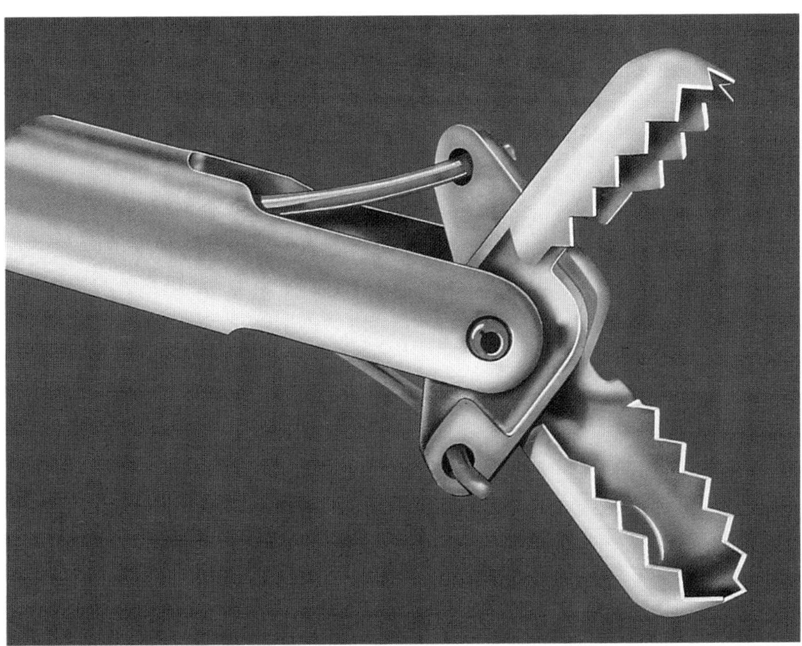

FIG. 19. Toothed (alligator) biopsy forceps. Figure courtesy of Microvasive Corp.

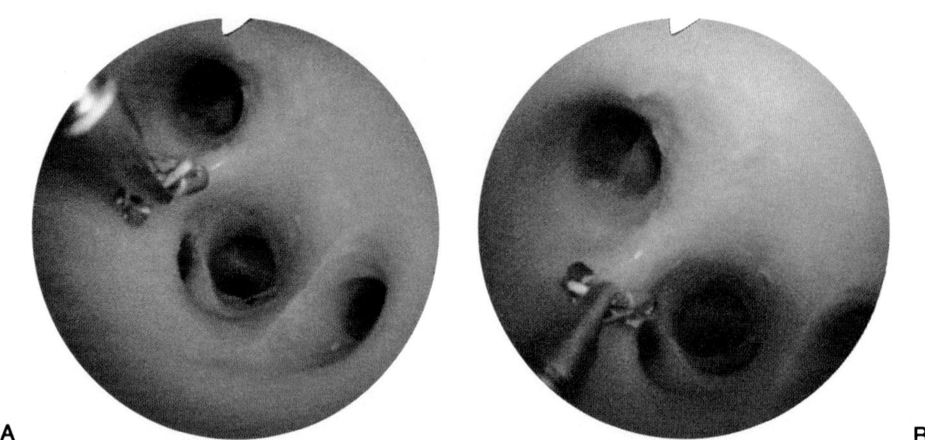

FIG. 20. Bronchoscopic view of simulated biopsy of a carinal lesion. Approaching a carina with the biopsy jaws in a parallel orientation results in easy skidding of the forceps **(A)**, whereas the perpendicular alignment of the jaws will permit easy biopsy **(B)**.

the handle of the forceps (the bronchoscopy assistant can accomplish this) than to twist the bronchoscope or the shaft of the biopsy forceps when it enters the bronchoscope. The former maneuver will enable the open forceps to approach the carina in a perpendicular manner (Fig. 20).

For the submucosal lesions in the trachea or main bronchi, a bronchoscopic needle can be used to obtain cytology aspirations. Multiple punctures of the mucosa can be attempted to raise a mucosal flap under which a biopsy forceps can be introduced to obtain deep submucosal biopsy.

Biopsy of Localized Lesions in Inaccessible Areas

As discussed above, the newer flexible bronchoscopes allow the operator to reach almost all bronchi without much difficulty. Even with the newer instruments, however, bronchoscopists occasionally find it difficult to introduce the bronchoscope into the bronchi leading to the apical segments of upper lobes and superior segments of lower lobes, and to other bronchi. Roentgenologically determined abnormalities in these inaccessible segments may necessitate bronchoscopic brushing and biopsy. Before attempting brush and biopsy procedures, the bronchoscopist should make sure that the results of other appropriate imaging studies (lateral chest roentgenogram, plain tomography, and computed tomography) are available to properly localize the lesion. If the lesion is peripheral and bronchoscopically invisible, then fluoroscopic guidance should be sought. The bronchoscopist should apply the techniques described above to enter the inaccessible bronchus.

First, a cytology brush should be used to obtain cytology smears if cancer is suspected. The brush itself can be used as a guide wire to direct the bronchoscope closer to the lesion. Then the brush can be removed and biopsy forceps introduced into the lesion under fluoroscopic guidance. The biopsy forceps is stiffer and more rigid than the cytology brush. As a result, the forceps tends to straighten the flexed tip of the bronchoscope, particularly in the upper lobes, and direct it away from the lesion (Fig. 21). To counter this, the cytology brush should be used to brush the lesion and to direct the tip of the bronchoscope toward the lesion. Using fluoroscopic guidance and tightly controlling the movement of the bronchoscope tip, the biopsy forceps should be gently but firmly threaded through the bronchoscope into the lesion. As long as the bronchoscope remains wedged within a segmental bronchus, the forceps can be advanced into a peripheral lesion, even if the bronchoscope tip is temporarily straightened during passage of the forceps. If the lesion is bronchoscopically invisible, the bronchoscopist should look at the fluoroscopy monitor and maneuver the tip of the bronchoscope with fluoroscopic guidance and biopsy forceps until an optimal biopsy is obtained from the lesion (Fig. 22).

Bronchoscopic Lung Biopsy

Bronchoscopic lung biopsy can be performed without fluoroscopic guidance if the pulmonary parenchymal disease is diffuse (29–31). Diffuse pulmonary infiltrate (Fig. 23, left), a localized lesion in the apical segments of upper lobes (Fig. 23, center), or well-defined infiltrates in middle lobe segments, well demonstrated by chest roentgenogram, can be approached without fluoroscopic guidance. When the pulmonary lesions are patchy or localized (Fig. 23, right), fluoroscopic guidance is highly desirable (32). A report on 231 bronchoscopists observed that the incidence of pneumothorax following bronchoscopic lung biopsy

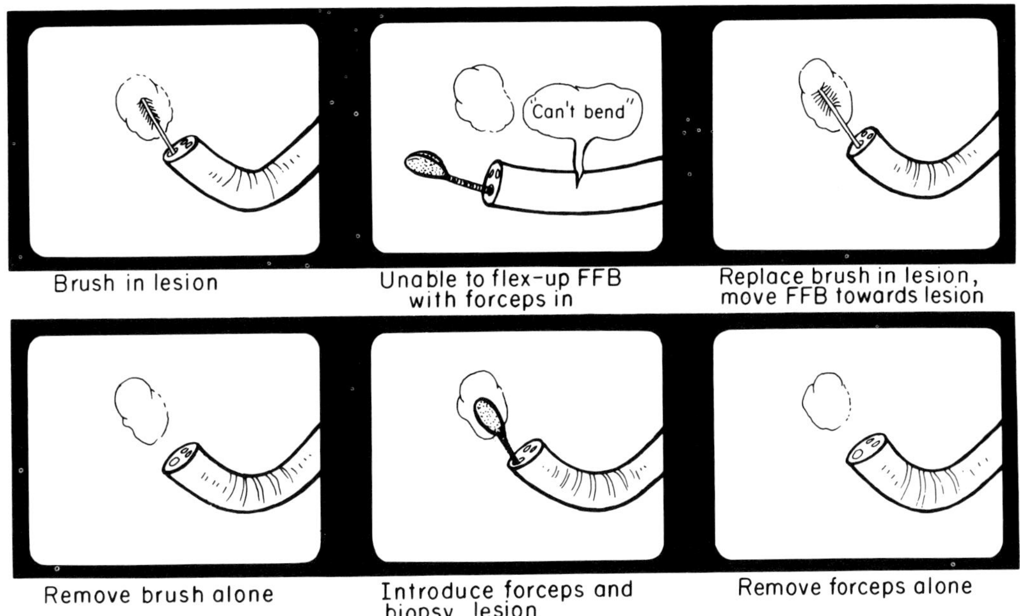

FIG. 21. Diagrammatic depiction of flexible bronchoscopic biopsy of apical and difficult-to-reach nodular lesions. FFB, flexible bronchoscope. See text for details of the technique.

was 1.8% when fluoroscopy was used and the incidence significantly increased to 2.9% when fluoroscopy was not used (33). Even if the roentgenologic abnormality is diffuse, we highly recommend the use of fluoroscopy because of the level of confidence it provides the bronchoscopist in selecting the maximally abnormal areas for biopsies. Additionally, fluoroscopic guidance permits precise placement of the forceps in the periphery of the lung for bronchoscopic lung biopsy near the pleura.

Several problems are associated with bronchoscopic lung biopsy, even when fluoroscopic guidance is used. Inability to obtain optimal specimens is a common problem. Proper functioning of biopsy forceps (see above), use of fluoroscopic guidance, and proper technique of biopsy will greatly increase the chance of obtaining good biopsy specimens. Opening the biopsy specimen cups closer to the area of parenchymal abnormality will prevent biopsy of the bronchial wall (Fig. 24). The biopsy forceps should be allowed to open

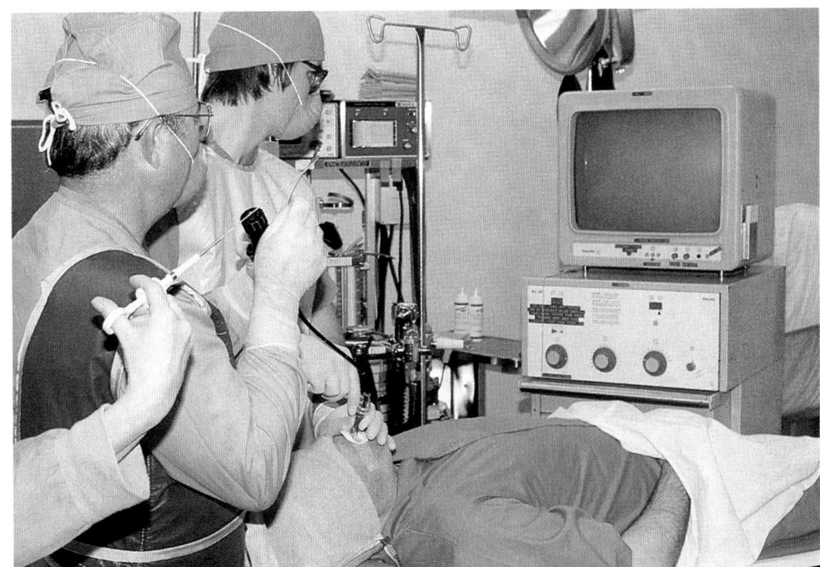

FIG. 22. Optimal use of fluoroscopy to obtain lung biopsy from abnormal areas. The bronchoscopist is visualizing the fluoroscopy screen to guide not only the tip of the bronchoscope but also the biopsy forceps to maximally abnormal areas. This technique is particularly useful when bronchoscopic visualization is poor for various reasons.

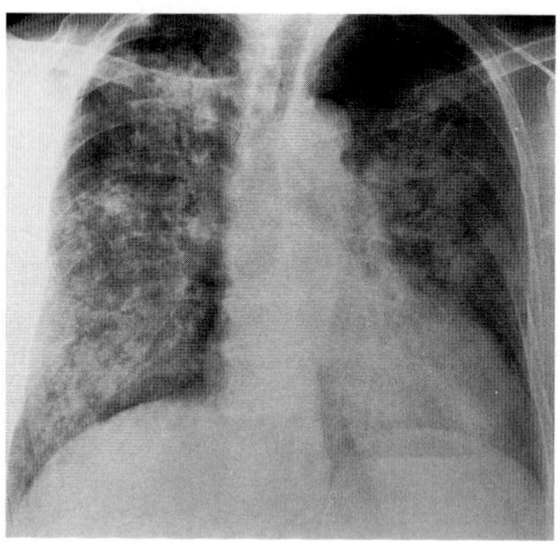

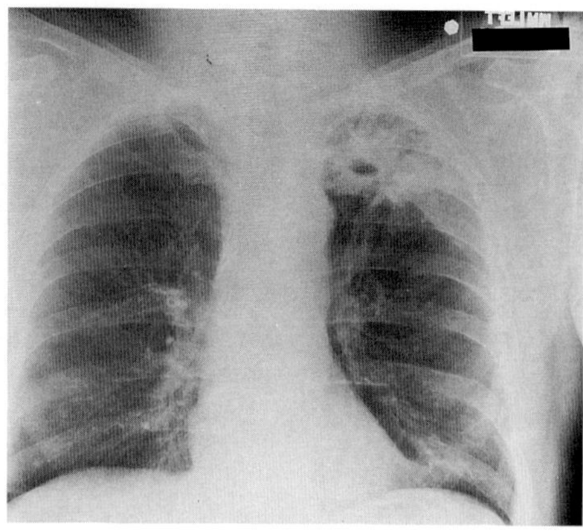

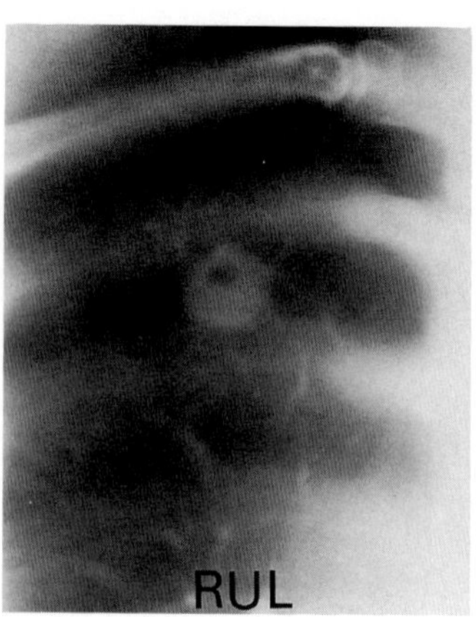

FIG. 23. Diffuse pulmonary parenchymal process **(left)** and localized processes in certain locations **(center)** may be biopsied without fluoroscopic guidance. A smaller localized lesion **(right)** requires fluoroscopic guidance for accurate localization.

fully before the assistant closes it, and to close fully before the forceps are withdrawn (34). Closing the forceps at the end of expiration may increase the size of the biopsy because the alveolar size at end-expiration is diminished and therefore a larger number of alveoli will be biopsied by the forceps. The use of toothed versus nontoothed biopsy forceps also has no bearing on the size of the biopsy or complications such as bleeding and pneumothorax. After the biopsy forceps is closed, gentle traction should be used to remove the biopsy specimen and avoid undue sudden traction on lung tissue and pleura.

If a biopsy forceps fails to obtain adequate samples, a new or different forceps should be employed. At times it is difficult to know if the biopsy forceps is open or not, even with fluoroscopic guidance. Rotation of the forceps, if fluoroscopy is used, may show the actual opening and closing of the cups (Fig. 25). If biopsy specimens cannot be obtained from one abnormal area, then biopsy of other abnormal areas should be attempted. If fluoroscopy is used, it should be used to direct the bronchoscope and biopsy forceps to another abnormal area for obtaining lung specimens. The number of bronchoscopic lung biopsies obtained will depend on the patient's cooperation, underlying disease process, the availability of immediate frozen section analysis, and the immediate (intraoperative) complications such as postbiopsy hemorrhage and pneumothorax. Further details regarding bronchoscopic lung biopsy can be found in Chapter 11 of this volume.

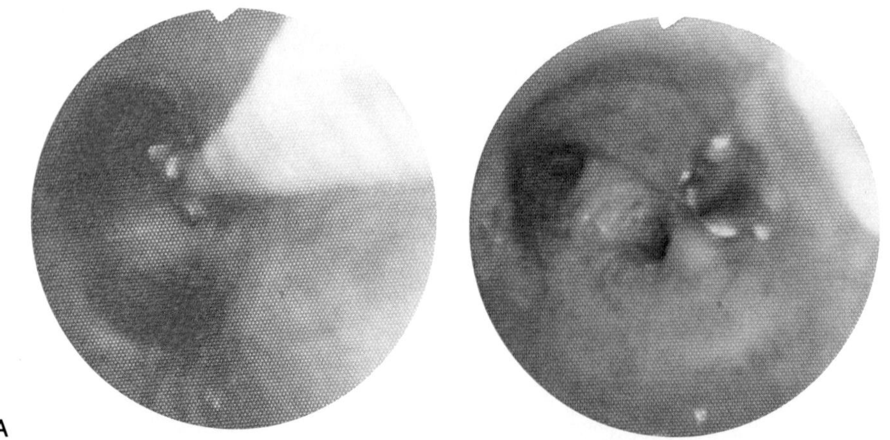

FIG. 24. Opening the jaws of biopsy forceps too proximally **(A)** to obtain bronchoscopic lung biopsy will result in biopsy of bronchial mucosa. The biopsy forceps should be advanced with its jaws closed **(B)** until reaching within 1 cm of area to be biopsied.

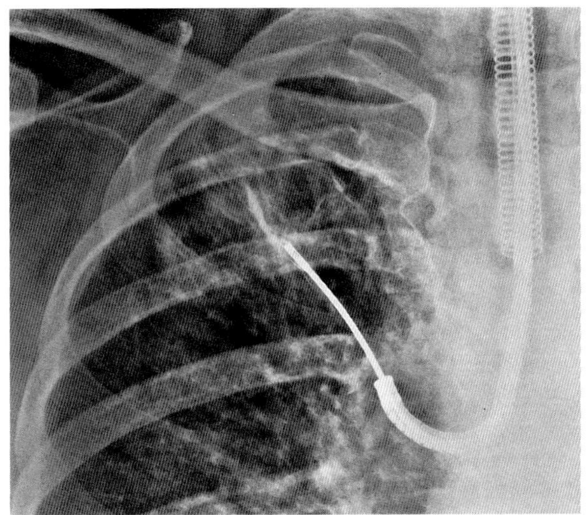
A

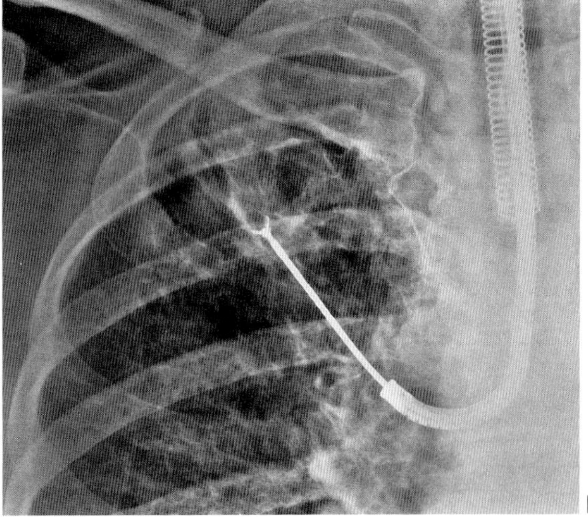
B

FIG. 25. Even the fluoroscopic monitoring (single plane) may not clearly show the open jaws of the biopsy forceps even when they are open **(A)**. Under fluoroscopic guidance, the bronchoscopy assistant turns the handle of the forceps until the open jaws are clearly visible on fluoroscopic monitor **(B)**.

Bronchoscopic Needle Aspiration and Biopsy

Bronchoscopic needle aspiration and biopsy are being used with increasing frequency in both malignant and benign lung diseases (Chapter 12, this volume) (35–38). The performance of the presently available needles is often unreliable. The novice as well as the experienced bronchoscopist will encounter several technical difficulties. It is not uncommon to use two or more needles in one patient because of the failure of the needle to function properly. One common obstacle we have observed is the inability of the needle to extrude out of the sheath once the apparatus has traversed the working channel of the bronchoscope. The plastic catheter frequently undergoes intussusception, thereby rendering the apparatus useless. The site of attachment of needle to catheter frequently bends and makes it difficult or impossible to aspirate. Another major problem is the well-documented high rate of needle-induced damage to the inner lining of the flexible bronchoscope (39). To avoid some of these problems, the bronchoscopist must ensure that the needle is not extruded before the catheter traverses the length of the working channel. Adequate lubrication is essential to prevent intussusception and acute bending of the plastic sheath. The acute bending is also common after inadvertent piercing of the tracheobronchial cartilage or aspiration of the high right paratracheal lymph node. This can be avoided by performing the puncture with a minimum length of the plastic catheter protruding from the bronchoscope channel. It is helpful to have the metal hub of the needle catheter located just at the distal tip of the bronchoscope and, with the needle in the visible field, insert the needle with a thrust of the bronchoscope and needle together, in one motion. Although fluoroscopy is not necessary for this procedure, its use, particularly in the aspiration and biopsy of paratracheal or hilar nodes, will not only ensure that the needle is in the suspected area of abnormality but also that it has pierced through the wall of the trachea or bronchus instead of its tip becoming lodged within the tracheobronchial wall.

If a computed tomographic scan of hilar, subcarinal, and paratracheal lymph nodes is available, the findings help in the accurate selection of areas to be aspirated.

Dynamic Bronchoscopy

Although bronchoscopy is by design a dynamic procedure, the dynamism applies more to the instrument and the bronchoscopist during the procedure. The patient is invariably a somewhat passive participant in almost all bronchoscopic procedures. We believe that more information can be gathered by patient participation during the procedure. Several abnormalities not detected by "routine" bronchoscopy can be uncovered by having the patient perform various maneuvers during the procedure. In patients presenting with obstructive disease of unknown cause, bronchoscopy and visualization of airway dynamics during forced breathing maneuver or coughing may reveal the unusual collapse of the large airways (Fig. 26). A normal-appearing bronchial tree may show an abnormality on deep inspiration (Fig. 27). When patients with suspected major airway lesions are referred to us for bronchoscopic evaluation, we routinely examine the upper airway (without an endotracheal tube) with the patient in supine and lateral decubitus postures. Additionally, we ask the patient to attempt to hyperflexion or hyperex-

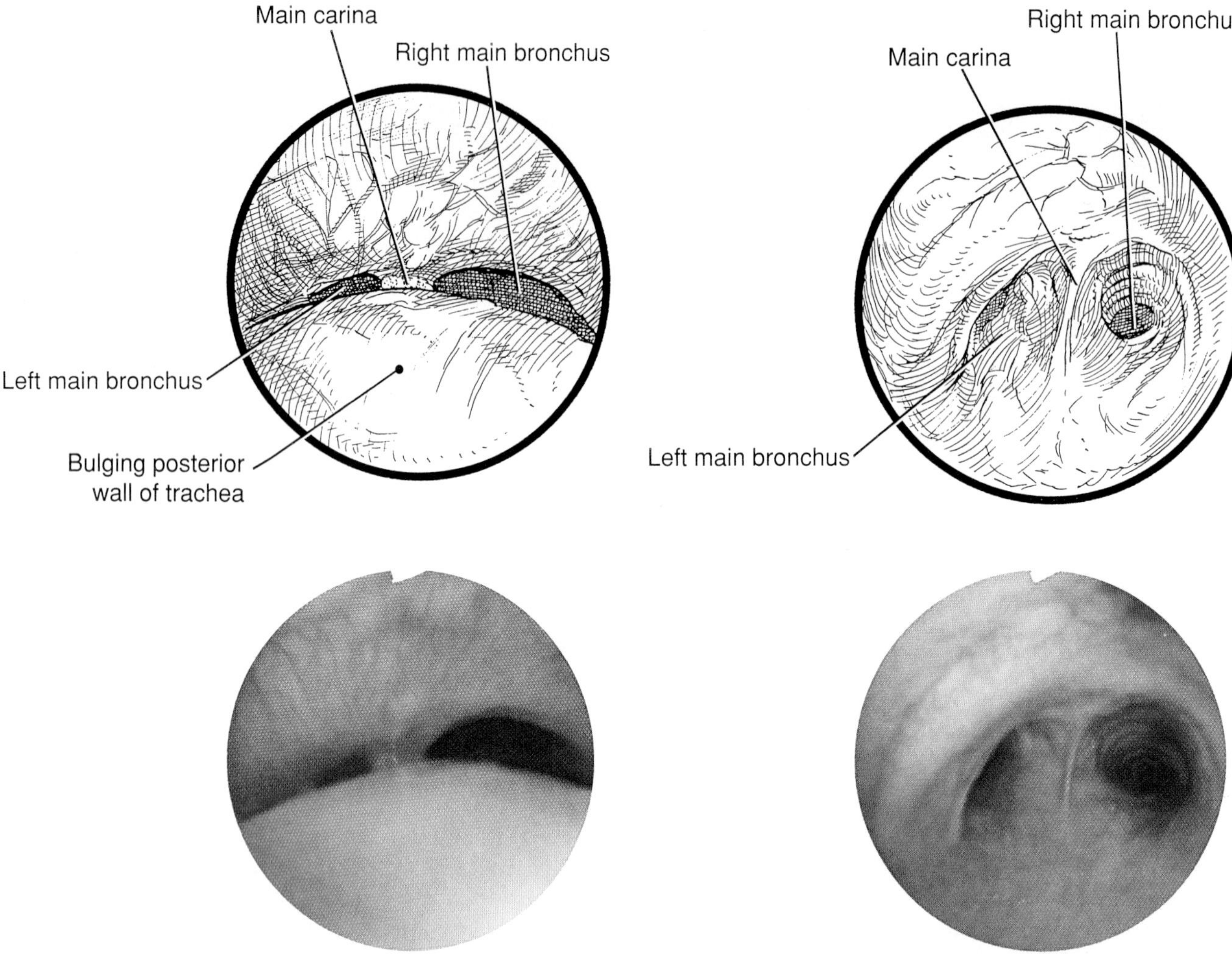

FIG. 26. An example of "dynamic bronchoscopy." Excessive collapse of the posterior membranous wall of trachea during forced expiration **(left)** and normal caliber of trachea during deep inspiration **(right)**.

tension of the neck to see if the upper trachea shows undue collapsibility. Careful examination of the larynx during phonation has resulted in the diagnosis of spastic dysphonia due to adductor spasm not detected by earlier bronchoscopy or clinical examination (see Chapter 32, this volume).

Dynamic bronchoscopy also includes the use of all available equipment to gather maximum information. For instance, a bronchial stenosis may be too narrow to permit the passage of a standard flexible bronchoscope through the stenotic segment. To estimate the length of the stricture and to plan appropriate therapy, one can consider tomography, bronchography, or a cine-computed tomography. On the other hand, if one has an ultrathin flexible bronchoscope, it can be used to examine the stricture and the distal bronchial tree and provide the necessary information (Fig. 28). A hurried bronchoscopic procedure that does not include contemplation of available options and an incomplete examination may easily miss an obvious endobronchial abnormality (Fig. 29).

SOLUTION TO OTHER PROBLEMS IN BRONCHOSCOPY

The reader is referred to other chapters in this book regarding the following topics: rigid bronchoscopy (Chapter 4), prevention and control of bronchoscopically induced bleeding (Chapter 17), different approaches to the extraction of a tracheobronchial foreign body (Chapter 18), other aspects of therapeutic bronchoscopy (Chapter 16), bronchoscopic lung biopsy (Chapter 11), bronchoscopic needle aspiration and biopsy (Chapter 12), bronchoalveolar lavage (Chapter 13), laser bronchoscopy (Chapter 19), bron-

Lt. Rt.

Bronchus to right middle lobe
RC2
RB6
Slit-like appearance during expiration
Bronchus to right lower lobe

Bronchus to right middle lobe
RC2
RB6
Bronchoesophageal fistula open during inspiration
Bronchus to right lower lobe

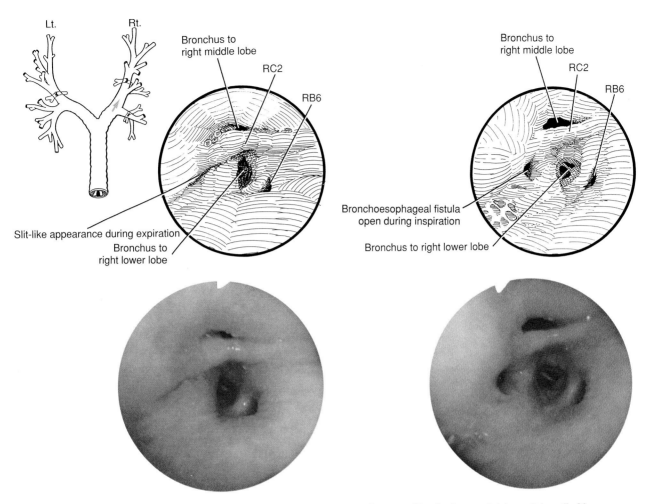

FIG. 27. Dynamic bronchoscopy shows no apparent abnormality during quiet breathing **(left)**. Deep inspiration reveals a bronchoesophageal fistula **(right)**.

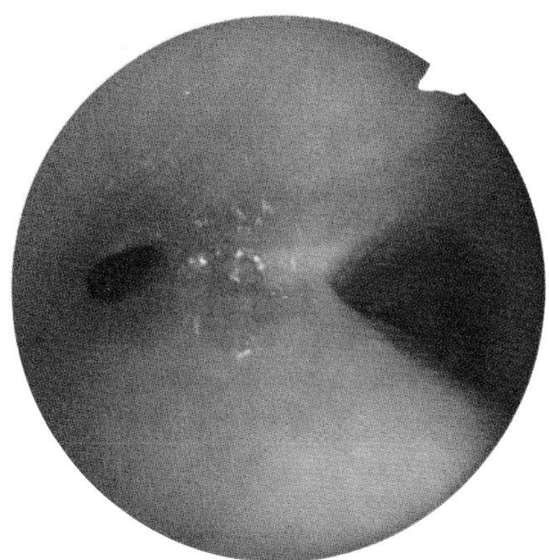

FIG. 28. Severe stenosis of the left main stem bronchus did not permit distal passage of a standard flexible bronchoscope. An ultrathin flexible bronchoscope was easily inserted into the distal bronchial tree to examine and determine the length of the stricture and to assess the distal bronchial anatomy.

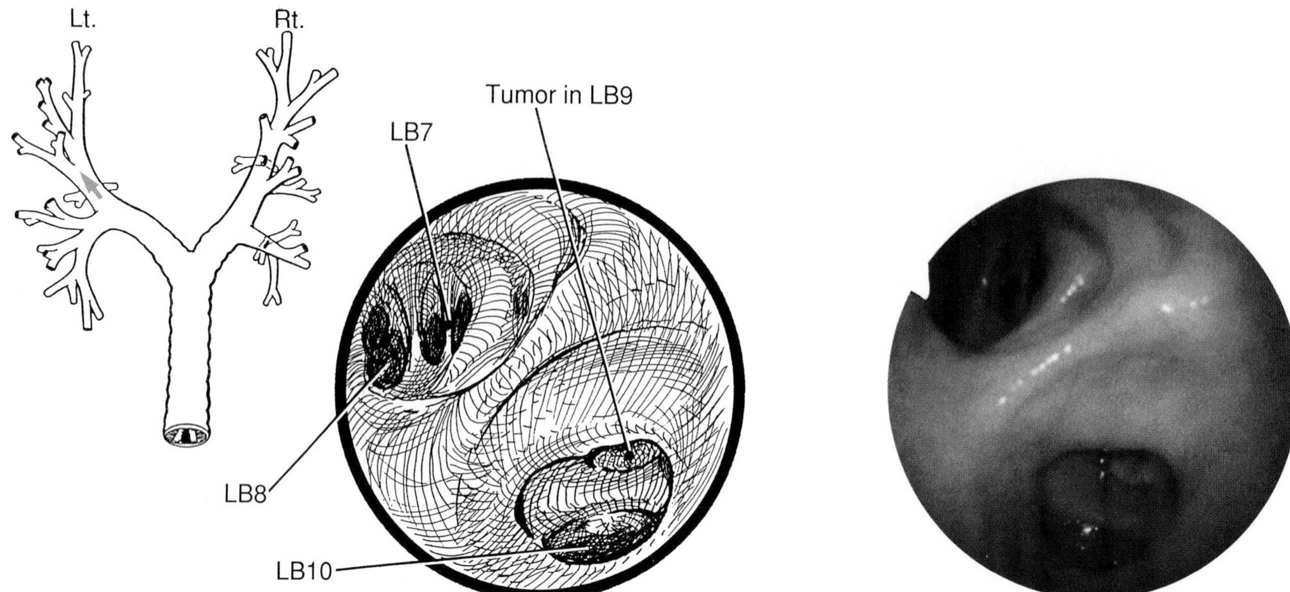

FIG. 29. A hurried bronchoscopic examination had originally overlooked the tumor in the bronchus to LB9.

choscopic brachytherapy (Chapter 20), dilatation of tracheobronchial stenosis (Chapter 21), and the handling of bronchoscopy specimens (Chapter 26).

We conclude by stressing that excellent communication between bronchoscopist and patient, and bronchoscopist and bronchoscopy team, is extremely important in avoiding many of the technical problems discussed above.

REFERENCES

1. Prakash UBS, Offord KP, Stubbs SE. Bronchoscopy in North America: the ACCP survey. *Chest* 1991;100:1668–1675.
2. Ikeda S. *Atlas of flexible bronchofiberscopy*. Baltimore: University Park Press; 1974.
3. De Kock MA. *Dynamic bronchoscopy*. Berlin: Springer-Verlag; 1977.
4. Zavala DC. *Flexible fiberoptic bronchoscopy: a training handbook*. Iowa City: University of Iowa Press; 1978.
5. Oho K, Amemiya R. *Practical fiberoptic bronchoscopy*. Tokyo: Igaku-Shoin; 1984.
6. Collins J, Goldstraw P, Dhillon P. *Practical bronchoscopy*. Oxford: Blackwell Scientific; 1987.
7. Du Bois RM, Clarke SW. *Fiberoptic bronchoscopy: in diagnosis and management*. Orlando: Grune and Stratton; 1987.
8. Becker HD, Kayser K, Schulz V, Tuengerthal S, Vollhaber H-H. *Atlas of bronchoscopy*. Philadelphia: B. C. Decker; 1991.
9. Stradling P, Stradling JR. *Diagnostic bronchoscopy: a teaching manual*. Edinburgh: Churchill Livingstone; 1991.
10. Kato H, Horai T. *A colour atlas of endoscopic diagnosis in early stage lung cancer*. London: Wolf; 1992.
11. Prakash UBS, Stubbs SE. Bronchoscopy: indications and technique. *Semin Resp Med* 1981;3:17–24.
12. American Thoracic Society. Guidelines for fiberoptic bronchoscopy in adults. *Am Rev Resp Dis* 1987;136:1066.
13. Colt HG, Morris JF. Fiberoptic bronchoscopy without premedication. A retrospective study. *Chest* 1990;98:1327–1330.
14. Pearce SJ. Fibreoptic bronchoscopy: is sedation really necessary? *Br Med J* 1980;281:779–780.
15. Simpson FG, Arnold AG, Purvis A, Belfield PW, Muers MF, Cooke NJ. Postal survey of bronchoscopic practice by physicians in the United Kingdom. *Thorax* 1986;41:311–317.
16. Goroszeniuk T. Premedication for fibreoptic bronchoscopy: fentanyl, diazepam, and atropine compared with papaveretum and hyoscine. *Br Med J* 1980;281:486.
17. Zavala DC. Complications following fiberoptic bronchoscopy. The "good news" and the "bad news." *Chest* 1978;73:783–785.
18. Rees PJ, Hay JG, Webb JR. Premedication for fiberoptic bronchoscopy. *Thorax* 1983;38:624–627.
19. Credle WF Jr., Smiddy JF, Elliott RC. Complications of fiberoptic bronchoscopy. *Am Rev Resp Dis* 1974;109:67–72.
20. Sandza JG Jr, Roberts RW, Shaw RC, Connors JP. Symptomatic methemoglobinemia with a commonly used topical anesthetic, cetacaine. *Ann Thorac Surg* 1980;30:187–190.
21. Douglas WW, Fairbanks VF. Methemoglobinemia induced by a topical anesthetic spray (cetacaine). *Chest* 1977;71:587–591.
22. Kotler RL, Hansen-Flaschen J, Casey MP. Severe methaemoglobinaemia after flexible fibreoptic bronchoscopy. *Thorax* 1989;44:234–235.
23. Christoforidis AJ, Tomashefski J, Mithell RI. Use of an ultrasonic nebulizer for the application of oropharyngeal, laryngeal, and tracheobronchial anesthesia. *Chest* 1971;59:629–632.
24. Reed AP. Preparation of the patient for awake flexible fiberoptic bronchoscopy. *Chest* 1992;101:244–253.
25. Adriani J, Campbell D. Fatalities following topical application of local anesthetics to mucous membranes. *JAMA* 1956; 162:1527–1530.
26. Weisel W, Tella RA. Reaction to tetracaine (pontocaine) used as topical anesthetic in bronchoscopy: a study of 1,000 cases. *JAMA* 1951;147:218–222.
27. Fulkerson WJ. Fiberoptic bronchoscopy. *N Engl J Med* 1984; 311:511–515.
28. Patterson JR, Blaschke TF, Hunt KK Jr, Meffin PJ. Lidocaine blood concentrations during fiberoptic bronchoscopy. *Am Rev Resp Dis* 1975;112:53–54.
29. De Fenoyl O, Capron F, Lebeau B, Rochmaure J. Transbronchial lung biopsy: a five year experience in outpatients. *Thorax* 1989;44:956–959.
30. Puar HS, Young RC, Armstrong EM. Bronchial and transbronchial lung biopsy without fluoroscopy in sarcoidosis. *Chest* 1985; 87:303–306.

31. Anders GT, Johnson JE, Bush BA, Matthews JI. Transbronchial lung biopsy without fluoroscopy. A seven year perspective. *Chest* 1988;94:557–560.
32. Prakash UBS, Stubbs SE. The bronchoscopy survey: some reflections. *Chest* 1991;100:1660–1667.
33. Simpson FG, Arnold AG, Purvis A, Belfield PW, Muers MF, Cooke NJ. Postal survey of bronchoscopic practice by physicians in the United Kingdom. *Thorax* 1986;41:311–317.
34. Zavala DC. Transbronchial lung biopsy in diffuse lung disease. *Chest* 1978;73(suppl):727–733.
35. Wang KP. Transbronchial needle biopsy for histology specimens. *Chest* 1989;96:226–227.
36. Shure D. Transbronchial biopsy and needle aspiration. *Chest* 1989;95:1130–1138.
37. Shure D. Transbronchial needle aspiration—current status. *Mayo Clin Proc* 1989;64:251–254.
38. Schenk DA, Strollo PJ, Pickard JS, Santiago RM, Weber CA, Jackson CV, Burgess RS, Dew JA, Komadina KH, Segarra J, et al. Utility of the Wang 18-gauge transbronchial histology needle in the staging of bronchogenic carcinoma. *Chest* 1989; 96:272–274.
39. Mehta AC, Curtis PS, Scalzitti ML, Meeker DP. The high price of bronchoscopy. Maintenance and repair of the flexible fiberoptic bronchoscope. *Chest* 1990;98:448–454.

Bronchoscopy,
edited by U. B. S. Prakash.
Mayo Foundation © 1994.
Published by Raven Press, Ltd., New York.

CHAPTER 10

Bronchoscopy in Peripheral and Central Lesions

Denis A. Cortese and John C. McDougall

The decision to perform bronchoscopy in patients is generally based on the clinical symptoms of acute or subacute airway disease or the detection of abnormalities on chest roentgenogram. The central airway lesions are more likely to produce respiratory symptoms than peripherally located pulmonary abnormalities. The possibility of both central and peripheral lesions in the same patient is also possible and should be considered prior to bronchoscopic examination. In this chapter, we discuss the role of bronchoscopy in the diagnosis of localized peripheral lesions and visible endobronchial lesions. The usefulness of bronchoscopy in the diagnosis of diffuse pulmonary parenchymal abnormalities and the technique of bronchoscopic lung biopsy are discussed in Chapter 11 of this volume.

PERIPHERAL LESIONS: BRUSHINGS AND BRONCHOSCOPIC BIOPSY

The bronchoscopic forceps are fairly standard with hinged cups and a cutting edge, or a serrated edge on the larger forceps (alligator forceps). Any biopsy forceps can be used to obtain tissue from peripheral nodules or lesions. Most forceps have a window on each cup reportedly to reduce artifact by limiting tissue crushing.

This procedure is usually performed using local anesthesia and with the patient in the supine position. The blood pressure and oxygen saturation are monitored throughout the procedure. An intravenous line is frequently in place for the purposes of providing mild intravenous sedation and to administer medication in case of a complication. An orotracheal tube facilitates the administration of supplemental oxygen and the repeated withdrawal and reinsertion of the bronchoscope as specimens are collected. The entire procedure can usually be performed in less than 30 min of bronchoscopic time (1,2).

Localized peripheral pulmonary lesions such as patchy infiltrates that are bronchoscopically invisible usually require fluoroscopic guidance so that the placement of the forceps or needle into the X-ray visible lesion can be confirmed. Using the same technique, bronchoscopic brushings can be obtained from the peripheral lesions for cytological examination. These brushings are usually smeared on a glass slide and fixed in alcohol for routine cytological examination.

For solitary nodular lesions, the position of the forceps can be confirmed using single-plane fluoroscopy while turning the patient, a rotating C-arm fluoroscope, or simultaneous biplane fluoroscopy. After confirming the position of the forceps, it can be opened, slightly advanced into the lesion, closed, and withdrawn through the channel of the bronchoscope (Fig. 1). Frozen section examination of biopsy specimens can be performed on the initial specimens whereas additional biopsies are placed in a formalin solution for preparation of permanent sections.

When dealing with lower lobe lesions, it is possible to time the biopsy to the respiratory cycle. The forceps is open, the patient inhales and then exhales deeply, and the forceps are closed at expiration. However, a study of transbronchoscopic lung biopsies done during inhalation and during exhalation found no significant difference in the number of alveoli obtained (3). In the diagnosis of pulmonary nodules, the timing to the respiratory cycle is not likely to be important for obtaining adequate tissue.

D. A. Cortese: Division of Thoracic Diseases and Internal Medicine, Mayo Clinic, Jacksonville, Florida 32224.
J. C. McDougall: Division of Thoracic Diseases and Internal Medicine, Mayo Clinic, Rochester, Minnesota 55905.

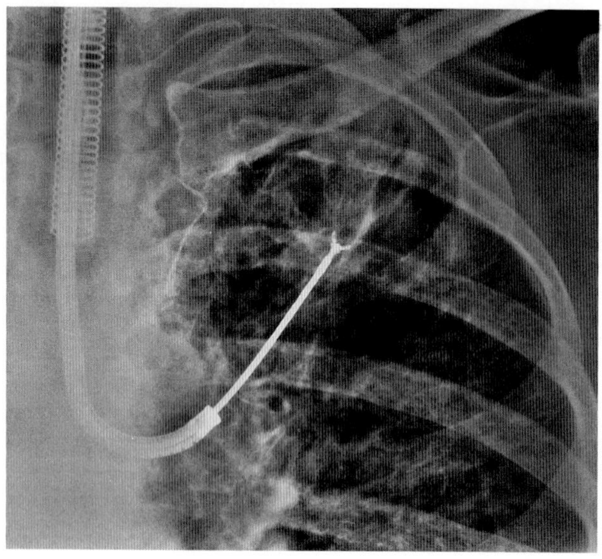

FIG. 1. Fluoroscopic guidance is invaluable in accurate placement of biopsy forceps into a bronchoscopically invisible, ill-defined nodular infiltrate in the periphery of lung. A soft wire-spiral endotracheal tube through which the flexible bronchoscope has advanced is also shown.

Complications

Insertion of the flexible bronchoscope with gentle pressure into the segmental bronchus is an important technique to reduce complications if bleeding develops. Wedging of the bronchoscope into the segmental bronchus as the biopsy forceps is withdrawn and leaving the bronchoscope in place for a period of time after the biopsy is helpful to maintain control of the bronchus, thereby preventing blood from spreading into other areas of the tracheobronchial tree and interfering with oxygenation.

Biopsy of a nodular lesion or localized process slightly increases the risk of bronchoscopy. The major complications are bleeding and pneumothorax. The risk of pneumothorax is less than 5% when performing bronchoscopic lung biopsies (2). In our experience with peripheral nodules and localized lesions, the risk is less than 3%. We use fluoroscopic guidance in every case, and the use of fluoroscopy has been reported to reduce the risk of pneumothorax by others (3–6).

The risk of serious hemorrhage (more than 50 ml during the procedure) is also less than 3% with higher rates reported in patients who are immunocompromised, have abnormal clotting, or uremia (2,4–6). In addition, the performance of a biopsy during mechanical ventilation has been reported to be associated with a 20% incidence of significant bleeding (7), and there is a reported increased incidence in bleeding following bronchoscopic lung biopsy in patients with pulmonary hypertension (8). Therefore, the procedure of bronchoscopic biopsy is relatively safe, but a potential increased risk exists for patients who are on mechanical ventilation, have coagulation disorders, have pulmonary hypertension, are uremic, and are immunocompromised.

PERIPHERAL LESIONS: BRONCHOSCOPIC NEEDLE ASPIRATION

A number of bronchoscopic aspirating needles are now available. They range in size from 18 to 21 gauge. The largest needles (18-gauge) are used for bronchoscopic needle aspiration and biopsies of mediastinal or hilar lesions.

To obtain a needle aspiration of a peripheral nodule, a plastic needle appears to be useful. The outer sheath is plastic and has no metal rigid section to interfere with the passage of the needle through the bronchoscope. This is particularly important in obtaining samples from apical segments of the upper and lower lobes where sharp bends are encountered and it is difficult to advance metal needles or forceps.

Whether using plastic or metal needles, the risk of penetrating the outer plastic sheath with a needle is minimized by passing the needle after straightening the tip of the bronchoscope and by placing the tip of the needle within 1 mm of the distal end of the sheath (9).

For peripheral lesions, the basic technique of bronchoscopy and use of fluoroscopy for bronchoscopic needle aspiration is the same as the procedure for obtaining biopsies (Fig. 2). The needle should be within its outer sheath as the sheath is advanced toward the lesion and withdrawn into the sheath as it is retracted through the bronchoscope channel after the aspiration.

A 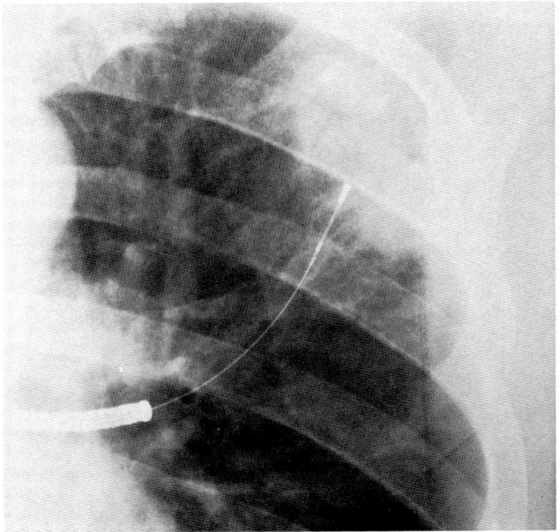 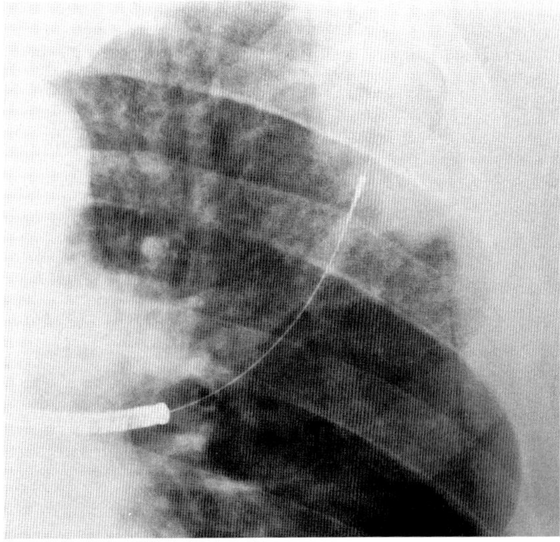 B

FIG. 2. **(A)** An aspiration needle, with needle retracted, is advanced through the flexible bronchoscope into the peripheral infiltrate under fluoroscopic guidance. **(B)** Protrusion of the needle into the center of the infiltrate. It is important to retract the needle into the sheath before withdrawal of the needle catheter out of the bronchoscope so that the delicate inner lining of the flexible bronchoscope is not damaged. Culture of the aspirate in the case shown grew *Blastomyces dermatides.*

Complications

The risk of this procedure seems to be lower than the risk of biopsy with no reports of pneumothorax or significant bleeding following aspiration of a peripheral lesion (10,11). However, we would still advise the wedging of the bronchoscope as described in connection to the technique for biopsy.

PERIPHERAL LESIONS: CURETTAGE

A double-hinged curette has been used to obtain tissue from peripheral nodules and lesions. This device is uncommonly used in the United States but has been used in Japan with success. The actual use and placement of the curette is similar to the use of the biopsy forceps (12–14). However, the technique of successful curettage involves the delineation of the bronchial pathway by selective bronchography whereas the bronchoscopic procedure is not performed until 2 weeks later after the inflammatory effects of bronchography have subsided (12–14). A double-hinged curette is guided to the lesion using the bronchogram as a map. Curettage is performed repeatedly until a suitable specimen is obtained. Considering the extraordinary effort in the increased time of the procedure, the time interval between the bronchogram and the bronchoscopy, and the increased cost, this procedure has not found wide application in the United States.

Peripheral Lesions: Results of Bronchoscopic Biopsy, Needle Aspiration, and Curettage

Biopsy and brushing of peripheral nodules and localized lesions under fluoroscopic guidance are complimentary procedures in the diagnosis of malignant disease. The biopsy has been reported to yield approximately a 60% diagnostic rate in primary lung cancer while brushing yield is approximately 50%. The procedures combined have been reported to result in a diagnosis in up to 80% of cases (6,15–24).

There is less information available regarding the diagnostic yield of fluoroscopic biopsy and brushing in metastatic cancer presenting as pulmonary nodules and nodular infiltrates. However, it appears that the biopsy may yield a diagnosis in up to 50% of cases while the brushings yield a diagnosis in 25–40% of cases. Overall, the combined diagnostic rate of using a biopsy and brushing in peripheral nodular metastatic disease yields a diagnosis in approximately 50% of patients (20,25–27).

The size of the lesion has a bearing on the result of the bronchoscopic procedure. Lesions smaller than 2 cm in size yield a diagnosis in less than 25% of cases, while for those lesions larger than 2 cm in size, the diagnostic yield is greater than 60% for both primary bronchogenic carcinoma and nodular metastatic cancer (22–27).

The use of the curette produces diagnostic material in greater than 70% of patients with peripheral lung cancer whose lesions were larger than 1 cm but less than 2 cm in diameter. The curette did not yield a diagnosis in any lesion less than 1 cm in diameter (12–14).

The addition of the transbronchoscopic needle aspiration of lesions larger than 2 cm in diameter is reported to result in a 50% greater yield than the transbronchoscopic biopsy (10,11). The needle aspiration appears to be useful in those patients with peripheral lesions that cannot be penetrated by the standard forceps. External compression of the bronchus by the tumor itself is a common problem with peripheral primary adenocarcinoma of the lung and metastatic carcinomas of the lung. It has been reported that needle aspiration obtains diagnostic material in 80% of such lesions (10).

ENDOBRONCHIAL LESIONS

Biopsy of visible endobronchial disease is easily accomplished via the flexible bronchoscope (Fig. 3). After satisfactory local or general anesthesia is established, the lesion is visualized, and the appropriate biopsy forceps is passed through the working channel of the flexible bronchoscope until the forceps is just beyond the tip of the bronchoscope. Accurate placement of the forceps is more difficult if the forceps is passed too far beyond the tip of the flexible bronchoscope. The forceps is opened, advanced into the area to be biopsied, and closed firmly. The forceps should be withdrawn slowly to avoid its slipping from the tissue. The forceps may then be withdrawn through the bronchoscope. Some bronchoscopists prefer to withdraw the bronchoscope and forceps together to avoid the possible shearing off of part of the specimen within the working channel of the bronchoscope.

Bronchial biopsy of all the major airways except for the upper lobes is simple to accomplish with standard forceps via the rigid bronchoscope. A special forceps fitted with a quartz rod telescope improves the visibility of lesions biopsied via the rigid bronchoscope, but is usually not needed.

Biopsy of lesions that are on the side wall of the bronchus may be difficult to engage with standard flexible forceps. A flexible forceps with serrated teeth (alligator forceps) or a special forceps with a needle between the jaws makes biopsies easier to obtain in this situation. If a rigid bronchoscope is used, side-biting forceps may be helpful in this situation.

The angle of deflection of the flexible bronchoscope is decreased when the forceps is in place, making entry into the upper lobes and the superior segments of the lower lobes difficult. Usually this difficulty can be overcome by positioning the bronchoscope in the lobe or segment to be biopsied prior to placement of the forceps. Care must be taken not to force the forceps and damage the lining of the working channel of the flexible bronchoscope.

Bronchoscopic Brushing

Bronchial brushing through the bronchoscope has been performed to collect specimens from bronchoscopically visible lesions. The technique is particularly helpful in providing cytological specimens for the diagnosis of lung cancer. Brushes are available in various sizes (2, 5, and 7 mm), types (sheathed and unsheathed), and reusable or disposable. The 5-mm brush is commonly used at most institutions. The sheathed brushes are usually disposable. The plastic sheath, with the brush enclosed, is advanced through the bronchoscope channel to the selected site. The brush is then advanced out of the sheath, collects the specimen, is withdrawn into the sheath, and the whole apparatus withdrawn from the bronchoscope.

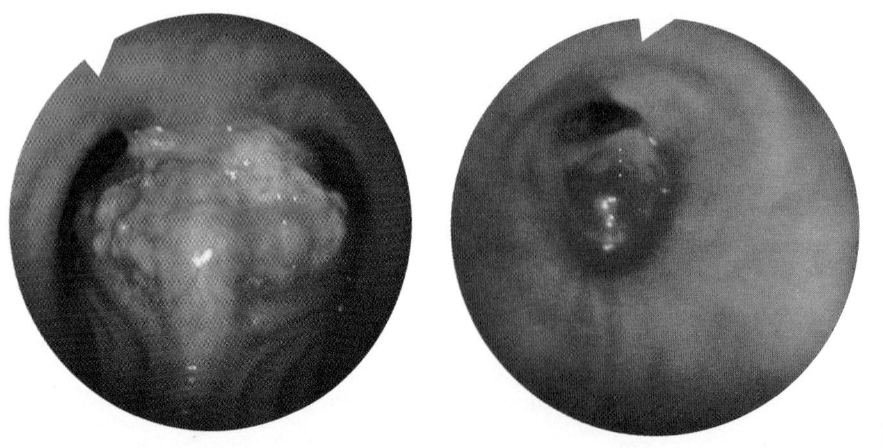

FIG. 3. Bronchoscopically visible lesions in either the central airways (**A,** squamous cell carcinoma of main carina) or peripheral airways (**B,** adenocarcinoma involving a branch of right lower lobe bronchus) are easy to brush or biopsy.

The reusable brushes are unsheathed and advanced unprotected through the channel of the bronchoscope. After the specimen is collected, the brush can be withdrawn through the bronchoscope. We prefer to withdraw the bronchoscope from the patient with the brush protruding from it to reduce the chance that cytological material will be left in the bronchoscope channel. This method is somewhat more cumbersome if the bronchoscopy is performed through the nares. Reusable brushes are less expensive than disposable brushes. However, care must be taken to clean them between cases to eliminate any possibility of cross-contamination. In addition, the brush should be inspected to ensure that the tip has not bent to the extent that it may break off during a procedure (41).

Complications

Bleeding is the most common complication of bronchial biopsy, but usually the amount of bleeding is small and easily controlled. If oozing of blood makes it difficult to see the lesion, topical application of 1:20,000 epinephrine will usually temporarily decrease the oozing, allowing accurate placement of the forceps.

Biopsy of very vascular lesions may result in life-threatening bleeding, and the bronchoscopist should always be prepared to manage the airway if this occurs. Many bronchoscopists prefer not to biopsy lesions that have the typical appearance of vascular carcinoid tumors, but they may usually be safely biopsied (28).

Endobronchial Lesions

Results of Biopsy

Bronchial biopsy of visible bronchogenic cancers is positive in 73–96% of cases (29–34). Studies have shown that three to five biopsies are needed to reach 90–100% sensitivity (34,44). The specificity of bronchial biopsy for lung cancer is reported to be 62–95% (35–37). Errors in cell type do occur, but usually they are among the non-small cell carcinoma types. Only 3 of 150 small cell carcinomas in one large series were later shown to be non-small cell carcinoma (37).

Bronchial biopsy is positive for noncaseating granulomata in 41–57% of patients with sarcoidosis (38–40). One study found a 91% sensitivity for noncaseating granulomata if bronchostenosis, mucosal nodularity, or hypervascularity was present at the biopsy site in this disease (40).

Results of Brushing

The cellular yield of cytological specimens obtained from small brushes is significantly increased when the brush is withdrawn with the bronchoscope. But the diagnostic yield is only slightly increased under this circumstance (42). Overall, the diagnostic yield with a brushing from a visible malignant process is as high as with biopsy. Furthermore, the brushing is occasionally complimentary, yielding a diagnosis when the biopsy is negative. A specific histological cell type is obtained more often from the combination of biopsy and brush cytology than from either technique alone (43).

REFERENCES

1. McDougall JC, Cortese DA. Transbronchoscopic lung biopsy for localized pulmonary disease. *Semin Resp Med* 1981;3:30–34.
2. Zavala DC. Pulmonary hemorrhage in fiberoptic transbronchial biopsy. *Chest* 1976;70:584–588.
3. Shure D, Abraham JL, Konopka R. How should transbronchial biopsies be performed and processed? *Am Rev Resp Dis* 1982; 126:342–343.
4. Herf SM, Suratt PM, Arora NS. Deaths and complications associated with transbronchial lung biopsy. *Am Rev Resp Dis* 1977; 115:708–711.
5. Pereira W Jr., Kovnat DM, Snider GL. A prospective cooperative study of complications following flexible fiberoptic bronchoscopy. *Chest* 1978;73:813–816.
6. Ellis JH Jr. Transbronchial lung biopsy via the fiberoptic bronchoscope: experience with 107 consecutive cases and comparison with bronchial brushings. *Chest* 1975;68:524–532.
7. Papin TA, Grum CM, Weg JG. Transbronchial biopsy during mechanical ventilation. *Chest* 1986;89:168–170.
8. Shulman LL, Smith CR, Drusin R, Rose EA, Enson Y, Reemtsma K. Utility of airway endoscopy in the diagnosis of respiratory complications of cardiac transplantation. *Chest* 1988; 93:960–967.
9. Shure D. Transbronchial biopsy and needle aspiration. *Chest* 1989;95:1130–1138.
10. Shure D, Fedullo PF. Transbronchial needle aspiration of peripheral masses. *Am Rev Resp Dis* 1983;128:1090–1092.
11. Schenk DA, Bryan CL, et al. Transbronchial needle aspiration in the diagnosis of bronchogenic carcinoma. *Chest* 1987;92:83–85.
12. Ono R, Loke J, Ikeda S. Bronchofiberscopy with curette biopsy and bronchography in the evaluation of peripheral lung lesions. *Chest* 1981;79:162–166.
13. Tsuboi E, Ikeda S, Tajima M, Shimosato Y, Ishikawa S. Transbronchial biopsy smear for diagnosis of peripheral pulmonary carcinoma. *Cancer* 1967;20:687–698.
14. Mori K, Yanase N, Kaneko M, Ono R, Ikeda S. Diagnosis of peripheral lung cancer in cases of tumors 2 cm or less in size. *Chest* 1989;95:304–308.
15. Richardson RH, Zavala DC, Munkerjee PK, et al. The use of fiberoptic bronchoscopy and brush biopsy in the diagnosis of suspected pulmonary malignancy. *Am Rev Resp Dis* 1974; 109:63–66.
16. Levin DC, Wick AB, Ellis JH Jr. Transbronchial lung biopsy by the fiberoptic bronchoscope. *Am Rev Resp Dis* 1974;110:4–12.
17. Solomon DA, Solliday NH, Gracy DR. Cytology in fiberoptic bronchoscopy: comparison of bronchial brushings, washings, and postbronchoscopic sputum. *Chest* 1974;65:616–619.
18. Schoenbaum SW, Koerner SK, Ramakrishna B, et al. Transbronchial biopsy of peripheral lesions with fluoroscopic guidance: use of the fiberoptic bronchoscope. *J Can Assoc Rad* 1974; 25:39–43.
19. Kovnat DM, Rath GS, Anderson WM, et al. Bronchial brushing through the flexible fiberoptic bronchoscope in the diagnosis of peripheral pulmonary lesions. *Chest* 1975;67:179–184.
20. Zavala DC. Diagnostic fiberoptic bronchoscopy: techniques ar results of biopsy in 600 patients. *Chest* 1975;3;68:12–19.
21. Kvale PA, Bode FR, Kini S. Diagnostic accuracy in lung canc comparison of techniques used in association with flexible beroptic bronchoscopy. *Chest* 1976;69:752–757.

22. Stringfield JT, Markowitz DG, Bentz RR, et al. The effect of tumor size and location on diagnosis by fiberoptic bronchoscopy. *Chest* 1977;72:474–476.
23. Cortese DA, McDougall JC. Biopsy and brushing of peripheral lung cancer with fluoroscopic guidance. *Chest* 1979;76:141–145.
24. Wallace JM, Deutsch AL. Flexible fiberoptic bronchoscopy and percutaneous needle lung aspiration for evaluating the solitary pulmonary nodule. *Chest* 1982;81:665–671.
25. Cortese DA, McDougall JC. Bronchoscopic biopsy and brushing with fluoroscopic guidance in nodular metastatic lung cancer. *Chest* 1981;79:610–611.
26. Mohsenifar Z, Chopra SK, Simmons DH. Diagnostic value of fiberoptic bronchoscopy in metastatic pulmonary tumors. *Chest* 1978;74:369–371.
27. Radke JR, Conway WA, Eyler WR. Diagnostic accuracy in peripheral lung lesions: factors predicting success with flexible fiberoptic bronchoscopy. *Chest* 1979;76:176–179.
28. Hurt R, Bates M. Carcinoid tumours of the bronchus: a 33 year experience. *Thorax* 1984;39(8):617–623.
29. Dierkesmann R: The diagnostic yield of bronchoscopy. *Cardiovasc Interven Radiol.* 1991;14(1):24–28.
30. Mak VH, Johnston ID, Hetzel MR, Grubb C. Value of washings and brushings at fibreoptic bronchoscopy in the diagnosis of lung cancer. *Thorax* 1990;45(5):373–376.
31. Zisholtz BM, Eisenberg H. Lung cancer cell type as a determinant of bronchoscopy yield. *Chest* 1983;84(4):428–430.
32. Lam WK, So SY, HSu C, Yu DY. Fibreoptic bronchoscopy in the diagnosis of bronchial cancer: comparison of washings, brushings and biopsies in central and peripheral tumours. *Clin Oncol* 1983;9(1):35–42.
33. Popovich J Jr, Kvale PA, Eichenhorn MS, Radke JR, Ohorodnik JM, Fine G. Diagnostic accuracy of multiple biopsies from flexible fiberoptic bronchoscopy. A comparison of central versus peripheral carcinoma. *Am Rev Resp Dis* 1982;125:521–523.
34. Gellert AR, Rudd RM, Sinha G, Geddes DM. Fibreoptic bronchoscopy effect of multiple bronchial bipsies on diagnostic yield in bronchial carcinoma. *Thorax* 1982;37(9):684–687.
35. Chuang MT, Marchevsky A, Teirstein AS, Kerschner PA, Kleinerman J. Diagnosis of lung cancer by fibreoptic bronchoscopy: problems in the histological classification of non-small cell carcinomas. *Thorax* 1984;39(3):175–178.
36. Rudd RM, Gellert AR, Boldy DA, Studdy PR, Pearson MC, Geddes DM, Sinha G. Bronchoscopic and percutaneous aspiration biopsy in the diagnosis of bronchial carcinoma cell type. *Thorax* 1982;37(6):462–465.
37. Marchevsky AM, Chuang MT, Teirstein AS, Nieburgs HE, Kleinerman J. Problems in the diagnosis of small cell carcinoma of the lungs by fiberoptic bronchoscopy. *Cancer Det Prev* 1984; 7(4):253–260.
38. Bjermer L, Thunnell M, Rosenhall L, Stjernberg N. Endobronchial biopsy positive sarcoidosis: relation to bronchoalveolar lavage and course of disease. *Resp Med* 1991; 85(3):229–234.
39. Stjernberg N, Bjornstad-Pettersen H, Truedsson H. Flexible fiberoptic bronchoscopy in sarcoidosis. *Acta Med Scand* 1980; 208(5):397–399.
40. Armstrong JR, Radke JR, Kvale PA, Eichenhorn MS, Popovich J Jr. Endoscopic findings in sarcoidosis. Characteristics and correlations with radiographic staging and bronchial mucosal biopsy yield. *Ann Otol Rhinol Laryngol* 1981;90(4 Pt 1):339–343.
41. Kinnear WJM, Wilkinson MJ, James PD, Johnston IDA. Comparison of the diagnostic yields of disposable and reusable cytology brushes in fiberoptic bronchoscopy. *Thorax* 1991; 46:667–668.
42. Parker RL, Haesaert SP, Kovnat DM, Bachus B, Snoder GL. Bronchial brushing in bronchogenic carcinoma. *Chest* 1977; 71:341–345.
43. Naryshkin S, Daniels J, Young NA. Diagnostic correlation of fiberoptic bronchoscopic biopsy and bronchoscopic cytology performed simultaneously. *Diag Cytopathol* 1992;8:119–123.
44. Shure D, Astarita RW. Bronchogenic carcinoma presenting as an endobronchial mass: optimal number of biopsy specimens for diagnosis. *Chest* 1983;865–867.

Bronchoscopy,
edited by U. B. S. Prakash.
Mayo Foundation © 1994.
Published by Raven Press, Ltd., New York.

CHAPTER 11

Bronchoscopic Lung Biopsy

John C. McDougall and Denis A. Cortese

The ability to obtain lung tissue without subjecting a patient to an open lung biopsy is a major advance in diagnostic bronchoscopy. Because bronchoscopic lung biopsy (also referred to as transbronchoscopic or transbronchial lung biopsy) is a procedure with low morbidity and mortality, patients who would not be candidates for open lung biopsy may have specific diagnoses made, thus allowing clinicians to withdraw potentially toxic "shotgun" therapy. The performance of lung biopsies in more patients allows for more accurate diagnoses, which contributes to our understanding of the clinical spectrum of lung diseases.

Early attempts at transthoracic needle biopsy of the lung (histology, not cytology) caused fatal bleeding (1). This resulted in a hiatus in efforts to biopsy the lung, except by open surgical methods. Bronchoscopic lung biopsy was first performed by Dr. Howard Andersen in 1963, using the rigid bronchoscope. He had noted that alveolar tissue was occasionally seen on tissue samples from attempts to biopsy peripheral lung masses. After practicing the procedure on a dog model, he performed the first bronchoscopic lung biopsy on a human patient in 1963. The patient had a 5-week history of shortness of breath. Chest roentgenogram showed diffuse miliary changes in both lungs. Biopsies from the anterior and posterior basal segments of the right lower lobe showed adenocarcinoma in the lung and lymphatics. Results in 13 patients were reported by Andersen and colleagues in 1965 (2). Pulmonary tissue was obtained in 11 of the 13 patients, and was considered clinically helpful in all 11. Over the next 7 years, Andersen and his colleagues reported 450 cases of bronchoscopic lung biopsy for diffuse lung diseases, and they obtained lung tissue in 84% of those cases (3).

J. C. McDougall: Division of Thoracic Diseases and Internal Medicine, Mayo Clinic, Rochester, Minnesota 55905.
D. A. Cortese: Division of Thoracic Diseases and Internal Medicine, Mayo Clinic, Jacksonville, Florida 32224.

There was some controversy regarding the need for fluoroscopic guidance during biopsies (4–7), but very few other technical differences were reported until 1974 when Levin and colleagues first reported their experience with bronchoscopic lung biopsy via the flexible bronchoscope (8). They reported positive biopsies in 82% of their initial series. These early favorable results (comparable to the rigid bronchoscopic lung biopsy experience) opened the door for the majority of pulmonary diseases specialists (not trained in rigid bronchoscopy) to perform bronchoscopic lung biopsy. Controversy still exists over the need for fluoroscopy (9,13–15) but most other technical details are similar from one report to another.

INDICATIONS

Bronchoscopic lung biopsy should be considered when a diffuse or localized interstitial, alveolar, miliary, or fine nodular pattern of disease is present on the chest roentgenogram, and when the diagnosis cannot reasonably be established by a less invasive diagnostic technique (12,16,17). Localized nodular disease may be diagnosed by bronchoscopic lung biopsy, especially if fluoroscopic guidance is used, but transthoracic needle aspiration or biopsy is more often successful, especially if the nodule is less than 2 cm in diameter (18–20). The indication for bronchoscopic lung biopsy must be carefully considered before the procedure is performed. For example, biopsy of localized disease should not be performed if the lesion will be resected regardless of the results of the biopsy.

CONTRAINDICATIONS

The only absolute contraindication to the performance of bronchoscopic lung biopsy is an uncooperative patient who cannot have a general anesthetic.

TABLE 1. *Contraindications to bronchoscopic lung biopsy*

Absolute:	Patient unable to cooperate with the procedure and unable to have general anesthesia
Relative:	Untreated bleeding diathesis (hemophilia, uremia, anticoagulant therapy, consumptive coagulopathy, thrombocytopenia)
	Severe pulmonary artery hypertension
	Patient's inability to control cough during the procedure

Relative contraindications (Table 1) include an untreated bleeding diathesis (21), thrombocytopenia (10), severe pulmonary artery hypertension (16), and inability to control the patient's cough during the procedure. Bleeding may be excessive if the patient has a platelet count lower than 50,000/μl (10), if the blood urea nitrogen is greater than 30 mg/dl (21), if the patient is on anticoagulant therapy, or if the patient has hemophilia, a consumptive coagulopathy, or other bleeding disorder.

TECHNIQUE

Safe and effective performance of bronchoscopic lung biopsy begins with proper selection and preparation of the patient. The patient should understand the goals and risks of the procedure, and should know how to communicate with the bronchoscopist during the procedure. A system of hand signals and head motion signals should be worked out with the patient in advance of the procedure. Identification of any special risk factors, and correction of those that can be corrected, will contribute to safer performance of bronchoscopic lung biopsy. The bronchoscopy and bronchoscopic lung biopsy procedure must be performed in a procedure room that is equipped with facilities for monitoring blood pressure, pulse, and O_2 saturation. Equipment to deliver supplemental oxygen therapy and for cardiopulmonary resuscitation should also be available. Trained staff should be available during the procedure to assist in monitoring the patient's condition, and to assist the bronchoscopist in the performance of bronchoscopy and bronchoscopic lung biopsy.

The use of fluoroscopy during bronchoscopic lung biopsy is still debated, but most bronchoscopists routinely use it during performance of bronchoscopic lung biopsy via the flexible bronchoscope, so the fluoroscopic equipment should be in place (22). The bronchoscopist should be trained in the use of fluoroscopic equipment or should have a trained person available during the procedure. The equipment may be fixed or portable, and may be single plane or biplane. If the equipment is single plane, the patient may be turned during the procedure to obtain more than one view of the chest. This will facilitate accurate placement of the biopsy forceps.

If a rigid bronchoscope is used, identify the segment to be biopsied and carefully advance the forceps into that segmental bronchus until the forceps moves in and out with the patient's respiratory motion (Fig. 1). Open the forceps as the patient takes a deep breath. Instruct the patient to breathe out fully, and close the forceps. Ask the patient if there is any chest pain. If the patient has no chest pain, slowly remove the closed forceps with the lung specimen. If the patient indicates that there is chest pain, ask the patient to point to the painful area. Pain in the appropriate chest wall location or in the ipsilateral shoulder should prompt the bronchoscopist to open the forceps, withdraw 2–3 cm, and reposition before completing the biopsy. If the patient indicates contralateral chest pain or pain in the throat area, the forceps need not be withdrawn and a biopsy can safely be taken.

If a flexible bronchoscope is used to perform bronchoscopic lung biopsy, the biopsies will be smaller because the forceps are smaller than those used with the rigid bronchoscope (Fig. 2). It is advantageous to pass an oral endotracheal tube to facilitate repeated removal and insertion of the bronchoscope. The endotracheal tube also enables the use of a large-suction catheter if brisk bleeding should develop. After the appropriate segmental bronchus is identified, wedge the tip of the bronchoscope firmly into that segmental orifice. The bronchoscope must not be removed from that position until after the biopsies of that segment are completed and there is no evidence of significant bleeding. If bleeding does develop, the bronchoscope should be

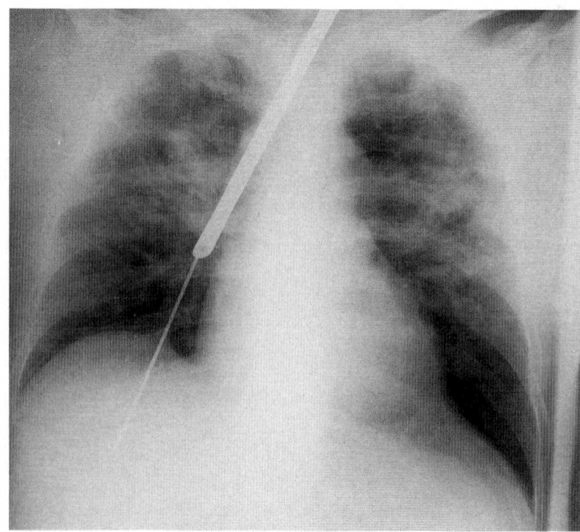

FIG. 1. Rigid bronchoscope with bronchoscopic lung biopsy forceps in place for biopsy.

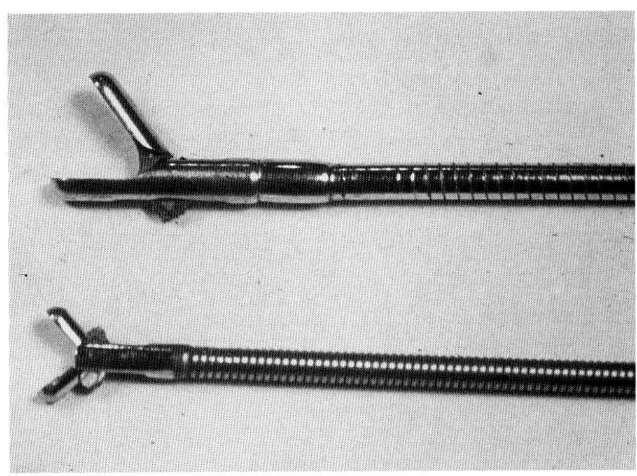

FIG. 2. Rigid (above) and flexible (below) bronchoscopic lung biopsy forceps.

held in the wedged position, to tamponade the segment, for at least as long as the patient's bleeding time. Advance the flexible forceps until it is just beneath the pleura. Withdraw the forceps 2–3 cm, open the forceps, and advance it to its subpleural position (Fig. 3). Close the forceps and ask the patient if there is any chest pain. If the patient indicates no pain, remove the forceps only (not the bronchoscope) with the lung specimen. The forceps should be withdrawn slowly to avoid sudden tearing of lung tissue. If the patient indicates ipsilateral chest or shoulder pain, open the forceps and withdraw it a few centimeters before closing it and repositioning for another attempt.

Fluoroscopic guidance during the performance of bronchoscopic lung biopsy is routinely used for localized infiltrates or lesions, and most bronchoscopists also use it for diffuse disease. If fluoroscopy is used, the position of the forceps should be checked during placement and just prior to removal of the forceps with the lung specimen. Many bronchoscopists routinely screen the lung for pneumothorax at the end of the procedure. If there has been no chest pain during biopsy attempts, if the patient is not short of breath, and if the patient has not coughed excessively while the forceps is placed peripherally, a roentgenogram of the chest is probably not necessary as the incidence of pneumothorax in these circumstances in exceedingly low. However, one should usually be done in the presence of any of the aforementioned three conditions. If the procedure is done with a rigid bronchoscope, the incidence of pneumothorax is high enough to warrant that a chest roentgenogram be done after the procedure whether or not these conditions exist.

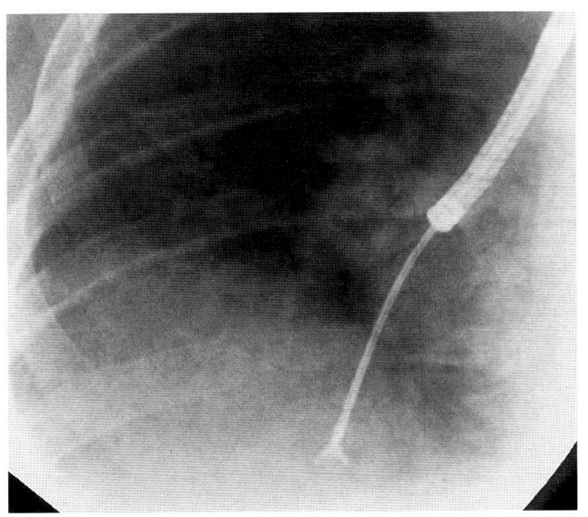

FIG. 3. Flexible bronchoscope with bronchoscopic lung biopsy forceps in place for biopsy.

It is unclear whether the bronchoscopic biopsy forceps pierces the distal bronchial or bronchiolar wall or nips the lung tissue in between two branching bronchi as envisioned by the developers of this technique (Fig. 4).

Controversy still exists over how many biopsies to obtain. Studies indicate that for sarcoidosis, four to five biopsies is enough (23). In other conditions, the yield increases even if six biopsies are taken (24). If the procedure is proceeding smoothly, a goal of five biopsies (good pieces of tissue, not attempts) is reasonable. More biopsies may be needed if some of the tissue is to be sent for cultures or special studies.

Proper handling of the specimens is crucial if optimal information is to be gained from the procedure. Tissue may be sent for frozen section if facilities are available. This allows the bronchoscopist to be confident that adequate samples have been obtained before the procedure is terminated. Tissue for routine histology is placed in formalin solution, and tissue for microbiological studies should be submitted according to guidance from the microbiologist (usually it is sent in sterile saline). Touch preparations of biopsies may be helpful if *Pneumocystis carinii* infection is suspected. Close communication among the bronchoscopist, laboratory

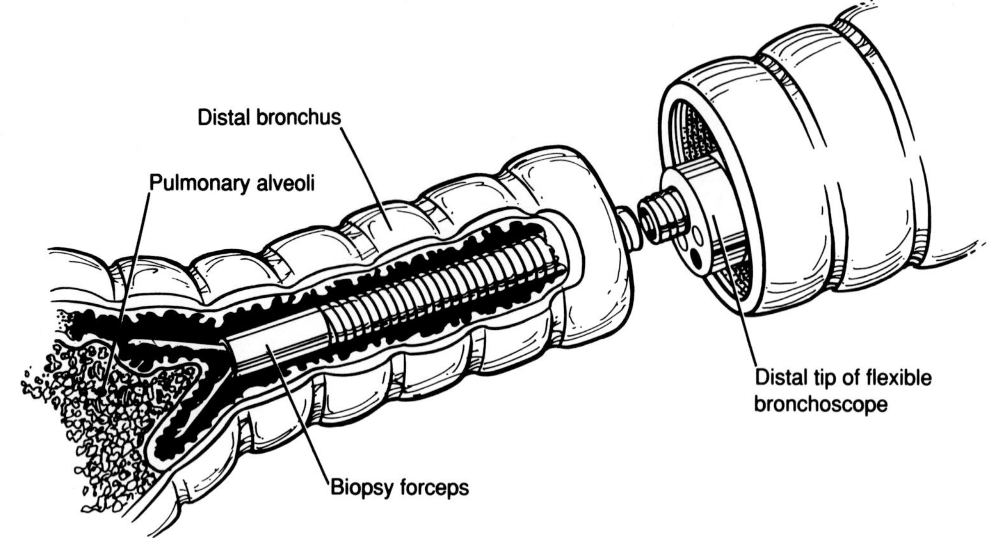

FIG. 4. Artist's rendering of the mechanism of bronchoscopic lung biopsy. The biopsy forceps pinches off the lung tissue located between two branches of terminal bronchi. It is unclear if the biopsy forceps truly pierces the bronchus to obtain lung tissue.

personnel, and the pathologist is essential if the best results are to be obtained.

RESULTS

The results of bronchoscopic lung biopsy depend on many factors, including the technical skill of the bronchoscopist, the type of disease being evaluated, the skill of the pathologist, and especially on the ability of the clinician and pathologist to use all the available information to properly evaluate the biopsy material (7,25–29).

Sarcoidosis is readily diagnosed by bronchoscopic lung biopsy (30–38). Diagnostic rates approaching 95% may be accomplished if adequate numbers of samples are obtained. The optimal number of lung biopsies is four to five (23). It should be noted that a simple bronchial mucosal biopsy may provide adequate tissue. If frozen section capability is available, a bronchial biopsy may be done at the start of the bronchoscopic procedure, and if it is positive, bronchoscopic lung biopsy may not be required (7). This will spare the patient even the small risk of bronchoscopic lung biopsy.

Lymphangitic carcinoma (39) and miliary tuberculosis (40) may also be diagnosed by bronchoscopic lung biopsy in a high proportion of cases. Less frequently, Goodpasture's syndrome may be diagnosed (41).

The diagnosis of usual interstitial pneumonitis (UIP) by bronchoscopic lung biopsy is somewhat controversial. Tissue consistent with the diagnosis is obtained in a large percentage of cases, but good biopsies may be difficult to obtain in advanced fibrotic disease. A nonspecific fibrotic pattern may be seen in other diseases such as scleroderma lung, rheumatoid lung, and radiation fibrosis. Nonspecific fibrosis may also be seen in biopsies from lungs of patients who have no significant lung disease. Careful correlation of historical data, physical findings, and other laboratory tests are needed to make the most of a bronchoscopic lung biopsy. If a patient has slowly progressive interstitial changes on chest roentgenogram, fine rales at the lung bases, digital clubbing, evidence of an altered immune state (elevated globulins, positive antinuclear antibodies, etc.), and a high-resolution CT scan of the lungs consistent with UIP, then a bronchoscopic lung biopsy consistent with the diagnosis may be adequate. If the clinical and laboratory picture are not consistent with the bronchoscopic lung biopsy diagnosis of UIP, then further diagnostic testing is indicated (40,42).

Diffuse nodular infiltrates (nodules >3–4 mm) are not easily diagnosed by bronchoscopic lung biopsy. There is far more normal lung volume than diseased lung volume in this instance, so that random biopsies of the lung are not likely to yield a diagnosis. Single or multiple larger nodules (>2 cm) are more likely to be diagnosed by bronchoscopic lung biopsy if fluoroscopic guidance is used (18,19).

Bronchoscopic lung biopsy is useful in diagnosing pulmonary disease in immune compromised patients (3,8–11,39,43–54,58). *Pneumocystis carinii* pneumonia may be diagnosed in nearly 100% of cases. The use of touch preparations increases the diagnostic efficacy of bronchoscopic lung biopsy in diagnosing this opportunistic infection. Fungal infections such as aspergillosis and cryptococcosis, and cytomegalovirus infections may also be diagnosed with bronchoscopic lung biopsy. The advent of bronchoalveolar lavage has added considerably to the diagnostic efficacy of bronchoscopy in the immune compromised patient, and bronchoscopic lung biopsy is done less frequently than in years past in this group of patients.

Noninfectious conditions that may be diagnosed in the immune compromised patient include radiation pneumonitis, cytotoxic pneumonitis from chemotherapeutic agents, malignant infiltration of the lung (lymphoma, leukemia, carcinomas, Kaposi's sarcoma), and vasculitis. Open lung biopsy is still necessary in some cases where bronchoscopic lung biopsy is unsuccessful (51,53–56).

COMPLICATIONS

Pneumothorax is the most frequent complication of bronchoscopic lung biopsy performed via the rigid bronchoscope, occurring in about 10% of cases (39). Chest tube placement is necessary in half of these instances. There have been deaths from pneumothorax that worsened many hours after lung biopsy (39). For this reason, careful observation is necessary for patients who are found to have a pneumothorax. Observation should take place in a facility where a chest tube can be placed if necessary. Pneumothorax occurs in less than 1% of cases following bronchoscopic lung biopsy performed via the flexible bronchoscope if fluoroscopic guidance is used (59). The incidence rises to 3.4% if fluoroscopic guidance is not used (13).

Moderate (>25 ml) to severe (>100 ml) bleeding occurs in 0.6–5.4% of cases (39,60). Preselection of cases may account for the differences in the reported incidence of bleeding in several large series. Death due to bleeding is rare (61), and bleeding is almost always controllable if careful patient selection and attendance to technical factors is observed. Clinical circumstances may not allow for exclusion of high-risk patients. In these cases, the risk of bronchoscopic lung biopsy must be weighed against the benefit of the procedure, and against the risk of not performing any diagnostic procedure or of performing another, more risky procedure.

Subcutaneous and mediastinal emphysema occur rarely following bronchoscopic lung biopsy, but no serious effects have been noted from these complications.

SUMMARY

The indications, results, and complications of bronchoscopic lung biopsy are well defined after only a 28-year history of this procedure. Patients with diffuse and localized pulmonary disease may now be given an accurate diagnosis in a high percentage of cases using this technique. However, this should not suggest that we have reached the pinnacle of knowledge with this procedure. As new instruments and new methods of laboratory analysis of the biopsies are found, and as new diseases develop, we will undoubtedly continue to build the fund of knowledge on the foundation of those who have taught us what we know today. It is especially important to remember and to teach the principles of safe and effective bronchoscopy if we and our successors are to continue to improve the practice of bronchoscopy and of bronchoscopic lung biopsy.

REFERENCES

1. Personal communication, Howard A. Andersen, M.D.
2. Andersen HA, Fontana RS, Harrison EG Jr. Transbronchoscopic lung biopsy in diffuse pulmonary disease. *Dis Chest* 1965; 48:187–192.
3. Andersen HA, Fontana RS. Transbronchoscopic lung biopsy for diffuse pulmonary diseases: technique and results in 450 cases. *Chest* 1972;62:125–128.
4. Piñeyro JA, Maseda MG, Casamayou E. Biopsia transbronquica dirigida por radioscopia. *Hoja Tisiol* 1969;26:103–112.
5. Palojoki A, Sutinen S. Transbronchoscopic lung biopsy as aid in pulmonary diagnostics. *Scand J Resp Dis* 1972;53:120–124.
6. Andersen HA, Miller WE, Bernatz PE. Lung biopsy: transbronchoscopic, percutaneous, open. *Surg Clin North Am* 1973; 53:785–793.
7. Anderson HA. Transbronchial lung biopsy in diffuse pulmonary disease. *Ann Thorac Surg* 1977;24:1.
8. Levin DC, Wicks AB, Ellis JH. Transbronchial lung biopsy via the fiberoptic bronchoscope. *Am Rev Resp Dis* 1974;110:4–12.
9. Scheinhorn DJ, Joyner LR, Whitcomb ME. Transbronchial forceps lung biopsy through the fiberoptic bronchoscope in *Pneumocystis carinii* pneumonia. *Chest* 1974;66:294–295.
10. Zavala DC. Diagnostic fiberoptic bronchoscopy: Techniques and results of biopsy in 600 patients. *Chest* 1975;68:12–19.
11. Hanson RR, Zavala DC, Rhodes ML, Keim LW, Smith JD. Transbronchial biopsy via flexible fiberoptic bronchoscope: Results in 164 patients. *Am Rev Resp Dis* 1976;114:67–72.
12. Stableforth DE, Knight RK, Collins JV, Heard BE, Clarke SW. Transbronchial lung biopsy through the fibreoptic bronchoscope. *Br J Dis Chest* 1978;72:108–114.
13. de Fenoyl O, Capron F, Lebeau B, Rochemaure J. Transbronchial biopsy without fluoroscopy: a five year experience in outpatients. *Thorax* 1981;44:956–959.
14. Anders GT, Johnson JE, Bush BA, Matthews JI. Transbronchial biopsy without fluoroscopy. *Chest* 1988;94:557–560.
15. Milligan SA, Luce JM, Golden J, Stulbarg M, Hopewell PC. Transbronchial biopsy without fluoroscopy in patients with diffuse roentgenographic infiltrates and the acquired immunodeficiency syndrome. *Am Rev Resp Dis* 1988;137:486–488.
16. Terry P, Marsh B, Heroy J. Transbronchial lung biopsy. *Ann Otol Rhinol Laryngol* 1977;86:115–121.
17. Shure D. Transbronchial biopsy and needle aspiration. *Chest* 1989;95:1130–1138.
18. Cortese DA, McDougall JC. Biopsy and brushing of peripheral lung cancer with fluoroscopic guidance. *Chest* 1979;75:141–145.
19. Cortese DA, McDougall JC. Bronchoscopic biopsy and brushing with fluoroscopic guidance in nodular metastatic lung cancer. *Chest* 1981;79:610–611.
20. Yuan A, Yuan PC, Chang DB, Yu CJ, Yee YC, Kuo SH, Lun KT. Ultrasound-guided aspiration biopsy of small peripheral pulmonary nodules. *Chest* 1992;101:926–930.
21. Zavala DC. Pulmonary hemorrhage in fiberoptic transbronchial biopsy. *Chest* 1976;70:584–588.
22. Prakash UBS, Offord KP, Stubbs SE. Bronchoscopy in North America: the ACCP survey. *Chest* 1991;100:1668–1675.

23. Roethe RA, Fuller PB, Byrd RB, Hafermann DR. Transbronchoscopic lung biopsy in sarcoidosis. Optimal number and sites for diagnosis. *Chest* 1980;77:400.
24. Popovich J Jr, Kvale PA, Eichenhorn MS, Radke JR, Ohorodnik JM, Fine G. Diagnostic accuracy of multiple biopsies from flexible fiberoptic bronchoscopy. *Am Rev Resp Dis* 1982; 125:521–523.
25. Fechner RE, Greenberg, SD, Wilson RK, Stevens PM. Evaluation of transbronchial biopsy of the lung. *Am J Clin Pathol* 1977; 68:17–20.
26. Chuang MT, Raskin J, Krellenstein DJ, Teirstein AS. Bronchoscopy in diffuse lung disease: Evaluation by open lung biopsy in nondiagnostic transbronchial lung biopsy. *Ann Otol Rhinol Laryngol* 1987;96:654–657.
27. Anders GT, Linville KC, Johnson JE, Blanton HM. Evaluation of the float sign for determining adequacy of specimens obtained with transbronchial biopsy. *Am Rev Resp Dis* 1991; 144:1406–1407.
28. Nagata N, Hirano H, Takayama K, Miyagawa Y, Shigematsu N. Step section preparation of transbronchial lung biopsy. *Chest* 1991;100:959–962.
29. Fraire AE, Cooper SP, Greenberg SD, Rowland LP, Langston C. Transbronchial lung biopsy. Histopathologic and morphometric assessment of diagnostic utility. *Chest* 1992;102:748–752.
30. Koerner SK, Sakowitz AJ, Appelman RI, Becker NH. Transbronchial lung biopsy for the diagnosis of sarcoidosis. *N Engl J Med* 1975;293:268–270.
31. Joyner LR, Schneinhorn DJ. Transbronchial forceps lung biopsy through the fiberoptic bronchoscope. *Chest* 1975;67:532–535.
32. Koontz CH, Joyner LR, Nelson RA. Transbronchial lung biopsy via the fiberoptic bronchoscope in sarcoidosis. *Ann Intern Med* 1976;85:64–66.
33. Teirstein AS, Chuang M, Miller A, Siltzbach LE. Flexible-bronchoscope biopsy of lung and bronchial wall in intrathoracic sarcoidosis. *Ann NY Acad Sci* 1976;278:522–527.
34. Smith CW, Murray GF, Wilcox BR, Starek PJ, Delany DJ. The role of transbronchial lung biopsy in diffuse pulmonary disease. *Ann Thorac Surg* 1977;24:54–58.
35. Valenti S, Scordamaglia A. Transbronchial lung biopsy with fiberoptic bronchoscope. *Scand J Resp Dis* 1978;59:243–548.
36. Mitchell DM, Mitchell DN, Collins JV, Emerson CJ. Transbronchial lung biopsy through fibreoptic bronchoscope in diagnosis of sarcoidosis. *Br Med J* 1980;280:679–681.
37. Armstrong JR, Radke JR, Kvale PA, Eichenhorn MS, Popovich J Jr. Endoscopic findings in sarcoidosis. *Ann Otol Rhinol Laryngol* 1981;90:339–343.
38. Stjernberg N, Thunell M, Lundgren R. Comparison of flexible fiberoptic bronchoscopy and scalene lymph node biopsy in the diagnosis of sarcoidosis. *Endoscopy* 1983;15:300–301.
39. Andersen HA. Transbronchoscopic lung biopsy for diffuse pulmonary diseases. *Chest* 1978;73:734–736.
40. Poe RH, Utell MJ, Israel RH, Hall WJ, Eshleman JD. Sensitivity and specificity of the nonspecific transbronchial lung biopsy. *Am Rev Resp Dis* 1979;119:25–31.
41. Abboud RT, Chase WH, Ballon HS, Brzybowski S, Magil A. Goodpasture's Syndrome: Diagnosis by transbronchial lung biopsy. *Ann Intern Med* 1978;89:635–638.
42. Haponic EF, Summer WR, Terry PB, Wang KP. Clinical decision making with transbronchial lung biopsies. *Am Rev Resp Dis* 1982;125:524–529.
43. Ellis JH. Transbronchial lung biopsy via the fiberoptic bronchoscope. *Chest* 1975;68:524–532.
44. Repsher LH, Levin DC, Matthay RA, Stamford RE. Transbronchial lung biopsy via the fiberoptic bronchoscope in the diagnosis of diffuse pulmonary infiltrates in the immunosuppressed host. *Natl Cancer Inst Monogr* 1976;43:127–132.
45. Mathay RA, Farmer WC, Odero D. Diagnostic fibreoptic bronchoscopy in the immunocompromised host with pulmonary infiltrates. *Thorax* 1977;32:539–545.
46. Ellis JH. Diagnosis of opportunistic infections using the flexible fiberoptic bronchoscope. *Chest* 1978;73:713–715.
47. Nishio JN, Lynch JP. Fiberoptic bronchoscopy in the immunocompromised host: the significance of a "nonspecific" transbronchial biopsy. *Am Rev Resp Dis* 1980;121:307–312.
48. Toledo-Pereyra LH, DeMeester TR, Kinealey A, MacMahon H, Churg A, Golomb H. The benefits of open lung biopsy in patients with previous nondiagnostic transbronchial lung biopsy. *Chest* 1980;77:647–650.
49. Williams D, Yungbluth M, Adams G, Glassroth J. The role of fiberoptic bronchoscopy in the evaluation of immunocompromised hosts with diffuse pulmonary infiltrates. *Am Rev Resp Dis* 1985;131:880–885.
50. Harcup C, Baier HJ, Pitchenik AE. Evaluation of patients with the acquired immunodeficiency syndrome (AIDS) by fiberoptic bronchoscopy. *Endoscopy* 1985;17:217–220.
51. Mones JM, Saldana MJ, Oldham SA. Diagnosis of *Pneumocystis carinii* pneumonia. *Chest* 1986;89:522–526.
52. Cockerill FR III, Wilson WR, Carpenter HA, Smith TF, Rosenow EC III. Open lung biopsy in immunocompromised patients. *Arch Intern Med* 1985;145:1398–1404.
53. Puska S, Hutcheon MA, Hyland RH. Usefulness of transbronchial biopsy in immunosuppressed patients with pulmonary infiltrates. *Thorax* 1983;38:146–150.
54. Leight GS Jr, Michaelis LL. Open lung biopsy for the diagnosis of acute, diffuse pulmonary infiltrates in the immunosuppressed patient. *Chest* 1978;73:477–482.
55. Catterall JR, McCabe RE, Brooks RG, Remington JS. Open lung biopsy in patients with Hodgkin's disease and pulmonary infiltrates. *Am Rev Resp Dis* 1989;139:1274–1279.
56. Wall CP, Gaensler EA, Carrington CB, Hayes JA. Comparison of transbronchial and open biopsies in chronic infiltrative lung diseases. *Am Rev Resp Dis* 1981;123:280–285.
57. Warner DO, Warner MA, Divertie MB. Open lung biopsy in patients with diffuse pulmonary infiltrates and acute respiratory failure. *Am Rev Resp Dis* 1988;137:90–94.
58. Mitchell DM, Emerson CJ, Collins JV, Stableforth DE. Transbronchial lung biopsy with the fibreoptic bronchoscope: analysis of results in 433 patients. *Br J Dis Chest* 1981;75:258–262.
59. Zavala DC. Transbronchial biopsy in diffuse lung disease. *Chest* 1978;73:727–733.
60. Flick JR, Wasson K, Dunn LJ, and Block AJ. Fatal pulmonary hemorrhage after transbronchial lung biopsy through the fiberoptic bronchoscope. *Am Rev Resp Dis* 1975;111:853–856.
61. Andersen HA, Harrison EG. Transbronchoscopic lung biopsy in diffuse pulmonary disease. *Ann Otol Rhinol Laryngol* 1965; 74:1113–1119.

Bronchoscopy,
edited by U. B. S. Prakash.
Mayo Foundation © 1994.
Published by Raven Press, Ltd., New York.

CHAPTER 12

Bronchoscopic Needle Aspiration and Biopsy

David E. Midthun and Denis A. Cortese

Bronchoscopic needle aspiration is one of the many techniques now available to the bronchoscopist to diagnose lung pathology and also offers a nonsurgical means to stage bronchogenic carcinoma. The desire to biopsy lymph nodes in the mediastinum lead to techniques for sampling tissue through the tracheal or bronchial wall. Initially, this was performed with the rigid bronchoscope and a long metal needle and later evolved to a short needle on a flexible catheter used through the flexible bronchoscope. In addition to the advances in the equipment used, the applications of bronchoscopic needle aspiration have expanded to include not only sampling of paratracheal or mediastinal lymph nodes but also peripheral, submucosal, and endobronchial lesions.

The original description of bronchoscopic puncture of subcarinal mediastinal lymph nodes is credited to Schieppati (1,2). The technique involved a rigid bronchoscope and a 50 cm × 1 mm needle; the bronchoscopist punctured the carina with the needle tip and advanced the needle 2–3 cm while suction was applied (2). In 1978, Wang et al. first described needle aspiration of paratracheal masses using a rigid bronchoscope and a long, rigid, esophageal varices needle (3). Although Ikeda introduced the revolutionary flexible bronchoscope in 1968, a number of years passed before the technique of needle aspiration was adapted to this bronchoscope. In 1979, Oho and colleagues reported use of the first needle adapted for the flexible bronchoscope and described its versatility as well as safety—no significant complications in over 800 procedures (4). Early adaptations of flexible needles varied in style and gauge and, for the most part, these were 20- to 23-gauge needles and allowed aspiration of lymph node tissue for cytological examination. Larger bore needles (18-gauge) have been developed in an attempt to obtain a histological specimen (5).

D. E. Midthun: Division of Thoracic Diseases and Internal Medicine, Mayo Clinic, Rochester, Minnesota 55905.

D. A. Cortese: Division of Thoracic Diseases and Internal Medicine, Mayo Clinic, Jacksonville, Florida 32224.

EQUIPMENT

As with any bronchoscopic procedure, the most important ingredient for successful bronchoscopic needle aspiration is a bronchoscopist knowledgeable in its application and skilled in its use. The needle itself must be designed to pass through a bronchoscope without causing damage and be pliant enough to negotiate flexion of the bronchoscope yet rigid enough to allow penetration of the airway wall. There are currently several types of needles available that incorporate these features. The exact details of available needles were excellently described by Wang in 1989 (6,7). Needle catheters currently in use are typically 120 cm long. One style consists of an inner stylet and an outer semitranslucent catheter with a 1- to 1.3-cm, 21- to 23-gauge needle fixed at its tip. Another style consists of an outer catheter with a smooth metal hub, an inner retractable catheter tipped with a similar needle, and a stylet to provide rigidity. Regardless of the needle and catheter configuration, suction is applied after withdrawal of the stylet and directly through the needle channel (6).

TECHNIQUE

The procedure of bronchoscopic needle aspiration begins with the review of the chest roentgenogram and other imaging materials to identify and select the anatomic location for needle aspiration and biopsy. The computed tomographic images of upper thorax are particularly helpful for selecting the location of paratracheal and subcarinal lymph nodes for the procedure. After standard bronchoscopic examination is completed to exclude obvious mucosal abnormalities, the location is selected for the needle puncture and extra amounts of topical anesthesia instilled through the bronchoscope to minimize cough. Then the selection of an appropriate needle is made. Most commonly, a 21- or 18-gauge needle is used depending on the size and location of the lesion and whether a cytology or a histology specimen is desired. The needle catheter is then introduced through the suction channel and the distal tip of the needle placed in a position just visible from the end of the bronchoscope to facilitate accurate placement (Fig. 1). When using a retractable needle, the distal tip of the outer catheter should be in view before the needle is extended to prevent damage to the working channel of the bronchoscope. Advancement of the needle through the tracheal or bronchial wall is facilitated by puncturing between the cartilaginous rings of the selected site (Fig. 2). The needle tip may be advanced by direct forward force on the catheter, by fixing the proximal aspect of the catheter on the bronchoscope and advancing the bronchoscope and catheter together, or by having the patient intentionally cough while maintaining the needle in a fixed position. If much of the flexible catheter extends beyond the tip of the bronchoscope, it may bend and make bronchial wall penetration difficult. The needle tip should be advanced so that its entire length is through the bronchial wall; assurance of this position may be noted by advancing the bronchoscope down the catheter to see that the hub is impaled against the mucosa (Fig. 3). Once the needle is embedded, suction is applied with a syringe connected to the distal port of the needle. While maintaining suction, the needle catheter is vigorously agitated to and fro, without removing the needle from the tracheobronchial wall, in an attempt to shear off cells in the impaled node or mass. While the needle is gradually withdrawn from the wall, suction is gently released. If possible, the needle tip is retracted to protect the working channel and the needle catheter is removed from the bronchoscope.

The specimen thus obtained is prepared by expelling a few drops of saline from the syringe through the catheter out the needle tip and onto a slide, smearing the fluid between two slides, and placing them in 95% ethanol for cytological review. Remaining fluid may be flushed through the catheter needle tip for additional cytological preparation. Studies have shown that two or three needle aspirations in the same site can be safely performed (8,9), although the optimal number of aspirations is yet to be clarified. When an 18-gauge needle is employed, there may be a core of tissue expelled from the needle, and this may be sent for histological preparation. Initial penetration and aspiration with a 21- to 23-gauge needle may allow identification of a vessel underlying the desired site and prevent puncture with the 18-gauge needle.

Slight alterations in technique allow needle aspirations of tissue from the submucosa, endobronchial lesions, and peripheral nodules or masses. In each case, it is important to protect the bronchoscope during needle manipulation as well as place the needle optimally to obtain the desired specimen. Advancing the needle tip incompletely and at an acute angle through the bronchial wall allows shearing off of cells from the submucosa. Endobronchial lesions are generally easily approached, and needle aspiration may avoid hemorrhagic complications resulting from forceps biopsy. With fluoroscopy to assure proper needle placement, peripheral lesions may be approached in a manner similar to bronchoscopic forceps biopsy.

Easy access to an excellent cytopathology laboratory is imperative for the success of bronchoscopic needle aspiration in the diagnosis of malignant and benign processes. The accuracy of diagnosis with a posi-

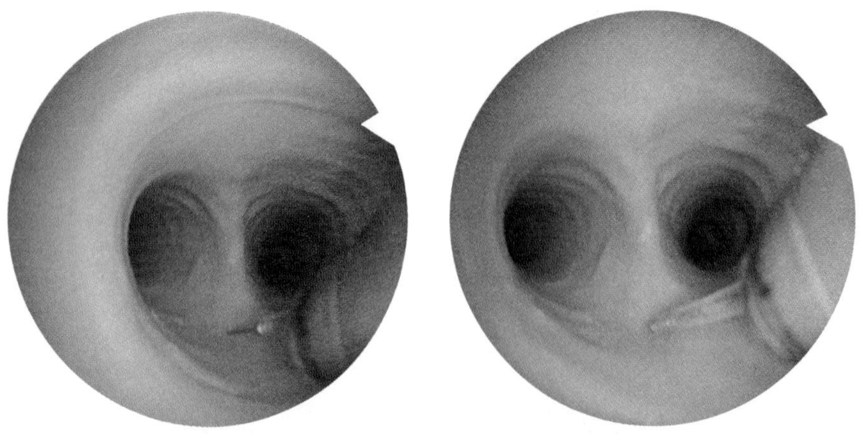

FIG. 1. **(A)** Bronchoscopic image of another bronchoscope in the process of performing transcarinal needle insertion in a model of a tracheobronchial tree. Note the ideal distance to which the needle has extended outside the flexible bronchoscope. **(B)** The needle has fully entered the carina.

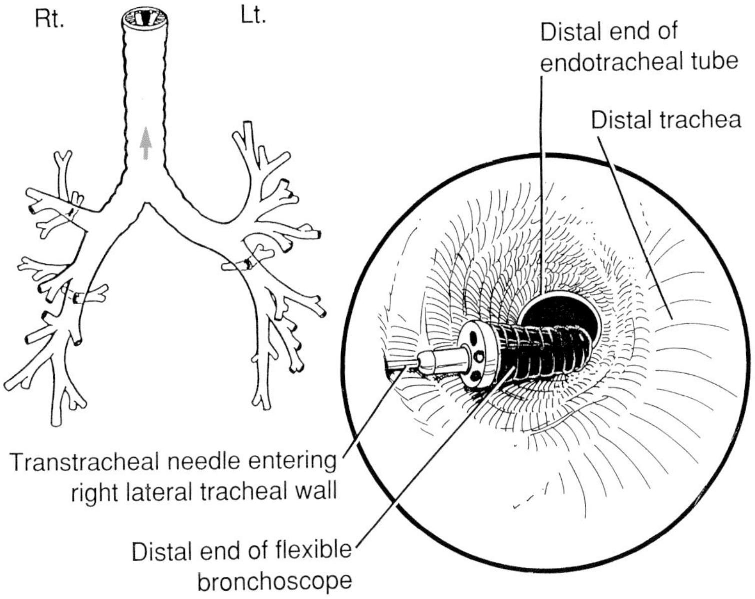

Rt.
Lt.
Distal end of endotracheal tube
Distal trachea
Transtracheal needle entering right lateral tracheal wall
Distal end of flexible bronchoscope

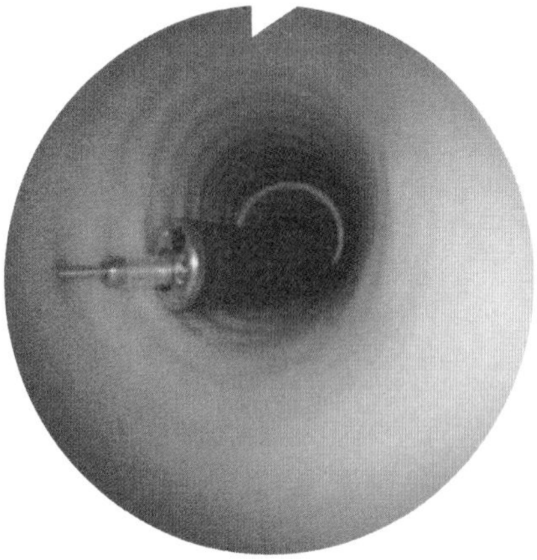

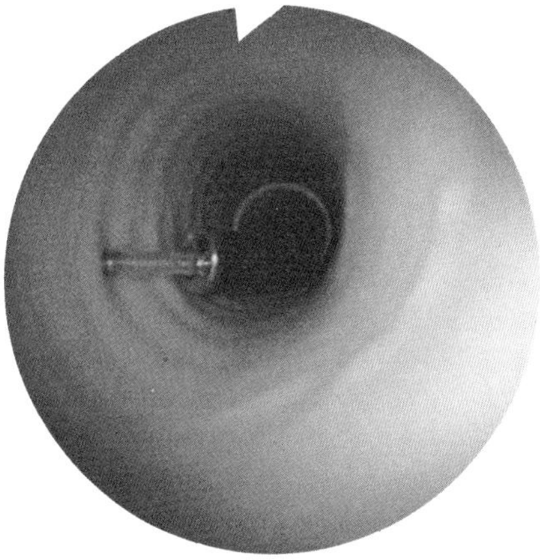

FIG. 2. Cephalad (reversed) view of right paratrache lymph node aspiration simulated in a model of the t cheobronchial tree. Ideally, the needle should be insert between cartilages as shown **(Top)**. The needle is fu inserted into the paratracheal area **(Bottom)**.

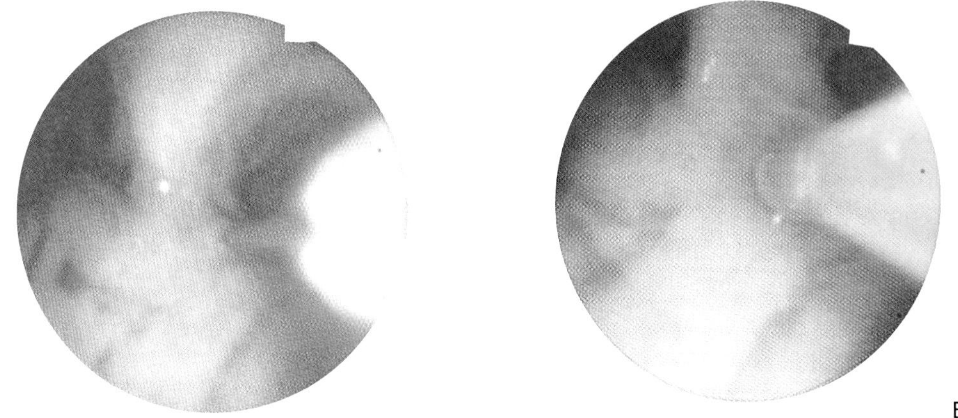

FIG. 3. Actual performance of subcarinal needle aspiration in a patient with significant subcarinal lymphadenopathy secondary to small cell carcinoma. **(A)** The needle is inserted half way. **(B)** The needle is inserted fully into the subcarinal lymph node before aspiration is begun.

tive cytology is very high, but a few false-positive cases have been reported (9–13). False-positive aspirations may be avoided by performing needle aspirations before brushings or biopsies are performed. Care needs to be taken to avoid contamination of the aspirate either with secretions in the airway or in the bronchoscope itself. Communication with the cytopathologist is important. Aspirates from lymph nodes should contain lymphocytes, and an aspiration containing few malignant cells in the absence of lymphocytes may represent contamination (11).

Although the accuracy of a positive cytology specimen is extremely high, the predictive value of a negative aspirate is quite low. The availability of immediate interpretation of bronchoscopic aspirates has been reported to result in a significant increase in the percentage of specimens containing malignant cells and a decrease in the percentage of specimens that were inadequate for diagnosis (14). If the patient has a separate mucosal lesion, inadvertent aspiration of abnormal cells from this area may results in false-positive cytology (13).

INDICATIONS

Diagnosis and Staging of Lung Cancer

Bronchoscopic needle aspiration is most commonly used in an attempt to establish the presence of malignancy in mediastinal lymph nodes. A positive aspirate from a mediastinal node assists in the staging of patients with bronchogenic carcinoma and may obviate the need for mediastinoscopy and/or thoracotomy. Considering the large number of patients with bronchogenic carcinoma, staging by bronchoscopic needle aspiration can result in considerable cost savings (15). The versatility of the needle allows node sampling in the paratracheal, subcarinal, hilar, and aortopulmonary regions. When computed tomography of the chest shows enlarged mediastinal lymph nodes and bronchoscopic needle aspirate is positive for malignancy, surgery is usually not indicated (11,16).

Surgical staging may still be required to determine operability when there is evidence of limited N2 disease (stage III), for which resection may still be a consideration. A negative needle aspiration of mediastinal lymph nodes does not exclude the possibility of nodal involvement even when the nodes are of normal size on computed tomography. Normal or small nodes are frequently involved with microscopic tumor. McKenna et al. showed that up to 40% of patients with bronchogenic carcinoma will have mediastinal lymph node involvement despite the fact that lymph nodes were less than 1 cm in size by computed tomography (17). Surgical staging is appropriate when bronchoscopic needle aspiration is negative. Results of bronchoscopic needle aspiration for staging of bronchogenic carcinoma vary considerably and correlate with the presence or absence of radiographic or bronchoscopic abnormalities.

Shure and Fedullo reported that bronchoscopic needle aspiration of the carina was positive in only 15% of 110 consecutive patients with bronchogenic carcinoma; however, 38% were positive if the carina appeared abnormal (15). In patients with a radiographically abnormal mediastinum and subsequently proven to have carcinoma, Gay and Brutinel reported positive needle aspirations in 37%; this increased to 88% if a mucosal abnormality or external compression was seen at bronchoscopy (18). In patients with malignancy and a normal mediastinum on chest roentgenogram, Harrow et al. reported positive transcarinal needle aspirations in 46% (16). Wang and Terry reported a 73% positive aspiration rate in patients with an abnormal mediastinum on roentgenogram (19). A recent series by Harrow showed the presence of N2 disease, as confirmed by positive bronchoscopic needle aspiration, correlated with three findings: adenopathy by chest roentgenogram or computed tomography, widening of the carina, and the presence of endobronchial disease, especially of the right upper lobe (12).

Peripheral Malignant Lesions

Bronchoscopic needle aspiration is a useful means to diagnose peripheral pulmonary lesions (see also Chapter 10, this volume). The placement of the needle is facilitated with fluoroscopic guidance. Shure and Fedullo reported an increase in yield from 48% to 69% in the diagnosis of peripheral bronchogenic carcinoma by adding needle aspiration to the combination of bronchoscopic biopsy, brush, and wash (20). The success of bronchoscopic forceps biopsy of peripheral lesions is dependent on lesion size with a very low yield in nodules less than 2 cm and 40–50% in nodules 2–4 cm (21). Bronchoscopic needle aspiration is similarly limited by lesion size but apparently less so than forceps biopsy. Wang et al. were able to establish a diagnosis of malignancy in 47% of nodules less than 3 cm in size, 80% in those greater than 3 cm, and bronchoscopy was nondiagnostic in three patients whose lesions were less than 2 cm in diameter (22). In this series, brush and forceps biopsy were performed prior to needle aspiration, and a needle aspiration was the only means of diagnosis in 35% of the lesions.

When approaching a peripheral lesion with a brush or biopsy forceps under fluoroscopy, one occasionally finds that the instrument can be passed to the border of the lesion but not into it. The ability of the needle to penetrate the bronchial wall offers an advantage under these circumstances when an extrabronchial or submucosal process produces narrowing of the bronchus and limits the approach of a brush or forceps. An additional attractive feature of needle aspiration over forceps biopsy in evaluating peripheral lesions is that the former generally produces less bleeding. The "needle brush," which is a brush with a sharpened tip that retracts into a flexible catheter, has shown promise with a higher diagnostic yield in malignant lung masses or nodules than bronchoscopic needle aspiration or forceps biopsy (23).

Submucosal Malignant Lesions

Bronchoscopic needle aspiration is also a helpful adjunct to forceps biopsy in diagnosing submucosal or peribronchial tumor (Fig. 4). Shure and Fedullo showed that bronchoscopic needle aspiration was positive in 71% of patients with bronchoscopic evidence of submucosal or peribronchial tumor, whereas forceps biopsy was positive in only 55% (8). The combination of needle aspiration and forceps biopsy provided a diagnosis of malignancy in 89% of the cases. York et al. used bronchoscopic needle aspiration to identify the submucosal tumor and found it useful in bronchoscopically defining the surgical resection line (24).

Endobronchial Malignant Lesions

Due to the diagnostic success attainable with brushing and forceps biopsy, there is little role for the bronchoscopic needle in diagnosing lesions visible through the bronchoscope. Kvale et al. reported a diagnostic yield of 86% using the combination of bronchial brushing and forceps biopsy in endobronchially visible lesions (25). In a study to determine the optimal number of biopsy specimens to be taken of an endobronchial mass lesion, Shure and Astarita obtained a diagnosis of bronchogenic carcinoma in 100% of consecutive cases by performing three forceps biopsies (26). In a direct comparison of forceps biopsy to bronchoscopic fine needle aspiration for visible tumors, Lundgren et al. obtained a diagnosis of malignancy in 85% of the cases with forceps biopsy and only 65% with needle aspiration (27). Forceps biopsy and brushing of visible lesions can usually be performed with minimal bleeding; however, the bronchoscopic needle may be helpful in safely obtaining a specimen from a high vascular tumor. The presence of endobronchial carcinoid tumor is one such instance in which forceps biopsy has been reported to have a high incidence of significant hemorrhage, and rigid bronchoscopy has been recommended as the preferred diagnostic approach (28). Givens and Marini reported the successful aspiration of a core of tissue from a bronchial carcinoid tumor using a bronchoscopic aspiration needle (29). If bronchial carcinoid is suspected, the use of a bronchoscopic needle may allow the bronchoscopist to obtain a diagnosis and avoid hemorrhagic complications.

Benign Diseases

In addition to its use in the diagnosis of pulmonary malignancy, bronchoscopic needle aspiration may be

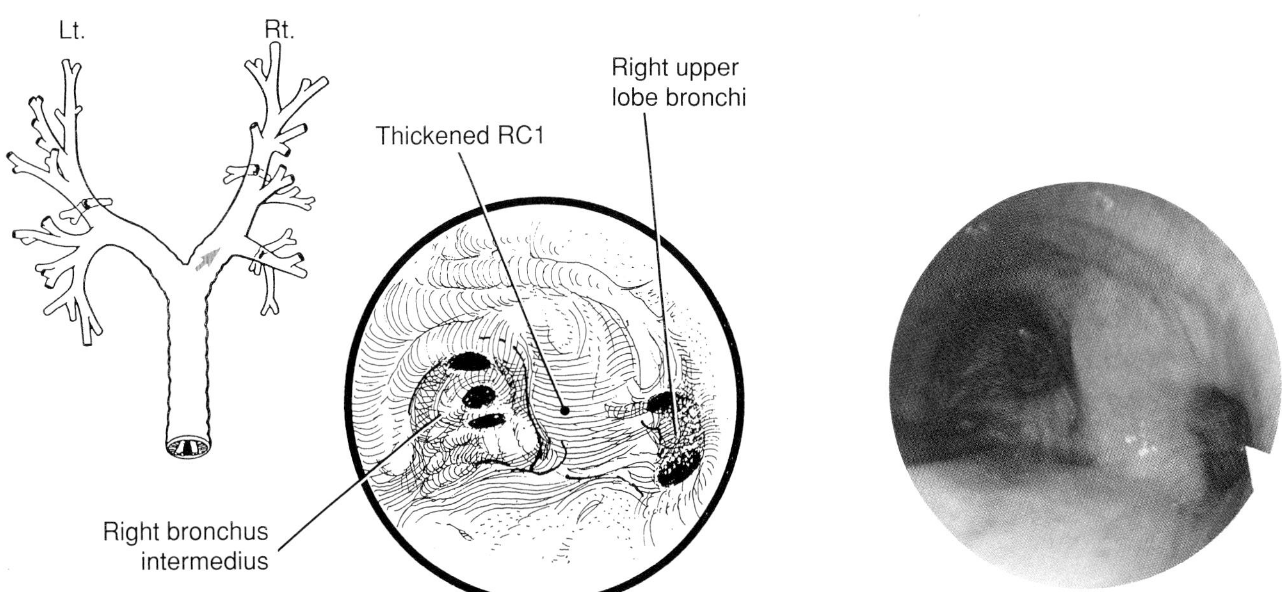

FIG. 4. An abnormally thickened RC1 carina. Even though the mucosa appears normal, this is an ideal location for submucosal and/or bronchoscopic needle aspiration and biopsy.

helpful in establishing a benign diagnosis. In a series of 193 patients with suspected sarcoidosis, Pauli et al. reported that bronchoscopic needle aspiration biopsies revealed noncaseating granulomas in 66% of patients (30). They used rigid bronchoscopy and a larger needle than is typically used with the flexible bronchoscope to aspirate lymph nodes in the right lobar carina, left lobar carina, and paratracheal regions. When they combined bronchoscopic needle aspiration with forceps biopsies of bronchial mucosa, the diagnosis of sarcoidosis increased to 78% (30). This is still considerably less than the 90% diagnostic rate in sarcoidosis reported with the combination of bronchial mucosal and bronchoscopic lung biopsies (31). Bronchoscopic needle aspiration has also been reported to be helpful in the diagnosis and treatment of bronchogenic cysts (32,33).

In an attempt to define a role for bronchoscopic needle aspiration in the diagnosis of pneumonia, Shure and Moser used a canine model of *Streptococcus pneumoniae* pneumonia but found that needle aspiration produced a poor yield compared to transthoracic needle aspiration, protected catheter brush, or bronchial biopsy (34). In a prospective study of 20 patients with acute bacterial pneumonia who had not received antibiotics, Lorch et al. reported no difference in the ability to diagnose pneumonia when comparing protected bronchoscopic needle aspiration to protected specimen brush (35). Baron reported the diagnosis of mediastinal mycobacterial lymphadenopathy by bronchoscopic needle aspiration (36).

CONTRAINDICATIONS

Contraindications to bronchoscopic needle aspiration and biopsy are similar to those for bronchoscopic lung biopsy. Absolute contraindications include the inability of the patient to cooperate, excessive coughing and movement of the body by the patient, and untreated hemorrhagic diathesis including thrombocytopenia and uremia. Pulmonary hypertension is a relative contraindication. Obstruction of the superior vena cava may result in increase in the number and size of paratracheal venous channels and a needle puncture in this region may result in paratracheal hemorrhage and formation of hematoma. The subcarinal region is devoid of major vascular structures and therefore the risk of bleeding is minimal.

COMPLICATIONS

Evaluation of clinical experience has established bronchoscopic needle aspiration as a safe and useful procedure with a very low incidence of complications (11,12,15,16,20,37). Removal of the needle from the bronchial wall commonly results in a small amount of bleeding, although this can hardly be considered a complication. Significant bleeding rarely occurs even after vascular puncture, as is indicated by a bloody return in the suction catheter. Harrow et al. reported no significant bleeding despite aspiration of blood in about 25% of cases (16). Hemomediastinum after bronchoscopic needle aspiration has been reported (38); however, in the past, cardiac and hemodynamic studies have been safely performed via placement of vascular needles through the bronchial wall into the aorta, pulmonary artery, and left atrium (39). In a series of 146 patients who underwent bronchoscopic needle aspiration for diagnosis or staging of mediastinal disease, Wang et al. reported one pneumothorax and one pneumomediastinum for a complication rate of 1.4% (40). In a different series, Wang et al. reported one pneumothorax that required a chest tube for resolution, although it was unclear whether the pneumothorax was a result of bronchoscopic needle aspiration or bronchoscopic forceps biopsy (22).

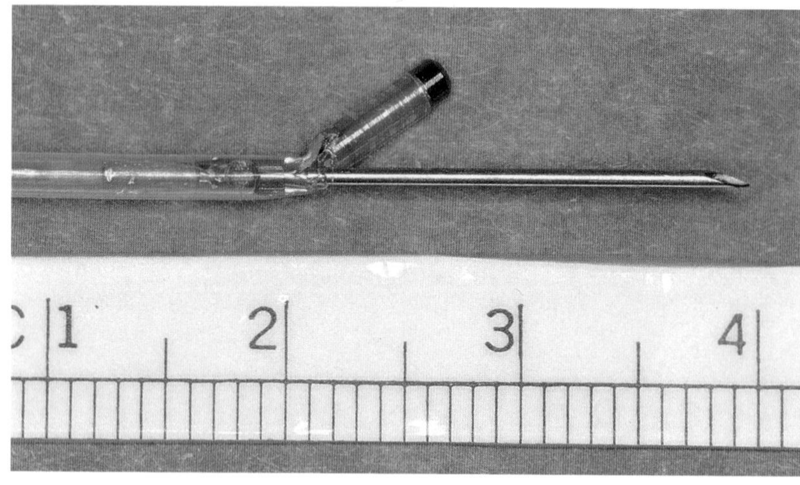

FIG. 5. Partial fracture of needle catheter by the sharp needle. The totally severed tip of the catheter has the potential to become an iatrogenic tracheobronchial foreign body.

Although the incidence is very low, fever and bacteremia have been reported following bronchoscopic needle aspiration (41,42), as has bacterial pericarditis (43). Most of the large series report use of bronchoscopic needles ranging in size from 20 to 23 gauge; however, use of an 18-gauge needle does not appear to significantly increase the rate of complications (5). To our knowledge, there has not been a death attributed to bronchoscopic needle aspiration. The plastic tip of the needle catheter can be severed by the sharp needle and become an iatrogenic tracheobronchial foreign body (Fig. 5).

SUMMARY

Bronchoscopic needle aspiration has evolved from subcarinal lymph node aspiration with a rigid bronchoscope to sampling of submucosal, peribronchial, and peripheral lesions, as well as mediastinal nodes with the flexible bronchoscope. Needle aspiration is generally easily performed and uncommonly results in significant hemorrhage or pneumothorax. Its greatest utility to the clinician remains the ability to sample paratracheal, subcarinal, and hilar nodes. Computed tomography directs the bronchoscopist in her or his approach, and the likelihood of a positive aspiration increases in the presence of carinal or endobronchial abnormalities. Although bronchoscopic needle aspiration of mediastinal nodes is frequently negative, a positive result establishes N2 disease and obviates surgical staging in most cases. False-positive results are rare and with precaution may be avoided.

REFERENCES

1. Schieppati E, La Punción Mediastinal a Través del Espolón Traqueal. *Rev As Med Angent* 1949;663:497.
2. Schieppati E. Mediastinal lymph node puncture through the tracheal carina. *Surg Gynecol Obstet* 1958;107:243–246.
3. Wang KP, Terry P, Marsh B. Bronchoscopic needle aspiration biopsy of paratracheal tumors. *Am Rev Resp Dis* 1978; 118:17–21.
4. Oho K, Kato H, Ogawa I, Hayashi N, Hayata Y. A new needle for transfiberoptic bronchoscope use. *Chest* 1979;76:492.
5. Wang KP. Flexible Transbronchial needle aspiration biopsy for histologic specimens. *Chest* 1985;88:860–863.
6. Wang KP. Flexible bronchoscopy with transbronchial needle aspiration: biopsy for cytology specimens. In: Wang KP, ed. *Biopsy techniques in pulmonary disorders*. New York: Raven Press; 1989.
7. Wang KP. Flexible bronchoscopy with transbronchial needle aspiration biopsy for histology specimens. In: Wang KP. *Biopsy techniques in pulmonary disorders*. New York: Raven Press; 1989.
8. Shure D, Fedullo PF. Transbronchial needle aspiration in the diagnosis of submucosal and peribronchial bronchogenic carcinoma. *Chest* 1985;88:49–51.
9. Harrow EM, Oldenburg FA Jr, Lingenfelter MS, Smith AM Jr. Transbronchial needle aspiration in clinical practice: a five-year experience. *Chest* 1989;96:1268–1272.
10. Cropp AJ, DiMarco AF, Lankerani M. False-positive transbronchial needle aspiration in bronchogenic carcinoma. *Chest* 1984; 85:696–697.
11. Schenk DA, Bower JH, Bryan CL, Currie RB, Spence TH, Duncan CA, Meyers DL, Sullivan WT. Transbronchial needle aspiration staging of bronchogenic carcinoma. *Am Rev Resp Dis* 1986;134:146–148.
12. Harrow E, Halber M, Hardy S, Halteman W. Bronchogenic and roentgenographic correlates of a positive transbronchial needle aspiration in the staging of lung cancer. *Chest* 1991; 100:1592–1596.
13. Carlin BW, Harrell JH II, Fedullo PF. False-positive transcarinal needle aspirate in the evaluation of bronchogenic carcinoma. *Am Rev Resp Dis* 1989;140:1800–1802.
14. Davenport RD. Rapid on-site evaluation of transbronchial aspirates. *Chest* 1990;98:59–61.
15. Shure D, Fedullo PF. The role of transcarinal needle aspiration in the staging of bronchogenic carcinoma. *Chest* 1984; 86:693–696.
16. Harrow EM, Oldenburg FA, Smith AM. Transbronchial needle aspiration in clinical practice. *Thorax* 1985;40:756–759.
17. McKenna RJ, Libshitz HI, Mountain CE, McMurtney MJ. Roentgenographic evaluation of mediastinal nodes for preoperative assessment in lung cancer. *Chest* 1985;88:206–210.
18. Gay PC, Brutinel WM. Transbronchial needle aspiration in the practice of bronchoscopy. *Mayo Clin Proc* 1989;64:158–162.
19. Wang KP, Terry PB. Transbronchial needle aspiration in the diagnosis and staging of bronchogenic carcinoma. *Am Rev Resp Dis* 1983;127:344–347.
20. Shure D, Fedullo PF. Transbronchial needle aspiration of peripheral masses. *Am Rev Resp Dis* 1983;128:1090–1092.
21. Cortese DA, McDougall JC. Biopsy and brushing of peripheral lung cancer with fluoroscopic guidance. *Chest* 1979;75:141–145.
22. Wang KP, Haponik EF, Britt EJ, Khouri N, Erozan Y. Transbronchial needle aspiration of peripheral pulmonary nodules. *Chest* 1984;86:819–823.
23. Wang KP, Britt EJ. Needle brush in the diagnosis of lung mass or nodule through flexible bronchoscopy. *Chest* 1991; 100:1148–1150.
24. York EL, Jones RL, King EG, Chaput MR, Nguyen GK. The value of submucous needle aspiration in the prediction of surgical resection line of bronchogenic carcinoma. *Chest* 1991; 100:1028–1029.
25. Kvale PA, Bode FR, Kini S. Diagnostic accuracy in lung cancer: comparison of techniques used in association with flexible fiberoptic bronchoscopy. *Chest* 1976;69:752–757.
26. Shure D, Astarita RW. Bronchogenic carcinoma presenting as an endobronchial mass: optimal number of biopsy specimens for diagnosis. *Chest* 1983;83:865–867.
27. Lundgren R, Bligman F, Angstrom T. Comparison of transbronchial fine needle aspiration biopsy, aspiration of bronchial secretion, bronchial washing, brush biopsy and forceps biopsy in the diagnosis of lung cancer. *Eur J Res Dis* 1983;64:378–385.
28. Hurt R, Bates M. Carcinoid tumors of the bronchus: A 33-year experience. *Thorax* 1984;39:617–623.
29. Givens CD Jr, Marini JJ. Transbronchial needle aspiration of a bronchial carcinoid tumor. *Chest* 1985;88:152–153.
30. Pauli G, Pelletier A, Bohner C, Roeslin N, Warter A, Roegel E. Transbronchial needle aspiration in the diagnosis of sarcoidosis. *Chest* 1984;85:482–484.
31. Koerner SK, Sakowitz AJ, Appleman RI, Becker NH, Schoenbaum SW. Transbronchial lung biopsy for the diagnosis of sarcoidosis. *N Engl J Med* 1975;293:268–270.
32. Schwartz AR, Fishman EK, Wang KP. Diagnosis and treatment of a bronchogenic cyst using tracheobronchial needle aspiration. *Thorax* 1986;41:326–327.
33. McDougall JC, Fromme GA. Transcarinal aspiration of a mediastinal cyst to facilitate anesthetic management. *Chest* 1990; 97:1490–1492.
34. Shure D, Moser KM. Transbronchial needle aspiration in the diagnosis of pneumonia in a canine model. *Am Rev Resp Dis* 1985;131:290–291.
35. Lorch DG, John JF Jr., Tomlinson JR, Miller KS, Sahn SA. Protected transbronchial needle aspiration and protected speci-

men brush in the diagnosis of pneumonia. *Am Rev Resp Dis* 1987;136:565–569.
36. Baron KM, Aranda CP. Diagnosis of mediastinal mycobacterial lymphadenopathy by tracheobronchial needle aspiration. *Chest* 1991;100:1723–1724.
37. Salathe M, Soler M, Bollinger CT, Dalquen P, Perruchoud AP. Tracheobronchial needle aspiration in routine fiberoptic bronchoscopy. *Respiration* 1992;59:5–8.
38. Kucera RF, Wolfe GK, Perry ME. Hemomediastinum after transbronchial needle aspiration. *Chest* 1986;90:466.
39. Crymes TP, Fish RG, Smith DE, Takaro T. Complications of transbronchial left atrial puncture. *Am Heart J* 1959;58:46–52.
40. Wang KP, Haponik EF, Gupta PK, Erozan YS. Flexible transbronchial needle aspiration: technical considerations. *Acta Otol Rhinol Laryngol* 1984;93:233–236.
41. Witte MC, Opal SM, Gilbert JG, Pluss JL, Thomas DA, Olsen JD, Perry ME. *Chest* 1986;89:85–87.
42. Watts WJ, Green RA. Bacteremia following transbronchial fine needle aspiration. *Chest* 1984;85:295.
43. Epstein SK, Winslow CJ, Brecher SM, Faling LJ. Polymicrobial bacterial pericarditis after tracheobronchial needle aspiration: case report with an investigation on the risk of bacterial contamination during fiberoptic bronchoscopy. *Am Rev Resp Dis* 1992; 146:523–525.

Bronchoscopy,
edited by U. B. S. Prakash.
Mayo Foundation © 1994.
Published by Raven Press, Ltd., New York.

CHAPTER 13

Bronchoalveolar Lavage

Richard A. Helmers and Richard J. Pisani

Although the technique of washing the lung with physiological saline to remove accumulated material and cells from the air space has been used for many years as a therapeutic approach to pulmonary alveolar (phospholipo) proteinosis, it was with the advent of widespread use of flexible fiberoptic bronchoscopy in the 1970s that instillation of smaller quantities of saline directly into the distal airways and recovering the aspirate for analysis—bronchoalveolar lavage (BAL)—became an important clinical and investigational tool (1,2). BAL allows the recovery of both cellular and noncellular components from the epithelial surface of the lower respiratory tract and differs significantly from bronchial washings, which refer to aspiration of either secretions or small amounts of instilled saline from the large airways (3). The conceptual basis of BAL is that cells and noncellular components present on the epithelial surface of the alveoli are representative of the inflammatory and immune system of the entire lower respiratory tract. In addition, BAL allows sampling of various components of the inflammatory and immune system at their site of action (1,4). In this chapter, we will describe the technique and the role of bronchoalveolar lavage in different pulmonary disorders.

TECHNIQUES AND PROCESSING

The techniques for performing BAL and processing the fluid are not standardized from one institution to another, which may account in part for the variability in reported results. The techniques described below are those used at the Mayo Clinic, which are identical to routine bronchoscopies except that the lavage procedure is also performed. BAL is performed after routine inspection/examination of the tracheobronchial tree and before biopsy and/or brushings in order to avoid contamination of the recovered fluid with excess blood, which would alter the concentrations of cellular and noncellular components. The suction channel of the bronchoscope is then thoroughly rinsed with saline, the suction trap changed, and the tip of the bronchoscope advanced distally until it is wedged into a subsegmental bronchus, usually at the level of the fourth to fifth branching. Care should be taken to avoid trauma and coughing as these may lead to excessive contamination of the recovered fluid with mucus and blood (5). Passing the bronchoscope through a previously inserted endotracheal tube has been shown to reduce oropharyngeal contamination when BAL specimens are cultured (6). There are no absolute contraindications to BAL, but one should be aware of high-risk situations and *relative* contraindications. These include an uncooperative patient, an FEV_1 less than 800–1000 cm^3, moderate to severe asthma, hypercapnia, hypoxemia uncorrected to an oxygen saturation of 90% with supplemental oxygen, serious cardiac dysrhythmia, myocardial infarction within 6 weeks, uncorrected bleeding diathesis, and hemodynamic instability (3).

In most cases, both segments of the lingula *and* the right middle lobe are routinely lavaged and analyzed separately. Other lobes may be lavaged (especially if radiographically abnormal); however, because of the upper lobe bronchial anatomy, returns from lavage of the upper lobe are significantly less than those from the middle and lower lobes (1,2,7).

In normals, the cell counts, cell differentials, and lavage proteins are similar between the right middle lobe, lingula, and lower lobes (7). However, when localized disease is apparent radiographically, lavage should be carried out in multiple sites, including the area with focal radiographic abnormalities, as the BAL results may be most abnormal from these areas (4,8,9).

R. A. Helmers: Division of Thoracic Diseases and Internal Medicine, Mayo Clinic, Scottsdale, Arizona 85259.

R. J. Pisani: Division of Thoracic Diseases and Internal Medicine, Mayo Clinic, Rochester, Minnesota 55905 (current address: 12911, 120th Avenue, NW, Seattle, Washington 98034).

There is not uniform agreement regarding interlobar variation in BAL results when the chest radiograph shows diffuse changes and, consequently, we routinely lavage both the right middle lobe and lingula. Garcia et al. (10) found significant interlobar variation in BAL cell differentials between the right middle lobe and lingula obtained from patients with idiopathic pulmonary fibrosis (IPF), pulmonary fibrosis associated with collagen vascular disease (PFCVD), and in a small group of mixed interstitial lung disorders; patients with sarcoidosis, however, had excellent bilobar agreement. In this study, the chest X ray was markedly insensitive to lavage interlobar variation (10). In contrast, Helmers et al. (11) found no significant differences in BAL cell concentration or differential from side to side (right middle lobe versus lingula) in patients with sarcoidosis, IPF, or PFCVD with nonfocal disease on chest radiograph.

In an average-sized person at total lung capacity, the typical lavaged zone represents about 165 ml and the residual volume of this zone is approximately 45 ml (12). It might be argued that pockets of residual gas may prevent BAL fluid from reaching some alveolar spaces and that BAL in these sites might be more bronchiolar than alveolar; however, animal studies have shown that although lavage of an air-free lobe recovers a larger number of cells than an air-filled lobe, the cell differentials remain the same (13).

After the bronchoscope is wedged, 20 ml of 0.9% sterile saline, preferably at 37°C, is infused with a syringe with or without a three-way stopcock into the suction port of the bronchoscope. The fluid is then removed from the lung by the use of 50–80 mm Hg of negative pressure from a usual suction apparatus and collected into 50- to 100-ml specimen traps. Prewarming the lavage fluid to 37°C may help prevent coughing and bronchospasm, especially in patients with hyperresponsive airways, and may increase fluid recovery and cellular yield in comparisons to instillations of fluid at room temperature (3,5,9). The traps should be made of material to which the cells are poorly adherent, such as polyethylene or polycarbonate; unsiliconized glass materials should not be used (5,9). The lavage procedure is repeated a total of 5 times in each site for a total of 100 ml per site. One should instruct the patient to inhale and exhale deeply during fluid aspiration and maintain the suction channel of the bronchoscope in the center of the airway lumen. If an adequate "wedge" is maintained throughout the lavage, the patient should not experience cough, since the lavage fluid should not "leak" proximal to the bronchoscope (4). Levels of applied suction greater than 50–80 mm Hg may cause distal airway collapse and lead to inadequate returns. Both during and for 2 hr following the BAL, all patients are routinely administered 2 L of nasal oxygen (12).

The lavage of a normal adult with 100 ml saline yields 40–60 ml fluid containing 5–10 $\times$ 10^6 cells and 1–10 mg protein (1). It has been estimated that a 100-ml lavage of a bronchial subsegment represents the sampling of about 10^6 alveoli (2,12). Lavage results are, in general, not considered valid if (a) the patient has purulent secretions in the airways, (b) the bronchoscope is not maintained in the wedge position during the lavage procedure, and (c) the volume of fluid recovery is less than 40% of the volume infused (4). In general, 40–60% of the infused volume is recovered and cell viability is generally greater than 80% (1,7,14). In patients with loss of elastic recoil, the recovery of fluid is usually less since the bronchial walls collapse when suction is applied (1,2,5). In general, the volume of fluid recovered decreases also with advancing age and with cigarette smoking; at least in normals, the percent of fluid recovery is greatest in young never-smokers (15). It has also been noted that the percentage of fluid recovered and total cell counts are significantly lower if the procedure is performed using general anesthesia versus local/topical anesthesia; the cell concentrations, proportions of various cells, and cell viability are not affected (16). Excessive lidocaine should be avoided primarily because of the theoretical argument that it may impair the in vitro function of the inflammatory and immune effector cells recovered; it is thought, however, that this effect is reversible by cell washing (17–19). BAL specimens have also been shown to not contain lidocaine concentrations high enough to inhibit the culture and growth of pathogens that may be inhibited by lidocaine (20).

The volume of fluid infused is an important variable between institutions. Often larger amounts of lavage fluid (up to 240–300 ml) have been used, particularly if a larger number of inflammatory cells is required; but it is generally agreed that increased patient morbidity may result, particularly local atelectasis and transient fevers (1,4,5). In contrast, smaller amounts of BAL fluid may sample only small bronchi and/or relatively few alveoli. Kelly et al. (21), by a digital subtraction imaging technique in normal volunteers, demonstrated that lavage volumes of 60 ml sampled only proximal airways but that a volume of 120 ml instilled into a single segment appeared to perfuse the entire segment (including distal airways and alveoli) and aspiration of this volume produced fluid movement from within the whole of the segment. Similar preliminary observations by magnetic resonance imaging (MRI) scanning in patients with interstitial lung disease (after lavage with 100 ml saline instilled into either the right middle lobe or lingula) support the concept that volumes of 100–120 ml adequately sample the alveolar surface (22). A recent study examined 55 patients with nonfocal interstitial lung disease in which both a 100-ml (20 cm^3 $\times$ 5) and a 250-ml (50 cm^3 $\times$ 5) BAL were performed in the same lobe of the lung along with a 100-ml BAL on the contralateral side (11). Although the percent fluid return was slightly higher with the large-volume BAL, there were no significant differences in cell differentials or cell concentrations between 100 and 250 ml BAL. For clinical purposes, then, a small-volume BAL of 100–150 ml is preferable since large-volume lavage may be associated with increased morbidity (see below).

Several investigators have evaluated cell differentials on sequential aliquots of recovered lavage fluid and have concluded that the initial aliquot (if the volume of infused fluid is small, i.e., 20 ml) is different from subsequent aliquots in that the initial aliquot is likely to recover cells and proteins from distal bronchi and not alveoli (5,23–26). For this reason, some suggest that the return from the initial aliquot should be discarded. Merrill et al. (27) evaluated protein recovery in successive aliquots of BAL fluid in normals and noted a decrease in the absolute concentration of all proteins in serial aliquots; however, the ratio of various proteins to an albumin standard did not change. They thus concluded that lung proteins are efficiently and homogeneously sampled with 100 ml of lavage instillate. Rennard et al. (26) processed the first 20-ml aliquot ("bronchial") separately from the return of the subsequent four 20-ml aliquots ("alveolar") in 109 patients and 18 normals. They found that pooling the "bronchial" and "alveolar" material will result in a sample that was mostly "alveolar" and concluded it is unlikely that including the first aliquot, which represents 10% or less of the total recovered cells, will affect the cellular analysis in the absence of significant inflammation. But if a patient has obvious airway inflammation, the analysis may be heavily influenced by bronchial airway secretions. Our policy is to pool all five aliquots in the absence of purulent bronchial secretions.

The problem of data standardization is also apparent with the quantification in lavage fluid of soluble, noncellular constituents of the lower respiratory tract such as proteins, lipids, and carbohydrates. The concentration of a soluble substance recovered with BAL depends on the lavage volume. However, as the lavage volume increases, the concentration of soluble factors decreases in a way that is not predicted by simple dilution (12). Quantitative expression of the noncellular constituents of BAL fluid is complex and controversial because of the variability of BAL return and the unavailability of satisfactory reference standards to control for the dilution of soluble components by the lavage fluid (3). However, comparison to a standard substance may be necessary if (a) a substance is present in the serum and also derived from local lung production, and (b) the percentage of recovery is markedly reduced by the underlying disease (9). Many investigators at present use albumin as the standard to normalize the concentration of soluble factors in BAL fluid. This relies on the assumption that the amount of albumin on the alveolar surface is not altered by various disease processes; this is clearly not the case in various interstitial lung diseases or in adult respiratory distress syndrome (ARDS) (14,63,64). If albumin is used as a standard in certain disease states, the concentration of certain components of lavage fluid may be underestimated (14). The use of urea or methylene blue as marker remains controversial (3,9,65). There is general agreement that no ideal denominator or method at calculation exists to quantitate the dilution factor; currently soluble components of the lower respiratory tract are expressed either as units per milliliter albumin or as units per milliliter of lavage fluid (3,9).

The concentration of glucose in BAL fluid is approximately 40 μg/ml and of protein is about 0.06 mg/μl, of which 30% is albumin (28). Rankin et al. (29) found that the viability of cells obtained by BAL was maintained when the lavage fluid was maintained at 25°C for up to 4 hr and that it is not necessary to add either culture medium or antibiotics to lavage specimens for transport to a centralized laboratory. Lavages performed at Mayo Clinic–Scottsdale and Mayo Clinic–Jacksonville are processed in Rochester. Immediately after the procedure is completed, the fluid is spun at 2,400 rpm for 5 min, the supernatant discarded, and the cell pellet resuspended in an equal volume of RPMI 1640 medium. The specimen is shipped on ice overnight to the Rochester laboratory and processed the next morning.

Kelly et al. (30), using tritiated water, technetium colloid, and methylene blue, performed a quantitative analysis of the complex fluid dynamics of a standardized BAL. They demonstrated a bidirectional flux of water occurred across the alveolar membrane. With the 5 × 20 ml technique, the net dilution of the aspirate was 20%; a 3 × 60 ml BAL produced a net dilution of 25%. But the final dilution was the net effect of fluid loss and gain and the total water gained contributed 45% of the total aspirated volume. Thus, for example, for every 180 ml of fluid introduced into a middle lobe segment, about 60 ml effluxed into the circulation, countered by an influx of about 105 ml from the circulation, giving a net dilutional volume of 225 ml (30).

PROCEDURE

At the Mayo Clinic, the processing of a BAL specimen involves the collaboration of physicians and technical support staff from pulmonology, hematopathology, cytopathology, and microbiology. Currently, there is not a standardized protocol for the analysis of BAL fluid. With that in mind, we will outline the interdisciplinary approach used at our institution and make reference to modifications that others have found useful.

Specimens obtained in the bronchoscopy suite are hand-carried to the microbiology area within 1–2 hr of being collected. Samples are designated as either "ICH" (immune compromised host) or "non-ICH," each of which activates a unique protocol. If the sample is ICH, 15 ml is decanted under sterile conditions in microbiology. This aliquot is then used to set up cultures for bacteria, legionella, mycobacteria (including *Nocardia*), fungi, and viruses. Some have recommended the use of quantitative cultures in diagnosing bacterial pneumonia (43), but other reports have downplayed the benefits of that technique (44). Preliminary data suggested that counting intracellular bacteria might distinguish colonization/contamination from lower respiratory infection (44), but more recent results from the same group raise questions about the sensitivity and specificity of this technique (45). Currently, we do not perform quantitative cultures or count intracellular bacteria on BAL specimens.

Viral cultures are set up from 2 ml of this aliquot. Cultures for cytomegalovirus (CMV), herpes simplex, varicella zoster, influenza A/B, enterovirus, parainfluenza, adenovirus, and respiratory syncytial virus are performed. A CMV shell vial assay employing a monoclonal antibody directed against CMV has been used at our institution for several years. This technique has been fully described elsewhere (46,47). The use of other monoclonal antibodies (48) and in situ hybridization (49) for the identification of CMV in BAL specimens has been well documented.

Once microbiology has removed 15 ml for the tests outlined above, the sample is promptly forwarded to the hematopathology lab for the preparation of cytospin slides and a cytology slide. The former can be stained by different methods to provide a differential count, microbiology stains, and immunocytological marker studies.

Cytology specimens are made by combining 2–5 ml of BAL fluid with 4–10 ml of Carbowax fixative in a 15-ml centrifuge tube. The sample is then plated on slides in the cytology area and reviewed by one of our cytopathologists for the presence of malignant cells.

The remainder of the BAL fluid is placed in 15-ml centrifuge tubes and centrifuged at 1,000 *g* for 5 min. The supernatant is decanted and stored at −70°C for future use. The pellets are inspected for the presence of red blood cells. If they are present, each pellet is briefly treated with 4 ml of lysing solution (1.09 g $KHCO_3$ and 8.12g NH_4Cl dissolved in 1 L of sterile water), recentrifuged, and resuspended in 1–2 ml of normal saline. Tubes are combined and saline is added until the combined sample contains 10 ml. Cells are counted in a Neubauer chamber and the sample is then diluted or concentrated to achieve a final working concentration of 1 million cells/ml. Two-hundred-microliter aliquots of this sample are placed in plastic cytospin funnels and centrifuged at 1,200 rpm for 5 min.

A differential count is done by air-drying one of the slides and staining with Wright's stain. If greater than 10% lymphocytes is identified by the technician performing the differential count, four slides are held over for possible immunophenotyping. If the sample is a non-ICH specimen, the differential count is reviewed by one of three hematopathology consultants for a final differential count. Some have suggested that the use of a cytocentrifuge selectively decreases the lymphocyte percentage on the differential count and recommended the use of a filter preparation to perform differential counts (50). Unfortunately, the use of a filter is time consuming and does not permit determination of lymphocyte subpopulations. Recently, a glass cover technique has been reported that circumvents these problems and does not diminish lymphocyte counts (51). Until the methodology for this portion of the BAL processing procedure is standardized, we plan to continue with cytocentrifugation.

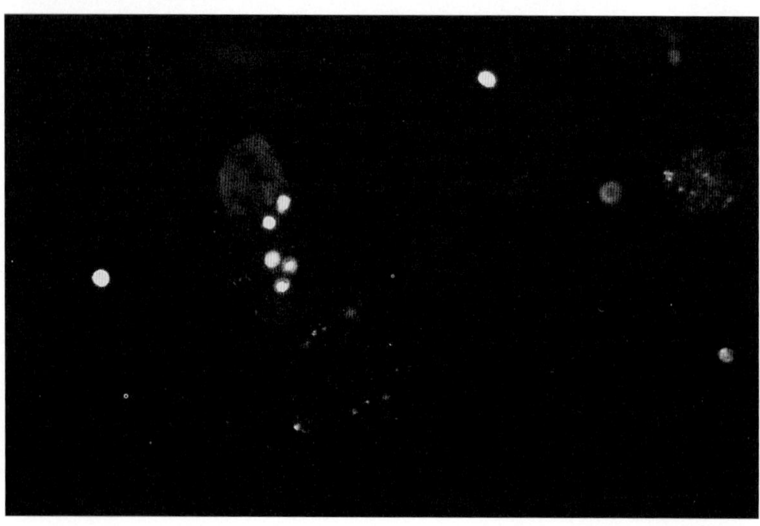

FIG. 1. *Pneumocystis carinii* cysts (white ovals) identified on BAL cytospin by calcifluor white staining.

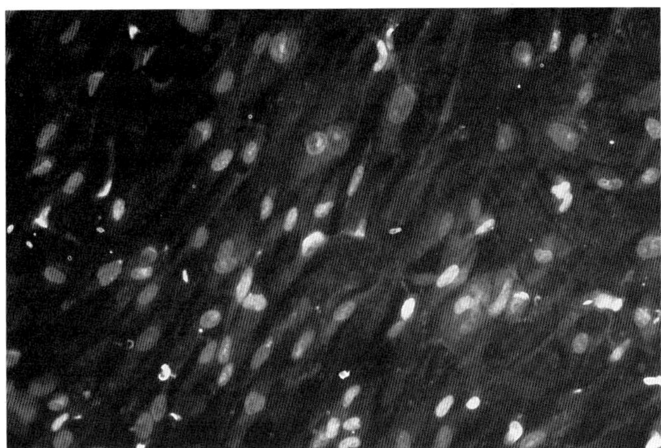

FIG. 2. Shell vial assay of BAL fluid showing positive immunofluorescence (white staining) for cytomegalovirus.

Ten of the cytospin slides are immediately sent back to microbiology for multiple staining procedures including Gram, *Nocardia,* direct fluorescent antibody (for legionella), AFB, KOH, and calcifluor white stains. The latter has replaced the methenamine silver stain in our microbiology laboratory as the preferred stain for *Pneumocystis carinii*. This is based on a study we reported recently demonstrating that the diagnostic yield with calcifluor white was comparable or superior to that of methenamine silver; BAL samples were examined using both (52). Calcifluor white is also less labor-intensive and time consuming. Numerous other techniques for detecting *Pneumocystis* have been described such as Papanicolaou (53), indirect fluorescent antibody (54), Diff-Quick (55), toluidine blue (56), Giemsa (57), and hematoxylin-eosin (58) stains. Dark field microscopy (59) and immunoblotting (60) have also been used successfully. At our institution, the results of rapid identification microbiology procedures are phoned back to the clinician requesting the BAL within 6–12 hr after bronchoscopy.

At least four cytospin slides are prepared for non-ICH processing. Along with the consultant-read differential, this protocol includes routine immunocytochemical staining for T cells (Leu 1 and Leu 4), B cells (HLA-DR or B1), and T-cell subsets (CD4 and CD8). In our experience, at least 10% lymphocytes must be present in the differential to permit high-quality immunocytochemical staining. A goat anti–mouse horseradish peroxidase secondary antiserum is used after a 30- to 60-min incubation with the primary antibody at room temperature. Exact details of this procedure have been described elsewhere (61). Some have favored the use of fluorescent second-step antibodies and, when applied to samples still in solution, this approach permits the application of flow cytometry to BAL samples (62).

In addition to these fairly regimented protocols for samples designated as ICH or non-ICH, physicians may request other tests that can be performed on BAL samples. If histiocytosis X is suspected, cytospins can be stained with OKT6 monoclonal antibody to detect Langerhans cells. If lymphoma or plasmacytoma is

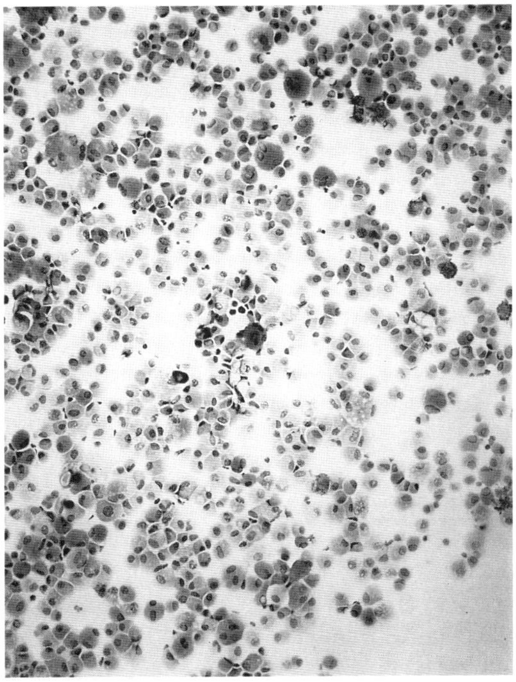

FIG. 3. Immunoperoxidase stain of BAL cytospin showing several CD6-positive (dark staining) cells in a patient with histiocytosis X.

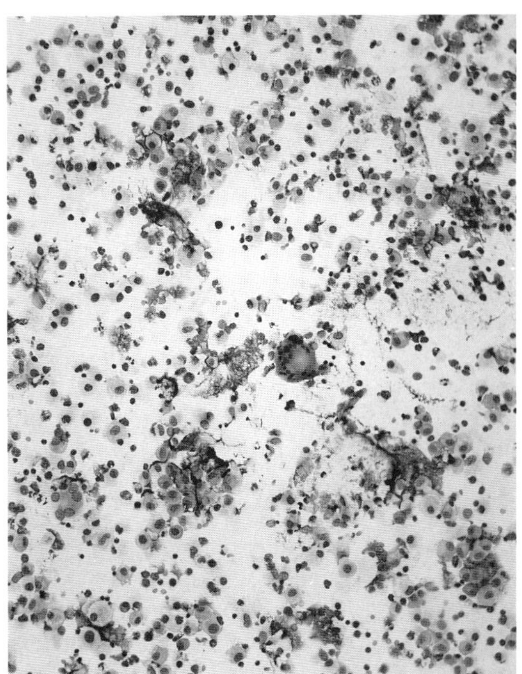

FIG. 4. Multinucleated giant cell seen in the BAL cytospin from a patient with sarcoidosis. BAL also showed 30% lymphocytes, consistent with sarcoidosis.

suspected, staining for λ and k surface antigens can be performed. At Mayo, we use an immunoperoxidase in both of these circumstances. Finally, if alveolar hemorrhage is suspected, cytospins can be stained with hemosiderin to establish the presence of hemosiderin-laden macrophages.

When the results of a lavage cell analysis are reported, BAL fluid cells should be expressed both as number/ml and as a percentage of the total cell population (plus an estimate of total cell numbers should be given), so that results are not misleading as these numbers provide complementary information (1,15). A normal cell differential does not always indicate that the lung is free of inflammation, e.g., a markedly increased number of cells with a normal differential may be associated with an inflammatory process in the lung (14).

SAFETY AND COMPLICATIONS

BAL is a relatively safe procedure that adds about 15 min to a routine flexible fiberoptic bronchoscopic examination. Strumpf et al. (31) reviewed 281 BAL procedures performed on 141 individuals. In >95% of the procedures, no complications or adverse reactions occurred. In the remaining procedures, only minor complications developed, none of which significantly compromised patient care. There were no episodes of pneumothorax, significant dysrhythmia, respiratory arrest, or mortality. The most frequently seen complication was post-BAL fever, which occurred in 7 (2.5%) patients and resolved with no therapy. Other studies have demonstrated that a delayed febrile response may occur in up to 10–50% of patients who undergo BAL; usually this does not represent pulmonary infection but a transient pyrogen effect that can be treated with antipyretics (28). Cole et al. (32) noted fever in approximately 20% of patients who underwent large-volume (300–500 ml) BAL and Pingleton et al. (7) noted fevers, chills, and myalgias in nearly 50% of normal volunteers who underwent extensive lavage of four lobes. The incidence of post-BAL fever thus seems to be related to both the number of lobes lavaged and the total volume of fluid instilled into each lavage site.

Tilles et al. (33) examined changes in pulmonary function 30 min after small-volume (175 ml) and large-volume (500 ml) BAL in normals and after small-volume lavage in patients with sarcoidosis. In normals, small-volume lavage produced no change in pulmonary function except for a small fall in peak expiratory flow rate (PEFR); large-volume lavage resulted in a significant fall in FEV_1, FVC, and PEFR. In patients with sarcoidosis FEV_1, FVC, and PEFR declined by 20 ± 4.8, 26.7 ± 7.3, and 15.2 ± 4.1%, respectively. Although these changes are greater than those found in our experience, they indicate that it is necessary to be cautious in performing BAL on patients with interstitial lung disease when this degree of reduction in pulmonary functions would be poorly tolerated (33). Ettensohn et al. (34) recently reported that pulmonary function in normals remains unchanged after multiple small-volume (120 ml) BAL procedures and concluded it was safe to perform repeated BAL in normal volunteers.

BAL may also result in a decrease in PaO_2. Cole et al. (32) noted an average fall in PaO_2 of 22.7 mm Hg, which persisted for at least 2 hr. Pirozynski et al. (35) noted that the degree of desaturation associated with BAL was related to the volume of fluid instilled. Lin et al. (36) performed 200-ml BAL in 27 young healthy individuals and found 1–2 hr following BAL that the PaO_2 fell 28.42 ± 6.2 mm Hg. They also found a significant fall in FEF_{25-75} when room temperature saline was instilled, but a fall in PaO_2 of 14.91 ± 5.04 mm Hg (and no change in FEF_{25-75}) if the saline instilled was 37°C.

Stover et al. (37) reviewed their results in 97 immunocompromised patients who underwent BAL in the evaluation of diffuse infiltrates. Eighteen patients were on assisted ventilation and 35 had severe thrombocytopenia at the time of BAL. There were no major complications; two thrombocytopenic patients had an increased amount of blood in their BAL fluid, but there was no persistent hemorrhage. Fifty percent of their patients had an increase in temperature post-BAL as well as a slight worsening of infiltrate in the area of lavage, but blood cultures were consistently negative and there were no adverse sequelae.

Multiple studies have looked at the safety of diagnostic BAL in AIDS patients. In general, most AIDS patients experience a transient increase in oxygen requirements, a transient increase in pulmonary infiltrates, and transient elevation in temperature post-BAL (38–40). In AIDS patients who were thrombocytopenic or who required mechanical ventilation, there was no significant morbidity or mortality with BAL and no episodes of serious hemorrhage. Similarly, in bone marrow transplant patients (even if thrombocytopenic or requiring mechanical ventilation) BAL has been judged safe (41). In studies of ARDS, BAL has also been well tolerated. In summary, multiple studies at different institutions have examined immunosuppressed and/or thrombocytopenic patients, in some cases requiring mechanical ventilation, and have concluded that BAL has an acceptable morbidity as a diagnostic tool.

Gurney et al. (42) prospectively evaluated the radiographic manifestations of lavage. In their study, 30 min after lavage, 90% (47 of 52) of lobes lavaged revealed homogeneous areas of new or increased consolidation, most often in the peripheral portion of the lobe. Usually, the margins were indistinct and prominent air bronchograms were absent. Resolution of these opacities was gradual, with opacities remaining in 91% (of the 47) at 90 min, 73% at 240 min, and all had cleared by 24 hr. The presence of these opacities correlated with the amount of retained saline solution, were limited to the area lavaged, and were not associated with clinical complications. The authors concluded that, following BAL, these benign fleeting opacities related to BAL should be considered in the differential diagnosis of new findings on chest X ray (42).

NORMAL VALUES

BAL fluid in a normal adult will be composed of approximately 92 ± 5% macrophages, 7 ± 1% lymphocytes, and less than 1% neutrophils, eosinophils, basophils, or mast cells (1,14). The high normal percentage of lymphocytes in lavage fluid is considered to be in the 10–15% range, with most normal individuals falling under 10%. However, Laviollette (66) reported 5 of 42 normal, healthy, nonsmoking volunteers who had a lymphocyte count greater than 20%, which then normalized to below 14% on follow-up BAL in four of the five. Ettensohn et al. (34) reported very similar findings. These observations suggest that normal subjects may have a transient increase in BAL lymphocytes with no clinically apparent reason.

Recently, a multicenter cooperative study (15) was conducted to evaluate the range of cellular and protein constituents of BAL fluid in healthy individuals. The findings were as follows:

1. Age, gender, and race had no significant effect on BAL fluid cell quantity or cell differential.
2. There were no significant differences in total cells in BAL fluid between ex-smokers and never-smokers (whether the results were expressed as total cells recovered or as cells/ml BAL fluid). The total number of cells obtained, however, was three times as high in current smokers.
3. The number of macrophages from current smokers was four times that of never-smokers and the increase in macrophages exceeded the increase in total cells so that the percentage of macrophages (92.5%) in smokers was significantly greater than that of never-smokers (85.2%). There were no differences between ex-smokers and never-smokers.
4. The number of neutrophils/ml in current smokers was approximately 6 times that in never-smokers, and in ex-smokers neutrophils were also significantly increased (twice that of never-smokers). But, when expressed as a percentage of total cells recovered, only the ex-smokers differed significantly from never-smokers. Also, the neutrophils remained significantly elevated in ex-smokers who had stopped smoking for more than 10 years, suggesting that the impact of smoking on the cell populations in the lung may not be entirely reversible. Smoking must be taken into account when comparing groups of subjects or patients with various diseases and ex-smokers should be differentiated from never-smokers.

In normals, the subtypes of lymphocytes found within the alveolar structures are similar to those of blood. Utilizing surface marker criteria, approximately 73% of alveolar lymphocytes are T cells, 7% are B cells, and the remaining 19% do not react with conventional agents and are thus classified as "null cells" (1,14). T-helper cells are reported to represent 39–48% of lymphocytes and T-suppressor cells 23–28%, so that the normal ratio of T-helper cells to T-suppressor cells is 1.6–1.8 (15,67). The National Institutes of Health (NIH) cooperative study findings included the following:

1. The percentage of T-helper cells in individuals >50 years old was, on the average, more than 10% higher than that in individuals <37 years old.
2. Total T-cells, T-suppressor cells, and B-cell percentages were significantly higher in men than in women and the H/S ratio was significantly lower in men.
3. T-helper cells were significantly lower (32.2%) in current smokers than in ex-smokers (46%) and in never-smokers (44.4%), and T-suppressor cells were higher in current smokers (29.2%) than in ex-smokers (20.7%) and never-smokers (20.7%). Thus, the H/S ratio was significantly lower in current smokers than in either ex-smokers or never-smokers.

Ciliated or squamous epithelial cells from the bronchi may also be present but usually do not exceed 3% of the total number of cells; higher counts may indicate bronchial inflammation (5). Again, polymorphonuclear leukocytes (PMNs) are rare in the alveoli of normal individuals and represent less than 1% of the total. When PMNs (particularly neutrophils) are in higher numbers in BAL fluid, one of the following is suggested:

1. There is blood contamination secondary to bronchoscopic trauma;
2. The patient is a smoker;
3. The patient has a chronic lung disease characterized by increased neutrophils in the alveolar strictures (see below); or
4. Inflammatory airway disease is present and the source of neutrophils is the bronchi and not the alveoli (1,4).

CLINICAL UTILITY OF BAL

In most situations, BAL by itself does not provide information to make specific diagnoses with absolute certainty. However, the BAL cell profile has important diagnostic value when considered in conjunction with other information. If patients cannot safely undergo open lung biopsy the BAL can provide supportive evidence for a diagnosis, and if a patient has respiratory symptoms but near-normal pulmonary functions and a normal chest X ray, an abnormal BAL result facilitates the decision to proceed with open lung biopsy (68).

INTERSTITIAL LUNG DISEASES

The interstitial lung diseases (ILDs) are a group of greater than 100 different disorders that are often disabling, sometimes fatal, and characterized morphologically by an increase in the number of inflammatory and immune effector cells within the lung parenchyma, i.e., a chronic alveolitis. It is believed that the alveolitis may precede and modulate the derangement of alveolar structures, including thickening and fibrosis of the adjacent interstitium, which may eventually lead to sufficient damage to the alveolar capillary membrane to interfere with proper gas exchange (1,69). If this observation is valid, knowledge of the presence and the intensity of the alveolitis is important in understanding these illnesses and may be of benefit in planning and/or evaluating therapeutic strategies, and the data that currently exist to address these questions in specific diseases are discussed below. Conventional studies, including chest X ray and pulmonary functions, do not specifically assess the alveolitis. The classical approach to evaluate the alveolitis of interstitial lung disease has been to biopsy the lung parenchyma and describe qualitatively the inflammatory and immune effector cells within the alveoli and the amount of fibrosis (70). However, this does not give information regarding type and function of the cells composing the alveolitis and practically cannot be performed serially during a patient's clinical course.

BAL is ideally suited to evaluate the alveolitis of interstitial lung diseases. Patients with interstitial lung disease usually have little associated inflammatory airway disease and the cells obtained by BAL are reflective of alveolar rather than airway processes. In addition, BAL permits functional evaluation of the inflammatory and immune effector cells involved in chronic lung diseases and is easily repeated. Thus, it can be used to follow the status of the alveolitis and its response to therapy (70).

It is essential that the inflammatory and immune effector cells collected by lavage accurately represent the effector cell within the alveolar structures; multiple studies illustrate this point. Haslam et al. (68) compared yields of cells obtained from BAL fluid with those observed using quantitative counts of cells extracted from open lung biopsy specimens in patients with idiopathic pulmonary fibrosis (IPF) and found that there was a correlation between the proportion of neutrophils obtained from lung lavage and tissue extraction ($p < .02$), but this correlation did not exist for eosinophils ($p < .07$) or lymphocytes ($p < .08$). They concluded that their data suggested that lung lavage reflects the cellularity of the peripheral parts of the lung in IPF patients without overt bronchial disease (68). Similarly, Hunninghake et al. (70) found that the proportions of BAL macrophages, neutrophils, eosinophils, basophils, and T and B lymphocytes were similar to those extracted from lung tissue in normal subjects and patients with either sarcoidosis or IPF. Similarly, Semenzato et al. (71) used monoclonal antibodies to compare cells in tissue sections to cells recovered by BAL in patients with sarcoidosis and hypersensitivity pneumonitis. A significant correlation between percentages of lymphocytes and macrophages in BAL and lung biopsies was found, supporting the concept that BAL correctly samples the alveolitis of these disorders (71).

IMPLICATIONS FOR DIAGNOSIS AND MANAGEMENT: SPECIFIC INTERSTITIAL LUNG DISEASES

Sarcoidosis

BAL cannot be used to make a definitive diagnosis of sarcoidosis, but analysis of helper (CD4) and suppressor (CD8) T lymphocytes may be of benefit in distinguishing sarcoidosis from other granulomatous diseases such as hypersensitivity pneumonitis. In sarcoidosis, the helper-to-suppressor T-cell ratio may be as high as 10–20/L; in hypersensitivity pneumonitis, the helper-to-suppressor T-cell ratio is decreased (14,72,73). An elevated neutrophil count (with or without an increased lymphocyte count) may also be present in the BAL fluid of patients with advanced sarcoidosis, but usually only in those whose disease has progressed to an extensively fibrotic and/or bullous radiographic pattern (74).

Although the clinical course of most sarcoid patients is relatively benign, 20–25% may suffer permanent loss of lung function, and in 5–10% of patients the disease may eventually be fatal (67,75). Obviously, the ability to predict by BAL which patients will have an unstable course would be helpful in decisions regarding therapy.

Keogh et al. (75) evaluated 19 untreated sarcoid patients without extrapulmonary manifestations and found subjects with a "high-intensity" alveolitis (defined as lavage T lymphocytes >28% and a positive gallium scan) had a greater (87% deteriorated) propensity to suffer significant deterioration in lung function over a 6 month period than subjects with a "low-intensity" alveolitis (8% deteriorated). Similar results would have been obtained if lavage itself had been used as the only criteria for active disease. However, the results of this study should be interpreted with caution since (a) "deteriorated" was defined as a 10% fall in only one pulmonary function parameter (total lung capacity, or TLC, FVC, FEV_1, or Dsb); (b) there was a significant difference in both the age and the duration of symptoms between the high- and low-intensity alveolitis patients (the "high-intensity" groups were younger and had disease of shorter duration, both important factors in the prognosis of sarcoidosis); (c) 75% of the episodes of high-intensity alveolitis spontaneously reverted to low-intensity, whereas 12% of all episodes of low-intensity alveolitis spontaneously reverted to high-intensity; and (d) the study was short term.

In contrast, Israel-Biet et al. (76) performed BAL on 94 untreated sarcoidosis patients with recent onset of the disease. All patients underwent repeat BAL at 1 year and 18 patients at 2 years. These investigators concluded that initial lymphocyte counts were "devoid of any predictive value" in predicting spontaneous "cure." However, to be considered "cured" in this study, all pulmonary functions as well as chest radiographs had to be considered totally normal on follow-up.

Foley et al. (77) evaluated by BAL 67 patients with sarcoidosis with a mean duration of disease of 60 months, none of whom had received corticosteroids for at least 6 months. Twenty-four subsequently required treatment with corticosteroids. The mean follow-up period was 25 (range 13–37) months. Repeat BAL at a mean of 8.4 months (range 4–20 months) was performed in 34 patients. On the basis of the initial lavage fluid, 42 patients had a total lymphocyte count of 28% or more of total cells, 25 patients had <28% total lymphocytes. There was no significant relation between initial lavage lymphocyte count and final outcome, whether judged by FVC_1, D_LCO, or radiological score. Most patients with chronic sarcoidosis who had pulmonary functional or radiographic deterioration belonged to the low-intensity alveolitis group at the initial assessment, so that the absence of lymphocytes did not indicate "burned-out" disease (77). Repeat BAL found a significant correlation between the fall in BAL fluid lymphocyte percentage and improvement in FVC (the more the lymphocytes fell, the greater the improvement in FVC), but appeared to have little to add to standard pulmonary function tests and chest radiograph in patient management.

Costabel et al. (78) examined 31 untreated sarcoid patients with disease of varying duration (range 0–108 months) and defined deterioration as the occurrence of any *one* of the following conditions: (a) new symptoms developed or old symptoms progressed; (b) values for *one* pulmonary function (VC, TLC, Dsb, or PaO_2 with exercise) fell 10%; or (c) successive radiographs indicated that the disease was progressive. With these criteria, lavage lymphocytes did not predict subsequent deterioration, but the T-lymphocyte helper-to-suppressor cell ratio did. A normal helper-to-suppressor cell ratio was highly predictive of a stable clinical course, whereas an elevated ratio was associated with deterioration during a 1-year follow-up period. In contrast, Cueppens et al. (79) found in nine untreated patients followed up from 2 to 16 months that the initial helper-to-suppressor T-cell ratio had no predictive value regarding spontaneous improvement of the disease. The same group more recently (80) examined 28 untreated patients with sarcoidosis after 22–36 months of follow-up. They found a significantly lower lymphocyte count in patients with stage III rather than stage I or II disease. The T_4/T_8(H/S) ratio was highest in stage I disease and correlated negatively with the radiological stage. No correlation was found between the total cell count or the percentage of lymphocytes in the baseline BAL fluid and the evaluation of any of the lung volumes or the D_LCO. But the evaluation of the D_LCO correlated positively with the proportion of BAL T_4 cells (as a percentage of lymphocytes) and with the BAL T_4/T_8 ratio and negatively with the proportion of BAL T_8 cells (as a percentage of lymphocytes) in the BAL sample obtained at the start of follow-up. All of the significances on the predictive value disappeared when only patients with stage I or II disease were considered, but the correlation between the D_LCO evolution and the baseline values of T-cell subsets in bronchoalveolar lavage fluid persisted if one excluded patients who presented with erythema nodosum (see below). The authors concluded that the total cell count and lymphocyte cell count in BAL fluid of untreated patients with sarcoidosis are not predictive of the evolution of the disease and that a high T_4/T_8 ratio is not an indicator of poor prognosis and may even be associated with a better prognosis (80).

Although there is not uniform agreement, BAL findings in sarcoidosis do not seem to correlate with disease duration. However, Ward et al. (81) found that two groups of patients with sarcoidosis presenting with acute inflammatory events (acute erythema nodosium or uveitis) had higher lavage T-lymphocyte percentages, T-helper cell percentages, and TH/TS ratios than patients with other presentations of sarcoidosis. They also found a progressive diminution over time in lavage T-lymphocyte percentage and TH/TS ratio for erythema nodosum patients not seen with patients with uveitis or respiratory symptoms, which is interesting because erythema nodosum is generally associated with a good prognosis. The authors concluded that the category of disease presentation may be crucial in the interpretation of individual lavage results and may explain the diversity of results in the literature. Widely varying results may be due to differences in the study population: if a particular study population has a large number of patients studied soon after an acute onset with erythema nodosum or uveitis, results may tend to show high lymphocyte counts and H/S ratios plus find them associated with a good prognosis.

In addition to the potential role of lavage lymphocyte counts in the management of patients with sarcoidosis, Bjermer et al. (82,83) examined lavage fluid mast cells. A significant increase in mast cells is ⩾0.5% of the total cells recovered. In 69 untreated sarcoid patients, they found (a) that a significant relationship exists between mast cell counts and both absolute and relative lymphocyte counts; (b) that mast cells in lavage fluid were inversely related to lung function; and (c) that mast cell counts tended to increase with radiographic stages. Hyaluronate (a potential marker for activated pulmonary fibroblasts) concentrations were also found to be strongly correlated with mast cell counts. In 45 newly diagnosed patients with sarcoidosis followed over a 2 year period, they found that the lymphocyte counts and/or the neutrophil count had limited prognostic value. In contrast, lavage mastocytosis was associated in general with lung disease deterioration, and lymphocytosis or neutrophilia plus mastocytosis had the highest specificity for prediction of deterioration. Increased mast cell counts were seen in 15/16 patients with more active and progressive disease, but in only 8/23 patients with inactive disease ($p < .02$). Exactly how the recruitment of mast cells would be linked to the established cellular immune events in the lung is not clear.

BAL has also been postulated to be of benefit to predict steroid responsiveness in sarcoidosis. Lawrence et al. (84) treated 12 patients with "clinically active disease" independent of the results of BAL and found no relationship between subsequent improvements and initial BAL lymphocyte counts. Hollinger et al. (85) followed up 21 treated patients for a mean of 22 weeks. They defined improvement as an increase in FVC. All patients with a pretreatment lavage lymphocyte count ⩾35% were stable or improved, whereas one half of patients with a pretreatment lavage lymphocyte count <35% worsened. In contrast, Baughman et al. (86) found no relationship in 16 patients treated for pulmonary symptoms between the percentage of lymphocytes obtained in initial lavage and the change in VC after 2 months of therapy. There was a positive correlation, however, between the change in VC and both the helper-to-suppressor T-cell ratio and the absolute numbers of helper cells in the BAL fluid. However, this group did not find the helper-to-suppressor ratio useful in predicting long-term (2-year) prognosis (87). Similarly, Turner-Warwick et al. (88) found that initial lavage lymphocyte counts were not predictive of radiographic improvement in 32 sarcoid patients. Thus, currently, there are also no conclusive data to demonstrate that lavage can accurately predict steroid responsiveness in sarcoidosis. To our knowledge there are no published studies to determine whether lavage cellular analysis can predict when therapy may be safely tapered and/or discontinued in sarcoidosis patients.

Others have recently evaluated the potential utility of noncellular substances in BAL fluid of patients with sarcoidosis. Ward et al. (89,90) measured initial BAL collagenase and subsequent disease course in 84 untreated patients with sarcoidosis. Those with significant collagenase activity in their BAL fluid had more severe physiological and radiographic impairment, were less likely to improve spontaneously, had a more prolonged disease duration, and had a greater need for steroid intervention than in the collagenase-negative group. The same group (91) also examined type 3 procollagen peptide concentrations in BAL fluid of 84 nontreated sarcoidosis patients. Procollagen type 3 is synthesized by fibroblasts as a precursor of collagen type 3 and thus type 3 procollagen peptides are potential markers of collagen secretion (92). Type 3 procollagen peptide levels were significantly elevated in this group compared to normals and usually correlated with increased T lymphocytes, but had no correlation with pulmonary function, mode of presentation, length of disease, or subsequent functional deterioration. Blaschke et al. (93) reported similar findings. Type 3 procollagen peptide levels thus do not appear to be of prognostic significance in sarcoidosis. Lavage lymphocyte activation markers also have not shown any correlation with disease duration or results of pulmonary function tests (94).

In summary, at the current time no BAL cellular or noncellular parameter has been shown to be definitely predictive in determining prognosis or making therapeutic decisions for individual patients with sarcoidosis.

Idiopathic Pulmonary Fibrosis (Cryptogenic Fibrosing Alveolitis)

In many patients, idiopathic pulmonary fibrosis (IPF) is usually fatal an average of 3–6 years after the onset of symptoms (67). IPF is a difficult disorder to manage because of its variable prognosis plus the fact that in some patients corticosteroids or cytotoxic agents can induce substantial subjective and objective improvement, whereas others show no improvement or deteriorate despite therapy (95,96). Due to potentially serious side effects of these medications, being able to predict which patients would respond to therapy would be very important. In contrast to sarcoidosis, there are no prospective studies of lavage in untreated IPF patients. Several studies suggest that BAL can predict response to therapy and prognosis in this disorder. Rudd et al. (31) studied 120 patients with IPF/cryptogenic fibrosing alveolitis (CFA), 74 with histological confirmation and 26 with an associated systemic disorder. All living patients were followed up for at least 12 months and for a mean of 38 months; 79 patients were treated with corticosteroids and 12 were treated with various cytotoxic drugs; response was defined as a 10% increase in FVC. Increased proportions of lymphocytes were associated with responsiveness to corticosteroids, whereas increased eosinophils or increased neutrophils without increased lymphocytes were associated with failure to respond. Increased eosinophils were also associated with a greater likelihood of progressive deterioration. Turner-Warwick and Haslam (97) showed by repeated lavage analysis in 32 patients with CFA (six with associated systemic disorders) that falls in neutrophils were significant in patients responding to prednisone, whereas falls in eosinophils were significant in those responding to cyclophosphamide. In patients who failed to improve, neutrophil and eosinophil counts tended to remain elevated. Interestingly, six patients with asymptomatic stable disease were not treated: four had raised neutrophil counts. Two of these remained completely stable, although their neutrophil counts remained substantially elevated.

In contrast, O'Donnell et al. (98) found that cyclophosphamide was much more effective than corticosteroids in suppressing the neutrophil component of the alveolitis (as assessed by BAL) despite the fact that the functional response to each drug was similar. Those patients treated with corticosteroids alone showed no suppression in the neutrophil components of the alveolitis after 3–6 months of therapy, whereas the cyclophosphamide group showed a marked reduction in the neutrophilic alveolitis at 3 months.

Recently, Watters et al. (99) reported that in 26 patients with IPF/CFA pretreatment lavage neutrophils or eosinophils were *not* related to the clinical response of patients after a year of corticosteroid therapy and would be an unreliable marker on which to base therapeutic decisions. There was an association, though, between the presence of BAL lymphocytosis prior to therapy and clinical improvement after 6 months of corticosteroid therapy. BAL lymphocytosis was also positively associated with biopsy findings of moderate-to-severe alveolar septal inflammation and negatively correlated with honeycombing and smooth muscle hypertrophy (advanced fibrosis). BAL neutrophil and eosinophil content did not correlate significantly with any of the histopathological architectural abnormalities. The absence of BAL lymphocytosis did not entirely preclude improvement with therapy, as two patients without this finding also improved. Lavage eosinophilia is frequently associated with more advanced IPF/CFA clinically but does not always predict a lack of responsiveness to therapy, especially if BAL lymphocytosis is also present. Interestingly, this group also followed three patients with neutrophil counts ranging from 1% to 25% and eosinophil counts ranging from 0% to 8% who remained stable 6 and 12 months after open lung biopsy without therapy.

Other more recent investigations have focused on noncellular components in the BAL fluid of patients with IPF/CFA and their potential usefulness, e.g., phospholipids. Pulmonary surfactant, which mainly consists of phospholipids such as dipalmitoylphosphatidylcholine (DPPC) and phosphatidylglycerol (PG), is synthesized in alveolar type II cells and secreted into alveolar spaces where it stabilizes the pulmonary alveoli against collapse (100). Thus, phospholipid analysis of BAL fluid is important in evaluating alveolar type II cells and metabolic changes in pulmonary surfactant in lung diseases (100). Phosphatidylinositol (PI) is formed from the same precursor as PG (100). The phospholipid profiles of BAL fluid are significantly altered in IPF (100–102). The prominent changes are (a) an overall decrease in the total phospholipid content and concentration; (b) a significant decrease in the PG-to-PI ratio; and (c) a relative decrease in DPPC, a main phospholipid component of pulmonary surfactant synthesized in alveolar type II cells (100,101). Robinson et al. (101) found no significant correlation between BAL fluid cellular constituents (either percentages or concentrations) or pulmonary function tests and BAL phospholipid content or composition. They did find that patients with IPF and relatively prominent alveolar septal inflammation tended to have a higher (more nearly normal) amount of phospholipid in BAL fluid plus the PG/PI ratio correlated better with histological alterations than total phospholipid amounts: PG/PI correlated negatively (was lower and more abnormal) with alveolar septal fibrosis and honeycombing, and was higher (closer to normal) in patients with more cellularity and less fibrosis and honeycombing (101). There was a significant increase in BAL total phospholipid content after 3 months of high-dose corticosteroids which fell again as the steroids were tapered. This increase in phospholipid content was not necessarily associated with clinical improvement. But the higher the *pretherapy* BAL phospholipid content, the greater the improvement in exercise gas exchange induced by 6 months of corticosteroid therapy, and a low pretherapy BAL phospholipid content was associated with a poor clinical outcome. The PG/PI ratio, on the other hand, did not predict clinical response nor did this ratio change with corticosteroid therapy in a statistically significant manner (101). In contrast, Hughes et al. (102) reported that although PG proportions were frequently reduced in the lavage of untreated IPF/CFA patients, an early and sustained increase in this component was associated with clinical improvement after corticosteroid therapy was instituted, whereas it did not increase in those who failed to improve. Thus, near-normal phospholipid levels and ratios in IPF/CFA may be representative of lung parenchyma not yet irreversibly damaged and thus more responsive to corticosteroid therapy (101,102).

As mentioned earlier, hyaluronate and type 3 procollagen peptide concentrations may be potential markers of activated fibroblasts or an expanded fibroblast mass associated with interstitial fibrosis (92). Bjermer et al. (92) found higher concentrations of hyaluronate and type III procollagen peptide in patients with IPF/CFA than in normal controls. Neutrophil and lymphocyte counts correlated with hyaluronate but not type 3 procollagen peptide levels. Diffusing capacity was inversely correlated with hyaluronate concentration. Patients who had deterioration in lung function and radiographic progression over 6 months had higher lavage fluid concentrations of hyaluronate and type 3 procollagen peptide levels than patients whose disease was stable. Increased levels of these substance may be linked to severity and activity of the lung disease.

All of these above studies clearly demonstrate that additional studies of both the cellular and noncellular components of BAL fluid are necessary to define the appropriate clinical use of BAL in patients with IPF/CFA as well.

Pulmonary Fibrosis Associated with Collagen Vascular Disease

The inflammatory process that develops in the lung in many of the collagen vascular diseases usually results in a diffuse interstitial disease similar to IPF/CFA (69). The findings in BAL fluid in patients with interstitial lung disease associated with collagen vascular disease (PFCVD) are also similar to those of patients with IPF/CFA (4). In general, in PFCVD, when there are increased numbers of lymphocytes present in BAL fluid, the lung disease is associated with a relatively good prognosis and response to therapy, whereas the presence of a predominantly neutrophilic or eosinophilic alveolitis is associated with a higher risk of functional and radiographic deterioration and a poor response to therapy (69,96,103–105).

Casale et al. (106) found in patients with rheumatoid arthritis and PFCVD, a good association between BAL histamine levels, BAL neutrophil and eosinophil numbers, pulmonary function tests, and chest radiographic findings. Similar to findings in IPF discussed above, Gilligan et al. (107) found increased neutrophils, collagenase levels, and increased concentrations of type 3 procollagen peptide in the BAL fluid of patients with rheumatoid arthritis and advanced PFCVD.

Silver et al. (108) examined 43 patients with systemic sclerosis. Nearly 50% had an alveolitis, usually characterized by increased numbers of macrophages and granulocytes (neutrophils and eosinophils), but without a lymphocytosis. The alveolitis persisted on serial studies. Those with an abnormal BAL had more dyspnea and greater abnormalities in pulmonary functions and chest radiographs and a faster rate of deterioration in pulmonary function than those with a normal BAL.

Several investigators also evaluated "subclinical" pulmonary involvement in the CVDs. Wallaert (109,110) performed BAL on 61 patients with various CVDs free of pulmonary symptoms with normal chest radiographs; 8/61 had abnormal pulmonary functions on entry into the study; 29/61 patients were found to have an abnormal BAL. A lymphocytic alveolitis was found in 11/25 patients with primary Sjögren's syndrome and 4/8 patients with Sjögren's associated with another CVD. A neutrophilic alveolitis with or without increased lymphocytes was found in patients with scleroderma (6/10), rheumatoid arthritis (1/4), dermatomyositis (2/3), and mixed connective tissue disease (3/8). Abnormalities in BAL were more common in patients with active and severe extrapulmonary disease. On 12-month follow-up, patients with either a normal BAL or a lymphocytic alveolitis had no functional deterioration, whereas 6/7 patients with an untreated neutrophilic alveolitis had deterioration in pulmonary function tests (PFTs). Four steroid-treated patients with a neutrophilic alveolitis did not deteriorate. The authors concluded that BAL allows early detection of a subclinical inflammatory alveolitis in CVD and that a neutrophilic alveolitis is associated with a higher risk of functional deterioration (109). Garcia et al. (111) in a similar manner examined BAL in patients with rheumatoid arthritis and found three distinct groups: (a) patients with definite interstitial involvement clinically; (b) patients with a normal chest X ray and PFTs but an abnormal BAL; and (c) patients with a normal chest X ray, PFTs, and BAL. Group 1 patients in general had increased BAL neutrophils, and group 2 patients had elevated lymphocytes. The above observations suggest that BAL may be useful in managing patients with PFCVD, but the exact manner in which it should be used is still not well defined (4).

Hypersensitivity Pneumonitis/Extrinsic Allergic Alveolitis

Hypersensitivity pneumonitis/extrinsic allergic alveolitis (HSP/EAA) is an inflammatory granulomatous response of the lungs to antigens in a wide range of inhaled organic dusts (112). The characteristic feature of BAL in HSP/EAA is increased numbers of lymphocytes, particularly suppressor T lymphocytes (in contrast to sarcoidosis). The percentage of lymphocytes may be strikingly increased (often ≥60%) compared to normal controls (113). Some of the lymphocytes have an atypical appearance suggestive of blast cells having markedly indented multiclefted nuclei and increased cytoplasmic area (112). The lymphocyte increases are a feature of the subacute or chronic phase of the inflammatory reaction and by the time of clinical presentation patients with HSP/EAA invariably show increased BAL lymphocytes. Macrophages account for a lower percentage of the total cells obtained by BAL in HSP/EAA (often <40%), but the actual numbers are comparable to controls (113). Neutrophils and eosinophils may also be present in the BAL in HSP/EAA, especially if there has been a recent exposure to antigen. Fournier et al. (114) found a marked increase in neutrophils in BAL lavage of patients with HSP/EAA who underwent antigen inhalation in an experimental setting. Twenty-four hours after exposure, 41.2% of the BAL cells were neutrophils compared to 8.3% prior to antigen challenge. The increased numbers of neutrophils returned to baseline 5–8 days later. In this study, the presence of neutrophils in BAL was associated with clinical symptoms. BAL samples from exposed patients with EAA/HSP also contain mast cells in increased numbers (as much as tenfold higher) in addition to lymphocytes (112,115). In most patients, the increased mast cells occur when individuals are currently or have been recently exposed and fall soon after removal from exposure, but the lymphocyte increases may (including the atypical forms) persist, often for years (112). Mast cells and neutrophils may remain elevated with continued exposure and symptoms (112). In this manner, serial studies of BAL mast cells and neutrophils may be useful in monitoring removal from exposure (112). During an acute episode of farmer's lung disease, markedly elevated concentrations of hyaluronate and type 3 procollagen peptide are recovered in BAL fluid and are closely related to mast cell levels.

The lymphocyte counts remain similarly high in patients with episodic and in those with chronic symptoms; even those who recover and become asymptomatic after removal retain persistently increased counts of total BAL lymphocytes (113). It remains unclear what the role of lung lymphocytes is in such asymptomatic patients with previous HSP/EAA; but an elevated percentage of BAL lymphocytes is a persistent finding for at least 2 years in patients with a history of previous farmer's lung disease who stay in contact with the farm environment (116). BAL lymphocytes may not constitute a sign of active disease and do not predict outcome or prognosis in patients with an established diagnosis of HSP/EAA (116). Increased levels of BAL lymphocytes and mast cells are also found in asymptomatic dairy farmers with positive serum precipitins who subsequently have not developed HSP/EAA over 6–7 years of follow-up: increased lymphocytes and mast cells are thus not a sign of lung disease or a predictor of eventual EAA/HSP (117).

Pneumoconioses

Asbestos-Related Interstitial Lung Disease

The assessment of asbestos exposure is often difficult because of the numerous jobs and hobbies in which asbestos is used and because the patient is usually unaware of its risk (118). The assessment of prior occupational exposure to asbestos can usually be accomplished through the clinical history; however, considering the large numbers of occupations in which asbestos is used and the long latency period between exposure and the development of disease, some patients may not be aware of or may fail to recall such exposure (119).

Asbestos body (AB) formation is an intracellular process that occurs as one or more alveolar macrophages engulfs an asbestos fiber. The fiber then becomes incorporated into an intracytoplasmic vacuole and is coated with an acid mucopolysaccharide (120). Iron accumulates in the coating initially as hemosiderin with only a small portion of asbestos fibers in the lung becoming coated as ferruginous bodies (120,121). Ferroprotein rarely develops on chrysotile and other short fibers; therefore, ABs are formed primarily on long fibers (e.g., amphibole) and represent only a fraction of the total asbestos burden in the lung and thus in BAL (120,122). The presence of ABs thus reflects primarily the burden of long amphibole fibers, which are considered to be most frequently associated with asbestosis and mesothelioma (118,122). In the population without occupational asbestos exposure but exposed to urban pollution, chrysotile constitutes the bulk of the asbestos fibers (123,124). These small fibers do not form ABs, which explains why finding ABs in BAL correlates well with occupational exposure, implying inhalation of long industrial fibers (123).

Measurement of ABs in lung parenchyma obtained at autopsy or surgery is a useful way of assessing exposure to asbestos, and a parenchymal concentration of greater than 1,000 AB per gram of dried lung tissue is generally associated with past specific exposure to asbestos (123,124). Data from both Sebastien et al. (125) and DeVuyst et al. (122) demonstrate that measuring the concentrations of AB in BAL fluid constitutes a useful test for predicting parenchymal concentrations: a measured BAL concentration of AB/ml would predict a parenchymal concentration ranging between 1,050 and 3,010 AB/gram (125). Thus, all measured BAL concentrations ≥1 AB/ml would correspond to lung concentrations in excess of 1,000 AB/g and thus indicate nontrivial and significant asbestos exposure (125).

DeVuyst et al. (122,123) recently published their experience in 563 subjects who underwent analysis of BAL for ABs. Of 215 patients, 84.3% with a definite exposure to asbestos had >1 AB/ml; 53.5% of 116 patients with probable or suspected asbestos exposure had >1 AB/ml; and 17.8% of 117 blue-collar workers with no known asbestos exposure and 6.9% of 115 white-collar workers with no known asbestos exposure had >1 AB/ml. All patients who had >1,000 AB/ml of BAL fluid and 36 of 37 with >100 AB/ml were in the definite exposure group. Their study also indicated that there is a definite relationship between asbestos exposure and BAL fluid AB counts: the greater or more definite the exposure, in general, the higher the number of ABs per ml of lavage fluid (118,123). Repeated lavages in ten patients showed that the AB remain at roughly the same concentration from one BAL to another. When ABs were compared to the categories of asbestos-related disease, in patients with radiographic findings consistent with asbestosis, 93.3% had >1 AB/ml; 70.4% of patients with asbestos-related pleural disease had >1 AB/ml; 62.5% of patients with malignant mesothelioma had >1 AB/ml; 78.3% of patients with lung cancer and occupational asbestos exposure had >1 AB/ml; and 63.5% of patients with occupational asbestos exposure and no evidence of lung cancer or asbestos-related disease had >1 AB/ml. The mean AB/ml recovery was significantly higher in the subjects with asbestosis (mean 120.5 AB/ml) than in subjects with benign pleural disease (mean 4.77 AB/ml, $p < .001$) or in workers with negative chest X rays (mean 3.57 AB/ml, $p < .001$). The presence or absence of ABs in BAL is most likely not a reliable indication of subpleurally deposited fibers involved in the development of asbestos-related pleural disease (effusion, fibrosis, malignancy). Of patients with an ill-defined occupational exposure and radiographic lesions consistent with an asbestos etiology, 83% (65/78) had a positive BAL for AB. There were also significant correlations between AB counts and duration of exposure (positive) and AB counts and time since the end of the last exposure (negative).

In another study of 93 asbestos-exposed patients, Garcia et al. (127) noted that ABs in BAL were significantly and inversely correlated with the diffusing capacity and directly correlated with profusion score abnormalities and BAL eosinophil levels.

The following can be concluded regarding ABs in BAL:

1. AB analysis of BAL fluid is probably of most value in patients with radiographic changes suggestive of an asbestos-related disease with an ill-defined exposure history (123).
2. Finding ABs in BAL fluid correlates with the occupational risk and can disclose unknown or forgotten exposure better than a questionnaire (118,121). AB in BAL is an excellent objective measure of asbestos exposure but in itself is not a good marker or proof of disease (118,121,123).
3. The absence of ABs in a correctly performed BAL does not exclude asbestos-related pleural disease but is significant evidence against the diagnosis of asbestosis (123).
4. In the presence of interstitial lung disease, the finding in BAL of numerous ABs tilts the balance of probabilities toward a diagnosis of asbestosis because ABs are not usually found in patients with other interstitial lung diseases, and when they are found in patients who do not have asbestosis, they do so in smaller numbers than are seen in asbestosis (119,128).
5. The concentration of ABs in BAL may correlate positively with length and intensity of exposure and may correlate negatively with time since last exposure.
6. The AB concentration in BAL correlates well with the lung tissue burden.

BAL fluid cellular analysis in patients with asbestosis is similar to that of patients with IPF/CFA. Geller et al. (128) evaluated 32 patients with documented previous occupational asbestos exposure and clinical and radiographic features of asbestosis. Forty-six percent (13/31) of the patients showed an increase in the percentage of neutrophils with or without an increase in the percentage of eosinophils; 29% (8/31) showed an increased proportion of lymphocytes. Multiple subsequent studies demonstrate that the helper/suppressor ratio of the T lymphocytes in the BAL fluid of patients with asbestosis probably is elevated (128). The numbers of neutrophils correlated positively with the length of history of the disease and higher percentages were associated with more severe impairment of lung function. Smokers more frequently had increased numbers of neutrophils than did nonsmokers. In nonsmokers, a negative correlation was found between the diffusing capacity and the percentages of PMNs, and a positive correlation between the diffusing capacity and the proportion of lymphocytes.

In a review of 27 patients with asbestosis, Robinson et al. (129) found that 70% had increased numbers of neutrophils in lavage fluid and 52% had increased numbers of eosinophils. They also found that there was no difference in the severity of the alveolitis in patients with radiographic and physiological evidence of asbestosis compared to those with asbestos exposure and crackles but no radiological or physiological evidence of asbestosis, suggesting that radiological or functional parameters do not reflect the severity of the alveolitis (129). Xaubet et al. (130), in contrast, found that the proportion of neutrophils in BAL correlated with the PaO_2 and $(A\text{-}a)O_2$.

Several studies have also suggested that a "subclinical" pulmonary involvement occurs in some asbestos-exposed workers. Begin et al. (131) found a significant increase in numbers of total cells, neutrophils, and lymphocytes in BAL of 17 of 42 exposed workers without the criteria for asbestosis; several of them developed full criteria for asbestosis within 3–5 years. The authors concluded that evidence of alveolitis on BAL should argue strongly against any further exposure to asbestos dust at any levels in such patients (131). Gellert et al. (128,132,133) also reported the presence of increased numbers of lymphocytes in BAL fluid in asbestos workers without clinical and radiographic evidence of asbestosis. Garcia et al. (126) also found that nonsmoking asbestos-exposed subjects without asbestosis had higher numbers of neutrophils in BAL than did nonexposed workers. Further follow-up, both functionally and by BAL, in this group with so-called subclinical involvement will determine if these abnormalities do indeed represent the early stages in the development of asbestosis.

For a more detailed discussion of BAL in asbestos-related lung diseases, the reader is referred to Ref. 127.

Silicosis

Begin et al. (134) evaluated with BAL 22 silica-exposed (average of 31 years of exposure) workers: 7 had no evidence of silicosis (group 1), 9 (group 2) had simple silicosis (no coalescence or large opacities), and 6 had silicosis with coalescence and/or large opacities. In all three groups there were twice as many total cells as controls with a prominent increase in macrophages and some increases in lymphocytes and neutrophils. The BAL cellularity did not differentiate the three groups of silica-exposed workers with different severity of disease. These data are not in agreement with those of Schuyler et al. (135), who noted only an increase in type II pneumocytes in the BAL of six silicotics compared to normal controls.

Christman et al. (136) evaluated nine healthy Vermont granite workers with normal spirometry and chest radiographs with BAL. Five of the nine workers had increased lymphocytes in BAL, significantly greater than controls, which was thought to represent a subclinical chronic inflammatory process (136). Polarizing particles were present in 5.8% of the alveolar macrophages in the controls compared with 75.7% of the workers' cells. There was also an increase in the percentage of alveolar macrophages that contained particulates with increasing duration of granite dust exposure and the percentage of lymphocytes in BAL also increased with longer duration of granite dust exposure. When clinical and radiographic data are consistent with silicosis, BAL is a noninvasive means to document silica exposure as birefringent particles are easily detected by polarized microscopy (136).

Bronchiolitis

Kindt et al. (137) performed BAL on 16 adult patients with bronchiolitis (confirmed by open lung biopsy evidence of prominent bronchiolar inflammation) both before and after 3 months of corticosteroid therapy. Neutrophils initially composed 54 ± 10% of the cells recovered by BAL from the patients with bronchiolitis compared with 3.9 ± 1% in smokers with chronic bronchitis ($n = 8$) and 0.8 ± 0.5% in normal nonsmoking volunteers ($n = 6$) ($p < .01$, both comparisons). BAL performed after 3 months of corticosteroids in 8 of 16 patients with bronchiolitis demonstrated a significant decrease in the percentage of BAL neutrophils (before: 57 ± 11% versus post: 26 ± 13%, $p < .05$). Of this group, the responder subset ($n = 5$) had a marked reduction in BAL neutrophil percentage after corticosteroids (46 ± 15% to 6 ± 3%, $p < .05$), whereas the non-responder subset (n = 3) did not (76 ± 11% to 59 ± 26%, = .391). This study suggests that BAL is useful for evaluating the inflammatory response at the level of the bronchioles in these patients as well as in patients in whom a high clinical suspicion of bronchiolitis exists. The finding of an elevated (>25%) percentage of neutrophils by BAL may be sufficient for a presumptive diagnosis of bronchiolitis (137).

Drug-Induced Lung Disease

Pulmonary drug toxicity can be suspected from the finding of bronchial and alveolar cell atypia (cytotoxic changes) in BAL fluid; however, these changes need to be interpreted with caution as they can appear similar to changes seen in some cases of malignancy (37,138). Consequently, the diagnosis of drug toxicity cannot be definitively made by BAL alone, but it is a valuable tool in examining the pathogenesis of these disorders.

BAL has potential, however, as an important adjunctive test in the evaluation of suspected amiodarone lung toxicity (139). Phospholipid accumulation in alveolar macrophages results in lamellar body formation, which gives the macrophages a foamy appearance because of these characteristic cytoplasmic inclusions (139). This is relatively characteristic for drug effect secondary to amiodarone. Lavage provides excellent cellular material for assessment of the foamy inclusions in alveolar macrophages. Its presence can be detected in up to 50% of patients receiving amiodarone and thus is not diagnostic of toxicity, but its absence makes the diagnosis of amiodarone pulmonary toxicity unlikely (139).

In a review of 14 subjects with amiodarone pulmonary toxicity from the Mayo Clinic, the cell differential counts from BAL grouped into three categories: (a) normal cell differential; (b) lymphocyte-predominant; and (c) polymorphonuclear leukocyte–predominant (139). The lymphocyte typing in the lymphocyte-predominant pattern showed a marked increase in CD8-positive lymphocytes (CD41/CD8 ratio of 0.4:1). Similar findings were noted by Israel-Biet et al. (140). When present, the finding of increased numbers of T-suppressor lymphocytes with or without polymorphonuclear leukocytes strongly supports the diagnosis of amiodarone pulmonary toxicity; a normal cell differential neither supports nor excludes the diagnosis (139).

IMPLICATIONS FOR DIAGNOSIS AND MANAGEMENT: RARER LUNG DISORDERS

Berylliosis

Beryllium has found widespread application in modern industry because of its physical properties, and it is used in the manufacture of products such as thermal coating for nuclear reactors, rocket heat shields, and brakes (141). Inhaled beryllium metal dusts, beryllium oxide, or beryllium salts can cause either acute or chronic lung disease. The acute form appears to be a toxic dose-related effect on the lungs and has largely been eliminated by controls on environmental exposure. The chronic form develops over 1–20 years in 1–3% of exposed persons and is a granulomatous interstitial disease remarkably similar, histopathologically and clinically, to sarcoidosis (14,141). The diagnosis of chronic berylliosis is usually based on a history of beryllium exposure, typical clinical and histological abnormalities, and elevated lung beryllium levels (14,141).

BAL may be extremely valuable in the evaluation of a patient with suspected berylliosis. BAL cells from patients with berylliosis are remarkably similar to those with sarcoidosis: the total numbers of macrophages and T cells are increased. The percentage of lymphocytes is increased, and most of these cells are helper T cells (14,141). BAL in berylliosis has its greatest use in showing a local immunological response to beryllium. Lymphocytes from the BAL of berylliosis patients proliferate when stimulated in vitro with soluble beryllium salts, with a sensitivity and specificity approaching 100% (14,141,142). This has become a valuable diagnostic tool in berylliosis and may replace open lung biopsy as a way to make a definitive diagnosis of chronic berylliosis (14,141,142).

Histiocytosis X (Eosinophilic Granuloma)

Histiocytosis X (HX) is a chronic granulomatous disorder that involves the mononuclear phagocytes of the reticuloendothelial system. With pulmonary involvement, there are reticulonodular infiltrates that progress to cystic changes and honeycombing, primarily in the upper lobes. Pathologically, there is an interstitial accumulation of atypical histocytes similar to Langerhans cells (14). Electron microscopic examination of these tissue histiocytes reveals an indented nucleus and small (40–45 nm diameter) elongated bodies scattered throughout the cytoplasm termed X bodies (1,14,143). Identification of HX cells by transmission electron microscopy is often time consuming and expensive (4).

BAL may be useful in the diagnosis of HX. In these patients, there is usually an increased total number of cells, the percentage of lymphocytes may be normal or elevated, and there may be a small increase in neutrophils and eosinophils (4). Chollet, et al. (144) evaluated the use of immunofluorescence of Langerhans cells using monoclonal antibodies to these cells (OKT6 monoclonal antibody) in BAL specimens. BALs from 131 patients with a variety of pulmonary diseases including HX (18 patients) were examined; fluorescent (OKT6-positive) cells were found in all patients with biopsy confirmed HX (range 1.8–25% of all BAL cells). In the other 113 patients, the fluorescent cells constituted only 0.2% of the total number of cells, significantly fewer than in the HX patients.

Casolero et al. (145) evaluated BAL fluid from five normal nonsmokers and ten normal smokers for the presence of Langerhans cells as identified by the OKT6 monoclonal antibody and by transmission electron microscopy. The OKT6 antibody identified 0.1 ± 0.1% of the cells from nonsmokers but labeled 1.1 ± 0.3% of the cells recovered from smokers ($p < .01$). By E.M., no Langerhans cells were demonstrated in nonsmokers while 0.4 ± 0.1% of the cells recovered from nonsmokers contained the characteristic intracytoplasmic inclusions of Langerhans cells. Xaubet et al. (146) evaluated BAL fluid for OKT6-positive cells in 70 subjects: 18 normal smokers, 14 normal nonsmokers, 15 patients with sarcoidosis, 12 patients with IPF, 3 patients with HX, and 8 patients with lung neoplasms. OKT6-positive cells were observed in 41 of 77 lavages (53.2%), accounting for 0.25–7% of alveolar macrophages. OKT6-positive cells were present in BAL from 12 of 18 control smokers, 7 of 14 control nonsmokers, 5 of 15 patients with sarcoidosis, 8 of 12 patients with IPF, and 3 of 8 cases of lung neoplasm.

The percentage of positive cells was significantly higher in smokers than nonsmokers. In all of these groups, however, the OKT6-positive cells composed less than 1% of alveolar macrophages, except in one case of IPF with 2% OKT6-positive cells. In contrast, OKT6-positive cells accounted for 3–7% of the alveolar macrophages in six BALs performed in the three patients with HX. These authors concluded that (a) normal smokers and nonsmokers as well as patients with various lung disorders rarely have more than 1% of positive cells in BAL fluid, and (b) a percentage of OKT6-positive cells equal to or greater than 3% suggests the diagnosis of HX (146). Whereas these are probably appropriate general guidelines, further studies with quantitative evaluation of Langerhans cells in BAL fluid are needed before there can be clearly defined criteria for the diagnosis of HX by BAL fluid analysis (3).

Pulmonary Alveolar Proteinosis

Pulmonary alveolar proteinosis (PAP) involves widespread filling of alveoli with a lipoprotein material that stains with a periodic acid-Schiff (PAS) reagent. Electron microscopic examination of the lipid material shows characteristic whorled lamellar bodies (14). In addition, the lipoprotein material has been demonstrated to stain with specific antibodies to surfactant apoprotein (14,147). Analysis of BAL may obviate the need for a diagnostic open lung biopsy in patients with PAP (3,148). The findings by BAL that have been reported in BAL in the PAP include the following: (a) the gross appearance is opaque and/or milky; (b) there are few alveolar macrophages and a normal cell differential; (c) alveolar macrophages occasionally contain eosinophilic granules identical to that seen in lung biopsies in PAP; (d) large acellular eosinophilic bodies against a background of small eosinophilic granules and amorphous debris are seen; and (e) there is predominant PAS staining of the proteinaceous material with a lack of significant Alcian blue staining (5,149). It is important that all of these conditions be satisfied before a diagnosis of PAP is considered because milky appearance and lipoprotein aggregates may occasionally occur in lavage fluid from patients with a variety of other interstitial lung disease; however, they are ultrastructurally and biochemically different from those from PAP (3,150). BAL may provide important diagnostic information in PAP, but an open lung biopsy may still be necessary in some instances for a definitive diagnosis.

Chronic Eosinophilic Pneumonia

BAL of patients with chronic eosinophilic pneumonia usually shows a marked increase in eosinophils (14,151,152). Dejaegher and Demendts (152) found that patients treated with steroids normalized their BAL along with improvements in clinical and radiological features.

Alveolar Hemorrhage

BAL may also be clinically useful in the diagnosis of occult pulmonary hemorrhage, which may cause radiographic abnormalities simulating other interstitial or infectious disorders. This is a particularly difficult problem in immunocompromised patients and hemoptysis is often absent. A grossly bloody appearance to BAL is not always diagnostic since it may be secondary to bronchoscopy-induced trauma, especially in the anticoagulated patient (4). Gold et al. (153), Finley et al. (154), and Drew et al. (155) reported that alveolar hemorrhage could be diagnosed safely in both immunocompromised thrombocytopenic patients and anticoagulated patients by staining alveolar macrophages obtained by BAL for the presence of hemosiderin. The episode of acute pulmonary hemorrhage probably has to occur at least 48 hr prior to BAL for the alveolar macrophages to demonstrate increased amounts of hemosiderin (37,156). Although the utility of BAL in the diagnosis of occult pulmonary hemorrhage has been recognized for some time, two important points must be remembered: (a) the cause of pulmonary hemorrhage is not diagnosed by BAL, i.e., other important pulmonary processes may be associated with occult pulmonary hemorrhage such as infection, particularly in immunocompromised patients, and (2) hemosiderin-laden macrophages have been found in a variety of other lung diseases including IPF, cardiac disease, sarcoidosis, carcinoma, vasculitis, PAP, and HX (4,14,137,154). Hemorrhage should be assumed to be the sole cause of pulmonary infiltrates if hemosiderin-laden macrophages predominate in lavage, pulmonary edema has been excluded, therapy is not altered, and the alveolar disease clears within 1–3 days (158).

Fat Embolism

The identification of neutral-fat droplets by staining with oil red O within cells recovered by BAL in patients with recent trauma may be a rapid and specific method for establishing the diagnosis of the fat embolism syndrome (159). Lipid staining of BAL specimens may also be useful in the diagnosis of lipoid pneumonia (160,161).

USE OF BAL IN THE DIAGNOSIS OF MALIGNANCY

The clinical value of BAL in the detection of pulmonary malignancy remains under study. The likelihood of a positive BAL cytology is heavily dependent on the prevalence of cancer in the population of patients being studied. In our own review of 250 BAL cytologies from ICH patients, only four were found to be positive for cancer (unpublished data). Two of these patients had a known history of nonpulmonary cancer (transitional cell and chordoma) prior to the discovery of malignant cells on BAL. Two others had primary lung cancers (bronchoalveolar and large cell). Other reports have suggested a higher yield from BAL cytology when it is used routinely in the evaluation of lesions suspected to be malignant (162). We will focus on the use of BAL cytology in three areas: (a) primary lung cancer, (b) metastatic lung cancer, and (c) lymphomatous or leukemic pulmonary involvement.

The application of BAL in the diagnosis of primary lung cancer is limited to peripheral (endoscopically nonvisible) lesions since visible lesions are usually readily diagnosed by conventional bronchoscopic techniques. BAL cytology is positive in 24–25% of patients with peripheral lesions that are eventually found to be malignant (163–165). Higher percentage yields, up to 70% (162), will be obtained if patients with endoscopically visible lesions are included. Yield also depends on radiographic appearance in that most studies show a higher percentage of positive cytologies in patients with infiltrates as compared to those with nodules. Cell type also influences the sensitivity of BAL cytology. Bronchoalveolar cell carcinoma appears to be the most readily identified primary lung cancer with a positive cytology frequency approaching 90% (166,167). Aside from cytology, other BAL measurements such as tumor marker concentrations (168) or immunoglobulin levels (169) remain investigational. This is primarily due to the inability of any particular "threshold" concentration to separate benign from malignant lesions with enough reliability to justify routine clinical use (170). From the above it is clear that BAL cytology is capable of detecting primary lung cancer. However, most authors have found that the number of cases in which BAL was the *exclusive* source of a malignant diagnosis is small. At this time, it would seem reasonable to reserve BAL cytology studies for patients in whom lung cancer is suspected but who do not have endoscopically visible lesions. It might be particularly useful in those with an infiltrative pattern on chest X ray or patients in whom transbronchial lung biopsy is contraindicated.

As noted above, metastatic malignancy can occasionally be detected by BAL cytology. Linder et al. reported identification of melanoma, soft tissue sarcoma, and malignancies of breast, gastrointestinal tract, and pancreas (162). Breast cancer metastases have been studied more thoroughly than other tumors. In one study, BAL cytology was positive in 7 of 20 (35%) breast cancer patients studied prior to the initiation of chemotherapy (171). Another report found BAL cytology to be positive in five of five patients examined who were eventually found to have lymphangitic carcinomatosis (four breast, one colon). The sensitivity of BAL cytology exceeded that of brushings of transbronchial biopsy (172). The routine use of BAL to evaluate

TABLE 1. *Bronchoalveolar lavage in the diagnosis of pulmonary hematological malignancy*

Study (1 patient each)	Involvement					Analysis of BAL fluid			
	Bone marrow	Other organ	SPEP†	TBLBx‡	OLBx§	% lymphocytes	Ig/ Alb#	PEP¶	Immuno-phenotype
Weynants et al.[2]	Neg	Neg	Monoclonal IgM	Neg	ND	44	IgG, IgM	Monoclonal IgM	ND
Davis & Gndek[3]	Neg	Neg	Monoclonal IgM	Suggestive of lymphoma	NHL	34	ND	ND	Monoclonal κ
Morgan et al.[4]	22% plasma cells	Fat aspirate neg	Monoclonal IgG-λ	Amyloidosis	ND	21	IgG	IgG-λ	ND
Oka et al.[5]	Neg	Neg	Monoclonal IgM-λ	Suspected NHL	ND	78	IgM	ND	ND
Menashe et al.[6]	10% plasma cells, IgG-κ	Neg	Monoclonal IgG-κ	Mild IF	ND	22	ND	ND	Monoclonal κ

* BAL = bronchoalveolar lavage; IF = interstitial fibrosis; ND = not done; neg = negative; NHL = non-Hodgkin's lymphoma.
† SPEP = serum protein electrophoresis.
‡ TBLBx = transbronchial lung biopsy.
§ OLBx = open-lung biopsy.
# Ig/Alb = immunoglobulin/albumin ratio in BAL fluid.
¶ PEP = protein electrophoresis on BAL fluid.

new lung lesions in patients with a history of extrapulmonary cancer is reasonable, particularly in those with a prior history of breast cancer.

Case reports dominate the literature regarding the use of BAL to diagnose lymphomatous and leukemic pulmonary involvement. The approach to these diagnoses differs from that for solid tumors. Cytology specimens should be reviewed by a hematopathologist accustomed to examining BAL and special immunohistochemical studies should supplement the routine Papanicolaou and Diff-Quik stains. We recently reported on the use of Southern blotting to supplement immunohistology in diagnosing pulmonary lymphoma (173). A summary of earlier case reports using BAL to diagnose lymphoma or myeloma in the lung is shown in Table 1. Only two of these reports utilized immunohistological techniques to confirm the presence of a monoclonal population of lymphoid cells. It is of interest that all reports of pulmonary lymphoma diagnosed by BAL have shown a BAL lymphocyte percentage greater than 20%. Hodgkin's lymphoma can be diagnosed by the identification of Reed–Sternberg cells in BAL cytology specimens. When BAL was performed routinely prior to bone marrow transplant in 50 patients with known Hodgkin's disease, 6 of 50 (12%) were found to have Reed–Sternberg cells (174). Although only three authors reported on the identification of leukemic cells in BAL fluid (175–177), further evaluation of BAL is justified since these patients are often gravely ill and thrombocytopenic. In this setting, BAL would be preferable to transbronchial or open lung biopsy even if its diagnostic sensitivity was fairly low. Currently, we frequently perform immunocytochemical studies on patients with a known history of non-Hodgkin's lymphoma, particularly if greater than 20% lymphocytes are noted on the BAL differential.

BAL IN THE DIAGNOSIS OF INFECTIOUS DISEASES

Nonimmunocompromised Hosts

It might be expected that BAL would provide an excellent sampling of the lower respiratory tract secretions that could be targeted toward the location of an abnormality seen on the chest X ray. Unfortunately, contamination of the bronchoscope as it traverses the naso- or oropharynx can produce misleading false-positive microbiological culture results. This is best exemplified by one study in which only one in ten normal volunteers had sterile BAL cultures (178). In this same study, when cultures of BAL were performed in nonimmunosuppressed individuals with interstitial lung disease that was presumably noninfectious, only 3 of 37 patients had sterile BAL cultures. Most BALs had more than one organism present and organisms were usually those that are part of the normal nasopharyngeal flora.

One approach to the problem of contamination is to employ quantitative bacterial cultures on BAL specimens. This has recently been done in eight healthy young (mean age 28) volunteers, and while six of eight specimens were nonsterile, all specimens contained <10,000 CFU/ml (179). It has also been shown that if a BAL sample obtained from a noninfected individual contains more than 1% squamous epithelial cells, even quantitative cultures will usually be falsely positive by these criteria (43). Special precautions, such as administration of lidocaine by inhalation rather than bolus injection and performance of BAL through a previously inserted endotracheal tube, have been shown to reduce the incidence of contamination (6). Even when quantitative cultures are used, the ability of BAL to correctly diagnose pneumonia remains equivocal. One group used >10,000 CFU/ml as the criteria for infection and found only a 7.4% (4 of 54) false-positive rate in their control group (180). While this seems attractive, it is likely that this represents an underestimate of the true percentage of false-positive results. Studies such as this one, which use criteria such as (a) fever, (b) new chest X ray infiltrate, (c) elevated white blood cell count, and (d) resolution with antibiotics as the gold standard for pneumonia, have been partially invalidated by the work of Fagon et al. (181) who showed that many patients who fulfill these criteria do not have bacterial pneumonia. When Chastre et al. studied BAL quantitative cultures applying more rigorous criteria for the diagnosis of pneumonia, 4 of 13 (31%) patients without pneumonia had >10,000 CFU/ml (44). In addition, among patients eventually found to have pneumonia, only three of five (60%) had >10,000 CFU/ml. These results undermine the credibility of BAL quantitative cultures as a means of diagnosing bacterial pneumonia.

Skepticism regarding quantitative cultures was briefly replaced by enthusiasm regarding the potential application of another BAL parameter, the percentage of cells containing intracellular bacteria, as a predictor of lower respiratory tract infection. In the article cited above, Chastre et al. noted that five of five patients found to have pneumonia had greater than 20% lavage cells containing intracellular bacteria (44). That was in 1988. The following year, in an update presented at the Aspen Lung Conference, 20% was no longer a suitable cutoff, since 7 of 13 patients with true pneumonia had < 20% (45). Changing the cutoff to 7% led to improvement in both sensitivity and specificity, but the trend that emerges as more experience is gained suggests that this parameter may travel the path of quantitative cultures.

TABLE 2. *Who is an immunocompromised host?*

Pharmacological Immunosuppression:
1) Use of a cytotoxic chemotherapeutic agent 1 month prior to BAL
2) Use of cyclosporine 1 month prior to BAL
3) Use of corticosteroids at a dose equivalent to >10 mg prednisone/day at any time during the 6 months prior to BAL

Immunodeficiency:
1) Immunoglobulin deficiency
2) Splenectomy
3) AIDS
4) Neutropenia (absolute neutrophil count <1,000)

Hematological Malignancy/Malfunction:
1) Leukemia
2) Lymphoma
3) Myeloma
4) Myelodysplastic syndrome, dysmyelopoietic syndrome with neutropenia

In mechanically ventilated patients suspected of having pneumonia, quantitative cultures of BAL have been compared with those from telescoping plugged catheters and the culture results of each technique agreed 89% of the time (182). False-positive cultures were rare for both techniques. Unfortunately, the criteria used to classify a patient as having pneumonia were as described above and therefore not stringent enough, particularly for ventilated patients. Another group, using a nonbronchoscopic method of performing BAL, also examined mechanically ventilated patients and documented pneumonia by performing an open lung biopsy within 1 hr of death (183). In ten patients with confirmed bacterial pneumonia, the BAL correctly identified one of the pathogens in ten of ten and all of them in nine of ten. In three patients without infection whose open lung biopsy was sterile, BAL cultures were also sterile. Quantitative culture techniques were not used. Although the numbers are small, these results suggest that the use of BAL cultures in mechanically ventilated patients suspected of having pneumonia may assist in the diagnosis of nosocomial pneumonia.

Immunocompromised Host

Reviews that provide an overview to the diagnosis of pulmonary disease (184, 185) and pulmonary infections (186) in immunocompromised hosts (ICHs) have been published over the last decade. Groups considered immunocompromised would usually be required to fulfill at least one of the criteria shown in Table 2. Although the specific criteria regarding steroid dose and degree of neutropenia are arbitrary, we have found them to be useful in predicting which patients are likely to have opportunistic lung infections.

More specifically, nine separate reports (Table 3) have examined the diagnostic utility of BAL in the ICH (37,187–194). The most frequent patient subgroup studied, the most common diagnosis made, and the estimated diagnostic yield are shown in Table 3. There is a wide variation in the diagnostic yield. There are many reasons for this variation. First, each center has a unique patient composition that will be determining factor in which pathogens are likely to be the cause of pulmonary disease. Therefore, a center primarily treating AIDS patients would be expected to have a high overall diagnostic yield from BAL that is quite effective at detecting *P. carinii*. Second, the yield will also be determined by what entities are considered capable of being diagnosed by BAL alone. While some authors might consider the identification of CMV, *Aspergillus, Candida, Cryptococcus,* or atypical mycobacteria in BAL as diagnostic, the American Thoracic Society recently published a position paper on BAL advising against such a practice (3). There are only a limited number of organisms that should routinely be considered pathogenic based on their detection in BAL fluid (Table 4). Third, estimates of BAL yields vary because studies use different denominators. We have shown that if one includes all patients considered to be ICH in the denominator, the diagnostic yield is 39% (194). However, if one includes only those patients who were truly immunocompromised (Table 2) and who eventually were diagnosed, yield improved to 62%. When reporting the yield for a specific diagnosis,

TABLE 3. *Utility of bronchoalveolar lavage (BAL)*

Author, year (Ref.)	No. of patients	Most common type of ICH	Most common (% PCP) organism detected[a]	Diagnostic yield (%)
Young, 1983 (52)	26	Renal transplant	*Pneumocystis* (27%)	93
Stover, 1984 (53)	97	Hematological malignancy	*Pneumocystis* (18%)	66
Linder, 1987 (54)	344	Hematological malignancy	*Candida* sp. (4%)	32
Abramson, 1987 (55)	50	Hematological malignancy	Cytomegalovirus (15%)	59
Martin, 1987 (56)	100	Hematological malignancy	*Pneumocystis* (17%)	30
Kahn, 1988 (57)	94	Hematological malignancy	*Pneumocystis* (18%)	62
Xaubet, 1989 (58)	96	Hematological malignancy	*Pneumocystis* (26%)	49
Sobonya, 1990 (59)	51	AIDS	*Pneumocystis* (54%)	87
Pisani, 1990 (60)	150	Hematological malignancy	*Pneumocystis* (50%)	39–62

[a] Percent (%) frequency with which BAL identified *Pneumocystis*; ICH, immunocompromised host.

TABLE 4A. *Criteria used to classify microorganisms obtained by bronchoalveolar lavage as pathogens*

1. Histopathological documentation of organism and typical tissue; cytopathological effects in non-BAL biopsy or autopsy specimens.
2. Special considerations indicating pathogenicity:
   a. *Candida*—Requires (1) due to the poor correlation of presence in blood cultures with pulmonary injection.
   b. *Viral*[a]—Cytopathic effect is demonstrated on BAL cytology or virus is identified in blood or other tissues with serological corroboration.
   c. *Aspergillus*[a]—When identified as the only potential pathogen in the appropriate clinical setting (leukopenia with hemoptysis or alveolar hemorrhage) or supported by simultaneous identification in normally sterile body fluids (blood, pleural fluid).
   d. *Cryptococcus*[a]—As per *Aspergillus*.
   e. *Bacteria*[a]—Cavitary progression on chest X ray or simultaneous isolation in blood, pleural fluid, or deep respiratory tract specimen (not sputum or tracheal secretions) without another more likely pathogen identified.
   f. *Atypical mycobacteria*[a]—Culture from respiratory specimens on more than one occasion without another more likely pathogen identified.

[a] Pathogenicity does not require histopathological documentation if special considerations are documented.

wide variations may also occur depending on the denominator selected. For example, if only four BAL cytologies were positive in 250 BALs examined, the diagnostic yield could be called 1.6%. However, if only six of these patients were eventually found to have lung malignancy, the BAL yield for the diagnosis of cancer could be 75% if only diagnosed cancer cases are used in the denominator.

Because the incidence and pathogenicity of certain organisms may differ between the ICH who has hematological malignancy and the immunosuppressed organ transplant patient, we will discuss the utility of BAL in each subgroup separately.

HIV/AIDS

BAL has recently been evaluated in HIV-positive patients who had not yet developed AIDS to determine if these patients harbored *P. carinii* in their lungs subclinically (195). Patients with chronic shortness of breath were included, but those with abnormal chest X rays, fever, cough, or acute dyspnea were not. None of the 35 BALs examined showed evidence of *P. carinii*. Specimens were not cultured for CMV, but a viral cytopathic effect was not seen in any of the samples. These findings suggest that there is not a colonization phase of *P. carinii* infection in HIV-positive patients.

On the other hand, HIV-positive pre-AIDS patients who develop fever, unexplained respiratory symptoms, or an abnormal chest X ray are just as likely to have an opportunistic pathogen identified as those with AIDS (196). *Pneumocystis carinii* (38%) and CMV (35%) were the most frequently identified pathogens, and were both found in 17% of 117 BALs. In patients who had respiratory symptoms or fever but normal chest X rays, 60% had at least one organism identified on the BAL. Other organisms identified included mycobacteria, herpes simplex, and various fungi. Each of these was seen with a frequency of less than 5%.

The largest study of BAL utility in AIDS involved 276 bronchoscopies in 171 patients with AIDS and pulmonary symptoms or abnormal chest X ray, gallium scan, or D_LCO (39). BAL diagnostic sensitivity (86%) was comparable to that of transbronchial lung biopsy (87%). When both were used, the sensitivity in detecting *P. carinii* was 100% and the negative predictive value was between 92% and 100%. A more recent study showed BAL to have a slightly greater sensitivity for detecting *P. carinii* than transbronchial biopsy (97.8% versus 83.6%) (197). In both of these studies, *P. carinii* was the most frequently identified pathogen, present in 50–57% of specimens examined. CMV grew in culture in 43–50% of BAL. *Mycobacterium avium-intracellulare* was seen in 10% of BAL in both studies, and all other pathogens were seen with frequencies less than 5%. At least one organism was identified with the same frequency in both studies (76% and 77%).

When BAL is performed in an AIDS patient with pulmonary symptoms or chest X ray changes, at least one organism is likely to be identified; and in approximately half of the cases, that organism will be *P. carinii*. In addition, BAL yield will be equal to or better than that of transbronchial lung biopsy.

TABLE 4B. *Pathogens (based on identification)*

Pneumocystis carinii
Mycobacterium tuberculosis
Legionella pneumophila
Histoplasma capsulatum
Coccidioides immitis
Blastomyces dermatiditis

BONE MARROW TRANSPLANT

In the first 2 years following bone marrow transplantation (BMT), roughly half of patients will develop some type of pulmonary problem. The most frequent diagnoses made in these patients are different from those of AIDS patients. The organisms most commonly identified by BAL are CMV, bacteria, and *Aspergillus* (198). Several other noninfectious diagnoses are frequently seen in BMT patients: idiopathic pneumonia, ARDS, and diffuse alveolar hemorrhage. BAL may provide support for the diagnosis of idiopathic pneumonia when no organisms are identified and the differential count contains increased numbers of lymphocytes or granulocytes. Although, as mentioned earlier, alveolar hemorrhage is not a specific diagnosis, some authors have described diffuse alveolar hemorrhage (DAH) syndrome that is unique to BMT (199). This entity usually occurs 2 weeks after transplant and is associated with thrombocytopenia, diffuse alveolar infiltrates, CNS dysfunction, and renal failure. BAL is characterized by the finding that each successive aliquot of lavage produces a bloodier sample while bronchial washing may not have any blood. This finding, coupled with the presence of typical clinical features and absence of BAL organisms, is diagnostic of DAH. The diagnostic yield of BAL was 52% in one study (198) and 80% in another (200). Although in most ICH the identification of CMV does not guarantee pathogenicity, one study of BMT patients correlating BAL with open lung biopsy noted that every time CMV was identified by BAL immunohistology, CMV pneumonia was also seen on the open lung specimens (201). CMV identified by conventional culture was not as specific. Therefore, it seems reasonable to treat these patients with antiviral therapy when the BAL identifies CMV by rapid diagnostic techniques. Often, due to thrombocytopenia, BAL will be the only bronchoscopic procedure that can be performed in BMT patients.

SOLID ORGAN TRANSPLANTS

The BAL yield in liver transplant patients with pulmonary complications is 53% (202). The most common pathogens identified in these patients are CMV and *P. carinii*. Mortality in those with no organisms identified is excellent. The mortality rate is similarly low in those whose BAL contained *P. carinii* and who were treated with trimethoprim/sulfamethoxazole. Unfortunately, 8 of 12 patients whose BAL contained CMV died despite antiviral therapy.

Pulmonary complications of renal transplantation are a major source of morbidity and mortality. The most common pathogen likely to affect the lung in these patients is CMV. CMV pneumonitis is most likely to occur 1–4 months after transplant but can occur much later (203). *Pneumocystis carinii* and *Legionella* occur less frequently and rarely appear outside of the 1- to 4-month time frame. Bacterial pneumonia may also be found but is more often noted after 4 months posttransplant. The diagnostic utility of BAL alone has not been assessed in this ICH group. However, two studies have shown that bronchoscopic evaluation that includes BAL is able to identify a pathogen in 80–93% of patients evaluated (203,204). When the BAL is nondiagnostic, congestive heart failure should be suspected since it is the most common noninfectious diagnosis accounting for pulmonary symptoms in these patients.

Heart and lung transplant recipients are subject to pharmacological immunosuppression similar to that used for other organ transplants. As a result, the same infectious agents cause pneumonia within analogous time intervals. Little has been written about the overall diagnostic utility of BAL in this particular transplant group. However, one group has made an interesting observation regarding the prevalence of *P. carinii* in these patients (205). During the course of post–lung transplant follow-up, serial BALs were performed in 16 lung transplant patients. Surprisingly, *P. carinii* was identified in 14 of 16 (88%) patients studies. Sixty-five percent of patients were asymptomatic when *P. carinii* was identified in the BAL. The incidence of symptomatic *P. carinii* infection (35%) was much greater in the lung transplants as compared to the heart transplants (4%) from the same institution. At the time this study was being done, prophylactic trimethoprim/sulfamethoxazole was not being used routinely. *Pneumocystis carinii* was not identified in the BAL of patients who had been receiving such prophylaxis. In lung transplant patients, major noninfectious causes of pulmonary infiltrates include reperfusion edema, lymphoproliferative disorders, and rejection. Some have suggested that BAL may be helpful in diagnosing the latter based on the presence of increased BAL lymphocytes that have donor-specific cytotoxicity (206). A lymphoproliferative process associated with immunosuppression can cause pulmonary infiltrates in both heart and lung recipients. As mentioned earlier, surface marker studies of BAL cells could help identify a clonal population of lymphocytes, but since many of these disorders are polyclonal in nature, negative BAL results do not rule out lymphoproliferation.

HEMATOLOGICAL MALIGNANCY

Although patients with Hodgkin's and non-Hodgkin's lymphoma would be expected to have a high incidence of opportunistic infections, two separate studies have found opportunistic infectious agents to be a rare cause of pulmonary infiltrates in these patients (207,208). These studies did not examine BAL specifically or its ability to make either infectious or noninfectious diagnoses. It has been established that the diagnosis of pulmonary involvement with lymphoma, which is estimated to occur at some point during the disease course in 60% of patients, can be diagnosed by BAL. However, the sensitivity of BAL for detection of lymphoma remains unknown. The diagnostic yield of BAL quoted in studies that combine patients with leukemia and lymphoma should not be applied to lymphoma patients since the nature of immunosuppression usually differs between these two groups. Other noninfectious pulmonary diseases common to lymphomas include drug-induced lung injury and radiation pneumonitis, neither of which can be diagnosed by BAL alone.

Up to 75% of deaths from leukemia are due to infection. Roughly half of such infections involve the lung and are most often due to one of three bacteria: *Klebsiella pneumonia, Pseudomonas aeruginosa,* and *Staphylococcus aureus* (209). The etiology of pulmonary infiltrates in patients with leukemia tends to depend on the chest X-ray pattern and the timing of infiltrate appearance. Infiltrates appearing before or within 72 hr of treatment initiation are not caused by opportunistic infections. Infiltrates appearing later tend to be caused by bacterial infection in patients with focal infiltrates. Those with diffuse lung involvement are more likely to have a noninfectious etiology (e.g., hemorrhage or leukemic lung), but of the 35% who develop infections, 93% are caused by opportunistic pathogens. One study has examined the efficacy of BAL in evaluating leukemia patients with infiltrates who eventually came to autopsy (210). BAL established a final diagnosis in only 3 of 20 patients (15%). All three diagnoses were *Candida* pneumonia. This is a difficult diagnosis to make based on BAL alone since *Candida* is a colonizer in the majority of cases in which the BAL detects it. Also interesting was the observation that BAL failed to diagnose all eight cases of autopsy-confirmed invasive aspergillosis. The low diagnostic yield may be due in part to the fact that most patients with leukemia have bacterial infection and are already on multiple antibiotics at the time BAL is done. Most authors feel that the identification of *Aspergillus* in the BAL from a leukemia patient with prolonged granulocytopenia (less than 3 weeks), hemoptysis, and infiltrate implies pathogenicity. Even if the sensitivity of BAL for the detection of *Aspergillus* is low, the BAL is still worth doing if it could potentially abrogate the need for open lung biopsy in a few patients.

BAL IN CHILDREN

Use of BAL in immunocompromised children has increased greatly over the last 5 years. Smaller volumes of lavage fluid (10–30 ml) are used in children, and the procedure appears to be as safe in children as it is in adults (211). BAL is able to make at least one diagnosis 58–71% of the time in this subgroup (211–213). The largest of these studies (211) divided patients into two groups: (a) those with acute pneumonia and (b) those with interstitial pneumonitis. The BAL yield was 90% in ICH children with acute pneumonia ($n = 11$) and the most common pathogens were respiratory syncytial virus and *Legionella pneumophila*. Overall diagnostic rate in the group ($n = 62$) with interstitial pneumonitis (IP) was 42%; however, the likelihood of making a diagnosis from BAL in children with IP increased with the severity of their illness (up to 85% in the children most ill). The most common organisms identified in children with IP were *Pneumocystis carinii* and CMV. Forty-six percent of the children in this study were considered to be ICH due to primary immune deficiency (e.g., severe combined immune deficiency), a group not often seen among adult ICH. Protected brush catheters and biopsy forceps cannot be passed through the lumen of the flexible bronchoscopes used in small children. Due to the inability to obtain specimens by these bronchoscopic techniques and the high diagnostic yield of BAL, BAL should see a marked increase in usage when an ICH child develops pulmonary problems.

SUMMARY

In conclusion, the appropriate clinical role of BAL in the various aspects of pulmonary medicine is continually evolving. In interstitial lung diseases such as sarcoidosis, IPF, and PFCVD, the precise role of BAL in determining therapeutic decisions or predicting response to therapy is currently unclear. In occupational lung diseases, particularly asbestos-related lung diseases and berylliosis, BAL may give very important information in assessing exposure. In malignancy, performing a BAL adds little risk or time to the bronchoscopic procedure but may give valuable diagnostic information that may not be provided by forceps biopsy or brushings (8). More studies are clearly needed to develop a clear consensus on the use of BAL in the diagnosis of nosocomial/bacterial pneumonia, but it is a valuable technique in immunocompromised patients, particularly those with AIDS.

In the future, hopefully, the role of BAL, especially in interstitial lung disease and bacterial/nosocomial pneumonia, will be more clearly elucidated. BAL will also in the future allow experimental manipulations of the lower respiratory tract and may even be used therapeutically: cells obtained by BAL could be subjected to "repair" mechanisms and reinfused into the lungs (214). BAL is one procedure whose potential will be most fully realized with continued cooperation between cellular and molecular biologists and clinicians.

REFERENCES

1. Hunninghake GW, Gadek JE, Kawanami O, Ferrans VJ, Crystal RG. Inflammatory and immune processes in the human in health and disease: evaluation by bronchoalveolar lavage. *Am J Pathol* 1979;97:149–198.
2. Reynolds HY, Newball HH. Analysis of proteins and respira-

tory cells from human lungs by bronchial lavage. *J Lab Clin Med* 1974;84:559–573.
3. American Thoracic Society. Clinical role of bronchoalveolar lavage in adults with pulmonary disease. *Am Rev Resp Dis* 1990;142:481–486.
4. Helmers RA, Hunninghake GW. Bronchoalveolar lavage. In: Wang KP, ed. *Biopsy techniques in pulmonary disorders*. New York: Raven Press; 1989;15–28.
5. Haslam PL. Bronchoalveolar lavage. *Semin Resp Med* 1984; 6:55–70.
6. Pang JA, Cheng AFB, Chan HS, French GL. Special precautions reduce oropharyngeal contamination in bronchoalveolar lavage for bacteriologic studies. *Lung* 1989;167:261–267.
7. Pingleton SK, Harrison GF, Stechschulte DJ, Wesselius LJ, Kerby GR, Ruth WE. Effect of location, pH, and temperature of instillate in bronchoalveolar lavage in normal volunteer. *Am Rev Resp Dis* 1983;128:1035–1037.
8. Helmers RA, Hunninghake GW. Bronchoscopy: bronchoalveolar lavage in the nonimmunocompromised patient. *Chest* 1989;96(5):1184–1190.
9. European Society of Pneumology Task Group on BAL. Technical recommendations and guidelines for bronchoalveolar lavage (BAL). *Eur Resp J* 1989;2:561–585.
10. Garcia JGN, Wolven RG, Garcia PL, Keogh BA. Assessment of interlobar variation of bronchoalveolar lavage cellular differentials in interstitial lung diseases. *Am Rev Resp Dis* 1986; 133:444–449.
11. Helmers RA, Dayton CS, Floerchunger C, Hunninghake GW. Bronchoalveolar lavage in interstitial lung disease: effect of volume of fluid infused. *J Appl Physiol* 1989;67(4):1443–1446.
12. Davis GS, Giancola MS, Constanza MC, Low RB. Analyses of sequential bronchoalveolar lavage samples from healthy human volunteers. *Am Rev Resp Dis* 1982;126:611–616.
13. Carre PH, Laviolette M, Belanger J, Cormier Y. Technical variations in bronchoalveolar lavage (BAL): influence of atelectasis and the lung region lavaged. *Lung* 1985;163:117–125.
14. Daniele RP, Elias JA, Epstein PE, Rossman MD. Bronchoalveolar lavage: role in the pathogenesis, diagnosis, and management of interstitial lung disease. *Ann Intern Med* 1985; 102:93–108.
15. BAL Cooperative Group Steering Committee. Bronchoalveolar lavage constituents in healthy individuals, idiopathic pulmonary fibrosis, and selected comparison groups. *Am Rev Res Dis* 1990;141:S169–S202.
16. Kuylenstiern R, Hernbrand R, Eklund A. Comparison of bronchoalveolar lavage fluid recovered during bronchoscopy with local or general anesthesia. *Arch Otolaryngol* 1988; 144:443–445.
17. Hoidal JR, White JG, Repine JE. Impairment of human alveolar macrophage oxygen consumption, and superoxide anion production by local anesthetics used in bronchoscopy. *Chest* (Suppl) 1979;755:2435–2465.
18. Rabinovitch M, DeStefano MJ. Cell shape changes induced by cationic anesthetics. *J Exp Med* 1976;143:290–304.
19. Hold PG. Alveolar macrophages. I. Simple technique for the preparation of high numbers of viable alveolar macrophages from small laboratory animals. *J Immunol Meth* 1979; 27:189–198.
20. Strange C, Barbarash RA, Heffner JE. Lidocaine concentrations in bronchoscopic specimens. *Chest* 1988;93(3):547–549.
21. Kelly CA, Kotre CJ, Ward C, Hendrick DJ, Walters EH. Anatomical distribution of bronchoalveolar lavage fluid as assessed by digital subtraction radiography. *Thorax* 1987;42:624–628.
22. Helmers RA, Galvin J, Dayton CS, Yuh W, Stanford W, Hunninghake GW. Small volume bronchoalveolar lavage (BAL) uniformly perfuses the lung segment in interstitial lung disease as assessed by magnetic resonance imaging (MRI). *Am Rev Resp Dis* 1989;139(4):A472.
23. Crystal RG, Reynolds HY, Kalica AR. Bronchoalveolar lavage. The report of an international conference. *Chest* 1986; 90:122–131.
24. Dohn MN, Baughman RP. Effect of changing instilled volume for bronchoalveolar lavage in patients with interstitial lung disease. *Am Rev Resp Dis* 1985;132:390–392.
25. Lam S, Leriche JC, Kijek K, Phillips D. Effect of bronchial lavage volume on cellular and protein recovery. *Chest* 1985; 88:856–859.
26. Rennard SI, Ghafouri M, Thompson AB, et al. Fractional processing of sequential bronchial and alveolar samples. *Am Rev Resp Dis* 1990;141:208–217.
27. Merrill W, O'Hearn E, Rankin J, Naegel G, Matthay RA, Reynolds HY. Kinetic analysis of respiratory tract proteins recovered during a sequential lavage protocol. *Am Rev Resp Dis* 1982;126:617–620.
28. Reynolds HY. Bronchoalveolar lavage. *Am Rev Resp Dis* 1987; 135:250–263.
29. Rankin JA, Naegel GP, Reynolds HY. Use of a central laboratory for analysis of bronchoalveolar lavage fluid. *Am Rev Resp Dis* 1986;133:186–190.
30. Kelly CA, Fenwick JD, Corris PA, Fleetwood A, Hendrick DJ, Walters EH. Fluid dynamics during bronchoalveolar lavage. *Am Rev Resp Dis* 1988;138:81–84.
31. Strumpf IJ, Feld MK, Cornelius MJ, Keogh BA, Crystal RG, Safety of fiberoptic bronchoalveolar lavage in evaluation of interstitial lung disease. *Chest* 1981;80:268–271.
32. Cole P, Twiton C, Lanyon H, Collins J. Bronchoalveolar lavage for the preparation of free lung cells: techniques and complications. *Br J Chest* 1980;74:273–278.
33. Tilles DS, Goldheim PD, Ginns LC, Hales CA. Pulmonary function in normal subjects and patients with sarcoidosis after bronchoalveolar lavage. *Chest* 1986;89:244–248.
34. Ettensohn DB, Jankowski MJ, Redondo AA, Duncan PG. Bronchoalveolar lavage in the normal volunteer subject. 2. Safety and results of repeated BAL, and use in the assessment of intrasubject variability. *Chest* 1988;94:281–285.
35. Pirozynski M, Sliwinski P, Zielinski J. Effect of different volumes of BAL fluid on arterial oxygen saturation. *Eur Resp J* 1988;1:943–947.
36. Lin C, Jen-Liang W, Huang W. Pulmonary function in normal subjects after bronchoalveolar lavage. *Chest* 1988; 93(5):1049–1053.
37. Stover DE, Zaman MB, Hajdu SI, Lange M, Gold J, Armstrong D. Bronchoalveolar lavage in the diagnosis of diffuse pulmonary infiltrates in the immunocompromised host. *Ann Intern Med* 1984;101:1–7.
38. Ognibene FP, Shelhamer J, Giu V, Masher AM, et al. The diagnosis of *Pneumocystis carinii* pneumonia in patients with the acquired immunodeficiency syndrome using subsegmental bronchoalveolar lavage. *Am Rev Resp Dis* 1984;129:929–932.
39. Broaddus C, Dake MD, Stulbarg MS, Blumenfeld W, Hadley K, Golden JA, Hopewell PC. Bronchoalveolar lavage and transbronchial biopsy for the diagnosis of pulmonary infection in the acquired immunodeficiency syndrome. *Ann Intern Med* 1985;102:747–752.
40. Stover DE, White DA, Romano PA, Gelleue RA. Diagnosis of pulmonary disease in the acquired immune deficiency syndrome (AIDS): role of bronchoscopy and bronchoalveolar lavage. *Am Rev Resp Dis* 1984;130:659–662.
41. Cordonnier C, Bomaddin JF, Fleury J, et al. Diagnostic yield of bronchoalveolar lavage in pneumonitis occurring after allogeneic bone marrow transplantation. *Am Rev Resp Dis* 1985; 132:1118–1123.
42. Gurney JW, Harrison WC, Sears K, Robbins RA, Dobry CA, Rennard SI. Bronchoalveolar lavage: radiographic manifestation. *Radiology* 1987;163:71–74.
43. Kahn FW, Jones JM. Diagnosing bacterial respiratory infection by bronchoalveolar lavage. *J Infect Dis* 1987;155:862.
44. Chastre J, Fagon JY, Soler P, et al. Diagnosis of nosocomial bacterial pneumonia in intubated patients undergoing ventilation: comparison of the usefulness of bronchoalveolar lavage and the protected specimen brush. *Am J Med* 1988;85:499.
45. Chastre J, Fagon JY, Soler P, et al. Quantification of BAL cells containing intracellular bacteria rapidly identifies ventilated patients with nosocomial pneumonia. *Chest* (Suppl) 1989; 95:1905.
46. Martin, II WJ, Smith TF. Rapid detection of cytomegalovirus in bronchoalveolar lavage specimens by a monoclonal antibody method. *J Clin Microbiol* 1986;23:1006–1008.

47. Paya CV, Wold AD, Ilstrup DM, Smith TF. Evaluation of number of shell vial cell cultures per clinical specimen for rapid diagnosis of cytomegalovirus infection. *J Clin Microbiol* 1988; 26(2):198–200.
48. Emanuel D, Peppard J, Stover D, Gold J, Armstrong D, Hammerbug U. Rapid immunodiagnosis of cytomegalovirus pneumonia by bronchoalveolar lavage using human and neurine monoclonal antibodies. *Ann Intern Med* 1986;104:476–481.
49. Hilborne LH, Nieberg RK, Cheng L, Levin KJ. Direct in situ hybridization for rapid detection of cytomegalovirus in bronchoalveolar lavage fluid. *Am J Clin Pathol* 1987;87:766–769.
50. Saltini, Hance AJ, Ferrans VJ, Bassett F, Bitterman PB, Crystal RG. Accurate quantification of cells recovered by bronchoalveolar lavage. *Am Rev Resp Dis* 1984;130:650–658.
51. Laviolette M, Carreau M, Coulombe R. Bronchoalveolar lavage cell differential on microscope glass cover: a simple and accurate technique. *Am Rev Resp Dis* 1988;138:451–457.
52. Kim YK, Parulekar S, Yu PKW, Pisani RJ, Smith TF, Anhalt JP. Evaluation of calcifluor white stain for detection of *Pneumocystis carinii*. *Diag Microbiol Infect Dis* 1990;13:307–310.
53. Dugan JM, Vaitabile AM, Rossman MD, Ernst CS, Atkinson BF. Diagnosis of *Pneumocystis carinii* pneumonia by cytologic evaluation of Papanicolaou-stained bronchial specimens. *Diag Cytopathol* 1988;4:106–112.
54. Baughman RP, Strohofer SS, Clinton BA, Nickol AD, Frame PT. The use of an indirect fluorescent antibody test for detecting *Pneumocystis carinii*. *Arch Pathol Lab Med* 1989; 113:1062–1065.
55. Chandra P, Delaney MD, Tuazon CU. Role of special stains in the diagnosis of *Pneumocystis carinii* infection from bronchial washing specimens in patients with the acquired immune deficiency syndrome. *Acta Cytologica* 1988;32(1):106–107.
56. Paradis IL, Ross C, Dekker A, Dauber J. A comparison of modified methenamine silver and toluidine blue stain for the detection of *Pneumocystis carinii* in bronchoalveolar lavage specimens from immunosuppressed patients. *Acta Cytologica* 1990;34(4):511–514.
57. Holten-Andersen W, Kolmos HJ. Comparison of methenamine silver and Giemsa stain for detection of *Pneumocystis carinii* in bronchoalveolar lavage specimen from HIV infected patients. *Acta Microbiol Pathol Immunol Scand* 1989;97:745–747.
58. Strigle SM, Gal AA, Koss MN. Rapid diagnosis of *Pneumocystis carinii* infection in AIDS by cytocentrifugation and rapid hematoxylin-eosin staining. *Diag Cytopathol* 1990;6:164–168.
59. Olling S. Rapid diagnosis of *Pneumocystis carinii* using dark field microscopy on bronchoalveolar lavage. *Acta Microbiol Pathol Immunol Scand* 1988;96:565–567.
60. Sethi KK. Application of immunoblotting to detect soluble *Pneumocystis carinii* antigen(s) in bronchoalveolar lavage of patients with *Pneumocystis* pneumonia and AIDS. *J Clin Pathol* 1990;43(4):584–586.
61. Li C-Y, Ziesmer SC, Yam LT, et al. Practical immunocytochemical identification of human blood cells. *Am J Clin Pathol* 1984;81:204–212.
62. Yamada M, Tamura N, Shirai T, Kira S. Fluorocytometric analysis of lymphocyte subsets in the bronchoalveolar lavage fluid and peripheral blood of healthy volunteers. *Scand J Immunol* 1986;24:559–565.
63. Baughman RP, Boskin CH, Loudon RG, Hurtubise P, Wesseler T. Quantification of bronchoalveolar lavage with methylene blue. *Am Rev Resp Dis* 1983;128:266–270.
64. Idell S, Kuchich U, Fein A, et al. Neutrophil elastase releasing factors in bronchoalveolar lavage from patients with adult respiratory distress syndrome. *Am Rev Resp Dis* 1985; 132:1098–1105.
65. Marcy TW, Merrill WW, Rankin JA, Reynolds HY. Limitations of using urea to quantify epithelial lining fluid recovered by bronchoalveolar lavage. *Am Rev Resp Dis* 1987; 135:1276–1280.
66. Laviolette M. Lymphocyte fluctuation in bronchoalveolar lavage fluid in normal volunteers. *Thorax* 1985;40:651–656.
67. Crystal RG, Bitterman PB, Rennard SI, Hance AJ, Keogh BA. Interstitial lung disease of unknown cause: disorders characterized by chronic inflammation of the lower respiratory tract. *N Engl J Med* 1984;310:154–166, 235–244.
68. Haslam PL, Turton GWG, Heard B, Lukozek A, Collins JV, Salsbury AJ, Turner WM. Bronchoalveolar lavage in pulmonary fibrosis: comparison of cells obtained with lung biopsy and clinical features. *Thorax* 1980;35:9–18.
69. Hunninghake GW, Gadek JE. Immunological aspects of chronic noninfectious pulmonary diseases of the lower respiratory tract in man. *Clin Immunol Rev* 1981–1982;1:337–374.
70. Hunninghake GW, Kawanai O, Ferrans VJ, Young RC, Robert WC, Crystal RG. Characterization of the inflammatory and immune effect or cells in the lung parenchyma of patients with interstitial lung disease. *Am Rev Resp Dis* 1981;123:401–412.
71. Semenzato G, Chilosi M, Ossi E, et al. Bronchoalveolar lavage and lung histology: comparative analysis of inflammatory and immunocompetent cells in patients with sarcoidosis and hypersensitivity pneumonitis. *Am Rev Resp Dis* 1985;132:400–404.
72. Hunninghake GW, Crystal RG. Pulmonary sarcoidosis: a disorder mediated by excess helper T-lymphocyte activity at sites of disease activity. *N Engl J Med* 1981;305:429–434.
73. Leathermann JW, Michael AF, Schwartz BA, Hoidal JR. Lung T-cells in hypersensitivity pneumonitis. *Ann Intern Med* 1984; 100:390–392.
74. Lin YN, Haslam PL, Turner-Warwick M. Chronic pulmonary sarcoidosis: relationship between lung lavage cell counts, chest radiograph, and results of standard lung function test. *Thorax* 1985;40:501–507.
75. Keogh BA, Hunninghake GW, Line BR, Crystal RG. The alveolitis of pulmonary sarcoidosis: evaluation of natural history and alveolitis-dependent changes in lung function. *Am Rev Resp Dis* 1983;128:256–265.
76. Israel-Biet D, Venet A, Chretien J. Persistent high alveolar lymphocytosis as a predictive criterion of chronic pulmonary sarcoidosis. *Ann NY Acad Sci* 1986;465:395–406.
77. Foley NM, Coral AP, Tung K, Hudspith BN, James DG, Johnson NM. Bronchoalveolar lavage cell counts as a predictor of short-term outcome in pulmonary sarcoidosis. *Thorax* 1989; 44:732–738.
78. Costabel U, Bross KJ, Guzman J, Nilles A, Ruhle KH, Matthys H. Predictive value of bronchoalveolar T-cell subsets for the course of pulmonary sarcoidosis. *Ann NY Acad Sci* 1986; 465:418–426.
79. Cueppens JL, Lacquet LM, Marien G, Demedts M, van den Eeckhout A, Stevens E. Alveolar T-cell subsets in pulmonary sarcoidosis: correlation with disease activity and effect of steroid treatments. *Am Rev Resp Dis* 1984;129:563–568.
80. Verstraeten A, Demedts M, Verwilghen J, van den Eeckhout A, Marien G, Larquet LM, Cueppens JL. Predictive value of bronchoalveolar lavage in pulmonary sarcoidosis. *Chest* 1990; 98:560–567.
81. Ward K, O'Connor C, Odlum C, Fitzgerald M. Prognostic value of bronchoalveolar lavage in sarcoidosis: the critical influence of disease presentation. *Thorax* 1989;44:6–12.
82. Bjermer L, Engstrom-Laurent A, Thune UM, Hallgren R. Hyaluronic acid in bronchoalveolar lavage fluid in patients with sarcoidosis: relationship to lavage most cells. *Thorax* 1987; 42:933–938.
83. Bjermer L, Rosenhall L, Angstrom T, Hallgren R. Predictive value of bronchoalveolar lavage cell analysis in sarcoidosis. *Thorax* 1988;43:284–288.
84. Lawrence ED, Teague RB, Gottlieb MS, Jhingran SG, Liebermann J. Serial changes in markers of disease activity with corticosteroid treatment in sarcoidosis. *Am J Med* 1983;74:747–756.
85. Hollinger WM, Staton GW, Fajman WA, Gilman MJ, Pine JR, Check IJ. Prediction of therapeutic response in steroid-treated pulmonary sarcoidosis: evaluation of clinical parameters, bronchoalveolar lavage, gallium-67 lung scanning, and serum angiotensin-converting enzyme levels. *Am Rev Resp Dis* 1985; 132:65–69.
86. Baughman RP, Fernandez M, Bosken CH, Mantil J, Hurtubise P. Comparison of gallium-67 scanning, bronchoalveolar lavage, and serum angiotensin-converting enzyme levels in pulmonary sarcoidosis. *Am Rev Respir Dis* 1984;129:676–681.
87. Baughman RP, Shipley R, Eisentrout CE. Predictive value of

gallium scan, angiotensin-converting enzyme level, and bronchoalveolar lavage in two-year follow-up of pulmonary sarcoidosis. *Lung* 1987;165:371–377.

88. Turner-Warwick M, McAllister W, Lawrence R, Britten A, Haslam PL. Corticosteroid treatment in pulmonary sarcoidosis: do serial lavage lymphocyte counts, serum angiotensin-converting enzyme measurements, and gallium-67 scans help management? *Thorax* 1986;41:903–913.
89. O'Connor C, Odlum C, Van Breda A, Power C, Fitzgerald MX. Collagenase and fibronectin in bronchoalveolar lavage fluid in patients with sarcoidosis. *Thorax* 1988;43:393–400.
90. Ward K, O'Connor CM, Odlum C, Power C, Fitzgerald MX. Pulmonary disease progress in sarcoid patients with and without bronchoalveolar lavage collagenase. *Am Rev Resp Dis* 1990;142:636–641.
91. O'Connor C, Ward K, Van Breda A, McIlgorn A, Fitgerald MX. Type 3 procollagen peptide in bronchoalveolar lavage fluid: poor indicator of course and prognosis in sarcoidosis. *Chest* 1989;96:339–344.
92. Bjermer L, Lundgren R, Hallgren R. Hyaluron and type III procollagen peptide concentrations in bronchoalveolar lavage fluid in idiopathic pulmonary fibrosis. *Thorax* 1989; 44:126–131.
93. Blaschke E, Eklund A, Hembrand R. Extracellular metrix components in bronchoalveolar lavage fluid in sarcoidosis and their relationship to signs of alveolitis. *Am Rev Resp Dis* 1990; 141:1020–1025.
94. Ainslie GM, Poulter LW, duBois RM. Relation between immunocytological features of bronchoalveolar lavage fluid and clinical indices of sarcoidosis. *Thorax* 1989;44:501–509.
95. Haslam PL, Turton CWG, Lukoszek A, Salsbury AJ, Dewar A, Collins JV, Turner-Warwick M. Bronchoalveolar lavage fluid cell count in cryptogenic fibrosing alveolitis and their relation to therapy. *Thorax* 1980;35:328–339.
96. Rudd RM, Haslam PL, Turner-Warwick M. Cryptogenic fibrosing alveolitis relationships of pulmonary physiology and bronchoalveolar lavage to response to treatment and prognosis. *Am Rev Resp Dis* 1981;124:1–8.
97. Turner-Warwick M, Haslam PL. The value of serial bronchoalveolar lavages in assessing the clinical progress of patients with cryptogenic fibrosing alveolitis. *Am Rev Resp Dis* 1987; 135:26–34.
98. O'Donnell K, Keogh B, Cantin A, Crystal RG. Pharmacologic suppression of the neutrophil component of the alveolitis in idiopathic pulmonary fibrosis. *Am Rev Resp Dis* 1987; 136:288–292.
99. Watters LC, Schwarz MI, Cherniack RM, Waldron JA, Dunn TL, Stanford RE, King TE. Idiopathic pulmonary fibrosis: pretreatment bronchoalveolar lavage cellular constituents and their relationships with lungs to pathology and clinical response to therapy. *Am Rev Resp Dis* 1987;135:696–704.
100. Honda Y, Tsunematsu K, Suzuki A, Akino T. Changes in phospholipids in bronchoalveolar lavage fluid of patients with interstitial lung diseases. *Lung* 1988;166:293–301.
101. Robinson PC, Walters LC, King TE, Maron RJ. Idiopathic pulmonary fibrosis: abnormalities in bronchoalveolar lavage fluid phospholipids. *Am Rev Resp Dis* 1988;137:585–591.
102. Hughes DA, Haslam PL. Changes in phosphatidylglycerol in bronchoalveolar lavage fluids from patients with cryptogenic fibrosing alveolitis. *Chest* 1989;95:82–89.
103. Silver RM, Metcalf JF, Stanley JH, LeRoy EC. Interstitial lung disease in scleroderma: analysis by bronchoalveolar lavage. *Arthritis Rheum* 1984;27:1254–1262.
104. Kallenberg CGM, Jansen HM, Elema JD, The TH. Steroid-responsive interstitial pulmonary disease in systemic sclerosis: monitoring by bronchoalveolar lavage. *Chest* 1984;86:489–491.
105. Greene NB, Solinger AM, Baughman RP. Patients with collagen vascular disease and dyspnea: the value of gallium scanning and bronchoalveolar lavage in predicting response to steroid therapy and clinical outcome. *Chest* 1987;91(5):698–703.
106. Casale TB, Little MM, Furst D, Wood D, Hunninghake GW. Elevated BAL fluid histamine levels and parenchymal pulmonary disease in rheumatoid arthritis. *Chest* 1989;96:1016–1021.
107. Gilligan DM, O'Connor CM, Ward K, Moloney D, Bresnihan B, Fitzgerald MX. Bronchoalveolar lavage in patients with mild and severe rheumatoid lung disease. *Thorax* 1990;45:591–596.
108. Silver RM, Miller KS, Kinsella MB, Smith EA, Schabel SI. Evaluation and management of scleroderma lung disease using bronchoalveolar lavage. *Am J Med* 1990;88:470–476.
109. Wallaert B, Hatron P, Grosbois J, Tonnel A, Devulder B, Voisin C. Subclinical pulmonary involvements in collagen vascular diseases assessed by bronchoalveolar lavage: relationship between alveolitis and subsequent changes in lung function. *Am Rev Resp Dis* 1986;133:574–580.
110. Wallaert B, Prin L, Hatron P, Ramon P, Tommel A, Voisin C. Lymphocyte subpopulations in bronchoalveolar lavage in Sjögren's syndrome: evidence for an expansion of cytoxic/suppressor subset in patients with alveolar neutrophilia. *Chest* 1987;92(6):1025–1031.
111. Garcia JGN, Parhami N, Killam D, Garcia PL, Keogh BA. Bronchoalveolar lavage fluid evaluation in rheumatoid arthritis. *Am Rev Resp Dis* 1986;133:450–454.
112. Haslam PL, Dewar A, Butcher P, Primett ZS, Newman-Taylor A, Turner-Warwick M. Mast cells, atypical lymphocytes and neutrophils in bronchoalveolar lavage in extrinsic allergic alveolitis. *Am Rev Resp Dis* 1987;135:35–47.
113. Haslam PL. Bronchoalveolar lavage in extrinsic allergic alveolitis. *Eur J Resp Dis* (Suppl) 1987;154:120–135.
114. Fournier E, Tonnel AB, Gossett P, Wallaert B, Ameisen JL, Voisin C. Early neutrophil alveolitis after antigen inhalation in hypersensitivity pneumonitis. *Chest* 1985;88:563–566.
115. Bjermer L, Engstrom-Laurent A, Hallgren R, Rosenhall L. Bronchoalveolar lavage in persons acutely exposed to dust in the farm environment. *Am J Ind Med* 1990;17(1):106.
116. Cormier Y, Belandger J, Laviollette M. Prognostic significance of bronchoalveolar lymphocytosis in farmer's lung. *Am Rev Resp Dis* 1987;135:692–695.
117. Gariepy L, Cormier Y, Laviollette M, Tardif A. Predictive value of bronchoalveolar lavage cells and serum perceptive in asymptomatic dairy farms. *Am Rev Resp Dis* 1989; 140:1386–1389.
118. DeVuyst P, Jedaub J, Dumortier P, Vandermoten G, Vande Meyer R, Yernault JC. Asbestos bodies in bronchoalveolar lavage. *Am Rev Resp Dis* 1982;126:972–976.
119. Roggli VL, Piantadosi CA, Bell DY. Asbestos bodies in bronchoalveolar lavage fluid: a study of 20 asbestos-exposed individuals and comparison to patients with other chronic interstitial lung diseases. *Acta Cytologica* 1986;30:470–476.
120. Rebuck AS, Brande AC. Bronchoalveolar lavage in asbestosis. *Arch Intern Med* 1983;143:950–952.
121. DuMortier P, DeVuyst P, Yernault JC. Mineralogical analysis of bronchoalveolar lavage fluids. *Z Erkrank Atmorg* 1988; 171:50–58.
122. DeVuyst P, DuMortier P, Moulin E, Yourassowski N, Roomans P, Yernault JC. Asbestos bodies in bronchoalveolar lavage reflect lung asbestos body concentration. *Eur Resp J* 1988; 1:362–367.
123. DeVuyst P, DuMortier P, Moulin E, Yourassowski N, Yernault R. Diagnostic value of asbestos bodies in bronchoalveolar lavage fluid. *Am Rev Resp Dis* 1987;136:1219–1224.
124. Churg A. Fiber counting and analysis in the diagnosis of asbestos-related disease. *Hum Pathol* 1982;13:381–392.
125. Sebastien P, Armstrong B, Monchaux G, Bignon J. Asbestos bodies in bronchoalveolar lavage fluid and in lung parenchyma. *Am Rev Resp Dis* 1988;137:75–78.
126. Garcia JGN, Griffith DE, Cohen AB, Callahan KS. Alveolar macrophages from patients with asbestos exposure release increased levels of leukotriene By. *Am Rev Resp Dis* 1989; 139:1494–1501.
127. Helmers RA. Bronchoalveolar lavage in asbestos-related lung disease. In: Peters CA and Peters BJ, eds. *Sourcebook of asbestos diseases*. London: Butterworth; 1991;6:89–124.
128. Gellert AR, Langford JA, Winter RJD, Uthayakumar S, Sinha G, Rudd RM. Asbestosis: assessment by bronchoalveolar lavage and measurement of pulmonary epithelial permeability. *Thorax* 1985;40:508–514.

129. Robinson BWS, Rose AH, James A, Whitaker D, Musk AW. Alveolitis of pulmonary asbestosis-bronchoalveolar lavage studies in crocidolite- and chrysotile-exposed individuals. *Chest* 1986;90:396–402.
130. Xaubet A, Rodriquez-Roisin R, Bombi JA, Marin A, Roca J, Agusti-Vidal A. Correlation of bronchoalveolar lavage and clinical and functional findings in asbestosis. *Am Rev Resp Dis* 1986;133:848–854.
131. Begin R, Bisson G, Boileau R, Masse S. Assessment of disease activity by gallium-67 scan and lung lavage in the pneumoconioses. *Semin Resp Med* 1986;7:271–280.
132. Gellert AR, Langford JA, Uthayakumar S, Rudd RM. Bronchoalveolar lavage and clearance of ^{99m}Tc-labelled DTPA in asbestos workers without evidence of asbestosis. *Thorax* 1985; 40:221.
133. Gellert AR, Macey MG, Uthayakumar S, Newland AC, Rudd RM. Lymphocyte sub populations in bronchoalveolar lavage fluid in asbestos workers. *Am Rev Resp Dis* 1985;132:824–828.
134. Begin RO, Cantin AM, Boileau RD, Bisson GY. Spectrum of alveolitis in quartz-exposed human subjects. *Chest* 1987; 92(6):1061–1067.
135. Schuyler MR, Gaumer HR, Stankus RP, Kaimal J, Hoffman E, Salvaggio JE. Bronchoalveolar lavage in silicosis-evidence of type II hyperplasia. *Lung* 1980;157:95–102.
136. Christman JW, Emerson RJ, Graham WGB, Davis GS. Mineral dust and cell recovery from the bronchoalveolar lavage of healthy Vermont granite workers. *Am Rev Resp Dis* 1985; 132:393–399.
137. Kindt GC, Weiland JE, Davis WB, Gadek JE, Dorinsky PM. Bronchiolitis in adults: a reversible cause of airway obstruction associated with airway neutrophils. *Am Rev Resp Dis* 1989; 140:483–492.
138. Huang M, Colby TV, Goellner JR, Martin II WJ. Utility of bronchoalveolar lavage in the diagnosis of drug-induced pulmonary toxicity. *Acta Cytol* 1989;33(4):533–538.
139. Martin WJ II, Rosenow EC III. Amiodarone pulmonary toxicity; recognition and pathogenesis. *Chest* 1988;93(5):1067–1075, 1242–1248.
140. Israel-Biet D, Venet A, Caubarrerre I, Bonan G, Danel C, Chretien J, Hance AJ. Bronchoalveolar lavage in amiodarone pneumonitis: cellular abnormalities and their relevance to pathogenesis. *Chest* 1987;91(2):214–221.
141. Epstein PE, Dauber JH, Rossman MD, Daniele RP. Bronchoalveolar lavage in a patient with chronic berylliosis: evidence for hypersensitivity pneumonitis. *Ann Intern Med* 1982; 97:213–216.
142. Rossman MD, Kern JA, Elias JA, et al. Proliferative response of bronchoalveolar lymphocytes to beryllium: a test for chronic beryllium disease. *Ann Intern Med* 1988;108:687–693.
143. Basset F, Soler P, Jaurand MC, Bignon J. Ultra-structural examination of bronchoalveolar lavage for the diagnosis of pulmonary histiocytosis X: preliminary report on 4 cases. *Thorax* 1977;32:303–306.
144. Chollet S, Soler P, Dournoro P, Richard MS, Ferraus VJ, Basset F. Diagnosis of pulmonary histiocytosis X by immunodetection of Langerhans cells in bronchoalveolar lavage fluid. *Am J Pathol* 1984;115:225–232.
145. Casolaro MA, Bernaudin J, Saltini C, Ferraus VJ, Crystal RG. Accumulation of Langerhans cells on the epithelial surface of the lower respiratory tract in normal subjects in association with cigarette smoking. *Am Rev Resp Dis* 1988;137:406–411.
146. Xaubet A, Agusti C, Picado C, Guerequiz S, Martos JA, Carrion M, Agusti-Vidal A. Bronchoalveolar lavage analysis with anti-T6 monoclonal antibody in the evaluation of diffuse lung diseases. *Respiration* 1989;56:161–166.
147. Singh G, Katyal SL, Bedrossian CWM, Rogers RM. Pulmonary alveolar proteinosis: staining for surfactant apoprotein in alveolar proteinosis and in condition simulating it. *Chest* 1983; 83:82–86.
148. Prakash UBS, Barham SS, Carpenter HA, Dines DE, Marsh HM. Pulmonary alveolar phospholipoproteinosis: experience with 34 cases and a review. *Mayo Clin Proc* 1987;62:499–518.
149. Martin RJ, Coalson JJ, Rogers RM, Horton FO, Manous IE. Pulmonary alveolar proteinosis: the diagnosis by segmented lavage. *Am Rev Resp Dis* 1980;121:819–825.
150. Haslam PL, Hughes DA, Dewar A, Pantin CFA. Lipoprotein macroaggregates in bronchoalveolar lavage fluid from patients with diffuse interstitial lung disease: comparison with idiopathic alveolar lipoproteinosis. *Thorax* 1988;43:140–146.
151. Lieske TR, Sunderrajan EV, Passamonte PM. Bronchoalveolar lavage and technetium-99m glucoheptonate imaging in chronic eosinophilic pneumonia. *Chest* 1984;85:282–284.
152. Dejaegher P, Demendts M. Bronchoalveolar lavage in eosinophilic pneumonia before and during corticosteroid therapy. *Am Rev Resp Dis* 1984;129:631–632.
153. Golde DW, Drew WL, Klein HZ, Finley TN, Cline MJ. Occult pulmonary hemorrhage in leukemia. *Br Med J* 1975;2:166–168.
154. Finley TN, Aronow A, Cosentino AM, Golde DW. Occult pulmonary hemorrhage in anticoagulated patients. *Am Rev Resp Dis* 1977;166:215–221.
155. Drew WL, Finley TN, Golde DW. Diagnostic lavage and occult pulmonary hemorrhage in thrombocytopenic immunocompromised patients. *Am Rev Resp Dis* 1977;166:215–221.
156. Sherman JM, Winnie G, Thomasseu MJ, Abdul-Karin FW, Boat TF. Time course of hemosiderin production and clearance by human pulmonary macrophages. *Chest* 1984;86:409–411.
157. Springmeyer SC, Hoges J, Hammar SP. Significance of hemosiderin-laden macrophages in bronchoalveolar lavage fluid. *Am Rev Resp Dis* 1984;131:A76.
158. Tenholder MF. Pulmonary infections in the immunocompromised host: perspective on procedure. *Chest* 1988; 94(4):676–678.
159. Chastre J, Fagon J, Soler P, et al. Bronchoalveolar lavage for rapid diagnosis of the fat embolism syndrome in trauma patients. *Ann Intern Med* 1990;113:583–588.
160. Silverman JF, Turner RC, West RL, Dillard TA. Bronchoalveolar lavage in the diagnosis of lipoid pneumonia. *Diag Cytopathol* 1989;5(1):3–8.
161. Spatafora M, Bellia V, Ferrara G, Genova G. Diagnosis of a case of lipoid pneumonia by bronchoalveolar lavage. *Respiration* 1987;52:154–156.
162. Linder J, Radio SJ, Robbins RA, Ghafouri M, Rennard SI. Bronchoalveolar lavage in the cytologic diagnosis of carcinoma of the lung. *Acta Cytol* 1987;31(6):796–797.
163. Bellmunt J, DeGracia J, Morales S, Orriols R, Tallada S. Cytologic diagnosis in bronchoalveolar lavage specimens. *Chest* 1990;98(2):513–514.
164. Shiner RJ, Rosenman J, Katz I, Reichart N, Hershko E, Yellin A. Bronchoscopic evaluation of peripheral lung tumors. *Thorax* 1988;43:887–889.
165. Sineway MJ, Francis PB, Honig EG, Boozer RM, Nassar VH. Bronchoalveolar lavage in the diagnosis of peripheral lung cancer. *Am Thorac Soc* 1984;129(4):A68.
166. Rennard SI. Bronchoalveolar lavage in the diagnosis of cancer. *Lung* 1990 (Suppl);1035–1040.
167. Springmeyer SC, Hackman R, Carlson JJ, McClellan E. Bronchoalveolar cell carcinoma diagnosed by bronchoalveolar lavage. *Chest* 1983;83:278–279.
168. Lemarie C, Lavandier M, Renoux M, Renoux G. Carcinoembryonic antigen in bronchoalveolar lavage fluid. *N Engl J Med* 1980;303(10):586–587.
169. Jain N, Kulpati DDS, Luthra UK, Gupta MM, Das DK. A study of bronchoalveolar lavage fluid (BALF) in lung cancer. *Indian J Chest Dis* 1988;30:103–110.
170. Pisani RJ, Cortese DA, Homburger HA, Grambsch PM. A prospective pilot study evaluating the effectiveness of secretory IgA measurements in bronchoalveolar lavage to detect non-small cell lung cancer. *Chest* 1990;97:586–589.
171. Radio SJ, Rennard SI, Kessinger A, Vaughan WP, Linder J. Breast carcinoma in bronchoalveolar lavage. *Arch Pathol Lab Med* 1989;113:333–334.
172. Levy H, Horak DA, Lewis MI. The value of bronchial washings and bronchoalveolar lavage in the diagnosis of lymphangitic carcinomatosis. *Chest* 1988;94:1028–1030.
173. Pisani RJ, Witzig TE, Li CY, Morris MA, Thibodeau SN. Confirmation of lymphomatous pulmonary involvement by immu-

nophenotypic and gene rearrangement analysis of bronchoalveolar lavage fluid. *Mayo Clin Proc* 1990;65:651–656.
174. Wisecarver J, Ness MJ, Rennard SI, Thompson AB, Armitage JO, Linder J. Bronchoalveolar lavage in the assessment of pulmonary Hodgkin's disease. *Acta Cytol* 1989;33:528–529.
175. Kovalski R, Hansen-Flaschen J, Lodato RF, Pietra GG. *Chest* 1990;97:674–678.
176. Rossi GA, Balbi B, Risso M, Repetto M, Ravazzoni C. Acute myelomonocytic leukemia: demonstration of pulmonary involvement by bronchoalveolar lavage. *Chest* 1985;87:259.
177. Young JA, Hopkin JM, Cuthbertson WP. Pulmonary infiltrates in immunocompromised patients: diagnosis by cytological examination of bronchoalveolar lavage fluid. *J Clin Pathol* 1984; 37:390–397.
178. Chamberlain DW, Braude AC, Rebuck AS. A critical evaluation of bronchoalveolar lavage: criteria for identifying unsatisfactory specimens. *Acta Cytol* 1987;31(5):599–605.
179. Kirkpatrick MB, Bass JB Jr. Quantitative bacterial cultures of bronchoalveolar lavage fluids and protected brush catheter specimens from normal subjects. *Am Rev Resp Dis* 1989; 139:546–548.
180. Thorpe JE, Baughman RP, Frame BT, Wessler TA, Staneck JL. Bronchoalveolar lavage for diagnosing acute bacterial pneumonia. *J Infect Dis* 1987;155:855–861.
181. Fagon JI, Chastre J, Hance AJ, et al. Detection of nosocomial lung infection in ventilated patients. Use of a protected specimen. *Am Rev Resp Dis* 1988;138:110–116.
182. Torres A, De La Bellacasa JP, Xaubet A, Gonzalez J, Rodriguez-Roisin R, Jimenez de Anta MT, Agusti Vidal A. Diagnostic value of quantitative cultures of bronchoalveolar lavage and telescoping plugged catheters in mechanically ventilated patients with bacterial pneumonia. *Am Rev Resp Dis* 1989; 140:306–310.
183. Gaussorgues P, Piperno D, Bachmann P, Boyer F, Jean G, Gerard M, Leger P, Robert D. Comparison of nonbronchoscopic bronchoalveolar lavage to open lung biopsy for the bacteriologic diagnosis of pulmonary infections in mechanically ventilated patients. *Intensive Care Med* 1989;15:94–98.
184. Rosenow EC III, Wilson WR, Cockerill FR III. Pulmonary disease in the immunocompromised host. Part I. *Mayo Clin Proc* 1985;60:473–487.
185. Wilson WR, Cockerill FR III, Rosenow EC III. Pulmonary disease in the immunocompromised host. Part II. *Mayo Clin Proc* 1985;60:610–631.
186. McCabe RE. Diagnosis of pulmonary infections in immunocompromised patients. *Med Clin North Am* 1988; 72:1067–1089.
187. Young JA, Hopkin JM, Cuthbertson WP. Pulmonary infiltrates in immunocompromised patients: diagnosis by cytological examination of bronchoalveolar lavage fluid. *J Clin Pathol* 1984; 37:390–397.
188. Linder J, Vaughan WP, Armitage JO, Ghafouri MA, Hurkman D, Mroczek EC, Miller NG, Rennard SI. Cytopathology of opportunistic infection in bronchoalveolar lavage. *Am J Clin Pathol* 1987;88:421–428.
189. Abramson MJ, Stone CA, Holmes PW, Tai EH. The role of bronchoalveolar lavage in the diagnosis of suspected opportunistic pneumonia. *Aust NZ J Med* 1987;17:407–412.
190. Martin WJ II, Smith TF, Brutinel WM, Cockerill FR III, Douglas WW. Role of bronchoalveolar lavage in the assessment of opportunistic pulmonary infections: utility and complications. *Mayo Clin Proc* 1987;62:549–557.
191. Kahn FW, Jones JM. Analysis of bronchoalveolar lavage specimens from immunocompromised patients with a protocol applicable in the microbiology laboratory. *J Clin Microb* 1988; 26(6):1150–1155.
192. Xaubet A, Torres A, Marco F, Puig-de la Bellacasa J, Faus R, Agusti-Vidal A. Pulmonary infiltrates in immunocompromised patients. Diagnostic value of telescoping plugged catheter and bronchoalveolar lavage. *Chest* 1989;95:130–135.
193. Sobonya RE, Barbee RA, Wiens J, Trego D. Detection of fungi and other pathogens in immunocompromised patients by bronchoalveolar lavage in an area endemic for coccidioidomycosis. *Chest* 1990;97:1349–1355.
194. Pisani R, Dupras DM. Clinical utility of BAL in non-AIDS immunocompromised host. *Chest* 1990;98:1015.
195. Johnson JE, Anders GT, Hawkes CF, LaHatte LJ, Blanton HM. Bronchoalveolar lavage findings in patients seropositive for the human immunodeficiency virus HIV. *Chest* 1990; 97:1066–1071.
196. Durand-Amat S, Zalcman G, Mazeron M-C, Sarfati C, Beauvais B, Gerber F, Perol Y, Hirsch A. Opportunistic agents in bronchoalveolar lavage in 99 HIV seropositive patients. *Eur Resp J* 1990;3:282–287.
197. Weldon-Linne CM, Rhone DP, Bourassa R. Bronchoscopy specimens in adults with AIDS. Comparative yields of cytology, histology and culture for diagnosis of infectious agents. *Chest* 1990;98:24–28.
198. Cordonnier C, Bernaudin J-F, Bierling P, Huet Y, Vernant J-P. Pulmonary complications occurring after allogeneic bone marrow transplantation. *Cancer* 1986;58:1047–1054.
199. Rennard SI. Role of bronchoalveolar lavage in the assessment of pulmonary complications following bone marrow and organ transplantation. *Eur Resp J* 1990;3(3):373–375.
200. Milburn HJ, Prentice HG, DuBois RM. Role of bronchoalveolar lavage in the evaluation of interstitial pneumonitis in recipients of bone marrow transplants. *Thorax* 1987; 42:766–772.
201. Springmeyer SC, Hackman RC, Holle R, Greenberg GM, Weems CE, Myerson D, Meyers JD, Donnall Thomas E. Use of bronchoalveolar lavage to diagnose acute diffuse pneumonia in the immunocompromised host. *J Infect Dis* 1986; 154(4):604–605.
202. Allen KA, Markin RS, Rennard SI, Shaw BW Jr, Thompson AB, Wood RP, Woods GS, Linder J. Bronchoalveolar lavage in liver transplant patients. *Acta Cytologica* 1989;33:539–541.
203. Heurlin N, Brattstrom C, Tyden G, Ehrnst A, Andersson J. Cytomegalovirus the predominant cause of pneumonia in renal transplant patients. *Scand J Infect Dis* 1989;21:245–253.
204. Johnson PC, Hogg KM, Sarosi GA. The rapid diagnosis of pulmonary infections in solid organ transplant recipients. *Semin Resp Infect* 1990;5(1):2–9.
205. Gryzan S, Paradis IL, Zeevi A, Duquesnoy RJ, Dummer JS, Griffith BP, Hardesty RL, Trento A, Nalesnik MA, Dauber JH. Unexpectedly high incidence of pneumocystis carinii infection after lung-heart transplantation. Implications for lung defense and allograft survival. *Am Rev Resp Dis* 1988;137:1268–1274.
206. Zeevi A, et al. Bronchoalveolar macrophage lymphocyte rejectivity in heart and lung transplant recipients. *Transpl Proc* 1987;19:2537–2540.
207. Campbell JH, Raina V, Banham SW, Cunningham D, Soukop M. Pulmonary infiltrates: diagnostic problems in lymphoma. *Postgrad Med J* 1989;65:881–884.
208. Phillips et al. Fiberoptic bronchoscopy and diagnosis of pulmonary lesions in lymphoma and leukemia. *Thorax* 1980; 35:19–25.
209. Tenholder MF, Hooper RG. Pulmonary infiltrates in leukemia. *Chest* 1980;78(3):468–469.
210. Saito H, Anaissie EJ, Morice RC, Dekmezian R, Bodey GP. Bronchoalveolar lavage in the diagnosis of pulmonary infiltrates in patients with acute leukemia. *Chest* 1988;94:745–749.
211. DeBlic J, McKelvie P, Le Bourgeois M, Blanche S, Benoist MR, Scheinmann P. Value of bronchoalveolar lavage in the management of severe acute pneumonia and interstitial pneumonitis in the immunocompromised child. *Thorax* 1987; 42:759–765.
212. Winthrop AL, Waddell T, Superina RA. The diagnosis of pneumonia in the immunocompromised child: use of bronchoalveolar lavage. *J Ped Surg* 1990;25:878–880.
213. Pattishall EN, Noyes BE, Orenstein DM. Use of bronchoalveolar lavage in immunocompromised children with pneumonia. *Ped Pulmonol* 1988;5:1–5.
214. Rennard SI. Future directions for bronchoalveolar lavage. *Lung* (Suppl) 1990;168:1050–1056.

Bronchoscopy,
edited by U. B. S. Prakash.
Mayo Foundation © 1994.
Published by Raven Press, Ltd., New York.

CHAPTER 14

Bronchoscopy in Pulmonary Infections

Denis A. Cortese and Udaya B. S. Prakash

Infections of the lungs caused by bacteria, mycobacteria, fungi, protozoa, and other organisms are very frequently encountered in clinical practice. The laboratory studies of expectorated sputum, gastric washings, pleural fluid, transtracheal aspirates, and transthoracic needle aspirates have been employed in the diagnosis of pleuropulmonary infections. Bronchoscopy allows direct access to the tracheobronchial tree for collection of bronchial and peripheral airway secretions and biopsy of parenchymal tissue. The use of the bronchoscope as a diagnostic tool in pulmonary infections has greatly expanded over recent years, particularly in immunocompromised patients who have pulmonary infiltrates. The bronchoscope traverses the oropharynx and thus the limitation to diagnose bacterial infections because of the contamination of the instrument in the upper airway by the oropharyngeal bacterial flora.

EFFECT OF TOPICAL ANESTHETIC AGENTS

The use of topical anesthetic agents appears to reduce the chance of reliably recovering and culturing bacteria from the lower respiratory tract (1). The topical anesthetic lidocaine has antibacterial properties even when used in 1% solution in vitro studies (2). In clinical practice topical lidocaine in both 2% solution and 4% solution does not significantly reduce the success in recovering aerobes and anaerobes from bronchoscopic aspirations (3,4). High concentrations of lidocaine, greater than 5,000 μg/ml, in bronchial secretions are sufficient to inhibit growth in culture of mycobacteria and fungi. Bronchial washing concentrations of lidocaine may be greater than this number whenever more than 250 mg of topical lidocaine are used. Therefore, judicious use of topical lidocaine is important if cultures are to be done in bronchial secretions. Bronchoalveolar lavage (BAL) specimens are suitable for culturing pathogens that may be inhibited by lidocaine because the lidocaine concentration in BAL aspirations has been shown to be low despite the use of more than 250 mg of topical lidocaine (5). Special procedures such as BAL and protected brush catheter, as well as careful attention to the conservative use of topical lidocaine, improve the sensitivity and specificity of bronchoscopy in reliably recovering bacteria from the lower respiratory tract.

Another reason for the reduction in the dose of topical lidocaine is the increased absorption of the drug in patients with candidiasis involving the oropharyngolaryngeal mucosa (6). Lidocaine has been shown to inhibit growth of *Blastomyces dermatidis* in vitro. High concentrations of lidocaine for topical anesthesia appear to adversely affect the recovery of the fungus from bronchoscopic specimens (7).

BACTERIAL INFECTIONS

The rate of nosocomial infections is approximately 6 per 1,000 hospitalized patients per year in the United States. Lower respiratory tract infections account for approximately 20% of the nosocomial infections with approximately 200,000 cases per year reported. Mortality in nosocomial pneumonia ranges from 15% to 50%. More than half of these pneumonias are due to gram-negative organisms, particularly *Pseudomonas aeruginosa, Klebsiella* species, *Enterobacter* species, *Escherichia coli, Serratia* species, and *Proteus* species. Seventeen percent are aerobic gram-positive organisms, most often coagulase-positive *Staphylococcus*. Other organisms include *Pneumocystis carinii,* cytomegalovirus, and *Candida* species in immunocompromised patients. The accurate diagnosis is difficult if sputum, peripheral blood, and pleural fluid cultures

D. A. Cortese: Division of Thoracic Diseases and Internal Medicine, Mayo Clinic, Jacksonville, Florida 32224.
U. B. S. Prakash: Division of Thoracic Diseases and Internal Medicine, Mayo Clinic, Rochester, Minnesota 55905.

are nondiagnostic. Pharyngeal cultures are not reliable since 45% of patients are colonized in the upper airway by the fourth hospital day. Flexible bronchoscopy is helpful, but since secretions may be contaminated from the upper airway, the clinician is uncertain whether or not the cultures obtained from bronchoscopic aspirates are reliably positive.

Protected Brush Catheter

The protected brush specimen technique was first described in 1979, and current techniques are similar (1). The bronchoscope, with no suction attached, is advanced into a bronchus leading to the involved area as determined by a recent chest roentgenogram. A triple-lumen protected brush is then advanced beyond the tip of the bronchoscope. With the tip of the protected brush within the visual field of the bronchoscopist, the gelatin plug is pushed out into a dependent bronchus. The inner catheter, containing the brush, is then advanced into a bronchial subsegment leading to the involved area. The brush is then advanced out of the inner catheter and the sample taken (Fig. 1). With the brush retracted into the inner sheath and the protected catheter still protruding through the distal bronchoscope channel the entire bronchoscope is removed from the airway. The outside of the sheath is cleaned with 70% alcohol and a 1-cm portion of the sheath cut off with a sterile scissors. The brush is then readvanced, cut off with sterile wire clippers, and placed in a sterile specimen tube containing a small quantity of sterile saline or sterile Ringer's lactate. The specimen can then be submitted for aerobic and anaerobic cultures.

The use of the protected brush catheter to collect secretions for culture reduces the chance of upper airway contamination and has improved the diagnostic accuracy of the bronchoscopic procedure. Quantitative cultures are needed since even secretions collected with the protected catheter brush may be contaminated to some degree. It is believed that cultures obtained from the protected brush catheter that provide greater than or equal to 10^3 colony-forming units (CFU) per ml indicate active infection, if initial specimens are diluted between 100–1,000 times with Ringer's lactate. This implies that the original secretions would have yielded greater than or equal to 10^5 or 10^6 CFU/ml if it were to be possible to collect the secretions directly from the lower respiratory tree and placed into culture undiluted (8–12). A culture result greater than to equal to 10^4 CFU/ml is required to indicate an infection if the secretions are collected by the nonprotected brush techniques.

Quantitative bacterial cultures of BAL fluids compared to protected brush catheter specimens obtained from normal subjects indicate that BAL specimens may frequently be contaminated. Seven of eight patients had BAL specimens that revealed one to four organisms, all of which grew in a concentration less than 10^4 CFU/ml. On the other hand, the protected brush catheter was sterile in seven of these patients while in one patient an organism was recovered on culture in a concentration less than 10^3 CFU/ml.

It appears that in normal subjects BAL fluid may frequently be contaminated by oropharyngeal bacteria and the quantitative cultures are less than 10^4 CFU/ml in this situation. With the protected brush catheter if contamination is present, the organism yield is less than 10^3 CFU/ml (13). The protected brush catheter method has been shown to be equivalent to the protected transbronchial needle aspiration technique in establishing the etiology of bacterial pneumonia. Both procedures permit quantitative cultures and are superior to nonquantitative methods. There does not seem to be an advantage in using the needle aspiration technique versus the brush technique (14). Furthermore, protected catheter brush is helpful in identifying multiple organisms in situations in which polymicrobial bacterial pneumonia is likely, such as bronchiectasis (15).

Even though the protected brush catheter is useful in diagnosing nosocomial infections, there are still some problems associated with interpreting the results. The protected brush catheter technique reveals organisms that are present where the brush is placed. It does not sample a large area of the tracheobronchial tree. On the other hand, cultures of tracheal aspirates reveal organisms that are found on the protected brush catheter and usually a few others that may be contaminants or represent organisms from other areas of pneumonia where the protected brush catheter was not placed. In a given patient, the tracheal secretions may be more representative of what may be a polymicrobial, multicentric, pneumonic process. In addition, cultures obtained by the protected brush catheter may not alter antimicrobial selection especially with the wider use of broad-spectrum antibiotics and the careful selection of these antibiotics based on the clinical situation. In any event, quantitative cultures should be used on protected brush catheter specimens to increase the clinician's confidence in the significance of the results (16).

In a prospective study of community-acquired pneumonia, bronchoscopy and protected catheter brushing in patients who demonstrated early therapy failure (less than or equal to 72 hr), late therapy failure (greater than 72 hr), or before start of antibiotic therapy in severely ill or immunocompromised patients has shown bronchoscopy with the use of quantitative cultures is a safe and specific diagnostic tool (17).

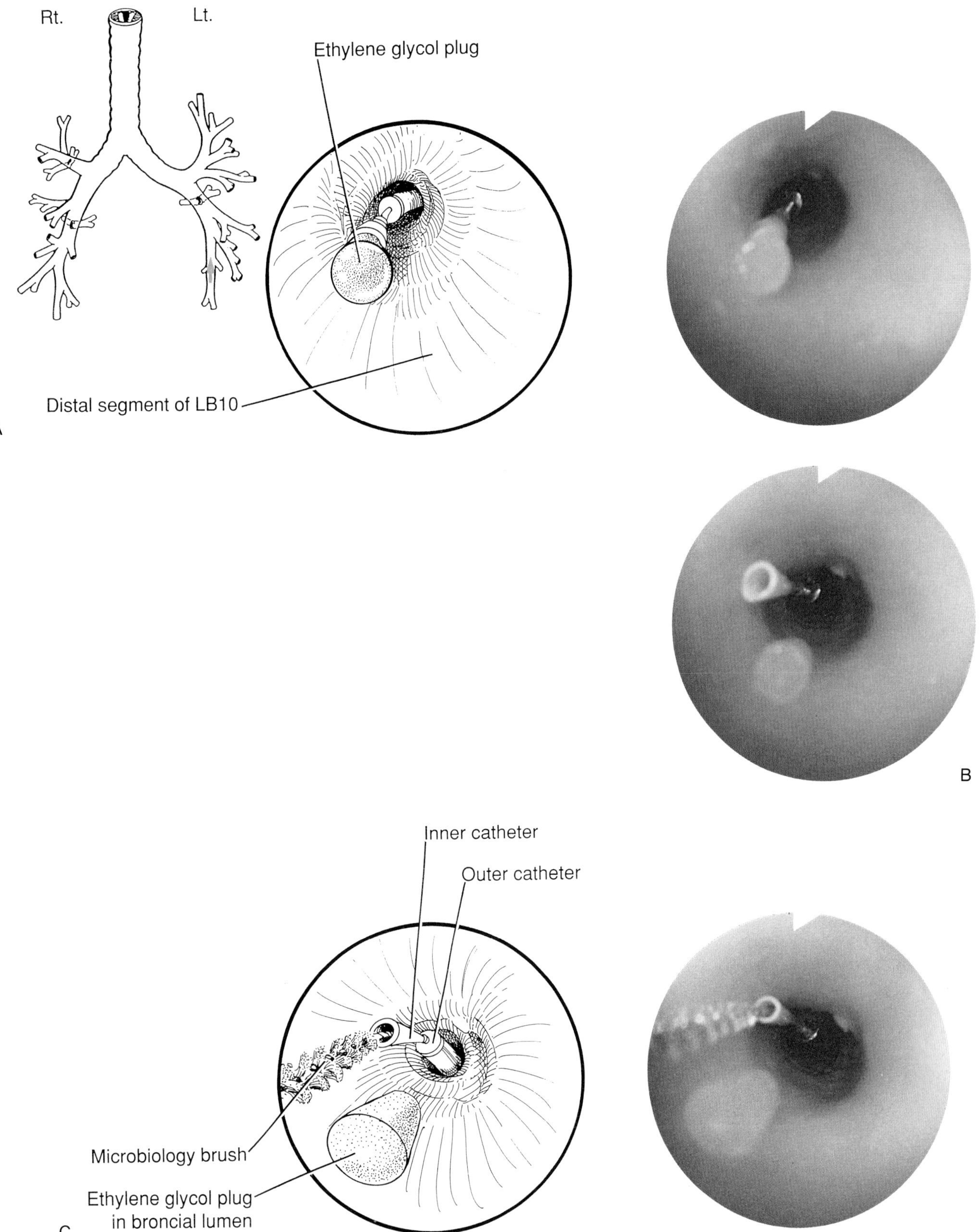

FIG. 1. (A) Cephalad view of protected catheter brush in a left lower lobe bronchus. **(B)** The inner catheter has pushed out the ethylene glycol plug, which will liquify and become absorbed or expectorated. **(C)** Microbiology brush has been pushed distally to obtain bacterial cultures.

Protected Brush Catheter in Patients on Mechanical Ventilation

Bacterial respiratory infections are common in patients undergoing prolonged mechanical ventilation, and antibiotic selection is generally based on the results of smears and cultures of tracheal aspirates (18). Specimens obtained by protected brush catheter have been shown to yield the same organisms as identified on culture and histological examination of open lung biopsy specimens in patients with pneumonia who were receiving mechanical ventilation (19). When the protected brush catheter specimen revealed less than 10^3 CFU/ml, pneumonia was not present. When the protected brush catheter revealed greater than or equal to 10^3 CFU/ml, all patients with pneumonia and all patients with greater than 10^4 CFU/g of lung tissue on open lung biopsy culture were identified.

In a report of ten patients with suspected pneumonia who were receiving mechanical ventilation, the results obtained by protected brush catheter correlated with the diagnosis of pneumonia. In the seven patients who had pneumonia, the offending organism was established by methods such as blood culture, pleural fluid culture, and open lung biopsy culture, and the same organisms were recovered by the protected brush catheter. In three additional patients in whom pneumonia was suspected, open lung biopsy showed no evidence of organisms and the protected brush catheter was sterile in all three. In seven other patients, pneumonia was not present; the protected brush catheter was sterile in each case, but the tracheal aspirates grew two or more organisms in each of the seven patients (20). It appears that the protected brush catheter can collect uncontaminated specimens in these patients. The organisms are the same as found by other techniques that demonstrate infection such as blood culture, pleural fluid culture, and open lung biopsy. Tracheal washing results in more organisms identified compared to protected brush catheter and it becomes a clinical decision as to which organisms recovered from tracheal washings are producing infection.

Quantitative culture techniques are important in patients receiving mechanical ventilation. When fewer than 10^3 CFU/ml organisms are identified, pneumonia is not present. On the other hand, when greater than or equal to 10^3 CFU/ml organisms have been identified on the material collected from a protected brush catheter, 76% of the patients had pneumonia (21,22).

The comparison between protected brush catheter and BAL in mechanically ventilated patients demonstrated that both reveal similar organisms (23,24). The protected brush catheter results are usually available within 24–48 hr while the results from BAL are available sooner based on microscopic examination aided by special stains and identification of intracellular organisms.

Some advocate the use of the protected brush catheter if the results of cultures from material collected from the lower respiratory tract using routine bronchoscopy or tracheal secretions show the presence of organisms. If the secretions from the lower respiratory tract are sterile, the diagnosis of pneumonia is unlikely. On the other hand, if the lower respiratory tract secretions reveal organisms, the possibility of pneumonia is approximately 50%. Protected brush catheter, particularly if the culture result reveals greater than or equal to 10^3 CFU/ml, would indicate the presence of pneumonia. However, the possibility of a false-negative protected brush catheter must be considered particularly in patients who have received antibiotics (25).

The complication of pneumothorax has been reported following the use of protected brush catheterization in ventilated patients in up to 8% of patients (20,26). In the setting of mechanical ventilation, tension pneumothorax can develop rapidly and lead to cardiorespiratory arrest. Hemorrhage of a very mild

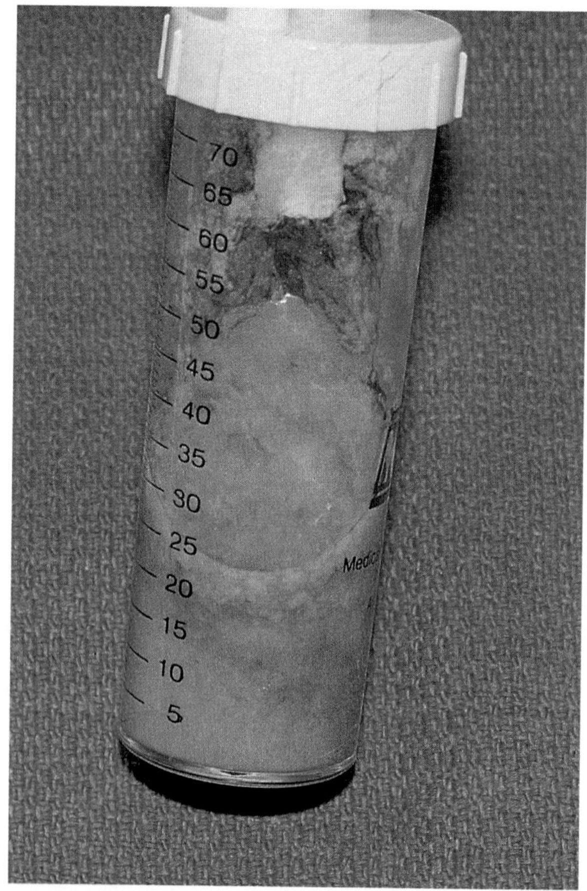

FIG. 2. Bronchoscopic drainage of purulent material from a lung abscess.

degree has rarely been mentioned and has not proven to be a significant problem.

Recently, a protected bronchoscopic balloon-tipped catheter was introduced for the purpose of collecting distal airway secretions for bacterial cultures (27). The balloon is wedged and inflated in a distal bronchus to isolate the distal airways. Then the diaphragm at the tip of the catheter is ejected and BAL performed. Using a growth threshold of 10^4 CFU/ml to diagnose pneumonia, quantitative bacterial cultures by this method have shown a sensitivity of 92% and a specificity of 97% (27,169).

Bronchoalveolar Lavage

The role of BAL in the diagnosis of pulmonary infections is discussed in the previous chapter. The efficacy and safety of BAL has been studied in mechanically ventilated patients. In one study, of the 30 patients with pneumonia who underwent BAL, 27 had one or more pathogens identified in the lavage specimen. Although no patient died as a result of lavage, significant hypoxemia was encountered in some patients undergoing lavage (28).

Recently, the rapid measurement of endotoxin in BAL effluent has been applied to accurately diagnose gram-negative bacterial pneumonia in patients on mechanical ventilators (29). Lymphocyte and lymphocyte subset numbers have been used to assess clinical response to the treatment of mycobacteriosis (30,31).

Bronchoscopy in Lung Abscess

In the preantibiotic era, open tube bronchoscopy resulted in a 50% cure rate if drainage was successfully established (32). Today most lung abscesses will resolve with long-term intravenous antibiotic therapy, particularly if the abscess is less than 4–6 cm in diameter. The presence of an air fluid level indicates communication with the bronchus and therefore postural drainage, antibiotics, and bronchodilators should suffice in most cases.

Flexible bronchoscopy with fluoroscope has been used to effect the drainage of pulmonary abscesses (Fig. 2). A technique that permits the intracavitary placement of brush forceps and fine arterial catheters has been described (33). However, massive intrabronchial aspiration of the contents of the abscess may occur (34). To prevent this complication, sedation should be minimized. Little or no topical anesthesia should be used, particularly in the trachea, to maintain an adequate cough reflex. The patient should be placed in the lateral decubitus position with the involved side down to prevent aspiration into the uninvolved lung. An orotracheal tube should be in place to provide rapid access with a large suction catheter if needed. A rigid bronchoscope should be available or should be used initially if this complication is anticipated, particularly if a foreign body is encountered at the beginning of the procedure.

In comparison to patients who have lung abscess without the presence of cancer, patients who have

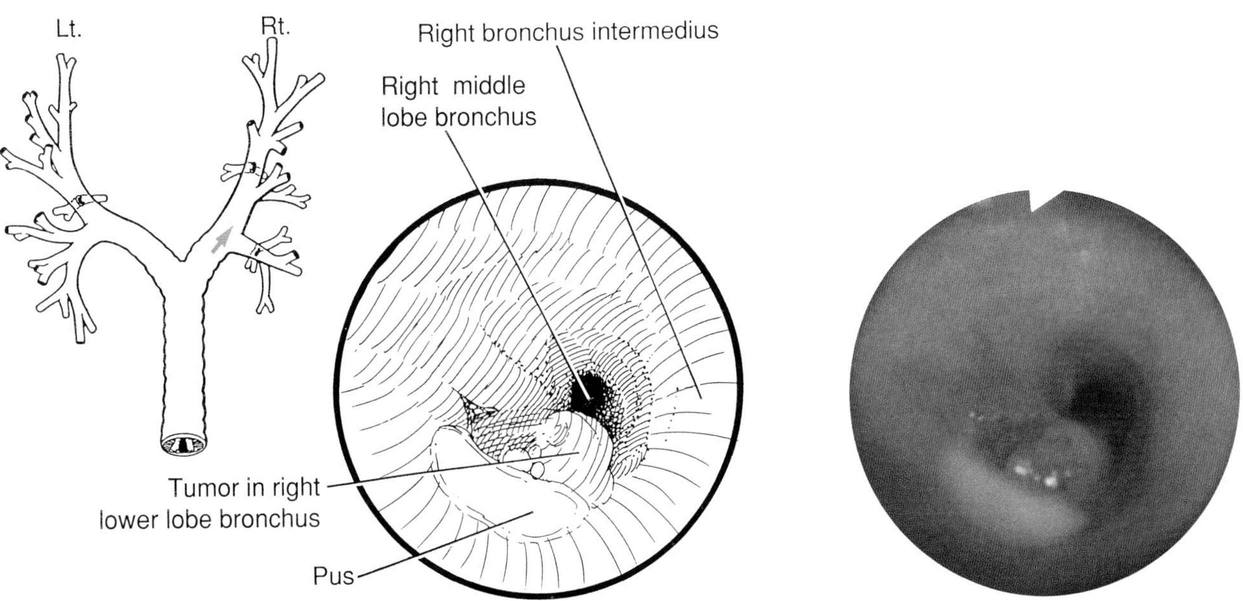

FIG. 3. Postobstructive pneumonitis caused by a neoplasm. Note the purulent material oozing out from behind the tumor.

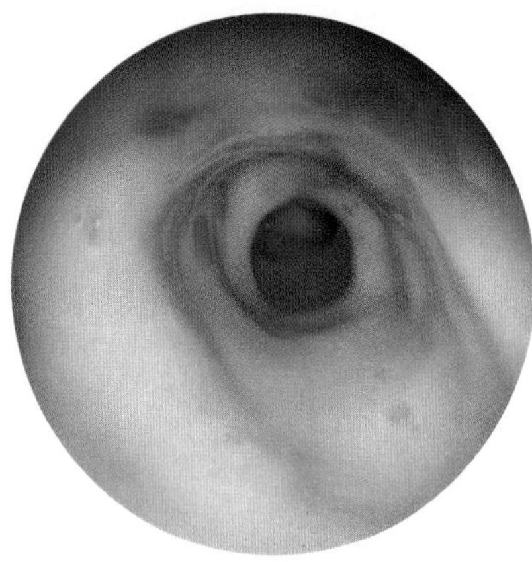

FIG. 4. Dilated bronchus with significant amount of pus in a patient with chronic bronchiectasis. (Courtesy of Lutz Freitag, MD)

bronchogenic carcinoma in association with a symptomatic lung abscess are reported to have a lower prevalence of systemic symptoms, a lower predisposition to aspiration pneumonia, a lower white blood cell count, a lower mean oral temperature, and less extensive pulmonary infiltration on initial chest roentgenogram (35). Routine bronchoscopy in all patients with lung abscess is not indicated. Indications for flexible bronchoscopy in patients with lung abscess would be to establish drainage for those who do not improve on antibiotics and to rule out an endobronchial lesion that may be benign, malignant (Fig. 3), or a foreign body.

Bronchoscopy in patients with bronchiectasis may reveal hemorrhage, submucosal vascular prominence, or dilated bronchi with outpouring of purulent material (Fig. 4).

MYCOBACTERIAL INFECTIONS

Diagnostic Value of Routine Mycobacterial Culture

Flexible bronchoscopy, including the culture results of material obtained by brushings, washings, and bronchoscopic lung biopsy in patients with known tuberculosis, will be successful in obtaining culture proof of tuberculosis in 58–96% of cases with an average rate of 72% (36–38). In a smaller number of patients, the bronchoscopic procedure will produce the only diagnostic cultures in 20–46% of cases with an average of 34% (36,38–42). In a review of the results of bronchial aspirate culture for mycobacteria sent routinely in a series of 1,734 patients who underwent flexible bronchoscopy, the incidence of tuberculosis was 8.3% (144 cases). Among the 144 cases, a positive bronchial aspirate culture was obtained in 82.6%, and it was the only means of diagnosis in 44.4%. Interestingly, in 66% of patients, tuberculosis was not suspected at the time of bronchoscopy even though the study was done in an area endemic to the disease (43). In another study, however, flexible bronchoscopy was used to investigate 35 patients who were considered to have tuberculosis but bronchoscopy confirmed the diagnosis in only 26% (44).

In a report of over 1,000 routine bronchoscopies, 6.6% of patients had tuberculosis and only 32% of those patients had a positive culture obtained by branchoscopy. In only 5% of tuberculosis patients was the bronchoscopy result the only diagnostic culture (45). The usual dose of lidocaine used was approximately 600 mg. In another series of over 4,000 routine bronchoscopies, the prevalence of tuberculosis was only 0.8%. However, the bronchoscopically obtained secretions revealed mycobacteria in 94% of the patients with proven tuberculosis. In 29% of the tuberculosis patients, the bronchoscopic examination was the only diagnostic procedure. The usual lidocaine dose in the latter report was less than 400 mg (46).

A report on flexible bronchoscopy in 65 patients who were either sputum smear–negative or had no sputum to test noted that bronchial aspirates were smear-positive in 38% of patients; interestingly, biopsy alone was positive in 12%. The overall definitive diagnostic rate was 94% (47).

One study demonstrated that bronchoscopy with BAL is far superior to gastric washing in identifying tuberculosis (48). Postbronchoscopy sputum should be studied in all patients suspected of tuberculosis. One study noted that among 30 cases of suspected pulmonary tuberculosis, prebronchoscopy sputum was negative for tubercle bacilli in all the patients, but a postbronchoscopy sputum smear detected tubercle bacilli in 73.3% of the cases (49).

Miliary Tuberculosis

Flexible bronchoscopy, including brushings, washings, and bronchoscopic lung biopsy, is helpful in the diagnosis of miliary tuberculosis in patients with a negative sputum smear (50). Under these conditions, bronchoscopy was diagnostic in 73% and 83% of patients with proven miliary tuberculosis while the bronchoscopic procedure provided the only positive culture material in up to 9% of patients (51,52). Significant spread of tuberculosis following bronchoscopy has been described in two cases but it is unclear if the extension of the disease was truly related to bronchoscopy (53).

Bronchoscopic Lung Biopsy in Tuberculosis

Bronchoscopic lung biopsy has a limited role, adding little to the diagnostic capabilities of brushings and washings. One study showed that in 16% of cases with tuberculosis bronchoscopic lung biopsy resulted in positive cultures, but in no case was it the only positive culture result (54). However, another study compared the diagnostic yields of bronchial washings, bronchial brushings, and lung biopsy specimens in 50 patients with positive cultures for *Mycobacterium tuberculosis* and reported that positive result obtained with cultures of bronchial brushings was significantly higher than that with bronchial washings and that the histological study of lung biopsy improved the rate of immediate or rapid diagnosis of tuberculosis (55). Identification of granuloma in bronchoscopic lung biopsy specimens is not diagnostic of tuberculosis, and the tissue should be cultured to document the presence of mycobacteria.

Bronchoscopic Appearance in Tuberculosis

The bronchoscopic examination can reveal a wide variety of appearances, including normal bronchial anatomy and mucosal appearance; mucosal and submucosal granulomas; mucosal ulcerations; endobronchial polyps; and bronchostenosis (36,56,57). Tuberculous lymph nodes occasionally erode into the tracheobronchial tree and mimic endobronchial malignancy. Airway obstruction secondary to erosion of tuberculous lymph node into the trachea and bronchoscopic treatment has been described (58). A publication on 16 adults with intrathoracic lymphadenopathy secondary to tuberculosis observed endobronchial involvement, proved by bronchoscopy, in 12 patients (59).

FUNGAL INFECTIONS

Pulmonary Histoplasmosis

Histoplasmosis is the most common fungal infection of the lungs in the United States. The role of the bronchoscope as a diagnostic aid in this mycosis has been studied. In a series of 469 patients with histoplasmosis, the diagnosis was established by bronchoscopy and other means in 71 patients. Bronchoscopy was the only diagnostic method that established the diagnosis in 11% of patients. However, in patients with pulmonary nodules due to histoplasmosis, bronchoscopy was not helpful (60).

Pulmonary Coccidioidomycosis

Coccidioidomycosis, caused by *Coccidioides immitis,* is an endemic disease in the southwestern United States. However, it is encountered in other areas of North America in immunocompromised patients. Bronchoscopy has been successfully used in the diagnosis of coccidioidomycosis (61,62).

Pulmonary Blastomycosis

Pneumonia secondary to blastomycosis, caused by the fungus *Blastomyces dermatiditis,* may produce patchy or diffuse pulmonary infiltrates. Occasionally, laryngeal involvement mimics carcinoma and if sputum examination is nondiagnostic, laryngoscopy or bronchoscopy is required to establish the diagnosis (63). Tracheal blastomycosis manifested by numerous white, streaky, nodular, and vesicular lesions has been described in the trachea and lobar bronchus (64). *Blastomyces dermatiditis* is one of the organisms whose growth is inhibited by lidocaine. A review of case records of 36 patients with pulmonary blastomycosis reported that when the fungus was present at microscopy, whether the specimen was sputum or bronchial washings, culture of the bronchoscopic specimen was more frequently negative than culture of the sputum specimen (7). Another report documented the usefulness of bronchoscopy in the diagnosis of blastomycosis (171). The inhibition of the fungus depends on the concentration of lidocaine and the duration of exposure.

Pulmonary Aspergillosis

Invasive Aspergillosis

The presence of hyphae in bronchoscopic specimens has a 53% sensitivity and a 95% specificity in the presence of invasive aspergillosis. However, culture of bronchoscopic specimens is positive for *Aspergillus* species in only 23% of patients with invasive aspergillosis (65). In patients with leukemia and invasive aspergillosis, 50% had bronchoscopic specimens (washings, brushings, or bronchoscopic lung biopsy) that revealed *Aspergillus* species on histological examination or culture. In only one patient was the diagnosis made by bronchoscopic lung biopsy alone (66). Bronchoscopy has a low diagnostic yield in the presence of invasive aspergillosis. BAL for the diagnosis of invasive aspergillosis carries a culture sensitivity of 40% and a specificity of 90% (67). Negative results do not exclude the diagnosis and further procedures or empiric therapy may be justified as indicated in the appropriate clinical setting. On the other hand, the finding of characteristic hyphae does not establish the diagnosis of invasive aspergillosis since saprophytic growth of *Aspergillus* is common.

Tracheobronchial Aspergillosis

Tracheobronchial invasive aspergillosis is a relatively new disease entity and has been described in immunocompromised patients, in patients with AIDS, and following heart–lung and lung transplantation (68–75). One subpopulation of immunocompromised patients at risk for developing tracheobronchial aspergillosis is the heart–lung and lung transplant recipients; the tracheobronchial anastomotic sites seem particularly affected by the process (73). The bronchoscopic findings consist of pseudomembrane formation of the mucosa of trachea and main stem bronchi. The pseudomembrane forms a thick cast and produces severe concentric narrowing of the tracheobronchial lumen. Bronchoscopic removal of the pseudomembrane reveals extensive shallow ulceration and denudation of the mucosa. Special stains of the pseudomembrane show *Aspergillus*. Relief of wheezing and dyspnea can be expected after bronchoscopic removal of the pseudomembrane. However, massive hemoptysis with death in one patient during bronchoscopic removal of the necrotic membrane from the airway has been described (74).

Allergic Bronchopulmonary Aspergillosis

Allergic bronchopulmonary aspergillosis is a complication observed in approximately 10% of asthmatics. One manifestation of this complication is the collection of thick and tenacious mucoid plugs in the lobar and segmental bronchi in the upper and mid-lung zones, leading to lobar and segmental atelectasis. The term *mucoid impaction syndrome* has been used to describe this (76,77). Resolution can be expected after aggressive therapy with bronchodilators and corticosteroids. However, a minority of patients develop persistent atelectasis and require bronchoscopic removal of the thick mucous plugs. The term *plastic bronchitis* has been used to describe formation of thick and tenacious mucous casts of the bronchial tree in patients with allergic bronchopulmonary aspergillosis, cystic fibrosis, asthma, bronchitis, bronchocentric granulomatosis, congenital tricuspid atresia, and chronic pericardial and pleural effusions (78–80). If flexible bronchoscopic removal of the bronchial casts is not possible, rigid bronchoscopy is indicated.

Pulmonary Aspergilloma

Pulmonary aspergilloma or mycetoma (fungus ball) is a complication that usually occurs in the upper lung zones chronically damaged by disease processes such as healed cavitary tuberculosis, mycoses, sarcoidosis, radiation pneumonitis, ankylosing spondylitis, or chronic obstructive pulmonary disease. Hemoptysis is a serious manifestation of pulmonary mycetoma and bronchoscopy is occasionally indicated to localize the lesion and to control severe hemoptysis. Biopsy of the fungus ball may reveal the presence of aspergillus. Rarely, the bronchoscopist may be able to enter the cavity and visualize the fungus ball (81).

Pulmonary Zygomycosis

Although rare, zygomycosis (mucormycosis) of the lungs presents life-threatening problems. Zygomycosis is more likely in patients with severe diabetes mellitus, diabetic ketoacidosis, leukemia, lymphoma, neutropenia, and those on immunosuppressive therapy or high-dose corticosteroid therapy (82). Host cell defense and leukocyte dysfunction seem to be important factors in predisposing patients to zygomycosis. One of the peculiar features of zygomycosis is its tendency to involve major airways (83). This is particularly true of patients with severe diabetes mellitus who develop zygomycosis (84). This leads to invasion of the tracheobronchial wall and hilar vessels with infarction or massive hemoptysis. Bronchoscopy is a reliable tool in the diagnosis of airway involvement in zygomycosis. Bronchial ulceration, necrosis of airway wall, endobronchial bleeding, and/or stenosis of lobar or segmental bronchi can be seen (170). A case of a 44-year-old man with poorly controlled diabetes mellitus who developed endobronchial zygomycosis that totally occluded the right lower lobe bronchus is described; the lesion was removed through a rigid bronchoscope. Two weeks later the bronchus was free of mucormycosis histologically and on culture (167).

IMMUNOCOMPROMISED PATIENTS

Bronchoscopy has a useful role in establishing the diagnosis of infection in immunocompromised patients with diffuse pulmonary infiltrates provided bronchial brushings, washings, BAL, and bronchoscopic lung biopsy are included in the procedure. Bronchoscopy can be 90% sensitive for infection in this setting (85). If results of bronchoscopy are negative, the probability that infection is not present may be as high as 94% (negative predicted value). The bronchoscopic lung biopsy is not helpful in establishing a nonfungal infectious diagnosis.

In 98 immunocompromised patients who had both a protected brush catheter and BAL performed during a bronchoscopy, the protected brush specimens revealed an infectious diagnosis in 22% of the patients while BAL demonstrated infection in 49% of these patients. Together the protected brush specimen and the BAL resulted in establishing an infectious etiology in

69% of patients (86). Another study reported that bilateral BAL provides a higher diagnostic yield in immunocompromised patients (173).

Bronchoscopy, including the use of BAL, bronchoscopic lung biopsies, and protected brush catheter, results in an overall disappointingly low yield of 27% of the diagnosis of pulmonary infiltrates in pediatric age patients with cancer. The low yield is for etiologies such as infection, leukemia, and lymphoma (87). The yield is also low for diagnosing infectious pulmonary infiltrates and may be due to the routine use of empiric antibiotics in these patients. However, subsequent procedures (open lung biopsy, transthoracic needle aspiration, autopsy) revealed infectious agents in several situations where the bronchoscopy and its associated procedures were previously negative. The organisms most frequently encountered include *Pneumocystis carinii*, *Candida* species, cytomegalovirus (CMV), and *Aspergillus* species. In the pediatric age group, a positive bronchoscopy is helpful; but a negative bronchoscopy should not delay further procedures or be a cause for discontinuation of antibiotics or antifungal therapy in children with cancer and pulmonary infiltrates.

ORGAN TRANSPLANTATION

Lung Transplantation

The major complications in long-term survivors of lung transplantation have been infection, rejection, and bronchial anatomotic strictures. The stenosis may be due to granulation and fibrotic tissue or dynamic compression with expirations to bronchomalacia. In either situation, bronchial dilatations and stent placement have been effective (161,162). To establish the presence of infection, BAL has proven sensitive and specific just as in other immunocompromised patients. However, the addition of multiple bronchoscopic lung biopsies has been of great use in establishing the presence of rejection as well as infections due to CMV, herpes simplex, and *Candida* species (163–166).

Cardiac Transplantation

It is possible to establish a diagnosis in up to 62% of patients who develop pulmonary infiltrates after cardiac transplantation. In the case of infections following cardiac transplantation, BAL is the most sensitive procedure establishing the infectious etiology in 63% of cases, while bronchoscopic lung biopsy established the diagnosis in 46% of the patients, and washings and brushings established the infectious etiology in 43% of patients. In the presence of pulmonary hypertension, there is approximately a 10% risk of mild hemorrhage (25–100 ml) (88). Pretransplant "surveillance" bronchoscopy has been done to evaluate the presence or absence of bronchitis (89), but we do not believe it is indicated.

Bone Marrow Transplant

In patients who undergo bone marrow transplant and develop pulmonary infiltrates, bronchoscopy with BAL and bronchoscopic lung biopsy has identified CMV, *Candida*, *Aspergillus*, general bacteria, adenovirus, and *P. carinii*. Overall, a diagnostic accuracy of 73% in defining the organisms has been reported in this group of patients (90). Since CMV is frequently isolated in the BAL effluent of bone marrow transplant recipients without pneumonia, the diagnosis of clinical illness due to this virus should not be based only on the isolation of the virus in BAL. Flexible bronchoscopy and BAL can be safely carried out in pediatric patients with pulmonary infiltrates following bone marrow transplant (92,168).

Renal Transplantation

Bronchoscopy with BAL and bronchoscopic lung biopsy has been reported to correctly establish the etiological organism in 93% of patients with renal transplants who develop infectious pulmonary processes. The most common organisms include CMV, general bacteria, *P. carinii*, and *Candida* species (93). One report described 39 flexible bronchoscopies performed in 51 renal allograft recipients who developed 52 episodes of fever and new pulmonary infiltrates. Specific etiological diagnoses were made in 77% of patients. The information obtained was clinically useful in 54% of patients and definitive but not clinically useful in 23%. Microbiology brush specimens were useful in detecting etiological diagnoses in 44% of the 27 patients in whom it was performed. Bronchoscopic lung biopsies yielded specific etiological diagnoses in 53% of the 17 biopsies obtained. Complications were minor and noted in 5% of all bronchoscopies (94).

ACQUIRED IMMUNODEFICIENCY SYNDROME (AIDS)

Infections

Infectious pneumonia is the most common pulmonary problem in patients with AIDS. The most common organisms include *Pneumocystis carinii*, CMV, *Mycobacterium avium-intracellulare*, *Cryptococcus neoformans*, *Mycobacterium tuberculosis*, *Coccidioides immitis*, and *Histoplasma capsulatum*. In one study of a large number of patients with acquired immunodeficiency syndrome, CMV was most often diagnosed from examination and culture of the BAL fluid (95).

Flexible bronchoscopy with BAL and with or without bronchoscopic lung biopsy frequently provides the diagnosis of the etiological agent of infectious pneumonia in these patients. Bronchoscopy may be considered up to 96% sensitive for diagnosing the organisms listed above if alveolar lavage and bronchoscopic biopsy are done at the same procedure. Diagnostic sensitivity falls to 86% with only alveolar lavage and 87% if only bronchoscopic lung biopsy is done (96). Bronchial brush biopsy carries with it a low diagnostic yield (97).

In a patient with AIDS, BAL and bronchoscopic lung biopsy have about equal sensitivity when used alone for diagnosing *P. carinii* (96,98,99). Alveolar lavage alone provides 95% sensitivity when cytological examination and special stains are performed (98,100). Bronchoscopic lung biopsy alone is sensitive in more than 94% of patients with *Pneumocystis* (98,101,102). Flexible bronchoscopy, using both alveolar lavage and bronchoscopic lung biopsy, has been reported to provide 100% sensitivity when the specimens are adequate (98). Occasionally, endobronchial mass caused by *P. carinii* may mimic carcinoma or endobronchial tuberculosis (103).

Bronchoscopic lung biopsy is useful in diagnosing *P. carinii* particularly if histology and touch preps are performed. Histology is reported to be up to 97% sensitive while touch preps are 88% sensitive (101,102). However, touch preps slightly increase the sensitivity of the overall procedure particularly if the patient has been on therapy and the alveoli are colonized with fewer organisms. Between two and four adequate bronchoscopic lung biopsies is the optimum number to provide a diagnostic sensitivity of 98% when both histology and touch preps are performed and examined simultaneously.

More and more patients with AIDS are undergoing empiric therapy for *P. carinii* without documentation of the infection. The role of bronchoscopy in every patient with acquired immunodeficiency syndrome and typical clinical features of *P. carinii* pneumonia has been questioned. In a prospective study of 73 patients with HIV-positive status, the authors estimated that 64% of bronchoscopies would have been saved by adopting an empiric approach to treatment for typical *Pneumocystis* pneumonia and thus cause a large reduction in the number of high-risk bronchoscopies performed (104). Persons who are positive for HIV and are asymptomatic are less likely to benefit from "routine" bronchoscopy to identify *P. carinii* (105).

Infections by *Mycobacterium tuberculosis* and *Mycobacterium avium-intracellulare* are very common in patients with AIDS (106). Recovery of *M. avium-intracellulare* is highest with culture of both washings and lavage (95). Since the lymphocyte function is abnormal in these patients, the biopsies may not show classic tuberculous granulomas. A retrospective study of 31 HIV positive patients who were proven to have *Mycobacterium tuberculosis* evaluated the role of bronchoscopy and reported that an immediate diagnosis of tuberculosis was made by bronchoscopy in 48% of patients. In 23%, bronchoscopic lung biopsy was the only positive specimen (107). Other studies have shown that bronchial brushings and bronchoscopic lung biopsy for the differential diagnosis of *M. tuberculosis* do not contribute to the diagnosis (108). Infection caused by *M. avium-intracellulare* can produce endobronchial lesions (109,110). The endobronchial lesions can enlarge and cause segmental or lobar atelectasis. Hemoptysis and bronchiectasis may result from this manifestation. The endobronchial lesions appear pale white or pale yellow and are firm to biopsy. Biopsy specimens may demonstrate caseous granulomata.

The role of repeat bronchoscopy in patients with AIDS and pulmonary infiltrates is also subject to question. In one study involving 286 patients with AIDS, the first group underwent repeat bronchoscopy within 30 days and the second group after 60 days. The repeat bronchoscopy provided a new treatable diagnosis in only 5% of the former group in contrast to 55% in the latter (111).

Culture of BAL fluid is particularly helpful in diagnosing CMV and *Mycobacterium* with little added benefit from bronchoscopic lung biopsy for these infections (100).

Noninfectious Disorders: *Kaposi's Sarcoma*

Kaposi's sarcoma is a noninfectious complication of AIDS. Approximately 6% of patients with Kaposi's sarcoma develop pulmonary involvement (112). Pulmonary involvement can manifest as parenchymal nodules or as endobronchial lesions (113). When pulmonary parenchyma alone is involved, the differentiation from *P. carinii* is difficult. Endobronchial Kaposi's sarcoma is characterized by bright red or violaceous raised mucosal lesions. Hemoptysis and hemorrhage of endobronchial biopsy are unusual. Bronchoscopic lung biopsy may be helpful in establishing the diagnosis of pulmonary Kaposi's sarcoma if the pulmonary process does not respond to treatment aimed at *P. carinii* (114). Bronchoscopic lung biopsy may be necessary to establish the diagnosis. Diagnostic yields of 34–56% have been described with bronchoscopy, endobronchial biopsy, and bronchoscopic lung biopsy (115,116).

OTHER INFECTIONS

Herpes simplex virus infection of the respiratory tract produces patchy pneumonia. Herpetic blisters are occasionally seen in the tracheobronchial mucosa. Tracheal stenosis from herpetic tracheitis has been described (117,118). They appear pale, raised, tense, and fluid-filled. Herpes simplex virus infection of the respiratory tract can be diagnosed by bronchial washings (119).

Bronchoscopic procedures, particularly BAL, have been successfully used in the diagnosis of other infections including chlamydia, cryptococcosis, nocardiosis, candidiasis, pulmonary strongyloidosis, and schistosomiasis (120–125). Unusual cases of actinomycosis producing an endobronchial mass mimicking cancer have been reported (126,127). BAL has been used to diagnose acute eosinophilic pneumonia caused by toxocariasis (128).

A report of necrotizing tracheitis caused by *Corynebacterium pseudodiphtheriticum* has been described in an immunocompromised patient (172).

DOES THE BRONCHOSCOPE PROPAGATE INFECTION?

All surgical procedures are potentially capable of transmitting infection from the surgical site to distant organs. Theoretically, bronchoscopic procedures are at greater risk of causing this complication because the instrument traverses the oropharyngeal area and carries with it the microorganisms to the distal tracheobronchial tree and pulmonary parenchyma. The bronchoscopy-induced infection may be a true infection or a pseudoinfection due to contaminated bronchoscopy equipment. The former produces clinical symptoms and signs of infection whereas the latter is characterized by laboratory isolation of organisms in the absence of clinical features of sepsis. The role of prophylactic antibiotic in the prevention of bacterial endocarditis is discussed in Chapter 8.

Bronchoscopy-Induced Infections

An earlier study of 249 flexible bronchoscopy procedures, specifically surveyed for the presence of bronchoscopy-related pneumonia, revealed no cases of pneumonia related to bronchoscopy (129). Another earlier prospective study of 100 flexible bronchoscopies assessed the frequencies of fever, parenchymal infiltration, and bacteremia after the procedure and observed fever after 16% and parenchymal infiltrations after 6% of the procedures. Most complications were mild and transient, but one patient developed rapidly progressive pneumonia and died. No organisms were isolated from cultures of blood drawn at the time of the procedure or during complications. The organisms most commonly isolated from the sputum of the patients who developed pneumonia were the aerobic and anaerobic bacteria normally found in the mouth (130). Others also reported the absence of significant incidence of infections related to bronchoscopy (131).

Several reports have described the clinical aspects of bronchoscopy-induced infections. Bacteremia, including fatality, following bronchoscopy has been described in several instances (132–136). Bacteremia and meningitis due to *Streptococcus pneumoniae* was reported in a 52-year-old man 28 hr after an otherwise uncomplicated flexible bronchoscopy; the patient responded to antimicrobial therapy and later underwent pneumonectomy for carcinoma (137). In another patient, bronchoscopy for the evaluation of hemoptysis was followed 2 weeks later by uveitis and 4 weeks later by endophthalmitis. Both sputum and vitreous cultures yielded *Pseudomonas aeruginosa*. Despite aggressive medical treatment, enucleation was eventually necessary (138). Fatal pneumococcal pneumonia and septicemia following flexible bronchoscopic examination and endobronchial biopsy is described in patient with severe chronic congestive heart failure, even though a causal relationship is unclear (139). Prophylactic (prebronchoscopic lung biopsy) antipseudomonadal antibiotic therapy in an immunocompromised patient believed to have bronchitis caused by *P. aeruginosa* with progressive pulmonary infiltrates did not prevent bacteremic *Pseudomonas* infection (140).

The transmission of *M. tuberculosis* from one patient to another by a bronchoscope that was disinfected with an iodophor solution has been documented (141). Anecdotal reports of development of pneumonia and lung abscess after transbronchial biopsy of a peripheral mass lesion are noteworthy (142,143).

Bronchoscopic Contamination

The cross-contamination of bronchoscopically obtained specimens is another potential problem. A large, tertiary care referral center reported the experience with recurrent episodes of mycobacterial cross-contamination of bronchoscopy specimens. One episode was followed by active pulmonary infection due to *M. tuberculosis*. In experiments, after bronchoscopy equipments were exposed to a saline suspension of *Mycobacterium fortuitum* (10^5–10^7/ml), they were readily sterilized by routine cleaning and disinfection procedures. The spring-operated suction valves, however, remained contaminated even after a 30-min exposure to 2% glutaraldehyde or after passage through a commercially available bronchoscope cleaner-washer (144). Bacterial contamination of the flexible bronchoscope, particularly by *Pseudomonas aeruginosa* and *Serratia marcescens*, has been described (145,146). In a report, the recovery of multiple isolates of *P. aerugi-*

nosa from bronchial lavage specimens was traced to contaminated bronchoscopes; four patients were involved and none became infected. Awareness of a cluster of *Serratia* cultures and immediate investigation and institution of control measures may have prevented the occurrence of true infections (145). Pseudo-outbreaks of infection by *Bacillus* species have also been traced to a contaminated automatic suction valve of the bronchoscope. It is likely that secretions became contaminated during passage through the valve en route to a collection device (147). The suction valves should be routinely autoclaved after each use. Another publication described a pseudoepidemic of infections caused by *Proteus* species, traced to bronchoscopy equipment; there was no definitive clinical illness in any patient (148).

Not all contaminations occur in the bronchoscopy equipment. In a report from a major medical center, 52 patients underwent flexible bronchoscopy by the same physician, one of four who performed the procedure during a 2.5-year period, and *Mycobacterium gordonae* was recovered from specimens obtained by bronchoscopy. Only this particular physician added one drop of green dye, stored in a bottle, to the cocaine used for topical anesthesia; cultures of the dye yielded *M. gordonae* (149). Another report described eight clinically uninfected patients whose bronchial washings showed growth of *Trichosporon cutaneum*. Interestingly, the source of the organism was the cocaine solution used for topical anesthesia during bronchoscopy; contamination was thought to have occurred during preparation of the solutions by pharmacy personnel (150). In a community hospital, *Rhodotorula rubra* was isolated from the bronchial washings of 54% of 56 patients who underwent bronchoscopy; pulmonary disease consistent with invasive fungal pneumonia was not apparent in any patient. Repeat sputum cultures were performed on 11 patients, none of whom were positive for *R. rubra*. Further investigation revealed fungal contamination of two brushes used to clean the bronchoscope channels (151). Bronchoscope-cleaning machines have been implicated in pseudoepidemics of noninfectious mycobacteriosis (152,153).

Appropriate mode of cleaning and disinfecting the bronchoscope should be mandatory to prevent true infections and pseudoinfections. Earlier studies reported that when the bronchoscope was disinfected with an iodophor solution, surveillance culture from a bronchoscope grew *Mycobacterium tuberculosis* (141). Several experiments demonstrated that iodophors failed to kill *M. tuberculosis* (141). Controlled studies have evaluated the efficacy of different disinfectants for cleaning of the flexible bronchoscope. Of the three disinfectants, glutaraldehyde, ethyl alcohol, and chlorhexidine, the most effective was chlorhexidine, with glutaraldehyde next and ethyl alcohol third (154). In another report, bronchoscopy specimens from three patients investigated during one week in a large teaching hospital were culture positive for the same sero variety of *Mycobacterium intracellulare*. Only the first patient was a genuine excretor of the mycobacterium; the isolates from the other two patients were false positives caused by inadequate disinfection of bronchoscopy equipment. The agent recommended for chemical disinfection of flexible bronchoscope is 2% glutaraldehyde solution; the instrument should be immersed in it for 20–30 min. Alternately, 5 hr exposure to ethylene oxide is recommended for sterilization. These procedures must be preceded by adequate mechanical cleaning (155,156). Detergent cleaning of the bronchoscope has been shown to remove all detectable HIV (157).

The bronchoscopist and bronchoscopy staff are at risk of being exposed to contagions. The evolution of the acquired immune deficiency syndrome (AIDS) has induced an extensive review of procedures for infection control. Epidemiological data indicate that transmission of human immunodeficiency virus (HIV) other than by direct inoculation or sexual contact is extremely rare. The HIV, however, has been found in flexible bronchoscopes used on patients with AIDS (158). Therefore, the theoretical risk of transmission of HIV by bronchoscopy exists. In providing medical care to patients who are suspected of harboring HIV, hepatitis B virus, mycobacteria, and other organisms, some medical centers have adopted "all-inclusive" precautions to prevent the spread of infections. Some argue that this policy of "overkill" precaution is not tenable, given the difficulty in identifying infected patients (159).

Even though our review of the literature suggests that the risk of transmitting infectious diseases through the bronchoscope is minimal, we suggest that, as far as the bronchoscopy practice is concerned, infection control policies should comply with the following: (a) infection control precautions should apply to all patients, whether the patient is deemed infectious or not; (b) all equipment used should be cleaned thoroughly in appropriate detergent immediately after use to remove respiratory secretions and reduce contamination; (c) there should be strict maintenance of "clean" and "infected" areas in bronchoscopy suite so that instruments used are separated from sterile and clean equipment; (d) medical personnel in contact with each patient should wear simple barrier clothing, masks, gloves, and goggles routinely; (e) contaminated bronchoscopes should be disinfected for at least 20 min in alkaline glutaraldehyde (2%) after cleaning; (f) bronchoscopy specimens for study should be handled appropriately; (g) the used disposable material must be disposed off properly; and (h) the bronchoscopist and personnel involved in the procedure should be administered hepatitis B vaccine (160).

REFERENCES

1. Bartlett JG, Alexander J, Mayhew J, Sullivan-Sigler N, Gorbach SL. Should fiberoptic bronchoscopy aspirates be cultured? *Am Rev Resp Dis* 1976;114:73–78.
2. Wimberley N, Willey S, Sullivan N, Bartlett JG. Antibacterial properties of lidocaine. *Chest* 1979;76:37–40.
3. Warnner A, Amikam B, Robinson MJ. Comparison between the bacteriologic flora of different segments of the airways. *Respiration* 1973;30:561–569.
4. Jordan GW, Wong GA, Hoeprich PD. Bacteriology of the lower respiratory tract as defined by fiberoptic bronchoscopy and transtracheal aspiration. *J Infect Dis* 1976;34:428–435.
5. Strange C, Barbarash RA, Heffner JE. Lidocaine concentrations in bronchoscopic secretions. *Chest* 1988;93:547–550.
6. Ameer B, Burlingame MB, Harman EM. Rapid mucosal absorption of topical lidocaine during bronchoscopy in the presence of oral candidiasis. *Chest* 1989;96:1438–1439.
7. Taylor MR, Lawson LA, Boyce JM, Lockwood WR. Inhibition of *Blastomyces dermatitidis* by topical lidocaine. *Chest* 1983; 84:431–435.
8. Wimberly N, Faling LJ, Bartlett JG. A fiberoptic bronchoscopy technique to obtain uncontaminated lower airway secretions for bacterial cultures. *Am Rev Resp Dis* 1979;119:337–343.
9. Wimberley N, Bass JB, Boyd BW, Kirkpatrick MB, Serio RA, Pollack HN. Use of a bronchoscopic protected catheter brush for the diagnosis of pulmonary infections. *Chest* 1982; 81:556–562.
10. Pollack HM, Hawkins EL, Bonner JR, Sparkman T, Bass J. Diagnosis of bacterial pulmonary infections with quantitative protected catheter cultures obtained during bronchoscopy. *J Clin Microbiol* 1983;17:255–259.
11. Glanville AR, Marlin GE, Hartnett BJ, Yap JM, Bradbury R. The use of fiberoptic bronchoscopy with sterile catheter in the diagnosis of pneumonia. *Aust NZ J Med* 1985;15:309–319.
12. Teague RB, Wallace RJ Jr. Awe RJ. The use of quantitative sterile brush culture and gram stain analysis in the diagnosis of lower respiratory tract infection. *Chest* 1981;79:157–161.
13. Kirkpatrick MB, Bass JB. Quantitative bacterial cultures of bronchoalveolar lavage fluids and protected brush catheter specimens from normal subjects. *Am Rev Resp Dis* 1989; 139:546–548.
14. Lorch DG, John JF, Tomlinson JR, Miller KS, Sahn SA. Protected transbronchial needle aspiration and protected specimen brush in the diagnosis of pneumonia. *Am Rev Resp Dis* 1987; 136:565–569.
15. Pang JA, Cheng A, Chan HS, Poon D, French G. The bacteriology of bronchiectasis in Hong Kong investigated by protected catheter brush in bronchoalveolar lavage. *Am Rev Resp Dis* 1989;139:14–17.
16. Winterbauer RH, Bass JB. Controversies in pulmonary medicine. Fiberoptic bronchoscopy with protected brush catheterization should be used for the specific diagnosis of nosocomial pneumonia. *Am Rev Resp Dis* 1988;138:1072–1074.
17. Ortqvist A, Kalin M, Lejdeborn L, Lundberg B. Diagnostic fiberoptic bronchoscopy and protected brush culture in patients with community-acquired pneumonia. *Chest* 1990;97:576–582.
18. Lambert RS, Vereen LE, George RB. Comparison of tracheal spirates and protected brush catheter specimens for identifying pathogenic bacteria in mechanically ventilated patients. *Am J Med Sci* 1989;297:377–382.
19. Chastre J, Lviau F, Brun P, Pierre J, Dauge MC, Bouchama A, Akesbi A, Gibert C. Perspective evaluation of the protected specimen brush for the diagnosis of pulmonary infections in ventilated patients. *Am Rev Resp Dis* 1984;130:924–929.
20. Villers D, Derriennic M, Raffi F, Germaud P, Baron D, Nicolas F, Courtieu AL. Reliability of the bronchoscopic protected catheter brush in intubated and ventilated patients. *Chest* 1985; 88:527–530.
21. Fagon J, Chastre J, Hance A, Guiguet M, Trouillet J, Domart Y, Pierre J, Gibert C. Detection of nosocomial lung infection in ventilated patients: use of a protected specimen brush and quantitative culture techniques in 147 patients. *Am Rev Resp Dis* 1988;138:110–116.
22. Fagon JY, Chastre J, Domart Y, Trouillet JL, Pierre J, Darne C, Gibert C. Nosocomial pneumonia in patients receiving continuous mechanical ventilation. Prospective analysis of 52 episodes with use of a protected specimen brush and quantitative culture techniques. *Am Rev Resp Dis* 1989;139:877–884.
23. Torres A, Bellacasa JP, Xaubet A, Gonzalez J, Rodriguez-Roisin R, Jimenez DeAnta MT, Vidal AA. Diagnostic value of quantitative cultures of bronchoalveolar lavage and telescoping plugged catheters in mechanically ventilated patients with bacterial pneumonia. *Am Rev Resp Dis* 1989;140:306–310.
24. Chastre J, Fagon JY, Soler P, Bornet M, Domart Y, Trouillet JL, Gibert C, Hance AJ. Diagnosis of nosocomial bacterial pneumonia in intubated patients undergoing ventilation: comparison of the usefulness of bronchoalveolar lavage and the protected specimen brush. *Am J Med* 1988;85:499–506.
25. Richard C, Pezzano M, Bouhaja B, Rottman E, Rimailho A, Riou B, Auzepy P. Comparison of non-protected lower respiratory tract secretions and protected specimen brush samples in the diagnosis of pneumonia. *Intensive Care Med* 1988; 14:30–33.
26. Torzillo PJ, McWilliam DB, Young IH, Woog RH, Benn R. Use of protected telescoping brush system in the management of bacterial pulmonary infection in intubated patients. *Br J Dis Chest* 1985;79:125–131.
27. Meduri GU, Beals DH, Maiju AG, Baselski V. Protected bronchoalveolar lavage. A new bronchoscopic technique to retrieve uncontaminated distal airway secretions. *Am Rev Resp Dis* 1991;143:855–864.
28. Guerra LF, Baughman RP. Use of bronchoalveolar lavage to diagnose bacterial pneumonia in mechanically ventilated patients. *Crit Care Med* 1990;18:169–173.
29. Pugin J, Auckenthaler R, Delaspre O, van Gessel E, Suter PM. Rapid diagnosis of gram negative pneumonia by assay of endotoxin in bronchoalveolar lavage fluid. *Thorax* 1992;47:547–549.
30. Ainsle GM, Solomon JA, Bateman ED. Lymphocyte and lymphocyte subset numbers in blood and in bronchoalveolar lavage and pleural fluid in various forms of human pulmonary tuberculosis at presentation and during recovery. *Thorax* 1992; 47:513–518.
31. Ozaki T, Nakahira S, Tani K, Ogushi F, Yasuoka S, Ogura T. Differential cell analysis in bronchoalveolar lavage fluid from pulmonary lesions of patients with tuberculosis. *Chest* 1992; 102:54–59.
32. Moersch HJ. Treatment of abscess by bronchoscopy. *Ann Surg* 1931;93:1126–1131.
33. Rowe LD, Keane WM, Jafek BW, Atkins JP Jr. Transbronchial drainage of pulmonary abscesses with the flexible fiberoptic bronchoscope. *Laryngoscope* 1979;89:122–128.
34. Hammer DL, Aranda CP, Galati V, Adams FV. Massive intrabronchial aspiration of contents of pulmonary abscess after fiberoptic bronchoscopy. *Chest* 1978;74:306–307.
35. Sosenko A, Glassroth J. Fiberoptic bronchoscopy in the evaluation of lung abscesses. *Chest* 1985;84:489–494.
36. Danek SJ, Bower JS. Diagnosis of pulmonary tuberculosis by flexible fiberoptic bronchoscopy. *Am Rev Resp Dis* 1979; 119:677–679.
37. Wongthim S, Udompanich V, Linthongkul S, Sharoenlap P, Nuchprayoon C. Fiberoptic bronchoscopy in diagnosis of patients with suspected active pulmonary tuberculosis. *J Med Assoc Thailand* 1989;72:154–159.
38. Baughman RP, et al. Bronchoscopy with bronchoalveolar lavage in tuberculosis and fungal infections. *Chest* 1991; 99:92–97.
39. Funahashi A, Lohaus GH, Politis J, Hranicka LJ. Role of fiberoptic bronchoscopy in the diagnosis of mycobacterial diseases. *Thorax* 1983;38:267–270.

40. Russell MD, Torrington KG, Tenholder MF. A ten-year experience with fiberoptic bronchoscopy for micobacterial isolation. *Am Rev Resp Dis* 1986;133:1069–1071.
41. Chawla R, Pant K, Jaggi OP, Chandrashekhar S, Thukral SS. Fiberoptic bronchoscopy in smear-negative pulmonary tuberculosis. *Eur Resp J* 1988;1:804–806.
42. Willcox PA, Benatar SR, Potgieter PD. Use of the flexible fiberoptic bronchoscope in diagnosis of sputum-negative pulmonary tuberculosis. *Thorax* 1982;37:598–601.
43. Ip M, Chau PY, So SY, Lam WK. The value of routine bronchial aspirate culture at fibreoptic bronchoscopy for the diagnosis of tuberculosis. *Tubercle* 1989;70:281–285.
44. Khoo KK, Meadway J. Fibreoptic bronchoscopy in rapid diagnosis of sputum smear negative pulmonary tuberculosis. *Resp Med* 1989;83:335–338.
45. Kvale PA, Johnson MC, Wroblewski DA. Diagnosis of tuberculosis: routine cultures of bronchial washings are not indicated. *Chest* 1979;76:140–142.
46. Jett JR, Cortese DA, Dines DE. The value of bronchoscopy in the diagnosis of micobacterial disease. A five-year experience. *Chest* 1981;80:575–578.
47. So SY, Lam WK, Yu DY. Rapid diagnosis of suspected pulmonary tuberculosis by fiberoptic bronchoscopy. *Tubercle* 1982; 63:195–200.
48. Norrman E, Keistinen T, Uddenfeldt M, Rydstrom PO, Lundgren R. Bronchoalveolar lavage is better than gastric lavage in the diagnosis of pulmonary tuberculosis. *Scand J Infect Dis* 1988;20:77–80.
49. Sarkar SK, Sharma GS, Gupta PR, Sharma RK. Fiberoptic bronchoscopy in the diagnosis of pulmonary tuberculosis. *Tubercle* 1980;61:97–99.
50. Burk JR, Viroslav J, Bynum LJ. Miliary tuberculosis diagnosed by fibreoptic bronchoscopy and transbronchial biopsy. *Tubercle* 1978;59:107–109.
51. Willcox PA, Potgieter PD, Bateman ED, Benatar SR. Rapid diagnosis of sputum-negative miliary tuberculosis using the flexible fiberoptic bronchoscope. *Thorax* 1986;41:681–684.
52. Pant K, Chawla R, Mann PS, Jaggi OP. Fiberoptic bronchoscopy in smear-negative miliary tuberculosis. *Chest* 1989; 95:1151–1152.
53. Rimmer J, Gibson P, Bryant DH. Extension of pulmonary tuberculosis after fibreoptic bronchoscopy. *Tubercle* 1988; 69:57–61.
54. Stenson W, Aranda C, Bevelaque FA. Transbronchial biopsy culture in pulmonary tuberculosis. *Chest* 1983;83:883–884.
55. Palenque E, Amor E, Bernaldo de-Quiros JC. Comparison of bronchial washing, brushing and biopsy for diagnosis of pulmonary tuberculosis. *Eur J Clin Microbiol* 1987;6:191–192.
56. Smith LS, Chillaci RF, Sarlin RF. Endobronchial tuberculosis. *Serial Fiberop Bronchosc Nat Hist* 1987;91:644–647.
57. Albert RK, Petty TL. Endobronchial tuberculosis progressing to bronchial stenosis. Fiberoptic bronchoscopic manifestations. *Chest* 1976;70:537–539.
58. Schwartz MS, Kahlstrom EJ, Hawkins DB. Airway obstruction secondary to tuberculosis lymph node erosion into the tracheal: drainage via bronchoscopy. *Otolaryngol Head Neck Surg* 1988;99:604–606.
59. Chang SC, Lee PY, Perng RP. Clinical role of bronchoscopy in adults with intrathoracic tuberculous lymphadenopathy. *Chest* 1988;93:314–317.
60. Prechter GC, Prakash UBS. Bronchoscopy in the diagnosis of pulmonary histoplasmosis. *Chest* 1989;95:1033–1036.
61. Sobonya RE, Barbee RA, Wiens J, Trego D. Detection of fungi and other pathogens in immunocompromised patients by bronchoalveolar lavage in an area endemic for coccidioidomycosis. *Chest* 1990;97:1349–1355.
62. Wallace JM, Catanzaro A, Moser KM, Harrell JH II. Flexible fiberoptic bronchoscopy for diagnosing pulmonary coccidioidomycosis. *Am Rev Resp Dis* 1981;123:286–290.
63. Onal E, Lopata M, Lourenco RV. Disseminated pulmonary blastomycosis in an immunosuppressed patient. Diagnosis by fiberoptic bronchoscopy. *Am Rev Resp Dis* 1976;113:83–86.
64. Kaufman J. Tracheal blastomycosis. *Chest* 1988;93:424–425.
65. Kahn FW, Jones JM, England DM. The role of bronchoalveolar lavage in the diagnosis of invasive pulmonary aspergillosis. *Am J Clin Pathol* 1986;86:518–523.
66. Albelda SM, Talbot GH, Gerson SL, Miller WT, Cassileth PA. Role of fiberoptic bronchoscopy in the diagnosis of invasive pulmonary aspergillosis in patients with acute leukemia. *Am J Med* 1984;76:1027–1034.
67. Levy H, Horak DA, Tegtmeier BR, Yokota SB, Forman SJ. The value of bronchoalveolar lavage and bronchial washings in the diagnosis of invasive pulmonary aspergillosis. *Resp Med* 1992;86:243–248.
68. Verea-Hernando H, Martin-Egana MT, Montero-Martinez C, Fontan-Bueso J. Bronchoscopy findings in invasive pulmonary aspergillosis. *Thorax* 1989;44:822–823.
69. Edmonds LC, Prakash UBS. A 70-year-old man with lymphoma, neutropenia, and upper airway wheezing. *Chest* 1993; 103:585–587.
70. Hall J, Heimann P, Costa C. Airway obstruction caused by *Aspergillus* tracheobronchitis in an immunocompromised patient. *Crit Care Med* 1990;18:575–576.
71. Hines DW, Haber MH, Yaremko L, Britton C, McLawhon RW, Harris AA. Pseudomembranous tracheobronchitis caused by *Aspergillus*. *Am Rev Resp Dis* 1991;143:1408–1411.
72. Clarke A, Skelton J, Fraser RS. Fungal tracheobronchitis: report of 9 cases and review of the literature. *Medicine* 1991; 70:1–14.
73. Kramer MR, Denning DW, Marshall SE, Ross DJ, Berry G, Lewiston NJ, Stevens DA, Theodore J. Ulcerative tracheobronchitis after lung transplantation: a new form of invasive aspergillosis. *Am Rev Resp Dis* 1991;144:552–556.
74. Berlinger NT, Freeman TJ. Acute airway obstruction due to necrotizing tracheobronchial aspergillosis in immunocompromised patients: a new clinical entity. *Ann Otol Rhinol Laryngol* 1989;98:718–720.
75. Pervez NK, Kleinerman J, Kattan M, Freed JA, Harris MB, Rosen MJ, Schwartz IS. Pseudomembrane necrotizing bronchial *Aspergillus*: a variant of invasive *Aspergillus* in a patient with hemophilia and acquired immune deficiency syndrome. *Am Rev Resp Dis* 1985;131:961–963.
76. Anderson WMcD. Mucoid impaction of upper lobe bronchi in the absence of proximal bronchiectasis. *Chest* 1990; 98:1023–1025.
77. Urschel HC, Paulson DL, Shaw RR. Mucoid impaction of the bronchi. *Ann Thorac Surg* 1966;2:1–16.
78. Muller W, von-der-Hardt H, Rieger CH. Idiopathic and symptomatic plastic bronchitis in childhood. A report of three cases and review of the literature. *Respiration* 1987;52:214–220.
79. Werkhaven J, Holinger LD. Bronchial casts in children. *Ann Otol Rhinol Laryngol* 1987;96:86–92.
80. Bowen A, Oudjhane K, Odagiri K, Liston SL, Cumming WA, Oh KS. Plastic bronchitis: large, branching, mucoid bronchial casts in children. *Am J Roentgenol* 1985;144:371–375.
81. Smith RL, Morelli MJ, Aranda CP. Pulmonary aspergilloma diagnosed by fiberoptic bronchoscopy. *Chest* 1987; 92:948–949.
82. Bigby TD, Serota ML, Tierney LM, Matthay MA. Clinical spectrum of pulmonary mucormycosis. *Chest* 1986; 89:435–439.
83. Benbrow EW, Bonshek RE, Stoddart RW. Endobronchial zygomycosis. *Thorax* 1987;42:553–554.
84. Hansen LA, Prakash UBS, Colby TV. Pulmonary complication in diabetes mellitus. *Mayo Clin Proc* 1989;64:791–799.
85. Williams D, Yungbluth M, Adams G, Glassroth J. The role of fiberoptic bronchoscopy in the evaluation of immunocompromised hosts with diffuse pulmonary infiltrates. *Am Rev Resp Dis* 1985;131:880–885.
86. Xaubert A, Torres A, Marco F, Puig-De-la-Bellacasa J, Faus R, Agusti-Vidal A. Pulmonary infiltrates in immunocompromised patients diagnostic value of telescoping plugged catheter and bronchoalveolar lavage. *Chest* 1989;95:130–135.
87. Stokes DC, Shenep JL, Parham D, Bozeman PM, Marienchek W, Mackert PW. Role of flexible bronchoscopy in the diagnosis of pulmonary infiltrates in pediatric patients with cancer. *J Pediatr* 1989;115:561–567.

88. Schulman LL, Smith CR, Drusin R, Rose EA, Enson Y, Reemtsma K. Utility of airway endoscopy in the diagnosis of respiratory complications of cardiac transplantation. *Chest* 1988;93:960–967.
89. Stahl M, Moulton A, Sears T, Linder J, Marriott SE, Rennard S. The role of surveillance bronchoscopy and bronchoalveolar lavage prior to heart transplantation. *Transpl Proc* 1988; 20(Suppl):747–750.
90. Heurlin N, Lonnqvist D, Tollemar J, Ehrnst A. Fiberoptic bronchoscopy for diagnosis of opportunistic pulmonary infections after bone marrow transplantation. *Scand J Infect Dis* 1989;21:359–366.
91. Ruutu P, Ruutu T, Tukiainen P, Ukkonen P, Hovi T. Cytomegalovirus is frequently isolated on bronchoalveolar lavage fluid of bone marrow transplant recipients without pneumonia. *Ann Intern Med* 1990;112:913–916.
92. McCray PB Jr, Wagener JS, Howe CW. Bronchoscopic diagnosis of cytomegalovirus pneumonia following pediatric bone marrow transplantation. *Am J Pediatr Hematol Oncol* 1986; 8:338–341.
93. Heurlin N, Brattstrom C, Tyden G, Ehrnst A, Andersson J. Cytomegalovirus the predominant cause of pneumonia in renal transplant patients. A two-year study of pneumonia in renal transplant recipients with evaluation of fiberoptic bronchoscopy. *Scand J Infect Dis* 1989;21:245–253.
94. Hedemark-LL, Kronenberg RS, Rasp FL, Simmons RL, Peterson PK. The value of bronchoscopy in establishing the etiology of pneumonia in renal transplant recipients. *Am Rev Resp Dis* 1982;126:981–985.
95. Stover DE, White DA, Romano PA, Gellene RA. Diagnosis of pulmonary disease in acquired immune deficiency syndrome (AIDS). Role of bronchoscopy and bronchoalveolar lavage. *Am Rev Resp Dis* 1984;130:659–662.
96. Broaddus C, Dake MD, Stulbarg MS, Blumenfeld W, Hadley WK, Golden JA, Hopewell PC. Bronchoalveolar lavage and transbronchial biopsy for the diagnosis of pulmonary infections in the acquired immunodeficiency syndrome. *Ann Intern Med* 1985;102:747–752.
97. Metersky ML, Harrell JH II, Moser KM. Lack of utility of bronchial brush biopsy in patients infected with the human immunodeficiency virus. *Chest* 1992;101:680–683.
98. Gal AA, Klatt EC, Koss MN, Strigle SM, Boylen CT. The effectiveness of bronchoscopy in the diagnosis of *Pneumocystis carinii* and cytomegalovirus pulmonary infections in acquired immunodeficiency syndrome. *Arch Pathol Lab Med* 1987; 111:238–241.
99. Pedersen U, Hansen IM, Bottzauw J. The diagnostic role of fiberoptic bronchoscopy in AIDS patients with suspected *Pneumocystis carinii* pneumonia. *Arch Otorhinolaryngol* 1989; 246:362–364.
100. Weldon-Linne CM, Rhone DP, Bourassa R. Bronchoscopy in adults with AIDS: comparative yields of cytology, histology, and culture for diagnosis of infectious agents. *Chest* 1990; 98:24–28.
101. Harcup C, Baier HJ, Pitchenik AE. Evaluation of patients with the acquired immunodeficiency syndrome by fiberoptic bronchoscopy. *Endoscopy* 1985;17:217–220.
102. Mones JM, Saldana MJ, Oldham SA. Diagnosis of *Pneumocystis carinii* pneumonia. Roentgenographic-pathologic correlates based on fiberoptic bronchoscopy specimens from patients with the acquired immunodeficiency syndrome. *Chest* 1986;89:522–526.
103. Gagliardi AJ, Stover DE, Zaman MK: Endobronchial *Pneumocystis carinii* infection in a patient with the acquired immunodeficiency syndrome. *Chest* 1987;91:463–464.
104. Miller RF, Millar AB, Weller IV, Semple SJ. Empirical treatment without bronchoscopy for *Pneumocystis carinii* pneumonia in the acquired immunodeficiency syndrome. *Thorax* 1989; 44:559–564.
105. Lundgren JD, Orholm M, Nielsen TL, Iversen J, Hertz J, Nielsen JO. Bronchoscopy of symptom free patients infected with human immunodeficiency virus for detection of pneumocystosis. *Thorax* 1989;44:68–69.
106. Barnes, et al. Tuberculosis in patients with human immunodeficiency virus infection. How often does it mimic *Pneumocystis carinii* pneumonia. *Chest* 1992;102:428–432.
107. Salzman SH, Schindel ML, Aranda CP, Smith RL, Lewis ML. The role of bronchoscopy in the diagnosis of pulmonary tuberculosis in patients at risk for HIV infection. *Chest* 1992; 102:143–146.
108. Miro AM, Gibilara E, Powell S, Kamholz SL. The role of fiberoptic bronchoscopy for diagnosis of pulmonary tuberculosis in patients at risk for AIDS. *Chest* 1992;101:1211–1214.
109. Packer SJ, Cesario T, Williams JH. *Mycobacterium avium* complex infection presenting as endobronchial lesions in immunosuppressed patients. *Ann Intern Med* 1988;109:389–393.
110. Mehle ME, Adamo JP, Mehta AC, Wiedemann HP, Keys T, Longworth DL. Endobronchial *Mycobacterium avium-intracellulare* infection in a patient with AIDS. *Chest* 1989; 96:119–200.
111. Barrio JL, Harcup C, Baier HJ, Pitchenik AE. Value of repeat fiberoptic bronchoscopies and significance of nondiagnostic bronchoscopic results in patients with acquired immunodeficiency syndrome. *Am Rev Resp Dis* 1987;135:422–425.
112. Garay SM, Belenko M, Fazzini E, Schinella R. Pulmonary manifestations in Kaposi's sarcoma. *Chest* 1987;91:39–43.
113. Zibrak JD, Silvestri RC, Costello P, Marlink R, Jensen WA, Robins A, Rose RM. Bronchoscopic and radiologic features of Kaposi's sarcoma involving the respiratory system. *Chest* 1986;90:476–479.
114. Purdy LJ, Colby TV, Yousem SA, Battifora H. Pulmonary Kaposi's sarcoma. Premortem histologic diagnosis. *Am J Surg Pathol* 1986;10:301–311.
115. Fouret PJ, Touboul JL, Mayaud CM, Akoun GM, Roland J. Pulmonary Kaposi's sarcoma in patients with acquired immunodeficiency syndrome: a clinicopathologic study. *Thorax* 1987;42:262–265.
116. Hanson PJV, Harcourt-Webster JN, Gazzard BG, Collins JV. Fiberoptic bronchoscopy in diagnosis of bronchopulmonary Kaposi's sarcoma. *Thorax* 1987;42:269–272.
117. St John RC, Pacht ER. Tracheal stenosis and failure to wean from mechanical ventilation due to herpetic tracheitis. *Chest* 1990;98:1520–1522.
118. Sherry MK, Klainer AS, Wolff M, Gerhard H. Herpetic tracheobronchitis. *Ann Intern Med* 1988;109:229–233.
119. Bedrossian CW, De Arce EA, Bedrossian UK, Kelly LV. Herpetic tracheobronchitis detected at bronchoscopy: cytologic diagnosis by the immunoperoxidase method. *Diag Cytopathol* 1985;1:292–299.
120. George RB, Jenkinson SG, Light RW. Fiberoptic bronchoscopy in the diagnosis of pulmonary fungal and nocardial infarctions. *Chest* 1978;73:33–36.
121. Sakowitz AJ, Sakowitz BH. Disseminated cryptococcosis. Diagnosis by fiberoptic bronchoscopy and biopsy. *JAMA* 1976; 236:2429–2430.
122. Malabonga VM, Basti J, Kamholz SL. Utility of bronchoscopic sampling techniques in cryptococcal disease in AIDS. *Chest* 1991;99:370–372.
123. Wheeler WB, Kurachek SC, Lobas JG, Einzig MJ. Acute hypoxemic respiratory failure caused by *Chlamydia trachomatis* and diagnosed by flexible bronchoscopy. *Am Rev Resp Dis* 1990;142:471–473.
124. Williams J, Nunley D, Dralle W, Berk SL, Verghese A. Diagnosis of pulmonary strongyloidosis by bronchoalveolar lavage. *Chest* 1988;94:643–644.
125. Shimazu C, Pien FD, Parnell D. Bronchoscopic diagnosis of *Schistosoma japonicum* in apt with hemoptysis. *Resp Med* 1991;85:331–332.
126. Lau K-Y. Endobronchial actinomycosis mimicking pulmonary neoplasm. *Thorax* 1992;47:664–665.
127. Ariel I, Breuer R, Kamal N, Ben-Dov I, Mogle P, Rosenmann E. Endobronchial actinomycosis simulating bronchogenic carcinoma. Diagnosis by bronchial biopsy. *Chest* 1991; 99:493–495.
128. Roig J, Romeu J, Riera C, Texido A, Domingo C, Morera J. Acute eosinophilic pneumonia due toxocariasis with bronchoalveolar lavage findings. *Chest* 1992;102:294–296.
129. Suratt PM, Gruber B, Wellons HA, Wenzel RP. Absence of

clinical pneumonia following bronchoscopy with contaminated and clean bronchofiberscopes. *Chest* 1977;71:52–54.
130. Pereira W, Kovnat DM, Khan MA, Iacovino JR, Spivack ML. Snider GL. Fever and pneumonia after flexible fiberoptic bronchoscopy. *Am Rev Resp Dis* 1975;112:59–64.
131. Kane RC, Cohen MH, Fossieck BE Jr. Tvardzik AV. Absence of bacteremia after fiberoptic bronchoscopy. *Am Rev Resp Dis* 1975;111:102–104.
132. Etzkorn ET, McAllister CK. Bacteremic pneumonia after fiberoptic bronchoscopy. *Milit Med* 1987;152:263–264.
133. Richardson AJ, Rothburn MM, Roberts C. Pseudo-outbreak of *Bacillus* species: related to fiberoptic bronchoscopy (letter). *J Hosp Infect* 1986;7:208–210.
134. Smith RP, Sahetya GK, Baltch AL, OHern J, Gort D. Bacteremia associated with fiberoptic bronchoscopy. *NY State J Med* 1983;83:1045–1047.
135. Pedro-Botet ML, Ruiz J, Sabria M, Roig J, Abad J, Carrasco I, Manterolas JM. Bacteremia after fibrobronchoscopy. Prospective study. *Enferm Infecc Microbiol Clin* 1991;9:159–161.
136. Timms RM, Harrell JH. Bacteremia related to fiberoptic bronchoscopy. A case report. *Am Rev Resp Dis* 1975;111:555–557.
137. Alexander WJ, Baker GL, Hunker FD. Bacteremia and meningitis following fiberoptic bronchoscopy. *Arch Intern Med* 1979; 139:580–583.
138. Boisjoly HM, Jotterand VH, Bazin R, Bergerson MG. Metastatic *Pseudomonas* endophthalmitis following bronchoscopy. *Can J Ophthalmol* 1987;22:378–380.
139. Beyt BE Jr. King DK, Glew RH. Fatal pneumonitis and septicemia after fiberoptic bronchoscopy. *Chest* 1977;72:105–107.
140. Robbins H, Goldman AL. Failure of a "prophylactic" antimicrobial drug to prevent sepsis after fiberoptic bronchoscopy. *Am Rev Resp Dis* 1977;116:325–326.
141. Nelson KE. Larson PA, Schraufnagel DE, Jackson J. Transmission of tuberculosis by flexible fiberbronchoscopes. *Am Rev Resp Dis* 1983;127:97–100.
142. Hsu JT, Barrett CR Jr. Lung abscess complicating transbronchial biopsy of a mass lesion. *Chest* 1981;80:230–232.
143. Muers M, Lane D. Acute pneumonia and pneumothorax as a complication of transbronchial biopsy. *Endoscopy* 1980; 12:183–187.
144. Wheeler PW, Lancaster D, Kaiser AB. Bronchopulmonary cross-colonization and infection related to mycobacterial contamination of suction valves of bronchoscopes. *J Infect Dis* 1989;159:954–958.
145. Siegman-Igra Y, Inbar G, Campus A. An "outbreak" of pulmonary pseudoinfection by *Serratia marcescens*. *J Hosp Infect* 1985;6:218–220.
146. Sammartino MT, Israel RH, Magnussen CR. *Pseudomonas aeruginosa* contamination of fibreoptic bronchoscopes. *J Hosp Infect* 1982;3:65–71.
147. Goldstein B, Abrutyn E. Pseudo-outbreak of *Bacillus* species: related to fibreoptic bronchoscopy. *J Hosp Infect* 1985; 6:194–200.
148. Weinstein HJ, Bone RC, Ruth WE. Contamination of a fiberoptic bronchoscope with *Proteus* species. *Am Rev Resp Dis* 1977; 116:541–543.
149. Steere AC, Corrales J, von-Graevenitz A. A cluster of *Mycobacterium gordonae* isolates from bronchoscopy specimens. *Am Rev Resp Dis* 1979;120:214–216.
150. Schleupner CJ, Hamilton JR. A pseudoepidemic of pulmonary fungal infections related to fiberoptic bronchoscopy. *Infect Control* 1980;1:38–42.
151. Hoffmann KK, Weber DJ, Rutala WA. *Rhodotorula rubra* in patients undergoing fiberoptic bronchoscopy. *Infect Control Hosp Epidemiol* 1989;10:511–514.
152. Gubler JGH, Slafinger M, von Graevenitz A. Pseudoepidemic of nontuberculous mycobacteria due to a contaminated bronchoscope cleaning machine. Report of an outbreak and review of literature. *Chest* 1992;101:1245–1249.
153. Fraser VJ, Jones M, Murray PR, Medoff G, Zhang Y, Wallace RJ Jr. Contamination of flexible fiberoptic bronchoscopes with *Mycobacterium chelonae* linked to an automated bronchoscope disinfection machine. *Am Rev Resp Dis* 1992; 145:853–55.
154. Kato H, Matsushima S, Smyth JP. Effect of disinfectants with and without usage of detergent for the flexible fiberoptic bronchoscope. *Jap J Exp Med* 1979;49:337–342.
155. Dawson DJ, Armstrong JG, Blacklock ZM. Mycobacterial cross-contamination of bronchoscopy specimens. *Am Rev Resp Dis* 1982;126:1095–1097.
156. Leers WD. Disinfecting endoscopes: how not to transmit *Mycobacterium tuberculosis* by bronchoscopy. *Can Med Assoc J* 1980;123:275–280.
157. Hanson PJV, Gor D, Clarke JR, Chadwick MV, Gazzrd B, Jeffries DJ, Gaya H, Collins JV. Recovery of the human immunodeficiency virus from fibreoptic bronchoscopes. *Thorax* 1991;46:410–412.
158. Hanson PJ, Collins JV. AIDS and the lung. 1. AIDS, aprons, and elbow grease: preventing the nosocomial spread of human immunodeficiency virus and associated organisms. *Thorax* 1989;44:778–783.
159. Hanson PJ, Jeffries DJ, Batten JC, Collins JV. Infection control revisited: dilemma facing today's bronchoscopists. *Br Med J* 1988;297:185–187.
160. Prakash UBS. Does the bronchoscope propagate infection? *Chest* 1993;104:552–559.
161. Schafers HJ, Haverich A, Wagner TO, Wohlers T, Alken A, Borst HG. Decreased incidence of bronchial complications following lung transplantation. *Eur J Cardiothorac Surg* 1992; 64:174–178.
162. Novick RJ, Ahmad D, Menkis AH, Reid KR, Pflugfelder PW, Kostuk WJ, McKenzie FN. The importance of acquired diffuse bronchomalacia in heart-lung transplant recipients with obliterative bronchiolitis. *J Thorac Cardiovasc Surg* 1991; 101:643–648.
163. Smyth RL, Scott JP, McGoldrick J, Wallwork J, Higenbottam T. Successful use of repeated transbronchial lung biopsies in a patient with multiple opportunistic infections. *Resp Med* 1989; 83:505–507.
164. Walts AE, Marchevsky AM, Morgan M. Pulmonary cytology in lung transplant recipients: recent trends in laboratory utilization. *Diag Cytopathol* 1991;7:353–358.
165. Scott JP, Fradet G, Smyth RL, Mullins P, Pratt A, Clelland CA, Higenbottam T, Wallwork J. Prospective study of transbronchial biopsies in the management of heart–lung and single lung transplant patients. *J Heart Lung Transpl* 1991; 10:626–636; discussion 636–637.
166. Trulock EP, Ettinger NA, Brunt EM, Pasque M, Kaiser L, Cooper J. The role of transbronchial lung biopsy in the treatment of lung transplant recipients. *Chest* 1992;102:1049–1054.
167. al-Majed S, al-Kassimi F, Ashour M, Mekki MO, Sadiq S. Removal of endobronchial mucormycosis lesion through a rigid bronchoscope. *Thorax* 1992;47:203–204.
168. McCubbin MM, Trigg ME, Hendricker CM, Wagener JS. Bronchoscopy with bronchoalveolar lavage in the evaluation of pulmonary complications of bone marrow transplantation in children. *Pediatr Pulmonol* 1992;12:43–47.
169. Meduri GU, Wunderink RG, Leeper KV, Beals DH. Management of bacterial pneumonia in ventilated patients. Protected bronchoalveolar lavage as a diagnostic tool. *Chest* 1992; 101:500–508.
170. Brown RB, Johnson JH, Kessinger JM, Sealy WC. Bronchovascular mucormycosis in the diabetic: an urgent surgical problem. *Ann Thorac Surg* 1992;53:854–855.
171. Frye MD, Seifer FD. An outbreak of blastomycosis in eastern Tennessee. *Mycopathologia* 1991;116:15–21.
172. Colt HG, Morris JF, Marston BJ, Sewell DL. Necrotizing tracheitis caused by *Corynebacterium pseudodiphtheriticum*: unique case and review. *Rev Infect Dis* 1991;13:73–76.
173. Meduri GU, Stover DE, Greeno RA, Nash T, Zaman MB. Bilateral bronchoalveolar lavage in the diagnosis of opportunistic pulmonary infections. *Chest* 1991;100:1272–1276.

Bronchoscopy,
edited by U. B. S. Prakash.
Mayo Foundation © 1994.
Published by Raven Press, Ltd., New York.

CHAPTER 15

Bronchoscopic Localization and Therapy of Occult Lung Cancer

Eric S. Edell and Denis A. Cortese

Lung cancer is currently the leading cause of cancer-related death in the United States (1). The overall therapeutic results have changed very little in the past decade in the face of an increasing incidence of this disease throughout the world. At diagnosis, most patients are found to have advanced disease and treatment of this population is disappointing, often only palliative. Several studies, however, have demonstrated that early detection, localization, and aggressive treatment of intrabronchial or preinvasive stages of lung cancer results in 5-year survival rates of 70–80% (2–4). The chest roentgenogram and sputum cytology tests are currently the only simple means available for detection of early asymptomatic lung cancer. In one study, 75% of patients with normal roentgenograms and abnormal sputum cytology tests had squamous cell cancer that was either in situ or early invasive (2). Detection at such an early stage should provide the best opportunity for long-term survival.

Once detected, localization of lung cancer at its earliest stage can generally be accomplished by direct visualization of the tracheobronchial tree using the flexible bronchoscope. Prior to the introduction of the flexible bronchoscope, by Ikeda in 1969, access to the tracheobronchial tree was limited to the proximal large airways (5). The flexible bronchoscope provides an avenue for inspection of peripheral airways including those of the upper lobes. Central carcinoma of the tracheobronchial tree can generally be localized after a single inspection with the flexible bronchoscope. Occasionally, localization of very early stage cancer can be difficult because it may not produce visibly detectable gross mucosal abnormalities. Such bronchoscopically occult carcinomas may require repeated examinations over many months before localization is accomplished.

Fluorescent compounds such as hematoporphyrin derivative (HpD) and dihematoporphyrin ether (DHE) have been shown to act as cancer tags (6). These compounds are retained in malignant tissue at higher concentrations than in normal tissue and emit a characteristic salmon red fluorescence when exposed to light of the proper wavelength (7). The fluorescent property of these compounds has been applied to the tracheobronchial tree as an aid in early localization of squamous cell carcinoma (8–10). More recently, spectral differences in autofluorescence of normal and cancerous tissue are being evaluated as an aid to localization (11,12).

Therapeutic options for early squamous cell carcinoma have traditionally been limited to surgical resection. The introduction of phototherapy provided a new therapeutic alternative to surgery (13,14). This form of therapy may be particularly helpful since patients with bronchogenic carcinoma are at risk for the development of a subsequent primary lung cancer. Any therapy that preserves lung parenchyma would be of benefit in the long-term management of these patients. The following is a brief discussion of the role of phototherapy using HpD or DHE in the bronchoscopic localization and treatment of occult lung cancer.

BRONCHOSCOPIC LOCALIZATION

Roentgenographically occult lung cancer is detected by sputum cytology. When a test is suspicious or positive, confirmation by two additional 3-day pooled collections of sputum is desirable. Once a roentgenographically occult cancer is strongly suspected, localization becomes the next challenge. Oral, pharyngeal, and laryngeal sources for neoplastic cells must

E. S. Edell: Division of Thoracic Diseases and Internal Medicine, Mayo Clinic, Rochester, Minnesota 55905.

D. A. Cortese: Division of Thoracic Diseases and Internal Medicine, Mayo Clinic, Jacksonville, Florida 32224.

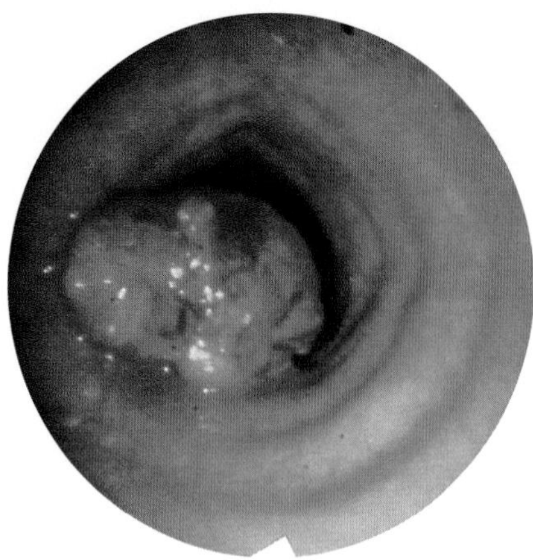

FIG. 1. Bronchogenic carcinoma causing obstruction of the midtrachea.

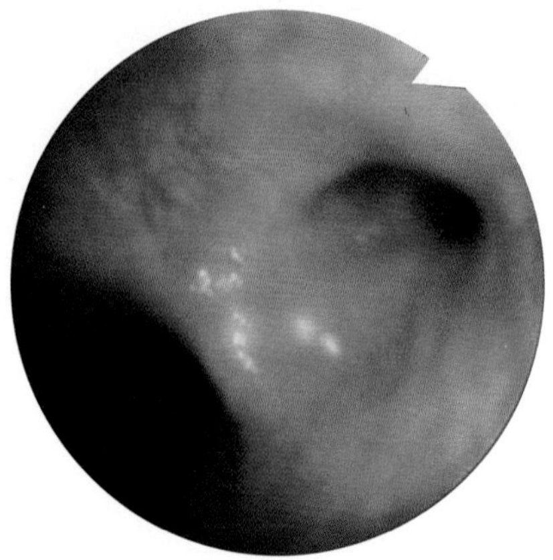

FIG. 2. Superficial squamous cell carcinoma involving right upper lobe spur.

be excluded by a thorough examination. The finding of a tumor in one of these sites, however, should not preclude a search elsewhere since this population of patients has a 7% rate of simultaneous cancers of the respiratory tract (15). After a thorough inspection of the upper airway, flexible bronchoscopy is required for localization of bronchogenic cancer. Over half of the roentgenographically occult cancers will be grossly visible at the first bronchoscopic inspection. The cancers range in appearance from obvious endobronchial masses (Fig. 1) to subtle mucosal irregularities (Figs. 2 and 3). Topical anesthesia is generally adequate for recognition and biopsy confirmation of these obvious carcinomas.

A more detailed and careful bronchoscopic examination under general anesthesia is necessary in the other half of patients in whom the cancer is not obviously visible. This allows the bronchoscopist time to inspect the mucosal surfaces for signs of early cancer, such as thickening, irregularity, erythema, or pallor. Ideally, all patients should discontinue smoking and have bronchitis treated with antibiotics and bronchodilator prior to bronchoscopic inspection to facilitate recognition of subtle mucosal changes. General anesthesia is used because it allows complete relaxation and control of respiration for the entire duration of the procedure.

The larynx and subglottic trachea should be carefully visualized before intubation since an endotracheal tube may obscure a small tumor in the upper trachea. Thorough inspection of the tracheobronchial tree is completed before any sampling begins. Multiple sheathed cytology brushes, preferably with bristles of 3–5 mm

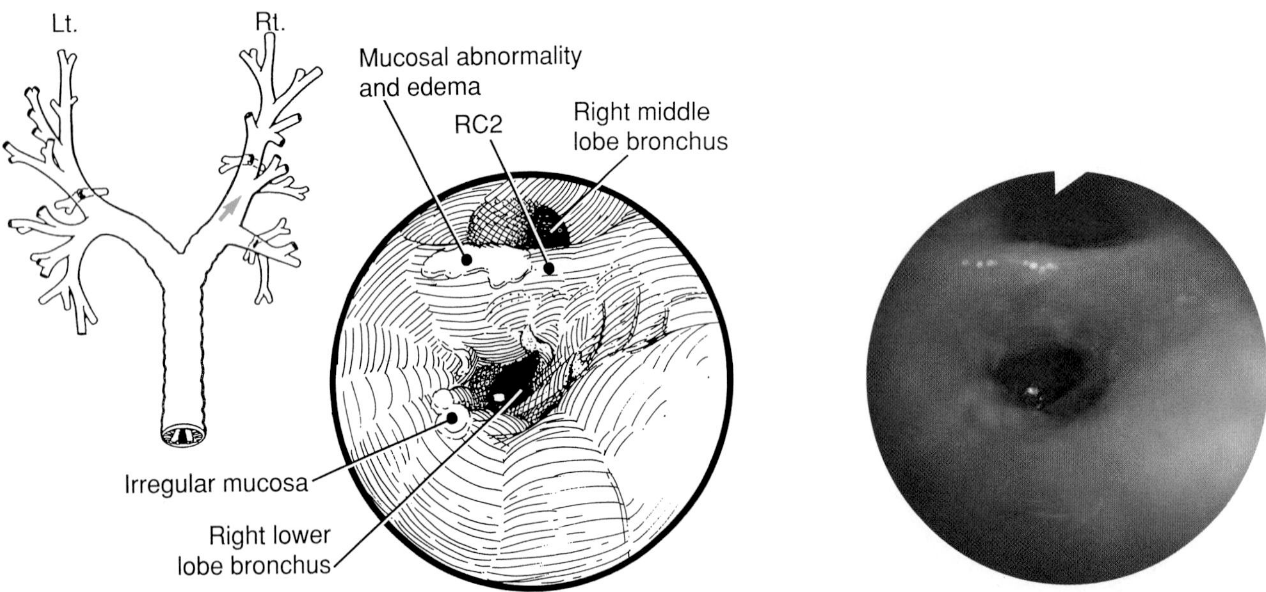

FIG. 3. Early squamous cell carcinoma involving RC2 carina and right lower lobe bronchus.

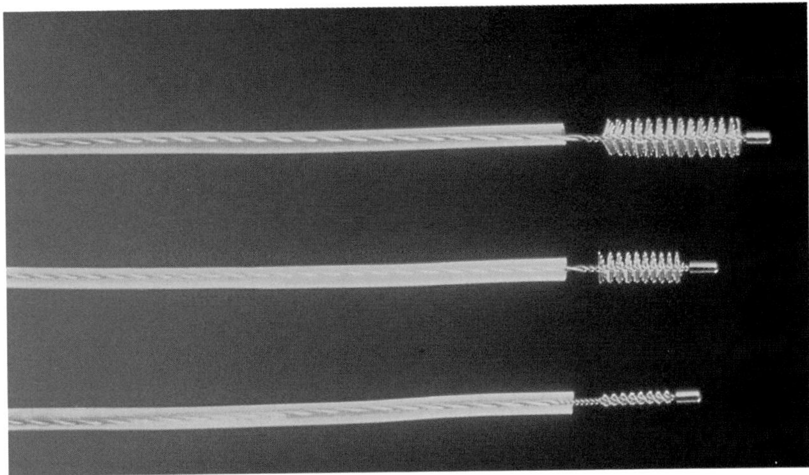

FIG. 4. Various sheathed cytology brushes used for selective specimen retrieval.

in diameter, are used for sampling each segmental and subsegmental bronchus (Fig. 4). Care should be taken to avoid withdrawing the brushes through the working channel of the bronchoscope. To avoid contamination, the working channel should be lavaged between each brushing. An assistant should prepare the bronchial brushing slide to make certain that all specimens are accurately labeled. Once brushings are collected, multiple biopsies from various sites are obtained. Localization is confirmed if at subsequent bronchoscopic examination, i.e., 1–2 weeks later, a brush from the same region is again positive for carcinoma. Rarely, the sequence described above also fails to confirm localization sufficiently to determine therapeutic options. Problems in localization of these early cancers are most often encountered when the cancer is either in situ or an early invasive squamous cell carcinoma. It may take several months with repeated bronchoscopic examinations before localization is accomplished.

To facilitate localization of bronchoscopically occult cancers, many chemicals have been evaluated as potential tumor markers including eosin, berberine sulfate, fluorescein, tetracycline, acridine orange, hematoporphyrin, and HpD. HpD, and more recently DHE, have received the most attention as compounds that are preferentially concentrated by malignant cells (6). Both compounds absorb light from the ultraviolet to the visible red region of the spectrum; however, the greatest absorption occurs around 405 nm (Figure 5). When exposed to light irradiation in this region. HpD and DHE are excited to a singlet state. Spontaneous decay results in the production of a characteristic red fluorescence whose wavelength is approximately 630 to 690 nm. Detection of the fluorescent light has been used to aid in the localization of some early carcinomas.[16,17] HpD and DHE are given intravenously at a dose of 2.5 mg/kg, 48 to 72 hours prior to bronchoscopy. Inspection of the tracheobronchial tree for occult

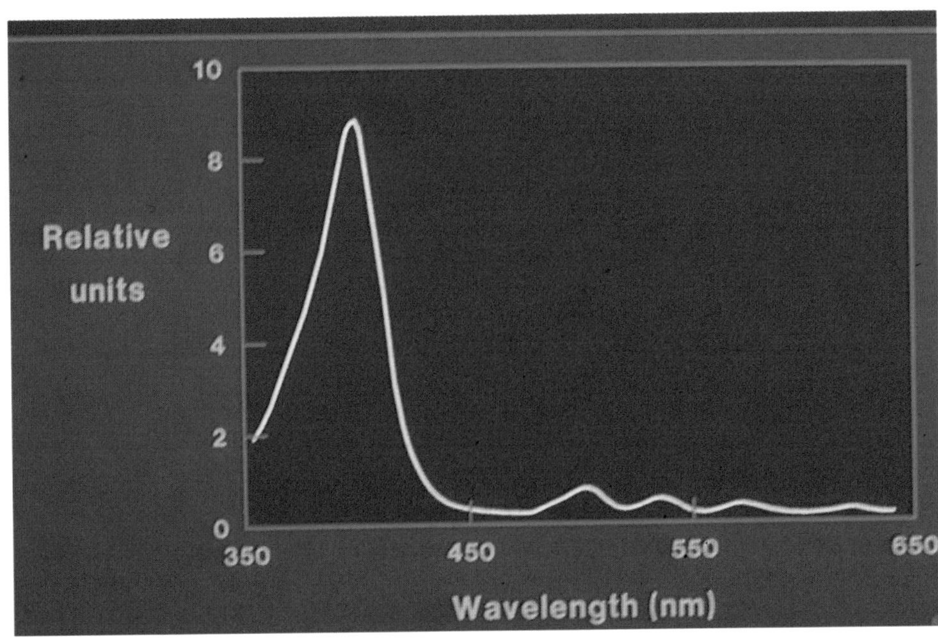

FIG. 5. Absorption spectrum of hematoporphyrin derivative.

cancer is then undertaken. However, in a situation of small superficial carcinomas of the tracheobronchial tree, HpD fluorescence is not consistently and reliably seen with conventional flexible bronchoscopes for several reasons; the small tumor size, the small quantity of chemical concentrated in the tumor, low fluorescence yield, and optical losses in the fiberoptic bundles. Special instrumentation has been developed to overcome the technical problems of fluorescence detection, and has resulted in the development of various detection systems.[9,16,18,19] Each system relies on amplification of a fluorescent signal which is then displayed as either an audio signal or visual image. The overall experience using these detection systems is that these compounds may be helpful in localization of tumors that are both roentgenographically and bronchoscopically occult. Fluorescence detection is, however, not specific for carcinoma. Areas of cellular atypia ranging from moderate to marked degrees have also been sites of low levels of fluorescence. Therefore, the bronchoscopist must rely on diagnostic biopsy material to confirm the presence of a cancer.

The flexible bronchoscopic detection system developed at Mayo Clinic, has been described in detail elsewhere.[9] In this system, a double lumen bronchoscope is used (Fig. 6). A fiberoptic detector guide that transmits fluorescence from the target region to a photomultiplier is placed in one lumen. The viewing and illumination guides are within the existing compounds of the bronchoscope. Alternate pulses of violet excitation light and unfiltered white light are transmitted to the target region via the illumination guide. The composite nature of the illumination light is provided by an electronically driven, constant-speed chopper wheel that alternates a clear aperture and a narrow band optical interference filter in a light beam produced by a 200-W, short arc mercury lamp. The chopper also alternately shutters and unshutters the face of the photomultiplier so that it can receive an incoming optical signal only when the violet excitation light has fallen on the target. The chopping rate is approximately 30 cycles/sec, and at this rate "flicker" does not disturb concurrent visual examination. A lock-in amplifier enhances the fluorescence signal. The output from the lock-in amplifier generates a frequency-modulated audio signal that indicates the amount of fluorescence emanating from a visual field. The audio pitch produced by this system is directly proportionate to the intensity of the fluorescence detected by the photomultiplier. This system therefore allows a bronchoscopist to perform routine flexible bronchoscopy while simultaneously searching for HpD fluorescence. The bronchoscopist does not actually see the fluorescence within the visual field. In this way, the fluorescence is used as a marker to attract the attention of the bronchoscopist to certain areas of the tracheobronchial tree where brushings and biopsies should be obtained.

A second detection system, developed by Doiran and Profio at the University of Southern California, Santa Barbara, consists of a flexible bronchoscope, an image intensifier, and a laser light source for excitation of HpD (10,18,19). The violet light is conducted via a small quartz fiber inserted through the channel of the bronchoscope. An image intensifier, which amplifies illumination more than 30,000 times, is attached to the eyepiece of the flexible bronchoscope. A krypton ion laser beam is then transmitted through a 400-μm quartz fiber inserted through the instrumentation channel or

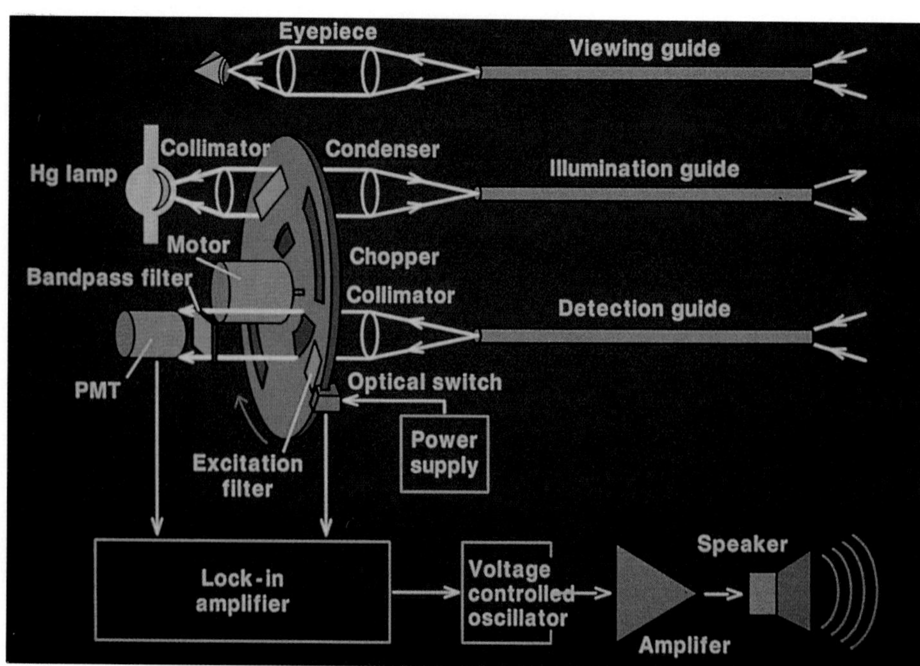

FIG. 6. Schematic design of the fluorescent detection system used at the Mayo Clinic. From Progress in Clinical Cancer, vol VIII, Grune & Stratton, 1982, page 200, with permission (fig 2).

via the fiber bundle of the bronchoscope. Fluorescence is displayed via the image intensifier on a cathode ray tube screen, where it appears as a white image on a green background. To make visible bronchoscopic examination more efficient, a flip-flop light source was developed to permit quick switching between white light and violet light illumination. To aid in localization and quantification of fluorescence, a nonimaging fluorometer probe was developed (10). The energy emitted from a tumor is picked up by the probe, split, passed through red and green filters, and then ratioed to make the signal strength independent of the distance and angle from the tumor. The autofluorescence of normal bronchial mucosa has a peak at approximately 580 nm wavelength while HpD fluorescence is longer than 630 nm. The bronchoscopic fluorescent spectroscope enables distinction between autofluorescence of normal bronchial mucosa and fluorescence of HpD. An audio signal is build in to herald red–green ratios that are above the background autofluorescence signal. The red–green ratio is directly proportional to the intensity of HpD fluorescence.

A third system, developed at the Tokyo Medical College, allows for direct viewing employing ultrasensitive solid state video cameras (16,17). This system is designed to display the wave pattern of light detected in order to distinguish between the fluorescence emitted by HpD and that of autofluorescence of the normal bronchial mucosa. A krypton ion laser is the light source for the excitation of HpD, and a white light is used for bronchoscopic observation. A 400-μm quartz fiber transmits light from both sources. A light transmission apparatus is designed to allow the operator to mechanically alternate between white light for bronchoscopic observation and laser light for excitation of HpD by operating a foot switch. The quartz fiberoptic guide is an integral part of a specially designed flexible bronchoscope. Fluorescence is transmitted through the bronchoscope's image guide and then separated by a half mirror for simultaneous observations and fluorescence spectroscopy analysis. This system can measure the intensity of fluorescence, which correlates with the quantity of HpD.

Clinical application of these fluorescence detection systems has resulted in the localization of bronchoscopically occult squamous cell carcinomas in a small, select population of patients. From 1978 to 1984, 16 patients were referred to the Mayo Clinic for localization of bronchoscopically and radiographically occult lung cancers. These patients were specifically referred for HpD fluorescence bronchoscopy because previous bronchoscopies were unsuccessful in localizing the tumor. Each of the 16 patients had sputum cytology that demonstrated squamous cell carcinoma. In these 16 patients, a total of 19 cancers were localized bronchoscopically (17). In five patients, the tumor was visible at the time of bronchoscopy. In each case, the cancer demonstrated HpD fluorescence and the biopsy from each site was positive for squamous cell carcinoma. In three patients, the cancer proved to be beyond the reach of the bronchoscope. In two of these patients, the fluorescent examination was negative. In one patient, low-level tissue fluorescence was detected over the orifice of the lingula. Biopsy from this site revealed moderate and marked squamous atypia. Brushings from the periphery of the lingula demonstrated squamous cell carcinoma and at resection the cancer was found to be beyond the reach of the flexible bronchoscope. Eleven cancers were localized in a central location, within the reach of the flexible bronchoscope, but were not visible at the time of bronchoscopy. In ten cancers, HpD fluorescence was detected, and in nine of these, biopsies were diagnostic of squamous cell carcinoma. In the tenth, however, the biopsy was negative for cancer but a biopsy obtained from the same site 2 months later was diagnostic for squamous cell carcinoma. In the eleventh cancer, a biopsy from the stump of a previous resection showed squamous cell carcinoma. This area showed no fluorescence at examination. This represents the only false-negative fluorescence examination noted in this group. Nine other patients were referred for fluorescence bronchoscopy during this period. Sputum cytology had demonstrated moderate and marked degrees of cellular atypia on repeated occasions. Fluorescence examination invariably revealed several sites of low-level HpD fluorescence. Biopsies from these sites were consistently interpreted as showing moderate and marked degrees of squamous atypia, but in no case was a squamous cell carcinoma found.

Other institutions have had similar results. Tissue fluorescence was noted in a wide range of tumors of the tracheobronchial tree including advanced carcinomas, early bronchoscopically occult carcinomas, and areas of cellular atypia (17,18). It is therefore imperative that the bronchoscopist rely only on biopsy tissue for diagnostic proof of the presence of cancer.

BRONCHOSCOPIC TREATMENT OF OCCULT PRIMARY BRONCHOGENIC CARCINOMA

Traditional management of early lung cancer has consisted of surgical resection of the involved region. Unfortunately, this results in the loss of functional pulmonary parenchyma. Studies have also shown that patients found to have squamous cell carcinoma are at risk of developing a second primary cancer at an annual rate of 5% per year (2,4). A method of treatment that is both safe and preserves functional lung parenchyma is therefore desirable. HpD and DHE not only produce fluorescence when exposed to the light of the proper wavelength but also mediate photodynamic chemical reactions that lead to cellular death through the production of toxic radicals including singlet oxygen and the hydroxyl ion (20). Experimental studies have shown that the photodynamic effect of these compounds may be useful in the treatment of small superficial cancers (21).

HpD was first used in the photodynamic treatment of lung cancer in 1980 (13). Subsequently, more than 200 patients with malignancies of the tracheobronchial tree have been treated with photodynamic therapy worldwide. Reports have demonstrated at least a 50% complete response in tumors that measured less than 3 cm^2 in the largest surface area (14,22,23). Between December 1980 and December 1990, 60 patients with 65 carcinomas were treated at the Mayo Clinic. The initial experience involved both early superficial carcinomas and large obstructive carcinomas of the tracheobronchial tree (14). Results have been categorized according to the therapeutic response after photodynamic therapy, the subsequent behavior of tumor growth, the long-term results, and the current status of each patient as of December 1990. Twenty-nine patients (with 31 carcinomas) demonstrated a complete response, defined as no evidence of carcinoma on follow-up bronchoscopy that included brushings, washings, and biopsy. An example is shown in Fig. 15–7. Twenty-three of these cancers had a complete response after a single course of treatment. Eight required a second treatment to achieve a complete response. Twenty-three cancers showed no local recurrence after follow-up periods that range from 4 to 63 months (means 28 months). Nineteen patients were alive at last follow-up. Fourteen of these demonstrated no local recurrence with follow-up ranging from 4 to 59 months (means 24 months). Two patients demonstrated local recurrence at 8 and 9 months, respectively. The first had a complete response to a second treatment, and the second demonstrated complete response after a third treatment. One patient had local recurrence at 46 months after treatment. Two patients have had local recurrence at 12 months; one received radiation therapy and the second underwent a completion pneumonectomy that on pathological analysis revealed no nodal involvement. Thirty-four cancers treated with photodynamic therapy showed evidence of persistent tumor on follow-up evaluation. In this group, eight patients remain alive, six with no evidence of cancer whose follow-up ranges from 10 to 93 months. Of this group of eight patients, each received additional combined therapy that included photodynamic therapy, external beam radiation, intraluminal radiation, and/or surgical resection of persistent disease.

The Tokyo Medical College group had similar results. Over 127 patients with lung cancer have been treated with photodynamic therapy since 1980. In their group, 30 patients had 31 cancers that were felt bronchoscopically to be early superficially squamous cancers. Treatment with photodynamic therapy resulted in a complete remission in 20 of these lesions (22). Kato et al. recently reported 5-year disease-free survival of a patient who was treated only by photodynamic therapy (24). At the Mayo Clinic, there is also one patient who has survived 5 years and several other patients who are beyond 4 years with no evidence of local recurrence after treatment with photodynamic therapy alone. Photodynamic therapy was recently reported as an alternative to surgical resection in early superficial squamous cell carcinoma (25). In this study, 12 patients had a complete response (93%) to treatment.

Complications from photodynamic therapy are relatively infrequent for occult lung cancer. Several patients have experienced a sunburn involving the face and/or hands. This occurred despite explicit instructions to avoid exposure to sunlight for up to 4 weeks after HpD phototherapy. Four patients from the Mayo Clinic series developed cough productive of blood-

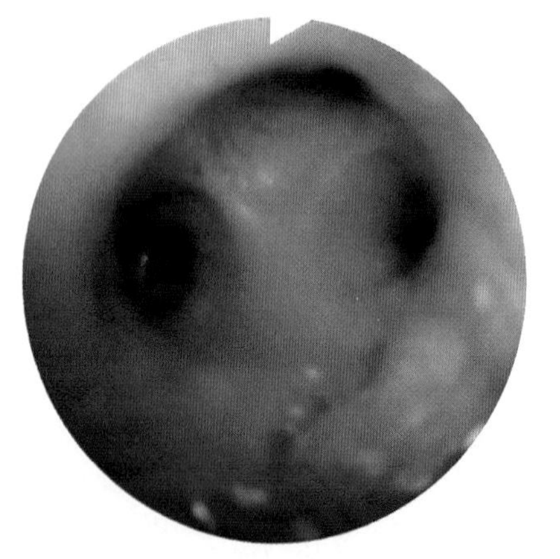

A

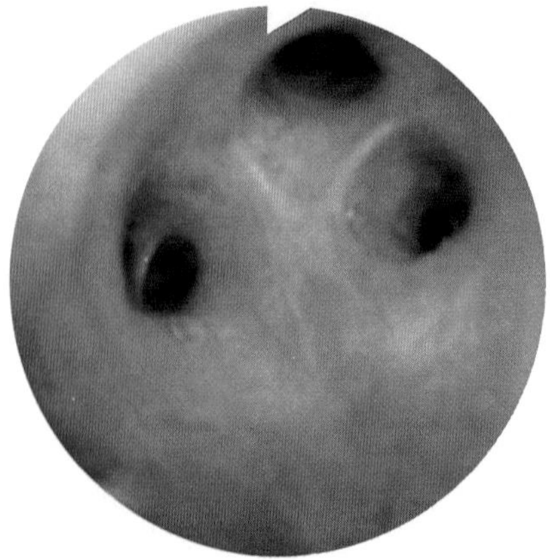

B

FIG. 7. Superficial squamous cell carcinoma before **(A)** and after **(B)** photodynamic therapy.

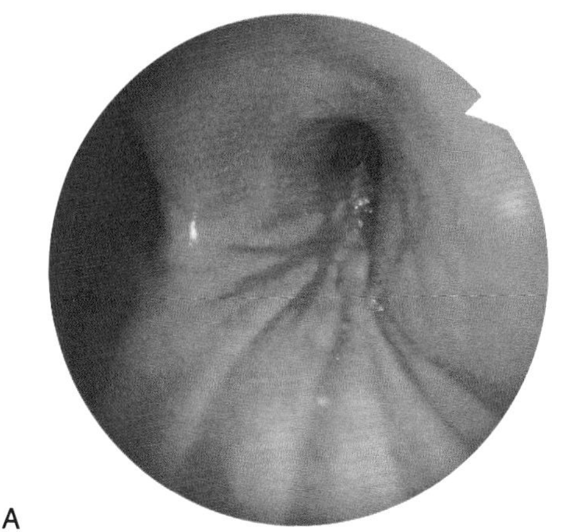

A

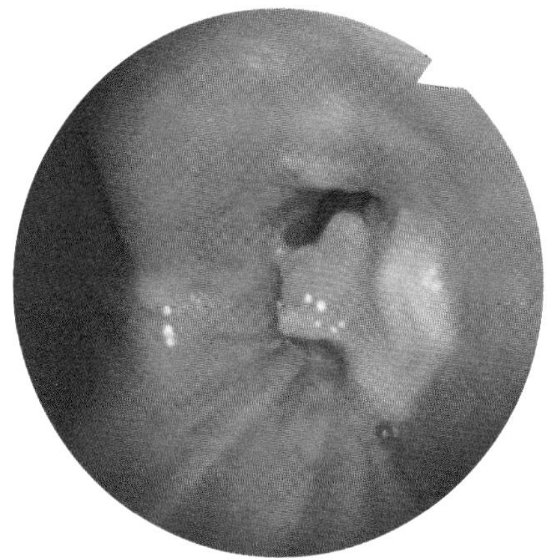

B

FIG. 8. (A) Carcinoma of right upper lobe before HpD therapy. **(B)** Thick necrotic pseudomembrane formation following therapy.

tinged sputum and gray necrotic material. Formation of thick necrotic debris following treatment can be a problem (Fig. 15–8). Five patients in our series had temporary airway obstruction that responded to intravenous administration of corticosteroid and inhaled bronchodilator. Three patients developed hypercapnic respiratory failure requiring mechanical ventilation. One had previously undergone left pneumonectomy and right upper lobectomy for two other squamous cell carcinomas, and a third superficial squamous cell carcinoma developed in the remaining bronchus. Four days after therapy the patient developed respiratory failure. Necrotic debris was removed without difficulty permitting prompt extubation of the patient (Fig. 15–9). The second patient had a previous right pneumonectomy and developed a second carcinoma in the left upper lobe. Respiratory failure developed 6 hr after photodynamic therapy. Necrotic debris was removed, but the patient died of a sudden tension pneumothorax. The third patient had three separate lesions treated simultaneously. Two days after treatment, respiratory failure ensued requiring mechanical ventilation. Necrotic debris was removed and extubation was accomplished without difficulty.

SUMMARY

The diagnosis and management of patients with malignancy of the tracheobronchial tree continues to present a formidable challenge to the practicing clinician. Data clearly indicate that early detection, localization, and treatment provide the best opportunity for long-term survival. Once detected, most cancers are readily localized by standard bronchoscopic evaluation. The earliest cancer, however, may require further evalua-

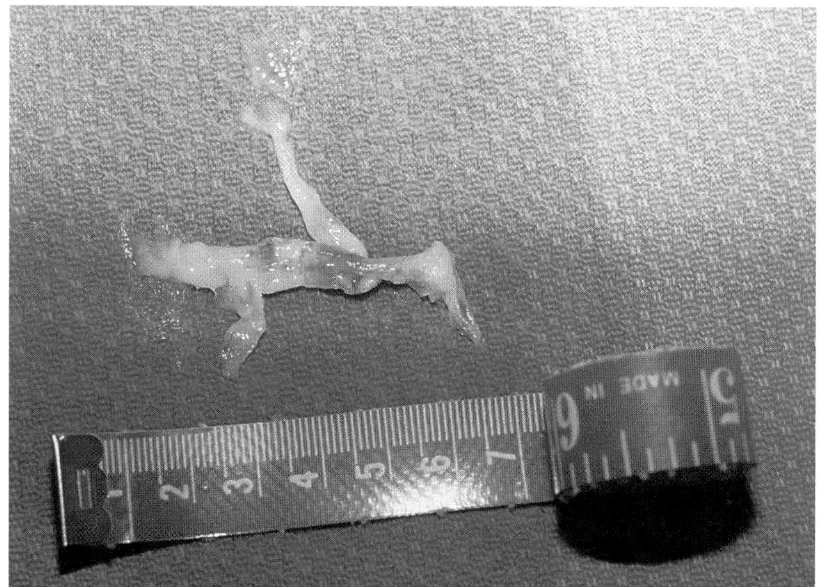

FIG. 9. Necrotic debris removed at clean-up bronchoscopy from right main stem bronchus after photodynamic therapy.

tion that includes repeated bronchoscopy and general anesthesia. Fluorescence compounds such as HpD or DHE, when used as tumor tags, may facilitate this process. More importantly, phototherapy with either HpD or DHE appears to be a valuable alternative to surgical resection. Patients with primary lung cancers are not only at increased risk for developing subsequent primaries, but also may be at a relatively higher risk for surgery because most have coexisting chronic obstructive pulmonary disease and ischemic heart disease (2,15). In properly selected patients, photodynamic therapy appears to be a reasonable alternative.

REFERENCES

1. Boring CC, Squires TS, Tong T. Cancer statistics, 1991. *Cancer* 1991;41:19–36
2. Cortese DA. Pairolero PC, Bergstralh EJ, Woolner LB, Uhlenhopp M, Peihler JM, Sanderson DR, Bernatz PE, Williams DE, Taylor WF, Payne WS, Fontana RS, Roentgenographically occult lung cancer: a ten-year experience. *J Thorac Cardiovasc Surg* 1983;86:376–380.
3. Tao L. Cytologic diagnosis of radiographically occult squamous cell carcinoma of the lung. *Cancer* 1982;50:1580.
4. Melamed MR, Felhinger BJ, Zaman MB, et al. Screening for early lung cancer. Results of Memorial Sloan-Kettering study in New York. *Chest* 1984;86:44.
5. Ikeda S. Flexible bronchofiberscope. *Ann Otol* 1970;79:916.
6. Lipson RL, Baldes EJ. The photodynamic properties of a particular hematoporphyrin derivative. *Arch Dermatol* 1960;82:508.
7. Profio AE, Doiron DR. A feasibility study of the use of fluorescence bronchoscopy for localization of small lung tumors. *Phys Med Biol* 1977;22:949–957.
8. Doiron DR, Svaasand LO, Profio AE. *Light dosimetry in tissue: application to photoradiation therapy*. New York: Plenum Press: 1983;63–76. (Kessel D, Dougherty TJ, eds; *Advances in experimental medicine and biology*; vol 160).
9. Cortese DA, Kinsey JH, Woolner LB. Clinical application of a new endoscopic technique for detection of in situ bronchial carcinoma. *Mayo Clin Proc* 1978;54:635–642.
10. King EG, Man G, LeRiche J, Amy R, Profio AE, Doiron DR. Fluorescence bronchoscopy in the localization of bronchogenic carcinoma. *Cancer* 1982;49:777–782.
11. Palcic B, Lam S, Hung J, MacAulay C. Detection and localization of early lung cancer by imaging techniques. *Chest* 1991; 99:742–743.
12. Hung J, Lam S, LeRiche JC, Palcic B. Autofluorescence of normal and malignant bronchial tissue. *Laser Surg Med* 1991; 11:99–105.
13. Hayata Y, Kato H, Konaka C, Ono J, Takizawa N. Hematoporphyrin derivative in laser photoradiation in the treatment of lung cancer. *Chest* 1982;81:269–277.
14. Edell ES, Cortese DA. Bronchoscopic Phototherapy with hematoporphyrin derivative for treatment of localized bronchogenic carcinoma: a five-year experience. *Mayo Clin Proc* 1987; 62:8–14.
15. Woolner LB, Fontana RS, Cortese DA, Sanderson DR, Bernatz PE, Payne WS, Pairolero PC, Piehler JM, Taylor WF. Roentgenographically occult lung cancer: pathologic findings and frequency of multicentricity during a ten-year period. *Mayo Clin Proc* 1984;59:453–466.
16. Kato H, Aizawa K, Ono J, et al. Clinical measurement of tumor fluorescence using a new diagnostic system with hematoporphyrin derivative, laser photoradiation, in a spectroscope. *Laser Surg Med* 1984;4:49–58.
17. Kato H, Cortese DA. Detection of lung cancer by hematoporphyrin derivative fluorescence and laser photoradiation. *Clin Chest Med* 1985;6(2):236–253.
18. Profio AE, Doiron DR, King EG. Laser fluorescence bronchoscopy for localization of occult lung tumors. *Med Phys* 1979; 6:523–525.
19. Doiron DR, Profio AE, Vincent RG, Dougherty TJ. Fluorescence bronchoscopy for detection of lung cancer. *Chest* 1979; 76:27–32.
20. Weishaupt KR, Gomer CJ, Dougherty TJ. Identification of singlet oxygen as the cytotoxic agent in photoactivation of a murine tumor. *Cancer Res* 1976;36:2326–2329.
21. Henderson BW, Dougherty TJ. Studies on the mechanism of tumor destruction by photoradiation therapy (PRT). In: Doiron DR, Gomer CJ, eds. *Porphyrin localization and treatment of tumors*. New York: Alan R. Liss: 1984;601–612.
22. Hayata Y, Kato H, Konaka C, Amemiya R, Ono J, Ogawa I, Kinoschita K, Sakai H, Takahashi H. Photoradiation therapy with hematoporphyrin derivative in early and stage I lung cancer. *Chest* 1984;86:169–177.
23. Ono R, Ikeda S, Suemasu K. Hematoporphyrin derivative photodynamic therapy in roentgenologically occult carcinoma of the tracheobronchial tree. *Cancer* 1992;69:1696–1701.
24. Kato H, Konaka C, Kawate H, Shinohara K, Kinoshita M, Naguchi M, Ootomo S, Hayata Y. Five-year disease-free survival of lung cancer patient treated only by photodynamic therapy. *Chest* 1986;90:768–770.
25. Edell ES, Cortese DA. Photodynamic therapy in the management of early superficial squamous cell carcinoma as an alternative to surgical resection. *Chest* 1992;102:1319–1322.

Bronchoscopy,
edited by U. B. S. Prakash.
Mayo Foundation © 1994.
Published by Raven Press, Ltd., New York.

CHAPTER 16

Therapeutic Bronchoscopy

Willane S. Krell and Udaya B. S. Prakash

The initial clinical application of the bronchoscope by Killian in 1889 was for the therapeutic purpose of removing a tracheal foreign body (1). Modifications in the rigid bronchoscope during the first 70 years of the twentieth century and the introduction of the flexible bronchoscope in the early 1970s increased the diagnostic role of both bronchoscopes. Recent developments have expanded therapeutic applications of the bronchoscope. Laser therapy of tracheobronchial lesions, dilatation of the strictures of the tracheobronchial tree, and stent placement to treat stenoses and strictures of the tracheobronchial tree have made therapeutic bronchoscopy as important as diagnostic bronchoscopy. Of the 871 bronchoscopists in North America who participated in a recent survey on bronchoscopy by the American College of Chest Physicians, 56% indicated that therapeutic bronchoscopy for lobar and segmental atelectasis was one of the five most common indications for bronchoscopy (2). Among patients in the intensive or critical care units, 47% to nearly 75% of bronchoscopies have been for therapeutic purposes (3–5).

The indications for therapeutic bronchoscopy are listed in Table 1. In clinical practice, however, it is common to simultaneously perform both diagnostic and therapeutic bronchoscopies. At times, performance of a single bronchoscopic procedure, e.g., the removal of an obstructing lesion of a lobar bronchus by a large biopsy forceps through the rigid bronchoscope, may accomplish both diagnostic and therapeutic objectives. The therapeutic roles of the bronchoscope in many of the clinical situations listed in Table 1 are discussed in detail in other chapters. Some aspects of therapeutic bronchoscopy in pediatric patients are discussed in Chapters 23 and 24. In this chapter we review other indications for therapeutic bronchoscopy and the techniques used.

W. S. Krell: Department of Pulmonary Medicine, Wayne State University, Detroit, Michigan 48201.

U. B. S. Prakash: Division of Thoracic Diseases and Internal Medicine, Mayo Clinic, Rochester, Minnesota 55905.

RETAINED SECRETIONS

Perhaps the most common indication for the therapeutic bronchoscopy is retained secretions. The retention of secretions is a common clinical complication in many patients, such as those with impaired cough mechanism due to altered level of consciousness, poor

TABLE 1. *Indications for therapeutic bronchoscopy*

- Airway clearance
  - Retained secretions
  - Mucous plugs
  - Pseudomembrane
  - Asthma
  - Cystic fibrosis
  - Blood clots
  - Necrotic tracheobronchial mucosa
  - Foreign bodies in the tracheobronchial tree (Chapter 18)
  - Hemoptysis (Chapter 17)
  - Obstructing neoplasms (Chapters 19–21)
- Intrinsic airway problems
  - Strictures and stenoses (Chapter 21)
  - Effects of intubation
- Artificial airways
  - Endotracheal tube placement
  - Difficult intubations
  - Intubation with cervicofacial trauma
- Parenchymal/mediastinal lesions
  - Pneumothorax
  - Bronchopleural fistula
  - Lung abscess
  - Hemoptysis
  - Bronchogenic cysts
  - Mediastinal lesions
  - Intralesional injection
  - Pulmonary alveolar proteinosis
- Following thoracic trauma

pulmonary function or weakness, recurrent aspiration, ventilator dependence, or postthoracotomy state. Patients with cystic fibrosis and allergic bronchopulmonary aspergillosis frequently develop respiratory distress from mucous plugs in the tracheobronchial tree. However, these patients rarely require therapeutic bronchoscopy.

The retained secretions may be made of mucus produced by the tracheobronchial mucosa or aspirated from the upper airway or upper gastrointestinal tract, gastroduodenal contents, or blood. Retained secretions in the tracheobronchial tree vary in consistency and volume. Thick, inspissated mucus assumes plug-like characteristics and can cause segmental or lobar atelectasis (Fig. 1). Large volumes of thin secretions in many bronchi may result in impaired gas exchange and hypoxemia. Patients with preexisting pulmonary disease can develop respiratory distress with smaller volumes of retained secretions in the tracheobronchial tree (Fig. 2).

An overwhelming majority of patients who develop retained secretions are hospitalized for other reasons. Retained mucus accompanies a wide variety of medical and surgical illnesses. Blood clots secondary to bleeding from intrinsic pulmonary lesions or after performance of complicated thoracic surgical procedures pose special problems in that the clots tend to be tenacious and much harder to remove than the mucoid secretions. Some uncommon types of clinical situations where therapeutic bronchoscopy is indicated include patients who develop pseudomembrane in the tracheobronchial tree following photodynamic therapy of tracheobronchial neoplasms and necrotic debris following chemical or thermal burns of the tracheobronchial mucosa (6–8). One study analyzed the results of initial bronchoscopy in 27 burned patients who had facial burns and reported that immediate bronchoscopy after burn injury neither indicates the level of respiratory support that will be required to maintain adequate oxygenation nor predicts its duration (9).

The initial clinical manifestations that indicate the need for therapeutic bronchoscopy include a gurgling, ineffective cough that fails to loosen secretions or progressive hypoxemia with or without chest roentgenographic evidence of relatively acute or subacute segmental or lobar atelectasis. Loss of lung volume, unilateral diaphragmatic elevation, and the abrupt cut-off of air bronchogram are the other roentgenographic signs that may indicate retained secretions.

Necrotizing tracheobronchitis is an uncommon complication of mechanical ventilation of newborns with respiratory failure. Despite the application of therapeutic bronchoscopy, 45% of the reported patients to date have died (10). Prolonged therapeutic bronchoscopies to remove the extensive tracheal debris are sometimes required (11).

We caution that each patient must be individually assessed before therapeutic bronchoscopy can take place. Careful examination of the patient and the appropriate use of chest physiotherapy are still indispensable in the optimal care of patients who develop the problem of retained mucous secretions and plugs.

The immediate performance of therapeutic bronchoscopy is indicated and indeed may be life saving in

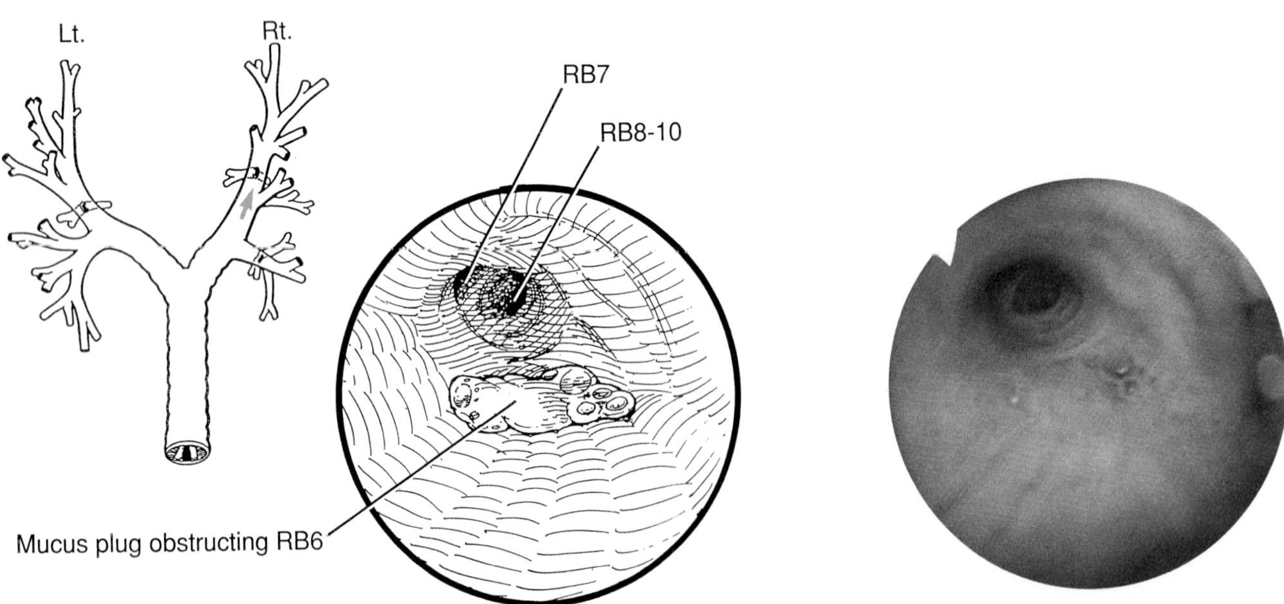

FIG. 1. Mucous plug obstructing a bronchus in the right lower lobe. This plug had assumed the shape of the bronchial tree (bronchial cast).

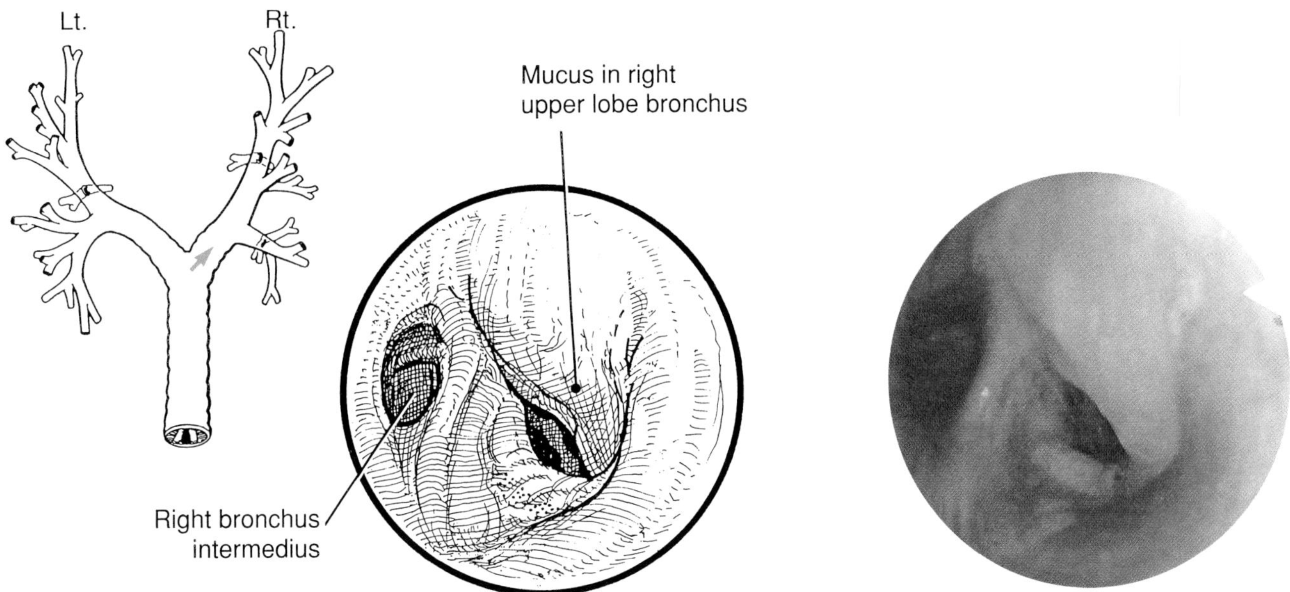

FIG. 2. Even smaller amounts of mucous secretions or mucous plugs can lead to respiratory distress in patients with preexisting hypoxemia.

some situations and therefore should not be withheld. The seriousness of retained secretions or blood clots is compounded in patients with underlying pulmonary diseases such as chronic obstructive pulmonary disease. However, it is sound clinical practice to attempt other means to dislodge the retained secretions and mucous plugs before proceeding with therapeutic bronchoscopy. These include mist therapy, nebulization of bronchodilator, chest percussion, and verbal encouragement of the patient to cough and expectorate (12–14). It has been recommended that therapeutic bronchoscopy be considered if there is any suspicion of aspiration, deterioration of blood gases, changes in chest roentgenograph, even in the absence of clinical symptoms of respiratory distress (15). Marini and associates (16) evaluated the usefulness of flexible bronchoscopy for the treatment of acute lobar atelectasis in 31 subjects who were randomly allocated to flexible bronchoscopy followed by respiratory therapy for 48 hr, or to respiratory therapy alone for the same period. The results suggested that flexible bronchoscopy did not add to respiratory therapy in the treatment of acute lobar atelectasis.

THE PROCEDURE

The preparation of the patient for therapeutic bronchoscopy is similar to that for diagnostic bronchoscopy (Chapter 8). Even though many of the patients who require therapeutic bronchoscopy are in the intensive care unit or too sick to cooperate with the application of topical anesthetic, every effort must be made to accomplish adequate local anesthesia and control of cough. The administration of narcotic agents prior to the procedure can reduce coughing. Sedative premedications may be indicated in very anxious or uncooperative patients, but must be used with caution. A short-acting or easily reversible agent is preferred. Sometimes, the spray-as-you-go type of instillation of topical anesthetic works as well.

In patients who are already intubated, the bronchoscopist must ensure that the internal diameter of the endotracheal tube permits the passage of the bronchoscope without interfering with adequate oxygenation. If an orotracheal tube is in place, a bite block is essential to guard against the possibility of damage to the flexible bronchoscope caused by the patient's bite. The minimum diameter endotracheal tube that can be safely used for bronchoscopy is somewhat controversial but generally an artificial airway of 8 mm or more will be acceptable (3,17,18). For performance of bronchoscopy in patients intubated with smaller diameter tubes, several options are available: changing the narrower tube to a larger one; passing the bronchoscope down the trachea next to the tube, then reinflating the tube's balloon to form a seal around the bronchoscope (not a good option for patient's using positive end-expiratory pressure); or ventilating the patient with a helium-oxygen mixture to reduce airway resistance to ventilation (18).

Monitoring of oxygen status is important in all patients undergoing bronchoscopy. Even in normal subjects, a 20 mm Hg decline in PaO_2 has been documented (3,19,20). In subjects with respiratory compromise, the decrease in oxygenation can be profound (20). Oxygen supplementation is an important part of the therapeutic bronchoscopy in these patients. For patients on mechanical ventilators, temporary removal of mechanical ventilation and delivery of oxygen by manual (Ambu bag) ventilation using high-flow oxygen may be necessary to assure optimal oxygenation.

When a flexible bronchoscope is used for removal of secretions and mucous plugs from the tracheobronchial tree, a large-channel instrument should be chosen so that thick and tenacious material can be aspirated without difficulty. An endotracheal tube also helps by allowing the bronchoscopist to remove the instrument from the tracheobronchial tree and clean the bronchoscope if the secretions totally block the channel of the instrument. One of the maneuvers that helps removal of the secretions is the rapid up-and-down movement of the flexible bronchoscope during simultaneous application of suction. For thick and "ropy" secretions, placing the tip of the instrument at the distal most visible portion of the mucous string and applying continuous suction may assist in clearing the mucus.

If a mucous plug is tightly impacted in a bronchus, we have used a "retrograde" wash to force the plug to move proximally in the tracheobronchial tree so that it can be removed easily. The tip of the flexible bronchoscope is gently nudged to enter the bronchial lumen distal to the mucous plug by sliding the tip of a flexible bronchoscope between the plug and the bronchial wall. Then an aliquot of about 10 ml normal saline is forcefully injected through the flexible bronchoscope. The saline then dislodges the mucous plug and pushes it up. Repeated bronchial washes are indicated when small particulate matter is lodged in the distal bronchi. A patient's coughing during the bronchoscopic suction also helps move the mucous secretions and plugs proximally. Occasionally, very thick and tenacious secretions and mucous plugs require removal by means of a biopsy forceps (Fig. 3). In this situation, the forceps should be applied to the base of the mucous plug so that the entire plug can be dislodged. Catching the proximal end of the plug usually results in the breakage of tiny pieces and this method can become time consuming. The use of the biopsy forceps and the rigid bronchoscope may be required to remove large pieces of necrotic mucosa, pseudomembrane, and necrotic debris in patients who develop the pseudomembrane following photodynamic therapy of tracheobronchial neoplasms and necrotic debris following chemical or thermal burns of the tracheobroncial mucosa (21). Caution is suggested in use of the forceps, as all that looks shiny like mucus may not be simple mucous plugs. In our institution over the past year, three patients who had been subjected to repeated "therapeutic" bronchoscopies were discovered to have the following: endobronchial metastatic tumor, endobronchial zygomycosis, and a tuberculous lymph node eroding into the bronchus. Failure to dislodge a plug may call for additional diagnostic studies in some patients.

In pediatric patients with retained tenacious secretions, it may be difficult to remove the secretions with the flexible bronchoscope. Therefore, rigid bronchos-

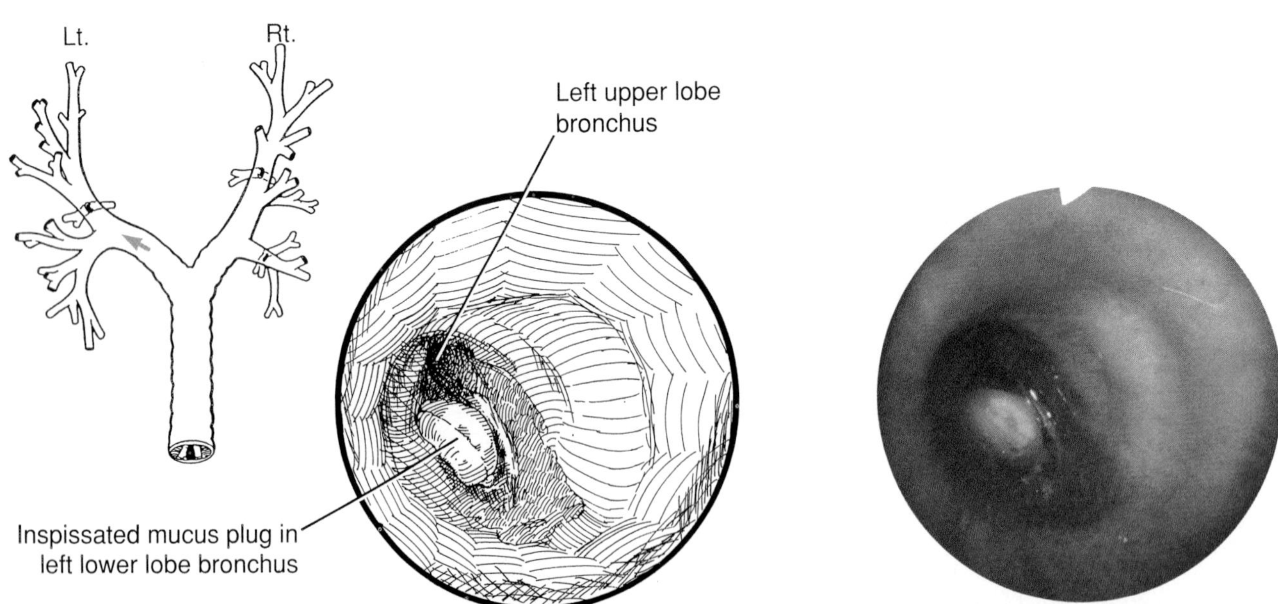

FIG. 3. Extremely thick and inspissated mucous plugs will require removal with a biopsy forceps. Occasionally, rigid bronchoscopic extraction may be necessary.

copy may be required (22). When appropriately used for aspiration of mucous plugs or bronchial secretions, pediatric flexible bronchoscopy is particularly helpful in children with segmental or lobar atelectasis. Nussbaum (23) described the details of 46 pediatric flexible bronchoscopies performed on 29 infants under 1 year of age, and 17 small children between 1 and 2 years of age with persistent unilobar or multilobar atelectasis and declining PaO_2 or rising $PaCO_2$. Therapeutic bronchoscopy resulted in the resolution of atelectasis in all infants. There was no mortality or significant morbidity. The therapeutic bronchoscopy effected the resolution of respiratory distress and cough within 24 hr, resulting in earlier hospital discharge in all patients regardless of complete or partial roentgenographic expansion.

In hypoxemic patients who require vigorous suctioning, the oxygenation should be carefully monitored by pulse oximetry so that the preexisting hypoxia is not worsened by the continuous suction of oxygen from the tracheobronchial tree (24). Large-channel flexible bronchoscopes are more likely to aggravate this problem because of their ability to suck large volumes of gas. Supplemental oxygen as indicated by pulse oximetry will generally allow the safe performance of therapeutic bronchoscopy.

BALLOON INSUFFLATION TO TREAT ATELECTATIC LUNG

The bronchoscope has been used for other therapeutic purposes, particularly in the critical or intensive care unit. In patients with refractory atelectasis, we have used endobronchial balloon occlusion with application of positive pressure ventilation delivered through the balloon catheter lumen with successful outcome. Initially, the bronchus leading to the collapsed segment or subsegment is thoroughly suctioned and washed to remove mucus. Then the bronchus is tamponaded by wedging the flexible bronchoscope, usually in a subsegmental bronchus. Room air is insufflated through the working channel of the bronchoscope into the atelectatic area of the lung. The air pressure is maintained for several minutes. Tsao and colleagues (25) used a similar technique and reported complete reexpansion in 12 of the 14 procedures and partial reexpansion in 2. The average alveolar-arterial oxygen pressure difference declined from 217.5 mm Hg before the procedure to 200.3, 150.0, and 152.2 mm Hg respectively at 30 min, 12 hr, and 24 hr after. There were no complications. Millen and colleagues (26), and others (27), reported similar experience in treating refractory atelectasis.

Harada and associates (28), using an inflator device consisting of a flexible bronchoscope with a small balloon cuff at the distal end, successfully performed insufflation in 14 of 15 patients with atelectasis who had failed to respond to conventional therapy. In 6 patients atelectasis recurred and the same treatment was successfully repeated.

The need for using the balloon insufflation techniques seldom arises. The risk of pneumothorax should be considered before applying this technique, even though Tsao and colleagues observed no complications following 14 procedures (25). The technique should be limited to segmental atelectasis rather than lobar atelectasis or the atelectasis of an entire lung. Chronic atelectatic areas are less likely to respond to this maneuver. If the maneuver is successful in opening the segment, the only definitive method to ascertain success is to obtain a chest roentgenograph.

BRONCHIAL TAMPONADE

Bronchial tamponade via the bronchoscope is aimed at isolating a pulmonary segment or subsegment distal to the site of tamponade. The bronchial tamponade technique has been used for the bronchoscopic treatment of bronchial or pulmonary hemorrhage, refractory pneumothorax, persistent air leaks following thoracotomy, and bronchopleural fistula. The bronchial tamponade technique is based on the principle that the bronchoscope can be used to isolate the pulmonary segment and then block the bronchus in which bleeding occurs or through which the air leak is occurring. In cases of hemorrhage, temporary tamponade may allow time to plan appropriate definitive treatment. Bronchoscopic modalities to treat bronchopleural fistula have included tissue glue, fibrin glue, gelfoam, lead plugs, balloon catheter, autologous blood patch, and sclerosing agents (29).

Bronchopleural fistulas are associated with high morbidity and mortality and are particularly challenging in the ventilated patient (30,31). Definitive therapy of the bronchopleural fistula by the bronchoscopic application of a sealing agent to occlude the fistula site can be used, particularly in the poor surgical candidate. If thoracotomy is planned to treat these clinical complications, bronchial balloon tamponade may aid the surgeon in isolating the segment responsible for the air leak so that the surgical procedure can be accomplished quickly. We point out that the tamponade procedures are generally time consuming and may require deep sedation and general anesthesia. Several methods, described below, can be used to tamponade the bronchus (32–34).

Successful application of the technique of transbronchoscopic endobronchial occlusion of a persistent bronchopleural fistula requires an accurate determination of the segmental location of the air leak. Lillington et al (35) injected of small boluses of xenon-133 into a number of segmental bronchi through a flexible bronchoscope and documented a marked increase in radioactivity in the intercostal drainage tube. Nagai and associates (36) used a different technique to detect the pulmonary parenchymal segment that was responsible for the air leak in refractory pneumothorax. A constant volume of 100% helium gas was introduced into each lobar bronchus of two patients with pneumothorax via a flexible bronchoscope. In both patients, only when helium gas was introduced into the bronchus communicating with a ruptured emphysematous bulla was a high concentration of helium detected in the intrathoracic gas. Some have used selective bronchography to identify the leaky bronchus (37).

Balloon Tamponade

Balloon tamponade can be accomplished with either a flexible or a rigid bronchoscope. A balloon catheter is inserted into the bronchus leading to the segment suspected to be causing the clinical problem and the balloon is inflated to tamponade the bronchus (Fig. 4). In a patient with persistent air leak, the tamponade will either stop or decrease the air leak through the chest tube if the correct segmental bronchus is tamponaded. Once the segmental bronchus is identified, further treatment, such as fibrin glue injection or surgery, can be undertaken. The problems associated with balloon tamponade include the slippage of the balloon due to coughing by the patient and loss of air in the balloon unless constant syringe pressure is maintained. Placement of the balloon in the upper lobe bronchi also tends to be a bit more difficult.

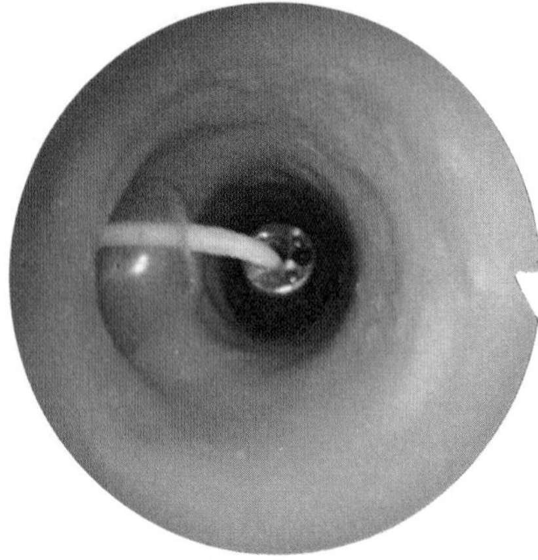

FIG. 4. Balloon tamponade of the bronchus. A cephalad view obtained in a model of tracheobronchial tree. The balloon is advanced via the working channel of a flexible bronchoscope and upon inflation of the balloon the abnormal segment is effectively isolated from the remainder of the tracheobronchial tree.

Fibrin Glue Tamponade

Application of fibrin glue to tamponade or close defects in the tracheobronchial tree has been tried in an effort to avoid major thoracic surgical procedures (30,32,34,38–41). In an experimental study on animals, endoscopic occlusion of infected bronchus stump fistulas was achieved with fibrin sealant (1 ml, 500 units/ml thrombin, 3,500 units/ml aprotinin) applied via a flexible bronchoscope. Necropsy studies after the second postoperative week showed that all bronchial stump fistulas had healed (42). Once identification of the bronchus leading the pulmonary segment responsible for the air leak, bronchopleural fistula, or hemorrhage is made, the fibrin glue can be injected through the bronchoscope. The fibrin glue is formed instantaneously when the cryoprecipitate and tissue thrombin come in contact with each other. The cryoprecipitate is easily obtainable from the blood bank and the tissue thrombin is commercially available in a powder form and can be reconstituted by adding normal saline according to the instructions provided in the package. It is not necessary to check the patient's blood group and type. Equal amounts of cryoprecipitate and thrombin should be loaded into separate syringes. Because the glue forms instantaneously, the channel of the bronchoscope should be protected from coming in contact with the glue. This can be managed by inserting a plastic catheter with double channel through the working channel of the bronchoscope.

We have successfully used the triple-channel pulmonary artery catheter, with the distal several centimeters cut off so that cryoprecipitate and the thrombin exude at the same level of the catheter, to simultaneously inject the cryoprecipitate and the thrombin (Chapter 17). The distal tip of the bronchoscope is then introduced into the bronchus to be tamponaded. Secretions, blood, or mucus should be fully suctioned before the application of the fibrin glue. The catheter is then introduced through the bronchoscope and the distal tip of the catheter pushed through so that it is at least 2 cm away from the distal end of the bronchoscope. The cryoprecipitate and the thrombin solution should be injected simultaneously, a few drops at a time, directly into the bronchial lumen or fistula. The fibrin clot forms within 5–6 sec. It is better to inject the mixture so that the fibrin clot forms in layers rather than a single lump. Once an adequate clot is formed, the bronchoscope with the catheter still projecting from its tip is removed and the catheter tip thoroughly cleaned before it is removed from the bronchoscope.

If the procedure is properly performed, the fibrin

clot effectively tamponades the bronchus for several days to weeks. The clot eventually disintegrates and is either absorbed by the bronchial mucosa or expectorated. Extremely large fibrin clots should be avoided because, should they become loose in the tracheobronchial tree, complications similar to those associated with the aspiration of a foreign body can ensue.

Some bronchoscopists have used a sclerosing agent (2–3 ml ethoxysclerol applied around the orifice of the fistula) in addition to the fibrin glue to stimulate fibrosis (42). The rate of success with the fibrin clot depends on the underlying pulmonary problems, the size of the fistula or the bronchus tamponaded, and the technique. Fibrin glue tamponade is more likely to succeed in patients with small air leaks following thoracic surgery and pneumothorax than in patients with more complicated problems such as an infected bronchopleural fistula or underlying malignancy. Although air trapping and infection distal to the site of tamponade are potential complications, these have not been reported. The few problems reported with the technique involved slippage of the glue into other airways due to inadequate tamponade, which is easily remedied once the problem is recognized.

Other Forms of Tamponade

To treat large bronchial fistulas following pneumonectomy or lobectomy, bronchoscopists have used other materials and fibrin glue to plug the hole. Heterologous spongy bone has been used to close large fistulous openings (30). Such procedures require rigid bronchoscopy and expertise in the use of various instruments. Recurrence of tracheoesophageal fistula after surgical repair for esophageal atresia occurs in approximately 5–15% of cases. The successful obliteration of recurrent tracheoesophageal fistula using diathermy through the bronchoscope has been reported (43). A patient with bronchopleural fistula has been successfully treated by selective intrabronchial injection of doxycycline and blood under flexible bronchoscopic guidance (44). Persistent bronchopleural fistula following treatment of fulminant pneumonia caused by *Staphylococcus aureus* has been successfully treated by instillation of tetracycline into the fistula via a flexible bronchoscope using a balloon catheter and blood clot occlusion technique (45). In complex cases of bronchopleural fistula in which the need for repeat thoracotomy is high, bronchoscopists have applied Super Glue (butyl or methyl methacrylate) through the flexible bronchoscope to seal large fistulas between the pleural cavity and a segmental bronchus (46). A tracheoesophageal fistula has been successfully closed with a fibrin adhesive applied by means of a flexible bronchoscope. To facilitate closure of the fistula, the technique was combined with decontamination of the oral cavity to avoid bacterial infection (47). With use of a flexible bronchoscope, vascular occlusion coils have also been used to seal large parenchymal bronchopleural fistula (48).

Gelfoam can be used through either flexible or rigid bronchoscope to occlude peripheral bronchopleural fistulas (49). After the leaky bronchus is identified, small strips of gelfoam ($0.25 \times 0.5 \times 2.0$ cm) are moistened with saline, placed in the flexible bronchoscopic channel with the aid of biopsy forceps or brush, and flushed with saline into the affected bronchus. This procedure is repeated until the bronchus is completely occluded with a gelfoam plug.

The use of the rigid bronchoscope and bronchial packing to control massive bronchial hemorrhage is discussed in Chapter 17.

BRONCHOSCOPIC TREATMENT OF INTRATHORACIC LESIONS

Lung Abscess

The presence of an acute lung abscess with clinical signs of fever, elevated white count, and systemic illness does not generally require a bronchoscopic examination. Bronchoscopic manipulation may effect rupture of the abscess and spillage of the infected contents into the tracheobronchial tree. However, with subacute or chronic clinical findings, the presence of a lung abscess may be a diagnostic indication for bronchoscopy to obtain material for culture and particularly to exclude an endobronchial obstructing (malignant) lesion that may be responsible for the formation of the abscess. The mainstays of therapy for acute abscesses are antibiotics and drainage by means of chest physiotherapy and coughing. Some bronchoscopists have used the rigid bronchoscope to effectively drain the abscess cavity while assuring that adequate visualization and suction are available to protect the remaining lung from the infected contents (Chapter 14).

Bronchogenic Cyst and Mediastinal Cysts

Occasionally, bronchogenic cysts and mediastinal cysts become filled with liquid and encroach on the tracheobronchial lumen and cause respiratory distress. Bronchoscopic drainage of these cysts has been accomplished in several cases (50,51). The bronchoscope has been used to drain lung abscesses, fluid-filled cysts, and other lesions in the mediastinum and the lung (52,53). Such procedures are usually unsuccessful in rapidly emptying the contents of the abscess cavity or the cyst. Patients who undergo bronchoscopic attempts to empty the contents of an abscess cavity may slowly expectorate the contents over a period of hours or days. Occasionally, however, the contents may massively drain into the tracheobronchial tree. If precautions are not taken, the putrid material may be aspirated into normal lung parenchyma (52).

Pulmonary parenchymal cysts and localized emphysematous lesions have been treated by selective bronchial tamponade. The balloon catheter, placed under direct visualization via the bronchoscope to occlude the bronchus, may be the safest method for selective bronchial occlusion (54). Either continuous or intermittent bronchial occlusion can be tried in such cases.

Broncholithiasis

Broncholithiasis represents the protrusion of a calcium phosphate stone into the lumen of the tracheobronchial tree. The majority of broncholiths begin as pulmoliths or pneumoliths in the pulmonary parenchyma. The formation of the stone is due to the localized deposition of dystrophic calcification within the lung parenchyma secondary to an inflammatory process. Common etiological causes include tuberculosis, mycotic infections, or other inflammatory processes. The pulmoliths seldom produce clinical problems. The symptoms of broncholithiasis, or erosion of a pulmolith into the airway, include sudden onset of cough, hemoptysis of varying degree, localized wheezing, lithoptysis, and postobstructive atelectasis and related symptoms. Clinical history, chest roentgenogram, and chest tomography may point to the diagnosis. Bronchoscopy remains the diagnostic method of choice to evaluate these lesions (55).

The bronchoscopic appearance of the broncholith may mimic a raised mucosal lump, granulation tissue, or a neoplastic lesion (Chapter 32). Occasionally, the white rock–like stone may be seen. The mucosa adjacent to the broncholith usually appears very friable. The procedure for removal of the broncholith is similar to that for tracheobronchial foreign bodies. However, the bronchoscopic removal of a broncholith should be attempted only if the stone is loose in the tracheobronchial tree and located in a relatively avascular area. If the broncholith is located adjacent to a bronchial artery, one should consider the possibility that the stone is also adherent to the artery and therefore forceful removal may be followed by massive bleeding. A gentle shaking and a to-and-fro motion of the stone with a biopsy forceps should be attempted before extraction from the tracheobronchial tree. Subcarinal broncholiths are usually situated in an avascular area and bronchoscopic removal may be attempted without the risk of severe hemorrhage.

Obstructing broncholiths that cannot be removed by bronchoscopic manipulation may require other types of instruments. Fragmentation of the large, impacted broncholith with the Nd:YAG laser eliminated the necessity for a thoracotomy in an elderly patient (56).

Intralesional Injections

Intralesional injections of chemicals and biological agents have been tried through the bronchoscope to treat tracheobronchial neoplasms and other abnormalities (57). The instrumentation and techniques used are similar to those used in transtracheal or transbronchial needle aspirations (Chapter 12). The intralesional injections of tracheobronchial tumors has remained experimental in application.

THERAPEUTIC BRONCHOALVEOLAR LAVAGE

Pulmonary Alveolar Phospholipoproteinosis

Diagnostic bronchoalveolar lavage to obtain material from the alveolar level in the diagnosis of infectious and noninfectious diseases is discussed in Chapter 13. Pulmonary alveolar phospholipoproteinosis or proteinosis is a disease in which a diffuse intraalveolar deposition of lipoproteinaceous material leads to progressive respiratory distress. The time-honored treatment for this rare disorder has been the insertion of the double-lumen endotracheal tube followed by instillation of massive amounts of normal saline to wash out the intraalveolar material (Fig. 5). This requires general anesthesia and special equipment and personnel (58). Several papers have described the use of a flexible bronchoscope to therapeutically wash individual segments (20,59,60). A 3.5-mm rigid bronchoscope has been used to treat pulmonary alveolar phospholipoproteinosis in a 15-week-old infant (61). A patient with a single lung has undergone successful therapeutic bronchoscopy for pulmonary alveolar phospholipoproteinosis (59). Such a procedure is time consuming and indeed may require deep sedation or general anesthesia. While the traditional therapeutic bronchoalveolar lavage can frequently accomplish treatment of both lungs in a single sitting, therapeutic bronchoscopy via a flexible bronchoscope will require several separate sessions to wash one lung. We believe that the patients who require therapeutic bronchoalveolar lavage for the treatment of pulmonary alveolar phospholipoproteinosis should be referred to medical centers equipped to provide total lung lavage.

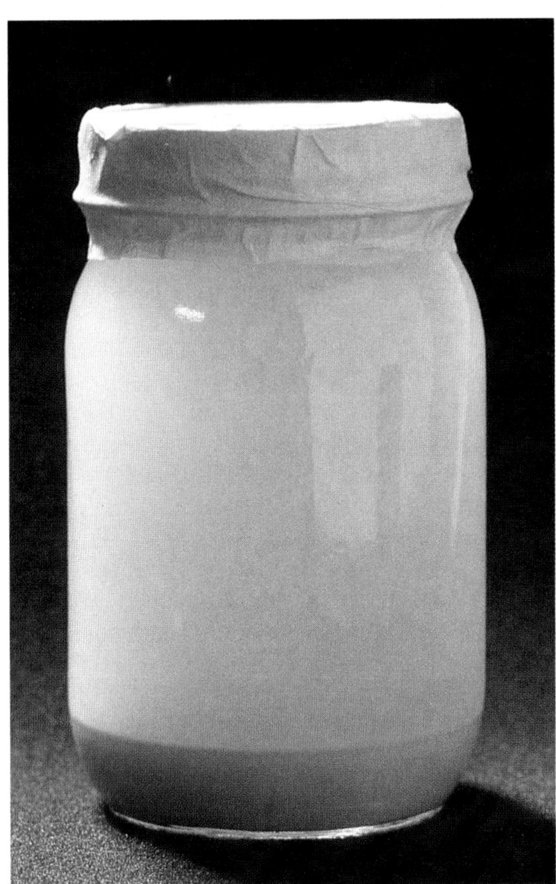

FIG. 5. Bronchoalveolar lavage effluent collected by flexible bronchoscopy from a patient with pulmonary alveolar (phospholipo)proteinosis. Note the sediment at the bottom of the container.

Cystic Fibrosis

The use of the therapeutic bronchoscopy to aspirate the purulent secretions from the tracheobronchial tree of patients with cystic fibrosis is controversial. Many different techniques have been described, and the results of such therapy are difficult to evaluate. Rothmann et al. (62) described their experience with 114 procedures with limited lavage using 4% acetylcysteine and saline via the rigid bronchoscope under general anesthesia. There were no deaths. The severity of cystic fibrosis is not a contraindication to bronchoscopy. In fact, therapeutic bronchoscopy is used not infrequently in patients with cystic fibrosis (62–66). Dahm et al. (67) performed 153 lung lavages on 81 patients with cystic fibrosis using the rigid bronchoscope under topical anesthesia in 24 lavages and using the flexible bronchoscope in 73 lavages. Subjective improvement was noted in 96% of the 56 patients who had lavage under general anesthesia. Objective improvement was apparent in 45% of the 24 patients who had lavage by rigid bronchoscopy and 64% of the 36 patients who had lavage by flexible bronchoscopy.

Asthma

Bronchoscopy is safe in persons with asthma. Rankin and associates (61) prospectively studied the safety of bronchoscopy and bronchoalveolar lavage with bilateral instillation of 300 ml of saline in ten adults with mild asthma and showed that there were no major complications.

Severe asthma is characterized by marked airway obstruction secondary to mucous plugging, airway edema and inflammation, and contractions of airway smooth muscle. Standard treatment includes bronchodilator and corticosteroids, and in some instances mechanical ventilation (68). The mucous plugs in asthmatic patients can be tenacious and difficult to expectorate in spite of aggressive medical therapy (Fig. 6). The inspissated mucus can produce obstructing

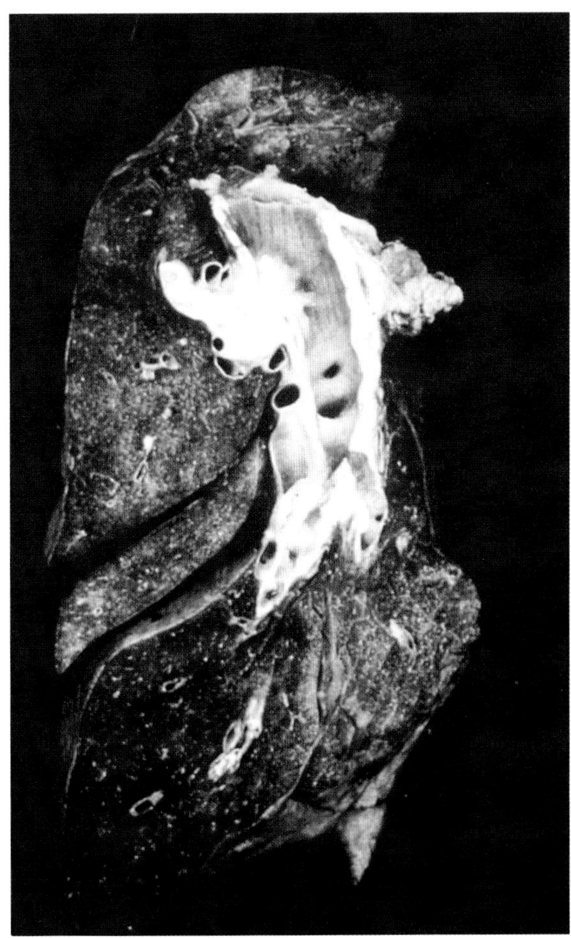

FIG. 6. Thick and tenacious mucous plugs in a patient with status asthmaticus. Note the obstruction of bronchi leading to all three lobes of the right lung.

bronchial casts and totally obstruct the bronchial lumen (Fig. 3). Bronchial asthma complicated by allergic bronchopulmonary aspergillosis is more likely to produce mucoid impaction of the bronchial tree. The term "plastic bronchitis" has been used to describe the formation of such casts (Chapter 32). Therapeutic bronchoscopy with forceps removal may be necessary in such cases (69). Lang and colleagues (70) assessed the value of 51 flexible bronchoscopic procedures with lavage in 19 patients during episodes of stabilized yet refractory asthma with mucous impaction. After the procedure, spirometric measurements of forced expiratory volume in 1 sec (FEV_1), forced expiratory flow ($FEF_{25\%-75\%}$), and forced vital capacity (FVC) increased significantly and correlated with relief of dyspnea and mobilization of secretions with cough. No significant complications were encountered. Others have used the bronchoscope to instill acetylcysteine, bronchodilator, and corticosteroids through the working channel of the instrument (71). Millman and colleagues (72) reported the case of a young woman, closely followed for 21 years, whose life was saved by repeated bronchoscopy and lavage to remove mucous plugs and casts from the tracheobronchial tree.

THORACIC TRAUMA

In the initial evaluation of patients with blunt chest trauma, therapeutic bronchoalveolar lavage on admission is reported to have reduced bacterial contamination and pneumonia in comparison to patients not lavaged (38). Pathological lesions of the lung parenchyma are often seen in association with blunt chest trauma. Diagnostic and therapeutic bronchoscopy is an integral part of the initial evaluation of such patients. This procedure helps to estimate the severity and extent of parenchymal lesions even before chest roentgenographic signs are noted (38). Often therapeutic bronchial lavage is needed for removal of aspirated particulate matter as well as larger foreign bodies, including loose teeth or pieces of denture materials.

ENDOTRACHEAL TUBE PLACEMENT

Therapeutic aspects of patients in the intensive or critical care unit include proper placement of the endotracheal tube for mechanical ventilation, particularly in cases with cervical spine trauma or massive facial injuries, and replacement or changing of such tubes. Faulty placement of endotracheal tubes was recognized among 15% of 92 diagnostic flexible bronchoscopies performed in the intensive or critical care unit by Stevens and coworkers (5). Others have used the flexible bronchoscope to assess the pathogenic factors leading to laryngotracheal injury due to tracheal intubation in the critically ill patients (73,74).

The upper respiratory tract of patients requiring long-term intubation should be assessed by flexible bronchoscopy and other modalities to prevent fatal late airway occlusion (75). In adult patients presenting with acute upper airway obstruction, the proper placement of the endotracheal tube under direct visualization through the flexible bronchoscope represents the approach of choice (76).

The flexible bronchoscope has been very helpful in replacing endotracheal tubes in patients on mechanical ventilation who require a change of tube. By threading the new or larger endotracheal tube over the instrument, the distal half of the flexible bronchoscope is used as the guide stent and passed next to the existing endotracheal tube, while the latter is removed and the new tube passed into the trachea over the bronchoscope. This ensures that the airway is not lost in a patient who is totally dependent on mechanical ventilation (77). This technique was used successfully in 27 of 29 attempts described by Halebian and Shires (78). These techniques are frequently used at the Mayo Clinic and have been effective in over 75% of cases (4). The flexible bronchoscope is very helpful in changing endotracheal tubes in patients with airway burns because the direct visualization aids in the protection of the already damaged tracheal mucosa (79). Verification of tracheal tube position by flexible bronchoscopy in critically ill patients has been compared with roentgenological techniques and found to be safe and accurate (80).

Problems with chronic tracheostomy tubes can also be addressed using the flexible bronchoscope (Fig. 7). If the tube fractures (usually at the proximal end due to manipulations of the tube during suctioning, etc.) or portions of the tube are aspirated, the flexible scope can be used to assess the problem and to retrieve tube-related foreign bodies, using a bronchoscopic basket or forceps (81).

The flexible bronchoscope is also helpful in assessing the placement of endotracheal tubes in neonates. A study evaluated the role of flexible bronchoscopy in 65 intubated neonates to ascertain the applicability of flexible bronchoscopy for assessment of endotracheal tube tip position. The results showed that the procedure was well tolerated in all cases and that 70 examinations in the 65 neonates were performed without interruption of mechanical ventilation. The accuracy of bronchoscopic measurement of endotracheal tube tip position improved markedly with user experience and closely correlated with the chest roentgenogram (82).

The flexible bronchoscope has been successfully applied to the evaluation of other airway problems in pediatric patients. Fan and associates performed 104 flexible bronchoscopies in 87 children (median age of 24

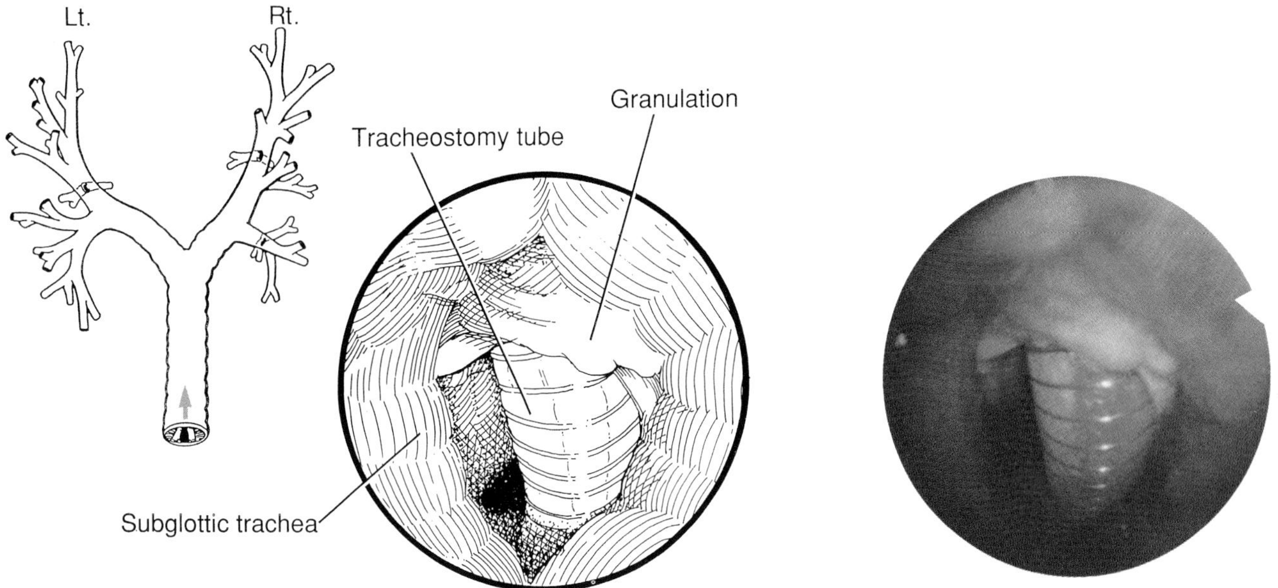

FIG. 7. Flexible bronchoscopy examining the tracheostomy tube and site in a patient with hemoptysis presumed to be arising from tracheostomy stoma.

months) over a 4-year period in a pediatric intensive care unit and reported success rates of 95% and 87% in diagnostic and therapeutic flexible bronchoscope, respectively (83). Rigid bronchoscopy using a ventilating bronchoscope provides a better control of the airway in very young children and infants, and is recommended in such situations (22).

The effectiveness of continuous positive airway pressure to treat severe respiratory distress in infants with bronchomalacia has been successfully accomplished with the aid of flexible bronchoscopy. Flexible bronchoscopy in four neonates described by Miller et al. (84) diagnosed the area of bronchomalacia, documented the effects of continuous positive airway pressure on the airway, and helped determine an effective level of continuous positive airway pressure.

The ultrathin flexible bronchoscope with an external diameter of less than 2 mm has been used to determine the position of endotracheal tube in newborns. Vigneswaran et al. (85) compared the utility of the ultrathin flexible bronchoscope in 20 intubated newborns to determine the position of the endotracheal tube with the roentgenographic studies and found that the bronchoscopic evaluation was comparable to that of roentgenography.

MANAGEMENT OF THE DIFFICULT AIRWAY

Bronchoscopists involved in airway management should have a plan of action to deal with the difficult airway or a failed intubation. When a difficult airway problem is anticipated, the equipment necessary for performing a difficult intubation should be immediately available. The flexible bronchoscope and accessory equipment for difficult intubation should be at hand (86). It also is prudent to have a surgeon skilled in performing a tracheotomy and a cricothyroidotomy stand by (87). The intubation should be attempted in the awake state, preferably using the flexible bronchoscope.

THERAPEUTIC BRONCHOSCOPY IN THE INTENSIVE OR CRITICAL CARE UNIT

The critically ill patients and patients in the intensive or critical care unit frequently require bronchoscopy for the removal of retained secretions, placement or change of endotracheal tubes, diagnostic bronchoalveolar lavage, and assessment of hemoptysis and other pulmonary problems. The following paragraphs address the bronchoscopic needs of this special group of patients.

The versatility of the flexible bronchoscope has enabled the bronchoscopist to utilize it frequently in the care of critically ill patients. As a result, flexible bronchoscopes have become part of the standard equipment in most intensive or critical care units (3–5,15,17,67,88–91). Rigid bronchoscopy, when used in the intensive or critical care unit, has been limited to situations where a flexible bronchoscope was unavailable or a mature tracheal stoma was present in a spontaneously breathing patient (90). Currently, an overwhelming majority of bronchoscopies performed in the intensive or critical care unit use the flexible bronchoscope.

In the Mayo Clinic series of 129 patients who underwent 198 flexible bronchoscopies, 75% were mechanically ventilated patients. Bronchoscopy was performed for therapeutic indications in 47%, diagnostic purposes in 44%, and for both diagnostic and therapeutic reasons in 9% (4). Of the 90 flexible bronchoscopies for retained secretions, 41% showed mucous plugs or significant secretions, but clinical improvement, as noted by the improved oxygenation or improved chest roentgenological findings up to 72 hr after the therapeutic bronchoscopy, was noted in only 19%. Among the 18 flexible bronchoscopies in which the procedure was done for both diagnostic and therapeutic purposes, 33% demonstrated mucous plugs or thick secretions but only 2% showed improvement in chest roentgenological findings after therapeutic bronchoscopy.

Lindholm and colleagues reported that of the 71 therapeutic bronchoscopies, 81% were successful in improving aeration as evaluated by chest roentgenogram (3). Stevens and colleagues (30) observed clinical improvement, as determined by oxygenation and physical examination, in 44% of 70 flexible bronchoscopies performed for retained secretions. Snow and Lucas reported that 58% of 51 patients in a surgical intensive care unit exhibited roentgenological improvement following therapeutic bronchoscopy (90).

Absolute contraindications for therapeutic bronchoscopy in the intensive or critical care unit include inexperienced personnel, inadequate facilities, severe hypoxemia and inability to oxygenate the patient adequately, and rapidly worsening hypercarbia. Clinical indications that increase the risk of therapeutic bronchoscopy include lack of cooperation by the patient, severe debilitation, recent myocardial infarction, unstable angina, unstable cardiac arrhythmias, worsening asthma or status asthmaticus, mechanical ventilation with positive end-expiratory pressure, thrombocytopenia, lung abscess, uremia, and pulmonary hypertension (Table 2) (92).

Based on the hypothesis that mucous plugs and secretions in smaller bronchi may be responsible for impaired exchange of gases and abnormal compliance in patients using mechanical ventilation, Weinstein and associates (93) performed 43 therapeutic bronchoalveolar lavage procedures using about 237 ml of physiological saline solution through the flexible bronchoscope in patients with respiratory failure. Eighty-one percent of the lavages were associated with a significant increase of the ratio of arterial to alveolar oxygen pressures and 63% of the lavages were associated with a significant increase in effective static compliance at 8 hr after lavage. There were no complications.

To evaluate a variety of suction catheters of various designs, the effect of a single suctioning procedure on the airway mucosa was observed in 20 patients undergoing diagnostic or therapeutic bronchoscopic examination and recorded by still and cinephotography through a flexible bronchoscope (94). Of the variety of catheter designs evaluated, all produced a negligible amount of trauma, and none was superior to bronchoscopy in efficiently evacuating mucus from the airways. Mucosal trauma with tracheobronchial suctioning procedures is more likely with repetitive or vigorous suctionings, or with high levels of suction applied, regardless of which type of catheter is used.

TABLE 2. *Factors associated with increased risk for complications during therapeutic bronchoscopy*

Severe
Lack of patient cooperation
Lack of skilled personnel
Lack of appropriate facilities
Refractory hypoxemia
Unstable angina
Uncontrolled arrhythmias
Moderate
Debility, advanced age, malnutrition
Partial tracheal obstruction
Hypercarbia
Mechanical ventilation
Severe asthma
Acute lung abscess (spillage)
Thrombocytopenia
Uremia (functional platelet defect)
Pulmonary hypertension
Superior vena caval obstruction

BRONCHOSCOPY IN THE MECHANICALLY VENTILATED PATIENTS

Mechanical ventilation is not a contraindication for either therapeutic or diagnostic bronchoscopy (95). More than 75% of bronchoscopies in the Mayo Clinic series of 198 patients were done in patients on mechanical ventilators (4). About two thirds of the flexible bronchoscopies reported by Lindholm and colleagues were carried out in patients with ongoing mechanical ventilation (3). Among the 297 flexible bronchoscopies performed by Stevens and associates, 65% were done while the patients were on mechanical ventilation (5). There is some risk involved in the bronchoscopy of mechanically ventilated patients. The addition of positive end-expiratory pressure breathing may contribute to more complications. Trouillet and colleagues, (96) assessed the complications of flexible bronchoscopy in 107 acutely ill patients who were mechanically ventilated and reported that a substantial decline in oxygen tension in arterial blood was consistently associated with the procedure, especially when midazolam was used for sedation. Hypoxemia, defined by PaO_2 lower than 60 mm Hg, was more frequent in patients with acute respiratory distress syndrome and in those who "fought" the ventilator.

Bronchoscopic lung biopsy has been accomplished in patients on mechanical ventilation. Pincus and associates (97) reported that bronchoscopic lung biopsy established a positive diagnosis in 6 of their 13 patients with progressive pulmonary infiltrates on mechanical ventilation. However, all their procedures were done in a bronchoscopy suite and not in the intensive or critical care unit. No mention is made regarding positive end-expiratory pressure breathing in this group of patients. Complications following bronchoscopic lung biopsy in the mechanically ventilated patients have included pneumothorax requiring chest tube drainage, pulmonary hemorrhage, and cardiac arrhythmias. Papin et al. (98) looked at the value and risk of bronchoscopic lung biopsy in 15 patients requiring mechanical ventilation for progressive pulmonary infiltrates. The results of the procedure significantly altered the management strategy in seven patients. The alveolar-arterial oxygen gradient widened by a mean of 110 mm Hg in nine patients but this alteration was transient and clinically insignificant. Complications consisted of three cases of reversible hypercapnia, three cases of self-limited bleeding, and one case of tension pneumothorax. It is not clear whether the procedures were done in the intensive care unit or the operating room.

Critically ill patients are frequently thrombocytopenic, uremic, or have other coagulation abnormalities. Further, their cooperation during bronchoscopic lung biopsy is less than satisfactory. These factors and the high frequency with which these patients are mechanically ventilated with positive end-expiratory pressure increase the risk of pneumothorax and bleeding following bronchoscopic lung biopsy. In high-risk patients, the safety and efficacy of bronchoscopic lung biopsy must be decided by the physician on an individual case basis. An open lung biopsy, which permits better control of bleeding and the pleural space, may be a more prudent option in some patients. We recommend that fluoroscopic guidance be used for bronchoscopic lung biopsies performed in the intensive care setting.

Complications of Bronchoscopy in the Intensive or Critical Care Unit

Complications from therapeutic bronchoscopy in critically ill patients have been mild and observed in less than 10% of the flexible bronchoscopies performed. For the most part, these have included tachycardia, cardiac arrhythmias, and mild degrees of aspiration during the procedure. Hypoxemia is one of the complications of flexible bronchoscopy, even in patients who are not critically ill (19,99). Careful monitoring of oxygen status by oximetry and appropriate supplementation should prevent this expected physiological occurrence during bronchoscopy.

Cardiac complications, particularly arrhythmias, can be noted in association with bronchoscopy. In large series, arrhythmias that could potentially compromise hemodynamics (sinus bradycardia, atrial fibrillation, supraventricular tachycardia, premature ventricular contractions, and other ventricular arrhythmias) are reported to occur in up to 11% of patients (17,100,101), but serious complications are rare, even in critically ill patients, if attention is given to monitoring the electrocardiogram and maintaining acceptable oxygen saturation. In one reported series, cardiopulmonary arrest occurred in less than 1% of critically ill patients undergoing bronchoscopy and deaths directly related to bronchoscopy were rare (17). Problems are more likely to occur in the face of unstable angina or severe preexisting hypoxemia (102).

Fever can develop after bronchoscopy in 10–20% of patients (103,104). Septicemia is generally not present. Age over 60 years seems to be the only consistent risk factor for this problem, which is usually a self-limited phenomenon (103). Other potential complications include severe bronchospasm, increased dyspnea, subcutaneous or mediastinal emphysema (3,5,90), sinusitis, nasal bleeding, or new chest roentgenologic infiltrates postprocedure (105).

Procedures added to therapeutic or diagnostic bronchoscopies carry an additional risk of complications. For example, instillation of large volumes of saline during bronchoalveolar lavage can result in a greater decrease in oxygen saturation than bronchoscopy alone (106). This abnormality will clear within 1–4 hr, but monitoring and supplemental oxygen may be needed after as well as during the procedure for the safety of the patient.

Bronchoscopic lung biopsy can lead to bleeding and pneumothorax. Factors that increase the risk of hemorrhagic complications have been previously outlined, including pulmonary hypertension, thrombocytopenia, and uremia. Immunocompromised patients with diffuse pulmonary infiltrates appear to be at especially high risk for bleeding, i.e., up to 29% incidence in one series (107–109). Pneumothorax, including tension pneumothorax, occurs in less than 5% of procedures and pulmonary fibrosis is an important risk factor for its occurrence (107,108).

In the Mayo Clinic series, complications were noted in 3.5% of 198 flexible bronchoscopies performed in the intensive or critical care unit (4). There were no deaths. Tachycardia up to 150 beats/min was present in almost all patients and was not considered a specific complication of flexible bronchoscopy. Only one patient had the procedure terminated because of severe arterial oxygen desaturation. Frequent premature ventricular contractions occurred in one patient. Increased dyspnea and cough occurred in one patient with *Pneumocystis carinii* pneumonia. Another patient with *P. carinii* had a temperature elevation to 40°C after the procedure. Tension pneumothorax requiring chest tube placement occurred in a fourth patient, following thoracotomy (thoracotomy done on opposite side) a few hours after flexible bronchoscopy. This patient had a Swan–Ganz catheter inserted on the same side as the pneumothorax 12 hr before therapeutic bronchoscopy.

Overall the rate of complications with bronchoscopy is low. Less than 5% of complications involve major morbidity. A review of patients described in seven publications (3–5,17,88–90) revealed that of the 1,150 flexible bronchoscopies performed in 804 patients in the setting of the intensive or critical care unit, there had not been a single death.

OTHER FORMS OF BRONCHOSCOPIC TREATMENTS

The role of bronchoscopy in the application of laser, phototherapy, brachytherapy, and other forms of endobronchial treatments is discussed in other chapters in this textbook. Three forms of bronchoscopic treatments deserve mention here: bronchoscopic cryotherapy, bronchoscopic electrocautery and balloon dilatation.

Cryotherapy

The basic principle of cryotherapy is to effect death of malignant cells by exposing them to extremely cold temperature. Liquid nitrogen or nitrous oxide is commonly used for this purpose (110,111). The technique utilizes a cryoprobe, introduced through a rigid bronchoscope. Most visible tumors are now reached with a flexible cryoprobe inserted in a flexible bronchoscope (112). Specially made channels carry the super-cooled liquid to the probe tip, which is kept in contact with the abnormal lesion. The contact with the tumor is maintained for several minutes or until formation of "frost" around the abnormal tissue is observed. The tumor undergoes necrosis during the next 48–72 hr and the tumor debris is usually coughed out by the patient. Bronchoscopic cryotherapy can be applied in patients who are not candidates for other forms of traditional therapy. Successful treatment of benign tracheobronchial lesions has been reported (112,113).

Walsh et al. (114) prospectively studied the value of 81 bronchoscopic cryotherapy procedures in 33 patients with inoperable bronchial carcinoma with bronchial obstruction and reported that most patients improved in terms of overall symptoms, stridor, hemoptysis, and dyspnea. Objective improvement in lung function was seen in 58% of patients. Bronchoscopic evidence of relief of bronchial obstruction was seen in 77% of patients. There were no serious complications. The results compared favorably with the results in published series of patients receiving laser therapy. Similar results have been reported by Maiwand, who treated 75 patients suffering from advanced carcinoma of the trachea or bronchi (115). Bronchoscopic cryotherapy has been successfully applied to pediatric patients (113,116).

Rodgers and associates (110) employed this technique (nitrous oxide cryoprobe measuring 3 mm in diameter and 43 cm in length) in the treatment of 29 refractory airway lesions in 27 patients ranging in age from 3 months to 42 years. The tip of the probe was applied directly to the stricture through the endoscope and cooled to −80°C for 45 sec. The frozen tissue was resected with biopsy forceps after the probe was removed. Cryotherapy successfully relieved the airway strictures in 20 of 24 lesions.

Electrocautery

Bronchoscopic electrocautery is an alternative to laser and cryotherapy for the treatment of tracheobronchial lesions. Electrocautery can be used for coagulation of bronchoscopically visible bleeding lesions (117). The equipment available is easier to use in combination with the rigid bronchoscope. The big channel of the rigid instrument allows simultaneous suctioning while the surface of the tumor or the mucosal vessels can be cauterized. Electrocautery probes are also available for larger flexible bronchoscopes (118). The major disadvantage of cauterization via the flexible bronchoscope is that the coagulation effect stops completely if carbonized tissue covers the surface of the electrode. Repetitive cleaning of the electrode is required, making it a time-consuming procedure.

Endobronchial electrocautery has been used successfully to treat patients with major airway obstruction resulting from bronchogenic carcinoma (119). As a result of high inspired oxygen concentration, a tracheal fire has occurred without injury to the patient (119). Electrocautery is an available economical tool that has potential value in the diagnosis and therapy of tracheobronchial tumors. Benign tracheobronchial lesions have been treated with electrocautery (120). The risk of formation of tracheobronchial stricture secondary to electrocautery therapy itself is a potential complication (121).

Bronchoscopic Balloon Dilatation

Acquired bronchial stenosis has been associated with sleeve resection, tracheobronchial anastomosis,

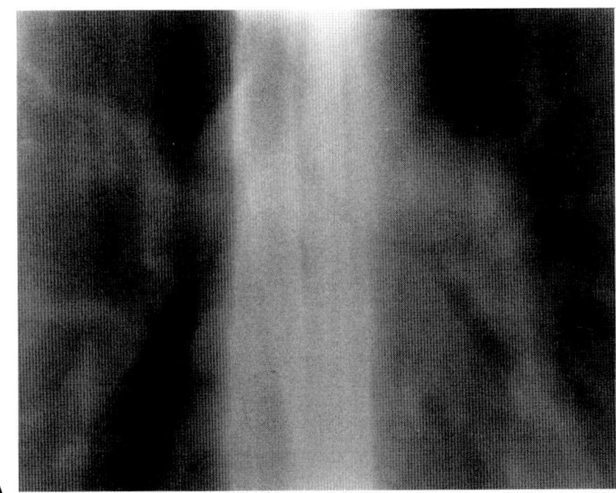

A

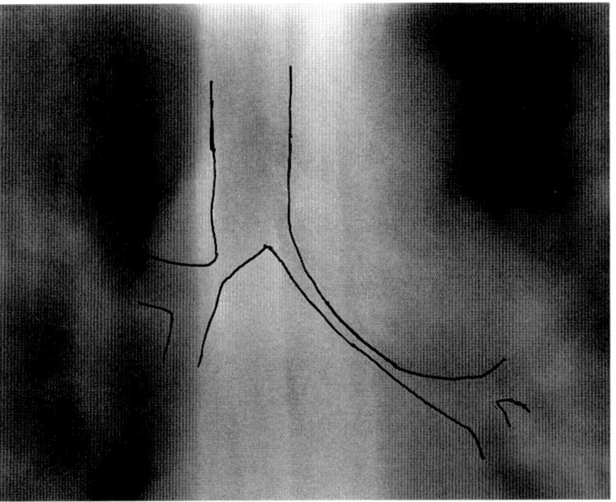

B

FIG. 8. An anteroposterior tomography shows a long stenotic segment of left main stem bronchus and a short stenosis of right main stem bronchus caused by an unknown process **(left)**; and a pencil enhancement better delineates the stenotic segments **(right)**.

tuberculosis, histoplasmosis, sarcoidosis, prolonged intubation, and chemical and thermal injuries of the tracheobronchial tree. Bronchostenosis is a well-recognized complication of pulmonary transplantation, occurring at the site of the anastomosis, and occasionally spreading distally from the original site of obstruction. Congenital tracheobronchial stenosis is encountered in pediatric bronchoscopy practice. The treatment of such stenoses or strictures has been accomplished by surgery, laser, electrocautery, and rigid bronchoscopy (the bronchoscope itself is used as a dilating instrument). In recent years, balloons have been used through the bronchoscope for this purpose (122–126). Balloons of different lengths and inflated diameters are available for the dilatation of such stenoses through either the rigid or the flexible bronchoscope. The balloons can be inflated with air or liquid (usually sterile saline) but liquid provides a more rigid dilating instrument.

Bronchoscopy, tomography, and bronchography may be necessary before attempting dilatation to assess the length and diameter of the stenotic lesion (Fig. 8). The information thus obtained will aid in selecting the appropriate equipment. Not all balloons can pass through the working channel of the flexible bronchoscope. In such situations, the balloon can be passed next to the flexible bronchoscope and directed by the tip of the bronchoscope through the stenotic segment. If an endotracheal tube is used, an ultrathin flexible bronchoscope will permit adequate ventilation as well as easy passage of the balloon next to it. Balloon dilatation through the rigid bronchoscope is much easier to perform because it allows the use of larger balloons. The balloon should be tested with liquid to assure that it is leak-proof and the stiffness is acceptable for dilatation (Figs. 9 and 10).

The external surface of the deflated balloon is slightly lubricated to permit its easy passage through the bronchoscope. After the patient takes several deep inhalations of oxygen, the tip of the deflated balloon is introduced through the stenotic lumen and positioned in such a manner that the middle of the balloon corresponds to the middle of the stenotic segment (Fig. 11). The balloon is gradually inflated to its maximum diameter by injecting the prescribed volume of liquid into the balloon or by using a manometer to measure and maintain a certain dilating pressure (Fig. 10). It is important to maintain the inflated balloon in place for

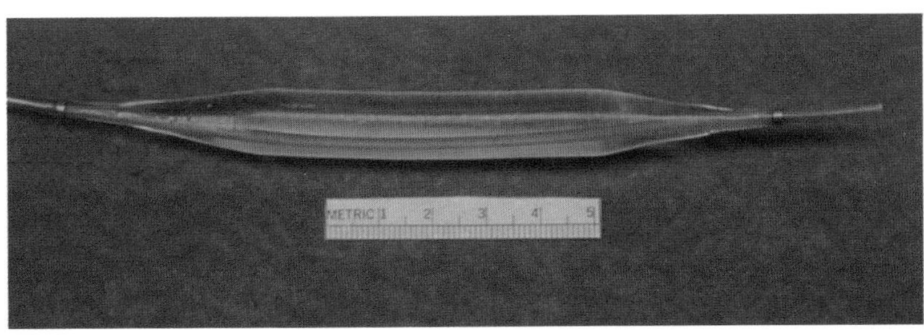

FIG. 9. A saline-inflated balloon. Such balloons are available in different lengths and outer diameters.

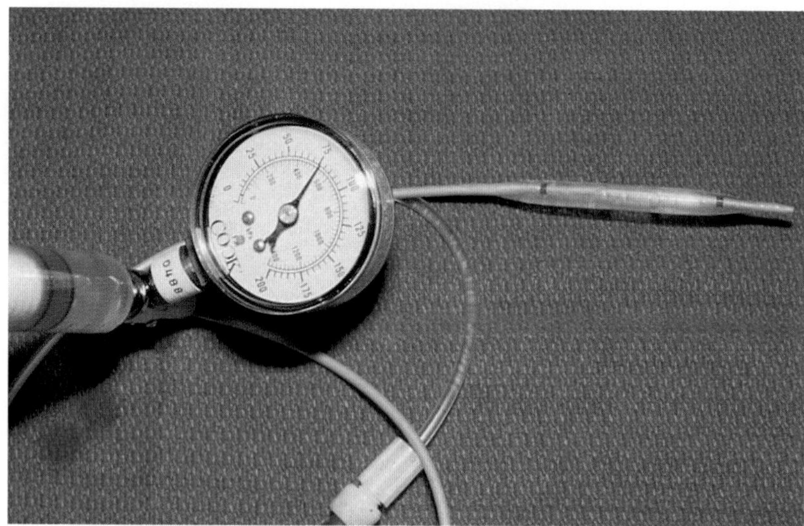

FIG. 10. A saline-inflated balloon with a manometer to measure the inflation pressure.

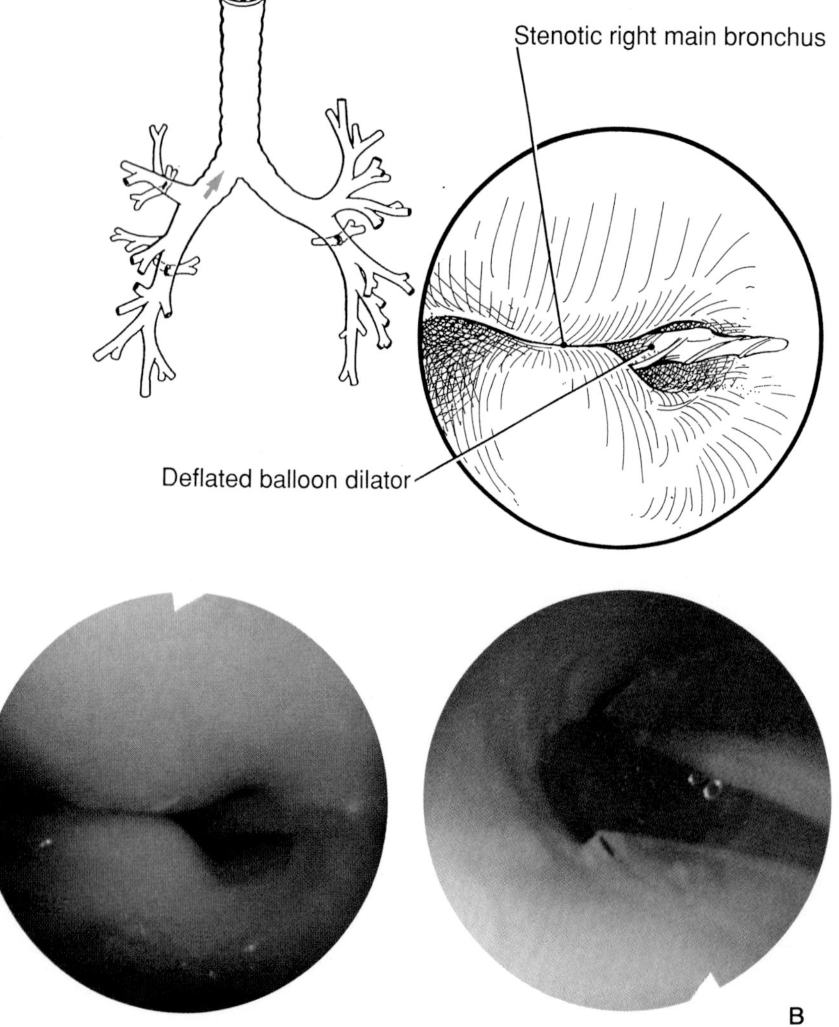

FIG. 11. Cephalad view of simulated bronchoscopic dilatation of bronchial stenosis in a model of the tracheo-bronchial tree. The deflated balloon's tip is passed through the stenotic bronchus **(A)**; and saline inflation of the balloon has dilated the stenosis **(B)**.

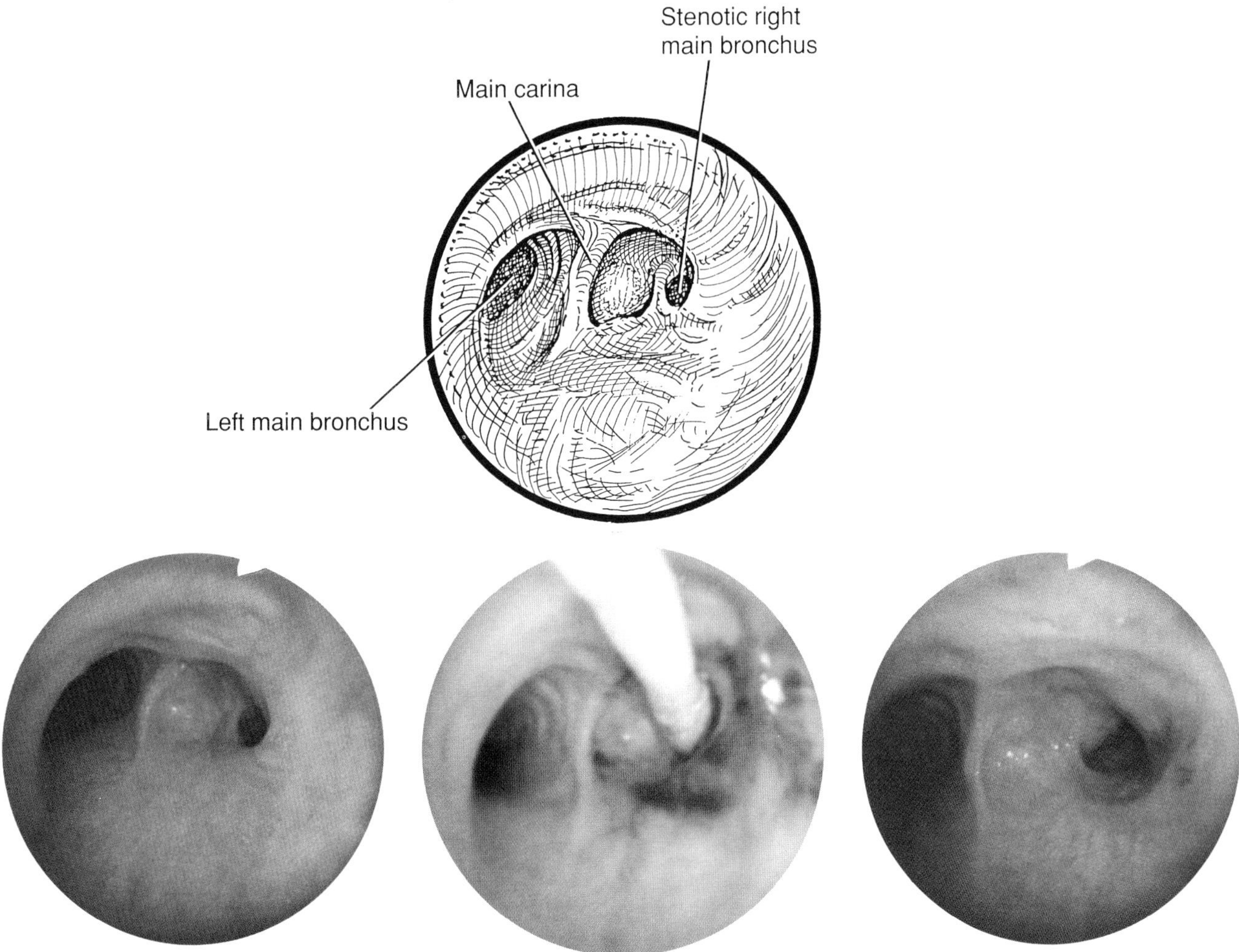

FIG. 12. Stenosis of the right main stem bronchus caused by inactive Wegener's granulomatosis **(left)**, balloon dilator is placed through the stenotic bronchus **(center)**, and enlarged lumen of the stenotic bronchus immediately after dilatation **(right)**.

90–120 sec so that the fibrotic process responsible for the stenosis is stretched and disrupted (Fig. 11). With good preoxygenation, it is possible to block a major bronchus for as long as 120 sec, even if the contralateral lung is not functioning properly. A gentle tug is applied to see if the stenotic segment is being stretched with adequate dilating force. The balloon is deflated and the effect of dilatation is assessed (Fig. 12). Depending on the result, successively larger balloons can be used to further dilate the stenotic bronchus.

Long-term results depend on the etiology and severity of the stricture. Slowly progressive benign strictures are more likely to respond than malignant stenoses (123). If the stricture is secondary to extrinsic compression, the response is poor in contrast to a stricture caused by a pathological process in the wall of the bronchus (Fig. 12). Congenital tracheobronchial stenoses have been successfully managed by balloon dilatation (125).

REFERENCES

1. Zollner F. Gustav Killian—father of bronchoscopy. *Arch Otolaryngol* 1965;82:656.
2. Prakash UBS, Offord KP, Stubbs SE. Bronchoscopy in North America: the ACCP survey. *Chest* 1991;100:1668–1675.
3. Lindholm CE, Ollman B, Snyder J, Millen E, Grenvik A. Flexible fiberoptic bronchoscopy in critical care medicine. Diagnosis, therapy, and complication. *Crit Care Med* 1974;2:250–261.
4. Olopade CO, Prakash UBS. Bronchoscopy in the intensive care critical care unit. *Mayo Clinic Proc* 1989;64:1255–1263.
5. Stevens RP, Lillington GA, Parsons GH. Fiberoptic bronchoscopy in the intensive care unit. *Heart and Lung* 1981; 10:1037–1045.
6. Schneider W, Berger A, Mailander P, Tempka A. Diagnostic and therapeutic possibilities for fibreoptic bronchoscopy in inhalation injury. *Burns. Incl. Therm. Inj.* 1988;14:53–57.
7. Eisenmenger W, Drasch G, von-Clarmann M, Kretschmer E, Roider G. Clinical and morphological findings on mustard gas [bis(2-chloroethyl)sulfide] poisoning. *J Forens Sci* 1991; 36:1688–1698.
8. Freitag L, Firusian N, Stamatis G, Greschuchna D. The role of bronchoscopy in pulmonary complications due to mustard gas inhalation. *Chest* 1991;100:1436–1441.

9. Bingham HG, Gallagher TJ, Powell MD. Early bronchoscopy as a predictor of ventilatory support for burned patients. *J Trauma* 1987;27:1286–1288.
10. Michael EJ, Zwillenberg D, Furnari A, Sheppard L, Desai HJ, Wolfson PJ, Robinson NB, Kornhauser M, Mobley S, Branca PA. Treatment of neonatal necrotizing tracheobronchitis with extracorporeal membrane oxygenation and bronchoscopy. *J Pediatr Surg* 1988;23:798–801.
11. Sauer PJ, v-d-Schans EJ, Lafeber HN. Bronchoscopic treatment of necrotising tracheo-bronchitis in a newborn [letter]. *Eur J Pediatr* 1986;144:596–597.
12. Kumar VA, Brandstetter RD. Chest physiotherapy vs. bronchoscopy (letter). *Crit Care Med* 1986;14:78–79.
13. Mahajan VK, Catron PW, Huber GL. The value of fiberoptic bronchoscopy in the management of pulmonary collapse. *Chest* 1978;73:817–820.
14. Passy V, Ermshar C. Bronchopulmonary lavage to remove pulmonary casts and plugs. *Arch Otolaryngol* 1976;102:193–197.
15. Groitl H. The flexible bronchofiberscope in the intensive care unit (ICU)—the optimal postoperative care for the bronchial system. *Endoscopy* 1981;13:100–103.
16. Marini JJ, Pierson DJ, Hudson LD. Acute lobar atelectasis: a prospective comparison of fiberoptic bronchoscopy and respiratory therapy. *Am Rev Resp Dis* 1979;119(6):971–978.
17. Barrett CR. Flexible fiberoptic bronchoscopy in the critically ill patients. *Chest* 1978;73(suppl):746–749.
18. Pingleton, SK, RC Bone, NK Ruth. Helium oxygen mixtures during bronchoscopy. *Crit Care Med* 1980;8:50–53.
19. Albertini RE, Harrell JH Jr, Kurihara N, Moser RM. Arterial hypoxemia induced by fiberoptic bronchoscopy. *JAMA* 1974; 230:1666–1667.
20. Brach BB, Harrell JH, Moser KM. Alveolar proteinosis. Lobar lavage by fiberoptic bronchoscopic technique. *Chest* 1976; 69:224–227.
21. Tan WC, Lee ST, Lee CN, Wong S. The role of fibreoptic bronchoscopy in the management of respiratory burns. *Ann Acad Med Singapore* 1985;14:430–434.
22. Muntz HR. Therapeutic rigid bronchoscopy in the neonatal intensive care unit. *Ann Otol Rhinol Laryngol* 1985;94:462–465.
23. Nussbaum E. Pediatric flexible bronchoscopy and its application in infantile atelectasis. *Clin Pediatr (Phila)* 1985; 24:379–382.
24. Arai T, Hatano Y, Komatsu K, Takada T, Miyake C, Harioka T, Reshad K. Real-time analysis of the change in arterial oxygen tension during endotracheal suction with a fiberoptic bronchoscope. *Crit Care Med* 1985;13:855–858.
25. Tsao TC, Tsai YH, Lan RS, Shieh WB, Lee CH. Treatment for collapsed lung in critically ill patients. Selective intrabronchial air insufflation using the fiberoptic bronchoscope. *Chest* 1990;97:435–438.
26. Millen JE, Vandree J, Glauser FL. Fiberoptic bronchoscopic balloon occlusion and reexpansion of refractory unilateral atelectasis. *Crit Care Med* 1978;6:50–55.
27. Lee TS, Wright BD. Selective insufflation of collapsed lung with fiberoptic bronchoscope and Swan–Ganz catheter. *Intens Care Med* 1981;7:241–243.
28. Harada K, Mutsuda T, Saoyama N, Taniki T, Kimura H. Reexpansion of refractory atelectasis using a bronchofiberscope with a balloon cuff. *Chest* 1983;84:725–728.
29. McManigle JE, Fletcher GL, Tenholder MF. Bronchoscopy in the management of bronchopleural fistula. *Chest* 1990; 97:1235–1238.
30. Baumann MH, Sahn SA. Medical management and therapy of bronchopleural fistulas in the mechanically ventilated patient. *Chest* 1990;97:721–728.
31. Powner DJ, Bierman MI: Thoracic and extrathoracic bronchial fistulas. *Chest* 1991;100:480–486.
32. Glover W, Chavis TV, Daniel TM, Kron IL, Spotnitz WD. Fibrin glue application through the flexible fiberoptic bronchoscope: closure of bronchopleural fistulas. *J Thorac Cardiovasc Surg* 1987;93:470–472.
33. Roksvaag H, Skalleberg L, Nordberg C, Solheim K, Hivik B. Endoscopic closure of bronchial fistula. *Thorax* 1983; 38:696–697.
34. Torre M, Chiesa G, Ravini M, Vercelloni M, Belloni PA. Endoscopic gluing of bronchopleural fistula. *Ann Thorac Surg* 1987; 43:295–297.
35. Lillington GA, Stevens RP, DeNardo GL. Bronchoscopic location of bronchopleural fistula with xenon-133. *J Nucl Med* 1982; 23:322–323.
36. Nagai A, Takizawa T, Konno K, Kawakami M. A new simple method to detect an air-leaking lung field in pneumothorax by a flexible bronchofiberscope. *Tohoku J Exp Med* 1982; 136:111–112.
37. York EL, Lewall DB, Hirji M, Gelfand ET, Modry DL. Endoscopic diagnosis and treatment of postoperative bronchopleural fistula. *Chest* 1990;97:1390–1392.
38. Regel G, Seekamp A, Aebert H, Wegener G, Sturm JA. Bronchoscopy in severe blunt chest trauma. *Surg Endosc* 1990; 4:31–35.
39. Regel G, Sturm JA, Neumann C, Schueler S, Tscherne H. Occlusion of bronchopleural fistula after lung injury—a new treatment by bronchoscopy. *J Trauma* 1989;29:223–226.
40. Walsh TE. Bronchial infusion therapy (BIT). A bit of caution (editorial). *Chest* 1989;96:456–457.
41. Matar AF, Hill JG, Duncan W, Orfanakis N, Law I. Use of biological glue to control pulmonary air leaks. *Thorax* 1990; 45:670–674.
42. Waclawiczek HW, Chmelizek F, Koller I. Endoscopic sealing of infected bronchus stump fistulae with fibrin following lung resections. Experimental and clinical experience. *Surg Endosc* 1987;1:99–102.
43. Rangecroft L, Bush GH, Lister J, Irving IM. Endoscopic diathermy obliteration of recurrent tracheoesophageal fistulae. *J Pediatr Surg* 1984;19:41–43.
44. Lan RS, Lee CH, Tsai YH, Wang WJ, Chang CH. Fiberoptic bronchial blockade in a small bronchopleural fistula. *Chest* 1987;92:944–946.
45. Martin WR, Siefkin AD, Allen R. Closure of a bronchopleural fistula with bronchoscopic instillation of tetracycline. *Chest* 1991;99:1040–1042.
46. Wood RE, Lacey SR, Azizkhan RG. Endoscopic management of large, postresection bronchopleural fistulae with methacrylate adhesive (Super Glue). *J Pediatr Surg* 1992;27:201–202.
47. Antonelli M, Cicconetti F, Vivino G, Gasparetto A. Closure of a tracheoesophageal fistula by bronchoscopic application of fibrin glue and decontamination of the oral cavity. *Chest* 1991; 100:578–579.
48. Salmon CJ, Ponn RB, Westcott JL. Endobronchial vascular occlusion coils for control of a large parenchymal bronchopleural fistula. *Chest* 1990;98:233–234.
49. Jones DP, David I: Gelfoam occlusion of peripheral bronchopleural fistula. *Ann Thorac Surg* 1986;42:334–335.
50. Crenshaw GL. Bronchial stenosis produced endoscopically to destroy space-consuming bullae. *Geriatrics* 1966;21:167–170.
51. Wang KP, Nelson S, Scatarige J, Siegelman S. Transbronchial needle aspiration of a mediastinal mass: therapeutic implications. *Thorax* 1983;38:556–557.
52. Hammer DL, Aranda CP, Galati V, Adams FV. Massive intrabronchial aspiration of contents of pulmonary abscess after fiberoptic bronchoscopy. *Chest* 1978;74:306–307.
53. Wanner A, Landa JF, Nieman RE Jr, Vevaina J, Delgado I. Bedside bronchofiberscopy for atelectasis and lung abscess. *JAMA* 1973;224:1281–1283.
54. Auerbach DA, Blackmon LR, Filston HC, Merten DF, Kirks DR. Localized pulmonary interstitial emphysema: treatment by bronchial occlusion. *Am J Perinatol* 1983;1:52–57.
55. Brantigan CO. Endoscopy for broncholith (letter). *JAMA* 1978; 240:1483.
56. Miks VM, Kvale PA, Riddle JM, Lewis JW Jr. Broncholith removal using the YAG laser. *Chest* 1986;90:295–297.
57. Millar JW, Hunter AM, Wightman AJ, Horne NW. Intralesional injection of BCG using the fibreoptic bronchoscope in the treatment of bronchogenic carcinoma. *Eur J Res Dis* 1980; 61:162–166.
58. Prakash UBS, Barham SS, Carpenter HA, Marsh HM, Dines DE. Pulmonary alveolar phospholipoproteinosis; experience with 34 cases and a review. *Mayo Clin Proc* 1987;62:499–518.

59. Heymach GJ 3d. Shaw RC, McDonald JA, Vest JV. Fiberoptic bronchopulmonary lavage for alveolar proteinosis in a patient with only one lung. *Chest* 1982;81:508–510.
60. Moazam F, Schmidt JH, Chesrown SE, Graves SA, Sauder RA, Drummond J, Heard SO, Talbert JL. Total lung lavage for pulmonary alveolar proteinosis in an infant without the use of cardiopulmonary bypass. *J Pediatr Surg* 1985;20:398–401.
61. Rankin JA, Snyder PE, Schachter EN, Matthay RA. Bronchoalveolar lavage. Its safety in subjects with mild asthma. *Chest* 1984;85:723–728.
62. Rothmann BF, Walker LH, Stone RT, Seguin FW. Bronchoscopic limited lavage for cystic fibrosis patients. An adjunct to therapy. *Ann Otol Rhinol Laryngol* 1982;91:641–642.
63. Ewing CW. Role of the fiberoptic bronchoscope in lung lavage of patients with cystic fibrosis. *Chest* 1978;73(Suppl):750–754.
64. Millis RM, Young RC Jr. Kulczycki LL. Validation of therapeutic bronchoscopic bronchial washing in cystic fibrosis. *Chest* 1977;71:508–513.
65. Quick CA, Warwick W. Bronchoscopy and lavage in management of pulmonary complications of cystic fibrosis. *Chest* 1978; 73(Suppl):755–758.
66. Sherman JM. Bronchial lavage in patients with cystic fibrosis: a critical review of current knowledge. *Pediatr Pulmonol* 1986; 2:244–246.
67. Dahm LS, Ewing CW, Harrison GM, Rucker RW. Comparison of three techniques of lung lavage in patients with cystic fibrosis. *Chest* 1977;72:593–596.
68. Hopewell PC, Miller RT. Pathophysiology and management of severe asthma. *Clin Chest Med* 1984;5:623–634.
69. Helm WH, Barran KM, Mukerjee SC. Bronchial lavage in asthma and bronchitis. *Ann Allergy* 1972;30:518–523.
70. Lang DM, Simon RA, Mathison DA, Timms RM, Stevenson DD. Safety and possible efficacy of fiberoptic bronchoscopy with lavage in the management of refractory asthma with mucous impaction. *Ann Allergy* 1991;67:324–330.
71. Millman M, Goodman AH, Goldstein IM, Millman FM, Van-Campen SS. Status asthmaticus: use of acetylcysteine during bronchoscopy and lavage to remove mucous plugs. *Ann Allergy* 1983;50(2):85–93.
72. Millman M, Goodman AH, Goldstein IM, Millman FM, Van-Campen SS. Treatment of a patient with chronic bronchial asthma with many bronchoscopies and lavages using acetylcysteine: a case report. *J Asthma* 1985;22:13–35.
73. Hovener B, Henneberg U. Limitation of prolonged nasotracheal intubation. *Anaesthesist* 1975;24:529–533.
74. Kastanos N, Estopa MR, Marin-Perez A, Xaubet MK, Agusti VA. Laryngotracheal injury due to endotracheal intubation: incidence, evolution, and predisposing factors. A prospective long-term study. *Crit Care Med* 1983;11:362–367.
75. Madden MR, Finkelstein JL, Goodwin CW. Respiratory care of the burn patient. *Clin Plast Surg* 1986;13(1):29–38.
76. Giudice JC, Komansky H, Gordon R, Kaufman JL. Acute upper airway obstruction—fiberoptic bronchoscopy in diagnosis and therapy. *Crit Care Med* 1981;9:878–979.
77. Rosenbaum SH, Rosenbaum LM, Cole RP, Askanazi J, Hyman AI. Use of the flexible fiberoptic bronchoscope to change endotracheal tubes in critically ill patients. *Anesthesiology* 1981; 54:169–170.
78. Halebian P, Shires GT. A method for replacement of the endotracheal tube with continuous control of the airway. *Surg Gynecol Obstet* 1985;161:285–286.
79. Lee KC, Weedman D, Peters WJ. Use of the fiberoptic bronchoscope to change endotracheal tubes in patients with burned airways: case report. *J Burn Care Rehabil* 1986;7(4):348–350.
80. Nielsen LH, Kristensen J, Knudsen F, Nielsen DT, Andersen PK. Fibre-optic bronchoscopic evaluation of tracheal tube position. *Eur J Anaesthesiol* 1991;8:277–279.
81. Slotnick DB, Urken ML, Sacks SH, Lawson W. Fracture, separation, and aspiration of tracheostomy tubes: management with a new technique. *Otolaryngol Head Neck Surg* 1987; 97:423–427.
82. Shinwell ES, Higgins RD, Auten RL, Shapiro DL. Fiberoptic bronchoscopy in the treatment of intubated neonates. *Am J Dis Child* 1989;143:1064–1065.
83. Fan LL, Sparks LM, Fix FJ. Flexible fiberoptic endoscopy for airway problems in a pediatric intensive care unit. *Chest* 1988; 93:556–560.
84. Miller RW, Pollack MM, Murphy TM, Fink RJ. Effectiveness of continuous positive airway pressure in the treatment of bronchomalacia in infants: a bronchoscopic documentation. *Crit Care Med* 1986;14:125–127.
85. Vigneswaran R, Whitfield JM. The use of a new ultra-thin fiberoptic bronchoscope to determine endotracheal tube position in the sick newborn infant. *Chest* 1981;80:174–177.
86. Dellinger RP. Fiberoptic bronchoscopy in adult airway management. *Crit Care Med* 1990;18:882–887.
87. Schwartz DE, Wiener-Kronish JP. Management of the difficult airway. *Clin Chest Med* 1991;12:483–495.
88. Gibney RTN, Brennan NJ, Davys RT, FitzGerald MX. Fibreoptic bronchoscopy in the intensive care unit. *Ir J Med Sci* 1984;153:416–420.
89. Milledge IS. Therapeutic fibreoptic bronchoscopy in intensive care. *Br Med J* 1976;2:1427–1429.
90. Snow N, Lucas AE. Bronchoscopy in the critically ill surgical patient. *Am Surg* 1984;50:441–445.
91. Jolliet P, Chevrolet JC. Bronchoscopy in the intensive care unit. *Inten Care Med* 1992;18:160–169.
92. Krell WS. Pulmonary diagnostic procedures in the critically ill. *Crit Care Clin North Am* 1988;4:393–407.
93. Weinstein HJ, Bone RC, Ruth WE. Pulmonary lavage in patients treated with mechanical ventilation. *Chest* 1977; 72:583–587.
94. Jung RC, Gottlieb LS. Comparison of tracheobronchial suction catheters in humans. Visualization by fiberoptic bronchoscopy. *Chest* 1976;69:179–181.
95. Prakash UBS, Stubbs SE. The bronchoscopy survey: some reflections. *Chest* 1991;100:1660–1667.
96. Trouillet J-L, Guiguet M, Gibert C, Fagon J-Y, Dreyfuss D, Blanchet F, Chastre J. Fiberoptic bronchoscopy in ventilated patients. Evaluation of cardiopulmonary risk under midazolam sedation. *Chest* 1990;97:927–933.
97. Pincus PS, Kallenbach JM, Hurwitz MD, Clinton C, Feldman C, Abramowitz JA, Zwi S. Transbronchial biopsy during mechanical ventilation. *Crit Care Med* 1987;15:1136–1139.
98. Papin TA, Grum CM, Weg JG. Transbronchial lung biopsy during mechanical ventilation. *Chest* 1986;89:168–170.
99. Karetsky MS, Graver JW, Brandstetter RD. Effect of fiberoptic bronchoscopy on arterial oxygen tension. *NY State J Med* 1974;74:62–63.
100. Credle WF, JF Smiddy, RC Elliot. Complications of fiberoptic bronchoscopy. *Am Rev Resp Dis* 1974;109:67–72.
101. Shrader DL, Lakshminarayan S. The effect of fiberoptic bronchoscopy on cardiac rhythm. *Chest* 1978;73:821–824.
102. Luck JC, Messender OH, Rubenstin MJ, et al. Arrhythmias from fiberoptic bronchoscopy. *Chest* 1978;74:139–149.
103. Pereira W, Kounat D, Zacovino J. Fever and pneumonia following fiberoptic bronchoscopy. *Am Rev Resp Dis* 1974; 109:692–693.
104. Witte MC, Opal JM, Gilbert JG, et al. Incidence of fever and bacteremia following transbronchial needle aspiration. *Chest* 1986;89:85–87.
105. Dreisin R, Albert RK, Talley PA, et al. Flexible fiberoptic bronchoscopy in the teaching hospital: yield and complications. *Chest* 1978;74:144–149.
106. Burns DM, Shure D, Francoz R, et al. The physiologic consequences of saline lobar lavage in healthy human adults. *Am Rev Resp Dis* 1983;127:695–701.
107. Hanson RR, Zavala DC, Rhodes ML, et al. Transbronchial biopsy via the flexible fiberoptic bronchoscope. *Am Rev Resp Dis* 1976;114:67–72.
108. Herf SM, Suratt PM, Arora NS. Deaths and complications associated with transbronchial lung biopsy. *Am Rev Resp Dis* 1977;115:708–711.
109. Zavala DC. Pulmonary hemorrhage in fiberoptic transbronchial biopsy. *Chest* 1976;70:584–588.
110. Rodgers BM, Moazam F, Talbert JL. Endotracheal cryotherapy in the treatment of refractory airway strictures. *Ann Thorac Surg* 1983;35:52–57.

111. Sanderson DR, Neel HB III, Fontana RS. Bronchoscopic cryotherapy. *Ann Otol Rhinol Laryngol* 1981;90:354–358.
112. Homasson JP, Renault P, Angebault M, Bonniot JP, Bell NJ. Bronchoscopic cryotherapy for airway strictures caused by tumors. *Chest* 1986;90:159–164.
113. Rodgers BM, Moazam F, Talbert JL. Successful cryotherapy of a benign tracheal neoplasm. *J Pediatr Surg* 1988;23:771–774.
114. Walsh DA, Maiwand MO, Nath AR, Lockwood P, Lloyd MH, Saab M. Bronchoscopic cryotherapy for advanced bronchial carcinoma. *Thorax* 1990;45:509–513.
115. Maiwand MO. Cryotherapy for advanced carcinoma of the trachea and bronchi. *Br Med J* 1986;293:181–182.
116. Cotton RT. Pediatric laryngotracheal stenosis. *J Pediatr Surg* 1984;19:699–704.
117. Gerasin VA, Shafirovsky BB. Endobronchial electrosurgery. *Chest* 1988;93(2):270–274.
118. Marsh BR. Bipolar cautery for the fiberoptic bronchoscope. *Ann Otol Rhinol Laryngol* 1987;96:120–121.
119. Hooper RG, Jackson FN. Endobronchial electrocautery. *Chest* 1985;87:712–714.
120. Davidoff AM, Filston HC. Treatment of infantile subglottic hemangioma with electrocautery. *J Pediatr Surg* 1992; 27:436–439.
121. Hooper RG, Spratling L, Beechler C, Schaffner S. Endobronchial electrocautery: a role in bronchogenic carcinoma? *Endoscopy* 1984;16:67–70.
122. Keller C, Frost A. Fiberoptic bronchoplasty. Description of a simple adjunct technique for the management of bronchial stenosis following lung transplantation. *Chest* 1992; 102:995–998.
123. Ball JB, Delaney JC, Evans CC, Donnelly RJ, Hind CR. Endoscopic bougie and balloon dilatation of multiple bronchial stenoses: 10 year follow up. *Thorax* 1991;46:933–935.
124. Nakamura K, Terada N, Ohi M, Matsushita T, Kato N, Nakagawa T. Tuberculous bronchial stenosis: treatment with balloon bronchoplasty. *Am J Roentgenol* 1991;157:1187–1188.
125. Bagwell CE, Talbert JL, Tepas JJ. Balloon dilatation of long-segment tracheal stenoses. *J Pediatr Surg* 1991;26:153–159.
126. Carlin BW, Harrell JH 2d, Moser KM. The treatment of endobronchial stenosis using balloon catheter dilatation. *Chest* 1988; 93:1148–1151.

Bronchoscopy,
edited by U. B. S. Prakash.
Mayo Foundation © 1994.
Published by Raven Press, Ltd., New York.

CHAPTER 17

Hemoptysis and Bronchoscopy-Induced Hemorrhage

Udaya B. S. Prakash and Lutz Freitag

Hemoptysis denotes the expectoration of blood that originates from the tracheobronchial tree or the pulmonary parenchyma. It is one of the most common symptoms in clinical practice. When the physician is challenged by the patient's complaint of "coughing" or "spitting" of blood, the first step is to determine if the bleeding is indeed originating in the respiratory system. It is not uncommon for patients to confuse true hemoptysis from pseudohemoptysis. The latter represents the expectoration of blood aspirated into the respiratory tract from supraglottic regions or the gastrointestinal tract. The major clinical differences between hemoptysis and pseudohemoptysis are listed in Table 1. Because hemoptysis is a fear-evoking symptom, the majority of patients who present with the first episode of hemoptysis are inclined to overestimate the amount of blood expectorated. This factor tends to inject a certain degree of urgency to the evaluation and treatment of the causative disease. The most common causes of significant hemoptysis worldwide are tuberculosis (Fig. 1), bronchiectasis, necrotizing pneumonia, and bronchogenic carcinoma (Fig. 2) (1–9). Chronic bronchitis is responsible for nearly 25% of all cases of hemoptysis (Fig. 3). Despite detailed evaluations, nearly 25% of all cases of hemoptysis remain undiagnosed. Table 2 lists the etiologies of hemoptysis.

ANATOMIC SOURCE OF HEMOPTYSIS

Hemoptysis can arise from four different vascular sources within the pulmonary system: bronchial arteries, pulmonary arteries, pulmonary veins, and pulmonary capillaries. In addition, acquired communications between the tracheobronchial tree and major vascular structures in the thoracic cage resulting from trauma, neoplasms, or radiation therapy can lead to massive

TABLE 1. *Differences between hemoptysis and pseudohemoptysis*

Clinical features	Hemoptysis	Pseudohemoptysis
Origin of blood	Respiratory tract	Oral cavity Larynx Esophagus and stomach Fictitious
Cough	More likely	Less likely
Respiratory symptoms	More likely	Less likely
Esophagogastric symptoms	Less likely	More likely
Alcohol use, hepatic disease	Less likely	More likely
Vomiting, nausea	Less likely	More likely
Hematemesis and melena	Less likely	More likely
Color of expectorated blood	Bright red	Brown or black
Consistency of expectorate	Clotted or liquid	Coffee ground appearance
Frothiness of expectorate	Usual	Never or seldom
pH of expectorate	Alkaline	Acidic
Pulmonary macrophages in expectorate	Present	Absent
Food particles in expectorate	Absent	Present

U. B. S. Prakash: Division of Thoracic Diseases and Internal Medicine, Mayo Clinic, Rochester, Minnesota 55905.
L. Freitag: Department of Bronchoscopy, Ruhrland Klinik, Center for Chest Medicine and Thoracic Surgery, Essen, Germany.

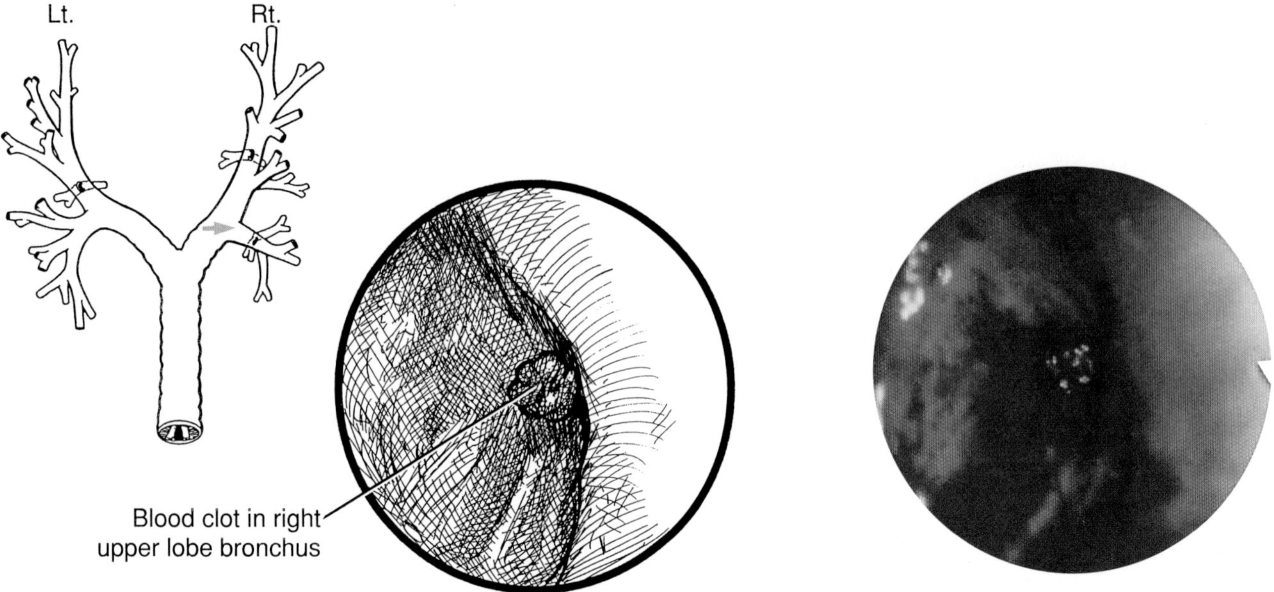

FIG. 1. Continuous oozing of blood from a tuberculous cavity in the right upper lobe. Tuberculosis remains the most common cause of significant hemoptysis worldwide.

life-threatening hemoptysis (10). Bronchial arterial bleeding tends to be brisk because of the systemic blood pressure in the bronchial arterial circulation (11,12). The submucosal plexus of arteries is made up of terminal branches of bronchial arteries (13). Most cases of bronchiectasis, bronchogenic carcinomas, bronchitis, trauma to the tracheobronchial tree, trauma caused by foreign bodies, mycetomas, and other cavitary diseases of the lung produce bronchial bleeding, even though bronchial and pulmonary circulations anastomose at several levels (12,14). The bleeding from the pulmonary arterial system, on the other hand, is

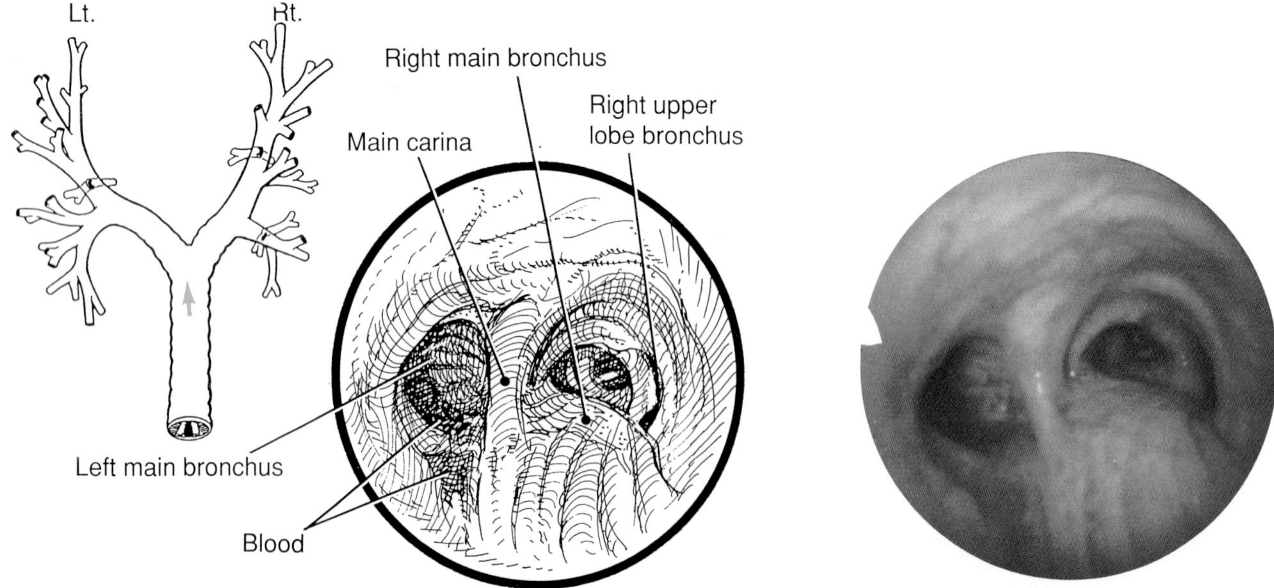

FIG. 2. Left main stem bronchial hemorrhage caused by primary bronchogenic carcinoma located distally.

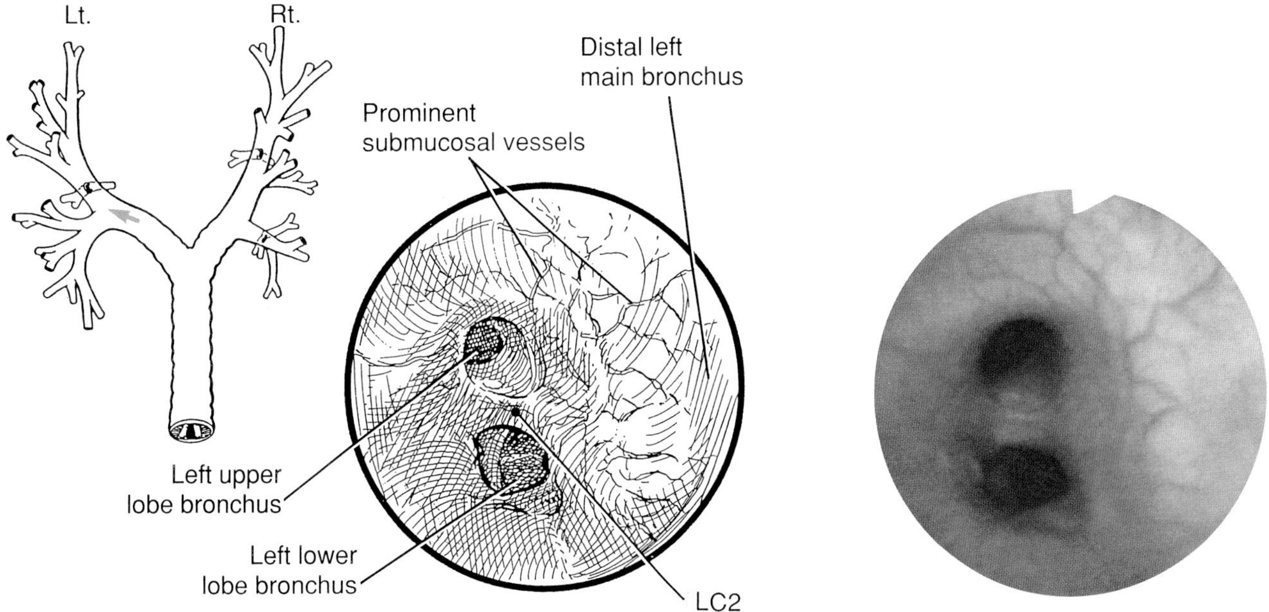

FIG. 3. Submucosal capillary proliferation secondary to chronic bronchitis. Chronic bronchitis is the most common cause of insignificant or streaky hemoptysis.

usually not brisk because of low pressure in the pulmonary artery tree. Severe bleeding, however, may develop in patients with pulmonary arteriovenous malformations (Osler–Rendu–Weber syndrome) or fistulas (Fig. 4) (15). Pulmonary capillary hemorrhage is secondary to disruption of the alveolocapillary integrity and may cause various amounts of bleeding and hemoptysis. Examples of alveolar hemorrhage syndrome are listed in Table 2 (16–22).

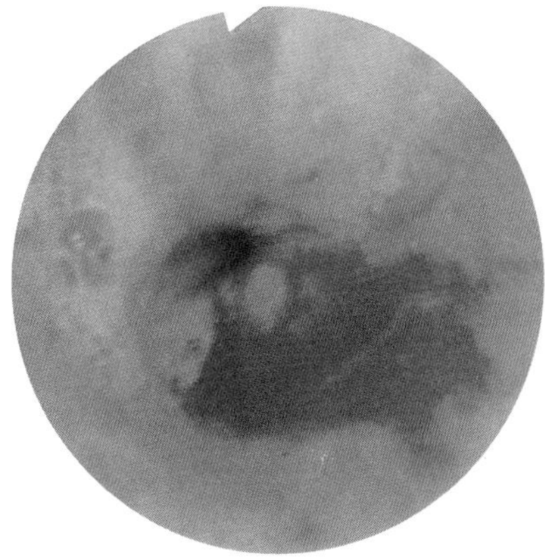

FIG. 4. Bleeding from the left lower lobe caused by pulmonary arteriovenous malformation.

HEMOPTYSIS

Diagnostic Evaluation

Hemoptysis Versus Pseudohemoptysis

The first information that must be obtained if a patient complains of blood-stained sputum is whether the blood originates from the respiratory tract (Table 1). Hematemesis is usually related to a long history of gastric complains or alcoholism. Nausea and vomiting usually precede gastrointestinal hemorrhage. The blood may contain food particles and has a pH of 7.0 or less. Bleeding from esophageal varices can be clearly distinguished from hemoptysis by the patient's history. Occasionally, blood originating in the esophagus or stomach is aspirated and coughed up. The clinical picture and an astute patient contribute to the determination of whether the blood originates from the respiratory or alimentary tract. Bleeding might also result from lesions in the nose, nasopharynx, oral cavity, or larynx. Rhinolaryngological examination can clear this issue (23).

Massive Hemoptysis

The definition of massive hemoptysis is somewhat arbitrary, with the criteria ranging from 100 to 600 ml in 24 hr (24). This definition, based on the volume of blood expectorated, can be misleading for two reasons. First, patients tend to overestimate the amount of blood coughed up. If the blood is mixed with mucus, it will be difficult for even the physician, let alone the patient, to provide a proper estimate. Second, even though the large volume of blood expectorated may indicate a serious pathology, it is uncommon to see patients who exsanguinate from this. Asphyxia from airway blockage by blood clot is more likely to produce serious respiratory insufficiency. Inadequate pulmonary reserve and other serious illnesses may effect respiratory distress with even smaller volumes of blood

TABLE 2. *Causes of hemoptysis*

1. Neoplastic Diseases of Lung
    - Bronchial/tracheal cancer (primary or metastatic)[a,b]
    - Carcinoid (adenoma)[b]
    - Hamartoma
    - Hematogenous metastases[b]
    - Leukemia
    - Lymphoma (primary or metastatic)
    - Parenchymal tumors (primary or metastatic)[a,b]
    - Tumor emboli[b]
    - Uncommon tumors

2. Infectious Diseases
    - Bacterial infections
        - Acute bronchitis[a]
        - Acute tracheitis[a]
        - Anaerobic pneumonia
        - Aspiration pneumonia
        - Bacterial endocarditis
        - Chronic bronchitis[a]
        - Lung abscess[b]
        - Necrotizing pneumonia[a]
    - Mycobacterioses
        - Endobronchial tuberculosis
        - Tuberculous cavity[a,b]
        - Tuberculous pneumonia
    - Mycoses
        - Actinomycosis
        - Aspergilloma[b]
        - Blastomycosis
        - Coccidioidomycosis
        - Cryptococcosis
        - Histoplasmosis
        - Nocardiosis
        - Sporotrichosis
        - Zygomycosis (mucor)[b]
    - Parasitic infections
        - Amebiasis
        - Ascariasis
        - Clonorchiasis
        - Hydatid disease
        - Paragonimiasis
        - Schistosomiasis
        - Strongyloidosis
        - Trichinosis
    - Viral pneumonitis

3. Cardiovascular Disorders
    - Amniotic fluid embolism
    - Aortic aneurysm (thoracic and abdominal)[b]
    - Bronchial telangiectasia
    - Congenital heart disease
    - Congestive cardiac failure[a]
    - Fat embolism
    - Hugh–Stovin syndrome
    - Mitral stenosis/insufficiency[b,c]
    - Neonatal pulmonary hemorrhage[b]
    - Post–myocardial infarction syndrome
    - Pulmonary arteriovenous fistula (congenital or acquired)[b]
    - Pulmonary embolism[a]
    - Pulmonary hypertension[b]
    - Pulmonary venoocclusive disease
    - Pulmonary venous varix
    - Superior vena cava syndrome

4. Vasculitides and Collagenoses
    - Behçet's disease[b]
    - Churg–Strauss syndrome[b]
    - Henoch–Schöenlein purpura
    - Lymphomatoid granulomatosis[b]
    - Mixed connective tissue disease
    - Mixed cryoglobulinemia
    - Scleroderma
    - Systemic lupus erythematosus[b,c]
    - Takayasu's arteritis[b]
    - Wegener's granulomatosis[b,c]

5. Trauma
    - Blunt chest trauma[b]
    - Penetrating injury[b]
    - Pulmonary contusion
    - Ruptured trachea/bronchus
    - Tracheobronchial foreign body[b]

6. Iatrogenic Procedures
    - Bronchoscopy
    - Cardiac catheterization
    - Endotracheal tubes
    - Pulmonary artery catheterization[b]
    - Radiation necrosis
    - Thoracic surgery
    - Tracheal suctioning
    - Tracheostomy
    - Transthoracic needle procedures[b]
    - Transtracheal needle procedures

7. Hemorrhagic Diatheses
    - Anticoagulant therapy
    - Disseminated intravascular coagulation[c]
    - Immune-suppressed patient
    - Renal failure
    - Thrombocytopenia
    - Other coagulopathies

8. Miscellaneous
    - Amyloidosis[b]
    - Bronchial stump granuloma
    - Bronchiectasis[a,b]
    - Broncholithiasis
    - Bronchial/pulmonary endometriosis[b]
    - Bronchopleural fistula
    - Bronchopulmonary sequestration
    - Congenital and acquired cysts
    - Cystic fibrosis[a,b]
    - Eosinophilic granuloma (histiocytosis-X)
    - Glomerulonephritis[b,c]
    - Goodpasture's syndrome[b,c]
    - Hydatid mole
    - Idiopathic pulmonary hemosiderosis[b,c]
    - IgA nephropathy[c]
    - Lymphangioleiomyomatosis
    - Sarcoidosis
    - Toxic fume inhalation
    - Tracheoesophageal fistula
    - Tracheopathia osteoplastica
    - Trimellitic anhydride[b,c]

9. Idiopathic Conditions[a]

[a] Common causes of hemoptysis.
[b] Causes of massive hemoptysis.
[c] Causes of alveolar hemorrhage syndrome.

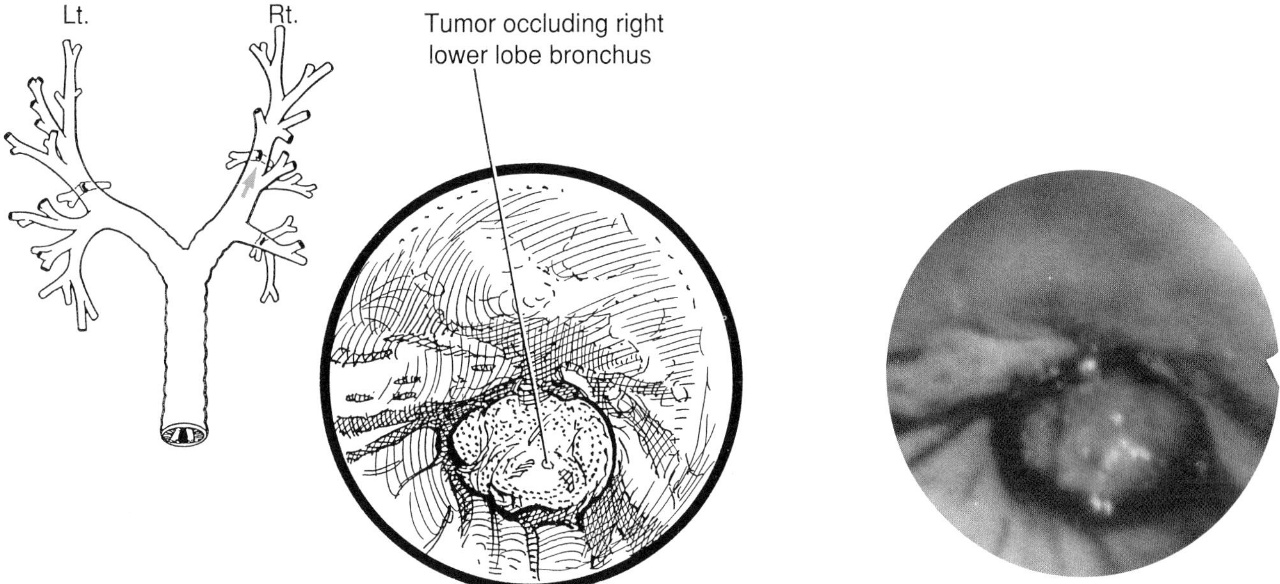

FIG. 5. Metastatic hypernephroma (involving right lower lobe bronchus) is frequently manifested by significant hemoptysis and expectoration of tumor fragments.

in the tracheobronchial tree or the alveolar spaces (25). Massive hemoptysis usually involves disruption of the high-pressure bronchial circulation or pulmonary circulation pathologically exposed to the high pressures of bronchial circulation (26,27). Massive hemoptysis can also occur from the disruption of alveolocapillary interphase, as seen in many of the alveolar hemorrhage syndromes (Table 2).

Worldwide, tuberculosis remains the most common cause of massive hemoptysis. The development of Rasmussen's aneurysm, an ectatic vessel typically found in tuberculous cavities and prone to rupture, has been responsible for the majority of cases of massive hemoptysis (3,28). Primary tracheobronchial neoplasms may occasionally produce significant hemoptysis. Among the metastatic tumors involving the tracheobronchial tree, hemoptysis is more likely from metastases secondary to hypernephroma (Fig. 5), thyroid carcinoma, and lymphoma (29). Bronchiectasis and cystic fibrosis are also responsible for a significant number of patients who present with massive hemoptysis (11,25). Aspergilloma (mycetoma) is complicated by significant hemoptysis in 50%–78% of patients (30–34). Zygomycetes (mucorale species) have a special propensity to invade vascular structures and can cause massive bleeding from bronchial or pulmonary arterial tree (7,8,35). Lung abscess, typically resulting from anaerobic bacterial infection, is a well-recognized cause of massive hemoptysis (36). Pulmonary embolism is also responsible for significant hemoptysis (37). Pulmonary vasculitides and disorders that cause pulmonary alveolar hemorrhage syndromes frequently result in significant hemoptysis (38,39). Both blunt and penetrating trauma to the thoracic cage and major airways can result in massive hemoptysis (40,41). Mitral stenosis is still a relatively common cause of massive hemoptysis in regions of the world where rheumatic fever and its cardiac complications are common (Fig. 6).

Clinical Examination

Obtaining an accurate history is of utmost importance. The presence of pulmonary and nonpulmonary diseases may provide the necessary information. The

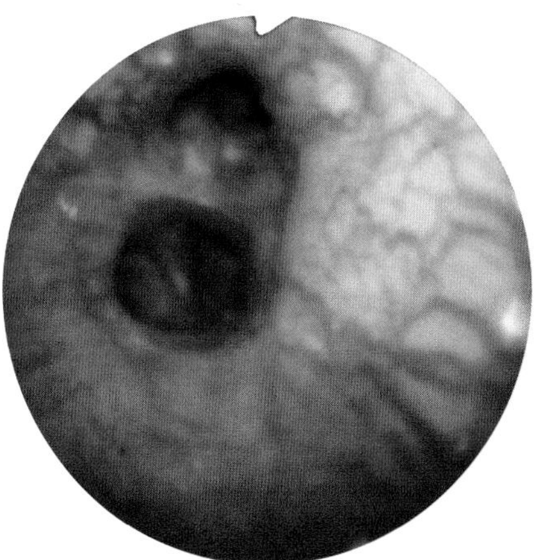

FIG. 6. Hemoptysis in this case was caused by mitral stenosis. Note the exuberant proliferation of submucosal vasculature in the distal left main stem bronchus.

patient can be helpful in determining the site of bleeding. Some patients obviously can sense where the blood comes from. Information about the frequency, timing, relation to activity and body position, etc., should be taken into consideration. Occasionally, the detection of unilateral or localized crackles or wheezes may point to the source of hemoptysis (42). Auscultation of lung may also reveal continuous bruits or hum related to an underlying arteriovenous malformation or cavernous (or amphoric) type of bronchial sounds arising from a cavitated lesion. Pleuritic chest pain, pleural friction rub, and hemoptysis can occur in pulmonary embolism. Cardiac examination may suggest the presence of significant valvular disease that may be responsible for the hemoptysis. Clinical signs of other disorders such as hereditary hemorrhagic telangiectasia, vasculitis, renal diseases, and hemorrhagic diseases may also provide clues.

Chest Roentgenograph

Chest roentgenography is perhaps the most important initial diagnostic test in the evaluation of hemoptysis. All patients who present with hemoptysis should be subjected to both a posteroanterior and a lateral chest roentgenography. Any chest roentgenological abnormality should be considered as a potential source for the hemoptysis. Large masses, cavitated lesions, and abnormalities that indicate postobstructive pneumonia are more likely to cause hemoptysis than ill-defined fibrotic infiltrates (1,2,4,7,8). Patients who had previously suffered from tuberculosis or inflammatory scar–type endobronchial lesions may present with hemoptysis even though their chest roentgenograms show chronic or inactive-looking lesions. Such findings should not be ignored because many cases of massive hemoptysis are encountered in patients with chronic, mild, and insignificant appearing roentgenological abnormalities. A normal chest roentgenogram does not exclude the respiratory tract as the source of hemoptysis. Indeed, neoplastic lesions of large airways may not be visible on the chest roentgenogram (43). However, one study of 45 patients with hemoptysis and normal or only nonlocalizing chest roentgenological abnormalities assessed the role of flexible bronchoscopy and found that in none of the patients was there evidence of malignant neoplasms found either at the time of the initial evaluation or at the time of follow-up 3 years later (44).

A significant number of chest roentgenograms in adults reveal calcified areas that are usually ignored during the viewing of the chest roentgenograph. In the presence of hemoptysis, such lesions should be carefully assessed because broncholithiasis, which they may represent, is a well-known cause of hemoptysis (Figs. 7 and 8).

Other Imaging Procedures

Plain tomography or computed tomography scans are invaluable diagnostic tools if the chest roentgenogram does not provide sufficient information. However, not every patient who present with hemoptysis requires a special imaging procedure. The high-resolu-

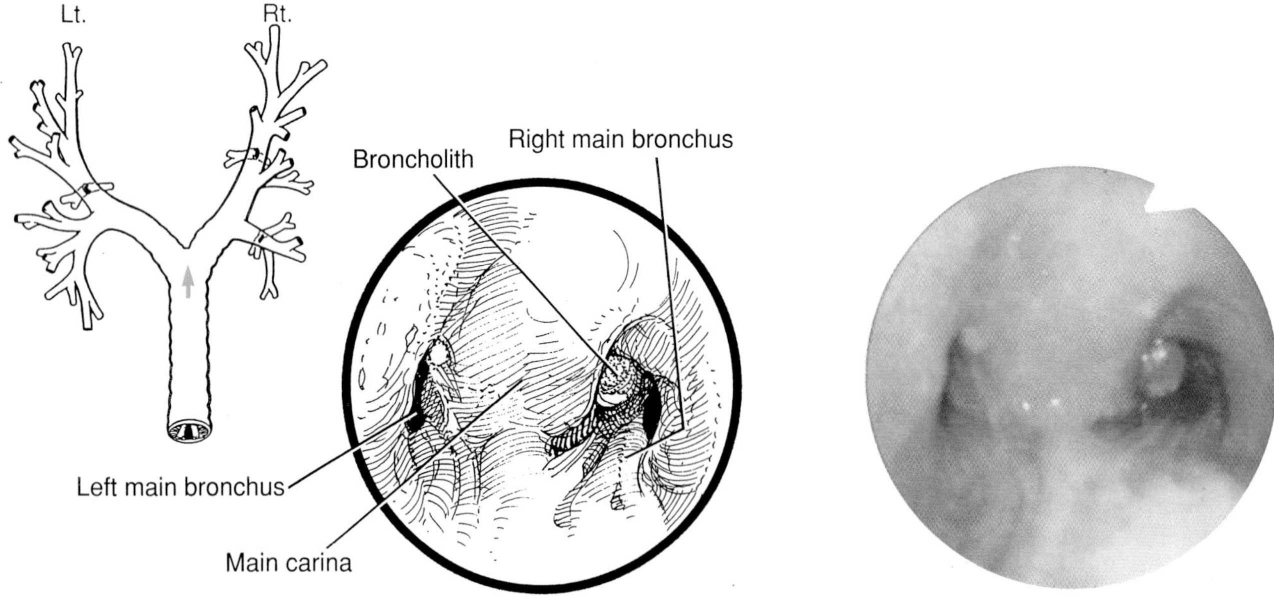

FIG. 7. Hemoptysis caused by broncholithiasis involving the medial wall of right main stem bronchus. Subcarinal lymph node calcification preceded the broncholithiasis.

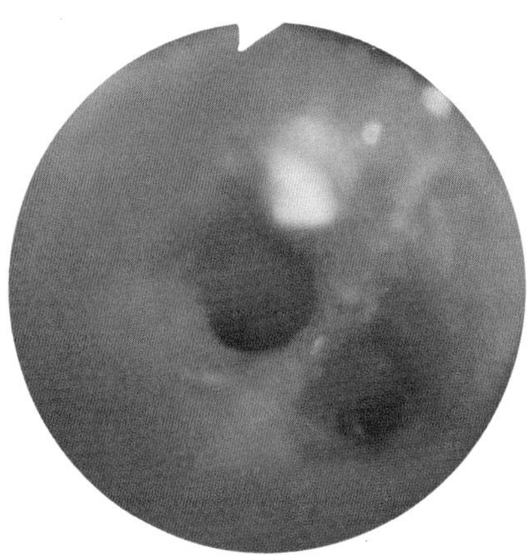

FIG. 8. Significant hemoptysis secondary to broncholithiasis involving right middle lobe bronchus.

tion computed tomography of the chest has supplanted bronchography for the diagnosis of bronchiectasis (45). At present, bronchography remains the "gold standard" and is recommended if surgical resection of bronchiectatic segments is contemplated (46).

Pulmonary arteriography is required for the definitive mapping of pulmonary arteriovenous malformations and fistulas (47). Bronchial angiography is sometimes needed to identify the blood vessel responsible for significant hemoptysis (48). Perfusion-ventilation scan aids in the diagnosis of pulmonary embolism. A study evaluated the role of bronchial arteriography in 36 patients during active hemoptysis and reported that positive arteriographies were observed in 56%; arteriography was positive in only two of the eight cases in which flexible bronchoscopy did not localize the site of bleeding (49). The indications should be carefully assessed before subjecting patients to these costly and invasive procedures.

Radionuclide scanning using technetium sulfur colloid and radiolabeled erythrocytes has been used for the localization of bleeding site (50,51). A prerequisite for application of these techniques is that the bleeding be active and at least at a rate of 6 ml/min. Such a rate of bleeding should be easily distinguished by bronchoscopy. The need for these techniques is somewhat limited in clinical practice.

Serial measurement of diffusing capacity for carbon monoxide has been reported to be helpful in the diagnosis of continuous pulmonary parenchymal bleeding in patients with alveolar hemorrhage syndrome (52). If the diffusing capacity for carbon monoxide increases from the baseline measurement, it signifies new uptake of carbon monoxide due to influx of new red blood cells into the alveoli. Our own experience has shown this to be an unreliable test.

Echocardiography is useful for the diagnosis of mitral valve stenosis and left ventricular dysfunction, both of which can lead to hemoptysis. The echocardiogram is also helpful in detecting cardiac from a noncardiac arteriovenous shunt, such as pulmonary arteriovenous malformations.

Laboratory Data

Laboratory tests are of limited help. The estimation of hematocrit and hemoglobin levels may or may not indicate loss of blood through the respiratory tract. Serial measurement of these parameters is important in the follow-up of patients who develop persistent or significant bleeding as in idiopathic pulmonary hemosiderosis and Goodpasture's syndrome. Tests to assess the coagulation mechanism are not routinely required unless the clinical features indicate the presence of such a problem. Hemorrhagic diathesis by themselves do not lead to spontaneous hemoptysis. In the presence of such disorders, trauma to the thoracic cage or instrumentation of the tracheobronchial tree or pulmonary parenchyma may induce bleeding. Immunological diseases such as Wegener's granulomatosis, systemic lupus erythematosus, and Goodpasture's syndrome can be diagnosed by serological markers. Immediate results cannot be expected from these tests. In the presence of active and brisk hemoptysis, these tests will have limited value.

Sputum specimens, if easily obtainable, can be assessed for infectious mircroorganisms, malignant cells, and hemosiderin-laden macrophage. In geographic areas where other tests are prohibitively expensive or unavailable, the physician has to depend on clinical examination and sputum analysis. Massive hemoptysis may not allow the luxury of waiting for the results of sputum cultures or serologic tests.

Diagnostic Bronchoscopy

The singularly important diagnostic test is bronchoscopy. Even if other diagnostic tests suggest a plausible cause of the hemoptysis, a bronchoscopic examination is mandatory in most patients. However, not every patient with hemoptysis requires a bronchoscopy. Chronic and streaky hemoptysis in a smoker with chronic bronchitis may not require bronchoscopy. Likewise, if the cause of hemoptysis is already established, as in mitral stenosis, Goodpasture's syndrome, systemic lupus erythematosus, or pulmonary vasculitis, bronchoscopy is unlikely to add to the management of the underlying problem. Rapid and complete resolution of hemoptysis following medical therapy is another reason for not performing bronchoscopy (53). On the other hand, persistent hemoptysis in the face of

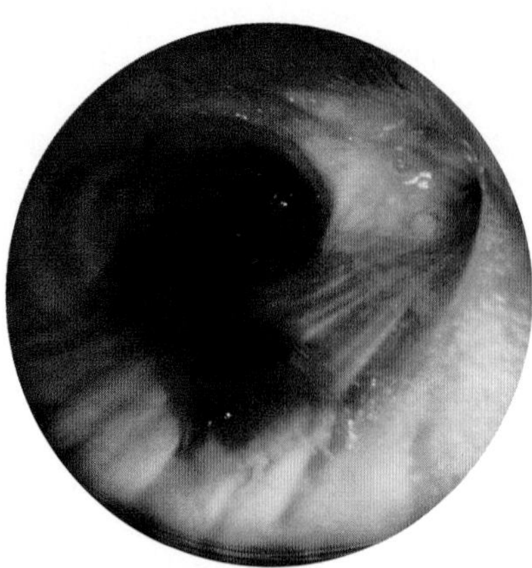

FIG. 9. A streak of old or dark blood in the right lower lobe bronchus suggests the likelihood of bleeding source on the right. Further bronchoscopic exploration is necessary to detect the etiology.

improvement of other clinical features should warn the physician that an unrelated cause may be responsible for the hemoptysis. It is of interest to note that in a survey of 114 physicians, 40% responded that a fear of litigation was one of the potential external factors influencing patient selection for bronchoscopy (54).

Some in the past have argued that bronchoscopy should not be done in the presence of active hemoptysis. We believe that to obtain as much information as possible regarding this symptom, bronchoscopy should be performed as soon as the patient presents with hemoptysis. In a study that analyzed the records of 129 consecutive patients with hemoptysis, early (during hemoptysis or during the 48 hr after hemoptysis stopped) flexible bronchoscopy more frequently localized and/or diagnosed the source of bleeding and influenced clinical outcome than delayed (48 hr or more after hemoptysis stopped) bronchoscopy (55). However, even though the likelihood of visualizing active bleeding (41% versus 8%) or its site (34% versus 11%) was significantly higher with early versus delayed procedure, respectively, neither active bleeding nor a bleeding site was visualized in at least 60% of the 92 patients who underwent early bronchoscopy. Definitive (bronchoscopic) diagnoses by early or delayed bronchoscopy occurred primarily in patients with neoplasm. Nevertheless, early, single bronchoscopy was generally neither diagnostic nor therapeutically decisive in those patients. Another study evaluated the role of bronchoscopy in 25 patients during active hemoptysis and reported that the bleeding site was identified in 68% (49). The likelihood of localizing the bleeding site was significantly higher with early (91%) versus delayed (50%) flexible bronchoscopy.

Indications for bronchoscopy in patients with hemoptysis and a normal or nonlocalizing chest roentgenogram is somewhat controversial. One study reviewed the records of 119 bronchoscopies performed for hemoptysis in patients with a normal or nonlocalizing chest roentgenogram and detected bronchogenic carcinoma in 2.5% of the bronchoscopies and other neoplasms in another 2.5%. Certain factors, namely,

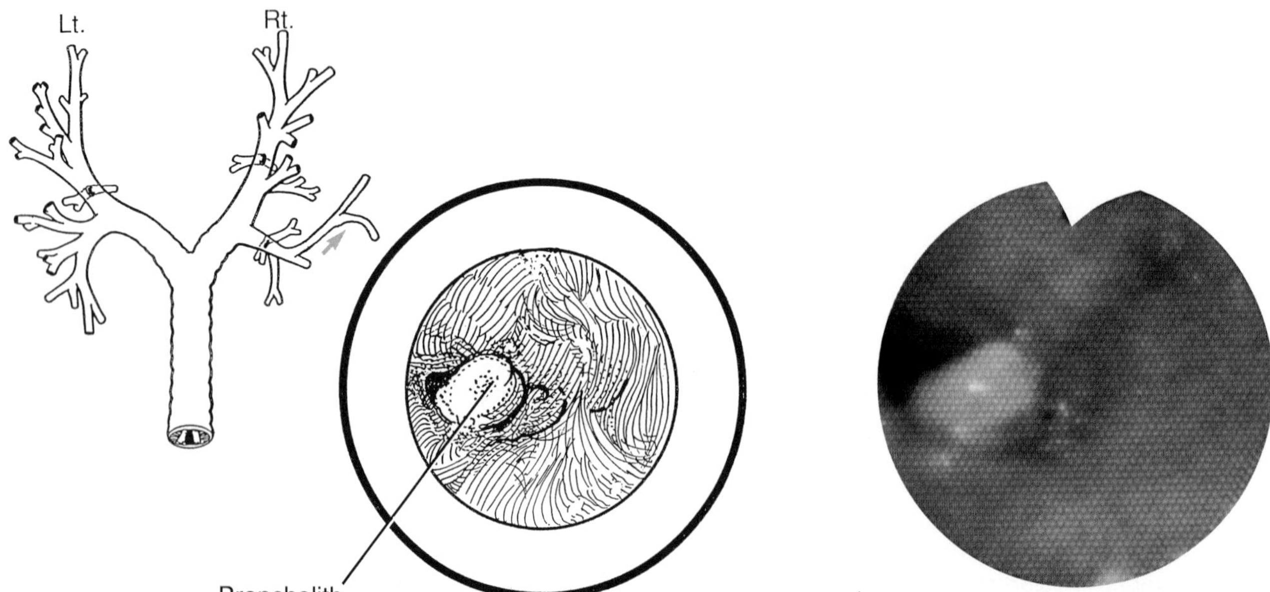

FIG. 10. Significant hemoptysis in this middle-aged male was investigated by three standard flexible bronchoscopies. Even though blood was seen exuding from the right upper lobe bronchus, the etiology could not be determined. Examination with a thin (pediatric) flexible bronchoscope revealed a broncholith in the seventh-generation branch of RB1.

the male sex, age above 40 years, and a more than 40-pack-a-year smoking history, appeared useful in identifying patients in whom the yield of bronchoscopy was likely to be high (56). Another study evaluated the role of flexible bronchoscopy in 196 patients with hemoptysis and nonlocalizing chest roentgenogram and reported that bleeding in excess of 30 ml daily, smoking of 40 pack-years or more, male sex, and age of 50 years or more were associated with an increase in overall diagnostic yield (57).

Very often a bronchoscopic examination shows that there is no directly visible source of bleeding. Sometimes only a "streak" of blood is found in the airway (Fig. 9). The task of the bronchoscopist is to track it down, as far as possible, preferably to a segmental, at least to a lobar, bronchus. In spite of an exhaustive bronchoscopic examination, it is common, especially if the chest roentgenogram is normal, to see traces of old blood without any hint as to the origin of the bleeding. If the standard flexible bronchoscope cannot identify the source of bleeding, an ultrathin bronchoscope may permit examination of the more distal bronchial tree. This technique has been used to identify the source of hemoptysis in patients with peripheral airway lesions (Fig. 10) (58). If no active bleeding is detected, the patient should be instructed to cough to see if this maneuver can induce bleeding. If a source cannot be identified, a diagnostic bronchoscopy has to be repeated as soon as new blood is coughed up.

If the bleeding from the respiratory tract is brisk and continuous, it is essential to use adequate topical anesthesia to control the cough. Excessive coughing by the patient not only clouds the objective lens of the bronchoscope but also spreads the blood to uninvolved areas of the tracheobronchial tree, thereby making it difficult to identify the exact source of bleeding. The bronchoscopist should pay special attention to the mucosa and the visible vessels. Obvious vascular abnormalities such as hemangiomas (Fig. 11), generalized inflammation, hypertrophy of vessels, and so forth are valuable findings. Biopsies for histological examination should be made from all visible neoplasms. Administration of vasoactive drugs prior to biopsy can reduce the risk of further heavy bleeding (see below). The risk of bleeding from the biopsy of bronchial carcinoid is frequently mentioned during bronchoscopy training,

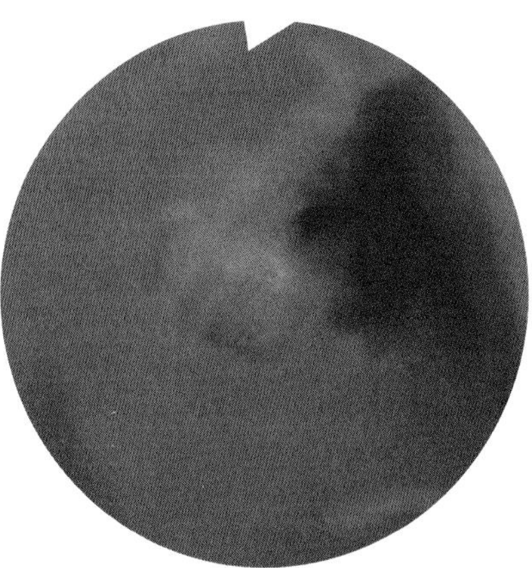

FIG. 11. Significant hemoptysis caused by hemangioma involving right middle lobe.

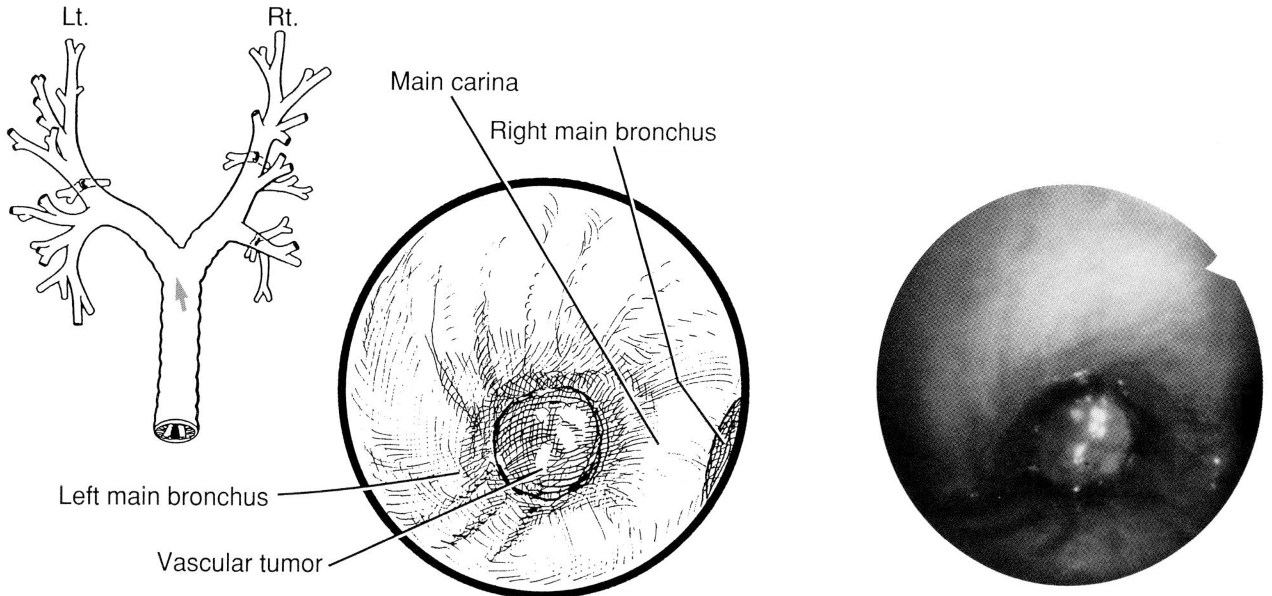

FIG. 12. Hemoptysis in this case was caused by carcinoid tumor of the left main stem bronchus. The high vascularity of this tumor should not persuade the bronchoscopist to abandon biopsy.

but we believe that a biopsy can be safely obtained from most carcinoid tumors without great risk of severe hemorrhage (Fig. 12). The use of vasoactive agents may minimize the bleeding.

Bronchial washing and brushing should be collected for cytological and microbiological studies if the bronchoscopic examination is nondiagnostic for visible tumors. Obviously, the need for these studies will depend on clinical aspects of each patient. In patients with suspected tuberculosis, immediate microscopic examination for acid-fast bacilli is recommended even if roentgenological changes are not typical. Bronchoalveolar lavage (BAL) may play an important role in the diagnosis of the alveolar hemorrhage syndrome, which can be found in immunocompromised patients, recipients of bone marrow transplantation, patients with immunological lung diseases, and vasculitis, etc. (59,60). Traces of blood can be found in the initial BAL effluent. In alveolar hemorrhage syndromes, however, the BAL effluent becomes progressively bloodier. Alveolar macrophages contain ingested erythrocytes and are filled with hemosiderin. In idiopathic hemosiderosis, in the absence of active hemorrhage, the supernatant shows a typical orange–brown color (Fig. 13). One problem with relying on the hemosiderin-laden macrophages is that there is no standardized method to quantify the number of cells in the sputum or the BAL effluent.

Despite all diagnostic efforts, the etiology of hemoptysis remains undiagnosed in 15–20% of patients. Patients with "idiopathic" hemoptysis require careful follow-up.

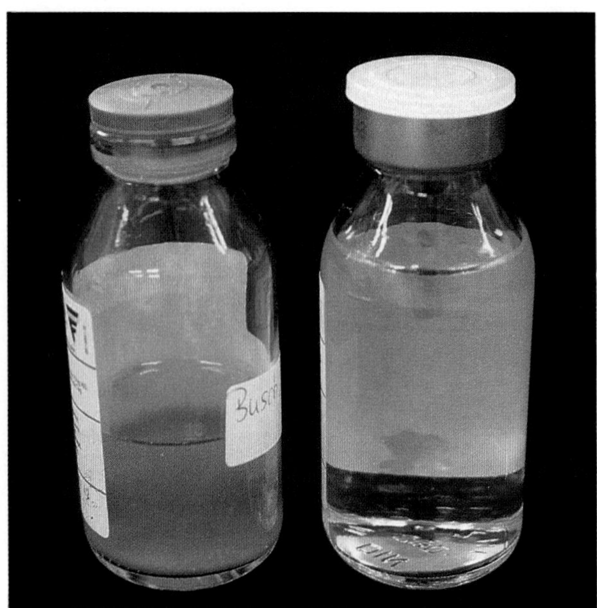

FIG. 13. Bronchoalveolar lavage effluent is clear in patients without chronic intraalveolar hemorrhage **(right)**. Bronchoalveolar lavage effluent in idiopathic pulmonary hemosiderosis appears orange–brown in color **(left)**.

BRONCHOSCOPY-INDUCED HEMORRHAGE

Predisposing Factors

A literature review of this complication noted bleeding rates to vary from less than 1% to approximately 20% (Table 3) (61–79). Life-threatening bleeding is rare. If a bronchoscopy is performed for the evaluation of hemoptysis, the risk of aggravating the preexisting respiratory hemorrhage is always present. However, such occurrence is also uncommon. In patients with tracheobronchial tumors, bleeding can occur following cytological brushing or forceps biopsy (61,62,65,66). Bronchoscopic brush- or biopsy-induced bleeding is more likely in the presence of underlying coagulation disorders. In the absence of such disorders, it is difficult to predict which patient is going to bleed. However, diagnostic bronchoalveolar lavage can be performed safely even in patients with severe coagulopathies (80,81). In general, neoplastic lesions of the tracheobronchial tree are more likely to bleed upon biopsy than benign mucosal lesions. Tracheobronchial carcinoid tumors are more vascular and tend to bleed more but this is not a contraindication to biopsy. Necrotic endobronchial tumors may expose newly developed vessels over the surface of the tumor, and a brush or a biopsy forceps can easily traumatize the vessel and provoke significant bleeding.

Bronchoscopic lung biopsy is more frequently followed by significant hemorrhage compared to biopsy of endobronchial lesions (62). Bronchcoscopic lung biopsy–induced bleeding occurs in 3–5% of patients. Inadvertent laceration of pulmonary vessels accompanying the "blind" bronchoscopic lung biopsy and the number of attempts at biopsy may contribute to the increased incidence of bleeding. Occasionally, it can be fatal (61,62). The risk of bleeding is not related to the type of biopsy forceps used. However, the larger the number of biopsies obtained, the higher the risk of bleeding.

Large cavitated lesions in the pulmonary parenchyma may also predispose to significant bleeding upon instrumentation (67). This is more likely in patients with aspergilloma (7,8), tuberculous cavities, and cavitated cancers. Highly vascular endobronchial lesions, such as those in endobronchial zygomycosis (mucormycosis), also result in serious hemorrhage after biopsy. Patients who present with hemoptysis due to severe bronchiectasis may bleed more during or after bronchoscopy. Bronchoscopic needle aspiration and biopsy may cause hematoma in the mediastinum but seldom produce tracheobronchial bleeding. Protected catheter brush used to obtain microbiological culture has occasionally, in our experience, resulted in considerable bleeding. The sharp edge of the outer catheter is perhaps the culprit in this.

TABLE 3. *Summary of literature reviews on bronchoscopy-induced hemorrhage*

Ref.	Year	Procedures	Coexisting illnesses	Final diagnosis	No. cases with bleeding	(%)	No. deaths
Levin et al. (73)	1974	33 Br 33 Bx	NA	NA	4	(12)	0
Pereira et al. (68)	1974	100 Br Bx-NA	NA	NA	6	(6)	0
Credle et al. (69)	1974	24,521 Br	NA	...	2	(0.008)	0
Flick et al. (61)	1974	1 Br 1 Bx	PDLL	LI	1 9	(100) (8.4/8.1)	1
Ellis (74)	1975	107 Br 111 Bx	NA	NA			0
Joyner and Scheinhorn (75)	1975	37 Br 37 Bx	ALT (1 patient)	NA	3	(8)	0
Koerner et al. (76)	1975	26 Br 26 Bx	...	...	1	(3.8)	0
Hanson et al. (64)	1976	507 Br 164 Bx	IS (9 patients: 7 renal tx 2 leukemia)	NA	15	(2.9/9.1)	0
Zavala (63)	1976	31 Br Br-NA	IS (31 patients)	NA	8	(26)	0
		164 Br Bx-NA	IS (9 patients)	NA	15	(9)	0
Surratt et al. (65)	1976	48,000 Br	NA	SCC (1 patient) OCC (1 patient)	5	(0.001/0.8)	0
Dreisin et al. (66)	1978	205 Br	SCC (1 patient) TP (1 patient)	NA	4	(1.9)	0
Stableforth et al. (77)	1978	55 Br 55 Bx	NA	NA	1	(1.8)	0
Burgher (71)	1979	76 Br 76 Bx	NA	NA	15	(19.7)	1
Mitchell et al. (78)	1981	456 Br 112 Bx	NA	NA	7	(1.5/6.3)	0
Prickett and LeGrand (67)	1984	112 Br	NA	NA	2	(1.6/3/1)	0
Rees (79)	1985	1 Br	None	FBR	1	(100)	0
Simpson et al. (72)	1986	39,564 Br Bx-NA	NA	NA	27	(0.7)	5
Ahmad et al. (70)	1986	688 Br 290 Bx	NA	NA	3	(0.4/1)	0
Cordasco et al. (62)	1991	6,969 Br 3,096 Bx	ALT IS, LI AIDS	[a]	58 59	(0.83) (1.9)	0 0

Table modified and updated from Cordasco et al. (62).

ALT, acute leukemic with thrombocytopenia; Br, bronchoscopies; Bx, biopsies; FBR, foreign body removal; IS, immunosuppressed; LI, leukemic infiltrate; NA, not available; OCC, oat cell carcinoma; PDLL, poorly differentiated lymphocytic lymphoma; SCC, squamous cell carcinoma; TP, thrombocytopenia; AIDS, acquired immunodeficiency syndrome.

[a] Several diagnoses were made by bronchoscopic procedures.

Significant bleeding is a common complication during YAG laser treatment of tracheobronchial tumors (82). This is one reason why many bronchoscopists, including ourselves, prefer the rigid bronchoscope for these procedures. Some of our patients have had hemoptysis after photodynamic therapy and brachytherapy. This usually indicates the last stage of the disease when the tumor has eroded major vessels.

The overall risk of bleeding following bronchoscopic procedures is low. One study (62) interpreted the experience with 6,969 flexible bronchoscopies and 3,096 bronchoscopically guided biopsies performed over a 9-year period and reported clinically significant bleeding (defined as more than 100 ml) in 0.83% of flexible bronchoscopies and 1.9% of bronchoscopic lung biopsies. A variety of underlying, coexisting nonpulmonary illnesses were present in 24% of cases with significant bleeding. These factors included metastatic carcinoma, renal dysfunction, and immunosuppression. Nevertheless, there was no consistent trend in the number of bronchoscopies, biopsies, or incidence of hemorrhage accompanying bronchoscopies. Earlier studies reported the rate of clinically significant bleeding in 15–26% of procedures performed in immunosuppressed patients (63,64).

Prevention of Bronchoscopy-Induced Hemorrhage

Even though spontaneous cessation of bleeding is the rule in almost all cases of bronchoscopy-induced hemorrhage (62), the bronchoscopist should be aware of the risks of bronchoscopy-induced bleeding and be prepared to manage it accordingly. The risk of hemorrhage should not deter the bronchoscopist from performing the appropriate procedure. During the preparation of the patient for the procedure, the bronchoscopist must ascertain underlying risk factors for bleeding. The presence of a clearly documented hemorrhagic diathesis is a contraindication to aggressive instrumentation such as brushing, biopsy of endobronchial lesions, and bronchoscopic lung biopsy.

Even though uremia is associated with a clinical bleeding tendency that can be quite severe, the correlation between abnormal platelet function and the risk of bleeding in patients with renal failure is unclear. Nevertheless, platelet dysfunction is common in patients with renal failure (83). A 45% incidence of hemorrhage following bronchoscopic lung biopsy has been documented in uremic patients, and a blood urea nitrogen of ≥45 mg/dl is considered a relative contraindication to bronchoscopic lung biopsy (63,84,85). Zavala stated that "any biopsy procedure is avoided, if at all possible, on a uremic patient because of hemorrhage" (84). In our practice, a serum creatinine level of ≥3 mg/dl is considered a relative contraindication to bronchoscopic lung biopsy (81). Platelet counts of at least 50,000/mm^3 for endobronchial biopsy and 75,000/mm^3 for bronchoscopic lung biopsy have been recommended (62). Some bronchoscopists routinely assess coagulation parameters as well as platelet counts in all patients undergoing flexible bronchoscopy and bronchial biopsy (62). This "routine" practice is unnecessary (81). Prebronchoscopy coagulation screening should be obtained in patients with active bleeding, known or clinically suspected bleeding disorders, liver disease, renal dysfunction, malabsorption, malnutrition, or other conditions associated with acquired coagulopathies (81,86).

Patients with platelet counts <50,000/mm^3 should receive six to ten packs of platelet transfusion before bronchoscopic lung biopsy (63,84). Patients with dysfunctional platelets (e.g., uremic patients) as determined by bleeding time testing may require a cryoprecipitate or deamino-8D-arginine–vasopressin (DDAVP) prior to biopsy (87–89). Immunosuppressed patients with bone marrow failure frequently require fresh-frozen plasma and platelets. Failure of the platelet count to "bump" significantly 1 hr past infusion of platelets implies the presence of platelet antibodies (62). Bronchoscopic lung biopsy should be avoided in these patients although bronchoalveolar lavage can be safely performed.

In anticipation of bleeding, the bronchoscopist should have at her or his disposal vasoactive agents, rigid bronchoscopy equipment, and other instruments (see below) as well as a well-prepared team. The most commonly used vasoactive agent is epinephrine, 1:20,000. To prepare this, epinephrine (1:1,000) 1.0 ml is thoroughly mixed with normal saline, 19 ml. An aliquot of 0.5–1.0 ml is used, making sure that excessive usage is avoided to prevent cardiovascular complications. To prevent coughing out the epinephrine, each aliquot can be mixed with an equal quantity of lidocaine, 2.0%. Prophylactic (just before biopsy) instillation of epinephrine or other vasoactive agent to minimize the bleeding at biopsy of large, polypoid, fleshy, or vascular-appearing endobronchial masses or bronchoscopic lung biopsy has not been proven effective. However, such a maneuver does produce immediate but transient blanching of overlying mucosa by producing vasoconstriction. Since there does not appear to be a maximal dose of epinephrine that can be safely administered, we recommend limiting the total dose to less than 3.0 ml (1:20,000).

Excessive suctioning following brush or biopsy can aggravate the bleeding. Brush and biopsy of bronchoscopically visible lesions is usually followed by immediate oozing of blood. Unless the hemorrhage is profuse, immediate suctioning close to the just-biopsied area is not necessary. In most situations, reflex vasoconstriction curtails bleeding and only minimal suctioning is required. Excessive manipulation of the abnormal area by the bronchoscope or accessories should be avoided. In patients with diffuse lung disease, some prefer biopsy of gravity-dependent portion of the lung (62). This is to prevent spillover of blood following biopsy from nondependent areas to dependent regions. To perform bronchoscopic lung biopsy, the tip of the flexible bronchoscope is wedged into the bronchus leading to the area to be biopsied, and following biopsy the instrument is maintained in the wedged position without suctioning in between the biopsies until the desired number of biopsies are obtained. Approximately 2–3 min after the completion of the biopsy procedure, the bronchoscope is gently withdrawn, without suctioning, and the blood is allowed to form a clot in the bronchus. If excessive bleeding occurs, continuous suctioning is applied so as to prevent aspiration of blood into other segments.

TREATMENT OF HEMOPTYSIS AND BRONCHOSCOPY-INDUCED HEMORRHAGE

General Measures

Even though hemoptysis is a relatively common complaint, less than 5% of patients present with massive bleeding. Nonmassive or non–life-threatening hemoptysis or bronchoscopy-induced bleeding may not require aggressive therapy. The step-by-step approach to the various techniques and treatments to control massive hemorrhage in the tracheobronchial tree is listed in Table 4.

Establishing and control of the airway and maintaining it free of blood is an important initial step. The life-threatening factor is not the loss of blood, but the danger of asphyxiation from blood and blood clots obstructing the airways. The easiest procedure is to position the patient in the reverse Trendelenburg position with the bleeding side down. The bleeding side may not be apparent unless a chest roentgenogram or clinical examination indicates it. Oxygen should be given, preferably during continuous monitoring of oxygen saturation with pulse oximetry. Antitussive drugs can help to stop the coughing but not the bleeding. However, overmedication with cough-suppressing sedatives can be harmful because the lack of cough may result in the pooling of blood and clotting in the tracheobronchial tree. An intravenous access must be secured. Typing and cross-matching of blood is required. The usual laboratory tests as well as eletrocardiogram and blood gas analysis should be ordered. The patient should refrain from eating and drinking and maintain bedrest. Consent for emergency anesthesia and surgery should be prepared (90–92). Whenever possible, treatment of etiological factors, e.g., substitution of coagulation factors in thrombocytopenia or plasmapheresis in immune complex–mediated hemorrhage, should be considered (93).

Bronchoscopic Therapy

Instruments

Bronchoscopy is the most important step not only in the diagnosis but also in the emergency management of hemoptysis. Localizing the source of bleeding is essential. An instrument with a large working channel is recommended. While flexible bronchoscopy is usually performed in most cases of hemoptysis, rigid bronchoscopy should be available if massive hemoptysis is present or anticipated. A large-diameter orotracheal tube is preferable so that the flexible instrument can be removed as often as necessary to clean the tip or to remove impacted blood clots. Furthermore, the endotracheal tube permits insertion of large-bore suction catheter for removing large quantities of blood from the tracheobronchial tree.

TABLE 4. *Therapeutic approach to hemoptysis or bronchoscopy-induced hemorrhage*

Airway control
Breathing (oxygenation)
Cardiovascular stabilization
Definitive therapy
- *Bronchoscopic treatment*
  - Repeated suctioning
  - Iced saline irrigation
  - Vasoactive drugs
  - Bronchoscopic tamponade
  - Balloon tamponade
  - Tamponade with gauze or gelfoam
  - Thrombin/fibrinogen instillation (Chapter 16)
  - Laser coagulation
  - Electrocautery
  - Isolation of bronchial tree (double-lumen endotracheal tube)
  - Bronchoscopic brachytherapy (Chapter 20)
- *Nonbronchoscopic therapy*[a]
  - Bed rest
  - Antitussive drugs
  - Vasoactive drugs (systemic administration)
  - Antibacterial, antituberculous, or antifungal agents
  - Anticoagulants
  - Corticosteroids
  - Cytotoxic agents
  - Plasmapheresis
  - Mitral valve replacement
  - Embolotherapy
  - Intracavitary therapy
  - Surgical resection

[a] Treatment for non-bronchoscopy–induced hemoptysis dependent on underlying disease or etiology.

Bronchoscopic Suction

Significant bleeding in the trachea or proximal bronchial tree requires continuous bronchoscopic suction using a large-channel flexible bronchoscope or a rigid bronchoscope. Continuous suctioning of blood prevents formation of clots in the airways and spilling of blood to distal airways. The latter effect is an important step to prevent excessive coughing by the patient. Repeated contact of the bleeding lesion by the bronchoscope should be avoided as much as possible. If the bleeding is arising from a very focal site, the rigid bronchoscope itself can be used to laterally compress the lesion, if the lesion is in the trachea or main stem bronchi. If continuous suctioning fails to control the bleeding, other measures may have to be considered. If bleeding slows down and a clot begins to form in a segmental or even a lobar bronchus, it is prudent to

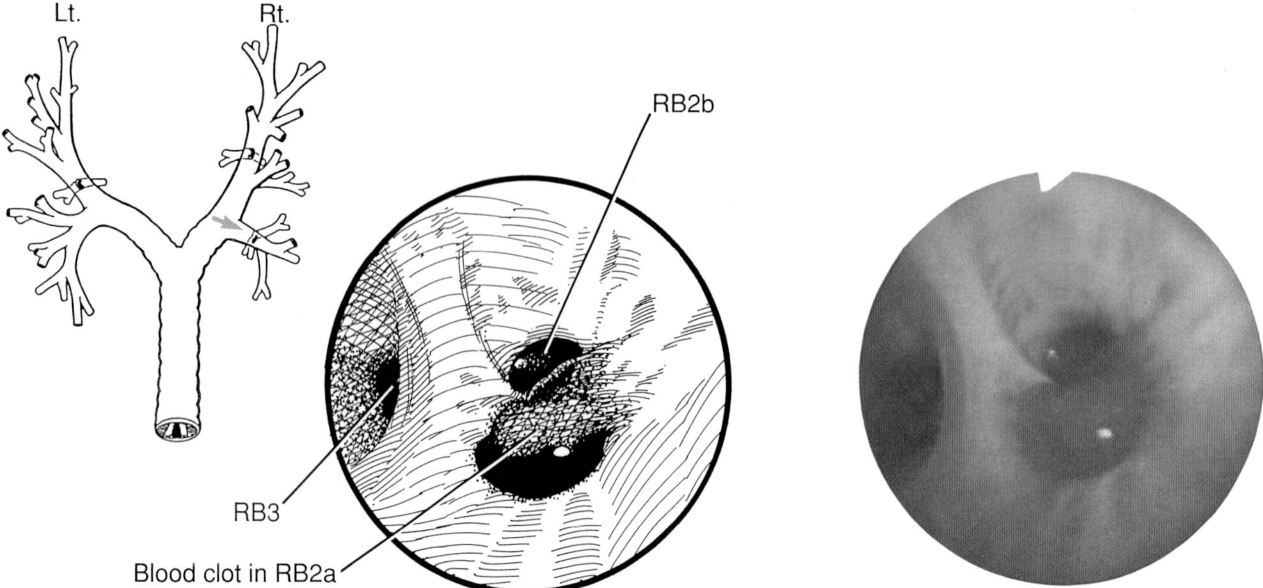

FIG. 14. Clot formation in RB2 following bronchoscopic lung biopsy and loss of about 80 ml of blood. It is prudent to leave the clot alone because suctioning may stimulate further hemorrhage.

allow the clot to fully form instead of suctioning and precipitating further hemorrhage (Fig. 14).

Iced Saline Lavage

One of the easier techniques to slow the rate of bleeding and to stop it is to instill ice-cold saline through the bronchoscope (94,95). The bronchoscopist should make sure that excessive saline is not used and that most of the saline is recovered by suction after each instillation. The saline can be used for control of bleeding from the proximal bronchial tree as well hemorrhage caused by bronchoscopic lung biopsy.

Vasoactive Drugs

Vasoactive drugs can be administered systemically or locally (96,97). If the bleeding is mild, epinephrine (1:10,000; up to 3 ml) can be instilled through the working channel of the flexible instrument. This drug is less expensive than glypressin, which has been used in those who do not respond to epinephrine. Usually a paling of the mucosa around the tumor indicates the vasoconstrictor effect on the supplying vessels. Serious effects of these agents on the systemic circulation, heart rate, or bronchomotor tone is minimal or negligible. Therapy using aerosolized ibuprofen has shown encouraging results in animal studies. A combination of glypressin and ibuprofen has been shown to be very effective in reducing blood flow in the bronchial arteries (98).

As noted above, vasoactive agents can be applied to the bleeding site by means of a cotton swab or gauze tape through a rigid bronchoscope.

Bronchoscopic Tamponade

If the bleeding is arising from a distal area, the tip of the bronchoscope should be wedged into the bronchus leading to the bleeding site and continuous suction applied. This wedge technique is effective in controlling the bleeding following bronchoscopic lung biopsy, or biopsy or manipulation of a lesion in the distal bronchial tree (63). The continuous bronchoscopic suctioning causes the distal bronchus to collapse, thus stopping the bleeding by compression.

A simpler, old-fashioned method is to use cotton swabs dipped in vasoactive drugs for tamponade through the rigid bronchoscope. Another method is to insert a long, narrow gauze tape (dipped in a vasoactive drug) through the lumen of a rigid bronchoscope, with the help of a forceps, to pack the bleeding bronchus. After several minutes, the gauze is gently pulled out.

Balloon Tamponade

Balloon catheters can be used for selectively blocking a lobe or a segment (99–103). Inserted via the working channel of a flexible bronchoscope or through a rigid instrument, the balloon blocks only the bleeding bronchus. Several types of catheters are available. The

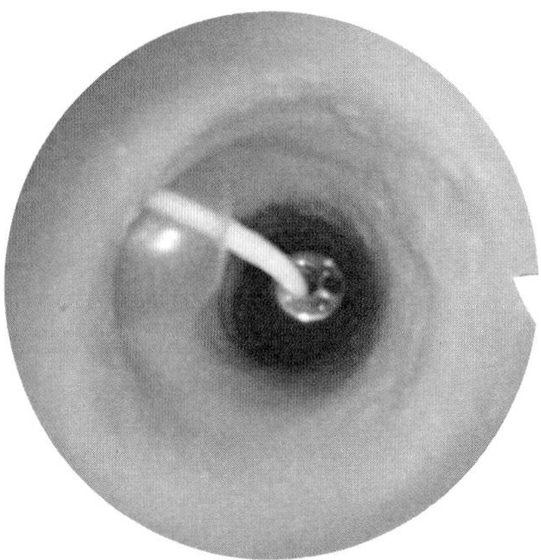

FIG. 15. A cephalad view of simulated endobronchial tamponade of right upper lobe with a Fogarty catheter passed through a flexible bronchoscope.

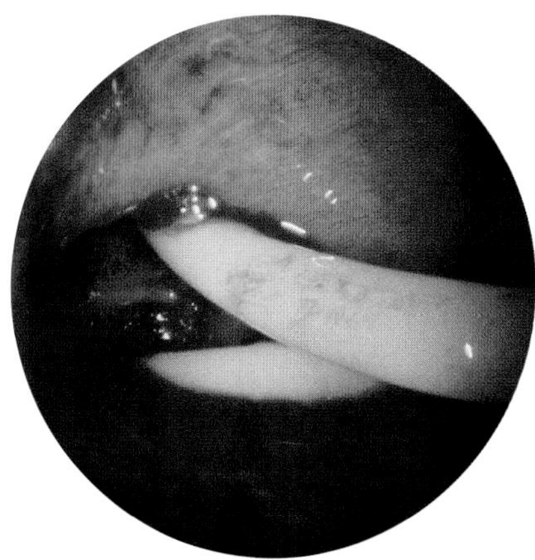

FIG. 17. Two Fogarty catheters inserted to control bleeding in a patient with thrombocytopenia and bleeding. Bleeding was from left lower lobe.

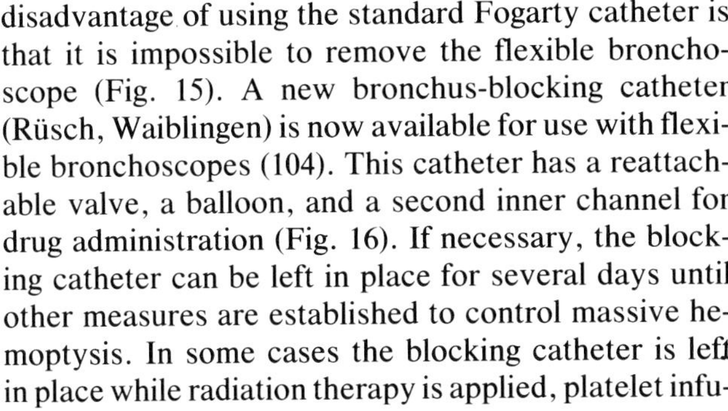

disadvantage of using the standard Fogarty catheter is that it is impossible to remove the flexible bronchoscope (Fig. 15). A new bronchus-blocking catheter (Rüsch, Waiblingen) is now available for use with flexible bronchoscopes (104). This catheter has a reattachable valve, a balloon, and a second inner channel for drug administration (Fig. 16). If necessary, the blocking catheter can be left in place for several days until other measures are established to control massive hemoptysis. In some cases the blocking catheter is left in place while radiation therapy is applied, platelet infusions are given (Fig. 17), or bronchial arterial embolization is performed.

Balloon catheters have certain limitations and inherent problems. They are well suited for use in patients whose rate of bleeding is slow and the location is at a segmental level or beyond. Bleeding at the origin of lobar bronchi is difficult to control with balloon tamponade. Insertion of the balloon into the upper lobe bronchi is more difficult because of the tendency of the catheter stem to straighten and slip out of the upper lobe bronchi. Excessive coughing by the patient can

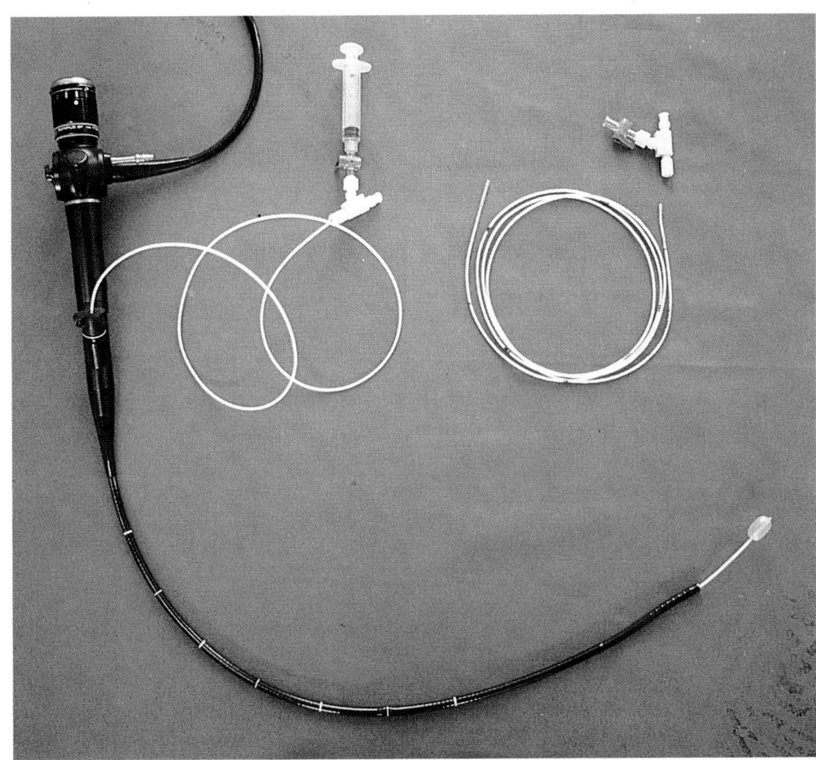

FIG. 16. Dedicated bronchus blocking catheter inserted through the working channel of a flexible bronchoscope.

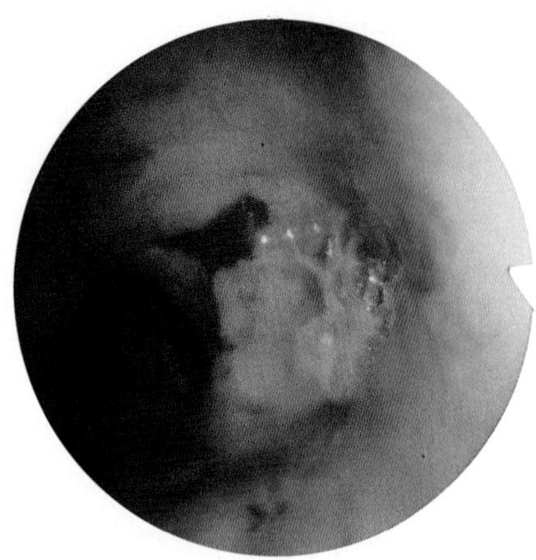

FIG. 18. Fibrin glue clot used to seal a bleeding right upper lobe bronchus.

dislodge the balloon. Blood or mucous in the bronchial tree can function as a lubricant and help move the balloon out of the tamponaded site. In patients who present with continuous massive bleeding, the presence of the catheter in the working channel of the flexible bronchoscope prevents the suctioning of blood. It also interferes with the bronchoscopic visualization of the tracheobronchial tree. Breakage of the balloon has resulted in an "iatrogenic foreign body" problem (see Chapter 18).

A Foley catheter, used for urethral catheterization, is valuable if the bleeding is severe and arises in the main stem bronchi. However, it cannot be introduced through the flexible bronchoscope. One technique involves the use of a flexible bronchoscope to guide the tip of an endotracheal tube into the bleeding main stem bronchus. The bronchoscope is quickly withdrawn and a Foley catheter introduced into the bleeding main stem bronchus. The tip of the endotracheal tube is brought back into the distal trachea and stabilized just above the main carina. The balloon of the Foley catheter is now inflated so that blood does not spill into opposite bronchial tree. Patient can continue to receive supplemental oxygen through the endotracheal tube. The blood loss can be accurately estimated by collecting it from the Foley catheter.

Fibrin Glue

Attempts have been made to use fibrin or fibrin precursors through the bronchoscope to treat hemoptysis (105–107). In a few cases we have managed to seal a segmental bronchus with fibrin glue (Fig. 18). In most cases, however, we have been less successful than those who have published excellent results in the literature. Topical thrombin alone, 5–10 ml (1,000 units/ml), or fibrinogen 2%, 5–10 ml followed by thrombin 5–10 ml, can be infused directly through the channel of the flexible bronchoscope. The bronchoscope is retained in place for about 5 min after which gentle suction is applied to confirm hemostasis (106). Alternatively, cryoprecipitate, with a lessened risk of hepatitis and human immunodeficiency virus (HIV) transmission, could be used if necessary (108,109). Persistent and significant bleeding tends to flush away the fibrin glue before a stable clot can form. The technique of fibrin glue application is described in Chapter 16.

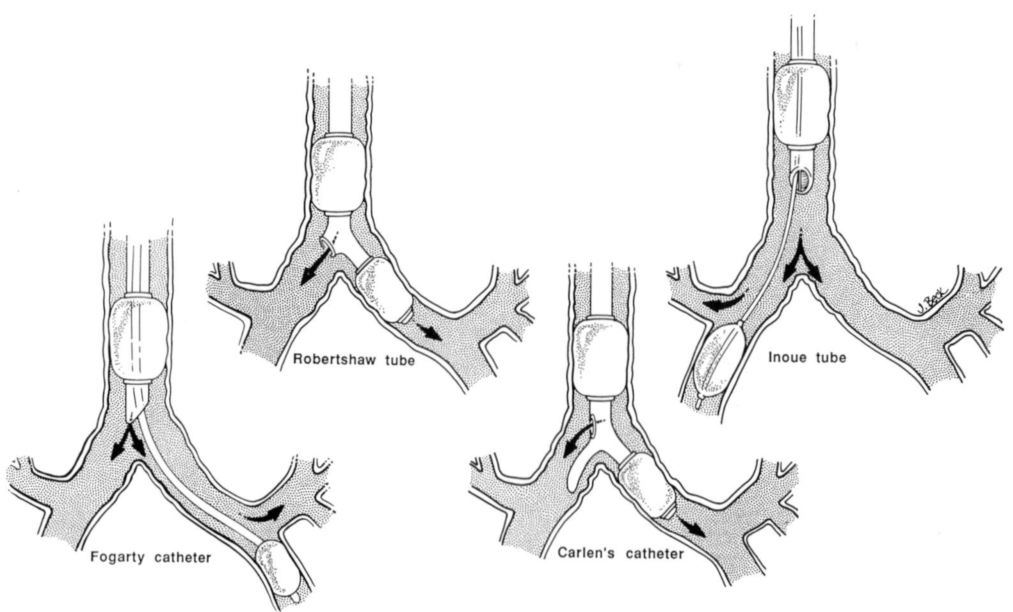

FIG. 19. Methods available to isolate one lung from another.

Isolation of Bronchial Tree

In patients with serious bleeding arising from one side, the danger of flooding the nonbleeding side and causing asphyxia is significant. Isolation of the nonbleeding side is an important consideration in such situations. The use of a Foley catheter, as described above, is one technique. The rigid bronchoscope is also useful in achieving this. The instrument is introduced into the nonbleeding bronchus so as to block the blood from spilling into the healthy side and to maintain sufficient ventilation. The most effective method, however, is the intubation with a double-lumen tube (Fig. 19). The original Carlens tube has a hook that sits on the carina. A modification of this is the Robertshaw tube. Some authors have reported that the plastic double-lumen endobronchial tube is superior to the Carlens tube in maintaining the airway in a patient with massive hemoptysis and nonresectable lung cancer (110). More recently, the Inoue endotracheal tube with blocking catheter was introduced into the market (Fig. 20). The lumens in the Carlens and Robertshaw tubes do not permit passage of a standard flexible bronchoscope. To assess the positioning of the distal ends of the tubes, it may be necessary to use an ultrathin flexible bronchoscope. The disadvantage is that the double-lumen endotracheal tubes block and thus "sacrifice" an entire lung even if the bleeding is segmental or subseg-

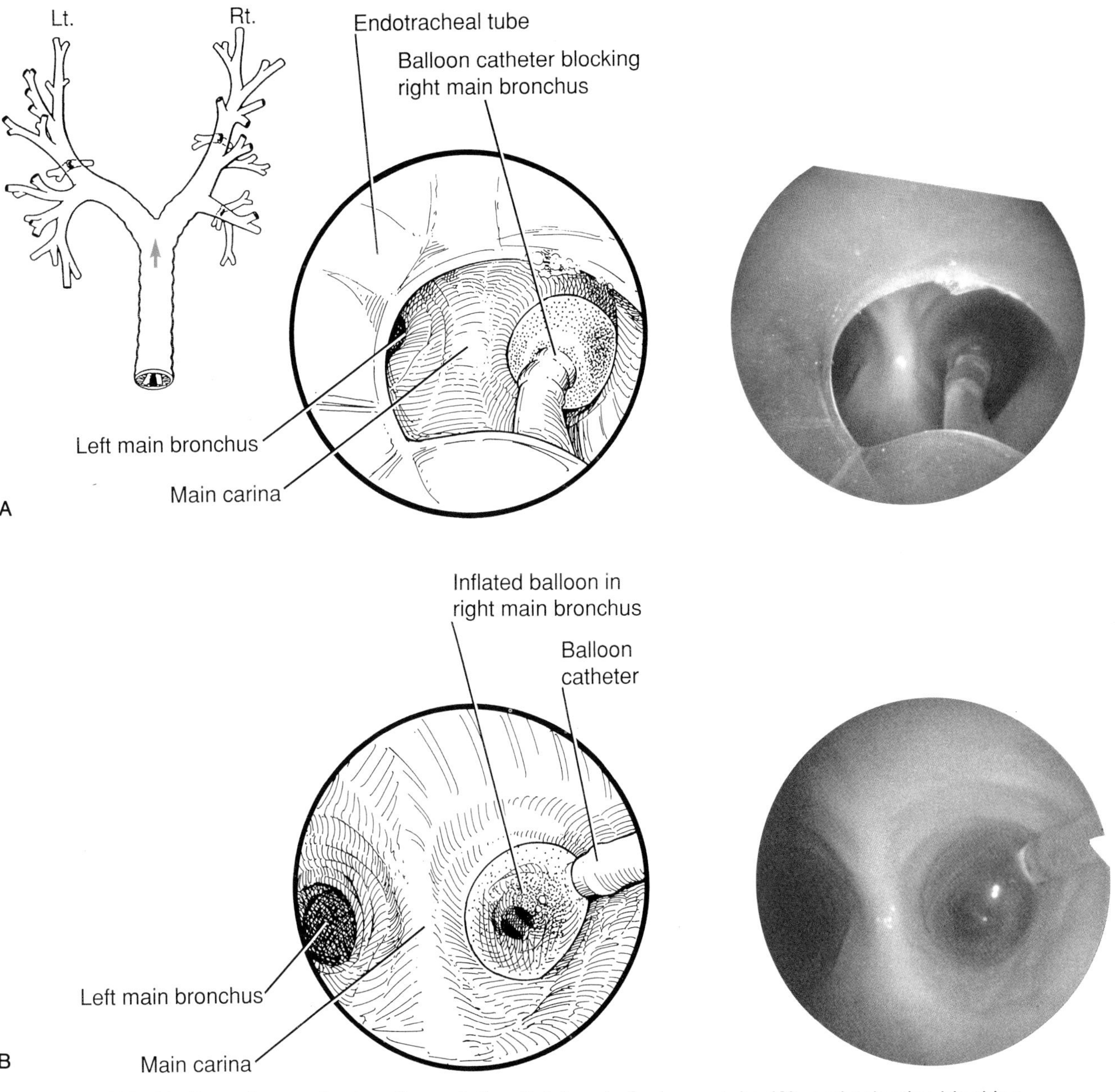

FIG. 20. Bronchoscopic view through the distal end of a Inoue tube **(A)**; and selective blocking (tamponade) of right main stem bronchus by the balloon **(B)**.

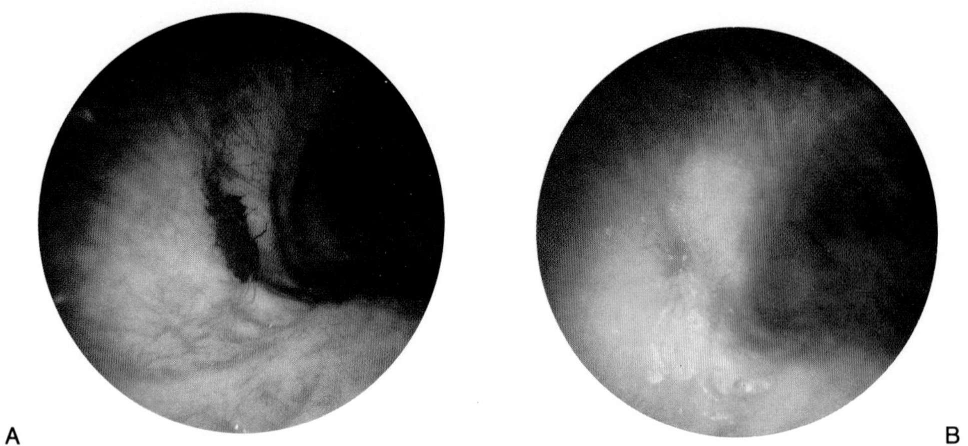

FIG. 21. Hemangioma in the trachea before treatment **(A)** and after laser coagulation **(B)**.

mental. Isolated ventilation with positive end-expiratory pressure reduces bronchial arterial blood flow and improves gas exchange (111).

Laser Coagulation

If the bleeding from a bronchoscopically visible lesion does not stop spontaneously, coagulation therapy may be necessary. Smaller lesions can be coagulated with the laser (Figs. 21 and 22). Lower energy (approximately 15 W) is suitable for coagulation. However, it is sometimes impossible to see the blood vessel supplying the lesion. Even to distinguish between tumor and blood clot can be difficult. Attempting to coagulate a heavily bleeding tumor with the laser results in boiling of blood without stoppage of bleeding.

Electrocautery

An alternative to laser coagulation is the electrocautery (112), especially in combination with the rigid bronchoscope. The big channel of the rigid instrument allows simultaneous suctioning while the surface of the tumor or the mucosal vessels can be cauterized. As soon as the heavy bleeding stops, final coagulation with the Nd:YAG laser should be done as this technique has a higher and more reliable depth of penetration. Electrocauters are also available for larger flexible

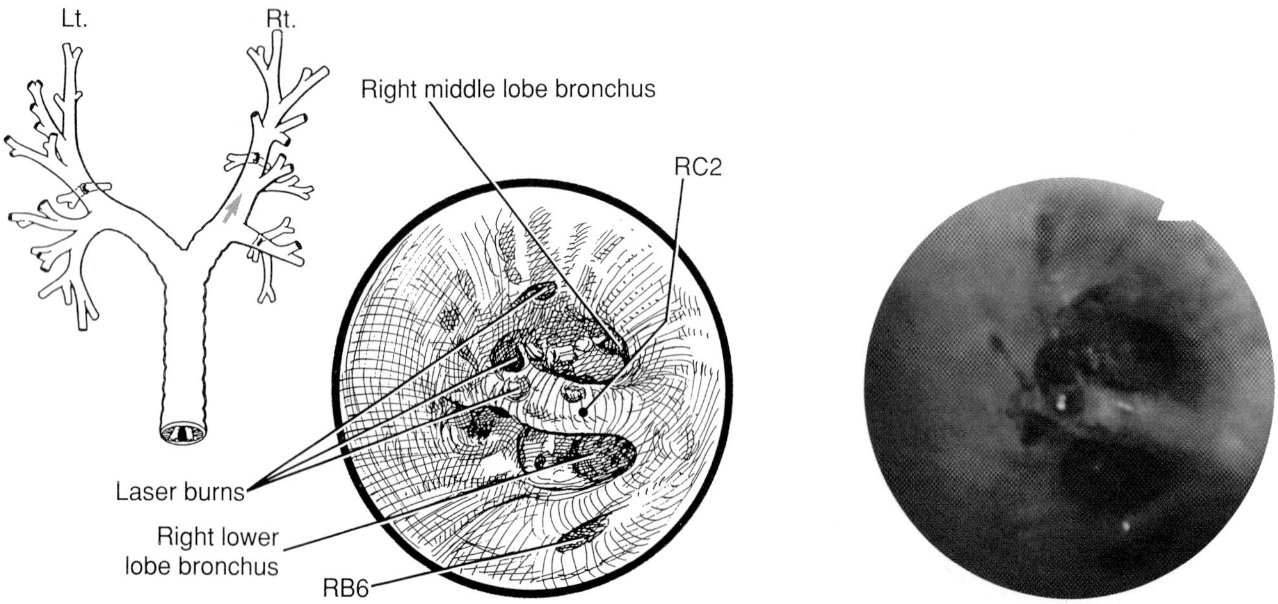

FIG. 22. Laser burns following coagulation of a small artery spurting blood from the medial aspect of RC2.

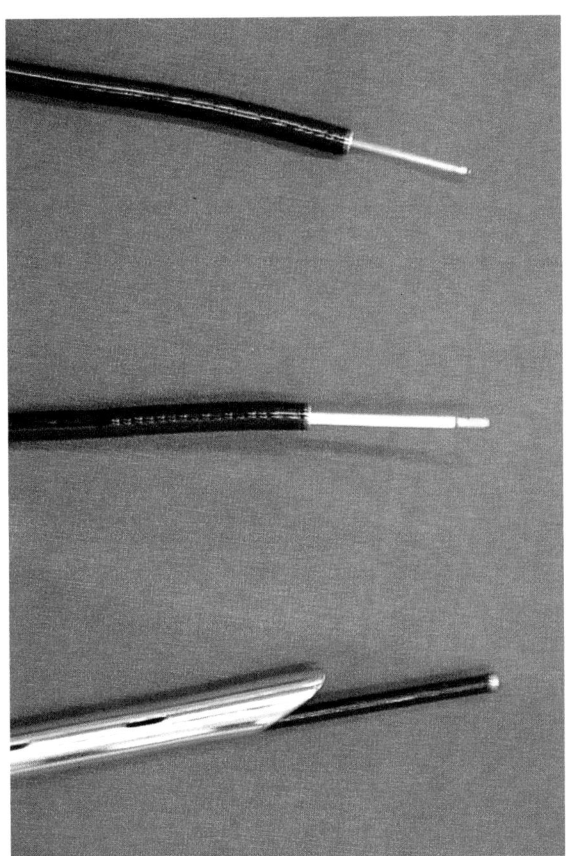

FIG. 23. Laser **(top)** and electrocauter **(middle)** through large-channel flexible bronchoscope and large electrocauter **(bottom)** through the rigid bronchoscope are the most appropriate coagulation instruments.

bronchoscopes (Gold Probe, Boston Scientific) (Fig. 23). However, the major disadvantage of cauterizing via the bronchoscope is the fact that the coagulation effect stops completely if carbonized tissue covers the surface of the electrode. Repetitive cleaning of the electrode is required, making it a time-consuming procedure in a situation where there is no time.

Other Bronchoscopic Treatments

Unusual cases of hemoptysis may require unusual bronchoscopic treatments. At the Mayo Clinic, we have used intrabronchial arterial clipping to stop hemorrhage caused by an artery in the bronchial lumen (Fig. 24) and injection of sclerosing agents to control bleeding from submucosal varices (Fig. 25).

Nonbronchoscopic Therapy

Embolization

If a patient is not a candidate for surgical therapy of massive hemoptysis, embolization therapy of bronchial or pulmonary arteries can be considered. The rate of success is about 85% accompanied by a low complication rate (30,83,113–118). Bronchial artery embolization, even though successful initially, may be followed by recurrent hemoptysis in 10–27% (30,49,119,120). Recurrent hemorrhage may require recurrent embolotherapy (121). A major complication of bronchial ar-

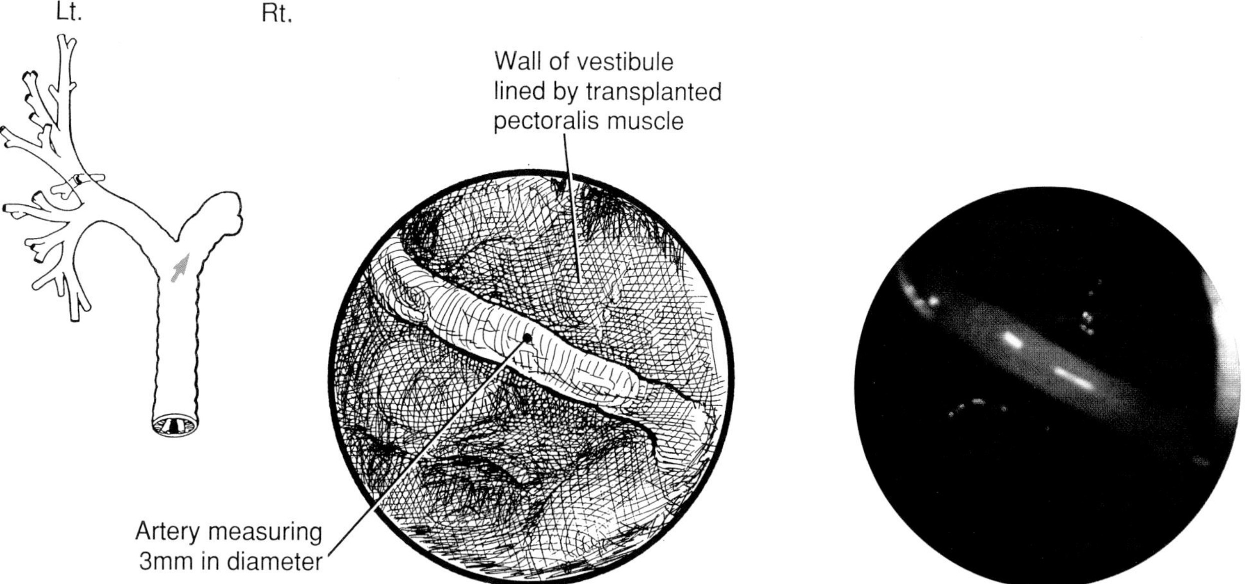

FIG. 24. Massive hemoptysis occurred 1 year after closure of right bronchopleural fistula (following right pneumonectomy for carcinoma) using pectoral muscle flap. A free artery measuring 3 mm in diameter was noted in the vestibule formed by the pectoral muscle. We theorize that the muscle atrophied and the intramuscular artery became free. We were able to apply vascular clips with a biopsy forceps through the rigid bronchoscope to control the bleeding.

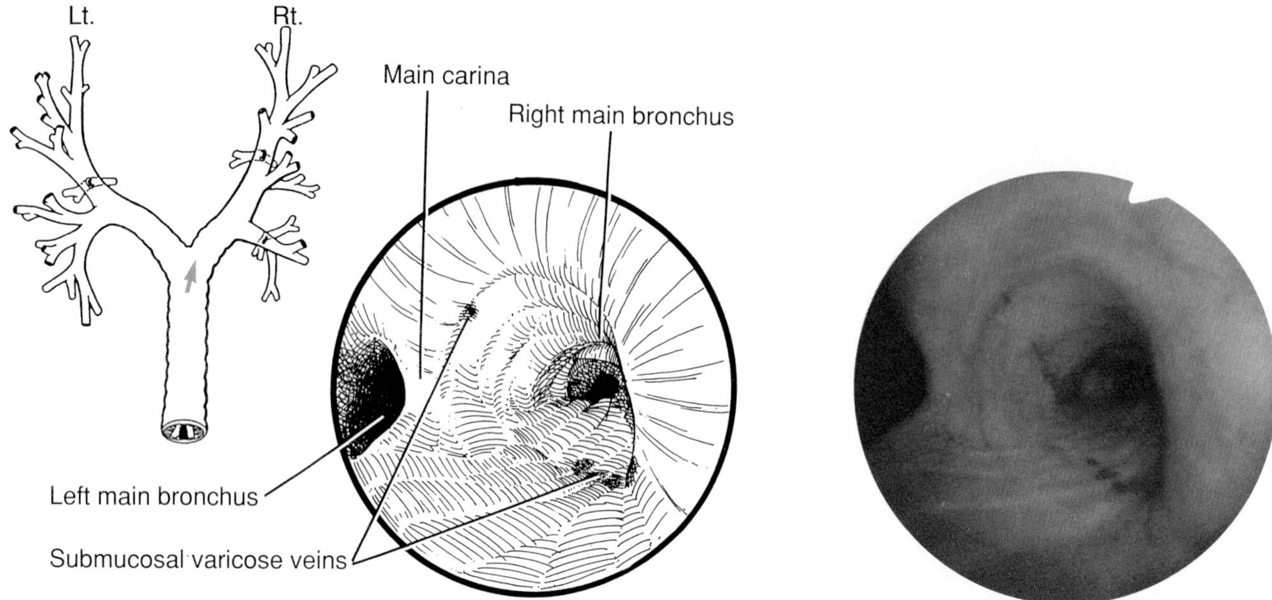

FIG. 25. Hemoptysis caused by multiple mucosal varicosities was controlled by flexible bronchoscopic needle injection of a sclerosing agent into the lesions.

tery embolization is the neurological sequelae, if spinal arteries, which frequently branch off the bronchial arteries, are accidentally embolized.

Pulmonary artery embolization is the treatment of choice in patients with significant bleeding or severe hypoxemia due to pulmonary arteriovenous malformations.

Surgery

In some cases of massive tracheobronchial bleeding, all bronchoscopic therapeutic approaches may fail. If the cause is clearly evident, no time should be wasted in considering surgical therapy (122–124). In such cases bronchoscopy is useful to identify the side and

TABLE 5. *Clinical studies advocating surgical therapy*

Ref.	Definition of massive hemoptysis	No.	Inoperable no. (mortality)	Surgical candidates no. (mortality): Surgically treated	Surgical candidates no. (mortality): Medically treated	Comments
Crocco et al. (126), 1968	600 ml/48 hr	67	26 (46.2%)	32 (18.8%)	9 (77.8%)	Medically treated group selected by opting to treat active infection or by patient refusal of surgery
Garzon and Gourin, (124), 1978	600 ml/24 hr	75	7 (71.4%)	106 (<1%)	27 (85.2%)	Follow-up of 59% of operated patients from 2 to 7 years disclosed only one recurrence
Sehhat et al. (128), 1978	600 ml/48 hr	146	13 (69.2%)	24 (25%)	NA	Patients selected for exsanguinating hemoptysis, 75% survival is compared to historical control of 25%
Garzon et al. (127), 1982	150 ml/hr	24	NA	68 (15.5%)	NA	Rate of blood loss and aspiration of blood into contralateral lung were major factors for morbidity and mortality

Adapted from Thompson et al. (24).

TABLE 6. *Clinical studies advocating medical therapy*

Ref.	Definition of massive hemoptysis	No.	Inoperable no. (mortality)	Surgical candidates no. (mortality)		Comments
				Surgically treated	Medically treated	
Yeoh et al. (99), 1967	200 ml/day	56	ND	13 (15.4%)	43 (23.3%)	All patients had tuberculosis. Eight of the 10 deaths in the medically treated group were due to sudden massive hemoptysis that preempted surgery. Bleeding usually stopped within 4 days
Stern et al. (6), 1978	300 ml/day	38	ND	1 (?)	37 (27.1%)	All patients had cystic fibrosis. Mortality was found to be comparable to another group of patients with equally severe lung disease. Bleeding stopped within 4 days
Yang et al. (91), 1978	200 ml/day	20	ND	3 (0%)	17 (17.6%)	Two of three fatalities occurred within minutes of the onset of hemoptysis. Surgery followed initial conservative management
Bobrowitz et al. (129), 1983	100 ml/day	113	31 (29%)	31 (12.9%)	51 (17.6%)	Eight of the nine fatalities in the medically treated group occurred within minutes of the onset of hemoptysis
Conlan et al. (1, 95), 1983	600 ml/day	123	ND	38 (15.8%)	85 (25.9%)	Bleeding that did not cease spontaneously was treated with iced saline bronchial lavage: surgery was always elective
Corey and Hla, (92), 1987	200 ml/day	59	28 (46.4%)	4 (50%)	27 (11%)	Patients with hemoptysis of >1000 ml/day had highest mortality. There was no mortality in patients with infections or inflammatory etiologies

Adapted from Thompson et al. (24).

site of bleeding, stabilize the patient, and minimize spilling of blood into the unaffected lung. Emergency pulmonary resection for massive hemoptysis requires protection of the contralateral lung from aspiration of blood. Flexible bronchoscopic placement of a double-lumen endotracheal tube or the use of a rigid bronchoscope to ventilate the unaffected lung during surgery permits safe conclusion of the surgical procedure (125).

Thompson and colleagues (24) reviewed the literature and noted that the series of publications (124,126–128) (Table 5) that advocated surgical therapy reported that the mortality in the groups of patients who underwent nonsurgical therapy for massive hemoptysis ranged from 78% to 85%. In contrast, the mortality in surgically treated groups ranged from 1% to 25%, with a median mortality of 17%. In the nonsurgical groups, patients were deemed inoperable if the bleeding site could not be localized, metastatic cancer was present, mediastinal vessels were involved, or if the patient had severe cardiovascular or respiratory disease. This subset of patients had mortality rates ranging from 46% to 71%. Thompson and associates (24) also analyzed the publications (1,6,91,92,95, 99,129) that recommended medical therapy (Table 6) and observed that the mortalities in the surgically treated and medically treated groups were 13–50% and 11–26%, respectively. In one study, it was reported that the mortality for actively hemorrhaging patients was 37% in contrast to 8% in whom bleeding had stopped (119).

Other Treatments

Treatment of alveolar hemorrhage syndromes will depend on the underlying etiology of the syndrome (Table 4). The therapies may include corticosteroids and/or cytotoxic agents (for vasculitis, systemic lupus erythematosus, Goodpasture's syndrome, and idiopathic pulmonary hemosiderosis), and plasmapheresis (Goodpasture's syndrome). Severe hemoptysis secondary to mitral stenosis is an indication for valvular surgery.

Pharmacological agents such as indomethacin, a cyclooxygenase inhibitor, and cimetidine, an H_2 blocker, have been documented to decrease bronchial blood flow by increasing bronchial vascular resistance in experimental animals (13,130). Control of hemoptysis in humans, following administration of cimetidine, 200 mg every 8 hr, has been reported (131).

In patients with aspergilloma complicated by non–life-threatening bleeding, intracavitary instillation of amphotericin B is an option.

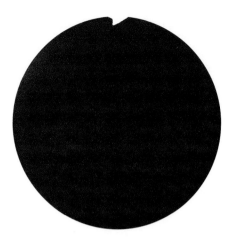

FIG. 26. A bronchoscopic image such as this can be caused by a small drop of blood stuck to the distal tip of the flexible bronchoscope or by massive hemorrhage. There are many bronchoscopic techniques to manage the latter.

PROGNOSIS

Irrespective of the underlying etiology, most cases of nonmassive hemoptysis can be controlled by one of the several methods discussed above. The prognosis for patients with idiopathic hemoptysis is generally good, usually with resolution of bleeding within 6 months of bronchoscopic evaluation (132).

Life-threatening hemoptysis is uncommon, occurring in less than 5% of all patients who present with hemoptysis (24). Fatal hemoptysis has been observed in 36% of patients with pulmonary malignancy and associated fungal pneumonia (133). Death from massive hemoptysis is usually due to aspiration of blood and asphyxia. The prognosis for the patients who present with massive hemoptysis is grave. The rate of blood loss from the respiratory system is the best predictor of mortality (24). However, inadequate pulmonary reserve and other serious illnesses may produce respiratory distress with smaller volumes of blood in the tracheobronchial tree or the alveolar spaces. Nevertheless, one study of 67 patients reported that mortality was directly proportional to the rate of blood loss, with expectoration of 600 ml over 4 hr resulting in a mortality of 71%, 600 ml in 4–16 hr with a 45% mortality, and 600 ml in 16–48 hr with a 5% mortality (126). Another study of 59 patients, 18 of whom died, observed expectoration of 1,000 ml or more in 24 hr in 15 patients (92). Yet another study of 123 cases with massive hemoptysis reported sudden catastrophic bleeding in 8 patients who were apparently stable and awaiting further evaluation (1).

SUMMARY

Hemoptysis is a relatively common clinical problem with myriad etiologies. In spite of extensive diagnostic evaluations, the etiology of hemoptysis remains undetected in up to 20% of patients. Bronchoscopy is the most important initial diagnostic test. Even though the initial bronchoscopic finding as shown in Fig. 26 may appear intimidating to the bronchoscopist, several bronchoscopic treatments are available to control bleeding in the respiratory system. Massive hemoptysis carries a high mortality unless prompt and aggressive therapy is undertaken. Failure of bronchoscopic methods to control hemorrhage may lead to other therapeutic approaches.

REFERENCES

1. Conlan AA, Hurwitz SS, Nicolaou N, Pool R. Massive hemoptysis. Review on 123 cases. *J Thorac Cardiovasc Surg* 1983; 85:120–124.
2. Middleton JR, Pernendu S, Lange M, Salaki J, Kapila R, Louria DB. Death-producing hemoptysis in tuberculosis. *Chest* 1977; 72–601.
3. Plessinger VA, Jolly PN. Rasmussen's aneurysm and fatal hemorrhage in pulmonary tuberculosis. *Am Rev Tuberc* 1949; 60:589–603.
4. Miller R, McGregor D. Hemorrhage from carcinoma of the lung. *Cancer* 1980;49:200–205.
5. Fajardo LF, Lee A. Rupture of major vessels after radiation. *Cancer* 1975;36:904–913.
6. Stern RC, Wood RE, Boat TE, Matthews LW, Tucker AS, Doershuk CF. Treatment and prognosis of massive hemoptysis in cystic fibrosis. *Am Rev Resp Dis* 1978;117:825–828.
7. Glimp RA, Bayer AS. Pulmonary aspergilloma: diagnostic and therapeutic considerations. *Arch Intern Med* 1983; 143:303–308.
8. Shapiro MJ, Albelda SM, Maycock RL, McLean GK. Severe hemoptysis associated with pulmonary aspergilloma. *Chest* 1988;94:1225–1231.
9. Santiago S, Tobias J, Williams AJ. A reappraisal of the causes of hemoptysis. *Arch Intern Med* 1991;151:2449–2451.
10. Dickman PS, Nussbaum E, Finkelstein JZ. Arteriotracheal fistula in patients treated for lymphoma. *Pediatr Pathol* 1989; 9:329–336.
11. Liebow AA, Hales MR, Lindskog GE. Enlargement of the bronchial arteries and their anastomoses with the pulmonary arteries in bronchiectasis. *Am J Pathol* 1949;25:211–227.
12. Pump KK. The bronchial arteries and their anastomoses in the human lung. *Dis Chest* 1963;43:245–252.

13. Deffebach ME, Charan NB, Lakshminarayan S, et al. The bronchial circulation. Small, but a vital attribute of the lung. *Am Rev Resp Dis* 1987;135:463–481.
14. Pump KK. Distribution of bronchial arteries in the human lung. Chest 1972;62:447–451.
15. Prakash UBS. Dermatological diseases. In: Murray JF, ed. *Pulmonary manifestations in systemic diseases*. New York: Marcel Dekker; 1992;421–516. (*Lung biopsy in health and disease*. vol 59).
16. Young KR. Pulmonary-renal syndromes. *Clin Chest Med* 1989; 10:655–675.
17. Buchanan GR, Moore GC. Pulmonary hemosiderosis and immune thrombocytopenia. *JAMA* 1981;246:861–864.
18. Leavitt RY, Fuci AS. Pulmonary vasculitis. *Am Rev Resp Dis* 1986;134:149–166.
19. Travis WD, Herschel AC, Lie JT. Diffuse pulmonary hemorrhage. An uncommon manifestation of Wegener's granulomatosis. *Am J Surg Pathol* 1987;11:702–708.
20. Soergel KH, Sommers SC. Idiopathic pulmonary hemosiderosis and related syndromes. *Am J Med* 1962;32:499–511.
21. Robboy SJ, Minna JD, Colman RW, Birndorf NI, Lopas H. Pulmonary hemorrhage syndrome as a manifestation of disseminated intravascular coagulation: analysis of ten cases. *Chest* 1973;63:718–721.
22. Prakash UBS. Rheumatological diseases. In: Murray JF, ed. *Pulmonary manifestations in systemic diseases*. New York: Marcel Dekker; 1992;385–430. (Lung biology in health and disease. vol 59).
23. Brewer D. Early diagnostic signs and symptoms of laryngeal disease. *Laryngoscope* 1975;85:499.
24. Thompson AB, Teschler H, Rennard SI. Pathogenesis, evaluation, and therapy for massive hemoptysis. *Clin Chest Med* 1992;13:69–82.
25. Wedzicha JA, Pearson MC. Management of massive hemoptysis. *Resp Med* 1990;84:9–12.
26. Pinet F, Clermont A, Michel C, et al. Embolization of the systemic arteries of the lung. *J Thorac Imag* 1987;2:11–17.
27. Stoll JF, Bettman MA. Bronchial artery embolization to control hemoptysis: a review. *Cardiovasc Intervent Radiol* 1988; 11:263–278.
28. Rasmussen V. Hemoptysis, especially when fatal, in its anatomical and clinical aspects. *Edinburgh Med J* 1868; 14:385–392.
29. Weiland JE, de-los-Santos ET, Mazzaferri EL, Schuller DE, Oertel JE. Hemoptysis as the presenting manifestation of thyroid carcinoma. A case report. *Arch Intern Med* 1989; 149:1693–1694.
30. Uflacker R, Kaemmerer A, Picon PD, Rizzon CFC, Neves CNC, Oliveira NJM, et al. Bronchial artery embolization in the management of hemoptysis: technical aspects and long term results. *Radiology* 1985;157:637–644.
31. Breuer R, Baigelman W, Pugatch RD. Occult mycetoma. *J Comput Assist Tomogr* 1982;6:166–168.
32. Butz RO, Zvetina JR, Leininger BJ. Ten-year experience with mycetomas in patients with pulmonary tuberculosis. *Chest* 1985;87:356–358.
33. Hughes CF, Waugh R, Lindsay D. Surgery for pulmonary aspergilloma: preoperative embolization of the bronchial circulation. *Thorax* 1986;41:324–325.
34. Jewkes J, Kay PH, Paneth M, Citron KM. Pulmonary aspergilloma: analysis of prognosis in relation to haemoptysis and survey of treatment. *Thorax* 1983;38:572.
35. Hansen LA, Prakash UBS, Colby TV. Pulmonary complications in diabetes mellitus. *Mayo Clin Proc* 1989;64:791–799.
36. Thoms NW, Wilson RF, Puro HE, Arbulu A. A life threatening hemoptysis in primary lung abscess. *Ann Thorac Surg* 1972; 14:347–358.
37. Dalen JE, Haffajee CI, Alpert JS. Pulmonary embolism, pulmonary hemorrhage and pulmonary infarction. *N Engl J Med* 1977;296:1431.
38. Prakash UBS: Vasculitides. In: Murray JF, ed. *Pulmonary manifestations in systemic diseases*. New York: Marcel Dekker; 1992;431–469. (Lung biology in health and disease. vol 59).
39. Leatherman JW, Davies SF, Hoidal JR. Alveolar hemorrhage syndromes: diffuse microvascular lung hemorrhage in immune and idiopathic disorders. *Medicine (Balt)* 1984;63:343–361.
40. Hara K, Prakash UBS. Fiberoptic bronchoscopy in the evaluation of acute chest and upper airway trauma. *Chest* 1989; 96:627–630.
41. Wilson RF, Soullier GW, Wiencek RG. Hemoptysis in trauma. *J Trauma* 1987;27:1123–1126.
42. American Thoracic Society. Statement on the management of hemoptysis. *Am Rev Resp Dis* 1966;93:471.
43. Shure D. Radiologically occult endobronchial obstruction in bronchogenic carcinoma. *Am J Med* 1991;91:19–22.
44. Heimer D, Bar-Ziv J, Scharf SM. Fiberoptic bronchoscopy in patients with hemoptysis and nonlocalizing chest roentgenograms. *Arch Intern Med* 1985;145:1427–1428.
45. Millar AB, Boothroyd AE, Edwards D, Hetzel MR. The role of computed tomography (CT) in the investigation of unexplained haemoptysis. *Resp Med* 1992;86:39–44.
46. Jone DK, Cavanagh P, Shneerson JM, Flower CD. Does bronchography have a role in the assessment of patients with hemoptysis? *Thorax* 1985;40:668–670.
47. Wagner RB, Baeza O, Stewart J. Active pulmonary hemorrhage localized by selective pulmonary angiography. *Chest* 1975;67:121–123.
48. Fellows KE, Stigos L, Shuster S, Khaw TK, Shwachman H. Selective bronchial arteriography in patients with cystic fibrosis and massive hemoptysis. *Radiology* 1975;114:551–556.
49. Saumench J, Escarrabill J, Padro L, Montana J, Clariana A, Canto A. Value of fiberoptic bronchoscopy and angiography for diagnosis of the bleeding site in hemoptysis. *Ann Thorac Surg* 1989;48:272–274.
50. Coel MN, Druger G; Radionuclide detection of the site of hemoptysis. *Chest* 1982;81:242–243.
51. Haponik EF, Rothfeld B, Britt EJ, Bleecker ER. Radionuclide localization of massive hemoptysis. *Chest* 1984;86:208.
52. Addleman M, Logan AS, Grossman RF. Monitoring intrapulmonary hemorrhage in Goodpasture's syndrome. *Chest* 1985; 87:119–120.
53. Berger R, Rehm SP. Bronchoscopy for hemoptysis. *Chest* 1991;99:1553–1557.
54. Haponik EF, Chin P. Hemoptysis: clinicians' perspective. *Chest* 1990;97:469–475.
55. Gong H Jr, Salvatierra C. Clinical efficacy of early and delayed fiberoptic bronchoscopy in patients with hemoptysis. *Am Rev Resp Dis* 1981;124:221–225.
56. ONeil KM, Lazarus AA. Hemoptysis. Indications for bronchoscopy. *Arch Intern Med* 1991;151:171–174.
57. Poe RH, Israel RH, Marin MG, Oritz CR, Dale RC, Wahl GW, Kallay MC, Greenblatt DG. Utility of fiberoptic bronchoscopy in patients with hemoptysis and a nonlocalizing chest roentgenogram. *Chest* 1988;92:70–75.
58. Prakash UBS. The use of pediatric fiberbronchoscope in adults. *Am Rev Resp Dis* 1985;132:715–717.
59. Danel C, Biet I, Costabel U, Rossi GA, Wallert B. The clinical role of BAL in pulmonary haemorrhages. *Eur Resp J* 1989; 2:951–952.
60. Drew L, Finley T, Golde D. Diagnostic lavage and occult pulmonary hemorrhage in thrombocytopenic immunocompromised patients. *Am Rev Resp Dis* 1977;116:215–221.
61. Flick MR, Wasson K, Dunn LJ. Fatal pulmonary hemorrhage after transbronchial biopsy via flexible bronchoscope. *Am Rev Resp Dis* 1975;111:853–856.
62. Cordasco EM Jr, Mehta AC, Ahmad M. Bronchoscopically-induced bleeding. A summary of nine years' Cleveland Clinic experience and review of the literature. *Chest* 1991; 100:1141–1147.
63. Zavala DC. Pulmonary hemorrhage in fiberoptic transbronchial biopsy. *Chest* 1976;70:584–588.
64. Hanson RR, Zavala DC, Rhodes ML. Transbronchial biopsy via flexible bronchoscope: results in 164 patients. *Am Rev Resp Dis* 1976;114:67–72.
65. Surratt DM, Smiddy JF, Bruber B. Deaths and complications associated with fiberoptic bronchoscopy. *Chest* 1976; 69:747–751.
66. Dreisin RB, Albert RR, Rabley PA. Flexible bronchoscopy in

the teaching hospital: yield and comparison. *Chest* 1978; 74:148–149.
67. Prickett C, LeGrand P. Complications of fiberoptic bronchoscopy in a community hospital. *Ala Med* 1984;53:25–27.
68. Pereira W, Kovnat DM, Snider GL. A prospective cooperative study of complications following flexible fiberoptic bronchoscopy. *Chest* 1978;73:813–816.
69. Credle WF Jr, Smiddy JF, Elliot RC. Complications of fiberoptic bronchoscopy. *Am Rev Resp Dis* 1974;109:67–72.
70. Ahmad M, Livingston DR, Golish JA, Mehta AC, Wiedemann HP. The safety of outpatient transbronchial lung biopsy. *Chest* 1986;90:403–405.
71. Burgher LW. Complications and results of transbronchoscopic lung biopsy. *Nebr Med J* 1979;64:247–248.
72. Simpson FG, Arnold AG, Purvis A, Belfield PW, Muers MF, Cooke NJ. Postal survey of bronchoscopic practice by physicians in the United Kingdom. *Thorax* 1986;41:311–317.
73. Levin DC, Wicks RB, Ellis JH Jr. Transbronchial lung biopsy via the fiberoptic bronchoscope. *Am Rev Resp Dis* 1974; 110:4–12.
74. Ellis JH Jr. Transbronchial lung biopsy via the fiberoptic bronchoscope: experience with 107 consecutive cases and comparison with bronchial brushing. *Chest* 1975;68:524–532.
75. Joyner LR, Scheinhorn DJ. Transbronchial forceps lung biopsy through the fiberoptic bronchoscope: diagnosis of diffuse pulmonary disease. *Chest* 1975;67:532–535.
76. Koerner DK, Sakowitz AJ, Appleman RI, Beckner NH, Schoenbaum SW. Transbronchial lung biopsy for the diagnosis of sarcoidosis. *N Engl J Med* 1975;293:268–270.
77. Stableforth DE, Knight RR, Collins JV, Heard BE, Clarke SW. Transbronchial lung biopsy through the fiberoptic bronchoscope. *Br J Dis Chest* 1978;72:108–114.
78. Mitchell DM, Emerson CJ, Collins JV, Stableforth DE. Transbronchial lung biopsy with the fiberoptic bronchoscope: an analysis of results in 433 patients. *Br J Dis Chest* 1981; 75:258–262.
79. Rees JR. Massive hemoptysis associated with foreign body removal. *Chest* 1985;88:475–476.
80. Olopade CO, Prakash UBS. Bronchoscopy in the intensive care critical care unit. *Mayo Clinic Proc* 1989;64:1255–1263.
81. Prakash UBS, Stubbs SE. The bronchoscopy survey: some reflections. *Chest* 1991;100:1660–1667.
82. Dumon JE, Shapshay S, Bourcereau J, Cavalieres S, Merc B, Garbi N, Beamis J. Principles for safety in application of Nd-YAG laser in bronchology. *Chest* 1984;86:163–168.
83. Ferris EJ. Pulmonary hemorrhage: vascular evaluation and interventional therapy. *Chest* 1981;80:710–714.
84. Zavala DC. Transbronchial biopsy in diffuse lung disease. *Chest* 1978;73:727–733.
85. Cunningham JH, Zavala DC, Corry RJ, et al. Trephine air drill, bronchial brush, and fiberoptic transbronchial lung biopsies in immunosuppressed patients. *Am Rev Resp Dis* 1977; 115:213–220.
86. Suchman AL, Mushlin AI. How well does the activated partial thromboplastin time predict postoperative hemorrhage? *JAMA* 1986;256:750–753.
87. Mannucci PM, Remozzi MD, Pusineri F, Lombardi R, Vlacchi C, Mecca G. Deamino 8D arginine vasopressin shortens the bleeding time in uremia. *N Engl J Med* 1983;308:8–11.
88. Mannucci PM, Vicente V, Vianello L, Cattaneo M, Alberca I, Coccato MP. Controlled trial of desmopressin in liver cirrhosis and other conditions associated with a prolonged bleeding time. *Blood* 1986;67:1148–1153.
89. Gerritsen SW, Akkerman JW, Sixma JJ. Correction of the bleeding time in patients with storage pool deficiency by infusion of cryoprecipitate. *Br J Haematol* 1978;40:153–160.
90. Bone RC. Massive hemoptysis. In: Sahn SA, ed. *Pulmonary emergencies*. New York: Churchill Livingstone; 1982;225–238.
91. Yang C-T, Berger HW. Conservative management of life-threatening hemoptysis. *Mt Sinai J Med* 1978;45:329–333.
92. Corey R, Hla KM. Major and massive hemoptysis: reassessment of conservative management. *Am J Med Sci* 1987; 294:301–309.
93. Drew PJT, Newland AC, Marsh FP. Immune complex mediated lung hemorrhage and nephritis—successful treatment with plasma exchange, haemodialysis and immunosuppressive drug therapy. *Postgrad Med J* 1984;60:52–55.
94. Sahebjami H. Iced saline lavage during bronchoscopy. *Chest* 1976;69:131.
95. Conlan AA, Hurwitz SS. Management of massive hemoptysis with the rigid bronchoscope and cold saline lavage. *Thorax* 1983;35:901–904.
96. Magee G. Williams MH Jr. Treatment of massive hemoptysis with intravenous Pitressin. *Lung* 1982;160:165–169.
97. Worth H, Breuer HWM, Charchut S, Trampisch HJ, Glaenzer K. Endobronchial versus intravenous application of glypressin for the therapy and prevention of lung bleeding during bronchoscopy. *Am Rev Resp Dis* 1987;135(4 part 2):A-108.
98. Long WM, Yerger LD, Marinez H. Modifications of bronchial blood flow during allergic airway responses. *J Appl Physiol* 1988;65:272–282.
99. Yeoh CB, Hubaytar RT, Ford JM, Wylie RH. Treatment of massive hemorrhage in pulmonary tuberculosis. *J Thoracic Cardiovasc Surg* 1967;54:503–510.
100. Hiebert CA. Balloon catheter control of life-threatening hemoptysis. *Chest* 1974;66:308–309.
101. Gottlieb LS, Hillberg R. Endobronchial tamponade therapy for intractable hemoptysis. *Chest* 1975;67:482–483.
102. Saw EC, Gottlieb LS, Yokahama Lee BC, et al. Flexible fiberoptic bronchoscopy and endobronchial tamponade in the management of hemoptysis. *Chest* 1976;70:589–591.
103. Swersky RB, Chang JB, Wisoff BG, Gorvoy J. Endobronchial balloon tamponade of hemoptysis in patients with cystic fibrosis. *Ann Thorac Surg* 1979;27:262–264.
104. Freitag L, Montag M. Development of a new balloon catheter for management of hemoptysis with bronchofiberscope. *Chest* 1993;103:593.
105. Schlehe H, Fritsche HM, Daum S. A new method for treatment of bronchial and lung bleeding. In: Nakhosteen JA, Maassen W, eds. *Bronchology* Haag:Nijhoff; 1984:111.
106. Tsukamoto T, Sasaki H, Nakamura H. Treatment of hemoptysis patients by thrombin and fibrinogen-thrombin infusion therapy using a fiberoptic bronchoscope. *Chest* 1989;96:473–476.
107. Bense L. Intrabronchial selective coagulative treatment of hemoptysis. Report of three cases. *Chest* 1990;97(4):990–996.
108. Lupinett FM, Stoney WS, Alford WC, Burrus GR, Glassford DM, Petracek MR. Cryoprecipitate-topical thrombin glue. *J Thorac Cardiovasc Surg* 1985;90:502–505.
109. Walsh TE: Bronchial infusion therapy (BIT). A bit of caution. *Chest* 1989;96:456–457.
110. Shivaram U, Finch P, Nowak P. Plastic endobronchial tubes in the management of life-threatening hemoptysis. *Chest* 1987; 92:1108–1110.
111. Baile EM, Albert RK, Kirk W, Lakshminarayan S, Wiggs BJR, Pare PD. Positive end-expiratory pressure decreases bronchial blood flow in the dog. *J Appl Physiol* 1984;56(5):1289–1293.
112. Gerasin VA, Shafirovsky BB. Endobronchial electosurgery. *Chest* 1988;93(2):270–274.
113. Wholey MH, Chamorro HA, Rao G, Gord WB, Miller WH. Bronchial artery embolization of the bronchial arteries. *Radiology* 1977;122:33–37.
114. Bredin CP, Richardson PR, King TKC, Sniderman KW, Sos TA, Smith JP. Treatment of massive hemoptysis by combined occlusion of pulmonary and bronchial arteries. *Am Rev Resp Dis* 1978;117:969–973.
115. Remy J, Lemaitre L, Lafitte JJ, Vilain MO, Saint Michel J, Steenhouwer F. Massive hemoptysis of pulmonary artery origin: diagnosis and management. *Am J Roentgenol* 1984; 143:963–969.
116. Muthuswamy PP, Akbik F, Franklin C, Spigos D, Barker WL. Management of major or massive hemoptysis in active pulmonary tuberculosis by bronchial arterial embolization. *Chest* 1987;92.1:77–82.
117. Pinet F, Clermont A, Michel C, Celard P, Lagrange C. Embolization of the systemic arteries of the lung. *J Thorac Imag* 1987; 2(2):11–17.
118. Ivanick MJ, Thoruvath W, Donohue J, et al. Infarction of the

left main-stem bronchus: a complication of bronchial artery embolization. *Am J Roentgenol* 1983;141:535–537.

119. Gourin A, Garzon And associates: Operative treatment of massive hemoptysis. *Ann Thorac Surg* 1974;18:52.
120. Sweezey NB, Fellows KE. Bronchial artery embolization for severe hemoptysis in cystic fibrosis. *Chest* 1990;97:1322–1326.
121. Katoh O, Yamada H, Hiura K, et al. Bronchoscopic and angiographic comparison of bronchial arterial lesions in patients with hemoptysis. *Chest* 1987;91:486.
122. McCollum WB, Mattox KL, Guinn GA. Immediate operative treatment for massive hemoptysis. *Chest* 1975;67:152–155.
123. Bodrowitz ID, Ramkrishna S, Shim Y. Comparison of medical vs surgical treatment of major hemoptysis. *Arch Intern Med* 1983;143:1343–1346.
124. Garzon AA, Gourin A. Surgical management of massive hemoptysis. *Ann Surg* 1978;187:267.
125. Gourin A, Garzon AA. Control of hemorrhage in emergency pulmonary resection for massive hemoptysis. *Chest* 1975; 68:120–121.
126. Crocco JA, Rooney JJ, Rankushen DS, DiBenedetto RJ, Lyons HA. Massive hemoptysis. *Arch Intern Med* 1968;121:495–498.
127. Garzon AA, Cerruti MM, Golding ME: Exsanguinating hemoptysis. *J Cardiovasc Surg* 1982;84:829.
128. Sehhat S, Oreizie M, Moinedine K. Massive pulmonary hemorrhage: surgical approach as choice of treatment. *Ann Thor Surg* 1978;25:12.
129. Bobrowitz ID, Ramakrishna S, Shim Y. Comparison of medical v surgical treatment of major hemoptysis. *Arch Intern Med* 1983;143:1343.
130. Long WM, Sprung CL, El-Fawal H. Effect of histamine on bronchial artery blood flow and bronchomotor tone. *J Appl Physiol* 1985;59:254–261.
131. Syabbalo NC. Medical management of hemoptysis. *Chest* 1989; 96:1441.
132. Adelman M, Haponik EF, Bleecker ER, Britt EJ. Cryptogenic hemoptysis. Clinical features, bronchoscopic findings, and natural history in 67 patients. *Ann Intern Med* 1985;102:829–834.
133. Panos RJ, Barr LF, Walsh TJ, Silverman HJ. Factors associated with fatal hemoptysis in cancer patients. *Chest* 1988; 94:1008–1013.

Bronchoscopy,
edited by U. B. S. Prakash.
Mayo Foundation © 1994.
Published by Raven Press, Ltd., New York.

CHAPTER 18

Tracheobronchial Foreign Bodies

Udaya B. S. Prakash and Denis A. Cortese

The first reported extraction of a tracheobronchial foreign body was in 1897 by Gustav Killian of Freiburg, Germany, who used an esophagoscope to extract a pork bone from the trachea of a 63-year-old farmer (1). Later, Killian modified the esophagoscope into a rigid bronchoscope. Chevalier Jackson of Philadelphia introduced a bronchoscope incorporating a suction tube as well as tip illumination in 1904 (2). The early years of bronchoscopy were exclusively dedicated to the extraction of tracheobronchial foreign bodies. The classic monograph on tracheobronchial foreign bodies by Jackson and Jackson in 1937 summarized the cases of several hundred patients with tracheobronchial and esophageal foreign bodies (3).

A review in 1982 (4) analyzed 141 fatalities associated with acute food asphyxiation, or the *cafe coronary* syndrome, but such cases are usually not considered in the discussion of tracheobronchial foreign bodies. Similarly, aspiration of gastric contents into the tracheobronchial tree and broncholithiasis are not considered foreign body problems. In this chapter, we discuss the diagnosis, various types, complications, and methods of extraction of tracheobronchial foreign bodies in children and adults.

TRACHEOBRONCHIAL FOREIGN BODIES IN CHILDREN

Clinical Features

For the purposes of discussion here, we will consider anyone below the age of 15 years a child. Aspiration of foreign bodies into the tracheobronchial tree is more common in children than in adults (5–12). Annual death rates from foreign body aspiration in the United States range from 500 to 2,000, with more than half of these occurring in children between the ages of 6 months and 4 years (13–17). Clinically unsuspected foreign bodies have been found in 1% of 1,054 pediatric patients who underwent flexible bronchoscopy for other reasons (18). In another report of 57 children who underwent bronchoscopy, tracheobronchial foreign bodies were found unexpectedly in 9% (19). The most likely candidate for inhalation of tracheobronchial foreign body is a boy around the age of 2 years. The commonly espoused reason for the high incidence of tracheobronchial foreign body aspiration in this age group, besides the bounding curiosity to bite and taste everything in sight, is the pattern of dental growth. Since the toddlers in this age group have yet to develop molars and premolars, all the biting is done by the incisors. When a child bites a hard object or a peanut, the object is forcefully squeezed between the upper and lower incisor teeth and instantaneously propelled backward toward the oropharynx and larynx. If the object is shattered, a piece of the object can do the same. The sudden and unexpected impact of the foreign body on the back of the throat elicits an inspiratory gasp during which the foreign object is aspirated into the tracheobronchial tree.

Elhassani (11) described the largest series of tracheobronchial foreign bodies in children living in the Middle East. Among the 2,170 children referred for bronchoscopy to exclude foreign bodies, 1,822 (83.7%) were found to have tracheobronchial foreign bodies. The commonest object was a watermelon seed, seen in 66.3% of patients. Bronchoscopy was successful in all but four patients. Mantel and Butenandt (8) studied 224 patients aged 7 months to 14 years who had aspirated foreign bodies. Eighty-one percent were younger than 3 years, 50% were in the second year of life, and there

U. B. S. Prakash: Division of Thoracic Diseases and Internal Medicine, Mayo Clinic, Rochester, Minnesota 55905.
D. A. Cortese: Division of Thoracic Diseases and Internal Medicine, Mayo Clinic, Jacksonville, Florida 32224.

were twice as many boys as girls. In a report from South Africa (20), 79% of 96 children were under 5 years old. Pasaoglu and associates (21) published their experience with 822 pediatric bronchoscopies performed from 1984 through 1990 at a Turkish university and reported that 65.3% were boys and 34.7% were girls, ranging in age from 1 month to 14 years. Definitive evidence of foreign body aspiration, as recorded from history, was obtained from 48% of patients and foreign bodies were found in 77.7%.

Vane et al. (22) performed rigid bronchoscopy in 131 children (79 boys and 52 girls, with a mean age of 2.1 years) for suspected aspiration of foreign bodies and found that all but two patients had evidence of a foreign body. Physical examination revealed diminished breath sounds in 99% and wheezing in 91% of patients. A report from Australia (23) noted that among 115 children who were found to have tracheobronchial foreign bodies, those between the ages of 1 and 3 years were the most commonly affected (75%) and boys outnumbered girls in the ratio 3:2. Mu and colleagues (24) conducted a retrospective review of 400 Chinese children who had inhaled foreign bodies and observed that nearly 90% of the patients were under 3 years of age, with the peak incidence of foreign body inhalation occurring between 1 and 2 years of age; the male/female ratio was about 1.2:1. Interestingly, a positive history of foreign body inhalation was obtained in 98% of cases.

Diagnosis

In the traditional teaching on clinical features of tracheobronchial foreign body, the classic diagnostic triad of sudden onset of coughing, wheezing, and decreased air entry is constantly mentioned. Yet during the early stage (within 24 hr) of foreign body aspiration, the complete triad is present in less than 30% of children (20,25). In delayed stage (beyond 24 hr), the triad may be seen in half the patients (25). Black and associates (17), in a review of 224 pediatric patients (ranging from 4 months to 13 years of age) with tracheobronchial foreign bodies, reported that coughing, choking, and wheezing were the presenting symptoms in 91% of patients. Inspiratory and expiratory roentgenograms were positive in 81%; fluoroscopy was positive in 41%.

It is not uncommon to miss the diagnosis of tracheobronchial foreign body in children. Nearly one fourth of children with tracheobronchial foreign body are treated initially on the basis of a different diagnosis (Fig. 1) (26). A delay of more than a week in the diagnosis as a result of patients' not seeking medical help is encountered in 16–50% of cases (23,27). One study of 157 children with tracheobronchial foreign bodies observed that, although there was a history of witnessed choking in 80% of patients, only 46% were diagnosed early (within 24 hr) (25). Of note is the finding from a Chinese study in 1991 that observed that even when there was a positive history of foreign body inhalation

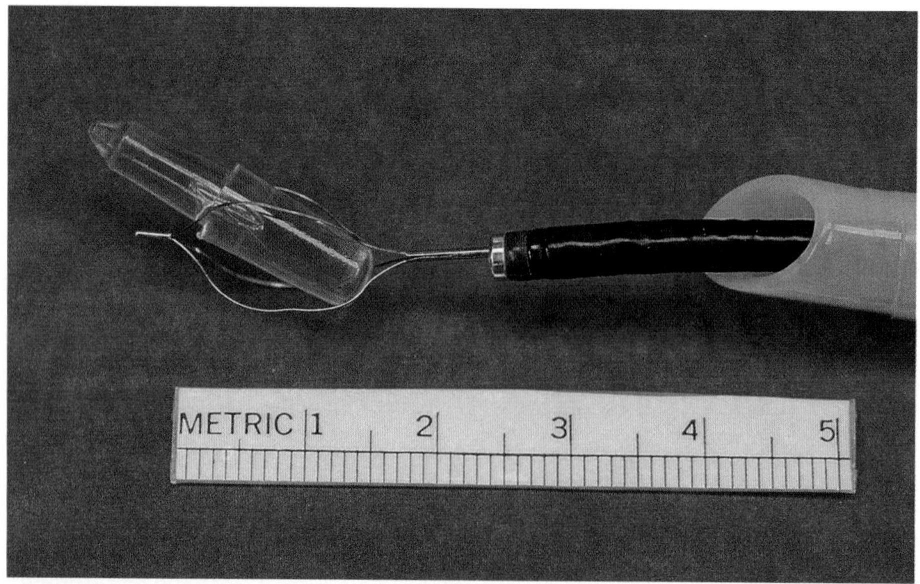

FIG. 1. A large foreign body (a plastic toy part) in a 2-year-old child was initially treated as upper respiratory infection because of the gurgly cough with no clinical evidence of bronchial obstruction. The possibility of a foreign body was considered only after 10 days of antibiotic therapy failed to resolve symptoms.

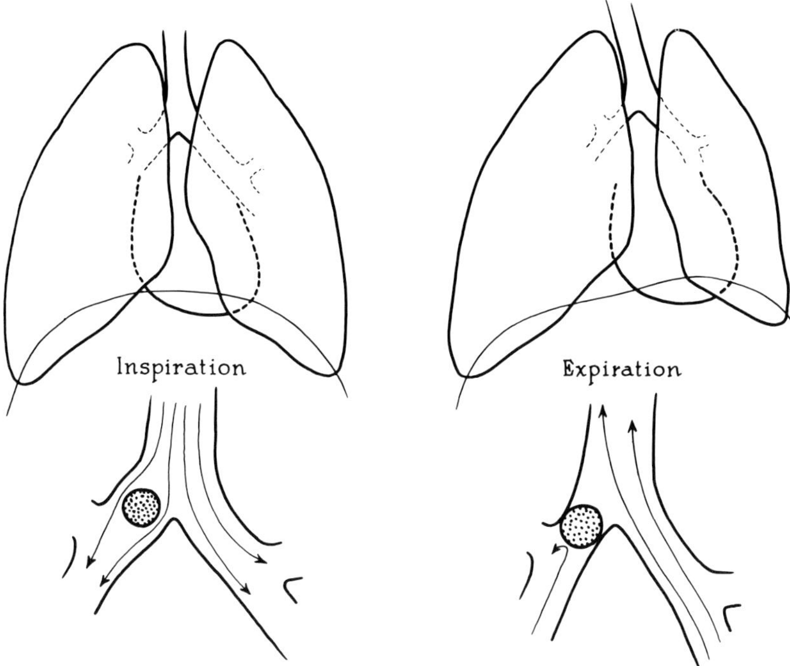

FIG. 2. The "ball-valve" mechanism of foreign body impaction in the right bronchial tree. During inspiration **(left)**, bronchial diameter increases and the inhaled air enters the alveoli by passing around the foreign body but during expiration **(right)**, bronchial narrowing does not allow the exhalation of air. This results in hyperinflation of lung on the side of foreign body impaction. The contralateral lung loses some volume because of mediastinal shift.

in 98% of 400 children, only 28% presented at the hospital within 24 hr, 71% within 1 week, and 29% more than 1 week after inhaling the foreign body (24). More than 30% of children are brought to the physician after 1–3 days following aspiration (21,26). Tracheal and right-sided foreign bodies are likely to be diagnosed earlier than the left-sided and peripherally lodged ones (25). Occasionally children who present with symptoms of foreign body inhalation may have other respiratory problems (28). A flexible bronchoscopy will be helpful in confirming the absence of a tracheobronchial foreign body.

Plain roentgenograms of chest are almost always obtained when foreign body aspiration is suspected. The size and shape of radiopaque objects are easily identified. Unilateral hyperinflation may suggest air trapping followed by hyperinflation (Fig 2). Lobar or segmental atelectasis may be present (Fig. 3). Mediastinal shift to the contralateral side is associated with hyperinflation (Fig. 3). Many studies have shown that a plain chest roentgenogram is not totally reliable. The inspiration chest roentgenogram is frequently normal even when the diagnosis is delayed. A retrospective study of 400 children with tracheobronchial foreign bodies showed

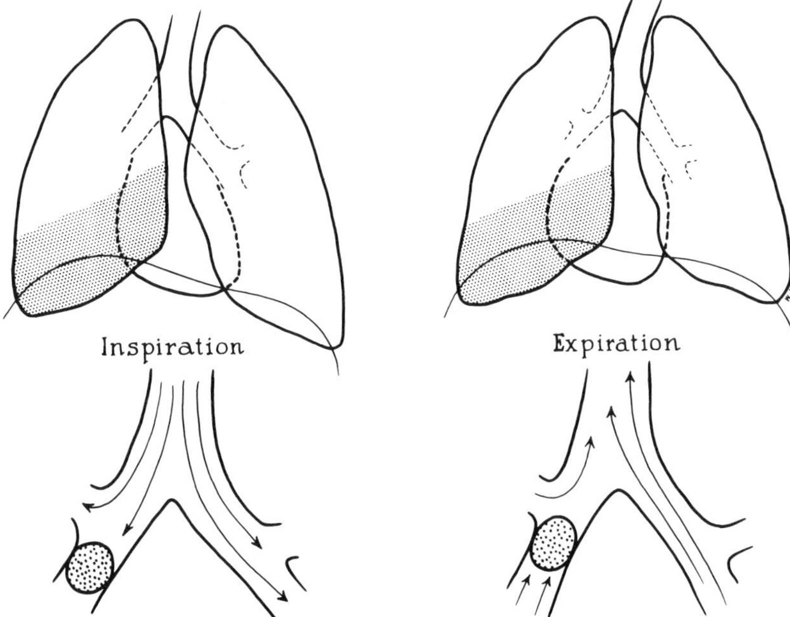

FIG. 3. A firm impaction of foreign body in a bronchus does not allow air to pass during inspiration **(left)** or expiration **(right)**. The oxygen in the obstructed lung segment is fully absorbed and the segment becomes atelectatic.

that approximately 65% of the children with laryngotracheal foreign bodies and 35% with bronchial foreign bodies had normal chest roentgenograms; the most common fluoroscopic findings in those children with bronchial foreign bodies were mediastinal shift in 36.8% and obstructive emphysema in 35.7% (24). One study noted normal chest roentgenograms in 24% of patients with documented tracheobronchial foreign bodies (29). Another study of 83 consecutive children with tracheobronchial foreign bodies demonstrated that the diagnostic accuracy of plain chest roentgenogram was 67%, sensitivity 68%, and specificity 67% (29). Therefore, it is strongly recommended that fluoroscopy or full-expiration films be obtained in any patient in whom the diagnosis is in doubt (30). Wiseman (25), during a 10-year period, treated 157 children for foreign body aspiration. The diagnostic accuracy of clinical and roentgenological findings was 83.5%. Others, however, reported higher diagnostic rates with plain chest roentgenograms. In one report on 129 children with tracheobronchial foreign bodies (22), the chest roentgenograms were diagnostic or suggestive of aspirated foreign bodies in 97%.

The timing of chest roentgenography in relation to foreign body aspiration may be a contributing factor for the differences in roentgenological findings. The chest roentgenogram tends to be normal in one third of the patients diagnosed early (within 24 hr of foreign body inhalation) but will exhibit atelectasis or consolidation in 50% of those diagnosed late (24 hr or longer after foreign body aspiration) (25).

Less than 25% of pediatric tracheobronchial foreign bodies are radiopaque (19,22,30,31). Unilateral hyperlucency on the chest roentgenogram may represent air trapping or be due to pulmonary vasoconstriction (30). In a retrospective review of 155 children with tracheobronchial foreign bodies, 6% exhibited pneumomediastinum on the initial chest roentgenogram (32). Roentgenological finding of pneumomediastinum in children should prompt further investigation for tracheobronchial foreign body.

Bronchoscopic Findings

The locations of foreign bodies in pediatric airways have been described in many reports. In one report on 224 children, 56% were localized to the right bronchial tree, 39% in the left, and 5% in the subglottic area or the trachea (8). Early bronchoscopy (within 24 hr of aspiration) may reveal mild mucosal inflammation in approximately 40% of patients, whereas delayed bronchoscopy (24 hr after aspiration) has shown severe inflammation in 36% (25).

The bronchoscopic findings depend on the type, size, and shape of the foreign body as well as the duration of its lodgement in the tracheobronchial tree. Often it is difficult to accurately identify the type of foreign body by bronchoscopic visualization even with a rigid bronchoscope and a Hopkins rod telescope system. The color of the inhaled object can cause difficulty in discriminating the object from the mucosa and the bronchial branchings. Aspirated raw carrot sticks, red or brown pencil erasers, and toy parts blend with the mucosa and may initially escape detection. Generally, an inorganic foreign body produces minimal or negligible mucosal inflammation or edema. Sharp objects may cause a mucosal tear and minor bleeding. Chronic retention of inorganic foreign body may provoke growth of granulation tissue. Rust produced by chronic retention of metallic foreign bodies such as pins and needles also induce granulation tissue. Bronchoscopy may reveal varying amounts of granulation tissue around the foreign body that may eventually become completely encased in the granulation tissue.

Organic foreign bodies, particularly peanut (ground nut) and other nuts that yield oil, produce severe mucosal inflammation within a short time. It is not uncommon to see significant mucosal edema and erythema within a few hours after aspiration (Fig. 4). Bronchoscopic extraction is more difficult once the inflammation and edema have set in because any manipulation is more likely to produce bleeding. Bronchial mucosal inflammation, edema, and formation of granulation tissue proximal to the foreign body can obscure the foreign object and increase the difficulty of extraction (Fig. 5). If not removed within 48 hr, purulent mucus will start collecting distally and bronchoscopy may reveal slow oozing of this material around the object (Fig. 5).

Treatment

The definitive treatment of tracheobronchial foreign body is removal at the earliest possible time. The reasons for early removal are mentioned above. The instrument of choice for extraction of a tracheobronchial foreign body in children is the rigid bronchoscope (8,33). Success rates exceeding 98% have been reported with a rigid bronchoscope (17,34). Black and associates (17) in a review of 224 pediatric patients (ranging from 4 months to 13 years) reported a bronchoscopic removal rate of 99%. Optically guided extraction instruments permit precise localization and removal. Several modifications of this system are available.

The flexible bronchoscope has been employed to extract pediatric foreign bodies. Monden and colleagues (35) used the flexible bronchoscope in conjunction with a Fogarty balloon catheter in 11 children with foreign bodies and reported a success rate of 82% in children

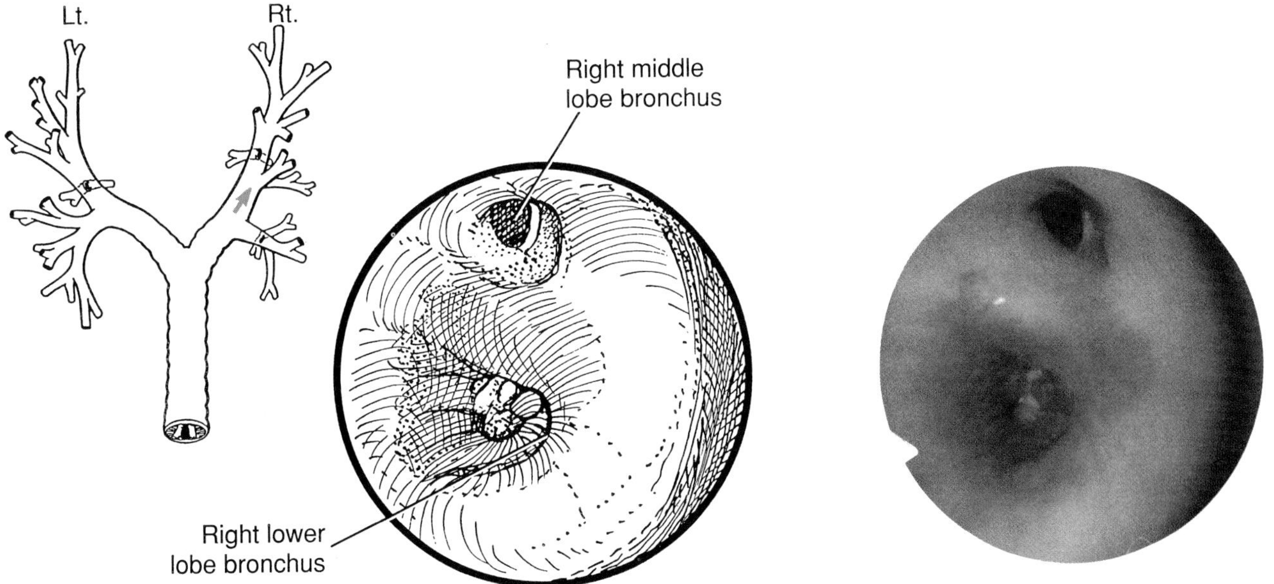

FIG. 4. Chemical reaction between bronchial mucosa and peanut oil following aspiration of a peanut produces intense inflammation, edema, and formation of granulation tissue within a short period. Hence the need for immediate removal of organic foreign body from the tracheobronchial tree.

who were 2 years of age or younger (Fig. 6). We have also used the flexible bronchoscope with an outer diameter of 3.2 mm to extract several foreign bodies from the pediatric tracheobronchial tree (Fig. 7). However, the bronchoscopist who wishes to use the flexible instrument for this purpose should be aware of the risk of loosing the foreign body in the narrow subglottic space and have the means to prevent the resultant asphyxia. If the foreign body is too small to cause total airway obstruction, even if it is lost in the upper trachea during removal, it is worth a try to use the suction to bring it out.

The diagnostic use of the pediatric flexible bronchoscope is safe, definitive, and cost-effective for the iden-

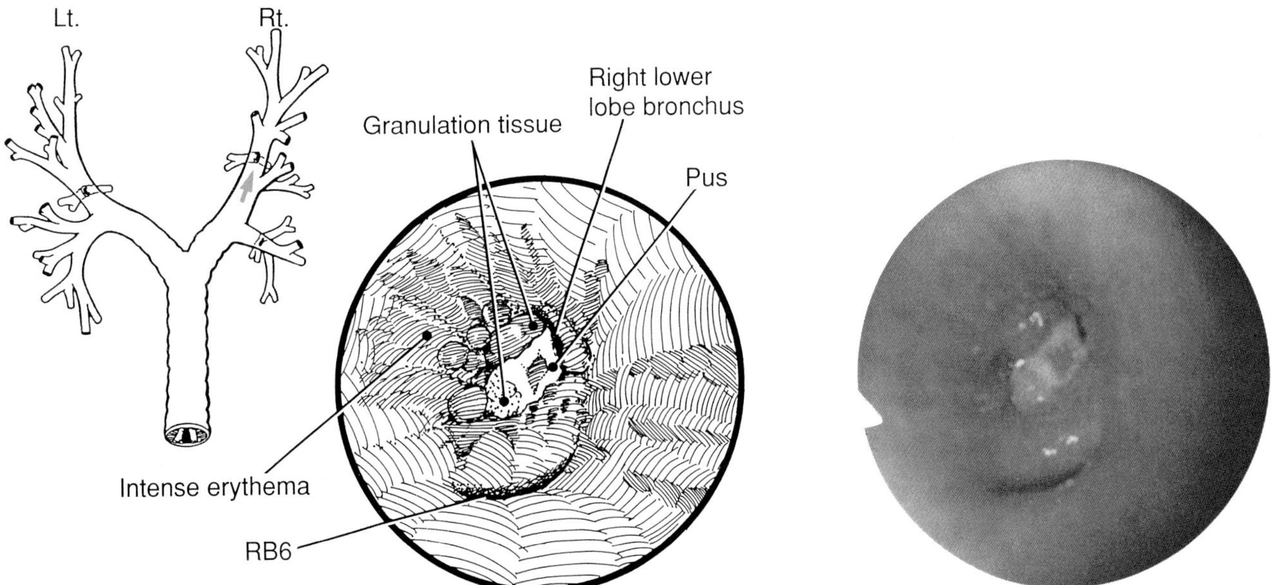

FIG. 5. Same case as in Fig. 4; close-up view reveals intense erythema, edema, formation of granulation tissue, and pus exuding from behind the foreign body. These changes occurred within 72 hr of aspiration of a peanut.

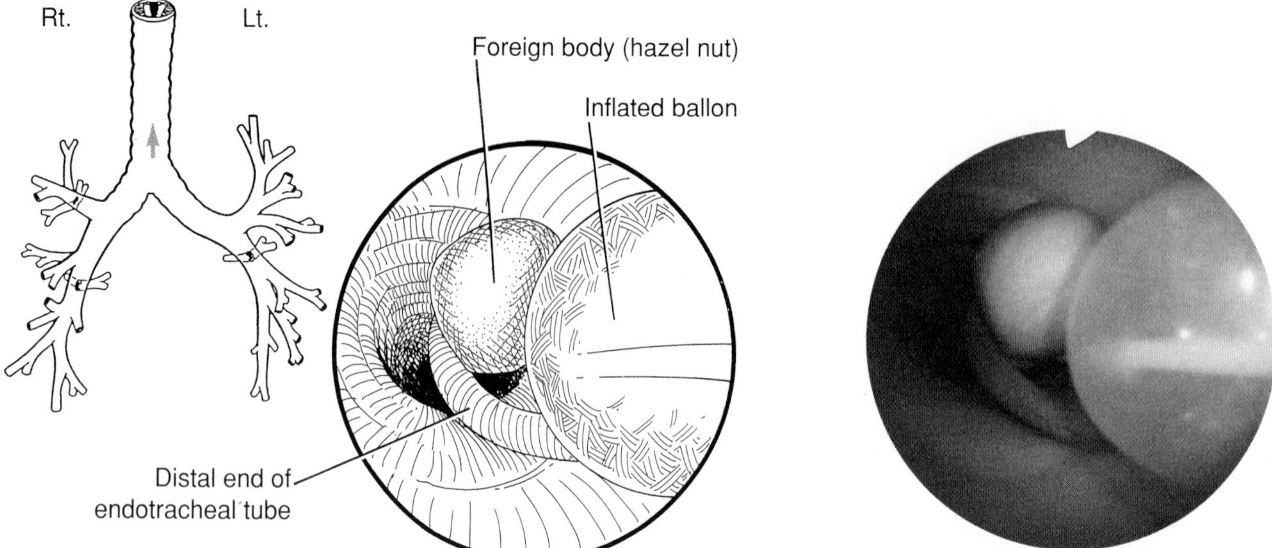

FIG. 6. Cephalad view of a simulated technique of foreign body (hazel nut) extraction using an endotracheal tube and a Fogarty balloon. Under direct view using an ultrathin flexible bronchoscope, the balloon is inflated distal to the foreign body, which is gradually withdrawn into the endotracheal tube and the entire combination (endotracheal tube, bronchoscope, foreign body, and inflated balloon) is removed en masse.

tification of tracheobronchial foreign bodies in pediatric patients when other techniques yield equivocal or negative results (18). Patients found to have a foreign body should undergo rigid bronchoscopy at the same time for foreign body removal. It is not cost-effective or safe to diagnose the foreign body by flexible bronchoscopy and then postpone the rigid bronchoscopic removal or transfer the patient to another area for rigid bronchoscopy.

TRACHEOBRONCHIAL FOREIGN BODIES IN ADULTS

Clinical Features

Tracheobronchial foreign bodies are uncommon in adults. In contrast to hundreds of publications pertaining to pediatric tracheobronchial foreign bodies, there are only a handful of reports on tracheobronchial for-

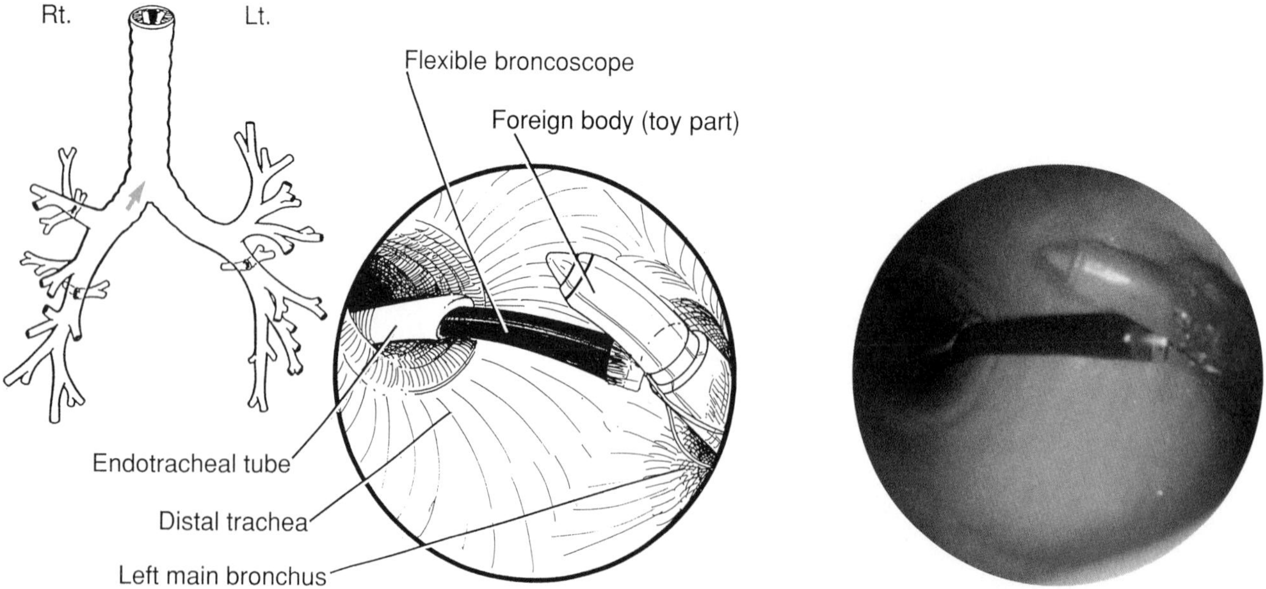

FIG. 7. Cephalad view of a simulated technique of foreign body (toy part shown in Fig. 1) extraction using a pediatric flexible bronchoscope (outer diameter 3.2 mm) and ureteral stone basket.

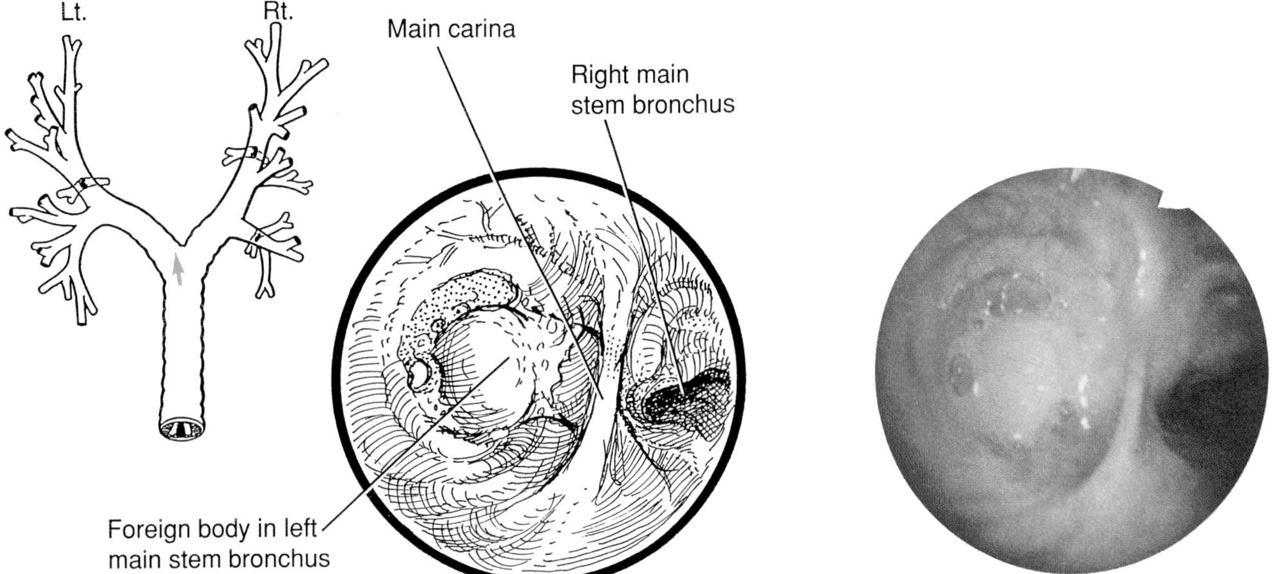

FIG. 8. Almost complete obstruction of left main stem bronchus by a foreign body (a large slippery segment of canned peach) in a 102-year-old edentulous female. We initially employed the flexible bronchoscope, but it was futile despite 30 min of flexible bronchoscopic procedure using various ancillary instruments. Ultimately we removed it in one piece in less than 3 min using a rigid bronchoscope.

eign bodies in adults (36–42). The monumental treatise by Jackson and Jackson (3) described extensive details of 191 adults with tracheobronchial foreign bodies; the right lower lobe was the site of foreign body impaction in 56%, followed by left lower lobe in 33%. Nearly half the foreign bodies were shawl pins, straight pins, and safety pins; the longest duration of foreign body retention in the tracheobronchial tree was 40 years.

The largest series of adults with tracheobronchial foreign bodies in recent years has been from the Mayo Clinic (42). Over a 33-year period, 60 adults (greater than 16 years of age) were identified; 42 patients were males, yielding a male-to-female ratio of 2.4:1. The median age was 60 years (range 18–88 years). Eighteen patients were in their seventh decade of life, with the remainder of cases evenly distributed among the other decades. In contrast to the common finding of metal pins in the series by Jackson and Jackson (3), the most commonly aspirated objects in the Mayo series were food items (24 patients) (Figs. 8 and 9), with peanuts leading the list (7 patients). The second predominant group of aspirations (19 patients) involved inadvertent loss of dental equipment or prostheses (Fig. 10), as well as tracheostomy tube segments and endotracheal tube appliances during dental or medical procedures. These aspirations were identified immediately at the time of the associated procedures. The final group of 17 patients had a wide variety of foreign bodies (Table 1) (42).

Occult aspiration of solid food pieces may not produce acute airway symptoms in some patients (43). This is particularly the case in elderly patients with chronic gastroesophageal reflux and neurological deficits (42).

Diagnosis

The singular diagnostic factor leading to the discovery of tracheobronchial foreign body aspiration in an

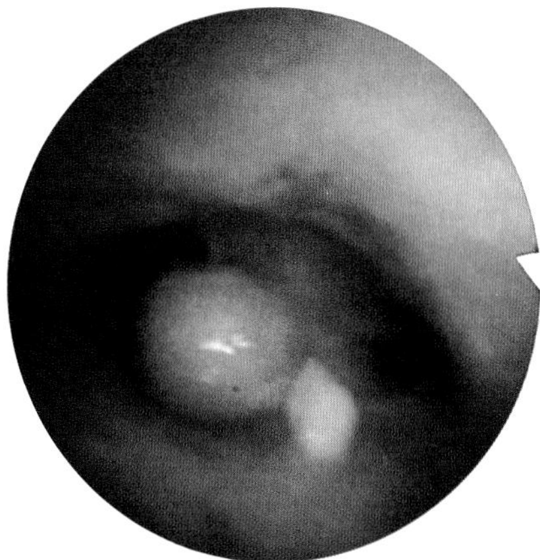

FIG. 9. A whole pea and a kernel of corn sitting on RC1 carina in 88-year-old edentulous male who aspirated a large number of peas, corn kernels, and bean segments. All were removed with a flexible bronchoscope.

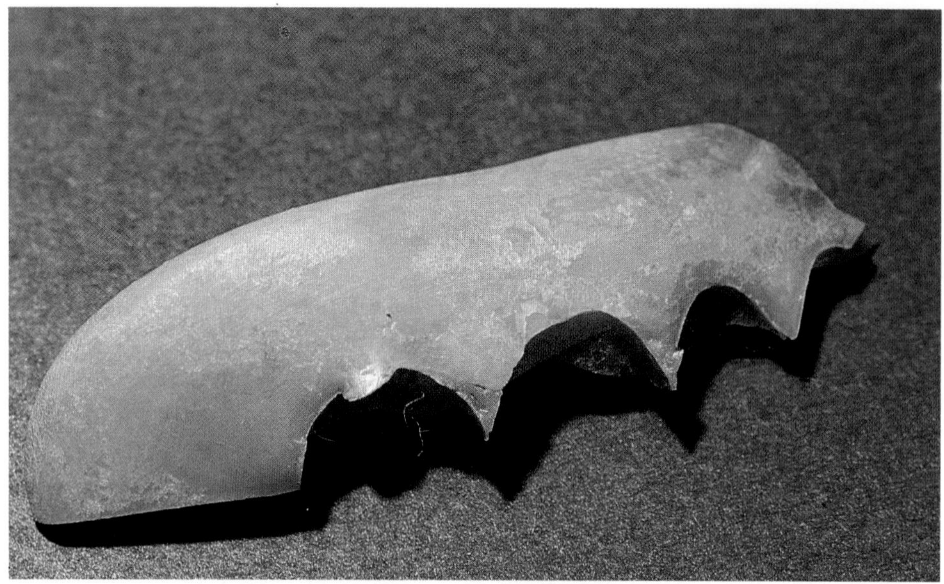

FIG. 10. A large piece of dental prosthesis removed from the right bronchus intermedius of a 40-year-old female who presented with chronic asthma that began soon after an automobile accident in which she had lost consciousness and presumably aspirated this foreign body. The diagnosis was not made until 9 years later when persistent unilateral wheezing was detected. The foreign body with surrounding granulation tissue was removed with a rigid bronchoscope.

TABLE 1. *Types of tracheobronchial foreign bodies aspirated by 60 adults*

Object	Cases (*n*)
Food particles	
Vegetable matter	17
Meat and bones	7
Total	24
Iatrogenic aspirations	
Dental appliances	10
Medical appliances	9
Total	19
Miscellaneous	
Straight pins	3
Safety pin	1
Piece of plastic drinking straw	1
Stone	1
Coin	1
Beverage can pull-tab	1
Tooth	1
Pine needle	1
Button	1
Grass inflorescence	1
Vitamin tablet	1
Metal toy	1
Denture fragment	1
Thermometer	1
Thumb tack	1
Total	17

From Limper AH, Prakash UBS (42), with permission.

adult is a high clinical index of suspicion. Foreign body inhalation is frequently suspected in children with acute or recurrent pulmonary symptoms. In adults, however, it is rarely considered unless a clear history of an aspiration event can be obtained. Nevertheless, certain clinical aspects should alert the physician to the possibility of foreign body inhalation. Predisposing factors in adults include neurological disorders, mental retardation, traumatic loss of consciousness, alcohol or sedative use, dental procedures, and medical procedures (particularly those involving cleaning, replacing, or manipulating tracheostomy or endotracheal tubes), including general anesthesia (Table 2). In most cases, the diagnosis was made with symptoms present for a median of 10 days prior to bronchoscopic examination (42). However, diagnosis can be delayed due to patients' disregarding their symptoms or failed attempts at diagnosis or treatment.

Occult foreign body aspiration in adults can remain undiagnosed for years and may lead to the wrong diagnosis of asthma, bronchitis, or chronic pneumonia (3,44,45). Abrupt onset of incessant cough should raise suspicion; hemoptysis has been observed in 15% of patients (42).

A chest roentgenogram (posteroanterior and lateral views) is very helpful in the diagnosis of more than 70% of patients (42). Radiopaque foreign bodies can

TABLE 2. *Factors predisposing adults to tracheobronchial foreign body aspiration*

Condition	Patients (*n*)
Primary neurological disorders	
Cerebrovascular accidents	3
Parkinson's disease	2
Seizures	2
Mental retardation	2
Primary brain neoplasm	1
Cerebral palsy	1
Total	11
Dental procedures	10
Medical procedures	9
Traumatic loss of consciousness	6
Alcohol or sedative use	5

From Limper AH, Prakash UBS (42), with permission.

be easily seen and anatomic locations identified (Fig. 11). Occasionally, it is difficult to ascertain whether the foreign body is in the trachea or esophagus. A non-radiopaque foreign body may be easily missed on chest roentgenogram but may be suggested by atelectasis or pneumonia or by air trapping, hyperinflation, and mediastinal shift (to the opposite side) on a postexhalation chest roentgenogram (8,11,12,42). Foreign bodies made of aluminum are radiolucent and may escape detection by standard chest roentgenogram (40,42). Many dental plates are made of materials that are radiolucent and hence are invisible on chest roentgenogram (46). Rarely, localized tomography, computed tomography, or bronchography may be required to identify an otherwise occult foreign body.

Bronchoscopic Findings

The most important procedure in the diagnosis and treatment of tracheobronchial foreign body in adults is bronchoscopy. The site of lodgement of the foreign body is dependent on the anatomic variations in the tracheobronchial tree and the body posture of the individual at the time of aspiration. In the Mayo series of 60 adults, the foreign body was in the right bronchial tree in 36, left side in 23, and trachea in 1 patient. The most common site was the right lower lobe bronchus (28%) followed by left lower lobe bronchus in 18%, and left main stem bronchus in 17% (42).

The types of foreign bodies recovered in the Mayo series of 60 adults are listed in Table 1. Some of the unusual foreign bodies included grass inflorescence, a piece of drinking straw, and stone. The stone was aspirated during a cave-in accident at a quarry (Fig. 11B), similar to other reported cases (47,48). Several cases of tracheobronchial aspiration of grass inflorescence (foxtail or cheat grass) have been reported (42,49–51). When aspirated with the spikes pointed backward, the grass inflorescence is almost impossible to dislodge by coughing.

Treatment

Management of tracheobronchial foreign body in adults has undergone substantial evolution mostly because of wider application of flexible bronchoscopy in clinical practice. Traditionally, rigid bronchoscopy has been the preferred treatment for adults (3). Many re-

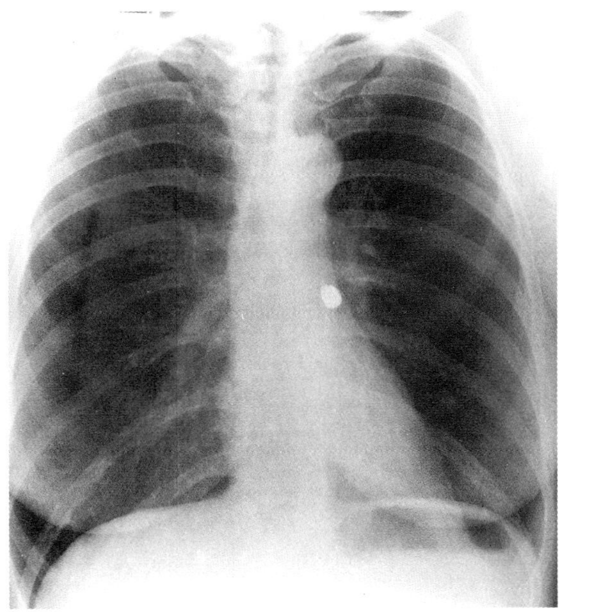

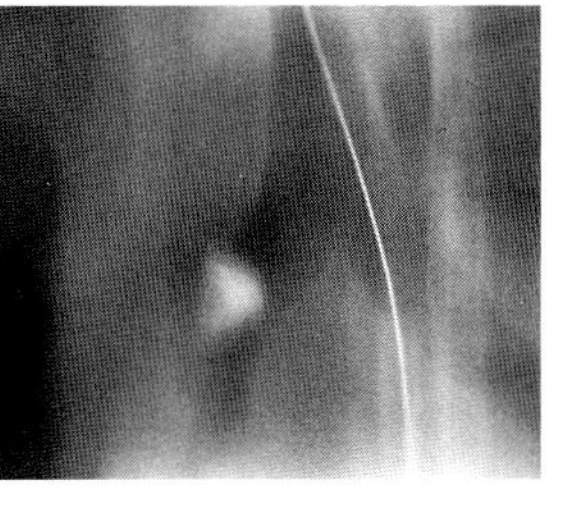

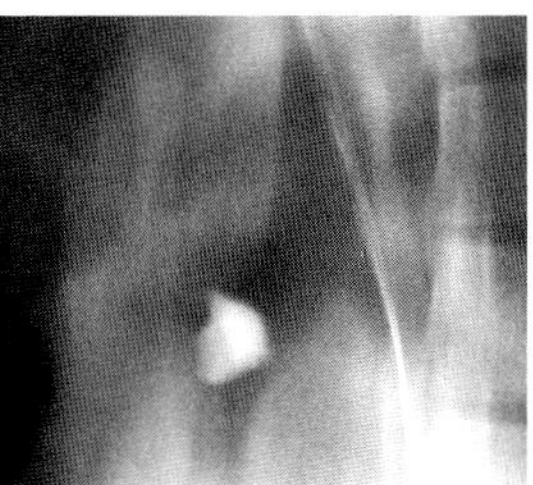

FIG. 11. (A) Chest roentgenogram showing a radiopaque foreign body in the left bronchial tree. **(B)** A large stone aspirated by a young male during a quarry cave-in was not well seen on routine chest roentgenogram but a tomography defined it. It was removed with a rigid bronchoscope.

ports have indicated that flexible bronchoscopy may be a valuable therapeutic option for adults (33,52–56). Lan and associates (57) described their experience using the flexible bronchoscope to treat chronically lodged tracheobronchial foreign bodies in 21 adults; the foreign bodies were recognized and removed by the first bronchoscopy in 85.7% of patients, but a second bronchoscopy was needed in the rest. Some authors have proposed that flexible bronchoscopy is preferable to rigid bronchoscopy in the evaluation and removal of tracheobronchial foreign bodies in adults (33,58). We disagree that the flexible instrument is superior to the rigid bronchoscope for extracting foreign bodies. In our own experience, flexible bronchoscopy has been successful in 60% of patients in contrast to a 98% success rate associated with rigid bronchoscopy (42). We recognize that flexible bronchoscopy is superior in specific cases where the foreign body is lodged too far distally to be reached with the rigid bronchoscope or in cases where instability of the cervical spine prevents rigid bronchoscopic manipulation. Other definitive indications for flexible bronchoscopy include foreign body in patients who are mechanically ventilated and patients with trauma or fractures of the jaw, cervical spine, or skull. There are many types of baskets, grasping claws, electromagnets, balloon catheters, suction tubes, and other instruments manufactured for use through the flexible bronchoscope (59–67). Our experience suggests that most of these instruments are flimsy, awkward to use, and ill-suited to grasp or extract all foreign bodies.

Bronchoscopists planning to use the flexible bronchoscope in foreign body removal should be aware of the problems and hazards that may ensue if improperly managed (68). Most notably, larger foreign bodies removed with a flexible bronchoscope may be sheared off from the extracting forceps while passing through the narrow subglottic trachea, with subsequent severe airway compromise. Such cases will require immediate removal with the rigid bronchoscope to restore airway patency (69).

Rigid bronchoscopy is highly effective in the extraction of foreign bodies. It is rapidly accomplished, usually within minutes, whereas flexible bronchoscopic removal tends to be a lengthy procedure. Additionally, a wide assortment of instruments are available for use with the rigid bronchoscope to extract virtually any shaped object from the tracheobronchial tree. Another major advantage is that the rigid bronchoscope provides the bronchoscopist with the ability to control the airway throughout the procedure (42). The risk of general anesthesia, if it is necessary, is minimal. The Mayo Clinic report on 60 adults stated that all but three were successfully treated by bronchoscopic retrieval of the foreign bodies. Two patients who failed bronchoscopic removal attempts and one patient in whom the foreign body was bronchoscopically invisible required thoracotomy; the foreign objects in all three were impacted in distal basilar segments of the lower lobes (42).

TYPES OF FOREIGN BODIES

Accidental Aspiration

The common foreign bodies in the tracheobronchial tree include nuts, seeds, pieces of vegetable, pins, needles, teeth, coins, tablets, and buttons. A review of the literature indicates many unusual types of tracheobronchial foreign bodies including hypodermic needles (70,71), bones of birds and small animals (37), toys (42,72), thermometer (42,72,73), piece of drinking straw (42,74), egg shell (75), dental polishing brush (76), golf tee (77), dental metal casting (78), pencil cap (79), polyurethane foam (80), and grass inflorescence (foxtail or cheat grass) (42,49–51). An unusual complication of aspiration of an intact four-unit metal bridge as a result of facial trauma has been reported (81). Aspiration of *Ascaris lumbricoides* (roundworm) from the gastric cavity to the tracheobronchial tree, while not a true example of accidental aspiration, can cause bronchial obstruction and is another "unusual" foreign body to be considered in the tropics (82).

The major tracheobronchial foreign body in children is a nut, with peanut (ground nut) being present in nearly half the children (8,20,23). Others (72) reported that more than two thirds of the foreign bodies are fruit and vegetable seeds and nuts. Al-Naaman and colleagues (10) described 40 pediatric cases of nonvegetable foreign bodies that included coins, washers, pins, reamers, nails, screws, wires, pencil caps, ball-point tip, worry beads, bones, broken tooth, small stones, and blades of broken foreign body forceps.

The type of foreign body may vary, depending on the geographic location. Among 639 Turkish children with tracheobronchial foreign bodies, the most commonly found foreign bodies were sunflower seeds (21.1%), beans (10.4%), watermelon seeds (10%), and hazelnuts (9.8%) (21). Prayer beads or distraction beads (worry beads) are commonly used in the Middle East and along with watermelon seeds are among the frequently aspirated objects (11,12). The fashions or occupations of different eras also dictate the type of foreign body. For instance, the common foreign bodies aspirated during the Jackson period (3) included shawl pins and hat pins, which were in vogue at that time.

Not all tracheobronchial foreign bodies are inhaled or aspirated. A case is described of a patient with a penetrating bullet wound of the chest in whom the 0.38 caliber bullet was unexpectedly found entirely within the lumen of the right lower lobe bronchus at bronchoscopy and was removed with a rigid bronchoscope (83).

Transtracheal migration of an intravertebral Steinmann pin to the left bronchus has been extracted with a rigid bronchoscope (84). Terasaki et al. (85) reported massive accidental inhalation of sawdust particles in a 17-year-old male that resulted in severe respiratory distress, subcutaneous emphysema, and left pneumothorax. The sawdust particles were removed by flexible bronchoscopy and bronchial lavage using venovenous extracorporeal lung assist with an artificial lung, with full recovery in 36 hr.

Iatrogenic Aspiration

Many instruments used in dentistry are small enough to be easily aspirated during dental procedures. The inadvertent aspiration of dental equipment or prostheses was recorded in 32% of 60 adults with tracheobronchial foreign bodies (42). Fracture, separation, and aspiration of parts of endotracheal or tracheostomy tubes is another iatrogenic cause of tracheobronchial foreign bodies (86).

Even though equipment malfunction is a rare complication of bronchoscopy, breakage of accessory instruments within the tracheobronchial tree results in the complication of iatrogenic tracheobronchial foreign body. The tip of the cytology brush, the cleaning brush, or a cup of the biopsy forceps may break off during the procedure (10,87–96). The use of the Fogarty catheter to remove tracheobronchial foreign body has resulted in the separation of the tip of the Fogarty catheter from the catheter body and resultant lodging of the catheter tip out of bronchoscopic range in the peripheral lower lobe of the lung (97). We have encountered a similar problem in a patient in whom a Fogarty catheter balloon was used to treat a bronchopleural fistula.

Metered dose inhalers that deliver aerosolized medications are frequently carried in the pockets of patients who use them. Other contents of the pocket, such as coins and loose materials, tend to accumulate in the mouthpiece. Several cases of tracheobronchial aspiration of coins and parts of inhalers themselves have been described (39,98).

An iatrogenic tracheobronchial foreign body may result from thoracic surgery. Surgical procedures involving pulmonary resections often employ metallic staples and sutures. Bronchoscopy in patients who have undergone lobectomy or pneumonectomy commonly reveal metallic staples or sutures in the resection stump or within the bronchial lumen. Although the majority of these remain asymptomatic and do not require removal, loose metal staples and sutures can cause cough, hemoptysis, and the formation of granuloma (99,100). Many patients cough out loose metal staples. Bronchoscopic removal with forceps is possible in most cases, although a Nd:YAG laser has been used to evaporate a nonmetallic suture (100,101). Plombage of the pleural cavity was one of the therapeutic procedures used in the past to treat pulmonary tuberculosis. The materials inserted into the pleural space to collapse the lung included paraffin and lucite balls, among other objects. We have encountered several patients presenting with expectoration of waxy bronchial casts and pieces of lucite.

TECHNIQUES OF REMOVAL

Nonbronchoscopic Methods

Should all tracheobronchial foreign bodies be removed? It is clear that many people aspirate foreign bodies into their tracheobronchial tree and remain asymptomatic for many years. The presence of a foreign body in such patients is detected by chest roentgenogram obtained for an unrelated reason. The lack of any symptom or the presence of only minimal symptoms is likely if the foreign body is small and lodged in the very small bronchi closer to lung parenchyma. The incidence of chronic complications in such cases is unknown. The risk of potentially serious complications is present in these subjects. Therefore, some have recommended removal of the foreign body even if the patient is asymptomatic (102). It is difficult to reconcile with this recommendation because if the bronchoscopic removal is not possible, then the patient has to be subjected to a major surgical procedure. Careful instruction to the patient to be on the lookout for symptoms and regular clinical and chest roentgenological follow-up seems more prudent.

Campbell and associates (103) attempted nonbronchoscopic treatment of tracheobronchial foreign bodies in 28 children in whom the foreign bodies were located in the segmental or lobar bronchi. The treatment consisted of inhalation of bronchodilator, pulmonary drainage, and thoracic percussion. Treatment was successful in 64% of patients who expectorated the foreign body; the remaining ten children underwent bronchoscopy, which was successful in eight and unsuccessful in two patients. Of the two patients, one required bronchotomy, and the other coughed out the foreign body. Another study on the efficacy of the inhalation therapy and postural drainage technique for removal of aspirated foreign bodies in 76 children documented that 25% coughed out the foreign body; the rest required bronchoscopy (104).

These studies suggest that a trial of inhalation-postural drainage, administered in a hospital, may be valuable in the initial management of aspirated foreign bodies. If unsuccessful after several treatments, however, the conservative treatment should be abandoned and bronchoscopy performed because delay of foreign body removal beyond 24 hr may be associated with increased morbidity and prolonged hospital stay (104).

Bronchoscopic Removal

Anesthesia

The majority of patients who undergo rigid bronchoscopy will require deep intravenous sedation or general anesthesia. The decision to use topical or general anesthesia is dictated by the patient's apprehension and clinical status as well as the size and location of the foreign body. A small, easily graspable foreign body in the proximal bronchial tree can be successfully removed under topical anesthesia with or without intravenous sedation. The removal process of a distally lodged or bronchoscopically invisible foreign body may become prolonged and therefore require deep intravenous sedation or general anesthesia. We recommend a reverse Trendelenburg position to let the foreign body, especially a spherical one, move proximally. This will also help in keeping the contralateral bronchial tree from flooding by blood or mucous generated during foreign body retrieval.

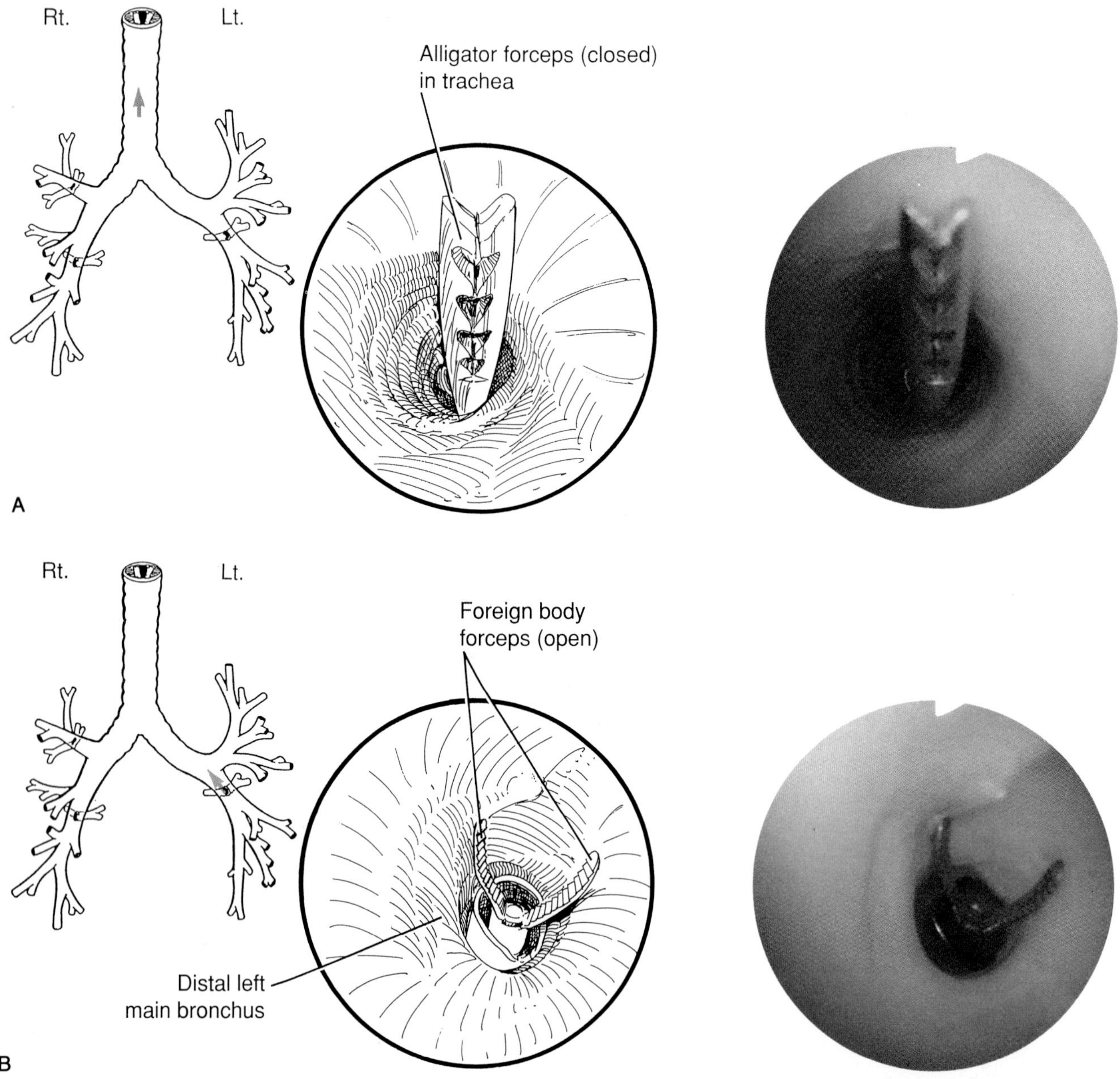

FIG. 12. (A) Cephalad view of a simulated tracheal entrance by a closed toothed (alligator) rigid bronchoscopy forceps. **(B)** A foreign body forceps has opened its jaws after exiting the distal end of a rigid bronchoscope located in the distal left main stem bronchus.

Instruments

If rigid bronchoscopy is to be used, the bronchoscopist should choose the instrument that can be easily inserted and manipulated in the airway of a given patient. The bronchoscopist should also make sure that the accessory instruments can be passed through the bronchoscope. The optically guided extraction forceps permit localization and removal of the foreign object. This is made possible by the use of modified optically directed extraction instruments. One such accessory is a flexible telescope with a diameter of 1.8 mm, and the other is a rigid telescope with a diameter of 1.6 mm, with each containing both image and light channels. Each telescope is easily inserted into the port of the conventional rigid bronchoscope. Advantages of using these optical telescopes are magnification of image and achievement of an unobstructed view during manipulation with forceps (105). The rigid bronchoscope can accommodate a wide variety of forceps, baskets, and other instruments to facilitate rapid extraction of an inhaled foreign body (Fig. 12). The use of a Hopkins telescope-guided foreign body grasper as opposed to traditional forceps guided by the naked eye has been shown to significantly lower the complication rates as well as the failure rate (106).

Any standard flexible bronchoscope (not ultrathin instruments) can be used for foreign body removal in adults. Larger channel bronchoscopes will permit easy insertion of forceps, Fogarty balloon, baskets, claws, and other grasping instruments (Fig. 13). The flexible bronchoscope has been successfully used to remove tiny foreign bodies lodged in the segmental and subsegmental bronchi (107). It has also been used in the intraoperative (thoracotomy) localization of an endobronchial foreign body (108). The ultrathin flexible bronchoscopes do not contain a working channel and therefore cannot accommodate biopsy forceps or other instruments. These instruments are helpful in the diagnosis of foreign body in small children but not in the removal.

Different types of removal accessories and methods of extraction can be used, depending on the shape and size of the foreign body. A Fogarty balloon is useful to extract spherical objects and the forceps technique for flat objects (Fig. 6) (10,34). An alligator forceps is helpful to grasp a flat and slippery metallic foreign body. Rigid bronchoscopic accessories provide the widest range of grasping forceps for almost any type of foreign body. Even a "safety pin–closing" forceps is available. Metallic foreign bodies can be retrieved using a magnetic extractor. A case is described of a patient in whom the biopsy forceps broke off during bronchoscopic lung biopsy; the broken fragment of the forceps was successfully retrieved by use of the magnetic extractor through a flexible bronchoscope under fluoroscopic guidance (87). Suction through the flexible bronchoscope has been used to retrieve a foreign body from the peripheral airway (109). The bronchoscopist should keep several types of accessory instruments handy so that he or she can change the technique as the situation dictates.

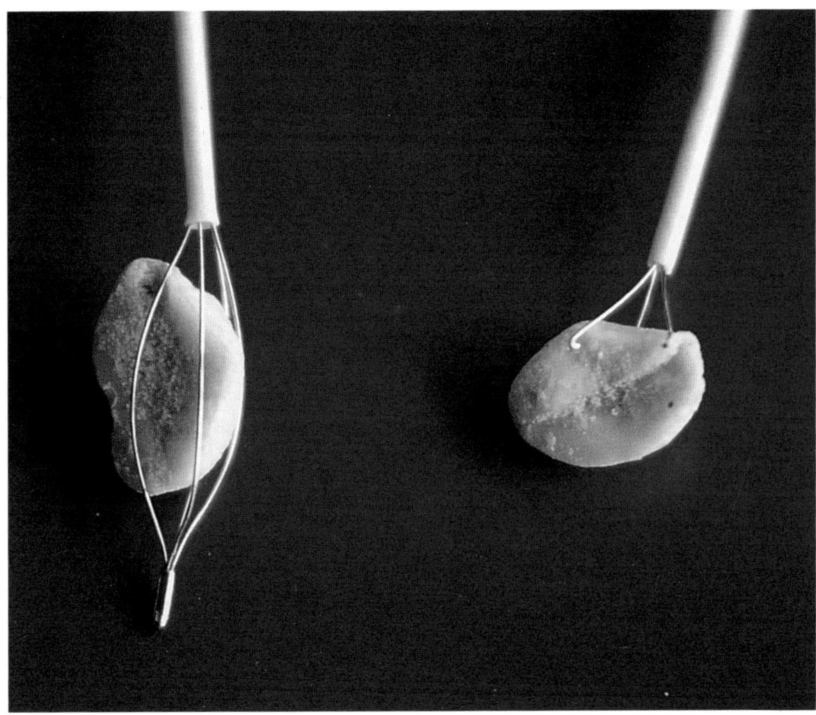

FIG. 13. A basket **(left)** and a three-toothed claw **(right)** designed for use with flexible bronchoscopes attempt to capture a foreign body (half peanut) during *in vitro* experiments. The performance of these instruments was less than satisfactory.

Fluoroscopy

Fluoroscopic guidance is essential for the removal of bronchoscopically invisible but roentgenologically visible foreign bodies (10,110). This is likely the case with foreign bodies located in the periphery of lungs or with foreign bodies that are small and made of densely radiopaque material such as pins and needles. In most reports on the retrieval of iatrogenic foreign bodies due to loss of bronchoscopic accessories in the pulmonary parenchyma, fluoroscopic guidance has been used. Foreign bodies made of aluminum and plastic are radiolucent and may not be seen on fluoroscopic screen.

Timing of the Procedure

The foreign body should be removed as soon as possible. This is particularly important in children and in anyone with significant symptoms. Once impacted in the peripheral airway, as is likely the case if the removal is delayed, the technical difficulties increase. If an organic foreign body such as a peanut is allowed to stay in the tracheobronchial tree for a prolonged period, intense mucosal inflammation followed by mucosal edema around the foreign body makes it difficult to manipulate the bronchoscope and to see the foreign body. The inflamed mucosa tends to bleed easily upon

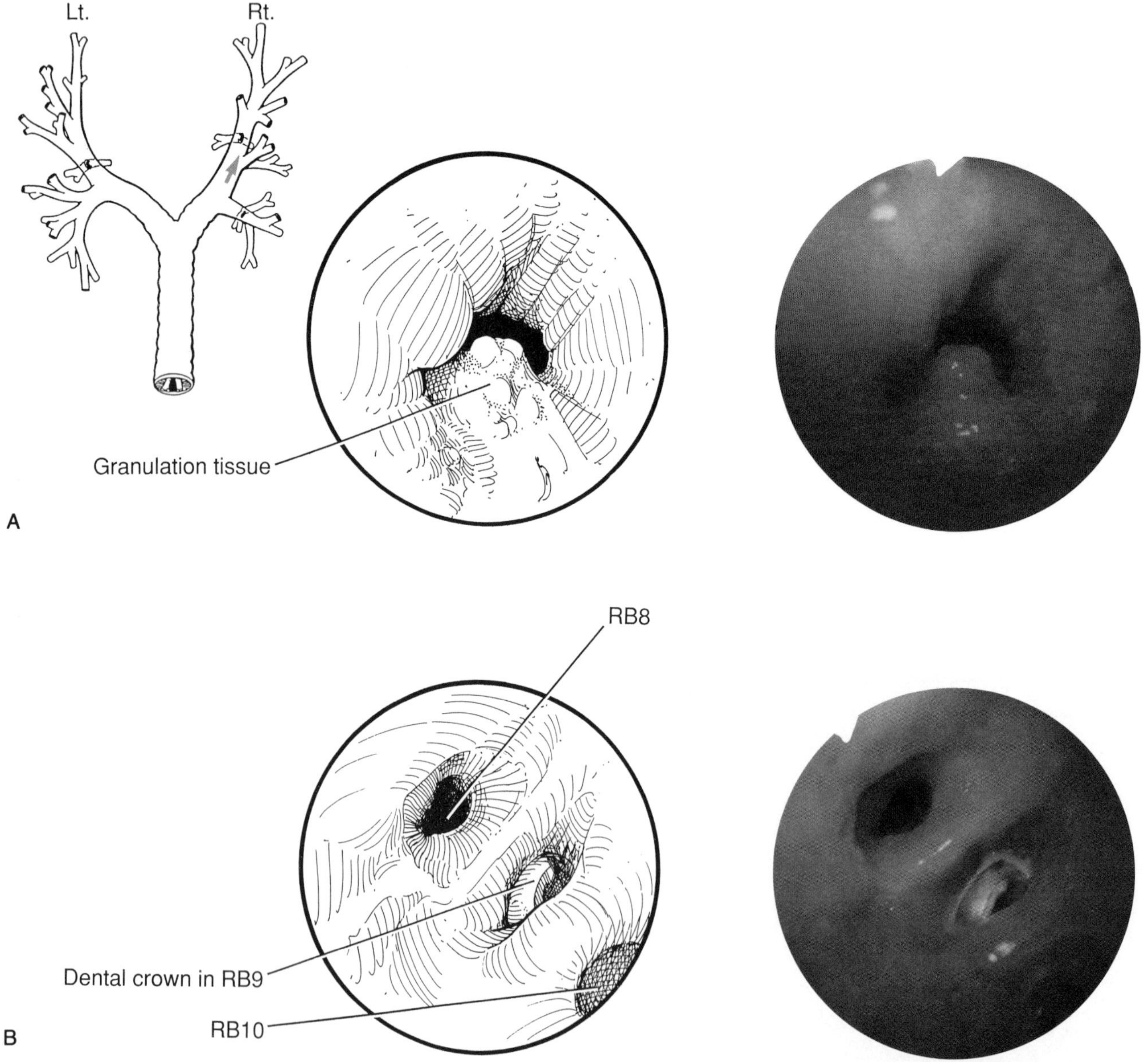

FIG. 14. Granulation tissue in distal bronchus intermedius where the dental crown had lodged for several months before diagnosis was made **(A)**. During three flexible bronchoscopic attempts at removal, the foreign body (dental crown) was pushed distally and became impacted in the distal right lower lobe bronchus **(B)**. Rigid bronchoscopy was used to remove the granulation tissue followed by extraction of the foreign body.

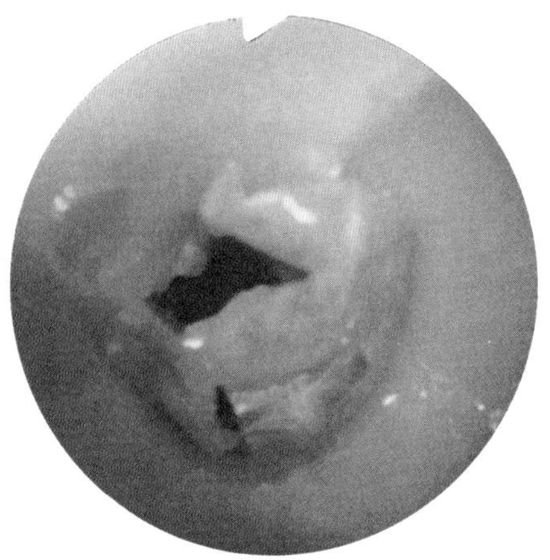

FIG. 15. An experimental attempt to remove an entire foreign body (peanut) from a model of a tracheobronchial tree shows that while the peanut was removed, its husk was left behind.

instrumentation. Topical application of racemic epinephrine and dexamethasone through the bronchoscope channel will diminish the edema and permit removal of the foreign body (111,112). Removal of a chronically retained endobronchial peanut has been facilitated by oral and topical steroid therapy of an obstructing, inflammatory polyp (113). The formation of granulation tissue and inflammatory polyps as a result of chronic retention of foreign body may cause technical difficulties in foreign body removal. The obstructing graulation tissue can be removed with biopsy forceps or laser therapy (Fig. 14). Excessive bleeding due to bronchoscopic resection of granulation may hinder foreign body extraction.

Postextraction Examination

It is important to reexamine the entire tracheobronchial tree immediately after the removal of the foreign body because retained fragments of the foreign body may necessitate repeat bronchoscopy (103). Wood and Gauderer (18) reported that 26% of patients who had previously had foreign bodies removed and who subsequently underwent flexible bronchoscopy for a variety of indications were found to have residual foreign bodies. Fragmentation of a foreign body in the tracheobronchial tree may result in "multiple" bilateral foreign bodies (Figs. 15 and 16). Simultaneous bilateral aspiration of foreign bodies can also occur (114). Once impacted into the peripheral airway, repeated attempts at removal may push these objects into segmental bronchi, causing endobronchial bleeding and prolonged anesthesia time (112).

Rigid Bronchoscopy

As soon as the foreign body is identified, the bronchoscopist may wish to proceed as described here. Make sure that the bronchoscope does not contact the object and push it distally. The secretions and blood, if present, should be aspirated without the suction tube touching the object. Visually estimate the approximate size, shape, and nature of the foreign body. Judge the

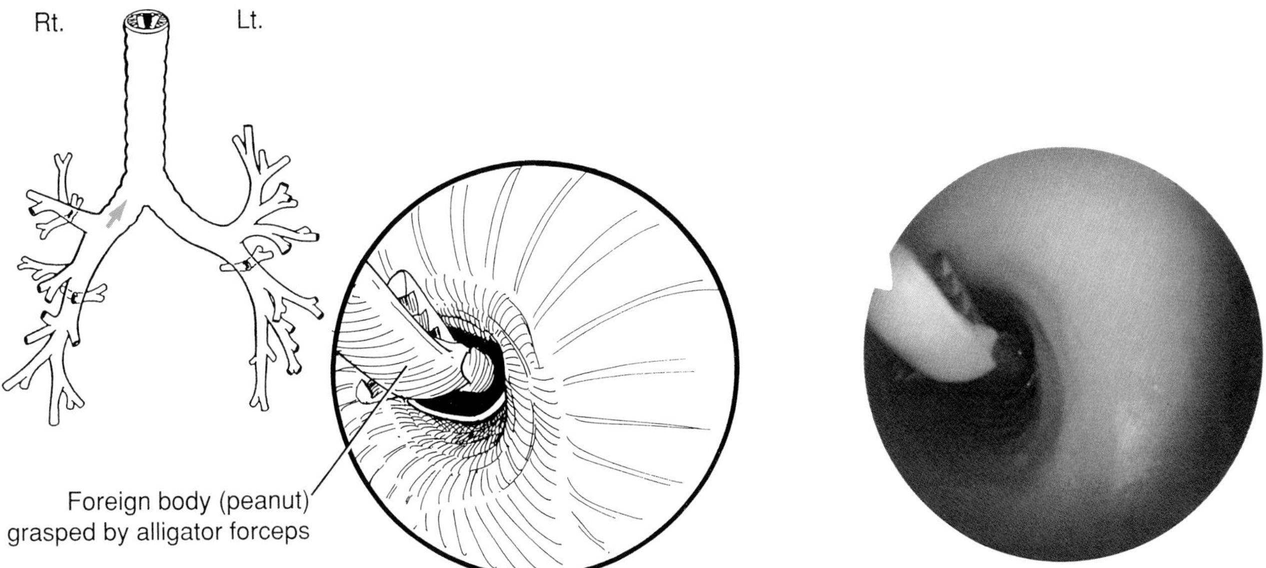

FIG. 16. Cephalad view of simulated extraction of a foreign body (half peanut) from the right main stem bronchus of a model of the tracheobronchial tree. Too tight a pressure on the forceps handle easily splintered the foreign body and produced "multiple" foreign bodies.

space available between the tracheal or bronchial wall and the foreign body to decide if the retrieval instrument (e.g., a Fogarty catheter) can be passed distally without pushing the foreign body. If the mucosa proximal to the foreign body is swollen and inflamed, instill racemic epinephrine (1.0 ml of 1 in 20,000) and liquid dexamethasone (2–4 mg) through the bronchoscope using a long metal cannula or a cotton swab attached to a long metallic staff. Manipulate the distal lumen of the bronchoscope so that the foreign body is in the center of the visual field and at least 1.5 cm distal to the tip of bronchoscope. Select the appropriate extraction forceps.

The distal tips of some forceps move forward (distally) on opening the cups and may push the foreign object distally. The bronchoscopist should open and close these several times to understand how much forward motion each forceps has. If an optically directed forceps is used, excellent vision is obtained and the foreign body can be grasped easily. If such an instrument is unavailable or cannot be passed through the bronchoscope, the bronchoscopist should manipulate the bronchoscope so the foreign body is in the center of the bronchoscopic visual field. The distance between the proximal tip of the bronchoscope and the foreign body should be estimated and the forceps slowly advanced until the estimated distance is reached. At this point the forceps is opened and gently advanced for 3–5 mm and then the cups closed slowly but firmly. If the foreign object is caught, it is easily recognized by the feel of the handles of the forceps. The bronchoscopist should try to peek through the narrow space between the wall of the bronchoscope and the forceps to see if the forceps has grasped the foreign body.

After the foreign body is securely grasped, the bronchoscope and the forceps are both withdrawn together into the distal trachea without attempting to bring the foreign body into the lumen of the bronchoscope. Once the distal tip of the bronchoscope is in the distal trachea, an attempt is made to withdraw the grasping forceps into the lumen of the bronchoscope so that the foreign body is encased by the bronchoscope. This maneuver, if successful, will permit the bronchoscopist to remove the bronchoscope, the forceps still grasping the foreign body en masse out of the trachea and mouth. If the foreign body appears larger than the diameter of the bronchoscope, this technique may in fact force the bronchoscope to shear off the foreign body from the forceps. An alternate method is to withdraw the forceps as close to the tip of the bronchoscope as possible and then remove the entire apparatus en masse from the trachea.

A chest roentgenogram may provide information regarding a sharp or a graspable edge that cannot be visualized by bronchoscopy. If the foreign body presents a smooth or rounded surface and cannot be grasped by the forceps, rotation of the foreign body is attempted in the lumen (Fig. 17). It is possible inadvertently to push the foreign body distally during this procedure. To rotate the foreign body, either a forceps or a balloon can be used. The distal portion of the forceps or the balloon is gently passed between the foreign body and the wall of the bronchus until 1–1.5 cm of the forceps or balloon is distal to the foreign object. The forceps is opened wide (or the balloon dilated) and withdrawn firmly. During this motion, the foreign body may change its orientation and present a sharp or graspable edge. If this strategy is unsuccessful, a foreign body basket is tried.

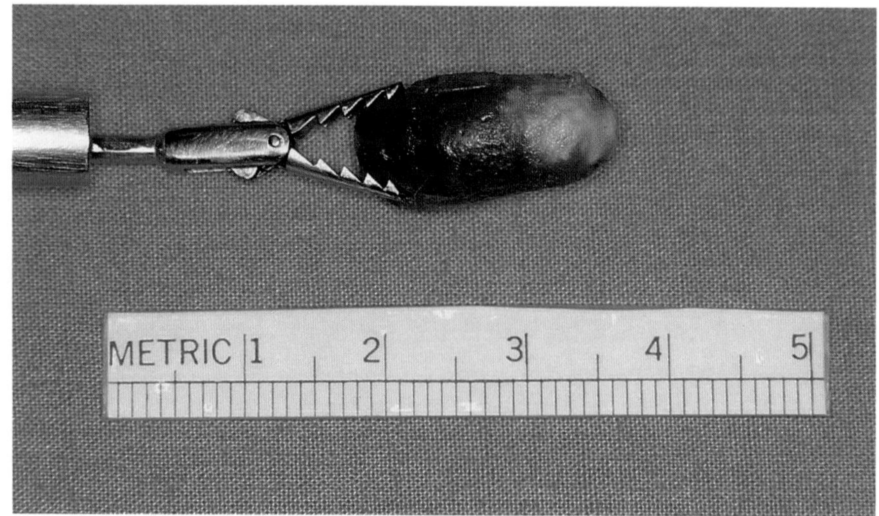

FIG. 17. A large round foreign body (hardened catheter balloon) had to be rotated inside the right main stem bronchus so that the rigid bronchoscopy forceps could grasp it (see Fig. 22).

Baskets used in retrieval of bladder stones or other specially designed baskets are helpful in the removal of a tracheobronchial foreign body. The basket should be opened and closed first to assess its mode of operation. It is introduced in the closed position and, as described above for the balloon, the entire basket part should be advanced beyond the object (Fig. 18). Then the assistant is instructed to open the basket. Since the basket is distal to the foreign object, the bronchoscopist may not be able to see the opening of the basket. Slight jiggling of the basket catheter will assure the opening. The catheter is gently pulled proximally so as to enable the wires of the open basket to snare the foreign body. This is not always effective at the first try and may necessitate repeated manipulation. Once the object is secured in the basket, the assistant is instructed to close the basket gently. Too forceful or complete a closure will expel the foreign body from the basket. The bronchoscopist has to decide how tightly the basket is closed, balancing the chance of releasing the foreign body with too tight a closure or too loose a closure. The ensnared object is pulled up to the distal end of the bronchoscope and then removed from the patient in the manner described above.

Various suction catheters can be tried to aspirate tracheobronchial foreign bodies. Small objects can be easily suctioned by using a straight metal catheter with a distal suction aperture and no side vents. Larger objects can be sucked onto the tip but during the withdrawal may get sheared off.

Lasers have been used to evaporate, break, or remove foreign bodies and broncholiths from the tracheobronchial tree (100,101,115,116). Lasers are helpful in removing granulation tissue blocking the

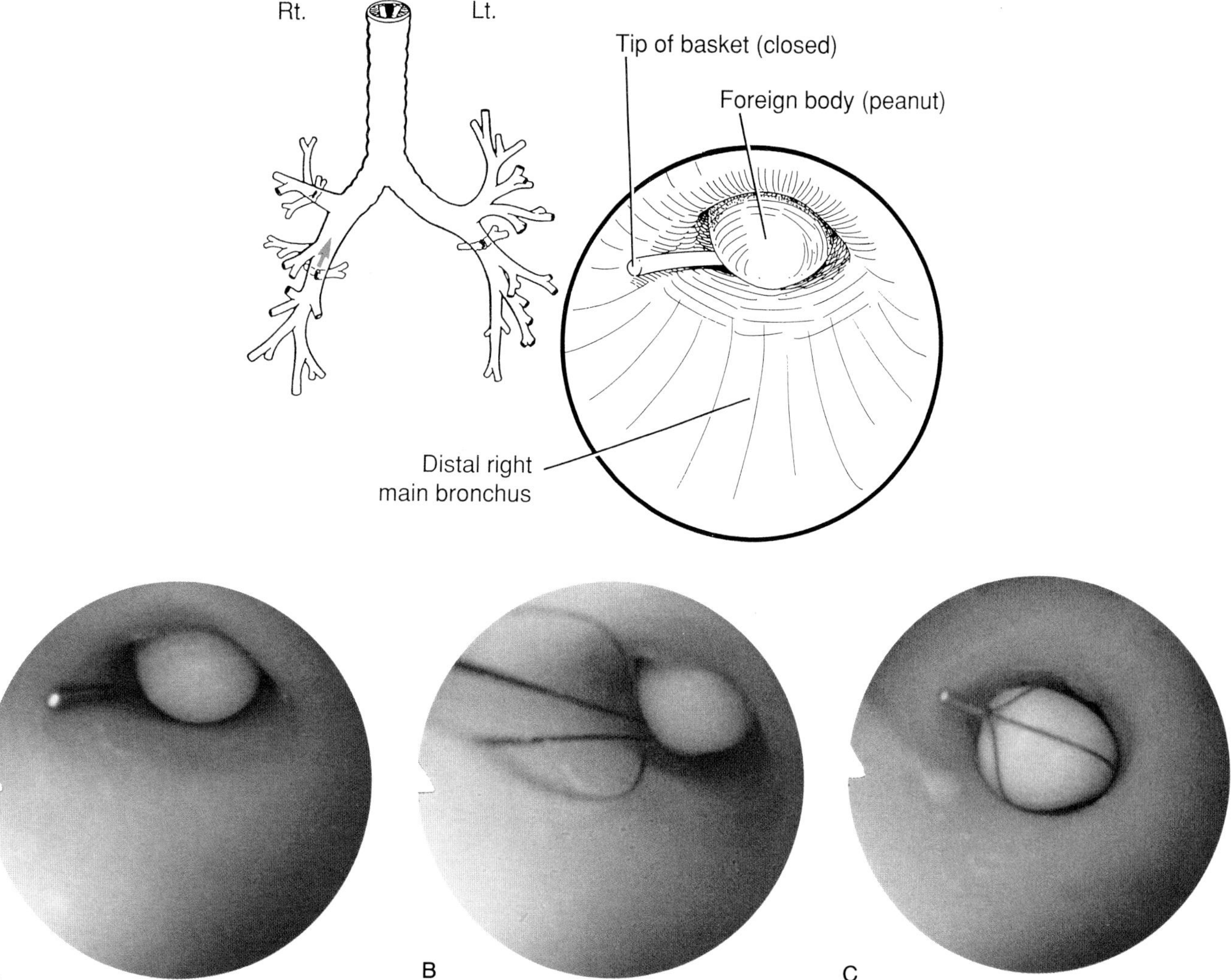

FIG. 18. Cephalad view of simulated extraction of a foreign body (peanut) from the right main stem bronchus of a model of the tracheobronchial tree. **(A)** The closed basket tip is passed distal to the foreign body, **(B)** the basket is opened distal to the foreign body, and **(C)** with gentle manipulation and twisting motion, the foreign body is captured by the basket.

approach to foreign body; a laser fiber can be passed through the pediatric rigid bronchoscope to accomplish this (116). An impacted cherry pit was removed by boring a hole through it with a laser after which a flexible biopsy forceps was passed through the hole and cups opened distally and the object extracted (117).

The functions and limitations of the varying grasping instruments should be studied thoroughly before their clinical application. Some are made to remove specific foreign bodies like open safety pins, objects with holes in them, round objects, and nuts. In vitro practice to grasp commonly encountered foreign bodies provides much information on their capabilities and limitations (Fig. 19). For instance, grasping a coin or a small object very close to the hinges of an alligator forceps will not permit complete closure of the forceps and tips of the cups will remain widely separated even though the foreign body is firmly grasped. During withdrawal, the wide open cups will make it difficult to bring the foreign body into the bronchoscope. In addition, this technique will allow only the proximal row of teeth in the alligator forceps to clutch the object. Another suggestion is to avoid contacting the bronchial wall with the foreign body. This may shear off the object. Balloon catheters can rupture if an attempt is made to remove foreign objects with sharp edges. Tightly impacted foreign bodies may not budge with balloons. It is not uncommon to see a fully inflated balloon quickly ooze out next to the foreign body, without moving it one bit, on attempting to move the object proximally.

Flexible Bronchoscopy

The accessory instruments include forceps (serrated and nonserrated), basket, claws, Fogarty balloon catheter, and laser. In the case of flexible bronchoscopy, the bronchoscopist should pass the accessory instruments in vitro through the working channel before clinical application to ascertain the feasibility of using the implements. Small objects can be removed using biopsy forceps. As outlined above, every effort should be made to prevent the distal migration of the foreign body during the attempt to remove it with the flexible bronchoscope. The bronchoscopist has less space to work and the visualization is not as good as it is with the rigid instrument. The vertical movement of the bronchoscope is minimized by instructing an assistant to hold the shaft of the bronchoscope at the point of its entrance into the mouth. If the patient is awake, additional amounts of topical anesthetic are used to minimize coughing. The patient is instructed not to cough. If the respiratory movements cause undue motion of the bronchus where the object is impacted, the bronchoscope should be advanced close to the object and, just before grasping it with a forceps or advancing distal to it with a balloon catheter, the patient is instructed to breathe in slowly and hold her or his breath as long as possible. During the breath holding, the object is grasped with the biopsy forceps.

If an endotracheal tube is used, the technique is identical to that described above for the rigid bronchos-

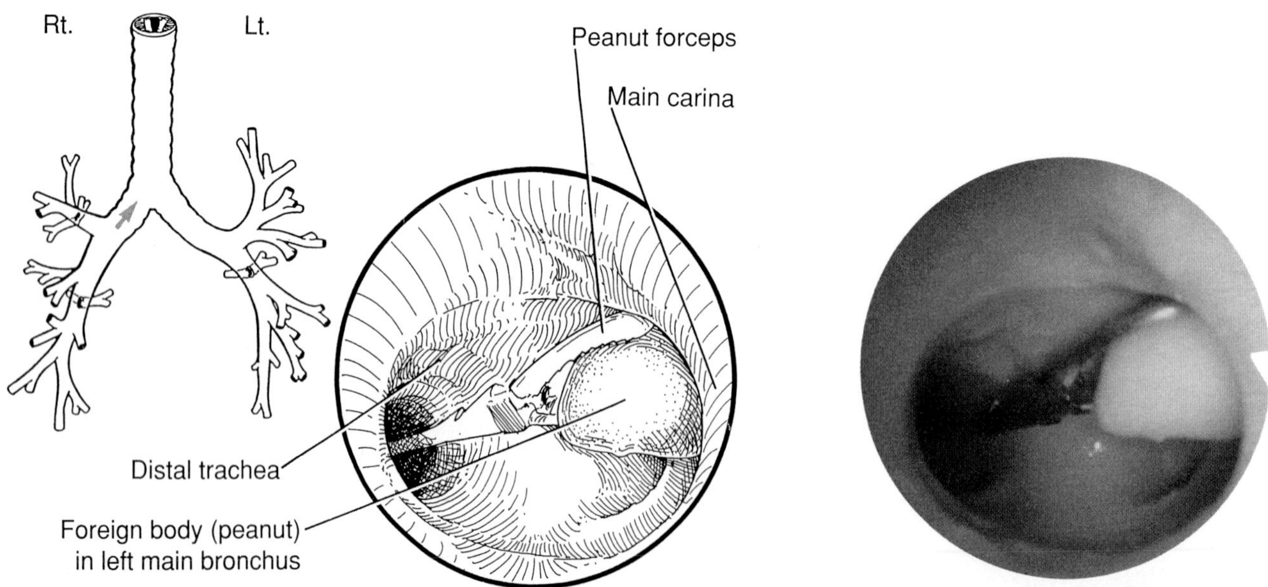

FIG. 19. Cephalad view of simulated extraction of a foreign body (peanut) from the left main stem bronchus of a model of the tracheobronchial tree. Repeated *in vitro* practice using models of tracheobronchial tree and various foreign bodies and bronchoscopic equipments will provide valuable information for clinical use.

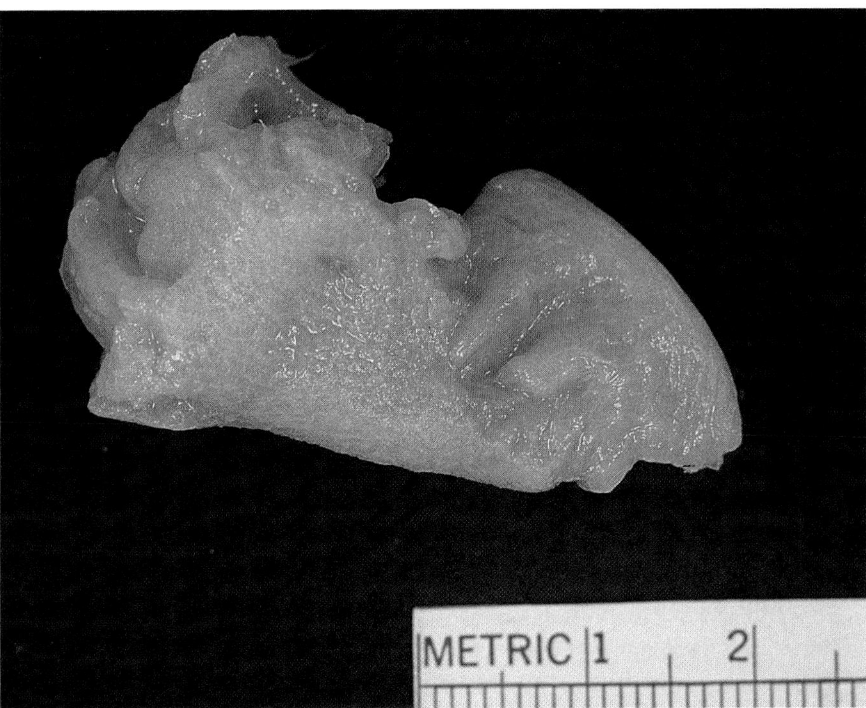

FIG. 20. Gross photography of a foreign body (a large segment of peach fruit) removed from the patient described in Fig. 8.

copy, the endotracheal tube being the surrogate to the rigid instrument to receive the foreign body into its lumen. If the foreign object is small it is possible·to retrieve it without removing the endotracheal tube. If the object is too large to be withdrawn through the endotracheal tube, the foreign body is brought as close to the distal lumen of the endotracheal tube as possible. At this point, the patient is instructed to slowly take in a deep breath and then exhale normally. During the exhalation, the endotracheal tube, bronchoscope, forceps, and foreign body are all withdrawn from the trachea as a single unit. The bronchoscopist must immediately check the contents of the biopsy forceps to ascertain that the foreign body has indeed been removed. If the forceps is empty, the bronchoscope is quickly reintroduced into the trachea while the upper airway is examined on the way down. Should the foreign body be identified in the subglottic area and if the patient is experiencing respiratory difficulty, the prudent step is to push the foreign body into the distal trachea or one of the main bronchi. This maneuver is also important during use of the rigid bronchoscope.

Removal of a foreign body by the nasal route without a nasotracheal tube is not advisable unless the object is small and can be grasped firmly by the forceps. The nasotracheal tubes are usually smaller in diameter and lengthier, thereby making it more difficult to extract the foreign body.

For most flexible bronchoscopic procedures to extract an airway foreign body, the bronchoscopist requires an assistant. The communication between the operator and the assistant during the procedure should be clear and timely. If videobronchoscopy is not used, the only instructional input an assistant gets is from the bronchoscopist.

Large tracheobronchial foreign bodies are best handle with a rigid bronchoscope and its ancillary instruments. We have encountered a significant number of patients, both adults and children, with tracheobronchial foreign bodies who underwent repeated flexible bronchoscopic procedures with each procedure lasting for more than 30–45 min or longer with unsuccessful results before being referred for rigid bronchoscopic treatment (Figs. 14 and 20) (42).

COMPLICATIONS OF TRACHEOBRONCHIAL FOREIGN BODIES

Complications Caused by Foreign Body

The complications from the foreign body itself can be acute or chronic. Acute complications are dependent on the size of the aspirated object, its location in the tracheobronchial tree, and preexisting pulmonary disease. Generally, acute and subacute complications are more common in children than in adults. Acute or early complications may include acute dyspnea, asphyxia, cardiac arrest, laryngeal edema, and pneumothorax. Acute transient cor pulmonale due to foreign body aspiration has been described in an adult (118). Acute obstruction of the subglottic space or the upper trachea by a foreign body is life threatening (119). Acute bronchial damage and subacute bronchial stenosis have resulted from aspiration of a ferrous sulfate tablet (120,121).

The delay in the diagnosis of tracheobronchial foreign body increases the incidence of complications. Mu and colleagues (122) observed that among 210 children the most common complications encountered as a result of delayed diagnosis (time between the aspiration event or onset of symptoms and the diagnosis exceeding 3 days) included obstructive emphysema in 41%, mediastinal shift in 34%, pneumonia in 24%, and atelectasis in 18% (122).

In a retrospective review of 155 children with tracheobronchial foreign bodies, 6% exhibited pneumomediastinum on the initial chest roentgenogram (32). Vane et al. (22) performed rigid bronchoscopy in 131 children for suspected aspiration of foreign bodies and found that all but two patients had evidence of a foreign body; postbronchoscopic complications included fever (21%), pulmonary infiltrate (8%), need for ventilatory support (3%), and pneumothorax (1.5%). However, most complications of removal of the foreign body in children have been minimal as a result of technical advances and improved safety of anesthesia (27).

Chronic complications consist of chronic cough, recurrent hemoptysis, bronchial stricture, development of inflammatory polyps at the site of lodgement of the foreign body, localized bronchiectasis (Fig. 21), chronic postobstructive pneumonia, lung abscess, bronchopleural fistula, and diminished perfusion to the ipsilateral lung (42,108,120,123–130). Growth of exuberant granulation tissue may lead to chronic cough, hemoptysis, wheezing, and lobar or segmental atelectasis. Noninvasive endobronchial epithelial papilloma associated with a foreign body (sunflower seed) and encasing it has been described in a 48-year-old man (131). An unusual complication of chronic tracheobronchial foreign body aspiration has been described in which a 66-year-old diabetic man presented with a bilobar pneumonia 2 months after aspiration of a chicken bone. Flexible bronchoscopy demonstrated a mass in the bronchus intermedius and the histological examination of endobronchial biopsy specimens revealed bone fragments, vegetable matter, and sulfur granules containing *Actinomyces* organisms. The patient responded to bronchoscopic removal of the foreign body and penicillin therapy (132).

Complications Caused by Treatment

A properly performed bronchoscopic removal should produce minimal complications. However, the complications caused by the foreign body may precipitate complications following therapy. Inflammatory polyps or granulation tissue may form with chronic im-

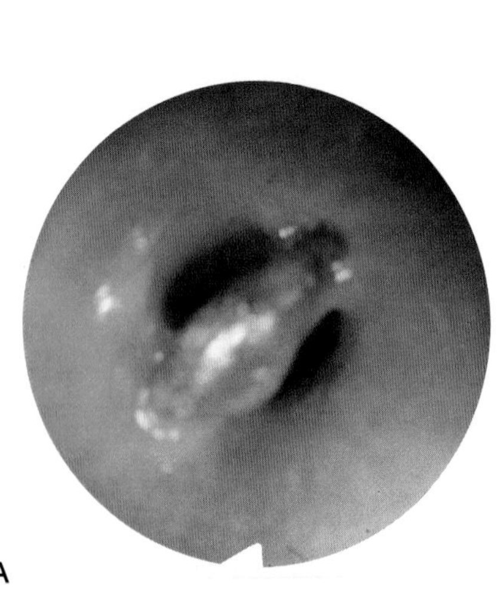

A

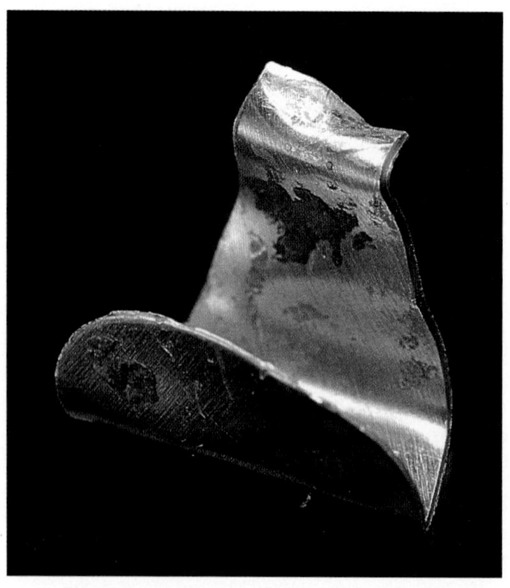

B

FIG. 21. A chronically impacted foreign body (thumb tack) in the right middle lobe bronchus resulted in bronchiectasis of right middle lobe; the foreign body was extracted with a rigid bronchoscope **(A)**. Bronchiectasis of left lower lobe and significant hemoptysis caused by this beer can pull-tab aspirated by an adult who was unaware of the aspiration; the foreign body was removed with flexible bronchoscope **(B)**.

paction and obscure the foreign body. Before the extraction of a foreign body in such cases, bronchoscopic resection of the granulation tissue is often necessary. Bronchial hemorrhage as a result of foreign body removal is generally mild. However, life-threatening hemorrhage has been reported (133). Among 60 patients who underwent foreign body extraction, bleeding due to bronchoscopy itself occurred in 3 patients, spontaneously abating in each case, and the bronchoscopic manipulation did not lead to acute airway compromise (42).

Prolonged attempts at bronchoscopic removal can induce nonpulmonary complications. In the Mayo series, one of the three patients who required thoracotomy for the removal of a foreign body sustained an acute myocardial infarction during a 2-hr attempt at the local hospital to retrieve an aspirated dental crown; after prolonged manipulation with the flexible bronchoscope, the foreign body, which had initially been in the left main stem bronchus, had slipped into the distal bronchi of the left lower lobe (42). Another patient we saw recently with an aspirated dental crown had undergone three flexible bronchoscopic procedures and the foreign body, which was originally located in the proximal bronchus intermedius, had been pushed down to the distal right lower lobe bronchus during these earlier procedures (Fig. 14).

Laryngeal edema was observed in 380 of 2,170 children referred for bronchoscopy to exclude tracheobronchial foreign body; 12 of the 380 children required tracheostomy (11). In a report on 639 children with tracheobronchial foreign body, 5 (0.6%) died after the bronchoscopic procedure (21). One fatality due to overwhelming aspiration of an unanticipated release of pus following the bronchoscopic removal of a chronically impacted foreign body was reported (20). Aytac and colleagues (129), in their series of 500 children with tracheobronchial foreign bodies, reported the inci-

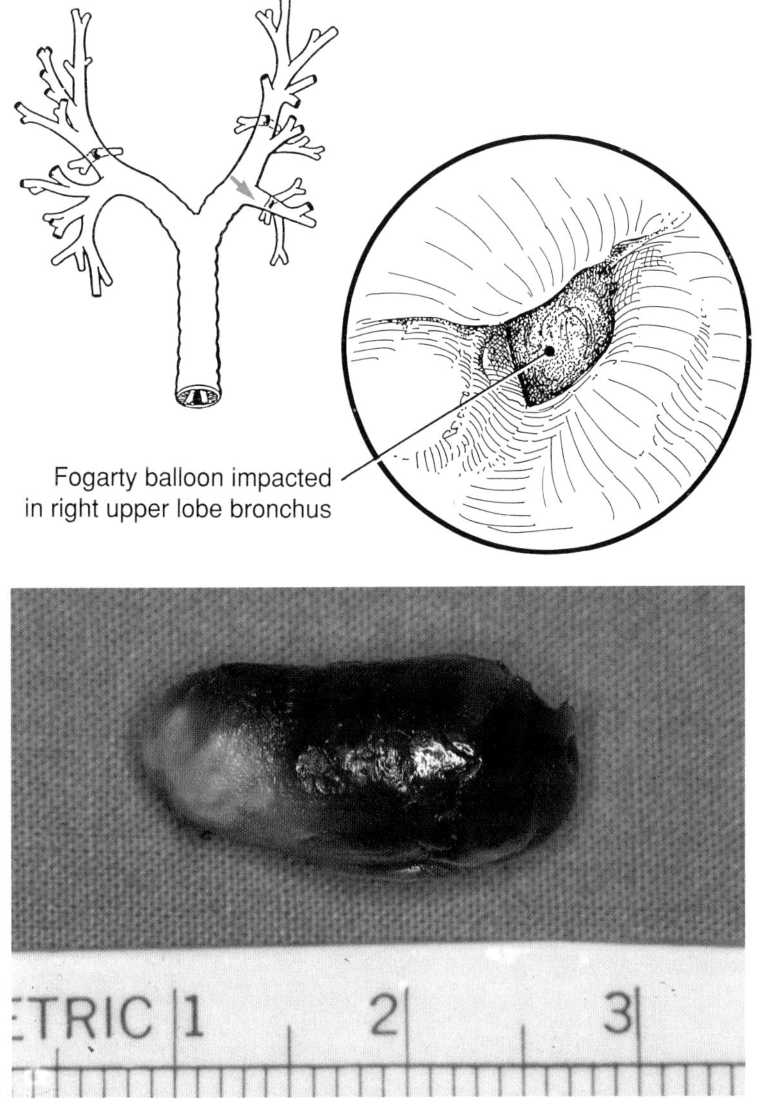

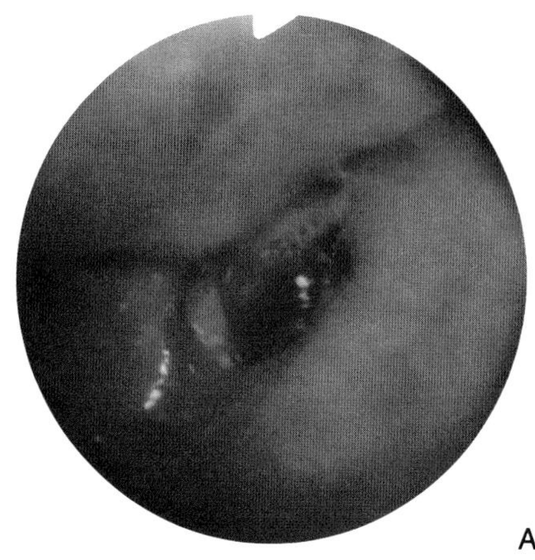

FIG. 22. A balloon (we had no information on the type or contents) was used in this patient to occlude a bronchopleural fistula, but it became impacted in the right upper lobe bronchus resulting in a bronchopleurocutaneous fistula. We were unable to remove it with a flexible bronchoscope and had to use a rigid bronchoscope to extract it **(A)**. Close-up of this foreign body, which felt hard to the touch and had no fluid inside it **(B)**.

dence of postbronchoscopic tracheostomy in 1.4% and a total mortality rate of 1.8%.

Unusual complications of mismanagement of ingested or inhaled foreign bodies have included pulmonary hemorrhage, tracheoesophageal fistula, mediastinitis resembling a mediastinal tumor, periesophageal infection from perforation, impaction in a bronchial tree of a balloon used to tamponade a bronchopleural fistula (Fig. 22), laryngeal stenosis, and the displacement of a foreign body into an almost inaccessible distal bronchus (Fig. 14) (134).

PREVENTION OF TRACHEOBRONCHIAL ASPIRATION OF FOREIGN BODY

Even though the possibilities of prevention of tracheobronchial foreign body inhalation are surmised to be limited (8), active involvement by the pediatricians in educating young parents should be stressed. Despite the fact that peanut is the most common foreign body in pediatric airways and constitutes 50% of all foreign bodies, it appears that many parents and others who care for young children are still unaware that peanut ingestion can be hazardous in the very young. A case report of a 6-month-old infant who arrived at the emergency room with severe respiratory distress after being spoon-fed with chicken soup points out the lack of understanding of the dangers of foreign body in infants; bronchoscopy revealed a hollow chicken bone lining the whole left main bronchus (135). Even disposable plastic diapers have been reported to pose a foreign body hazard (136).

Another problem is the delay in diagnosis and treatment. One study of 210 children with tracheobronchial foreign bodies listed the causes for the delays as follows: parental negligence in 50%, misdiagnosis by the fellow professionals and pediatricians in 19%, normal chest roentgenological findings in 14%, lack of typical symptoms and signs in 12%, mismanagement in 4%, and a negative bronchoscopic finding in 1%. The incidence of major complications was 64% (48/75) in the children who were diagnosed within 4–7 days; however, the complication rate was 70% (39/56) in those with a delay in diagnosis of 15–30 days, and 95% (20/21) in the cases with a delay in diagnosis of over 30 days after aspiration of the foreign body (122).

In an interesting study, Puterman and associates (137) provided a postgraduate educational program to medical practitioners in order to increase their awareness of tracheobronchial foreign bodies in children. A survey of the participants before and after the program revealed that the percentage of cases in which a positive history of aspiration was obtained increased from 47.6% to 84% respectively; the mean number of hospitalizations due to tracheobronchial foreign bodies decreased from 1.9 to 1.04 per infant, and the mean number of hospital days required for final diagnosis decreased from 17.6 to 5.3. Similar ongoing programs are important for the early detection and treatment of tracheobronchial foreign bodies.

SUMMARY

Tracheobronchial foreign body will remain a common problem among young children. It should be suspected in every child who develops acute or abrupt onset of respiratory symptoms. If the clinical suspicion is strong, immediate bronchoscopic evaluation should be considered. Since general anesthesia, if necessary, can be safely administered and the ultrathin flexible bronchoscope is widely available for diagnostic purposes, it is highly advisable to proceed with bronchoscopy to exclude the possibility of inhaled foreign body when the clinical features indicate even a small likelihood of this diagnosis. The rigid bronchoscope remains the instrument of choice for the extraction of tracheobronchial foreign body in children.

Tracheobronchial foreign bodies are uncommon in adults. A high clinical index of suspicion, imaging procedures, and bronchoscopy are essential for the diagnosis and treatment. Since foreign bodies are not usually suspected in adults, their frequently unanticipated discovery by flexible bronchoscopy tempts the bronchoscopist to proceed with attempts to extract the foreign body with the flexible instrument. This is more likely the case in the absence of training in rigid bronchoscopy. As the popularity of flexible bronchoscopy continues to increase, the use of the rigid bronchoscope may be limited to laser bronchoscopy, placement of airway stents, tracheobronchial dilatation, and removal of tracheobronchial foreign bodies. Clearly, continued training in the techniques of rigid bronchoscopy and the development of better designed instruments for use via the flexible bronchoscope for extraction of tracheobronchial foreign bodies in adults is needed (42).

The overall success rate of bronchoscopy in the removal of tracheobronchial foreign bodies is in excess of 95% (31). The failure of bronchoscopy to extract the foreign body is reported in 2–10% of patients (5,16,42,72). If the foreign body cannot be removed by bronchoscopy, thoracotomy followed by bronchotomy or segmental resection may be necessary (138–140).

REFERENCES

1. Killian G. Meeting of the Society of Physicians of Freiburg. Dec 17, 1897, *Munchen Med Wschr* 1898;45:378.
2. Jackson C. Foreign bodies in the trachea, bronchi, and esophagus. *Laryngoscope* 1905;15:527–539.

3. Jackson C, Jackson CL. *Diseases of the air and food passages of foreign body origin*. Philadelphia: WB Saunders; 1936.
4. Mittleman RE, Wetli CV. The fatal cafe coronary; foreign-body airway obstruction. *JAMA* 1982;247:1285–1288.
5. Banerjee A, Rao KS, Khanna SK, Narayanan PS, Gupta BK, Sekar JC, Retnam CR, Nachiappan M. Laryngotracheobronchial foreign bodies in children. *J Laryngol Otol* 1988; 102:1029–32.
6. Puhakka H, Kero P, Erkinjuntti M. Pediatric bronchoscopy during a 17-year period. *Int J Pediatr Otorhinolaryngol* 1987; 13:171–180.
7. Kramer TA, Riding KH, Salkeld LJ. Tracheobronchial and esophageal foreign bodies in the pediatric population. *J Otolaryngol* 1986;15:355–358.
8. Mantel K, Butenandt I. Tracheobronchial foreign body aspiration in childhood. A report on 224 cases. *Eur J Pediatr*. 1986; 145:211–6.
9. Blazer S, Naveh Y, Friedman A. Foreign body in the airway. A review of 200 cases. *Am J Dis Child* 1980;134:68–71.
10. Al-Naaman YD, Al-Ani MS, Al-Ani HR. Non-vegetable foreign bodies in the bronchopulmonary tract in children. *J Laryngol Otol* 1975;89:289–297.
11. Elhassani NB. Tracheobronchial foreign bodies in the Middle East. *J Thorac Cardiovasc Surg* 1988;96:621–625.
12. Abdulmajid OA, Ebeid AM, Motaweh MM, Kleibo IS. Aspirated foreign bodies in the tracheobronchial tree: report of 250 cases. *Thorax* 1976;31:635–640.
13. National Safety Council. *Accident facts*. Chicago: National Safety Council Press; 1980:7.
14. Sanford CC. Aspiration of foreign bodies in children. *Ann Fam Physician* 1970;20:150–154.
15. Cohen SR, Herbert WI, Lewis GB Jr, Geller KA. Foreign bodies in the airways. Five-year retrospective study with special attention to management. *Ann Otol Rhinol Laryngol* 1980; 89:437–442.
16. Svensson G. Foreign bodies in the tracheobronchial tree. Special references to experience in 97 children. *Int J Pediatr Otorhinolaryngol* 1985;8:243–251.
17. Black RE. Choi KJ. Syme WC. Johnson DG. Matlak ME. Bronchoscopic removal of aspirated foreign bodies in children. *Am J Surg* 1984;148:778–781.
18. Wood RE. Gauderer MW. Flexible fiberoptic bronchoscopy in the management of tracheobronchial foreign bodies in children: the value of a combined approach with open tube bronchoscopy. *J Pediatr Surg* 1984;19:693–698.
19. Kero P. Puhakka H. Erkinjuntti M. Iisalo E. Vilkki P. Foreign body in the airways of children. *Int J Pediatr Otorhinolaryngol* 1983;6:51–59.
20. Linegar AG, von-Oppell UO, Hegemann S, de-Groot M, Odell JA. Tracheobronchial foreign bodies. Experience at Red Cross Children's Hospital, 1985–1990. *S Afr Med J* 1992;82:164–167.
21. Pasaoglu I, Dogan R, Demircin M, Hatipoglu A, Bozer AY. Bronchoscopic removal of foreign bodies in children: retrospective analysis of 822 cases. *Thorac Cardiovasc Surg* 1991; 39:95–98.
22. Vane DW, Pritchard J, Colville CW, West KW, Eigen H, Grosfeld JL. Bronchoscopy for aspirated foreign bodies in children. Experience in 131 cases. *Arch Surg* 1988;123:885–888.
23. Brown TC, Clark CM. Inhaled foreign bodies in children. *Med J Aust* 1983;2:322–326.
24. Mu L, He P, Sun D. Inhalation of foreign bodies in Chinese children: a review of 400 cases. *Laryngoscope* 1991; 101:657–660.
25. Wiseman NE. The diagnosis of foreign body aspiration in childhood. *J Pediatr Surg* 1984;19:531–535.
26. Steen KH, Zimmermann T. Tracheobronchial aspiration of foreign bodies in children: a study of 94 cases. *Laryngoscope* 1990; 100:525–530.
27. Hamilton AH, Carswell F, Wisheart JD. The Bristol Children's Hospital experience of tracheobronchial foreign bodies 1977–87. *Bristol Med Chir J* 1989;104:72–74.
28. Winter PH, Koopmann CF Jr. Juvenile myasthenia gravis: an unusual presentation. *Int J Pediatr Otorhinolaryngol* 1990; 19:273–276.
29. Svedstrom E, Puhakka H, Kero P. How accurate is chest radiography in the diagnosis of tracheobronchial foreign bodies in children? *Pediatr Radiol* 1989;19:520–522.
30. Reed MH. Radiology of airway foreign bodies in children. *J Can Assoc Radiol* 1977;28:111–118.
31. Puhakka H, Svedstrom E, Kero P, Valli P, Iisalo E. Tracheobronchial foreign bodies. A persistent problem in pediatric patients. *Am J Dis Child* 1989;143:543–545.
32. Burton EM, Riggs W Jr. Kaufman RA, Houston CS. Pneumomediastinum caused by foreign body aspiration in children. *Pediatr Radiol* 1989;20:45–47.
33. Case 48, case records of the Massachusetts General Hospital. *N Engl J Med* 1983;309:1374–1381.
34. Kosloske AM. Bronchoscopic extraction of aspirated foreign bodies in children. *Am J Dis Child* 1982;136:924–927.
35. Monden Y, Morimoto T, Taniki T, Uyama T, Kimura S. Flexible bronchoscopy for foreign body in airway. *Tokushima J Exp Med* 1989;36:35–39.
36. McGuirt WF, Holmes KD, Feehs R, Browne JD. Tracheobronchial foreign bodies. *Laryngoscope* 1988;98:615–618.
37. Casson AG, Guy JRF. Foreign-body aspiration in adults. *Can J Surg* 1987;30:193–194.
38. Brischetto MJ, Malouf J, Taylor RW. Foreign-body pneumonitis associated with tracheostomy. *Crit Care Med* 1984; 12:689–690.
39. Hannan SE, Pratt DS, Hannan JM, Brienza LT. Foreign body aspiration associated with the use of an aerosol inhaler. *Am Rev Resp Dis* 1984;129:1025–1027.
40. Rogers LF, Igini JP. Beverage can pull-tabs: inadvertent ingestion or aspiration. *JAMA* 1975;233:345–348.
41. Kullbom TL, Adwers J. Unusual complication associated with severe maxillofacial trauma. *Oral Surg* 1974;37:355–358.
42. Limper AH, Prakash UBS. Tracheobronchial foreign bodies in adults [see comments]. *Ann Intern Med*. 1990;112:604–609.
43. Ristagno RL, Kornstein MJ, Hansen-Flaschen JH. Diagnosis of occult meat aspiration by fiberoptic bronchoscopy. *Am J Med* 1986;80:154–156.
44. Hussain A. Neglected foreign body in the right bronchial tree. *Int Surg* 1976;61:366–367.
45. Abrol BM, Chattopadhyay AK. Forgotten bronchial foreign body. *J Indian Med Assoc* 1973;61:224.
46. Knowles JE. Inhalation of dental plates—a hazard of radiolucent materials. *J Laryngol Otol* 1991;105:681–682.
47. Wales J, Jackimczyk K, Rosen P. Aspiration following a cave-in. *Ann Emerg Med* 1983;12:99–101.
48. Van Dyke JJ, Lake KB. Survival after asphyxia secondary to gravel aspiration. *Arch Intern Med* 1976;136:471–473.
49. Jackson C. Grasses as foreign bodies in therapy bronchus and lung. *Laryngoscope* 1952;62:897–923.
50. Woolley PV Jr. Grass inflorescence as foreign bodies in respiratory tract. *J Pediatr* 1955;46:704–706.
51. Hilman BC, Kurzweg FT, NcCook WW Jr, Liles AE. Foreign body aspiration of grass inflorescences as a cause of hemoptysis. *Chest* 1980;78:306–309.
52. Zavala DC, Rhodes ML. Experimental removal of foreign bodies by fiberoptic bronchoscopy. *Am Rev Resp Dis* 1974; 110:357–360.
53. Lillington GA, Ruhl RA, Peirce TH, Gorin AB. Removal of endobronchial foreign body by fiberoptic bronchoscopy. *Am Rev Resp Dis* 1976;113:387–391.
54. Ikeda S. *Atlas of flexible bronchoscopy*. Baltimore: University Park Press; 1974.
55. Barrett CR Jr, Vecchione JJ, Bell AL Jr. Flexible fiberoptic bronchoscopy for airway management during acute respiratory failure. *Am Rev Resp Dis* 1974;109:429–434.
56. Wanner A, Landa JF, Nieman RE Jr, Vevaina J, Delgado I. Bedside bronchofiberscopy for atelectasis and lung abscess. *JAMA* 1973;224:1281–1283.
57. Lan R-S, Lee C-H, Chiang Y-C, Wang WJ. Use of fiberoptic bronchoscopy to retrieve bronchial foreign bodies in adults. *Am Rev Resp Dis* 1989;140:1734–1737.
58. Whitlock WL, Brown CR, Young MB. Tracheobronchial foreign bodies (letter). *Ann Intern Med* 1990;113:482–483.

59. Moss R, Kanchanapoon V. Stone basket extraction of a bronchial foreign body (letter). *Arch Surg*. 1986;121:975.
60. Inhaled foreign bodies (editorial). *Br Med J* 1980; 282:1649–1650.
61. Dajani AM. Bronchial foreign-body removed with a Dormia basket. *Lancet* 1971;1:1076–1077.
62. Kosloske AM. The Fogarty balloon technique for the removal of foreign bodies from the tracheobronchial tree. *Surg Gynecol Obstet* 1982;155:72–73.
63. Zavala DC, Rhodes ML. Foreign body removal: a new role for the fiberoptic bronchoscope. *Ann Otol Rhinol Laryngol* 1975; 84:650–656.
64. Heinz GJ III, Richardson RH, Zavala DC. Endobronchial foreign body removal using the bronchofiberscope. *Ann Otol Rhinol Laryngol* 1978;87:50–52.
65. Fieselmann JF, Zavala DC, Keim LW. Removal of foreign bodies (two teeth) by fiberoptic bronchoscopy. *Chest* 1977; 72:241–243.
66. Zavala DC, Rhodes ML, Richardson RH, Bedell GN. Fiberoptic and rigid bronchoscopy: the state of the art (editorial). *Chest* 1974;65:605–606.
67. McCullough P. Wire basket removal of a large endobronchial foreign body (letter). *Chest* 1985;87:270–271.
68. Hiller C, Lerner S, Varnum R, Bone R, Pingelton W, Kerby G, Ruth W. Foreign body removal with the flexible fiberoptic bronchoscope. *Endoscopy* 1977;9:216–222.
69. Limper AH, Prakash UBS. Tracheobronchial foreign bodies (letter). *Ann Intern Med* 1990;113:482–483.
70. Nussbaum M, Nash M, Cho H, Cohen J, Pincus R. Hypodermic needles: an unusual tracheobronchial foreign body. *Ann Otol Rhinol Laryngol* 1987;96:698–700.
71. Coutras S. Hypodermic needles: an unusual tracheobronchial foreign body (letter). *Ann Otol Rhinol Laryngol* 1988;97:330.
72. Weissberg D, Schwartz I. Foreign bodies in the tracheobronchial tree. *Chest* 1987;91:730–733.
73. Dhar GJ, Pierach CA.: Aspiration of thermometer fragment (letter). *Br Med J* 1973;4:737–738.
74. Kollef MH, Winn RE. Occult coiled drinking straw aspiration. *Heart and Lung* 1990;19:24–26.
75. Naveh Y, Friedman A, Altmann M. Eggshell aspiration in infants. *Am J Dis Child* 1975;129:498–499.
76. Rafferty P, Fergusson RJ, Gaddie J. Polished off: an inhaled dental brush. *Br J Dis Chest* 1985;79:390–392.
77. Abdel Salam AS, Gibb AG. Undiagnosed bronchial foreign body-golf tee. *J Laryngol Otol* 1980;94:671–675.
78. Seals ML, Andry JM, Kellar PN. Pulmonary aspiration of a metal casting: report of case. *J Am Dent Assoc* 1988; 117:587–588.
79. Yuksek T, Solak H, Odabas D, Yeniterzi M, Ozpinar C, Ozergin U. Dangerous pencils and a new technique for removal of foreign bodies. *Chest* 1992;102:965–967.
80. Wager GC, Williams JH Jr. Flexible bronchoscopic removal of radiooccult polyurethane foam, with pneumonitis in a hyperventilated lobe. *Am Rev Resp Dis* 1990;142:122–124.
81. Loh HS, Rauff A. "A bridge too far." Case report. *Aust Dent J* 1991;36:29–31.
82. Ramchander V, Ramcharan J, Muralidhara K. Fatal respiratory obstruction due to *Ascaris lumbricoides*—a case report. *Ann Trop Paediatr* 1991;11:293–294.
83. Choh JH, Adler RH. Penetrating bullet wound of chest with bronchoscopic removal of bullet. *J Thorac Cardiovasc Surg* 1981;82:150–153.
84. Richardson M, Gomes M, Tsou E. Transtracheal migration of an intravertebral Steinmann pin to the left bronchus. *J Thorac Cardiovasc Surg* 1987;93:939–941.
85. Terasaki H, Higashi K, Takeshita J, Tanoue T, Morioka T. Resuscitation by extracorporeal lung assist of a patient suffocating after inhalation of sawdust particles. *Crit Care Med* 1990; 18:239–240.
86. Slotnick DB, Urken ML, Sacks SH, Lawson W. Fracture, separation, and aspiration of tracheostomy tubes: management with a new technique. *Otolaryngol Head Neck Surg* 1987; 97:423–427.
87. Saito H, Saka H, Sakai S, Shimokata K. Removal of broken fragment of biopsy forceps with magnetic extractor. *Chest* 1989;95:700–701.
88. Credle WF Jr, Smiddy JF, Elliott RC. Complications of fiberoptic bronchoscopy. *Am Rev Resp Dis* 1974;109:67–72.
89. Suratt PM, Smiddy JF, Gruber B. Deaths and complications associated with fiberoptic bronchoscopy. *Chest* 1976; 69:747–751.
90. Fuentes-Otero F, Garcia-Vinuesa G, Tellez F, Rincon P, Perez-Miranda M. Unusual complication during bronchial brushing through the flexible fiberoptic bronchoscope. *Chest* 1980; 78:901–902.
91. Sanders DM. Needle in a haystack (letter). *Chest* 1983; 83:935–936.
92. Oleson LL, Thorshauge H, Nielsen BA. Breakage of the wire cytology brush during fiberoptic bronchoscopy (letter). *Chest* 1987;92:188.
93. Malik SK, Behera D. Breakage of alligator biopsy forceps: an unusual complication during fiberoptic bronchoscopy. *Chest* 1984;85:837–838.
94. Masa-Jimenez JF, Verea-Hernando R, Martin-Egana MT, Fontan-Bueso J. Breakage of alligator forceps in transbronchial biopsy (letter). *Chest* 1985;88:156.
95. Weissberg D. Breakage of alligator forceps in transbronchial biopsy (letter). *Chest* 1985;88:156.
96. Roach JM, Ripple G, Dillard TA. Inadvertent loss of bronchoscopy instruments in the tracheobronchial tree. *Chest* 1992; 101:568–569.
97. Carpenter RJ III, Snyder GG III. A complication in the use of a Fogarty catheter for foreign body removal during bronchoscopic management. *Otolaryngol Head Neck Surg* 1981; 89:998–1000.
98. Polosa R, Finnerty JP. Inhalation of the propeller from a spinhaler. *Eur Resp J* 1991;4:236–237.
99. Shure D. Endobronchial suture. A foreign body causing chronic cough. *Chest* 1991;100:1193–1196.
100. Mitchell I. Chronic cough caused by endobronchial sutures (letter). *Chest* 1992;102:1637.
101. Unger M. Neodymium: YAG laser therapy for malignant and benign endobronchial obstructions. *Clin Chest Med* 1985; 6:277–290.
102. Savage PJ, Dellinger RP. Inability to remove an aspirated straight pin by flexible fiberoptic bronchoscopy. *South Med J* 1984;77:930–931.
103. Campbell DN, Cotton EK, Lilly JR. A dual approach to tracheobronchial foreign bodies in children. *Surgery* 1982; 91:178–182.
104. Law D, Kosloske AM. Management of tracheobronchial foreign bodies in children: a reevaluation of postural drainage and bronchoscopy. *Pediatrics* 1976;58:362–367.
105. Kobayashi T, Shima K. Removal of bronchial foreign bodies in children. Use of a new minioptical telescope. *Arch Otolaryngol* 1982;108:265–256.
106. Inglis AF Jr, Wagner DV. Lower complication rates associated with bronchial foreign bodies over the last 20 years. *Ann Otol Rhinol Laryngol* 1992;101:61–66.
107. Papamichael EE. Removal of foreign bodies from subsegmental bronchi with the fiberbronchoscope. *Endoscopy* 1976; 8:192–195.
108. Rubenstein RB, Bainbridge CW. Fiberoptic bronchoscopy for intraoperative localization of endobronchial lesions and foreign bodies. *Chest* 1984;86:935–936.
109. Thorburn JR, Levy H, Schlosberg M, Feldman C, Kallenbach JM. A technique for foreign body removal from the airway. *Endoscopy* 1986;18:71–72.
110. Rohde FC, Celis ME, Fernandez S. The removal of an endobronchial foreign body with the fiberoptic bronchoscope and image intensifier (letter). *Chest* 1977;72:265.
111. Bready LL, Orr MD, Petty C, Grover FL, Harman K. Bronchoscopic administration of nebulized racemic epinephrine to facilitate removal of aspirated peanut fragments in pediatric patients. *Anesthesiology* 1986;65:523–525.
112. Hight DW. Philippart AI. Hertzler JH. The treatment of retained peripheral foreign bodies in the pediatric airway. *J Pediatr Surg* 1981;16:694–699.

113. Moisan TC. Retained endobronchial foreign body removal facilitated by steroid therapy of an obstructing, inflammatory polyp. *Chest* 1991;100:270.
114. Rubio PA, Farrell EM, Ayers LN. Simultaneous bilateral aspiration of foreign bodies. *South Med J* 1979;72:1499–1500.
115. Miks VM, Kvale PA, Riddle JM, Lewis JW Jr. Broncholith removal using YAG laser. *Chest* 1986;90:295–297.
116. Hayashi AH, Gillis DA, Bethune D, Hughes D, O'Neil M. Management of foreign body bronchial obstruction using endoscopic laser therapy. *J Pediatr Surg* 1990;25:1174–1176.
117. Gillio R. Personal communication.
118. Aronson RJ. Acute transient cor pulmonale due to foreign body asphyxia. *Am J Cardiol* 1986;58:379.
119. Steichen FM, Fellini A, Einhorn AH. Acute foreign body laryngo-tracheal obstruction: a cause for sudden and unexpected death in children. *Pediatrics* 1971;48:281–285.
120. Tarkka M, Anttila S. Sutinen S. Bronchial stenosis after aspiration of an iron tablet. *Chest* 1988;93:439–441.
121. Godden DJ, Kerr KM, Watt SJ, Legge JS. Iron lung: bronchoscopic and pathological consequences of aspiration of ferrous sulphate. *Thorax* 1991;46:142–143.
122. Mu L, He P, Sun D. The causes and complications of late diagnosis of foreign body aspiration in children. Report of 210 cases. *Arch Otolaryngol Head Neck Surg* 1991;117:876–879.
123. Poukkula A, Ruotsalainen EM, Jokinen K, Palva A, Nuorviita J. Long-term presence of a denture fragment in the airway (a report of two cases). *J Laryngol Otol* 1988;102:190–193.
124. Berman DE, Wright ES, Edstrom HW. Endobronchial inflammatory polyp associated with a foreign body. Successful treatment with corticosteroids. *Chest* 1984;86:483–484.
125. Karnik AS, Deresinski S, Lourenco RV. Decreased pulmonary perfusion with bronchial foreign body. *Am Rev Resp Dis* 1973; 107:127–129.
126. Chopra S, Simmons DH, Cassan SM, Becker S, Ben-Isaac FE. Bronchial obstruction by incorporation of aspirated vegetable material in the bronchial wall. *Am Rev Resp Dis* 1975; 112:717–720.
127. Kovnat DM, Anderson WM, Rath GS, Snider GL. Hemoptysis secondary to retained transpulmonary foreign body. *Am Rev Resp Dis* 1974;109:279–282.
128. Pattison CW, Leaming AJ, Townsend ER. Hidden foreign body as a cause of recurrent hemoptysis in a teenage girl. *Ann Thorac Surg* 1988;45:330–331.
129. Aytac A, Yurdakul Y, Ikizler C, Olga R, Saylam A. Inhalation of foreign bodies in children. Report of 500 cases. *J Thorac Cardiovasc Surg* 1977;74:145–151.
130. Merchant SN, Kirtane MV, Shah KL, Kernik PP. Foreign bodies in the bronchi (a ten year review of 132 cases). *J Postgrad Med* 1984;30:219–223.
131. Greene JG, Tassin L, Saberi A. Endobronchial papilloma associated with a foreign body. *Chest* 1990;97:229–230.
132. Dicpinigaitis PV, Bleiweiss IJ, Krellenstein DJ, Halton KP, Teirstein AS. Primary endobronchial actinomycosis in association with foreign body aspiration. *Chest* 1992;101:283–285.
133. Rees JR. Massive hemoptysis associated with foreign body removal. *Chest* 1985;88:475–476.
134. Cohen SR. Unusual presentations and problems created by mismanagement of foreign bodies in the aerodigestive tract of the pediatric patient. *Ann Otol Rhinol Laryngol* 1981; 90:316–322.
135. Avital A, Springer C, Meyer JJ, Godfrey S. Hollow bone in the bronchus or the danger of chicken soup. *Respiration* 1992; 59:62–63.
136. Johnson CM III. Disposable plastic diapers: a foreign body hazard. *Otolaryngol Head Neck Surg* 1986;94:235–236.
137. Puterman M, Gorodischer R, Lieberman A. Tracheobronchial foreign bodies: the impact of a postgraduate educational program on diagnosis, morbidity, and treatment. *Pediatrics* 1982; 70:96–98.
138. Carter R. Bronchotomy: the safe solution for an impacted foreign body. *Ann Thorac Surg* 1970;10:93–94.
139. Steelquist JH. Transpleural bronchotomy in the treatment of intractable foreign bodies in children. *Am J Surg* 1969; 118:188–193.
140. Salomon JS, Shindel J, Levy MJ. Bronchotomy for removal of aspirated foreign bodies. *Dis Chest* 1968;54:39–41.

Bronchoscopy,
edited by U. B. S. Prakash.
Mayo Foundation © 1994.
Published by Raven Press, Ltd., New York.

CHAPTER 19

Laser Bronchoscopy

Eric S. Edell and Stanley M. Shapshay

The increase in the prevalence of bronchogenic carcinoma during the latter half of the twentieth century was followed shortly after by the clinical observation that a significant number of patients with lung cancer could not be treated either surgically or by external beam radiation with or without chemotherapy. This finding led to the application of alternate modes of therapy. The light-amplified simulation of emitted radiation (laser), photodynamic therapy, and brachytherapy are among the newer forms of treatment available as palliative measures. Bronchoscopic brachytherapy is discussed in Chapter 20. In this chapter, we will describe the various laser and photodynamic therapies available for treatment of tracheobronchial malignancies.

Introduction of the first operational laser by Maiman in 1960 led to a rapid increase in the biological applications of this device (1). By the end of that decade, hundreds of materials had been found capable of laser action. Subsequent development of fiberoptics expanded the use of laser energy by providing an avenue to areas previously inaccessible (2). This is particularly true for the use of laser energy as a tool in the management of tracheobronchial pathology. The first application of laser energy for management of airway diseases was by Strong et al. in 1974 (3). In this paper, Strong et al. reported the removal of an airway papilloma. In 1981 Toty et al. (8) described the use of a neodymium: yttrium-aluminum garnet (Nd:YAG) laser for resection of a bronchial tumor (8). The argon laser has been used in combination with the photosensitizer for both early detection and treatment of lung carcinoma (4,5). This chapter will review the use of these laser systems and their application in various disorders of the trachea and bronchi.

E. S. Edell: Division of Thoracic Diseases and Internal Medicine, Mayo Clinic, Rochester, Minnesota 55905.
S. M. Shapshay: Department of Otorhinolaryngology, Lahey Clinic Foundation, Burlington, Massachusetts 01805.

LASER–TISSUE INTERACTION

Laser systems used in the management of tracheobronchial pathology are selected depending on their tissue interaction. The optimal use of these laser devices requires some basic understanding of the interaction of laser radiation with biological tissue. It is not the purpose of this chapter to discuss this very complicated topic in depth but rather to provide information so that operators may select the safest and most effective laser systems available. For a more detailed description of this interaction, the reader is referred to the *Endoscopic Laser Surgery Handbook* (6). The distribution of optical energy and the depth of penetration is determined by laser wavelength since attenuation is a function of wavelength. Ultraviolet (UV) wavelengths and far-infrared (IR-C) wavelengths do not have the depth of penetration that is seen in the visible and near-infrared regions (IR-A). Wavelengths <300 nm are poorly absorbed and are therefore suitable for superficial treatment. The argon laser has wavelengths ranging from 457 to 514 nm and can penetrate to a depth of 1 mm in most tissues that are not heavily vascularized. Nd:YAG lasers have a wavelength of 1,064 nm. This wavelength is the most penetrating radiation available for medical use. The carbon dioxide laser has a wavelength of 10,600 nm and a depth of penetration of approximately 10 nm. Below is a description of each of the laser sources and the most commonly used application in the management of tracheobronchial lesions.

TYPES OF LASERS

Carbon Dioxide (CO_2) Laser

The carbon dioxide (CO_2) laser was the first laser used for treatment of tracheobronchial lesions. The CO_2 laser is a gas laser emitting a wavelength of 10,600 nm (3). The active medium is a mixture of CO_2, helium, and nitrogen. Because the wavelength is in the deep infrared range and not visible, most CO_2 laser systems are equipped with a low-power red helium–neon laser system that aids in aiming the laser. The long wavelength of the CO_2 laser prevents transmission with current fiberoptic systems. A series of mirrors and tubes mounted in swivel joints on an articulating arm is required. Fiberoptic systems are under development that would allow transmission of this system to regions that are now only accessible with this technology. As a result the carbon dioxide laser is currently used in the upper airway for management of laryngeal and proximal tracheal lesions.

Nd:YAG Laser

The Nd:YAG is a glass laser. An yttrium–garnet glass is coated with neodymium to produce an energy band capable of lasing. The YAG laser has 13 possible emissions, the major being 1,060 nm. Kiefhaber's use of the Nd:YAG laser to control massive gastrointestinal bleeding was the first clinical application of this laser system. Toty et al. reported the first endoscopic treatment of tracheobronchial lesions by Nd:YAG in 1981 (7). Since its early introduction, several individuals, particularly Dumon, have developed the Nd:YAG as a preferred modality for palliative treatment of obstructing malignant tumors of the airway (8). Clinical YAG systems are set to operate at 1,060 nm, which is invisible, and penetrate tissue maximally at approximately 1.5 cm. Typical systems produce 100 W of laser power and are officially transmitted via commercially available fiberoptics. Such fibers allow application of the Nd:YAG laser through both rigid and flexible endoscopes.

Argon Laser

The argon laser is a gas laser that produces energy in the blue–green region of visible light. These wavelengths penetrate only 1–2 mm. The major use of the argon laser in chest medicine is in pumping of dye laser systems. Dye lasers in the red range are used to activate photochemicals such as hematoporphyrin derivative or dihematoporphyrin ether treatment of both obstructive and superficially invasive carcinomas of the tracheobronchial tree.

CLINICAL APPLICATIONS OF LASER BRONCHOSCOPY

The use of laser energy in the tracheobronchial tree has been shown to be effective in the management of both benign and malignant lesions. The majority of these utilize either the Nd:YAG or CO_2 laser systems. Benign processes include properly selected strictures of the airway and cases of airway hemorrhage due to mucosal arteriovenous malformations. Most cases of laser bronchoscopy involve the management of malignant processes of the tracheobronchial tree. Two distinct types of malignant lesions can be managed with laser bronchoscopy: (a) radiographically occult squamous cell carcinoma; and (b) advanced or recurrent malignancies that cause significant airway obstruction. We will discuss the management of each of these categories individually.

Benign Lesions

The ideal laser for the treatment of benign lesions of the subglottic larynx and trachea should have the features of very precise soft tissue interaction that would preferably be in a non–contact mode, with adequate hemostasis and a fiberoptic delivery system. The CO_2 laser, as discussed previously, has an extremely precise interaction with soft tissue with very little scatter and penetration beyond the impact site. Of all the clinically available lasers, the CO_2 laser is the one of choice for the precise removal of benign lesions such as scar tissue and selected benign neoplasms. Unfortunately, however, the CO_2 laser cannot be transmitted through commonly available flexible quartz fibers, limiting its application to rigid bronchoscopic coupling systems or semiflexible wave guides. The first bronchoscopic application of the CO_2 laser followed the development of a micromanipulator system for laryngeal applications. Coupling the CO_2 laser to an operating microscope gave the endoscopist an unparalleled precision for removal of laryngeal lesions through an operating fiberoptic laryngoscope. The first bronchoscopic application of the CO_2 laser occurred in 1974 with the development of a coupling system allowing laser application through modified rigid bronchoscopes. This prototypic system was at times difficult to align down through smaller rigid bronchoscopes and, in fact, the original prototype lacked an aiming light and a dependable steering mechanism. Ossoff and Karlan in 1983 presented their clinical experience with an improvement to this system featuring quick coupling devices to the rigid bronchoscopes, which were modified as well for suction, evacuation, and better ventilation control during general anesthesia by providing a good seal at the glottic level (9). This improved bronchoscopic coupler also featured a helium neon aiming light and a steering device (Fig. 1). Although this system provides a coherent laser beam in the preferable transverse electromagnetic mode (Gaussian-shaped vaporization impact) problems with the system included only 2–3 times magnification on the proximal part of the

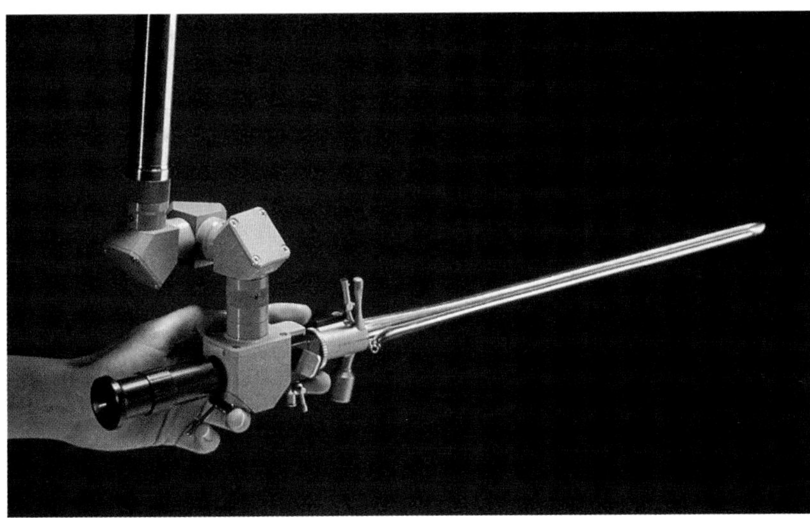

FIG. 1. Carbon dioxide laser system with improved coupler and steering device.

endoscopic coupler and the necessity for a completely closed system. This closed system prevents the simultaneous use of endoscopic suction catheters so necessary during laser application for the evacuation of smoke and clearing of secretions. This system also does not allow simultaneous usage of the excellent optics associated with Hopkins rod–type telescopes. An additional problem associated with the CO_2 laser transmission through articulated arm bronchoscopic system is difficulty in aligning and passing the CO_2 laser through smaller pediatric-sized bronchoscopes. Despite these shortcomings, the bronchoscopic coupler system still remains in widespread use around the world. The development of a hollow waveguide system for the CO_2 laser wavelength has obviated some of the shortcomings associated with the bronchoscopic coupling system. This evolving technology features a metallic semirigid delivery mechanism attached to the articulated arm mechanism (10,11). Suitable flexible fiberoptic fibers for the transmission of CO_2 wavelength are currently in the development stage and are not yet available for clinical application (12,13).

CO_2 LASER BRONCHOSCOPY: INDICATIONS

The earliest and perhaps still the most common application of the CO_2 laser in bronchoscopy is for the treatment of recurrent respiratory papillomatosis (Fig. 2). Although the CO_2 laser does not reduce the frequency of recurrence, it is the safest and most precise technology for the removal of this recurrent tumor. Since the papilloma is often pale in color with small blood vessels, the CO_2 laser is the laser of choice since

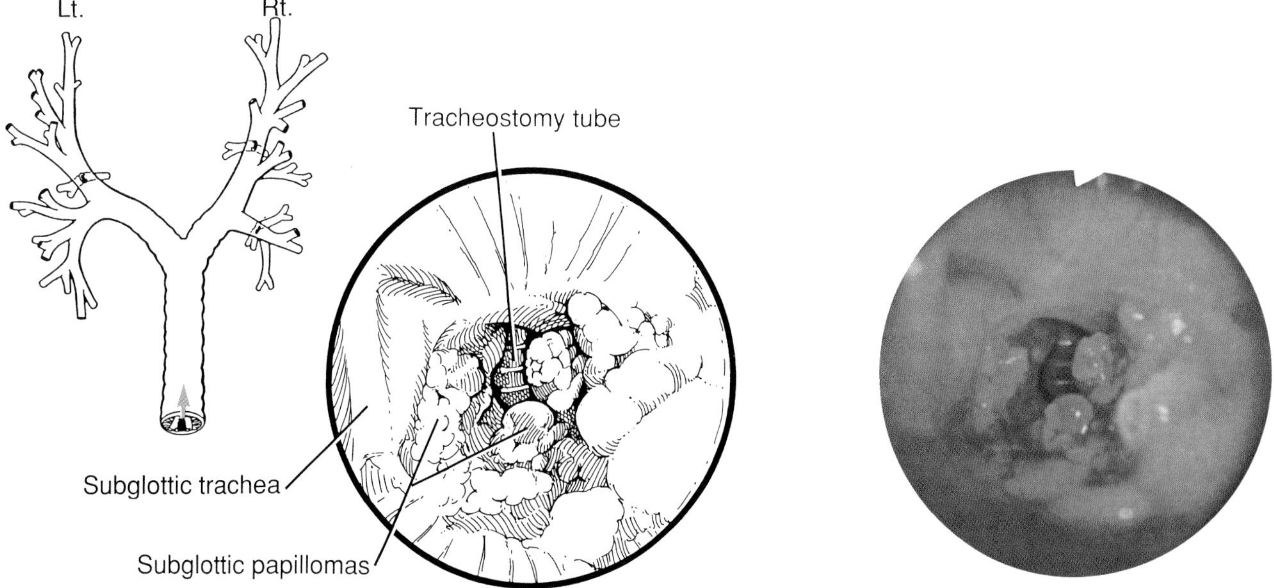

FIG. 2. Extensive subglottic papillomatosis. Tracheostomy tube can be seen.

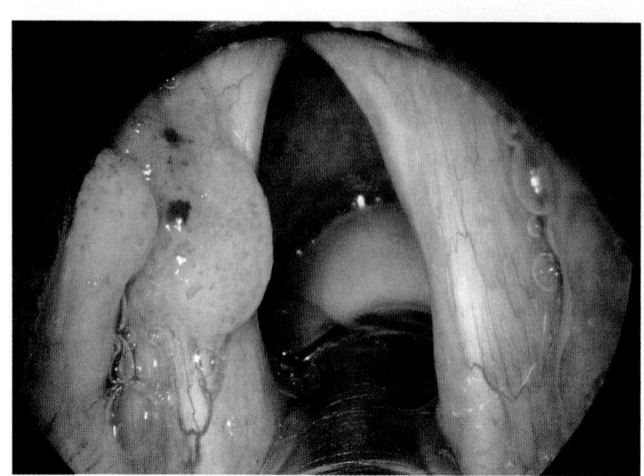
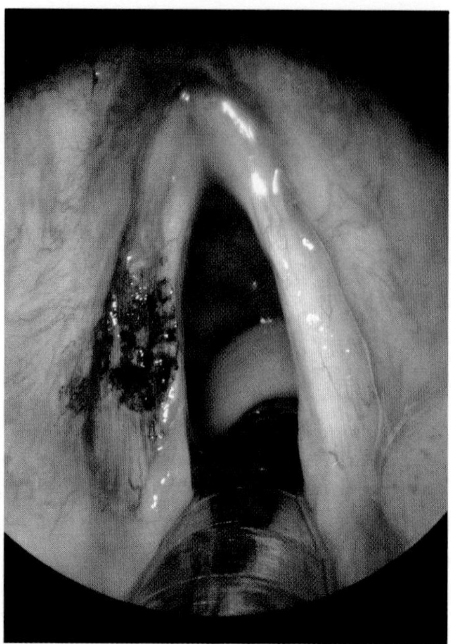

FIG. 3. Laryngeal papilloma before **(A)** and after **(B)** treatment with CO_2 laser.

both the Nd:YAG and argon lasers are dependent on pigment for their absorption into tissue. Since the CO_2 laser has minimal scatter and deep coagulation effects, less collateral damage to surrounding tissue occurs with the CO_2 laser than with the more deeply penetrant Nd:YAG laser. The goal of treatment, particularly in the pediatric patient, is to preserve the airway, maintain a functional voice, and avoid a tracheotomy. It is generally accepted that a tracheotomy in a patient with recurrent respiratory papillomas will induce seeding of the papillomas into the tracheobronchial airway. Papillomas in the tracheobronchial tree involving the pediatric airway is usually a result of a preexisting tracheotomy. Isolated tracheal/bronchial papillomas are more common in the adult airway, although laryngeal involvement is definitely overall more common. The CO_2 laser is used to vaporize the papilloma through the bronchoscope limiting the laser application to the mucosa and submucosa without damaging the underlying perichondrium or cartilage (Fig. 3). Other laser wavelengths such as the KTP/532 and the argon are available and are probably most useful in the smaller pediatric airways in which the CO_2 laser is definitely more difficult to apply. Although these are not the wavelengths of choice for soft tissue application, a higher power density available with thin fiberoptics allow fairly accurate tissue removal without a great deal of surrounding tissue damage. The CO_2 laser energy is usually used at a power setting of 10–15 W at intermittent exposures of ½–1 sec. The disadvantage of the CO_2 laser system in the tracheobronchial tree is the need for a fairly dry field since the CO_2 laser is very well absorbed in water. It is important to note that prior to any lasing of papillomatous lesions, a biopsy would always be obtained to confirm the pathology. Malignant degeneration of tracheobronchial papillomas is distinctly rare; however, there have been reported cases of this occurring (Fig. 4). Other benign tracheobronchial neoplasms such as lipomas, hamartomas, and fibrous histiocytomas have been removed with the CO_2 laser with satisfactory results. If the lesion is deeply invasive into the wall of the trachea, recurrence is probable, making tracheal resection a more desirable alternative. Certainly, an attempt to remove a benign tumor endoscopically first does not preclude a later tracheal resection. Although not technically a neoplasm, amyloidosis affecting the trachea can be a most difficult problem to treat. These

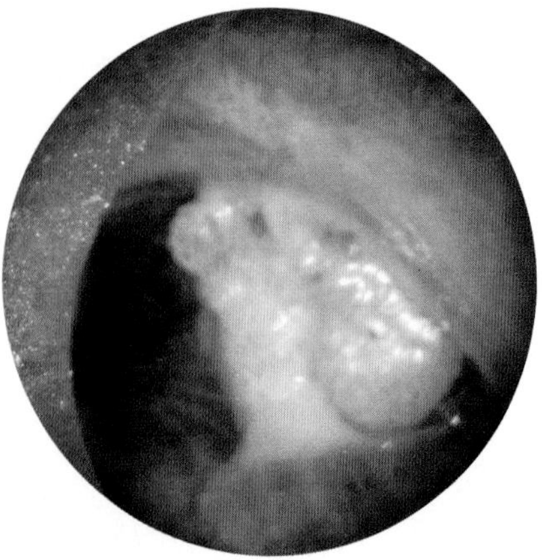

FIG. 4. Left main stem bronchial papilloma with malignant degeneration.

pale infiltrates of amyloid can cause severe respiratory distress if not treated. The CO_2 laser can be used to vaporize these lesions, restoring an adequate airway. Unfortunately, amyloidosis may extend into the more distal bronchi as well as throughout the tracheal wall making treatment in these cases almost impossible.

Subglottic and Tracheal Stenosis

Subglottic and tracheal stenosis had been treated endoscopically for many years with electrocautery, cryosurgery, and, more recently, since the mid-1970s with the CO_2 laser. Early series using prototypic first generation CO_2 laser instrumentation documented moderate success in about 60% of cases (14). Successful management usually necessitated multiple procedures and factors generally associated with poor results included circumferential scarring with contracture, scarring greater than 2 cm in the vertical dimension, previous history of severe bacterial infection associated with tracheotomy, loss of cartilage or tracheomalacia, and scarring of the posterior glottic airway often with arytenoid fixation. In general, a higher success rate has been reported for subglottic stenosis (77%) than for tracheal stenosis (57%) (15,16). In the pediatric airway, Healy reported excellent results in 30 of 39 patients with acquired subglottic stenosis. Decanulation of their tracheotomy was achieved by using the CO_2 laser with a microsurgical approach (17). In cases with severe stenosis a small silastic stent was placed and fixed over a through-and-through laryngeal wire suture. These stents were usually left in place for 4–6 weeks. To improve the somewhat disappointing success rate using the CO_2 laser for treatment of subglottic and tracheal stenosis, Dedo and Sooy reported the use of a "micro–trap-door" flap in the posterior glottic region for posterior glottic stenosis and web-like tracheal stenosis (18). Elevation of this flap with the CO_2 laser permits vaporization of the underlying scar tissue without sacrificing the epithelial lining. Eight of nine patients treated in this fashion had successful outcomes. Successful outcome would appear to be related to elevation of the subglottic epithelium over the scar tissue using a small spot (0.3 mm) CO_2 laser through a microsurgical approach. This technique becomes much more difficult when attempted in the tracheal airway using a bronchoscopic approach. Avoidance of a circumferential laser–induced injury was stressed by Shapshay et al. using a technique of CO_2 laser radial incision and gentle atraumatic dilatation with the level of rigid scopes (Fig. 5) (19). Immediate airway patency was achieved in 11 of 12 patients without complications. Five patients went on to require open tracheal resection because of recurrence of stenosis several months after the procedure. The CO_2 laser waveguide (LaserSonics), 3 mm in diameter, was used in this series. The use of the waveguide allowed an open bronchoscopic system with simultaneous use of a 0° Hopkins rod telescope and a semiflexible heat-resistant polyethylene catheter. The key to successful endoscopic treatment appears to be careful selection of patients with a relatively thin web-like stenosis, atraumatic incision, and dilation of the stenotic tissue. Postoperatively these patients were given broad-spectrum antibiotics for 3 weeks. Systemic steroids were avoided due to the potential for delay in epithelization. It must be stressed that prior to any consideration for treatment of subglottic and tracheal stenosis, a careful evaluation of laryngeal function should be undertaken. It makes little sense to attempt to repair subglottic or tracheal stenosis in the presence of vocal cord paralysis, particularly bilateral. In addition, a direct laryngoscopy is often necessary to assess arytenoid mobility by

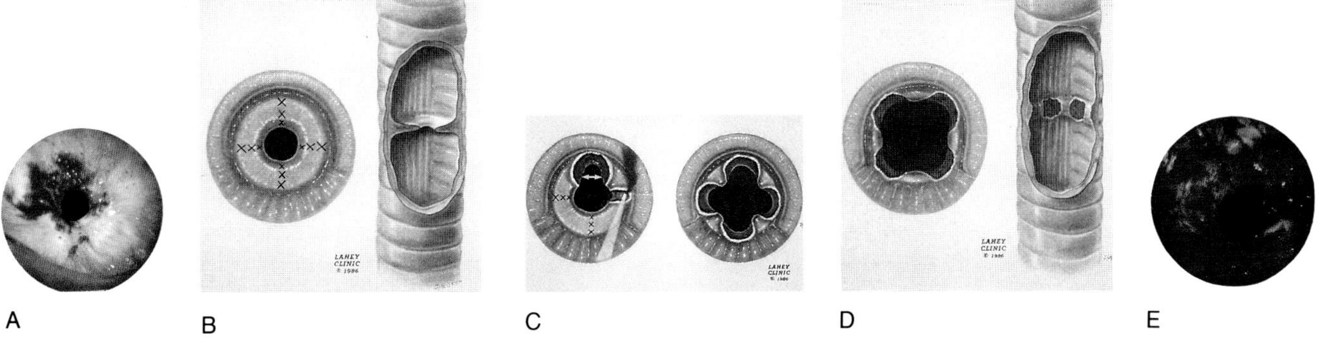

FIG. 5. Diagrammatic illustration of tracheal lumen from bronchoscopic view, and tracheal cross-section. **(A)** tracheal stenosis, **(B)** fibrous concentric tracheal stenosis with lumen size of 3–4 mm x-radial laser incisions, **(C)** lumen of airway is enlarged by radial laser incision and subsequent retraction (arrows) of scar tissue, **(D)** tracheal size after radial laser incision and progressive dilatation of lumen with 7.5- and 8.5-mm rigid bronchoscopes, and **(E)** islands of epithelium are depicted between laser incisional areas. From Shapshay et al., with permission (35).

palpation. This would be extremely important if trauma was associated with the etiology of the stenosis. A flexible examination of the upper and lower airway is essential prior to the repair done under general anesthesia. Laryngeal function and the presence of tracheomalacia with collapse of the airway can only be determined with the patient breathing spontaneously. It is also extremely important in assessing the results of treatment for subglottic and tracheal stenosis to attempt to classify the stenosis appropriately. The literature is replete with comparisons of "apples to oranges," mixing adult and pediatric airway stenosis as well as fibrous stenosis with tracheomalacia. It is also important to consider those patients needing tracheotomy as a separate category since they often have more severe stenosis and are almost universally associated with some degree of infection from the tracheotomy site.

Adult Subglottic Stenosis

In general, the easiest and best indication for CO_2 laser endoscopic treatment is web-like or fibrous stenosis without an existing tracheotomy. These patients are best treated if the subglottic stenosis is just below the vocal cords with an anterior commissure Dedo-type laryngoscope with the tip placed just between the cords. A small spot micromanipulator (0.3 mm impact spot) can be used for laser incision of this subglottic web. If the stenosis is somewhat distant to this area, a subglottic laryngoscope placed on the usual laryngeal suspension system can be utilized. Alternatively, a tracheoscope designed without ventilating ports on the side of the scope will sustain adequate ventilation at the vocal cord level and still allow usage of shortened, rigid telescopes for excellent visualization. Shorter waveguides can be used for transmission of the CO_2 laser through this instrument. If the patient does not have a tracheotomy, a Venturi jet type of ventilation system should be utilized either on the posterior lip of the laryngoscope or built into the laryngoscope or tracheoscope. This system avoids an endotracheal tube in the airway, which interferes with visibility and is a potential source of ignition with the laser. Preoperatively, the patient should have anteroposterior and lateral tracheal tomograms to assess the integrity of the tracheal cartilages, as well as flexible bronchoscopy to assess lumen stability and laryngeal function. If complete subglottic stenosis exists necessitating a tracheotomy for airway maintenance, a T-tube silicon stent may be useful after endoscopic laser resection of the stenosis (20). Endoscopic therapy, of course, does not preclude future open resection and in fact may facilitate tracheotomy extubation by removing a potential source of infection prior to open surgery. The largest possible T-tube stent should be placed after the trachea is dilated, using rigid bronchoscopes with gradually increasing diameters for maximum dilation. Size 12–14 mm Montgomery T-tube stents are usually satisfactory. The technique of T-tube placement through the tracheotomy site is well described in the literature. However, it is important to stress that the T tube should be plugged externally to avoid drying of secretions and mucous plugging. Meticulous postoperative care of the T tube is absolutely necessary. The T tubes are generally left in place for a minimum of 6 months. If persistent stenosis occurs or recurs after removal of the stent, open surgical resection is indicated. Excellent results, namely, decanulation and good voice, were achieved in 8 of 12 patients with multiple laser and dilation treatments often necessary. It is important to note, however, that T-tube stents are more dangerous in the pediatric airway because of their smaller size and a potential for displacement. Tracheal resection and anastomosis is the treatment of choice should the endoscopic route fail or if the stenosis is primarily a tracheomalacia with loss of cartilaginous support. Tracheal resection is preferred, even for cases of subglottic stenosis, in preference over open cricoid split and grafting techniques. It is important to remove the tracheotomy at the time of definitive treatment so as to remove a source of infection and ultimate restenosis. If endoscopic laser treatment or tracheal resection are not possible due to the age and medical condition of the patient, tracheal dilation and insertion of a T tube may suffice for long-term palliation. If well cared for, the T tube may be left in place for over a year without changing the tube. Of course, it must be kept in mind that long-term or permanent tracheotomy is always a viable alternative to the aforementioned techniques.

OTHER INDICATIONS

An important use of the CO_2 laser is treatment of subglottic hemangioma in the pediatric airway. Healy et al. reported the use of the CO_2 laser to treat 41 patients with subglottic hemangioma (21). If patients had not had a previously placed tracheostomy, it was not usually necessary to perform this procedure either before or after laser therapy. The patient could be intubated with a small endotracheal tube and the subglottic larynx exposed with a pediatric laryngoscope. The endotracheal tube is then removed and a Venturi jet ventilation system is used while biopsy specimens of the subglottic hemangioma are taken prior to vaporization of the hemangioma. It is important to note that this is a compact capillary-type hemangioma and not a venous malformation of the cavernous type, which is best and is treated with the noncontact Nd:YAG laser. The latter type of venous malformation is usually found in adults and is located in the supraglottic region as opposed to the subglottic airway with the capillary-type subglottic hemangioma. For other vascular lesions in the smaller pediatric airway, such as granulomas and superficial vascular malformations, the KTP laser (potassium titanyl phosphate) can be very useful. It can be transmitted through a 600-μm fiber and precisely manipulated through rigid pediatric bronchoscopes as small as 3 mm. The Hopkins rod telescopic lens system may also be used for improved visibility and visual control during laser application.

Malignant Lesions

The management of patients with malignancies of the tracheobronchial tree continues to present a formidable challenge to the practicing clinician. Treatment of these patients has been disappointing and is often only palliative. Many patients are not candidates for surgical treatment because of underlying medical problems. Radiotherapy and chemotherapy have a limited effect on tumor responsiveness and can produce serious side effects. Studies have demonstrated that early diagnosis of bronchogenic carcinoma provides the best opportunities for long-term survival (22). Studies sponsored by the National Cancer Institute evaluated the effectiveness of sputum cytology in the detection of occult bronchogenic carcinoma. These studies showed that carcinomas could be detected at an earlier stage, but subsequent follow-up showed no changes in mortality between groups that were detected when they were radiographically occult as compared to those in the later stage (23). The reason for this difference may be that this group of patients had a high incidence of multicentricity with 7–15% of patients having simultaneously occult carcinoma at the time of initial diagnosis and a subsequent primary tumor developing at a rate of 5% per year (22). Additionally, operative mortality is increased in patients with occult disease compared with all patients undergoing surgery for lung cancer (22). Therefore, a method of treatment that is safe and preserves pulmonary parenchyma may lead to further increase in length of survival in patients with early superficial occult squamous cell carcinoma of the lung. Bronchoscopic phototherapy is a combination of photosensitizing agents that can be activated by a laser energy of the proper wavelength. A number of photosensitizing agents have been considered for treatment of malignant tumors. In 1960, Lipson developed a derivative of hematoporphyrin (HpD) that was found to accumulate in malignant and dysplastic tissue (24). When HpD was exposed to light, a photodynamic reaction occurred with destruction of malignant cells, which was demonstrated in both cell culture and animal models. This observation led to the application of HpD phototherapy (HpD-PT) in the management of several human malignancies including radiographically occult cancer of the tracheobronchial tree. HpD-PT was first used to treat malignancies of the tracheobronchial tree in 1980 by Hayata et al. (4). Since its introduction, photodynamic therapy has been used in the management of occult squamous cell carcinoma in nearly 200 patients. Complete remission has been reported between 65% and 75% of patients treated. An argon-pumped rhodamine B dye laser with an emission of 630 nm is used to activate the photosensitizer, hematoporphyrin derivative or dihematoporphyrin ether (Fig. 6). Patients who have radiographically occult central

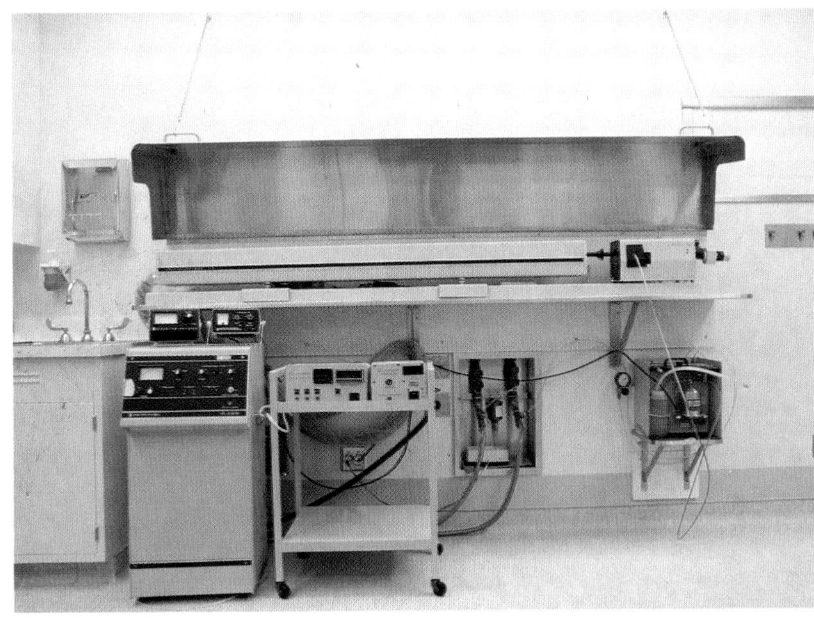

FIG. 6. Argon-pumped rhodamine B dye laser equipment (Spectra-Physics).

FIG. 7. Quartz optical fiber (400 nm) with microlens tip **(left)** or diffuser tip **(right).**

superficial squamous cell carcinoma are selected for therapy. Those lesions that appear to be most amenable are superficial in nature. Patients receive the photosensitizer 40–50 hr before laser therapy. The tumor is then treated, via a flexible bronchoscope, with either the argon dye laser or an excimer dye laser tuned to 620–630 nm. The total energy and fiber used depends on the configuration of the lesion. The total energy for effective treatment appears to be 200–250 J/cm^2 using the argon dye laser or 100–150 J/cm^2 using the excimer laser. For well-localized lesions, a microlens emitting 200 mW of power appears to be most effective. For more diffuse lesions, diffusing fibers emitting 400 W/cm are most effective (Fig. 7).

Laser Bronchoscopy for Advanced or Recurrent Obstructing Malignancies

Patients with bronchogenic carcinomas that obstruct the central airway have traditionally been treated by surgical resection, radiotherapy, chemotherapy, or a combination of these modalities. Bronchoscopic debulking of tumor using the Nd:YAG laser provides a second application of laser bronchoscopy in the management of malignancies in the tracheobronchial tree. The Nd:YAG laser delivers radiation at 1,064 nm, allowing transmission via quartz monofilament fiber through a flexible or rigid bronchoscope. The Nd:YAG laser allows deep-tissue penetration and provides coagulation of vessels several millimeters in diameter. This system has been used successfully by several groups to treat airways obstructed by inoperable malignant carcinomas (7,8). It acts directly on malignant tissue causing thermonecrosis and vaporization of tissue (Figs. 8 and 9). This system allows debulking of large obstructive tumors and simultaneously provides photocoagulation that helps control bleeding during treatment. The proper selection of patients for Nd:YAG laser treatment is important to decrease risk of complications that include hemorrhage from tumor necrosis, perforation of large blood vessels, bronchopleural fistulas, airway combustion, and hypoxemia (25). Candidates should meet most if not all of the following criteria: (a) tumor is unresponsive to all of the reasonable therapy; (b) tumor should protrude into the bronchial lumen without obvious extension beyond the cartilage; (c) the actual length of tumor is smaller than 4 cm; (d) the bronchoscopist is able to see a bronchial lumen; (e) there is functioning lung parenchyma beyond the obstruction; and (f) the symptoms of the malignancy are primarily respiratory (26). As mentioned above, the YAG laser can be applied through either a flexible bronchoscope or a rigid bronchoscope. Several authors have discussed the pros and cons of each instrument (8,22). Most laser bronchoscopists believe that the rigid bronchoscope is the instrument of choice in the treatment of malignant airway obstruction (8,25).

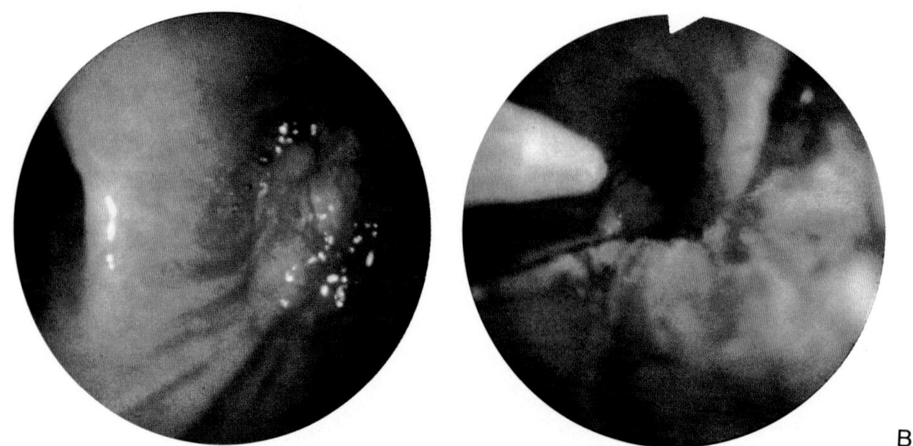

FIG. 8. Squamous cell carcinoma before **(A)** and after **(B)** Nd:YAG resection using rigid bronchoscope. From Cortese DA, Edell ES. *Clin Chest Med* 1993;14:149–159, with permisison.

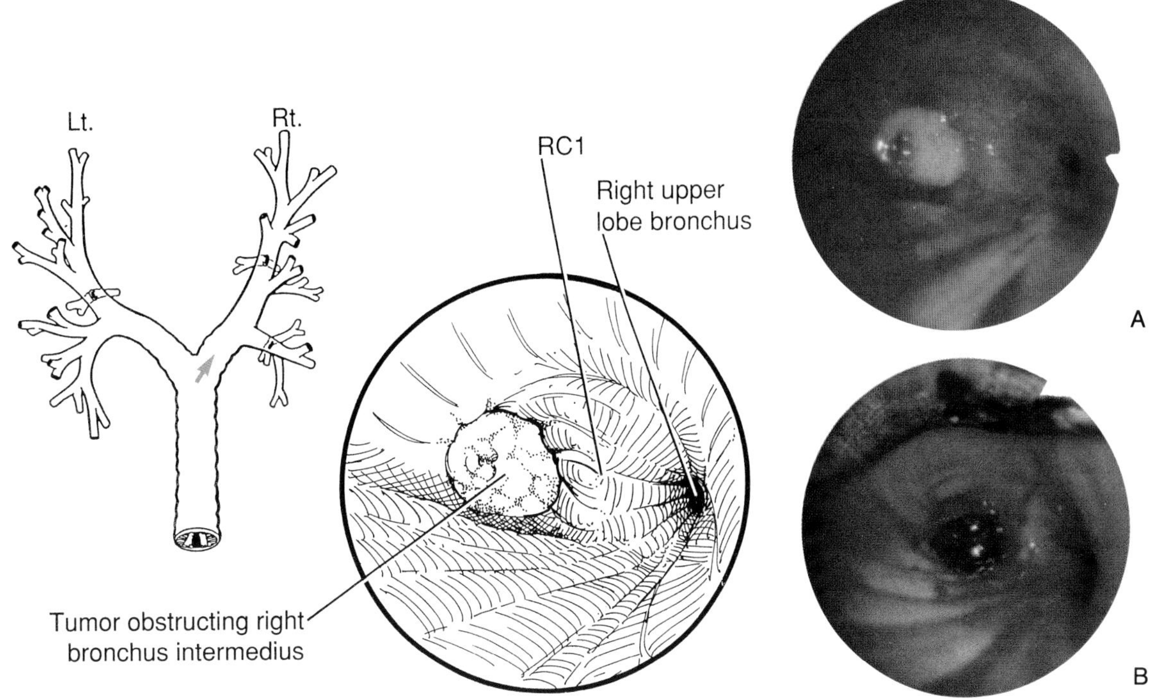

FIG. 9. (A) Malignant tumor with complete obstruction of right bronchus intermedius. **(B)** Charring of tumor following initial application of laser therapy. Tip of the rigid bronchoscope is seen.

The advantages of the rigid system include superior airway control, ease of removal of necrotic tissue, ease of ventilation, and a shorter operation time (Fig. 10). In patients with more distal obstruction, the flexible bronchoscope allows access for treatment (Fig. 11) (28). Indications for treatment of the distal airway include obstructive pneumonitis and recurrent or persistent hemoptysis. Both primary and metastatic airway lesions can be effectively palliated (Figs. 12–14). To ensure optimal patient safety, laser bronchoscopists should be trained in both rigid and flexible bronchoscopic systems (29). A second laser system is available and currently under investigation in the management of a malignant airway obstruction. Several authors have reported the use of photodynamic therapy using HpD or dihematoporphyrin ether with an argon-pumped dye

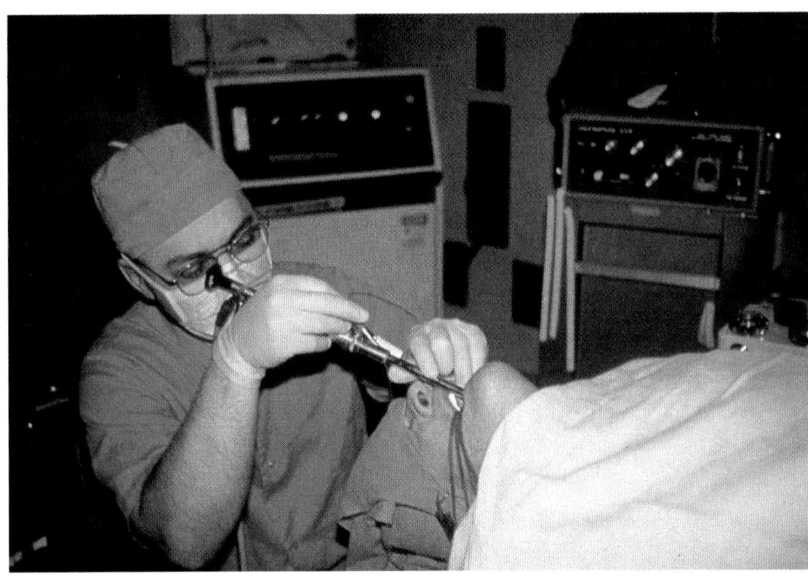

FIG. 10. Nd:YAG laser treatment via rigid bronchoscope.

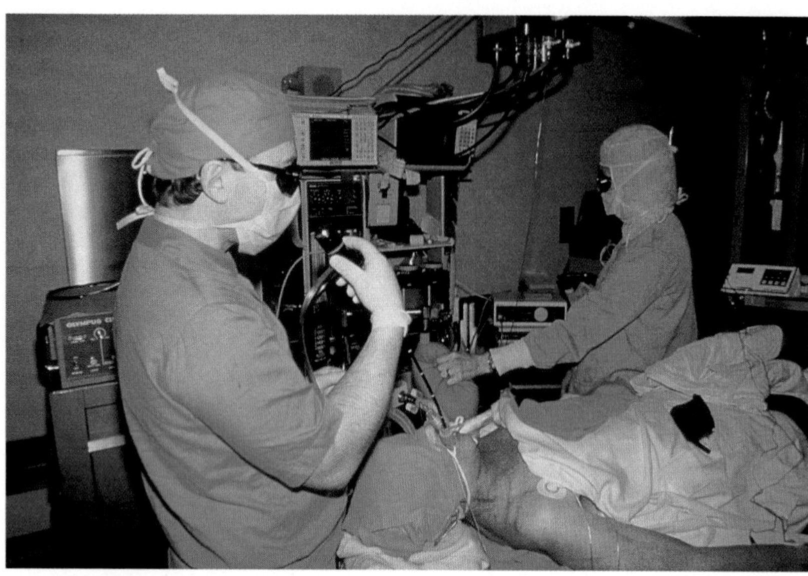

FIG. 11. Nd:YAG laser treatment via flexible bronchoscope.

laser (30–33). In these patients, a flexible system can be used for treatment of these lesions. Obstructing tumors are treated by direct implantation of a diffusing fiber into the bulk of the tumor (Fig. 15). This is followed by a clean-up bronchoscopy at which time necrotic tissue is removed with the flexible bronchoscope or an open rigid tube bronchoscope (Fig. 15B and C). Whether this system provides an advantage over the Nd:YAG laser has yet to be determined.

SUMMARY

The development and subsequent application of laser energy has provided the bronchoscopist a valuable new tool. As we have outlined, management of both benign and malignant lesions of the tracheobronchial tree may be facilitated with the proper application of these laser systems. It is important that bronchoscopists realize the various tissue interactions encoun-

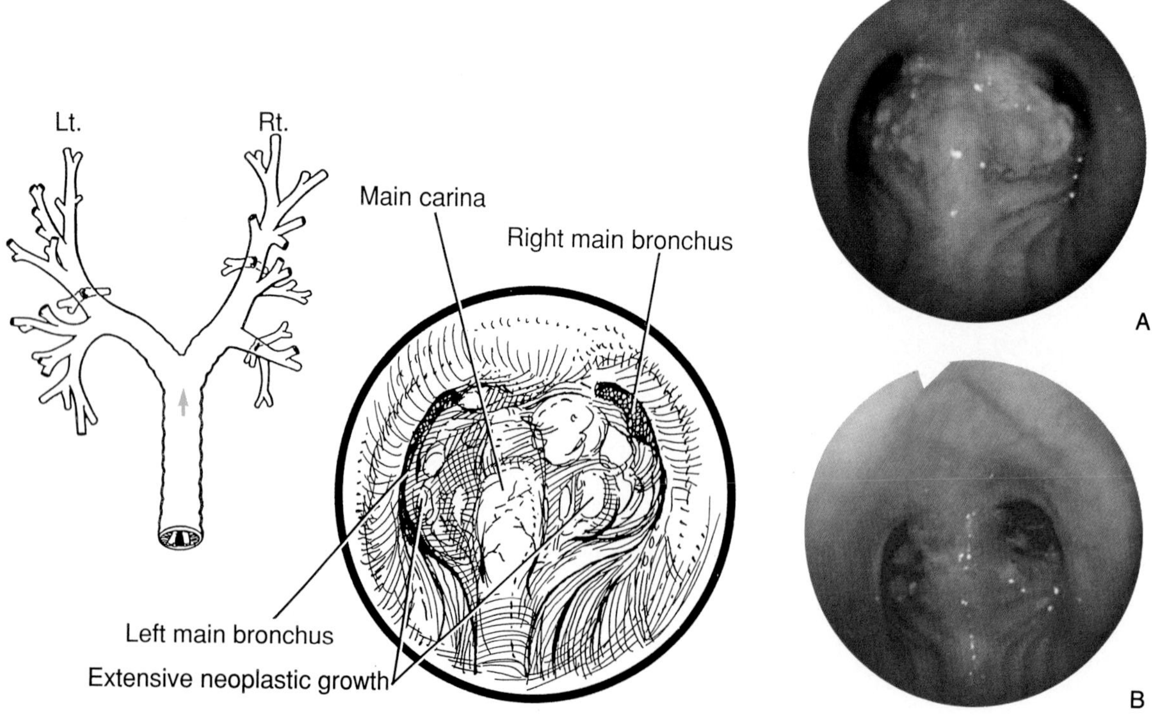

FIG. 12. (A) Extensive squamous cell carcinoma of main carina. **(B)** Partial palliation of obstruction with beginning stages of laser therapy.

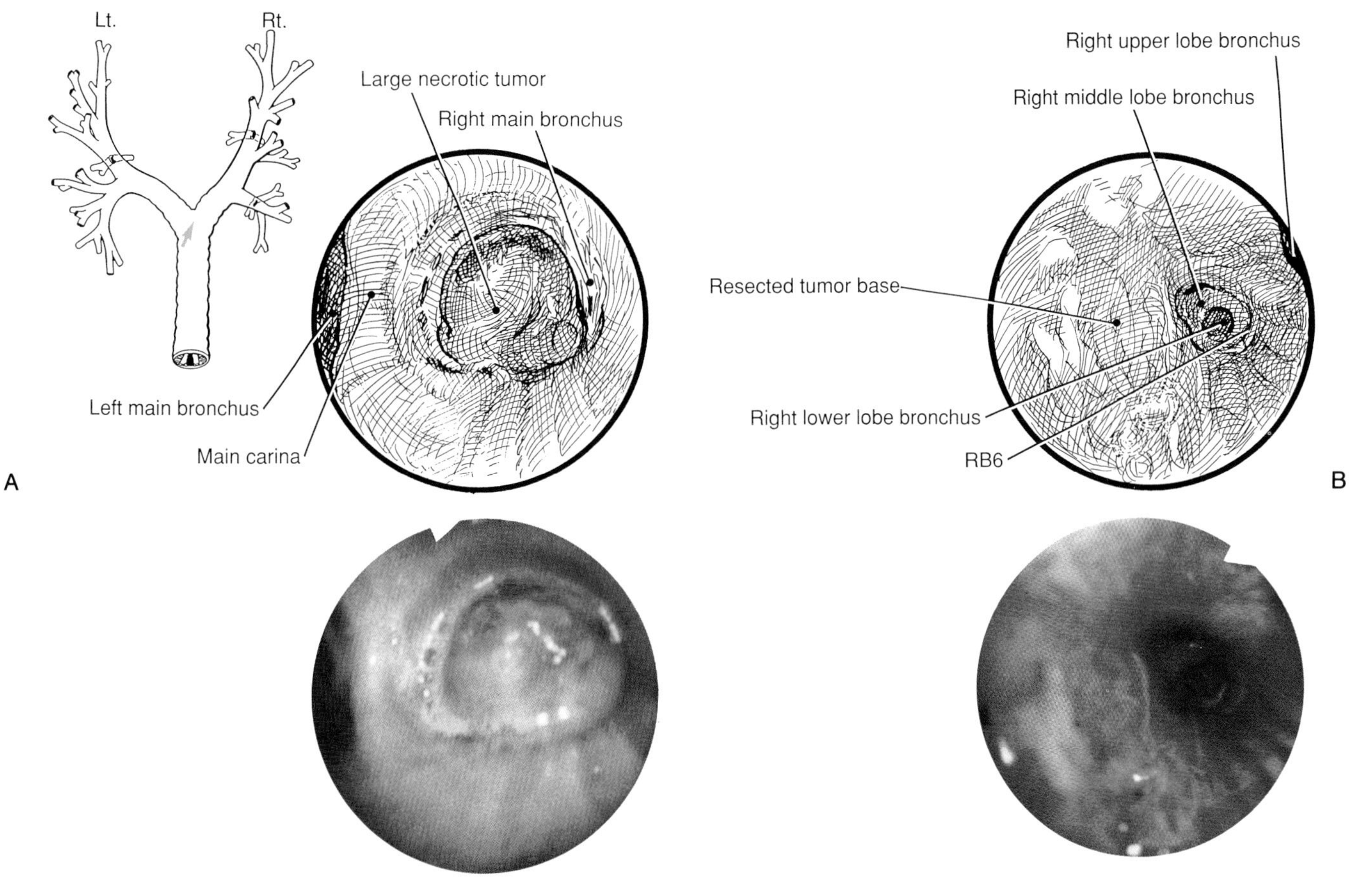

FIG. 13. (A) Complete obstruction of right main stem bronchus by metastatic leiomyosarcoma. **(B)** View following laser resection shows distal bronchial tree.

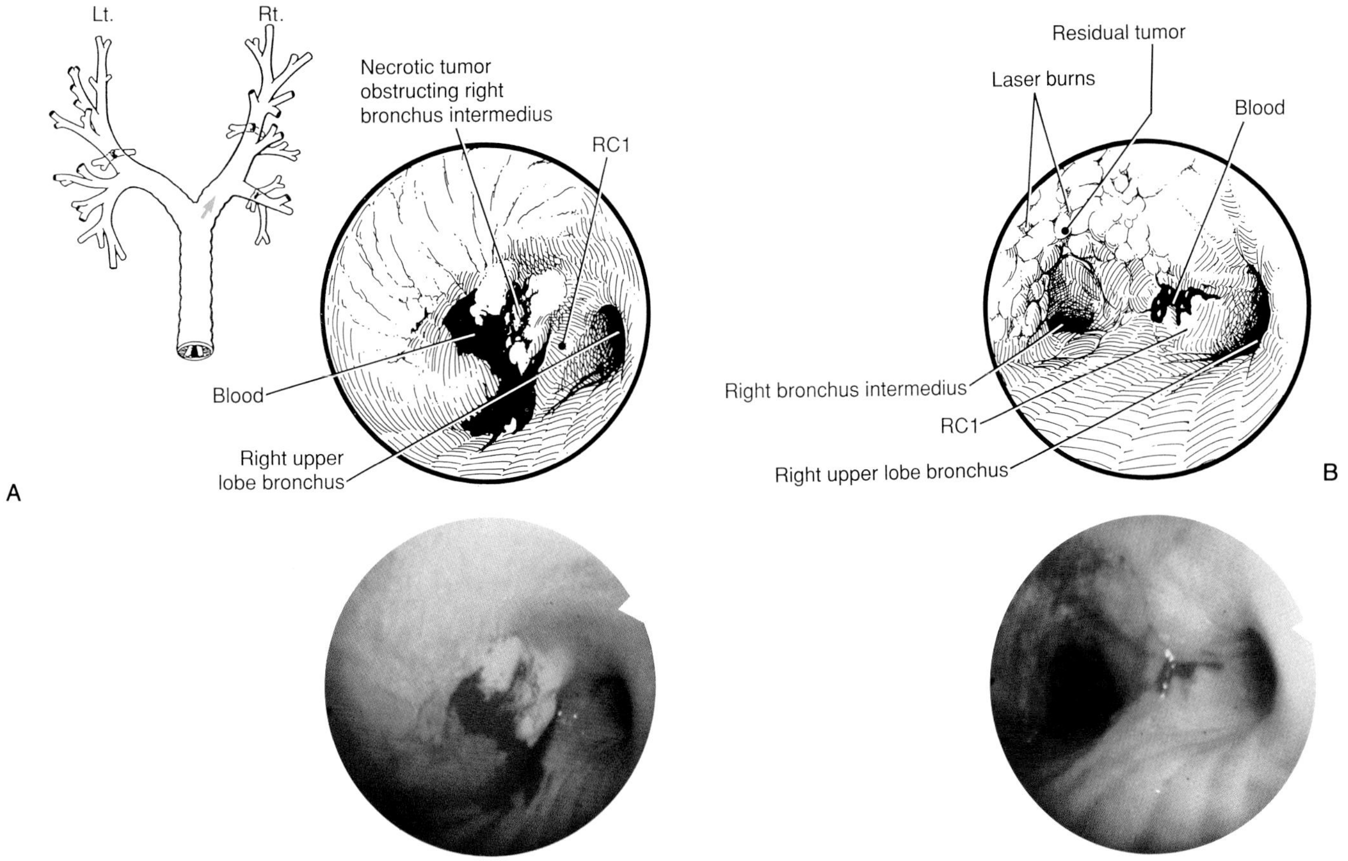

FIG. 14. (A) Total occlusion of right main stem bronchus by squamous cell carcinoma. **(B)** Bronchoscopic view immediately after laser therapy.

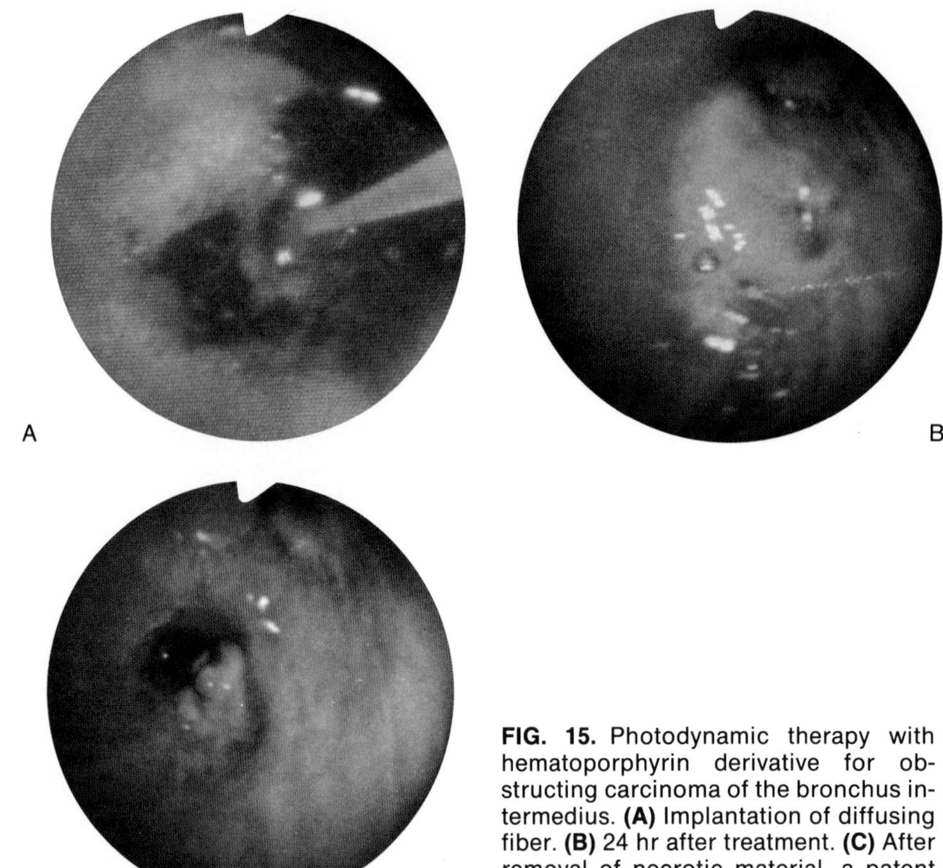

FIG. 15. Photodynamic therapy with hematoporphyrin derivative for obstructing carcinoma of the bronchus intermedius. **(A)** Implantation of diffusing fiber. **(B)** 24 hr after treatment. **(C)** After removal of necrotic material, a patent lumen is seen.

tered with these laser systems. The CO_2 laser appears best suited to application in the proximal trachea. Absorption of the CO_2 laser limits its application to superficial hemangiomas and benign strictures. The absorption characteristics of the CO_2 laser enables it to act as a precise cutting tool. Unfortunately, the wavelength of the carbon dioxide laser prevents application to fiberoptic systems. The Nd:YAG laser is capable of deeper tissue penetration. It is best suited for photocoagulation of malignant lesions of the tracheobronchial tree. The argon dye laser and excimer lasers can be used to excite various photochemicals that may be useful for management of both early superficial squamous carcinoma and late obstructing or recurrent carcinoma of the tracheobronchial tree. Proper selection of laser systems to fit the clinical application is important not only to provide the best opportunity for satisfactory outcome but also to ensure safety. Other measures such as proper eye protection, shielding of flammable endotracheal tubes, and education of paramedical personnel are imperative for the function of a cohesive laser unit. When the above guidelines are followed, these various laser systems provide an invaluable tool to the bronchoscopist.

REFERENCES

1. Maiman TH. Stimulated optical radiation in ruby. *Nature* 1960;187:493.
2. Van Heel ACS. A new method of transporting optical images without abberation. *Nature* 1954;173–179.
3. Strong MS, Vaughan CW, Polany TG. Bronchoscopic CO_2 laser surgery. *Ann Otol Rhinol Laryngol* 1974;83:769–776.
4. Hayata Y, Kato H, Konaka C, Ono J, Takizawa N. Hematoporphyrin derivative in laser photoradiation in the treatment of lung cancer. *Chest* 1982;81:269–277.
5. Cortese DA, Kinsey JH, Woolner LB. Clinical application of a new endoscopic technique for detection of in situ bronchial carcinoma. *Mayo Clin Proc* 1979;54:635–642.
6. Shapshay S, ed. *Endoscopic laser surgery handbook.* New York: Marcel Dekker; 1991;1–131.
7. Toty L, et al. Bronchoscopic management of tracheal lesions using Nd:YAG laser. *Thorax* 1981;36:175–178.
8. Dumon JF, Shapshay S, Bourcerean J, Cavaliere S, Meric B, Garb N, Beams J. Principles for safety in application of neodymium-YAG laser in bronchology. *Chest* 1984;86:163–168.
9. Ossoff RH, Karlan MS. Universal endoscopic coupler for carbon dioxide laser surgery. *Ann Otol Rhinol Laryngol* 1982;91:608–609.
10. Shapshay SM. Laser application in the trachea and bronchi: a comparative study of soft tissue effects using contact and noncontact delivery systems. *Laryngoscope* 1987;97(suppl 41):1–26.
11. Shapshay SM, Setzer S, Aretz HT. Clinical options in the delivery of the CO_2 laser in the tracheobronchial tree. *SPIE Proc* 1988;906:205–209.

12. Katzir A. Optical fibers in optics medicine and biology. *SPIE Proc* 1985;906:576.
13. Rontal M, Fuller T, Rontal E, Jacob HJ. Flexible nontoxic fiberoptic delivery system for the carbon dioxide laser. *Ann Otol Rhinol Laryngol* 1985;94:357–360.
14. Simpson GT, Strong MS, Healy GB, Shapshay SM, Vaughan CW. Predictive factors of success or failure in the endoscopic management of laryngeal and tracheal stenosis. *Ann Otol Rhinol Laryngol* 1982;91:384–388.
15. Koufman JA, Thompson JN, Kohut RI. Endoscopic management of subglottic stenosis with the CO_2 laser. *Otolaryngol Head Neck Surg* 1981;89:215–220.
16. Ossoff RH, Tucker GF Jr, Duncavage JA, Toohill RJ. Efficacy of bronchoscopic carbon dioxide laser surgery for benign strictures of the trachea. *Laryngoscope* 1985;95:1220–1223.
17. Healy GB. Laser surgery in the pediatric airway. In: Shapshay SM, ed. *Endoscopic laser surgery Handbook*. New York: Marcel Dekker; 1987:453–462.
18. Dedo HH, Sooy CD. Endoscopic laser repair of posterior glottic, sub-glottic and tracheal stenosis by division of microtrap door flap. *Laryngoscope* 1984;94:445–450.
19. Shapshay SM, Beamis JF Jr, Hybels RL, Bohigian RK. Endoscopic treatment of subglottic and tracheal stenosis by radial laser incision and dilation. *Ann Otol Rhinol Laryngol* 1987; 99:661–664.
20. Shapshay SM, Beamis JF Jr, Dumon JF. Total cervical tracheal stenosis: treatment by laser, dilation and stenting. *Ann Otol Rhinol Laryngol* 1989;98:890–895.
21. Healy GB, McGill T, Friedman EM. Carbon dioxide laser management of subglottic hemangioma—an update. *Ann Otol Rhinol Laryngol* 1984;93:370–373.
22. Cortese DA, Pairolero PC, Bergstralh EJ, et al. Roentgenographically occult lung cancer: a ten-year experience. *J Thorac Cardiovasc Surg* 1983;86:373–380.
23. Melamed MR, Felhinger BJ, Zamen MB. Screening for early lung cancer. Results of Memorial Sloan-Kettering Study in New York. *Chest* 1984;86:44.
24. Lipson RL, Baldes EJ. The photodynamic properties of a particular hematoporphyrin derivative. *Arch Dermatol* 1960;82:508.
25. Brutinel WM, Cortese DA, Edell ES, McDougall JC, Prakash UBS. Complications of Nd:YAG laser therapy. *Chest* 1988; 94:902–903.
26. Brutinel WM, Cortese DA, McDougall JC, Gillio RG, Bergstralh EJ. A two-year experience with the neodymium-YAG laser in endobronchial obstruction. *Chest* 1987;91:159–165.
27. Brutinel WM, Cortese DA, Edell ES, McDougall JC, Prakash UBS. Complications of Nd:YAG laser therapy. *Chest* 1988; 94:902–903.
28. Unger M. Neodymium: YAG laser therapy for malignant and benign endobronchial obstructions. *Clin Chest Med* 1985; 6:277–290.
29. Kvale PA. Training in laser bronchoscopy and proposals for credentialling. *Chest* 1990;97:983–989.
30. McCaughan JS, Williams TE Jr, Bethel BH. Photodynamic therapy of endobronchial tumors. *Lasers Surg Med* 1986;6:336–345.
31. Pass HI, Delaney T, Smith PD, Bonner R, Russo A. Bronchoscopic photo-therapy at comparable dose rates: early results. *Ann Thorac Surg* 1989;47:693–699.
32. Lam S, Muller NL, Miller RR, et al. Predicting the response of obstructive endobronchial tumors to photodynamic therapy. *Cancer* 1986;58:2298–2306.
33. LoCicero J III, Metzdorff M, Almgren L. Photodynamic therapy in the palliation of late stage obstructing non-small cell lung cancer. *Chest* 1990;98:97–100.
34. Shapshay SM, et al. Endoscopic treatment of subglottic and tracheal stenosis by radial laser incision and dilatation. *Ann Otol Rhinol Laryngol* 1987;96:661–664.

Bronchoscopy,
edited by U. B. S. Prakash.
Mayo Foundation © 1994.
Published by Raven Press, Ltd., New York.

CHAPTER 20

Bronchoscopic Brachytherapy

Edward G. Shaw and John C. McDougall

Bronchogenic carcinoma is the most common malignancy and the number one cause of cancer mortality in both men and women in the United States (1). Curative surgical treatment is possible in only one third of patients (2,3). The remaining patients present with locally advanced, inoperable, or metastatic disease. Local tumor progression affecting the airways, i.e., endobronchial disease, or nodal disease in the mediastinum or hilum causing extrinsic compression occurs in approximately 20% of patients following curative surgery (4–6) and up to 80% of patients following external beam thoracic radiation therapy for inoperable lung cancer (7). Major causes of morbidity and mortality in these patients include obstructive pneumonitis, dyspnea, cough, and hemoptysis. Many modalities of local therapy have been devised over the years for curative and palliative treatment of bronchogenic carcinoma—cryotherapy, neodymium–YAG (Nd:YAG) laser therapy, CO_2 laser therapy, argon laser therapy, hematoporphyrin phototherapy, mechanical removal of endobronchial tumor tissue, stent placement, and brachytherapy. Brachytherapy has become popular and its use is now widespread.

Brachytherapy is defined as the delivery of ionizing radiation therapy from a source of ionizing radiation placed within or very near the tissue being treated. The main advantage of brachytherapy is the rapid fall-off of dose [as a function of 1/distance (d) or $1/d^2$] resulting in a concentration of dose to the tissue surrounding the implant with a relative sparing of adjacent normal tissues including lung parenchyma, esophagus, heart, great vessels, and spinal cord. For the purposes of this chapter, only those forms of brachytherapy which involve the use of the bronchoscope to place radioactive sources or an afterloading device for the subsequent placement of radioactive sources into the affected airway will be discussed.

E. G. Shaw: Department of Radiation Oncology, Mayo Clinic, Rochester, Minnesota 55905.
J. C. McDougall: Division of Thoracic Diseases and Internal Medicine, Mayo Clinic, Rochester, Minnesota 55905.

HISTORY OF BRACHYTHERAPY

The first written report of endoscopic placement of radioactive sources was by Yankaur (8) in 1921, who placed radon-222 (^{222}Ra) seeds within endobronchial tumors. In 1961, endobronchial placement of ^{222}Ra sources was again described by Pool (9) while Johnston et al. (10) introduced the use of radioactive gold (^{198}Au) in endobronchial tumors. Gibbons and Baker (11) subsequently described a large series of 198 patients treated by bronchoscopically placed ^{198}Au into endobronchial tumors. Hilaris and colleagues then described the use of iodine-125 (^{125}I) in patients with primary or recurrent endobronchial tumors (12,13). All of these reports feature permanent placement of radioactive seeds directly into endobronchial tumor via the rigid bronchoscope. In the late 1970s and into the early 1980s, flexible bronchoscopic placement of devices designed for the afterloading of temporary radioactive iridium-192 (^{192}Ir) sources was described. Mittal et al. (14) and Moylan et al. (15) reported a flexible implantation system for endobronchial ^{198}Au brachytherapy in 1984.

The most commonly utilized technique for endobronchial irradiation involves the use of ^{192}Ir. The use of this radioactive source, temporarily inserted within a plastic afterloading catheter by flexible bronchoscopy, was first reported by Percarpio et al. (16) and was subsequently reported by Mendiondo et al. (17) and Schray et al. (18,19). Other radioactive sources used for afterloading include cesium-137 (^{137}Cs) as reported by Boedker et al. (20), and cobalt-60 (^{60}Co) as described by Seagren et al. (21).

Since these reports, numerous others have described their experience primarily with afterloaded ^{192}Ir with or without the concomitant use of Nd:YAG laser therapy. The results of these reports will be the focus of the latter portion of this chapter.

RADIOISOTOPES USED

The most common radioactive source used for endobronchial irradiation is ^{192}Ir. Iridium-192 is a γ-ray emitter. The γ rays primarily interact with water molecules in the surrounding tissues, generating free radicals that damage the DNA of dividing cells, resulting in cell death. Figure 1 shows a typical ^{192}Ir source or "wire" used for low-dose-rate brachytherapy. The wire contains multiple ^{192}Ir sources or "seeds" that are spaced so that there are two seeds per centimeter, fixed in a nylon ribbon. The strength of the ^{192}Ir seeds, measured in millicuries (mCi), can be varied and classified as either low, medium, or high dose rate. The γ energy of ^{192}Ir is 380 keV, which means that for a 10-cm wire that delivers 100% of its dose at a distance of 0.5 cm, only 48% of the dose is present at 1 cm away, and 21% 2 cm away (22). Low-dose-rate brachytherapy is defined as a dose rate of 40–200 cGy (rad) per hour, while high-dose-rate brachytherapy utilizes a dose rate of greater than 1,200 cGy per hour (23,24). Low- and high-dose-rate brachytherapy are most commonly used for endobronchial irradiation, although at least one series has described intermediate-dose-rate brachytherapy (200–1,200 cGy) (25). Typical low-dose-rate endobronchial implants involve a total dose of 1,500–5,000 cGy, typically 3,000 cGy, resulting in a total implant time of 20–30 hr (assuming 100–150 cGy/hr). This requires an inpatient hospitalization. On the other hand, high-dose-rate applications involve 600–1,000 cGy total dose for a total implant time under 1 hr. These applications can be performed on an outpatient basis, although multiple (up to four) high-dose-rate applications are usually administered, typically at weekly intervals, necessitating repeat bronchoscopy. Both low-dose-rate and high-dose-rate applications minimize personnel exposure because the ^{192}Ir wires are afterloaded into hollow plastic tubes that have been previously placed under flexible bronchoscopic guidance into the involved airway. The low-dose-rate applications require manual afterloading, although the personnel exposure from such is minimal (26). Most high-dose-rate applications are remotely afterloaded from outside the treatment room, essentially eliminating personnel exposure. The remote afterloading systems also offer greater flexibility in customizing the dosimetry [or dose distribution around the catheter(s)] of the implant. The cost of remote afterloading equipment is considerable. Both the low-dose-rate and high-dose-rate approaches are well tolerated by the patient. When selecting one of the approaches for clinical use, the technical aspects as well as the efficacy and toxicity of each approach must be considered.

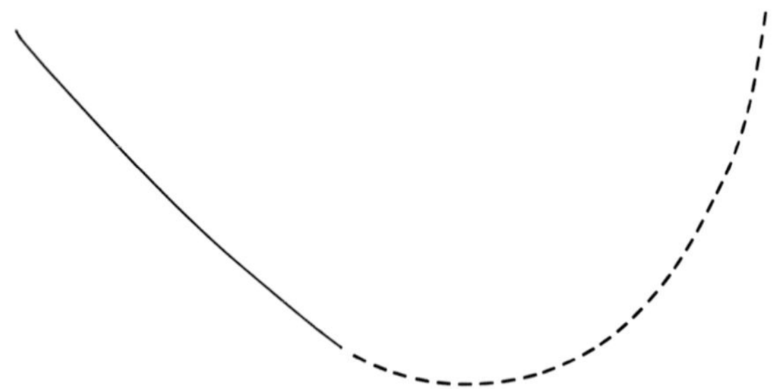

FIG. 1. Typical ^{192}Ir source or "wire" used for low-dose-rate brachytherapy. The wire would be afterloaded into a bronchoscopically placed hollow plastic catheter.

Other sources used for endobronchial irradiation include ^{198}Au and ^{125}I. These sources come in the form of small seeds that can be directly inserted into endobronchial tumors using specialized insertion devices. This approach, called interstitial brachytherapy, is not widely used at the present time for the treatment of endobronchial tumors, other than perhaps in the setting of complete obstruction. Disadvantages of the approach include potential dislodging and displacement of the radioactive seeds, which may migrate distally and lodge in a subpleural location, or may be coughed out into the environment, creating a radiation safety concern. More detailed overviews of this approach can be found elsewhere (27–29).

The majority of patients who undergo endobronchial irradiation will have received prior high-dose fractionated external beam thoracic radiation therapy (TRT). A bronchoscopic diagnosis of recurrent tumor will have been made. The extent of the tumor may be endobronchial alone, endobronchial plus extrinsic (presumable from extraluminal mediastinal or hilar nodal disease), or extrinsic only. If the endobronchial component of tumor is completely or nearly completely obstructing such that an afterloading catheter cannot be placed beyond the obstruction, Nd:YAG laser therapy can be helpful not only to establish a lumen to permit the safe placement of an afterloading catheter, but also to provide immediate relief of symptoms for the patient. When Nd:YAG laser therapy is not possible, as in the setting of significant extrinsic compression, dilation, stent placement, or a short course of fractionated external beam TRT utilizing off-cord oblique fields is warranted. Typically, with additional TRT, an additional 3,000 cGy in 15 fractions is given to treatment fields that encompass the trachea, main stem bronchi, and adjacent mediastinal and ipsilateral hilar lymph nodes. A computed tomography scan of the chest is particularly helpful not only in diagnosing the extent of the extrinsic nodal disease but also for the planning of the radiation fields. When Nd:YAG laser therapy alone is employed prior to brachytherapy, a 1-week interval between the laser therapy and the brachytherapy is employed. When additional fractionated external beam TRT is given, a 1-month break is typically employed to allow maximum tumor shrinkage to facilitate subsequent afterloading catheter placement.

BRONCHOSCOPIC TECHNIQUE

Transnasal flexible bronchoscopy is performed in the usual manner (Fig. 2). The first step in the implant procedure is to determine where the plastic afterloading catheter will be placed within the affected large airways (Fig. 3). The proximal and distal extent of gross tumor involvement should be measured in centimeters and referenced in terms of fixed landmarks that will be readily identifiable to the radiation oncologist on the subsequent treatment planning plain roentgenograph of the chest. The main carina is usually the best landmark. The afterloading catheter should then be threaded into the bronchoscope. The end of the catheter should be placed 3–6 cm beyond the most distal visible extent of gross tumor to minimize the risk of inadvertent coughing out of the catheter by the patient. The bronchoscope is carefully withdrawn and reinserted transorally to ensure the proper seating of the afterloading catheter. The proximal end of the catheter is then taped to the patient's nose.

The radiation treatment planning process then begins with an anteroposterior and sometimes a lateral roentgenograph of the chest. A decision is made as to the length of the radioactive ^{192}Ir wire necessary to encompass the grossly visible tumor plus a 2- to 3-cm margin both proximal and distal to the gross tumor (e.g., an endobronchial segment involved over a 4-cm length would require an 8- to 10-cm active length). Usually, a spacer is necessary in the distal portion of the catheter. The radioactive source is then placed into the afterloading catheter and secured into place by either a clip or a piece of tape. Another plain chest roentgenograph is then taken to ensure proper placement. The patient must be confined to a radiation-protected room during the course of the implant. Once the treatment is completed, the source and the afterloading catheter can be removed in a matter of a few seconds. Although the implant is well tolerated in nearly all cases, narcotic analgesics or cough suppressants may be necessary to maximize patient comfort.

The length of time the implant is to be left in place depends on the dose rate of the ^{192}Ir source and the dose prescription point. For tracheal applications, the dose is typically prescribed to a radius of 1 cm from

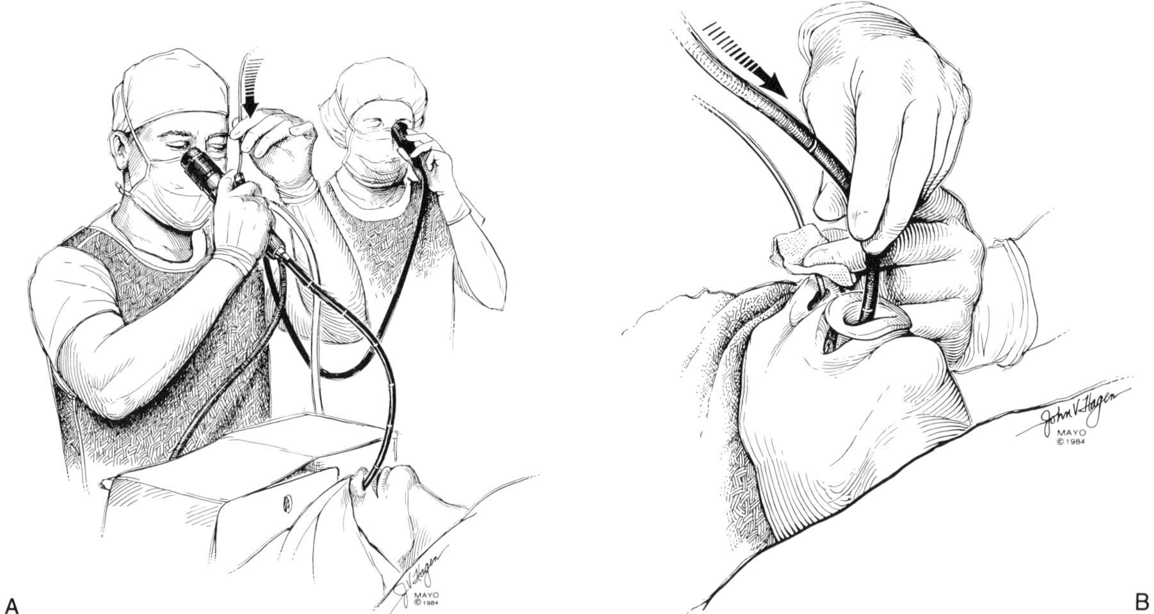

FIG. 2. (A) Under bronchoscopic visualization and control, the blind-end nylon catheter is advanced through the working channel of the flexible bronchoscope to the appropriate position while the radiation oncologist watches the extent of the tumor and the placement of the catheter. **(B)** Following removal of the bronchoscope over the catheter, the bronchoscope is reintroduced orally (or through the other nostril) to confirm and adjust the catheter position. From ref. 18, with permission.

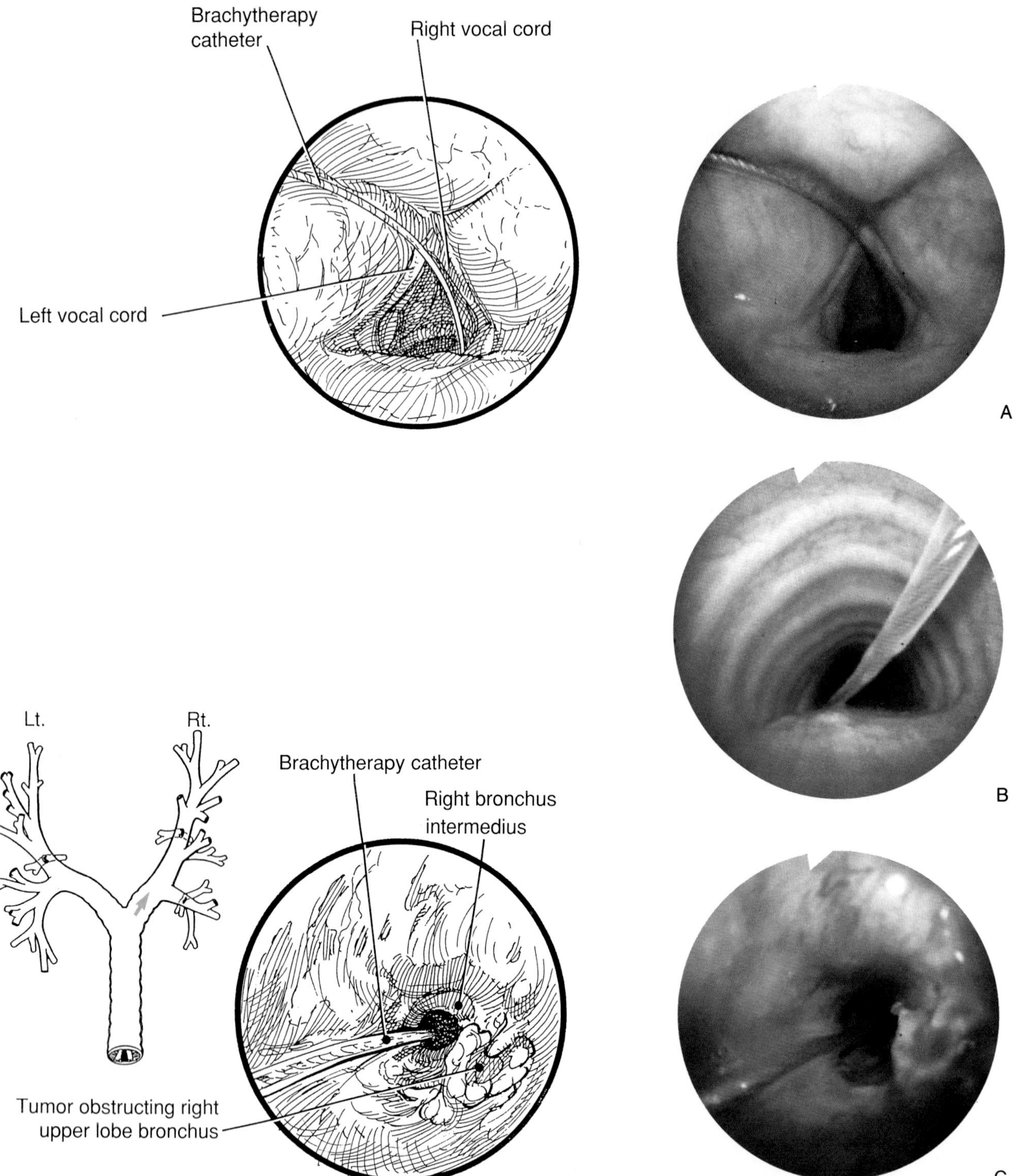

FIG. 3. (A) Brachytherapy catheter traversing the vocal cords after being inserted into tracheobronchial tree via the flexible bronchoscope. **(B)** Catheter in the midtrachea.**(C)** Catheter introduced into right main stem bronchus affected by malignancy.

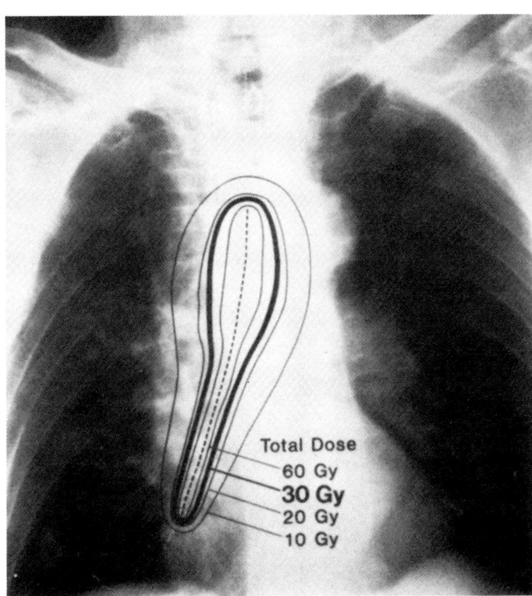

FIG. 4. Dose distribution superimposed over a chest radiograph from a trachea and right main stem bronchus placement delivering 30 Gy (3,000 cGy or rad) to a 0.5- to 1.0-cm radius from the ^{192}Ir wire.

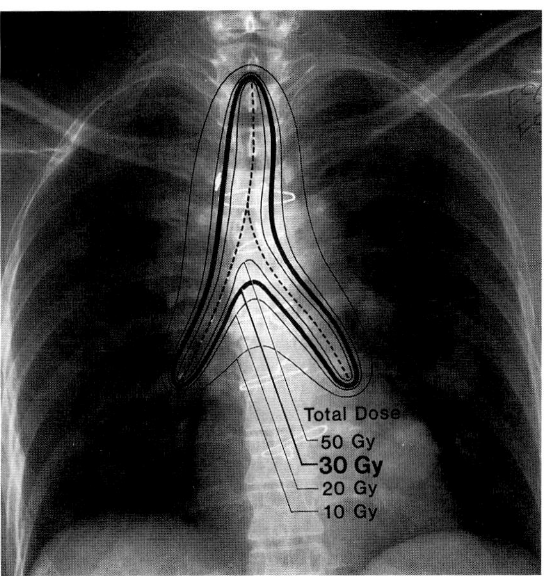

FIG. 5. Dose distribution superimposed over a chest radiograph from a combined trachea and bilateral mainstem bronchi placement delivering 30 Gy (3,000 cGy or rad) to a 0.5- to 1.0-cm radius form the ^{192}Ir wire.

the source (assuming that the catheter will lie in the middle of the trachea, which has a typical diameter of 2 cm). For bronchial placements, dose is usually prescribed to a radius of 0.5 cm. The distribution of radiation dose is cylindrical about the ^{192}Ir wire, with some tapering at the ends. Figure 4 shows a typical single-catheter implant treating endobronchial disease in the trachea and right main stem bronchus. Figure 5 shows another common application involving two catheters, both of which treat the trachea and then each treating one main stem bronchus.

RESULTS

Table 1 summarizes the patient characteristics and technical aspects of 14 series published within the last

TABLE 1. *Patient characteristics and technical aspects of 14 series utilizing afterloaded ^{192}Ir for palliation of malignant airway obstruction*

Series	# Pt / # Imp	Lung CA (%)	Prior EBRT (%)	Concomitant Tx (%) Laser	Concomitant Tx (%) EBRT	Dose rate[a]	# Impl	Total dose (Gy)	Dose Rx radius (cm)
Allen et al. (30)	15/18	100	100	33	20	LDR	1	20–40	0.5–1.5
Schray et al. (31)	65/93	88	91	62	20	LDR	1	30	0.5–1.0
Roach et al. (26)	15/17	100	13	0	33	LDR	1	30	0.5
Lo et al. (34)	77/95	69	87	40	0	LDR	1	25	2.0
Mehta et al. (32,33)	66/70	92	55	18	ns	LDR	1	48	1.0
Paradelo et al. (35)	32/38	100	97	22	56	LDR	1	25	1.0
Speiser and Spratling (25)	45/128	96	44	31	56[b]	IDR	3	30	0.5
Seagren et al. (21)	20/22	90	100	20	0	HDR	1	10	1.0
Macha et al. (36)	106/383	100	ns	54	0	HDR	4	30	1.0
Nori et al. (27)	15/45	100	ns	ns	ns	HDR	4–5	20	1.0
Bedwinek et al. (37)	38/38	100	38	ns	0	HDR	3	18	1.0
Khanavkar et al. (38)	12/66	92	92	42	ns	HDR	5.5	43.6	0.5
Mehta et al. (33)	31/124	77	30	0	ns	HDR	4	32	1.0
Sutedja et al. (39)	31/86	100	100	45	ns	HDR	3	30	1.0

Abbreviations: Pt, patients; Impl, implants; CA, cancer; EBRT, external beam radiation therapy; Tx, treatment; DR, dose rate (L, low; I, intermediate; H, high); Gy, Gray (1 Gy = 100 rad); cm, centimeters; ns, not stated.

[a] Radioactive source was ^{192}Ir in all series except Seagren et al. (21), which used ^{60}Co.

[b] Concomitant EBRT only given to patients who did not have prior EBRT.

TABLE 2. *Results of 14 series described in Table 1*

Series	Median or mean survival (mos)	Improvement (%)		Complication rate (%)[a]	Incidence hemorrhage (%)
		Overall symptoms	Re-bronch		
Allen et al. (30)	ns	100	ns	0	0
Schray et al. (31)	4.0	50–79	60	6	11
Roach et al. (26)	6.5	67	60	7	0
Lo et al. (34)	5.1	59[c]	76	5	3
Mehta et al. (32,33)	5.5	78	73	3	6
Paradelo et al. (35)	6.6	66	85	3	9
Speiser and Spratling (25)	5.8[b]	98	69	2	0
Seagren et al. (21)	9.0	94	100	0	28
Macha et al. (36)	ns	78	75	ns	ns
Nori et al. (27)	ns	80	ns	ns	ns
Bedwinek et al. (37)	ns	76	81	ns	32
Khanavkar et al. (38)	ns	67	ns	42	50
Mehta et al. (33)	4.0	79	ns	0	3
Sutedja et al. (39)	3.0/7.0	58	71	10	32

[a] Complication rate excludes hemorrhages.
[b] Mean survival was 5.8 months for patients treated with palliative intent.
[c] FEV_1 improved from 1.47 to 1.88 L and FVC from 2.21 to 3.09 L in 12 patients with PFTs.
Abbreviations: mos, months; CXR, chest X ray; PFT, pulmonary function tests; Re-bronch, repeat bronchoscopy; ns, not stated in publication.

10 years utilizing afterloaded ^{192}Ir for the palliative treatment of malignant airway obstruction. The majority of patients had lung cancer, and most of them had received prior fractionated external beam radiation therapy. Some patients also received Nd:YAG laser therapy or additional fractionated external beam TRT prior to their endobronchial implant. In six series, low-dose-rate brachytherapy was utilized, always with a single implant and using total doses of 2,000–4,800 cGy to radii of 0.5–2 cm. Intermediate dose rate was used in one series. High dose rate was employed in the other seven, typically involving multiple implants (usually three to five) to deliver total doses of 1,900–4,360 cGy, most commonly at a 1-cm radius. The results of these series are shown in Table 2. Overall improvement in symptoms occurred on average in 75% of patients. Schray et al. (31) found that the response rate depended on the interval between the initial course of fractionated external beam TRT and the brachytherapy procedure used to treat the recurrence. Patients with an interval of greater than a year had an 83% response rate, those with an interval between 6 months and 1 year had a 50% response rate, and only 31% of those treated at an interval of under 6 months responded. Bedwinek et al. (37) found that the extent of the extrabronchial disease affected response rate, with 100% response in patients with less than 5-cm-diameter extrabronchial disease compared to 26% in those with more than 5 cm. He also found the median duration of symptom relief to be 7.5 months. Chest roentgenographs show clearing of obstructive pneumonitis in about one quarter (26,35,40) to two-thirds (32,37) of patients. Improvement in pulmonary function tests have occurred in one quarter to three quarters of patients in whom this information was available (30,36–38). In most of the reported series, repeat bronchoscopy was performed at a fixed time following the endobronchial irradiation, usually 1 month. Response rates based on the bronchoscopic findings are 75% on average (Table 2).

COMPLICATIONS

Major complications, including fistula formation (tracheo- or bronchopleural or esophageal) and abscess formation, have been reported in less than 10% of patients (Table 2). The incidence of massive hemorrhage has been similar in those series utilizing low- or intermediate-dose-rate brachytherapy. Hemorrhage rates have been higher (between 28% and 50%) in four of the high-dose-rate series (21,38,39). It is difficult to necessarily equate hemorrhage with complication, since Seagren et al. noted tumor recurrence in 28% of their patients who had hemorrhage (21).

Both efficacy and nonhemorrhagic complication rates appear comparable among the low-, intermediate-, and high-dose-rate experiences. Similar results between low- and high-dose-rate brachytherapy have been obtained in other disease sites as well (23). Longer term follow-up and additional reports will be necessary to assess the trend of a higher incidence of massive hemorrhage after high-dose-rate endobronchial brachytherapy.

UPDATE OF MAYO CLINIC EXPERIENCE

Between March 1983 and July 1990, 114 adult patients were treated with palliative intent utilizing low-dose-rate brachytherapy. Eighty-two percent of patients were males, and 89% had recurrent lung cancer (most were squamous cell carcinoma). All patients underwent initial bronchoscopy to define the disease extent. Five percent of patients had tracheal disease, 67% bronchial, and 28% tracheobronchial. The bronchoscopic disease extent was further characterized as endobronchial in 77%, extrinsic in 10%, and both endobronchial and extrinsic in 13%. The symptoms included cough in 72% of patients, dyspnea in 82%, and hemoptysis in 45%. Most patients had multiple symptoms. Ninety-three percent of patients had received prior fractionated external beam thoracic radiation therapy with a median dose of 5,900 cGy (range 3,000–11,000 cGy). The median time interval between the completion of prior external beam radiation therapy and the brachytherapy was 8 months. Nd:YAG laser therapy preceded brachytherapy in 68% of patients. An additional course of fractionated external beam radiation therapy was given to 25% of patients (median dose 2,000 cGy).

Eighty-six patients had one catheter placed, 28 had two catheters, and 1 patient had three, for a total of 145 catheter placements, which form the basis of this review. An additional 14 patients, who had a subsequent catheter placed for tumor progression, are not included in the review. The dose rate used was generally 80–150 cGy/hr. All patients were treated with ^{192}Ir. The total dose prescribed for bronchial disease was 3,000 cGy at a 0.5-cm radius and for tracheal disease 3,000 cGy at a 1-cm radius. The active length of the ^{192}Ir wire encompassed the grossly visible tumor plus a 2- to 3-cm margin proximally and distally.

One hundred patients had sufficient follow-up information to document the clinical response of their symptoms. Eighty-five percent of patients had improvement, which was from a combination of Nd:YAG laser therapy and brachytherapy in patients who underwent both and from the brachytherapy alone in patients who were not treated with the laser. Ninety-three percent of patients who underwent Nd:YAG laser therapy prior to the implant had symptomatic improvement compared to only 63% of those who did not. Palliation of symptoms was otherwise independent of whether or not the patient received additional external beam radiation therapy, the time between the initial course of fractionated external beam radiation therapy and the implant, the location of the disease (tracheal vs. bronchial or tracheobronchial), or the bronchoscopic extent of the disease (intrinsic vs. extrinsic vs. both). Repeat bronchoscopy was performed in 56% of patients. Early in the experience, a routine postimplant bronchoscopy was performed regardless of the patient's clinical status. For the majority of patients in the series, however, bronchoscopy was performed for recurrence or worsening of symptoms at a median of 2 months following brachytherapy. Results demonstrated persistent and progressive tumor in 72% of patients, regression or absence of tumor in 17%, necrotic debris in 8%, fistula in 5%, and abscess in 2% (several patients had multiple findings). Patients with necrotic debris symptomatically benefitted from its mechanical removal. Patients with persistent or progressive tumor were noted to have this finding within the implant volume in all but one case.

Ten percent of patients experienced minor complications, including implant in the wrong position, implant pulled out or coughed out by the patient, implant removed because of acute dyspnea, and desquamation of the skin of the anterior neck. Major complications occurred in 11% of patients, and included fistula formation in 7%, bronchial necrosis in 3%, and lung abscess in 2%. Eleven percent of patients experienced massive and ultimately fatal hemorrhages from either progressive tumor or as a complication of treatment (impossible to distinguish in most cases). Hemorrhage was not significantly more common in patients with upper lobe involvement (14%) compared to other sites of involvement (11%).

Median survival for the entire group was 4 months. Only 13% of patients survived more than 1 year. The longest survivor was a patient with recurrent squamous cell carcinoma of the lung who survived 42 months following brachytherapy.

SUMMARY

The majority of patients who undergo endobronchial brachytherapy are those with recurrent non–small cell carcinoma of the lung who have failed prior fractionated external beam thoracic radiation therapy. Its use as an adjunct to primary treatment has yet to be fully defined. Either low- or high-dose-rate brachytherapy may be used, typically with afterloaded ^{192}Ir. There are advantages and disadvantages to both approaches. Efficacy and toxicity appear similar between the two. Eighty percent of patients will have significant palliation of their symptoms. Significant nonhemorrhagic complications occur in 10% or less of patients, but fatal hemorrhage rates of up to 30% have been noted either from tumor progression or as a complication of treatment, with a trend toward more fatal hemorrhages in patients undergoing high-dose-rate brachytherapy. This technique will remain in the armamentarium of the pulmonologist and oncologist for palliative treatment of large-airway obstruction due to recurrent cancers, and possibly for initial therapy as well.

REFERENCES

1. Boring CS, Savires TS, Tong T. Cancer statistics, 1991. *CA* 1991;41:19–36.
2. Holmes EC. Surgical adjuvant chemotherapy in non-small cell lung cancer. *Sem Oncol* 1988;15:255–260.
3. Mountain CF, Hermes KE. Management implications of surgical staging studies. In: Muggia F, Rozensweig M, eds. *Lung cancer: progress in therapeutic research*. New York: Raven Press; 1979: 233–242.
4. Thomas P, Feld R. Preliminary report of a clinical trail comparing post resection adjuvant chemotherapy versus no therapy for T2N1, T2NO non-small cell lung cancer (Abstract). *Lung Cancer* 1988;4(Suppl):A160.
5. Weisenberger T, for the Lung Cancer Study Group. Effects of postoperative mediastinal radiation on completely resected stage II and stage III epidermoid cancer of the lung. *N Engl J Med* 1986;315:1377–1381.
6. Holmes CE, Gail M, for the Lung Cancer Study Group. Surgical adjuvant therapy for stage II and stage III adenocarcinoma and large cell undifferentiated carcinoma. *J Clin Oncol* 1986; 4:710–715.
7. Perez CA. Non-small cell carcinoma of the lung: dose–time parameters. *Cancer Treat Symp* 1985;2:131–142.
8. Yankauer S. Two cases of lung tumor treated bronchoscopically. *NY Med J* 1921;115:741–74.
9. Pool JL. Bronchoscopy in the treatment of lung cancer. *Ann Otol Rhinol Laryngol* 1961;70:1172–1178.
10. Johnston MS, Cleland WP, Howard N. Treatment of carcinoma of the bronchus by interstitial irradiation. *J Thorac Cardiovasc Surg* 1961;42:527–539.
11. Gibbons JR, Baker R. Treatment of carcinoma of the bronchus by interstitial irradiation. *Thorax* 1969;24(4):451–456.
12. Hilaris BS, et al. A new endobronchial implanter. *Clin Bull* 1979; 9(1):21–23.
13. Hilaris BS, Martini, N, Loumanen RK. Endobronchial interstitial implantation. *Clin Bull* 1979;9(1):17–20.
14. Mittal BB, Matuschak G, Culpepper J. Endobronchial interstitial brachytherapy using a bronchofiberscope with a flexible injector system. *Radiology* 1984;152(1):219–20.
15. Moylan D, et al. Transbronchial brachytherapy of recurrent bronchogenic carcinoma: a new approach using the flexible fiberoptic bronchoscope. *Radiology* 1983;147:253–254.
16. Percarpio B, Price JC, Murphy P. Endotracheal irradiation of adenoid cystic carcinoma of the trachea. *Radiology* 1978; 128:209–210.
17. Mendiondo OA, Dillon M, Beach JL. Endobronchial irradiation in the treatment of recurrent non–oat cell bronchogenic carcinoma. *J Ky Med Assoc* 1983;81(5):287–290.
18. Schray MF, et al. Management of malignant airway obstruction: clinical and dosimetric considerations using an iridium-192 afterloading technique in conjunction with the neodymium-YAG laser. *Int J Radiation Oncol Biol Phys* 1985;11:403–409.
19. Schray MF, et al. Malignant airway obstruction: management with temporary intraluminal brachytherapy and laser treatment. *Endocuriether Hypertherm Oncol* 1985;1:237–245.
20. Boedker A, Hald A, Kristensen D. A method for selective endobronchial and endotracheal irradiation. *J Thorac Cardiovasc Surg* 1982;84:59–61.
21. Seagren SL, Harrell JH, Horn RA. High dose rate intraluminal irradiation in recurrent endobronchial carcinoma. *Chest* 1985; 88:810–814.
22. Kline RW, Gillin MT, Grimm DF, Niroomand-Rad A. Computer dosimetry of the ^{192}Ir wire. *Med Phys* 1985;12:634–638.
23. Foo KF, Phillips TL. High dose rate versus low dose rate intracavitary brachytherapy for carcinoma of the cervix. *Int J Radiat Oncol Biol Phys* 1990;19:791–796.
24. Speiser B. Advantages of high dose rate remote afterloading systems: physics or biology. *Int J Radiat Oncol Biol Phys* 1991; 20:1133–1135.
25. Speiser B. Spratling L. Intermediate dose rate remote aferloading brachytherapy for intraluminal control of bronchogenic carcinoma. *Int J Radiat Oncol Biol Phys* 1990;18:1443–1448.
26. Roach M, Leidholdt EM, Talera BS, et al. Endobronchial radiation therapy (EBRT) in the management of lung cancer. *Int J Radiat Oncol Biol Phys* 1990;18:1449–1454.
27. Nori D, Hilaris BS, Martini N. Intraluminal irradiation in bronchogenic carcinoma. *Surg Clin North Am* 1987;67(5):1093–1102.
28. Law MR, et al. Bronchoscopic implantation of radioactive gold grains into endobronchial carcinomas. *Br J Dis Chest* 1985; 79(2):147–151.
29. Rabie T, et al. Palliation of bronchogenic carcinoma with ^{198}Au implantation using the fiberoptic bronchoscope. *Chest* 1986; 90(5):641–645.
30. Allen MD, Baldwin JC, Fish VT, et al. Combined laser therapy with endobronchial radiotherapy for unresectable lung carcinoma with bronchial obstruction. *Am J Surg* 1985;150:71–77.
31. Schray MF, et al. Management of malignant airway compromise with laser and low dose rate brachytherapy. *Chest* 1988; 93(2):264–269.
32. Mehta MP, et al. Endobronchial irradiation for malignant airway obstruction. *Int J Radiat Oncol Biol Phys* 1989;17(4):847–851.
33. Mehta MP, et al. Sequential comparison of low dose rate and hyperfractionated high dose rate endobronchial radiation for malignant airway occlusion. *Int J Radiat Oncol Biol Phys* 1992; 23:133–139.
34. Lo TCM, et al. Intraluminal low dose rate brachytherapy for malignant endobronchial obstruction. *Radiother Oncol* 1992; 23:16–20.
35. Paradelo JC, et al. Endobronchial irradiation with ^{192}Ir in the treatment of malignant endobronchial obstruction. *Chest* 1992; 102:1072–1074.
36. Macha HN, et al. Neue Wege der Strahlentherapie des Bronchialkarzinoms. *Dtsch Med Wochenschr* 1986;111(18):687–691.
37. Bedwinek J, Petty A, Bruton C, Sofield J, Lee L. High dose rate endobronchial brachytherapy and fatal pulmonary hemorrhage. *Int J Radiat Oncol Biol Phys* 1990;19(Suppl 1):161.
38. Khanavkar B, et al. Complications associated with brachytherapy alone or with laser in lung cancer. *Chest* 1991;99:1062–1065.
39. Sutedja G, et al. High dose rate brachytherapy in patients with local recurrences after radiotherapy of non-small cell lung cancer. *Int J Radiat Oncol Biol Phys* 1992;24:551–553.
40. Chetty KG, et al. Effect of radiation therapy on bronchial obstruction due to bronchogenic carcinoma. *Chest* 1989; 95(3):582–584.

Bronchoscopy,
edited by U. B. S. Prakash.
Mayo Foundation © 1994.
Published by Raven Press, Ltd., New York.

CHAPTER 21

Tracheobronchial Prostheses

Eric S. Edell, Henri G. Colt, and Jean-François Dumon

Obstruction of the trachea or main stem bronchi results from various causes and presents perplexing therapeutic problems to bronchoscopists. The most common lesion is malignant airway obstruction either by endobronchial tumor or by extrinsic compression from tumor or mediastinal lymph nodes. Benign stenoses can result from various inflammatory processes including injury from tracheal intubation of crushing injuries of the neck. New surgical techniques such as cryosurgery and laser therapy may severely injure the airway mucosa and lead to tracheal or bronchial narrowing. Whether from a malignant or a benign process, obstruction of major airways cause progressive dyspnea and eventual hypoxemia if not treated.

The bronchoscopist must select a method of treatment that is appropriate for the lesion encountered. Surgical removal of the narrowed lesions followed by reconstruction is the treatment of choice, but unfortunately, patients with malignant airway obstruction have often exhausted such therapeutic options. Others have severe underlying cardiopulmonary dysfunction or lesions that are too advanced to allow surgical resection. Laser photoresection is useful in those patients who present with malignant endobronchial obstructing lesions. Unfortunately, there is a large population of patients who have extrinsic narrowing or localized tracheomalacia or bronchomalacia. Other bronchoscopic methods including dilatation of narrowed regions by rigid bronchoscopy or balloon dilatation may be useful but provide only temporary palliation. Tracheal and endobronchial prostheses have gained increasing acceptance as an additional means for establishing and maintaining patent airways. Prosthetic devices have been used in the management of both malignant and benign disorders of the tracheobronchial tree.

The role of the bronchoscope in the diagnosis and treatment of tracheobronchial obstructions caused by both benign and malignant lesions is discussed in this chapter. The application of various types of lasers for relief of tracheobronchial obstruction is addressed in Chapter 19. Discussions on the balloon dilatation are also included in Chapter 16, this volume.

ETIOLOGY OF TRACHEOBRONCHIAL OBSTRUCTION

Primary malignancies of the trachea are relatively rare. Squamous cell carcinoma and adenocystic carcinoma (cylindroma) comprise over two thirds of all primary tumors of the trachea (1). Both may present as well-localized lesions and, if so, are best managed by surgical resection. Unfortunately, one third of the patients examined by Grillo had mediastinal or pulmonary metastasis at the time of initial diagnosis (2). Adenocystic carcinoma tends to infiltrate the airway submucosally and is therefore often not amenable to surgical resection. Flexible bronchoscopy is essential in determining whether surgical resection is a viable option.

The majority of patients present with main stem lesions or recurrent carcinoma from previously resected tumors. Extrinsic compression is a frequent cause of airway narrowing. Most patients have received maximum doses of external beam radiation and have few therapeutic alternatives remaining. Narrowing of the trachea and main stem bronchi can also occur from various inflammatory processes. Postinfectious obstruction of the trachea is quite rare but has been reported as a complication of tuberculous infection,

E. S. Edell: Division of Thoracic Diseases and Internal Medicine, Mayo Clinic, Rochester, Minnesota 55905.
H. G. Colt: Department of Medicine, Pulmonary Division, University of California at San Diego, San Diego, California 92103.
J.-F. Dumon: Laser Bronchoscopy Center, University of Marseille, Marseille, France.

diphtheria, syphilis, or typhoid fever. Fibrosing mediastinitis may also involve the trachea and main stem bronchi. Other inflammatory processes such as Wegener's granulomatosis or relapsing polychondritis can cause stenoses or areas of tracheomalacia resulting in major airway obstruction (3). Penetrating injuries to the trachea as well as blunt trauma to the thorax may result in lesions that subsequently become stenotic (4).

The most common cause of benign narrowing of the trachea is likely related to injury from an endotracheal tube (5). Originally, these injuries were a function of the cuff rather than the endotracheal tube itself. The introduction of the low-compliance, high-volume cuff resulted in a decrease in these iatrogenic tracheal lesions. The endotracheal tube may produce various lesions related primarily to pressure necrosis. Injury of the posterior commissure with subsequent fusion, or mucosal erosion at the level of the cricoid may result from pressure of the endotracheal tube. The nares may be eroded. The vocal cords may become irritated and granulomas may form. Most laryngeal lesions are reversible with time, but subglottic granulation tissue may require removal.

The most serious complication of endotracheal tubes or tracheostomy tubes results from the increased pressure of the sealing cuff. Many etiological factors have been invoked including hypotension, bacterial infection, and toxicity from materials used in the tubes. Andrews and Pearson showed that the single most common denominator (both clinically and experimentally) was due to direct-pressure necrosis by high-pressure cuffs (6). If tissue is injured to a certain depth, cicatrization produces circumferential stenosis (Fig. 1). If full-thickness injury results, a tracheoesophageal fistula or trachea-innominate artery fistula may occur. Tracheomalacia is another consequence of injury from intubation. The inflammatory changes lead to thinning of the cartilage without mucosal ulceration. Softening of the segment results in a functional type of obstruction with tracheal collapse on forced expiration.

Patients with either malignant or benign obstructing lesions present primarily with symptoms of increasing dyspnea, wheezing, and cough. Often patients complain of worsening dyspnea in the supine position. It is not unusual for patients to have received several courses of corticosteroid or β agonist for a presumed diagnosis of asthma. One should be concerned about a patient who develops symptoms of airway obstruction that has either undergone general anesthesia or has had prolonged mechanical ventilation. Pulmonary function tests are very helpful in patients with symptoms of worsening dyspnea and presumed major airway obstruction. Clues to diagnosis include disproportionate decreases in the maximum voluntary ventilation and forced expiratory volume in 1 sec. Additionally, the flow volume loop has been shown to be diagnostic of either intra- or extrathoracic major airway obstruction (7). The flow volume loop is less helpful in those patients who present with either left or right main stem bronchial obstruction. The chest roentgenogram is often normal in patients with major airway obstruction (8). Tomography, however, is quite useful in determining the extent of disease of either trachea or main stem bronchi. In patients with suspected areas of tracheomalacia or bronchomalacia, cine-computerized tomography has been very helpful in determining the presence and extent of abnormalities (9).

Flexible bronchoscopy remains the main tool for evaluating the presence of major airway obstruction. It provides direct visualization of the area of involvement as well as the opportunity to obtain pathological specimens for diagnosis.

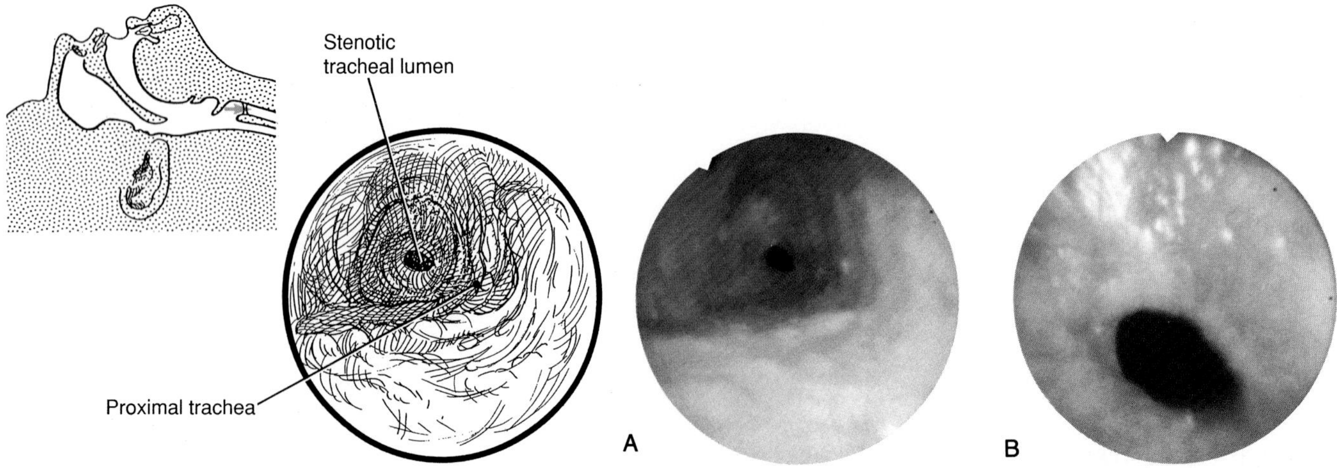

FIG. 1. (A) Cicatricial benign upper tracheal stenosis from previous endotracheal intubation. **(B)** Close-up view of the stricture.

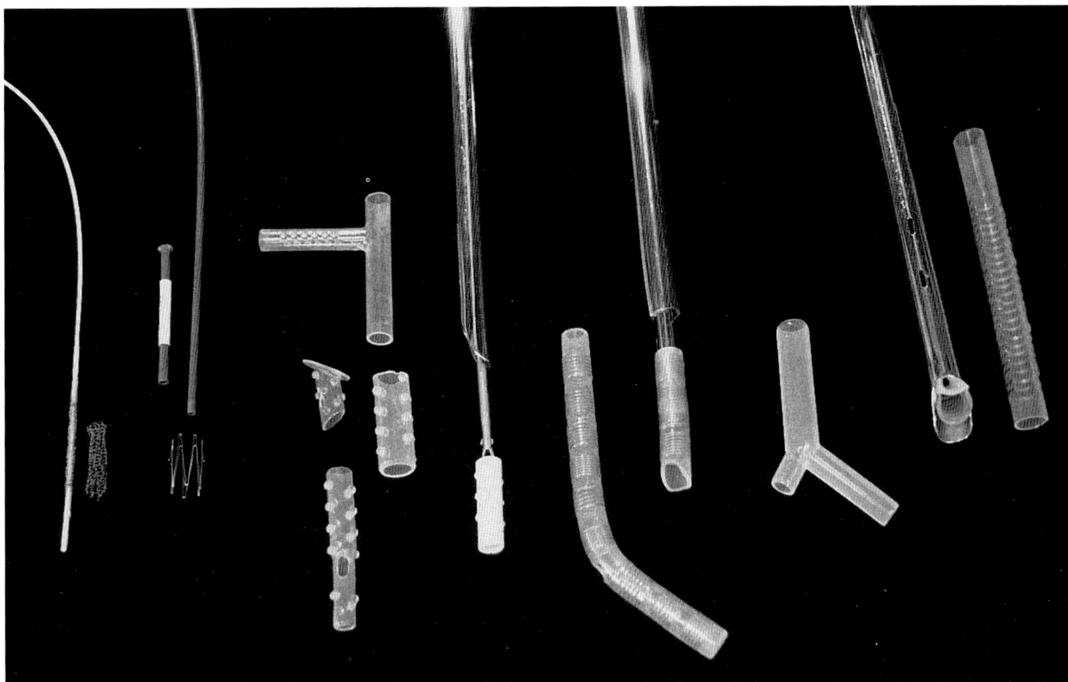

FIG. 2. Various tracheobronchial prostheses currently used. Figure courtesy of Lutz Freitag, M.D.

MANAGEMENT

Patients with obstructing lesions of the trachea or main stem bronchi are best managed by surgical resection. Unfortunately, this is not feasible in a significant number of patients. Neodymium–YAG (Nd:YAG) laser resection is effective in the treatment of patients with malignant endobronchial obstruction, simple stoma granulomas, or thin web-like stenoses (10–13). A growing number of patients presenting with obstruction of the major airway are not amenable to surgical or endobronchial laser resection. This includes patients with malignant extrinsic compression, stenosis from tracheal intubation or another inflammatory process, and patients with areas of tracheobronchomalacia. An alternative for this group of patients may be a tracheobronchial stent.

Several types of tracheobronchial prostheses are currently available and include products of expandable metal wire, molded silicone, or combinations of both (Fig. 2) (14–18). The use of endobronchial prosthesis for lesions of major airways is not new. Unfortunately, the materials and techniques for insertion have previously been unsatisfactory. During the past several years, advances have been made that resulted in the development of products that are easier to insert and more tolerable to the patient.

William Montgomery designed a silicone rubber T tube in 1965 (19), which has been widely used as an adjunct for management of subglottic and tracheal stenosis (Fig. 3) (20,21). This prosthesis requires permanent maintenance of a tracheotomy orifice (Fig. 4). Several operators have modified the Montgomery tube by removing the external side-limb, thereby eliminating the need for a tracheotomy orifice. Westaby designed a straight silicone stent with a Y-shaped distal

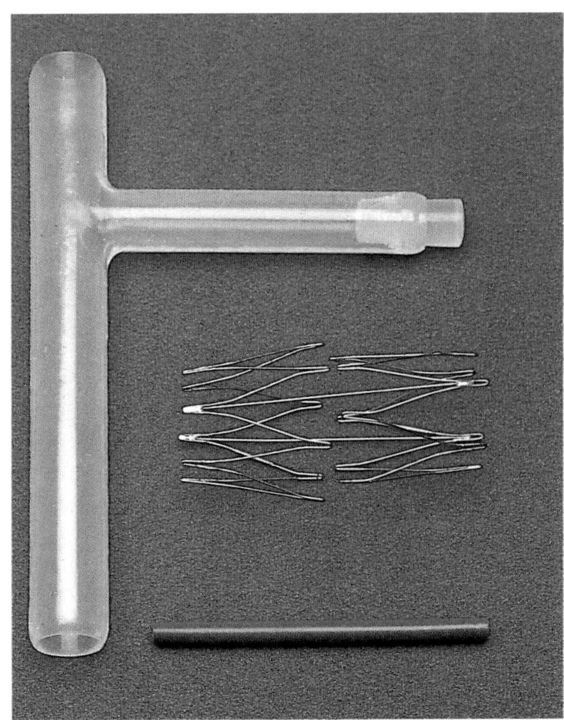

FIG. 3. Montgomery silicone T tube and Gianturco Z stent with plastic loading sleeve.

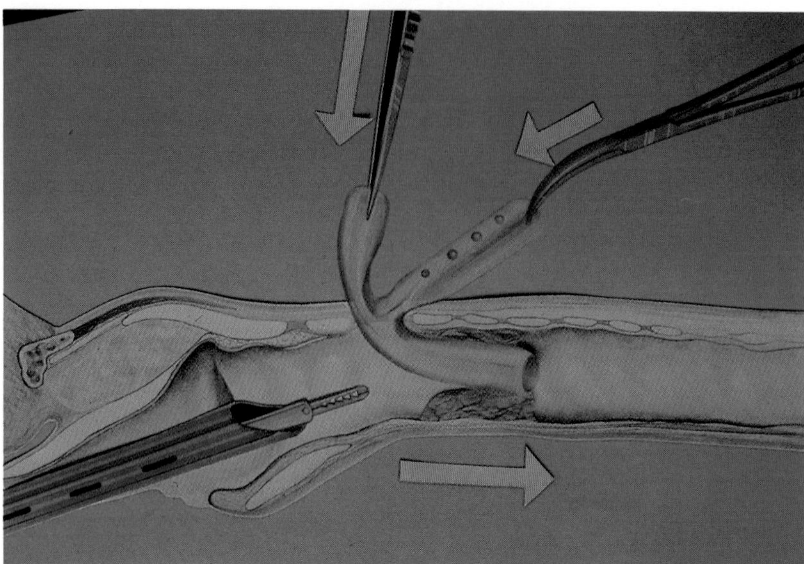

FIG. 4. Insertion of a Montgomery T tube through a tracheostomy. Placement is facilitated with the aid of forceps and a rigid bronchoscope.

A

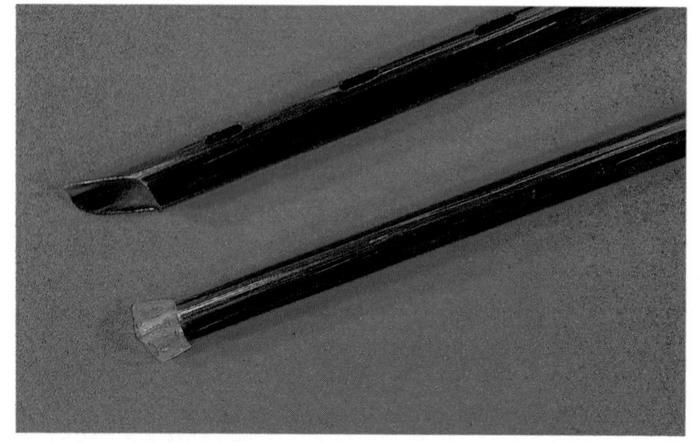

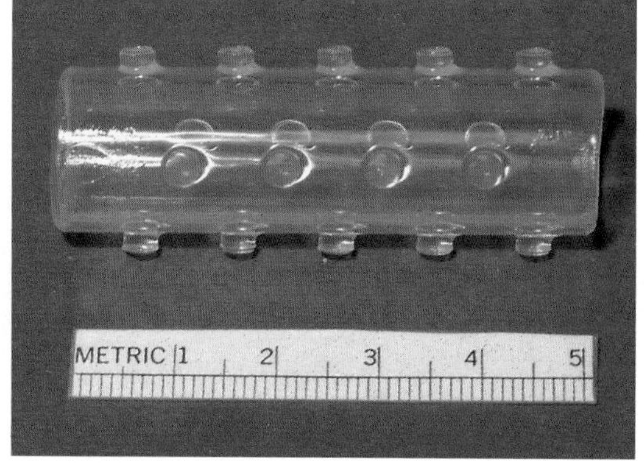

B

FIG. 5. **(A)** Dumon prosthesis with rigid bronchoscope and introducer system. **(B)** Close-up view of the stent shows plastic nipples to hold to tracheobronchial wall.

A

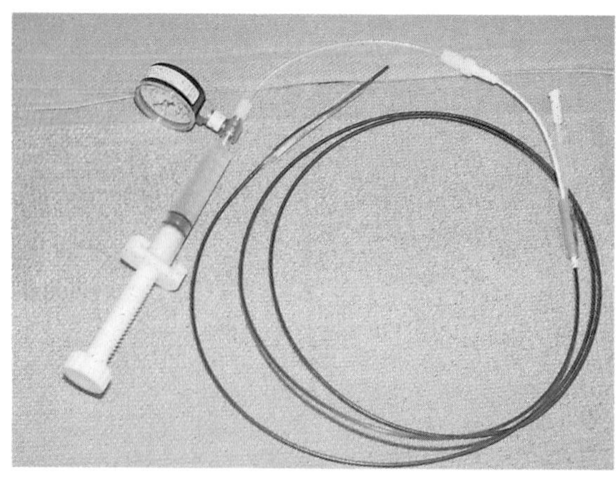

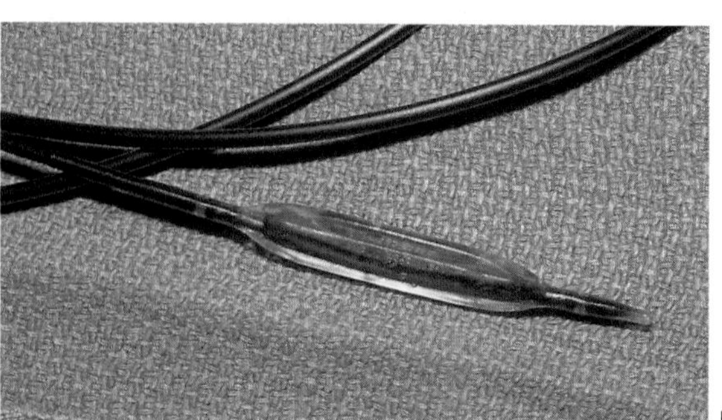

B

FIG. 6. **(A)** Esophageal balloon dilator with manometer. **(B)** Close-up of the distal end of deflated balloon.

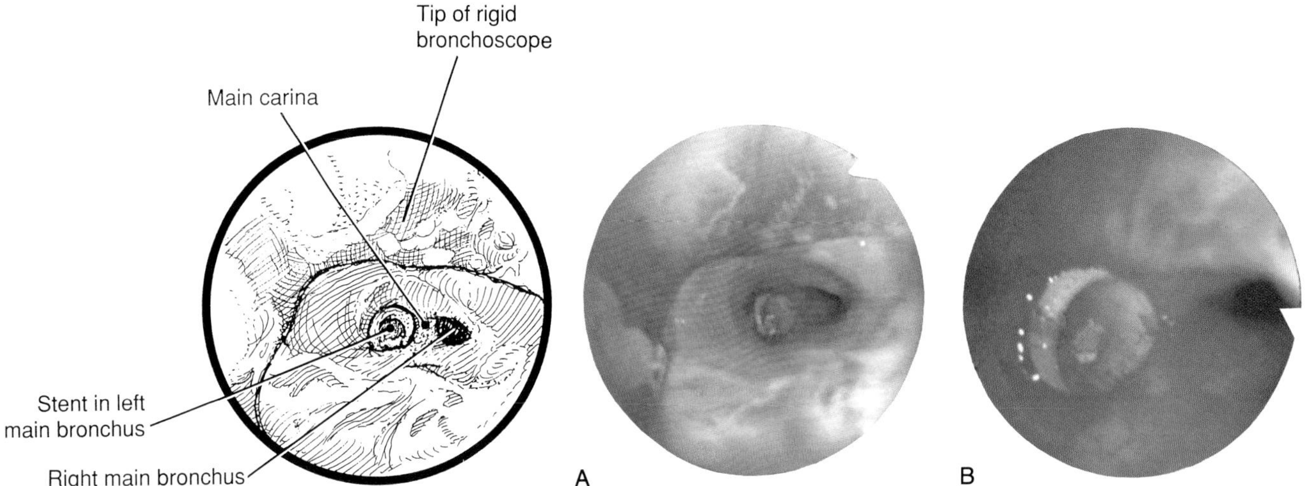

FIG. 7. (A) View of distal trachea and main stem bronchi as well as the tip of rigid bronchoscope. **(B)** Close-up view of main stem bronchi showing stent in proximal left main stem bronchus.

segment to intubate both left and right main bronchi at the level of the carina (22). Neville et al. (23) incorporated Dacron. Dumon experimented with modified Montgomery T tubes in the 1980's, using both long and short prostheses, and main bronchial stents with sideholes to ventilate the upper lobes. Results, however, were often unsatisfactory. Trimmed stents tended to provoke excessive growth of inflammatory tissue around the cut ends of the prosthetic tubes. Migration was also an occasional problem, and stents with sideholes tended to rotate, obstructing the otherwise patent upper lobe bronchial orifice. Insertion was also problematic because stents were placed onto the tip of a small-diameter rigid bronchoscope, patients were intubated, and a tube of larger diameter was used to push the stent into place. Using this technique, stents of maximal size could not always be inserted, and use of larger stents risked injury to the larynx and vocal cords during intubation.

In 1990, results were published of Dumon's use of a straight silicone stent with studs on its external surface to prevent migration (24). Several predetermined diameters and lengths of these stents are available, and a specially designed Stent Introducer System was manufactured (Fig. 5). Using this syringe-plunger system, stents are loaded into, then pushed into place through, rather than over, the rigid bronchoscopes. Luminal diameter can be maximized by either laser resection or, in some cases, balloon dilatation (Fig. 6) (25). There are several devices available to assist dilatation of the trachea or bronchus. These include bougie, rigid bronchoscopes, and various balloon dilators (Fig. 6). Whatever the technique, one must be careful not to rupture the tracheal or bronchial wall. After dilatation, the placement and positioning of the airway prosthesis becomes much easier for the bronchoscopist. Stents can be placed in different sites in the trachea or bronchial tree (Figs. 7–12). Further, a patient may require place-

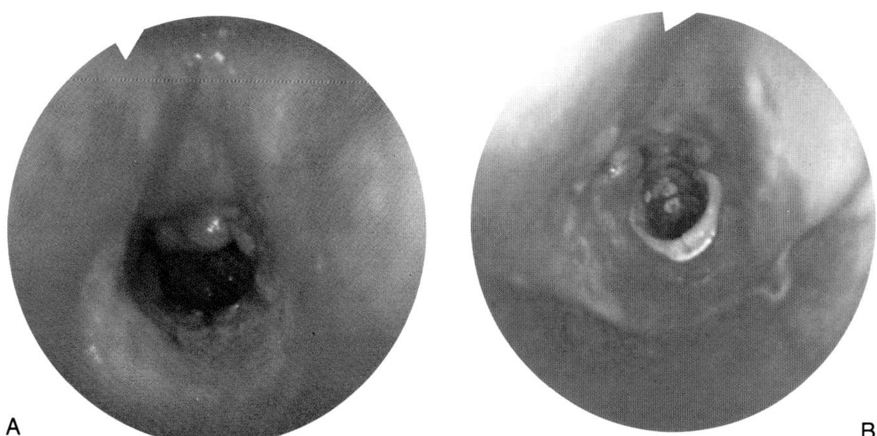

FIG. 8. (A) Subglottic tracheal obstruction caused by squamous cell carcinoma. **(B)** Stent in the upper trachea.

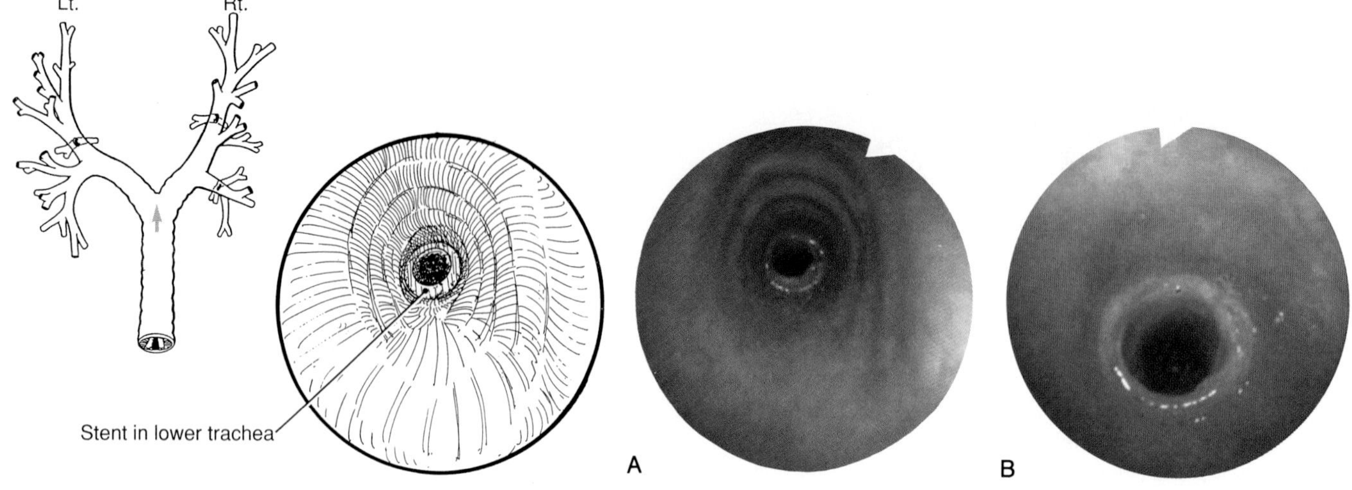

FIG. 9. (A) A well-placed stent in the midtrachea. **(B)** Close-up view of the proximal end of the stent.

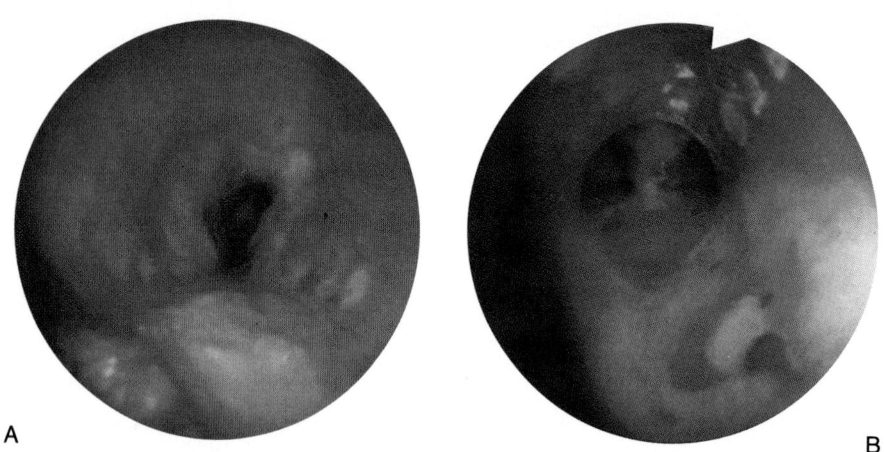

FIG. 10. (A) Stricture of distal trachea caused by Wegener's granulomatosis. **(B)** View through the distal end of the tracheal stent.

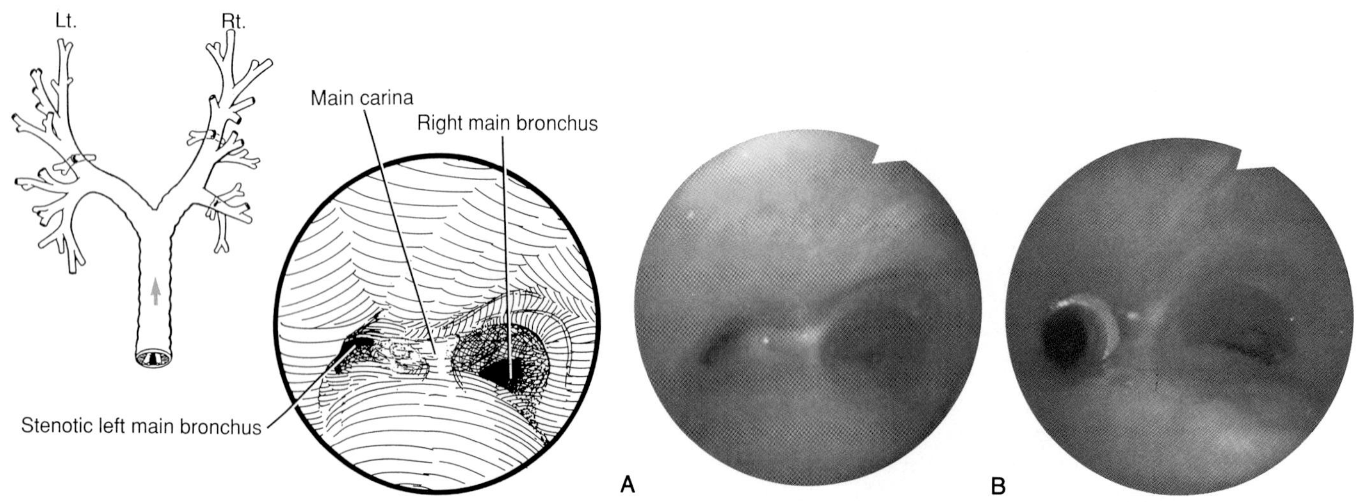

FIG. 11. (A) Benign stricture of left main stem bronchus. **(B)** Well-placed left main stem bronchial stent.

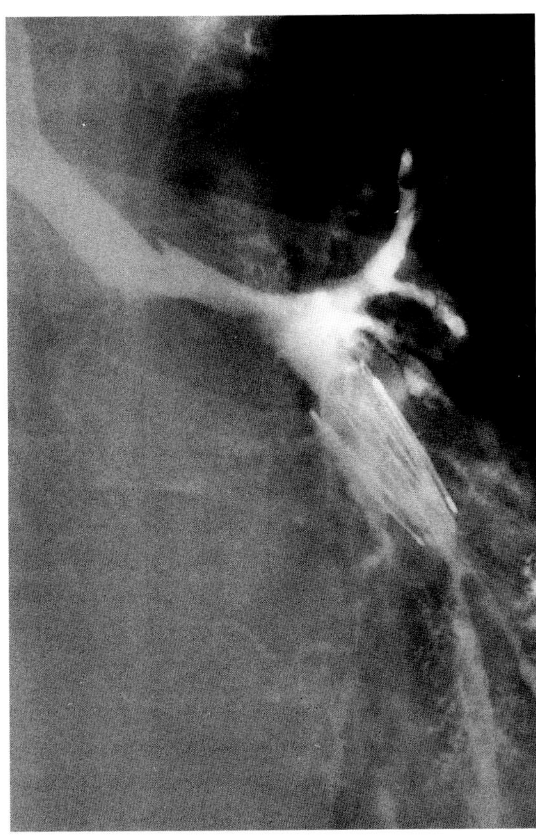

FIG. 12. Gianturco Z stent in left lower lobe bronchus (see Fig. 3); bronchographic medium shows patency of distal bronchi. Figure courtesy of Lutz Freitag, M.D.

ment of multiple stents for treatment of strictures at more than one site in the tracheobronchial tree (Fig. 13). Results have been promising, although some complications may occur (26). These are more frequent in benign disease than in malignant stenosis due to intraluminal tumor and extrinsic compression. Migration occurs most frequently when stents are inserted for palliation of tracheomalacia, but it should also be expected in patients with malignant disease undergoing radiation or effective tumor shrinking chemotherapy (Fig. 14). Obstruction by dried secretions can usually be avoided if patients adhere to large-drop aerosol treatments (Fig. 15). However, randomized studies of the efficacy of such aerosol treatments are lacking. Granulomas occur occasionally and are easily removed by Nd:YAG laser therapy. An understanding of factors affecting granuloma formation as well as why certain patients develop inflammatory tissue when others do not requires further study.

Many other types of stents are also used (Fig. 2). Modified tracheotomy cannulas, silicone-coated stainless steel wire springs, steel wire coil, and modified steel Souttar tubes previously used for esophageal stenosis have all been successfully employed (27–30). Stainless steel stents originally designed for intravascular use have been employed as well. The Gianturco Z stent (Figs. 3 and 16) (31,32) and, more recently, the Schneider prosthesis (previously known as the Wallstent) are frequently inserted (33). These stents can be placed through a flexible catheter under fluoroscopic guidance, but many experts prefer placement under direct visual control. Once inserted, metal stents are often impossible to remove. Also, granulomas may occur through wire struts occluding the airway lumen (34). Indications for metal stents should therefore be limited to patients with malignant airway disease and short expected survival.

Silicone stents are easily removed and are also the most popular. These include studded Dumon stents, cuffed Hood stents, and custom-made silicone prostheses. More recently, Freitag (personal communication) developed a stent with metallic ribs (to resemble tracheal cartilages) and a collapsible posterior wall to mimic normal tracheobronchial dynamics during respiratory movements (Fig. 17). Although malignancy remains the most frequent indication for placement (Fig. 18), stents are used to palliate benign stenosis from iatrogenic causes, connective tissue disorders, tuberculosis, amyloidosis, Wegener's granulomatosis, and, less successfully, tracheomalacia and bronchomalacia. Several reports of successful management of stenosis at the level of airway anastomoses after lung transplantation have been published (34–36).

Physicians working with patients who have stents must be aware of potential problems and of the need for careful, frequent clinical, radiographic, and bron-

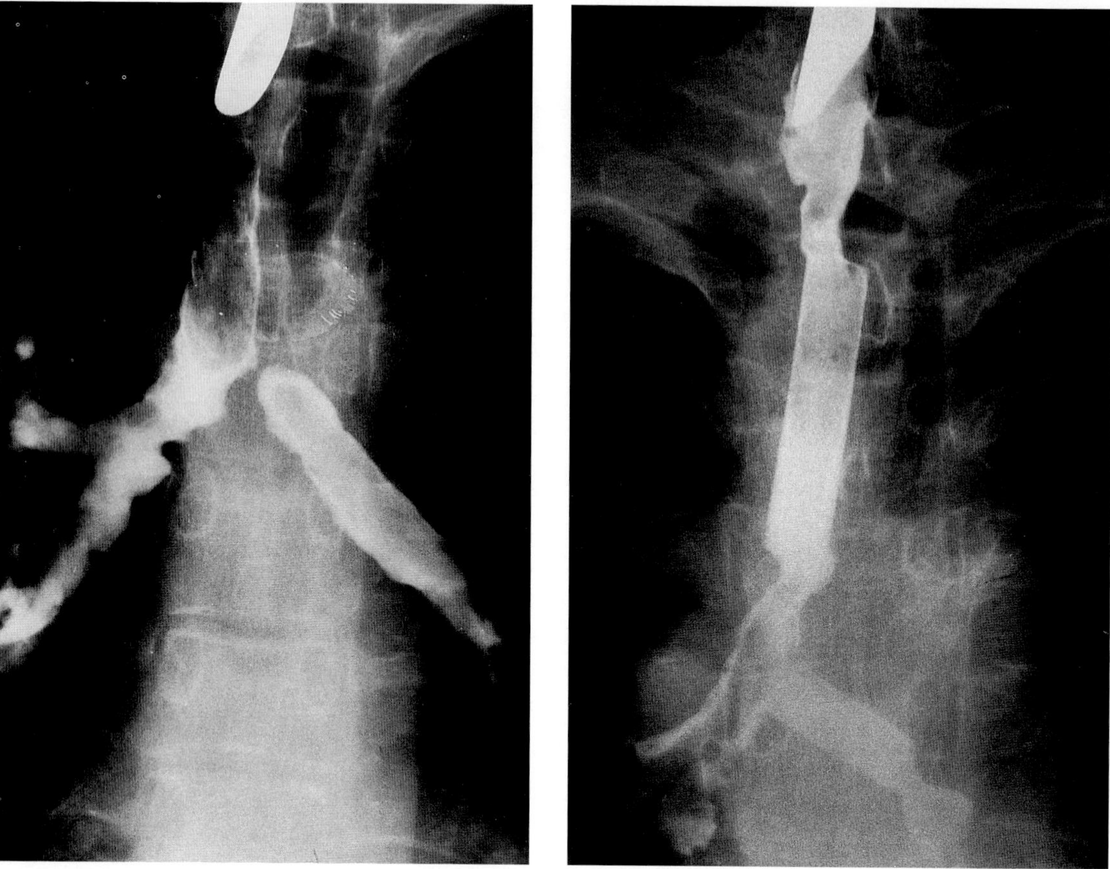

FIG. 13. Bronchography shows stricture of lower trachea and proximal left main stem bronchus **(left)**; stents in lower trachea and left main stem bronchus **(right)**. Figure courtesy of Lutz Freitag, M.D.

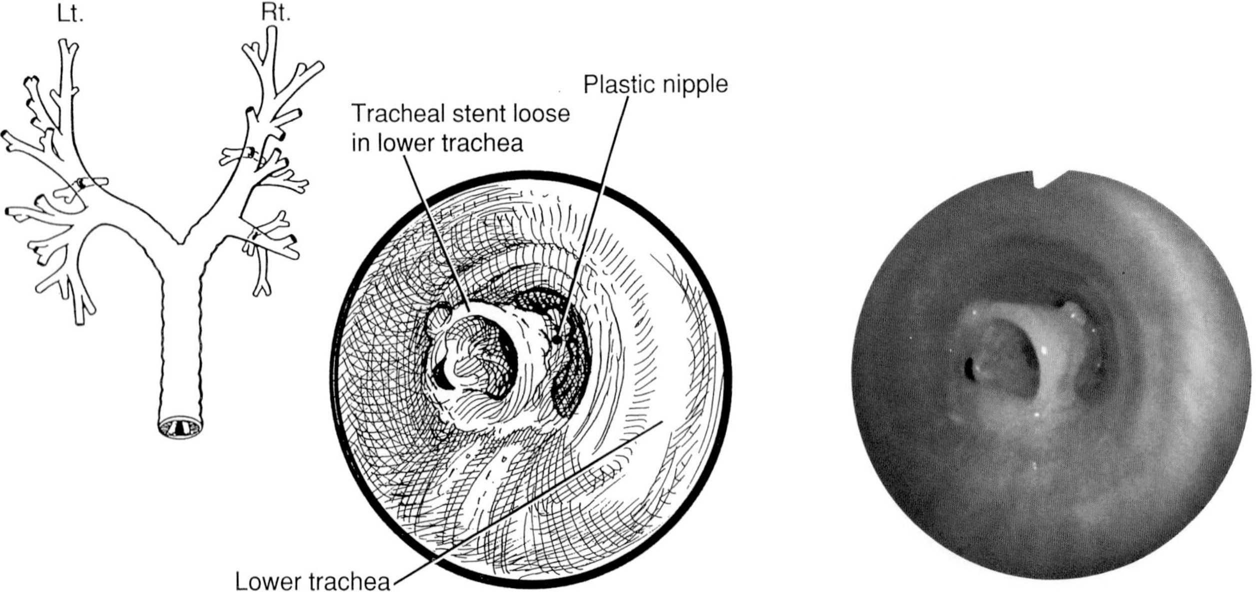

FIG. 14. Dislodged (from proximal trachea) tracheal stent located in distal trachea. Patient was completely asymptomatic.

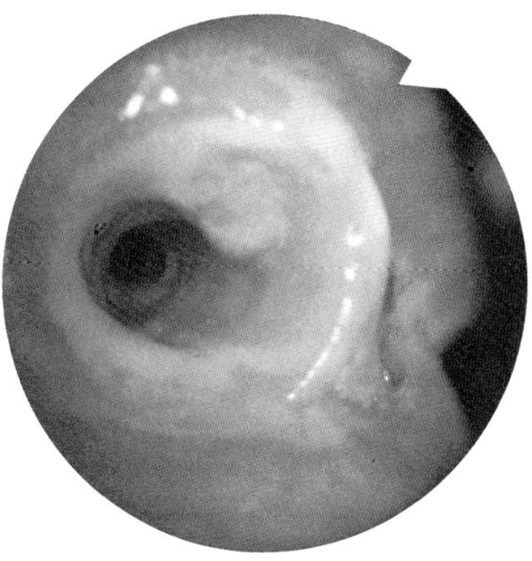

FIG. 15. Retained secretions in left main stem prosthesis. These are easily removed by flexible bronchoscopy.

choscopic follow-up examinations. Any patient with increased or new-onset cough, sputum production, or dyspnea should be suspected of having a stent-related complication. If a patient with an indwelling tracheal stent requires endotracheal intubation, only smaller (below 8 mm) diameter endotracheal tubes should be used, and bronchoscopy should always be performed immediately after intubation, and shortly following extubation.

Airway stent insertion has rapidly become an important procedure, often complementary to laser resection. Knowledge and extensive experience with both of these procedures is necessary for the bronchoscopist. Many as yet unanswered questions remain. What is the optimal duration for stents to be left in place? How does one decide to remove a stent, and on what clinical and subjective criteria should this decision be based? Which patients with benign disease should be offered airway stents, and for how long, prior to considering open surgical repair? Further refined indications, newer materials, and improvements on already available prostheses should make complications even less

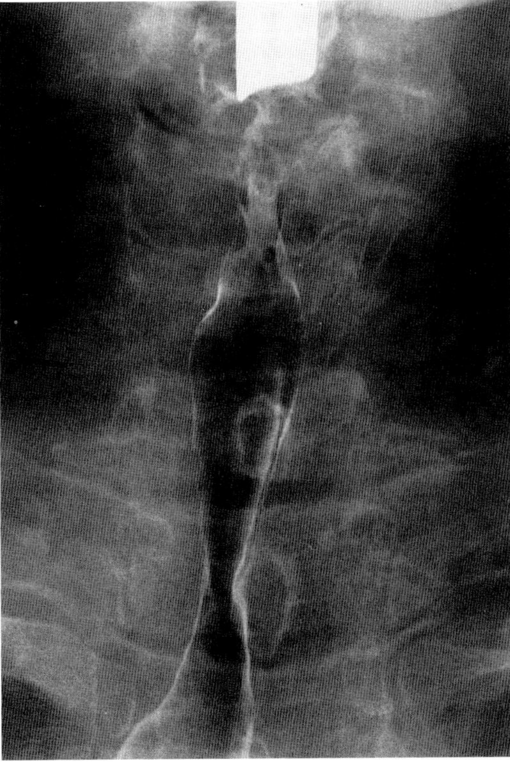

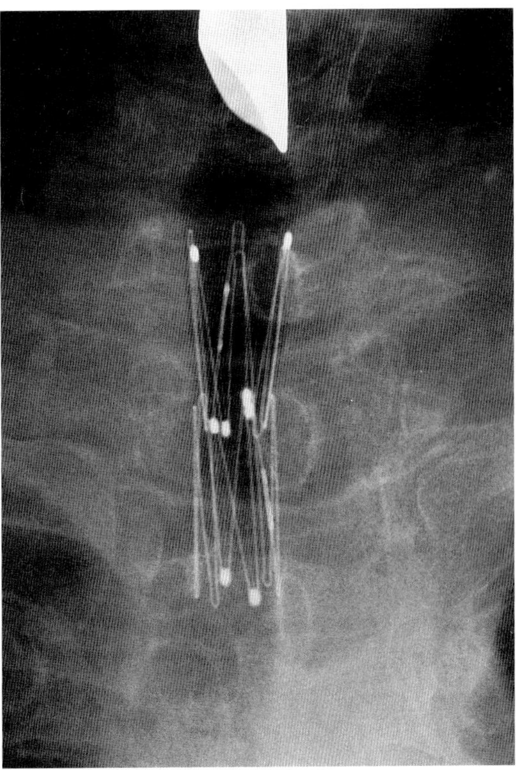

FIG. 16. Bronchography showing stricture of upper trachea **(left)** and Gianturco Z stent in place **(right)**. Figure courtesy of Lutz Freitag, M.D.

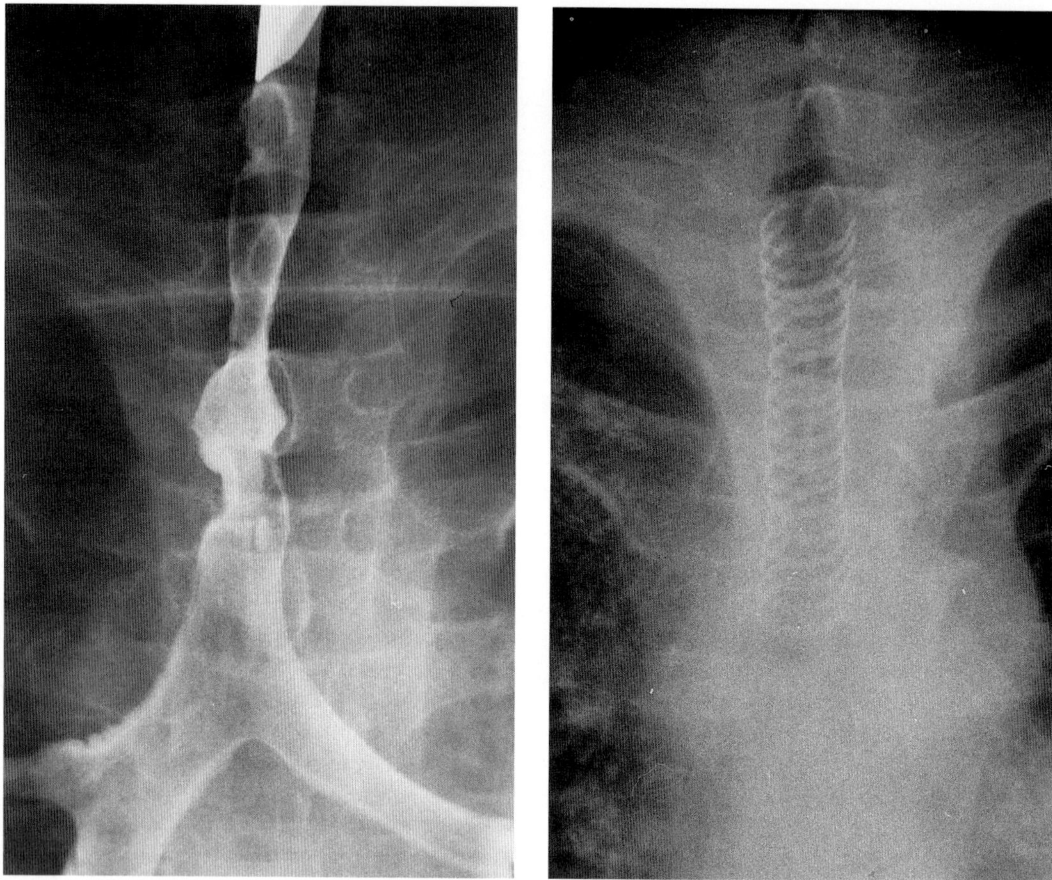

FIG. 17. Bronchographic depiction of upper tracheal stricture **(left)**, and Freitag stent in place **(right)**. Horseshoe-shaped metallic rings are designed to mimic normal physiological motion of tracheal cartilages. Figure courtesy of Lutz Freitag, M.D.

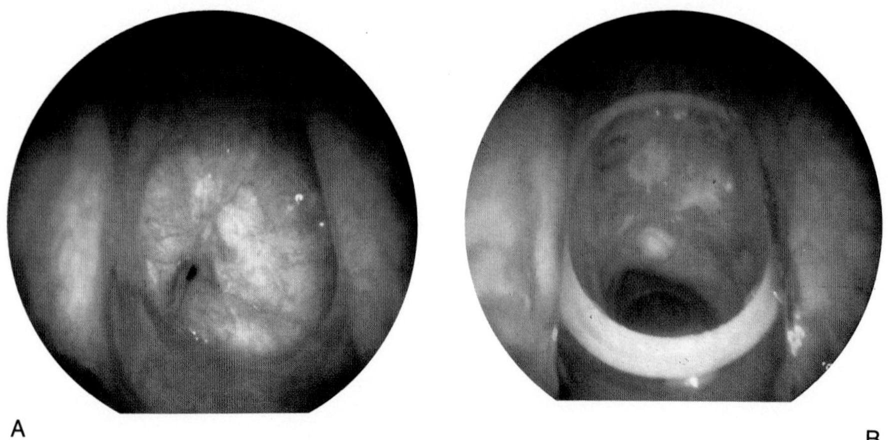

FIG. 18. (A) Severe subglottic narrowing by extrinsic compression in a patient with small cell cancer. **(B)** After placement of a Dumon silicone stent.

frequent, but bronchoscopists must continue to investigate any and all methods that may provide satisfactory palliation and cure of tracheobronchial obstruction.

REFERENCES

1. Pearson FG, Todd TRJ, Cooper JD. Experience with primary neoplasms of the trachea and carina. *J Thorac Cardiovasc Surg* 1984;88:511.
2. Grillo HC. Congenital lesions, neoplasms, and injuries of the trachea. In: Sabiston DC, Spencer FC, eds. *Surgery of the chest.* 5th ed. Philadelphia: WB Saunders; 1990:335–371.
3. Michet CJ, McKenna CH, Luthra HS, O'Fallon WM. Relapsing polychondritis: survival and predictive role of early disease manifestations. *Ann Intern Med* 1986;104:74–78.
4. Mathison DJ, Grillo HC. Laryngotracheal trauma. *Ann Thorac Surg* 1987;43:254.
5. Grillo HC. Surgical treatment of postintubation tracheal injuries. *J Thorac Cardiovasc Surg* 1979;78:860.
6. Andrews MJ, Pearson FG. The incidence and pathogenesis of tracheal injury following cuffed tube tracheostomy with associated ventilation: analysis of a two-year prospective study. *Ann Surg* 1971;173:249.
7. Miller RD, Hyatt RD. Evaluation of obstructing lesions of the trachea and larynx by flow-volume loops. *Am Rev Resp Dis* 1973;108:475–481.
8. Shure D. Radiographically occult endobronchial obstruction in bronchogenic carcinoma. *Am J Med* 1991;91:19–22.
9. Ell SR, Jolles H, Galvin JR. Cine CT demonstration of non-fixed upper airway obstruction. *Am J Roentgenal* 1986;146:669–677.
10. Dumon JF, Shapshay S, Bourcerean J, Cavaliere S, Meric B, Garb N, Beams J. Principles for safety in application of neodymium-YAG laser in bronchology. *Chest* 1984;86:163–168.
11. Shapshay SM. Laser application in the trachea and bronchi: a comparative study of soft tissue effects using contact and noncontact delivery systems. *Laryngoscope* 1987;97(Suppl 41):1–26.
12. Brutinel WM Cortese DA, McDougall JC, Gillio RG, Bergstrath EJ. A two-year experience with the neodymium-YAG laser in endobronchial obstruction. *Chest* 1987;91:159–165.
13. Kvale PA. Training in laser bronchoscopy and proposals for credentialling. *Chest* 1990;97:983–989.
14. Simonds AK, Irving JD, Clarke SW, Dick R. Use of expandable metal stents in the treatment of bronchial obstruction. *Thorax* 1989;44:680–681.
15. Wallace MJ, Charnsangavej C, Ogawa K, et al. Tracheobronchial tree: expandable metallic stents used in experimental and clinical applications. *Radiology* 1986;158:309–312.
16. Westaby S, Shepard MP. Palliation of intrathoracic tracheal compression with silastic tracheobronchial stent. *Thorax* 1983; 38:314–315.
17. Dumon JF. A dedicated tracheobronchial stent. *Chest* 1990; 97:328–332.
18. Orlowski TM. Palliative intubation of the tracheobronchial tree. *J Thorac Cardiovasc Surg* 1987;94:343–348.
19. Montgomery WW. T-tube stent. *Arch Otolaryngol* 1965; 83:71–75.
20. Montgomery WW. The surgical management of supraglottic and subglottic stenosis. *Ann Otol Rhinol Laryngol* 1968;77:534–546.
21. Cooper JD, Todd TRJ, Ilves R, Pearson FG. Use of the silicone tracheal T-tube for the management of complex tracheal injuries. *J Thorac Cardiovasc Surg* 1981;82:559–568.
22. Westaby S, Jackson JW, Pearson FG. A bifurcated silicone rubber stent for relief of tracheobronchial obstruction. *J Thorac Cardiovasc Surg* 1982;83:414–417.
23. Neville WE, Hamouda F, Anderson J. Dwan FM. Replacement of the intra-thoracic trachea and both stem bronchi with a molded silastic prosthesis. *J Thorac Cardiovasc Surg* 1972; 63:569–576.
24. Dumon JF. A dedicated tracheobronchial stent. *Chest* 1990; 97:328–332.
25. Carlin BW, Harrell JH, Moser KM. The treatment of endobronchial stenosis using balloon catheter dilatation. *Chest* 1988; 93:1148–1151.
26. Colt HG, Dumon JF. Airway obstruction in cancer: pros and cons of stents. *J Resp Dis* 1991;12(8):741–749.
27. Orlowski TM. Palliative intubation of the tracheobronchial tree. *J Thorac Cardiovasc Surg* 1987;94:343–348.
28. Leoff DS, Filler RM, Gorenstein A, et al. A new intratracheal stent for tracheobronchial reconstruction: experimental and clinical studies. *Pediatr Surg* 1988;23:1173–1177.
29. Pagliero KM, Shepherd MP. Use of stainless-steel wire coil prosthesis in treatment of anastomotic dehiscence after cervical tracheal resection. *J Thorac Cardiovasc Surg* 1974;67:932–935.
30. Clarke DB. Palliative intubation of the trachea and main bronchi. *J Thorac Cardiovasc Surg* 1980;80:736–741.
31. Uchida BT, Putnam JS, Rosch J. Modifications of Gianturco expandable wire stents. *Am J Roentgenol* 1988;150:1185–1187.
32. Wallace MJ, Charnsagaveg C, Ogawa K, et al. Tracheobronchial tree: expandable metallic stents used in experimental and clinical applications. *Radiology* 1986;158:309–312.
33. Rousseau H, Puel J, Joffre F, et al. Self-expanding endovascular prosthesis: an experimental study. *Radiology* 1987; 164:709–714.
34. Colt HG, Janssen JP, Dumon JF, Noirclerc MJ. Endoscopic management of bronchial stenosis after double lung transplantation. *Chest* 1992;102:10–16.
35. Schafers HJ, Haydock DA, Cooper JD. The prevalence and management of bronchial anastomotic complications in lung transplantation. *J Thorac Cardiovasc Surg* 1991;101:1044–1052.
36. Patterson GA, Todd TR, Cooper JD, Pearson FG, Winton TL, Maurer J. Airway complications after double lung transplantation. *J Thorac Cardiovasc Surg* 1990;99:14–21.

Bronchoscopy,
edited by U. B. S. Prakash.
Mayo Foundation © 1994.
Published by Raven Press, Ltd., New York.

CHAPTER 22

Bronchoscopy and Thoracic Surgery

Udaya B. S. Prakash and Peter C. Pairolero

Bronchoscopy is an integral element of many surgical procedures involving the thoracic organs. Prior to the introduction of the flexible bronchoscope into clinical practice in the early 1970s, the majority of the rigid bronchoscopic procedures were performed by thoracic surgeons. Currently, most of the bronchoscopic procedures utilize the flexible instrument and the majority of flexible bronchoscopies are performed by pulmonary physicians (1,2). The American College of Chest Physicians (ACCP) conducted a mail survey of bronchoscopists in North America, and of the 871 respondents, 98.2% (855) were pulmonary physicians and the rest were thoracic surgeons and specialists in critical care medicine. If a substantial number of general thoracic surgeons who also perform a significant number of bronchoscopies were included in the survey, the results may have differed (1). It is unclear at present as to how many general thoracic surgeons perform bronchoscopic procedures as part of their surgical practice, but the assumption is that nearly all do. This supposition stresses the importance of the role of bronchoscopy in thoracic surgery. Indeed, the American Board of Thoracic Surgery requires its candidates to have performed at least "25 bronchoscopy and esophagoscopy" procedures to become "board-eligible" (3).

Irrespective of which specialist performs the bronchoscopic procedures, it is mandatory that the bronchoscopist communicate with the thoracic surgeon regarding bronchoscopic findings if bronchoscopy is included as part of the preoperative evaluation. If bronchoscopy, whether diagnostic or therapeutic, is needed after a thoracic surgical procedure, again it is imperative that the bronchoscopist and the thoracic surgeon discuss the indication before the procedure is scheduled. To better communicate with the surgeon, if the surgeon and the bronchoscopist is not the same person, documentation of bronchoscopic findings on diagrams or videotape by the bronchoscopist is very advantageous (Chapter 27). We recognize that the setup of bronchoscopy and thoracic surgery varies from one medical center to another, and the arrangements, however diverse they are, must be amicable to all parties concerned, including the patient.

While the bronchoscope is one of the most important diagnostic tools used by the thoracic surgeon, other diagnostic tests such as pulmonary function tests, analysis of arterial blood gas measurements, chest roentgenograph, electrocardiogram, and computed tomography of chest are also used to evaluate the patient's ability to withstand major surgical procedures within the thoracic cage. The bronchoscopist should recognize that bronchoscopy by itself is not the ultimate procedure in the diagnosis or treatment of thoracic diseases. It is obvious that if bronchoscopy fails to accomplish the purported goal, the surgeon has other avenues to consider, such as mediastinoscopy, mediastinotomy, thoracoscopy, or thoracotomy.

The role of bronchoscopy in surgical procedures involving the thoracic organs can be broadly classified into preoperative, intraoperative, and postoperative bronchoscopies. Often, all three types of bronchoscopic procedures are required in the same patient and it is difficult to classify each indication into one of these three categories. The part played by the bronchoscope in the diagnosis of bronchogenic cancer is discussed in Chapter 15. In this chapter, we discuss the other major applications of bronchoscopy in various thoracic surgical procedures.

U. B. S. Prakash: Division of Thoracic Diseases and Internal Medicine, Mayo Clinic, Rochester, Minnesota 55905.
P. C. Pairolero, Section of Thoracic Surgery, Mayo Clinic, Rochester, Minnesota 55905.

PREOPERATIVE BRONCHOSCOPY

Diagnosis of Thoracic Malignancy

Perhaps the most important role played by the bronchoscope is in establishing the diagnosis of malignancy of the tracheobronchial tree and pulmonary parenchyma. The documentation of a particular type of carcinoma, e.g., small cell carcinoma, may entirely preclude any therapeutic surgical resection (Fig. 1). Similarly, a diagnosis of metastatic malignancy in the pulmonary parenchyma or pulmonary nodule may drastically alter the surgical approach.

Staging of Bronchogenic Carcinoma

Precise staging of primary lung cancer is important in predicting the survival. Bronchoscopy plays a major role in the staging of primary bronchogenic carcinoma. In addition to the visual staging of tracheobronchial involvement by the tumor, bronchoscopy may also help in identifying clinically unsuspected abnormalities such as vocal cord paralysis due to primary lung cancer and the presence of another neoplastic (multicentric) process or other abnormalities of the tracheobronchial tree that may alter the management options (Fig. 2). Bronchoscopic visualization of a bronchogenic cancer will help in deciding the extent of surgical resection that is feasible. For instance, the proximity of the tumor to the main carina may place a patient in "T3" stage (Fig. 3). Similarly, the bronchoscopic identification of a clinically occult vocal cord paralysis denotes a worse prognosis.

Intrathoracic Lymphadenopathy and Mass

Bronchoscopy should be considered in any patient with roentgenological diagnosis of intrathoracic lymphadenopathy or mass and symptoms of tracheobronchial involvement (4). Extrinsic compression or mucosal involvement of the trachea or bronchial tree should be excluded. Many surgeons routinely perform diagnostic bronchoscopy prior to mediastinoscopy in such cases.

Esophageal and Mediastinal Tumors

Esophageal and mediastinal tumors may produce extrinsic compression of the tracheobronchial tree, invade the major airways (Fig. 4), or result in tracheobronchoesophageal fistula (4,5). One study reported the experience with 27 patients with malignant respiratory tract fistula related to carcinoma of the thoracic esophagus and observed that the fistula involved the trachea in 11, left main bronchus in 7, right main bronchus in 3, and was more distal in 6 patients (6). Bronchoscopy in 13 patients prior to the development of fistulas showed tracheobronchial invasion or impingement in all. Another tumor that can produce similar problems is cancer of thyroid (Fig. 5) (7). Bronchoscopy is invaluable in these situations, particularly if surgical treatment is contemplated. It is advisable to

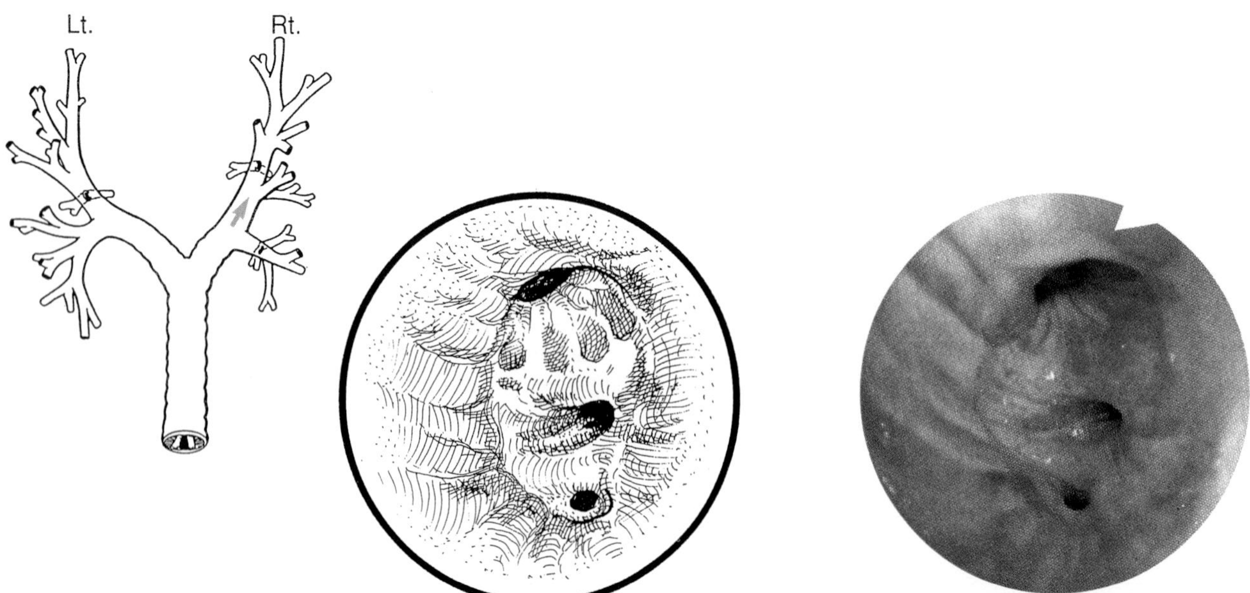

FIG. 1. Involvement of distal aspect of bronchus intermedius and bronchi to right middle and lower lobes by mucosal abnormality. Bronchoscopic biopsy in this patient who was referred for right pneumonectomy established the diagnosis of small cell carcinoma and precluded surgery.

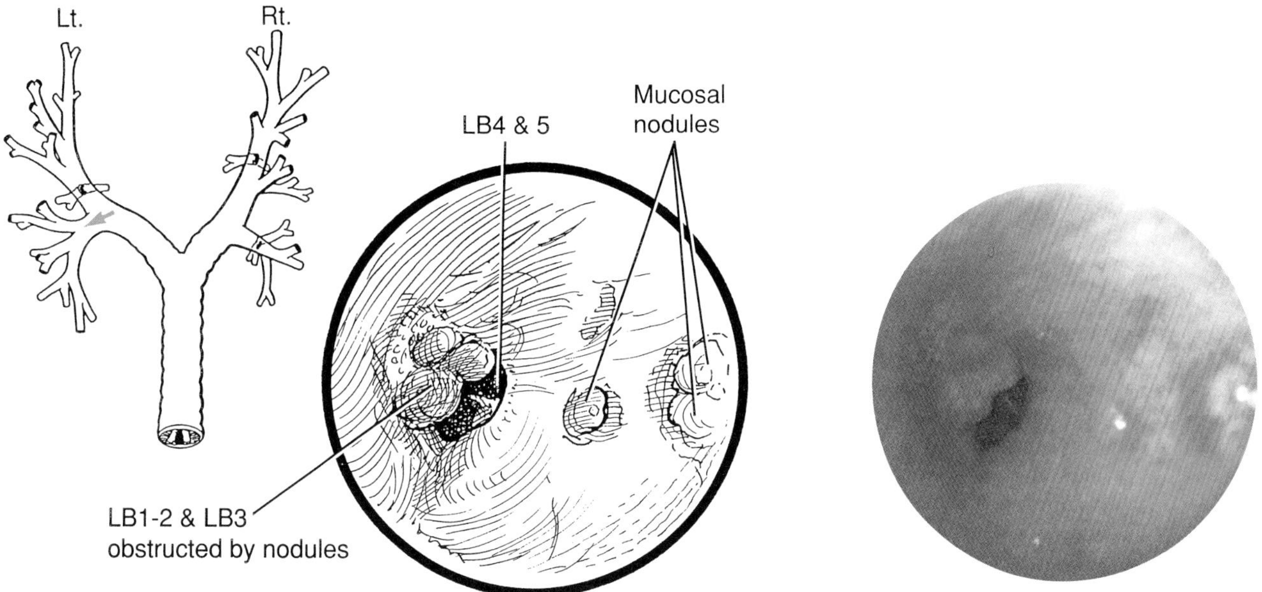

FIG. 2. Multicentric bronchial malignancy in a patient who was referred for left upper lobectomy following an earlier bronchoscopy that was reported to show the involvement of only the bronchus leading to left upper lobe. Repeat bronchoscopy indicated that the patient required more than a lobectomy.

perform bronchoscopy before extensive surgical resections are undertaken.

Bronchoscopic Needle Aspiration and Biopsy

Bronchoscopic needle aspiration and biopsy has been studied in the staging of bronchogenic carcinoma (Chapter 12). The diagnosis of malignancy in the paratracheal, hilar, or subcarinal lymph nodes by this procedure may place the patient in a worse stage and therefore preclude extensive thoracic surgical procedure. In the survey of North American bronchoscopists by the American College of Chest Physicians (1), the low rates of routine use of the transtracheal/bronchial needle aspiration in malignant and nonmalignant

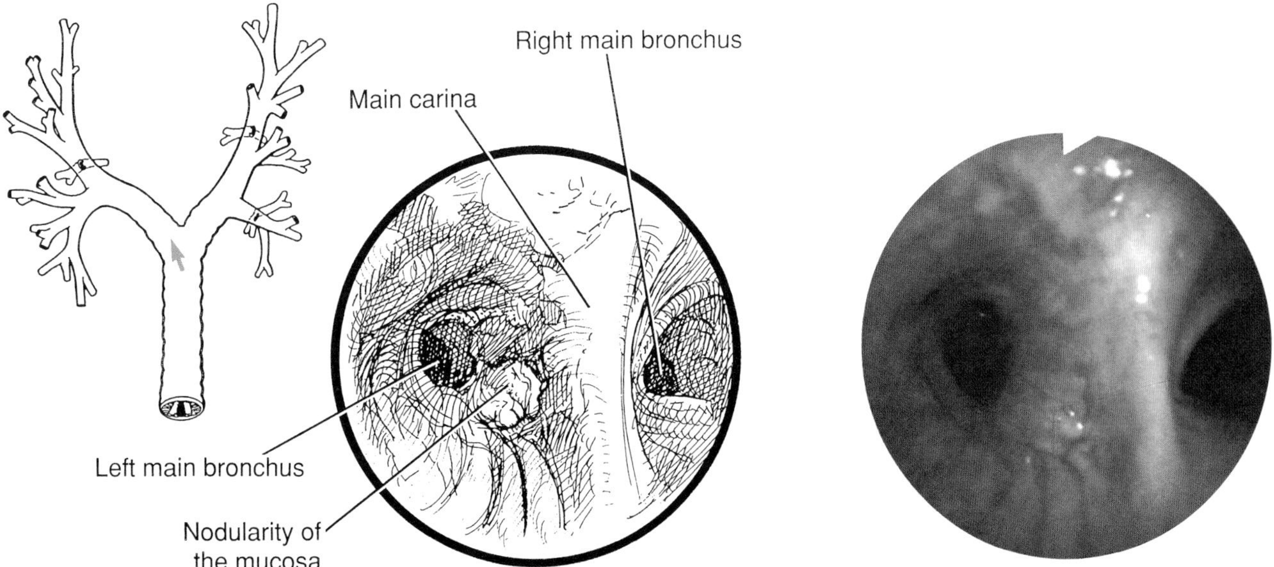

FIG. 3. Bronchoscopic staging of bronchogenic carcinoma. Involvement of either main stem bronchus (left proximal main stem bronchus involved in this case) within 2.5 cm of the main carina by non–small cell carcinoma places the cancer in "T3" stage.

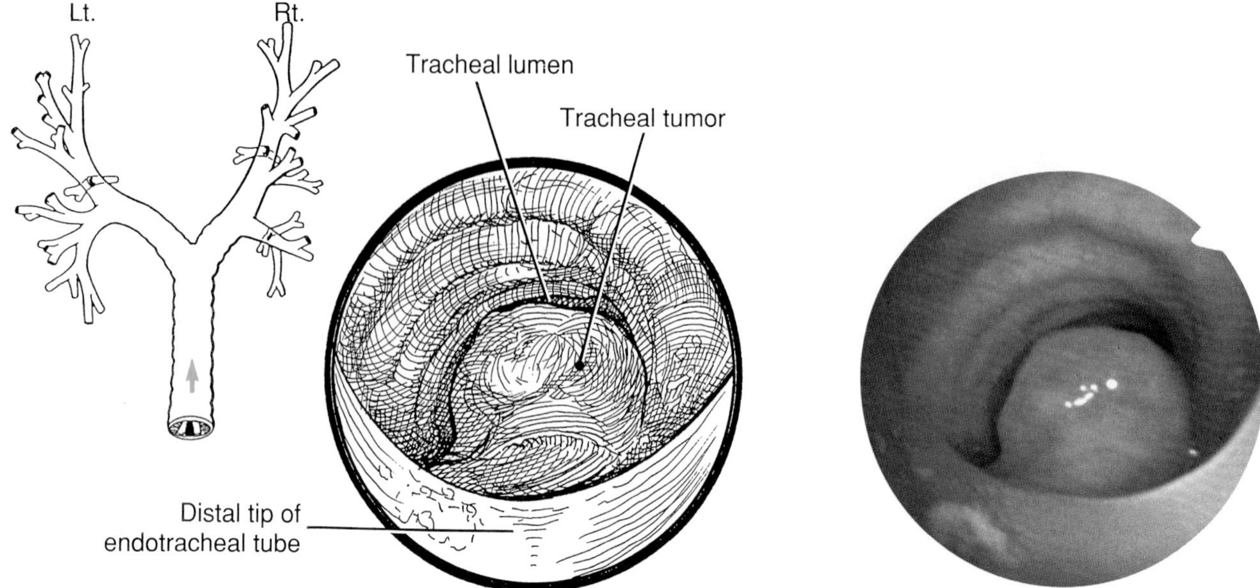

FIG. 4. Bronchoscopy in esophageal neoplasms. Tracheal involvement by esophageal cancer may remain subclinical unless bronchoscopy, along with other imaging procedures, is undertaken.

diseases and the large number of negative comments regarding this procedure suggest that the procedure had not gained popularity among the bronchoscopists who participated in the survey. This is in spite of several studies that have reported on the clinical usefulness of this procedure (8–11). Nevertheless, as observed by many survey participants, we too find the performance of the instruments available for transtracheal or transbronchial needle aspiration to be unreliable too often. Our experience with needles made by various manufacturers has shown several technical obstacles. It is not uncommon to use two or more needles in one patient because of the failure of the needle to function properly. Another major problem is the well-documented high rate of needle-induced damage to the inner lining of the flexible bronchoscope (12). In spite of the proliferation of publications on this procedure, the role of transbronchial needle aspiration/biopsy in

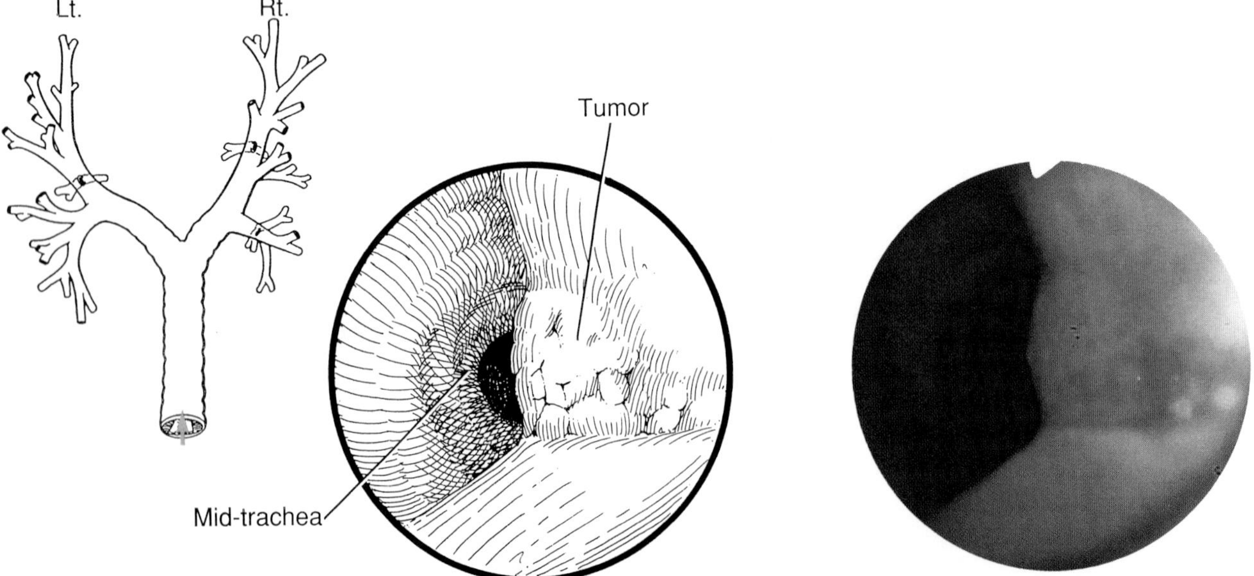

FIG. 5. Bronchoscopy prior to planned thyroid surgery in this case (minimal cough was the only symptom) precluded radical surgery.

the diagnosis of pulmonary diseases seems unclear to many. Unquestionably, one can sample malignant nodules, masses, or lymph nodes. This can be very useful in preoperative staging of a patient with lung cancer who is a poor surgical risk. The finding of small cell cancer may obviate surgical intervention. In an otherwise healthy individual without evidence for metastatic disease, however, one must weigh the experience of the bronchoscopist, pathologist, and surgeon acting as a team in their desire to offer the patient the best chance for good results. In many cases, a direct surgical approach seems appropriate (2).

Diagnosis of Pulmonary Parenchymal Disorders

The diagnosis of benign thoracic diseases, e.g., pulmonary sarcoidosis, by performing bronchoscopic biopsy may also prevent or alter other surgical procedures. The establishment of infectious processes by bronchial washings or bronchoalveolar lavage and lymphangitic carcinomatosis and unusual pulmonary disorders by bronchoscopic lung biopsy may obviate the need for open lung biopsy. Chapter 11 provides further details on the role of bronchoscopic lung biopsy.

Diagnosis of Benign Disorders of the Airway

Bronchoscopy plays a significant role in the diagnosis and planning of surgical treatment of several benign disorders of the tracheobronchial tree. The two main aims of bronchoscopy are to assess the extent of the airway involvement and the feasibility of surgical therapy. The following are some of the clinical disorders where preoperative bronchoscopy greatly assists in surgical planning.

Tracheobronchial Strictures and Stenoses

Tracheobronchial strictures and stenoses are caused by benign as well as malignant diseases. In the majority of patients with significant stenoses, clinical information should point to the diagnosis although the wrong diagnosis of asthma is sometimes made. The luminal narrowing can be intrinsic or can be caused by extrinsic compression. The most common etiology of both intrinsic and extrinsic narrowing of the tracheobronchial tree is malignant disease. Benign strictures can result from diverse processes including injury from tracheal intubation, crush injury of neck, infectious diseases such as histoplasmosis and tuberculosis, mediastinal granulomatosis, and Wegener's granulomatosis. Bronchoscopic examination is very helpful in establishing the diagnosis of malignant disease. In benign strictures, the bronchoscopic examination may show atrophic mucosa, mucosal edema, or granularity, and multiple biopsies should be obtained to exclude malignancy. The presence of granulomas in biopsy specimens will indicate an infectious process or sarcoidosis. Often the etiology of benign strictures cannot be established.

In patients in whom surgical options are impractical or not feasible, bronchoscopic dilatation should be considered (Chapter 16). Both benign and malignant airway lesions can be treated. In benign strictures, the passage of the rigid bronchoscopes of gradually increasing diameters may dilate the trachea and main

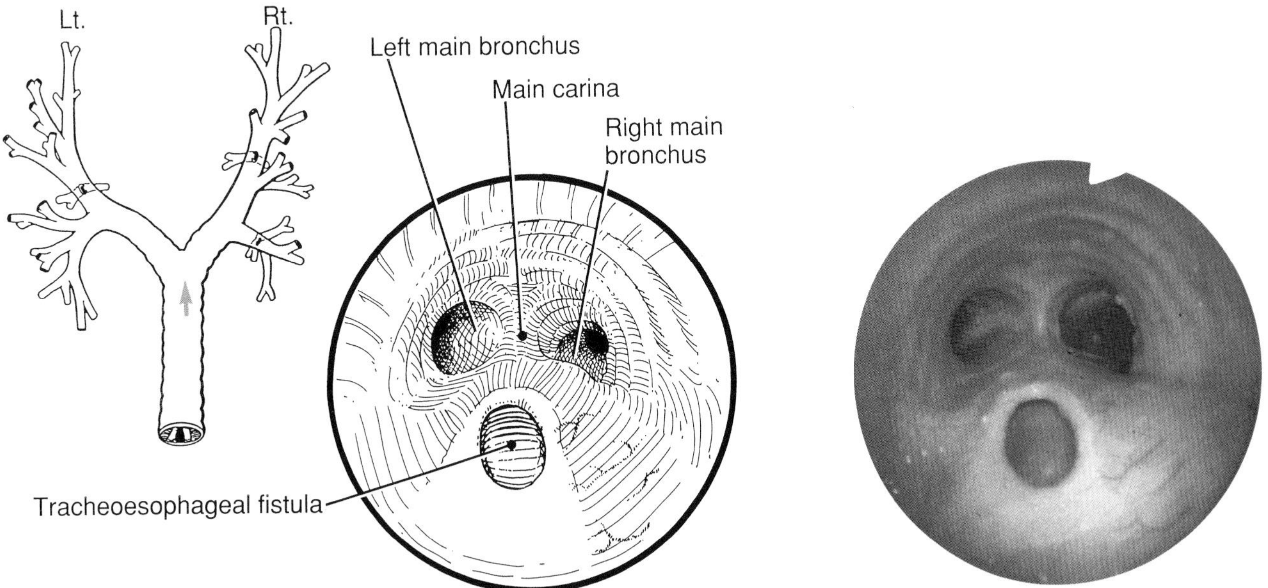

FIG. 6. Fistula connecting distal trachea and esophagus resulting from radiation therapy to a mediastinal neoplasm. Bronchoscopy aided the surgeon to plan appropriate procedure.

stem bronchi. Balloon dilatation through either the flexible or rigid bronchoscope can be accomplished if the stenosis is limited to a shorter segment of the airway. Repeated dilatations are often required because of the recurrence of airway stenosis. Bronchoscopic dilatation is more likely to be effective if the stenosis is intrinsic rather than extrinsic.

Tracheoesophageal Fistula

Bronchoscopy is extremely helpful in the diagnosis of tracheoesophageal and bronchoesophageal fistula. Prior to definitive surgical treatment, bronchoscopy provides information regarding the location, size, and other details regarding the fistula (Fig. 6) (13). In children with congenital tracheoesophageal or bronchoesophageal fistulas, both bronchoscopy and esophagoscopy should be performed to assess the anatomic derangement (14). Intraoperative bronchoesophagoscopy in these patients is frequently used to guide the surgeon.

Bronchopleural Fistula

Bronchopleural fistula is a complication of thoracic trauma, extensive radiation therapy, inflammatory or infectious disease, or previous thoracic surgical procedure. It is one of the most difficult disorders to manage medically and often requires recurrent surgical procedures to cure. Bronchoscopy aids in locating the site and size of the fistula and provides the surgeon with the necessary outline of the tracheobronchial tree so that an appropriate treatment can be planned. In our experience, it is somewhat difficult to locate a tiny fistula even when the location, such as the necrotic lobectomy or pneumonectomy stump, is suspected. We have used a cytology to brush to gently probe the suspicious area to see if a communication exists between the airway and distal anatomic areas. Asking the patient to inhale and exhale deeply may also reveal a fistula not apparent during quiet breathing. Instillation of small amounts of normal saline over the suspicious location and appearance of bubbles on deep-breathing maneuvers may suggest the presence of the fistula. When bronchopleurocutaneous fistula is suspected, we have used methylene blue through the bronchoscope (to avoid discoloration of the inner lining of the flexible instrument, we use a plastic catheter through the bronchoscope). Examination of the skin wound during the next 6–24 hr may reveal exudation of greenish effluent, thereby establishing the communication between the airway and the skin wound (Fig. 7). A large bronchopleural fistula is usually obvious and in fact the bronchoscope can be easily introduced into the fistulous tract.

Broncholithiasis

Bronchoscopic treatment of broncholithiasis is controversial. The major symptoms include cough, wheeze, and hemoptysis. Lithoptysis may be observed by 26–60% of patients (15–18). Of all the tests (chest roentgenograph, tomography, computed tomography), bronchoscopy provides the highest diagnostic yield in broncholithiasis (16). Even though bronchoscopic stone removal is successful in 20–45% of patients, many patients require thoracotomy and operations varying from simple lung wedge resection to repair of a bronchoesophageal fistula. Bronchoscopy not only establishes the diagnosis but also aids in the planning of surgical treatment.

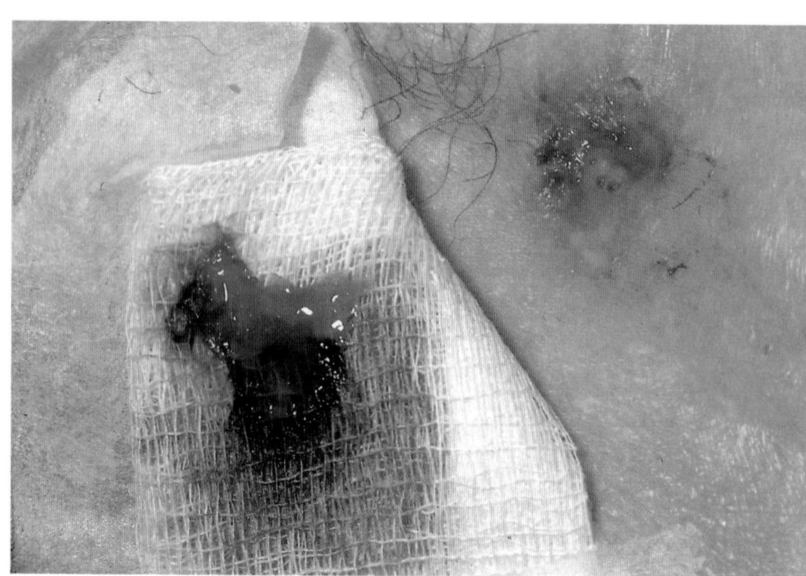

FIG. 7. Bronchopleurocutaneous fistula with the cutaneous opening in right axilla. Bluish green discoloration of the dressing gauze represents methylene blue injected earlier into the bronchial tree through a flexible bronchoscope.

Lung Abscess

The reasons for bronchoscopy in patients with lung abscess include establishing drainage for those patients who do not improve on antibiotics and ruling out an endobronchial lesion that may be benign, malignant, or a foreign body. Bronchoscopy can be used to drain lung abscess (Chapters 14 and 16). However, massive intrabronchial aspiration of the contents of the abscess may occur. To prevent this complication, sedation and excessive topical anesthesia should be avoided. An orotracheal tube should be in place to provide rapid access with a large-suction catheter if needed. A rigid bronchoscope should be available or should be used initially if this complication is anticipated, particularly if a foreign body is encountered at the beginning of the procedure.

Thoracic Trauma

Traumatic rupture of the tracheobronchial tree is an increasingly occurring complication of blunt chest trauma. Early detection and surgical repair are important for definitive and successful reconstruction. Bronchoscopy is the most reliable diagnostic procedure in these patients (19). Diagnostic bronchoscopy should be considered in all cases of major thoracic trauma (20–22). The main reason for diagnostic bronchoscopy in patients with recent chest trauma is to exclude serious airway injury (22,23). Bronchoscopy is useful in the assessment and management of other trauma-related problems such as atelectasis of lung, lobe, or segment. Bronchoscopy may also reveal aspirated material or thick secretions and mucous plugging, which can be removed at the time of diagnostic bronchoscopy. Bronchoscopy for evaluation of hemoptysis following chest trauma may suggest pulmonary contusion and hemorrhage. Hara and Prakash reviewed their experience and documented that bronchoscopy was helpful in 30% of patients with chest trauma (22). The bronchoscopic findings were helpful in planning the nonsurgical and surgical treatment. Flynn and associates reviewed their experience with tracheal and bronchial injury due to penetrating and blunt trauma and reported that all blunt injuries were diagnosed by bronchoscopy (24). Occasionally, bronchoscopy may fail to reveal signs of traumatic airway lesions and because of the possibility that a lesion might be overlooked by initial bronchoscopy, repeat bronchoscopic examination should be performed if the clinical situation suggests such a lesion (22,25). Diagnostic bronchoscopy should be considered in patients who present with bullet wounds of the thoracic cage. In addition to locating the site of tracheobronchial hemorrhage, bronchoscopy may help in identifying other problems such as aspirated foreign body or bullets within the airways. Indeed, bronchoscopic removal of a bullet unexpectedly found entirely within the lumen of the right lower lobe bronchus has been described (26).

Tracheobronchial Foreign Bodies

Tracheobronchial foreign bodies are usually removed by either flexible or rigid bronchoscopic procedures (27). However, in 3–5% of instances, thoracotomy and bronchotomy or segmental resection is required to extract the foreign body (27,28). Chapter 18 provides a detailed discussion on the diagnosis and treatment of tracheobronchial foreign bodies.

INTRAOPERATIVE BRONCHOSCOPY

Tracheal Intubation

Bronchoscopy during a surgical procedure in the thoracic cage is often required in patients with major airway trauma, in reconstruction procedures involving the tracheobronchial tree, to aid in the placement of an endotracheal tube, and to assess the immediate outcome of bronchoplasty procedures. Endotracheal intubation in patients with unstable neck, microstomia, and maxillofacial injury frequently precludes flexion of the neck and the use of laryngoscope-guided endotracheal intubation. Under such circumstances, endotracheal intubation with a flexible bronchoscope is indicated (29,30).

It is often necessary to use a double-lumen endotracheal tube prior to lung surgery. Many anesthesiologists recommend the use of an ultrathin flexible bronchoscope to ascertain the location of each opening of the endotracheal tube. An important point to remember is that the standard flexible bronchoscope commonly used in adult patients has too large a diameter to traverse the lumen of the double-lumen endotracheal tube and therefore an ultrathin flexible bronchoscope should be available for this procedure.

Bronchoscopy and Anesthesia

Several reports have described the unusual occurrence of acute tracheal obstruction, with fatal outcome in some, in patients with large anterior mediastinal masses who are subjected to general anesthesia (4,31–34). Flexible bronchoscopy in such cases has demonstrated near-total obstruction of the distal half of the trachea secondary to an extrinsic compression (Fig. 8). This type of acute tracheal obstruction is more common in children than in adults.

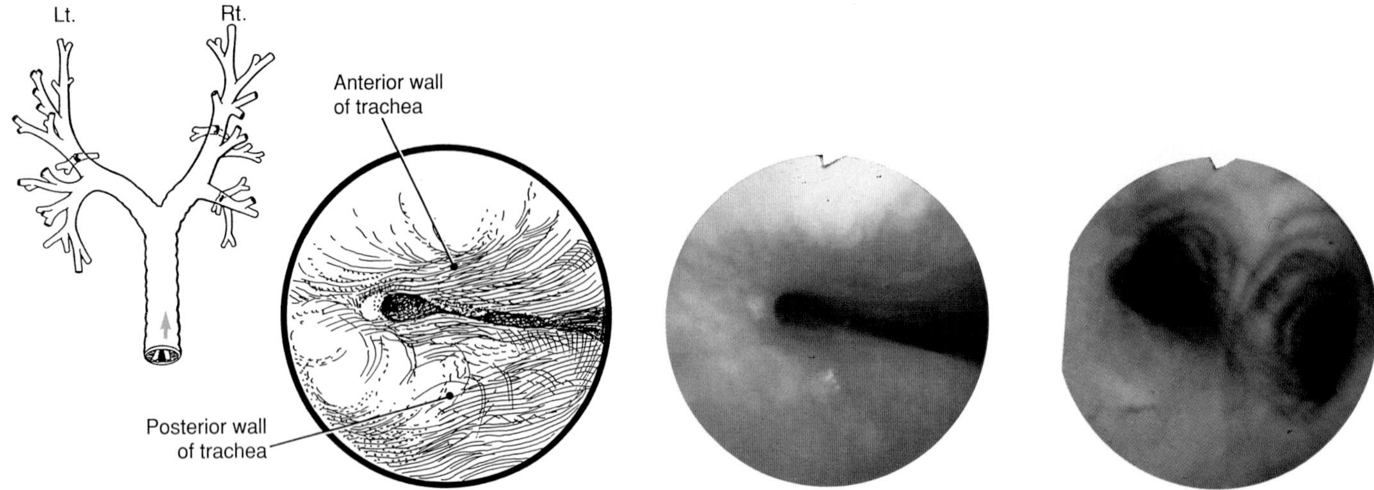

FIG. 8. Acute airway obstruction during induction of anesthesia for mediastinoscopy to biopsy a large anterior mediastinal mass **(left)**; turning patient to prone position removed the extrinsic compression by the large mass **(right).** From Prakash et al. (4), with permission.

Pretracheostomy Bronchoscopy

Patients who present with acute stridor and severe respiratory distress secondary to glottic or subglottic pathology (including tracheal foreign body) may require tracheostomy on an emergent basis. If an endotracheal tube cannot be inserted to relieve the respiratory distress before tracheostomy can be performed, then a rigid bronchoscope should be used to intubate the trachea and provide a temporary airway until tracheostomy is carried out.

Chronic complications of tracheostomy include bleeding, stenosis at the tracheostomy site, and formation of granuloma at the stoma or along the tracheal wall in close contact with the tracheostomy tube. Bronchoscopic examination can identify all of these complications and provide the information that is necessary to plan appropriate therapy. Bronchoscopic treatment of subglottic strictures and tracheobronchial bleeding is discussed in Chapters 16, 17, and 21 of this volume. Students of bronchoscopy should recognize that the rigid bronchoscope can be passed through the tracheostomy stoma and can be used as dilator of tracheal stenosis.

Compression of Major Airways

In addition to mediastinal and hilar masses that can squeeze the major airways, compression of the tracheobronchial tree with symptoms of airway compromise can also be caused by vascular abnormalities such as right-sided aortic arch and anomalous intravascular structures (35,36). If surgical correction is contemplated to correct the vascular abnormality, intraoperative bronchoscopy is useful in gauging the effect of surgery on the tracheobronchial tree.

Bleeding into the Airway

During thoracic surgery, particularly in the procedures involving resection of airway or lung parenchyma, a negligible quantity of blood commonly seeps into the airway lumen and may clot within the lumen and induce postoperative atelectasis of a lung segment or lobe. Occasionally, a significant amount of blood is seen coming out of the endotracheal tube. This usually suggests major bleeding in the surgical field with flooding of the airways with potential for fatal asphyxia. We have encountered this problem when the intrapulmonary artery balloon catheter caused inadvertent rupture of the pulmonary artery. Unless controlled immediately, the hemorrhage can be lethal. Bronchoscopy in such circumstances is very helpful in identifying the side (right vs. left), site, and intensity of bleeding. Depending on the patient's oxygenation status, bronchoscopic tamponade using bronchial balloon catheter or rigid bronchoscopic control of hemorrhage has to be considered.

Bronchoscopy during thoracic surgery is usually performed under suboptimal conditions because of the smaller or double-lumen endotracheal tube used, the frequently used lateral decubitus position of the patient's body, the need to stay away from the sterile surgical field, and the large number of instruments and machinery surrounding the operating table. Because of the patient's body position, it is easy to become disoriented with regard to the tracheobronchial anatomy. However, proper communication among surgeon, anesthesiologist, and bronchoscopist should make it easier. At times the bronchoscopists will have to adapt to the given situation and provide the needed assistance (Fig. 9).

Resection and Reanastomosis of Airway Stricture and Stenosis

In surgical procedures designed to resect tracheobronchial strictures and stenoses, bronchoscopy has been helpful in estimating the site and the length of strictures and stenoses (Fig. 10). After the thoracic cage is opened and the trachea exposed, the bronchoscopist introduces the bronchoscope (either flexible or rigid) into the trachea through the endotracheal tube and identifies the proximal extent of the airway narrowing. The surgeon pierces the trachea with thin needles to identify the proximal and distal sites of intended resection. The bronchoscopist, by directly visualizing the needles and their relation to the proximal and distal extent of the airway narrowing, will assist the surgeon in identifying the exact sites of stricture and anastomosis (Fig. 11).

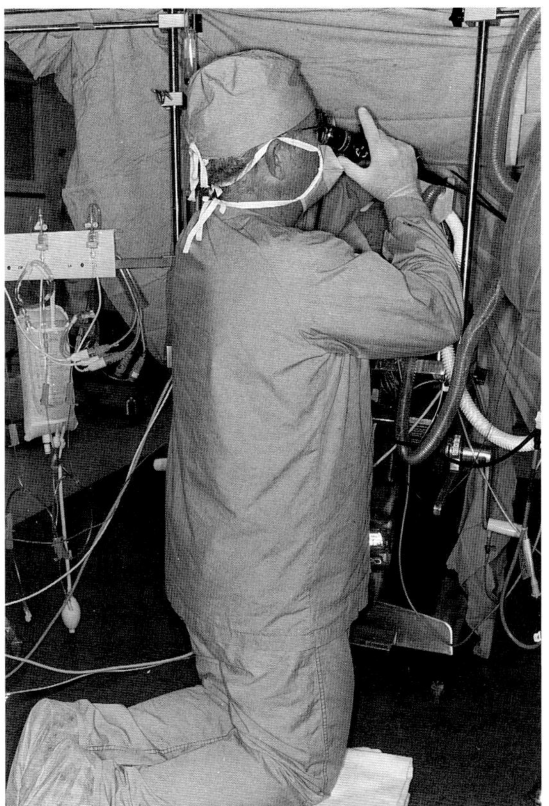

FIG. 9. Bronchoscopy in a patient who is undergoing thoracic surgery. The bronchoscopist is kneeling on the floor to perform the procedure because of the patient's lateral decubitus position.

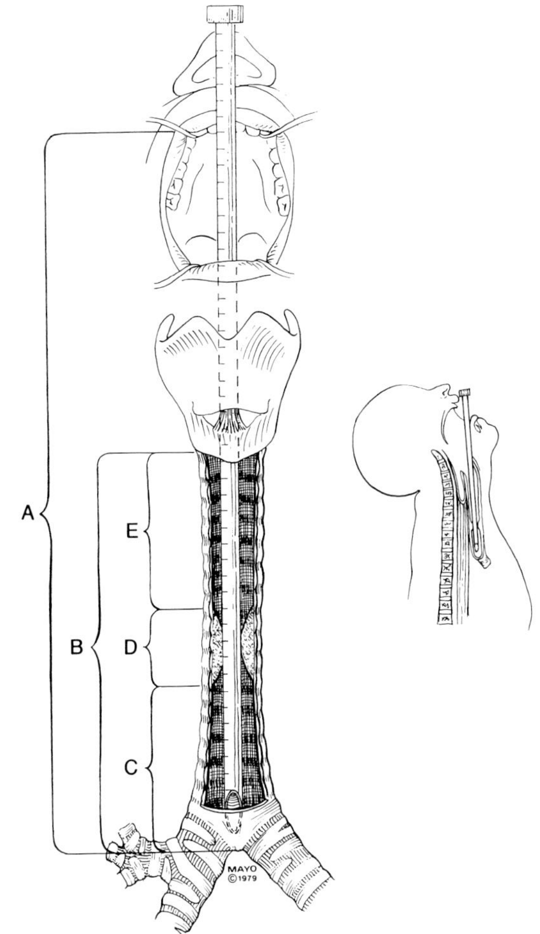

FIG. 10. Estimation of tracheobronchial dimensions before tracheoplasty procedures. **(A)** Distance from incisors to carina. **(B)** Distance from cricoid cartilage to carina. **(C)** Distance from lower level of stricture to carina. **(D)** Length of stricture. **(E)** Distance from cricoid cartilage to proximal suture.

Identification of Airway Abnormalities

During the repair of tracheoesophageal or bronchoesophageal fistula, bronchoscopic examination assists in evaluating the efficacy of the surgical procedure (Figs. 12 and 13). To simplify the intraoperative identification of the tracheoesophageal fistula a new technique has been described; the surgeons have used a flexible bronchoscope to pass a flexible vascular guidewire across the tracheoesophageal fistula (37). Others have used the telescope rod system with the bronchoscope to identify the fistula and thread a balloon catheter. The balloon is inflated and the bronchoscope re-

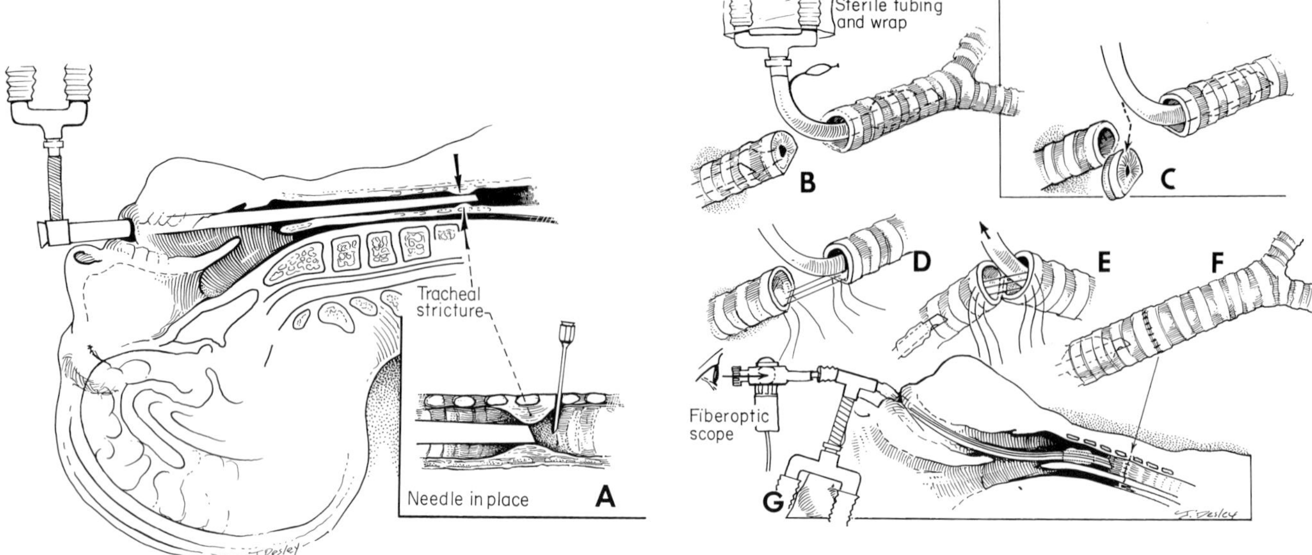

FIG. 11. A technique of airway control and surgical repair of tracheal stricture. Rigid bronchoscope in place and caudad extent of stricture defined by placing transbronchial needle just distal to lower limit of stricture at time of repair **(A)**. Tracheal resection caudad to stricture and sterile endotracheal tube **(B)**. Stricture is resected **(C)**. Anastomosis of trachea; note orotracheal tube advanced with removal of tubing from surgical field **(D–F)**. Flexible bronchoscope used in assessment of anastomosis and adequacy of airway as orotracheal tube is removed **(G)**. From *Surg Clin North Am* 1973;53:875–884, with permission.

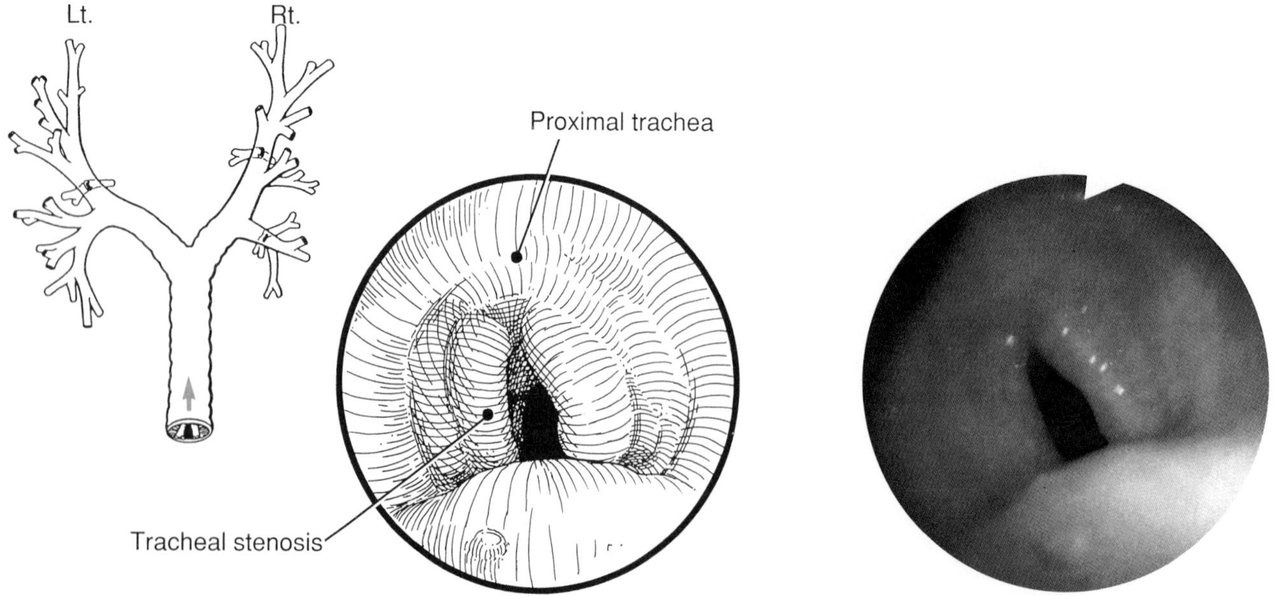

FIG. 12. Stricture of proximal trachea requiring resection and anastomosis.

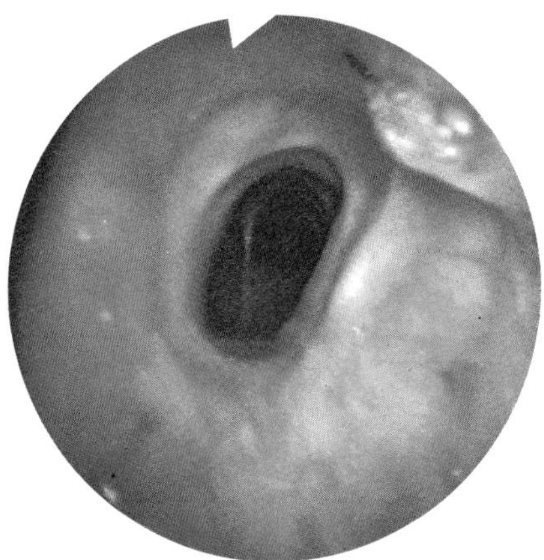

FIG. 13. Postoperative bronchoscopic view to assess the anastomosis. Same case as in Fig. 12.

moved, leaving the catheter in place, so that the surgeon is able to identify the location and plan appropriate procedure (38).

POSTOPERATIVE BRONCHOSCOPY

Therapeutic Bronchoscopy

One of the most important indications for postoperative bronchoscopy is the common occurrence of segmental or lobar atelectasis following lung surgery. The atelectasis may result from bronchial luminal obstruction secondary to thick secretions, mucous plugs, or blood clots related to the surgical procedure itself. While the common postoperative maneuvers such as chest physiotherapy, incentive spirometry, proper humidification of inspired air, and encouragement of the patient to cough and expectorate the mucus are extremely important, therapeutic bronchoscopy to remove the obstructing mucous plugs and clots should not be withheld. Patients who cannot cough or expectorate airway secretions, plugs, and blood clots due to weakness of respiratory muscles, underlying illness, and generalized weakness may require an almost daily therapeutic bronchoscopic procedure. Further discussion regarding this topic is included in Chapter 16.

Before proceeding with bronchoscopy, it is important for the bronchoscopist to know the details of the thoracic surgical procedure performed. Undue stress or pressure on the fresh lobectomy or pneumonectomy stump can result in "stump blowout" and predispose to tension pneumothorax. The suction and pressure applied on the anastomotic site and the stump should be gentle and minimal.

Follow-up of Tracheobronchoplasty Procedures

In patients who undergo resection and anastomosis of trachea or bronchial tree, particularly sleeve resection, airway reconstruction using pericardial patch, resection of the main carina, and repair of bronchopleural fistula, the risk of anastomotic dehiscence and retention of secretions distal to the site of anastomosis becomes greater. Many of these patients are left intubated for several days after surgery. To ensure that the endotracheal tube is in proper position without the cuff impinging on the anastomotic site, remove secretions and mucous plugs, and to assess the viability and intactness of the anastomosis, we perform flexible bronchoscopic examinations on a daily basis during the first 2–3 days after surgery (Fig. 13). Some patients require long-term endotracheal intubation and mechanical ventilation. Complications in such patients include tracheoesophageal fistula and airway stenosis (39). Repeat bronchoscopic examinations may be necessary to assess airway damage and prevent serious complications. The onset of new respiratory symptoms in these patients may indicate a new problem or a complication secondary to tracheobronchial surgery. Bronchoscopy may show the reason (formation of granulation or development of a fistula) for the pulmonary symptoms and aid in the treatment of the complication (Fig. 14).

Follow-up of Lung Cancer Resection

Patients with lung cancer who have undergone various types of treatments often require bronchoscopic examination to ascertain the effectiveness of therapy. In such patients, repeat brushings and biopsies will be required to document the recurrence or persistence of malignancy. Surgical treatment involving complicated procedures, such as tracheoplasty and reanastomosis, will often require intraoperative or immediate postoperative bronchoscopy to assess the technical results of the surgical procedure.

Patients who undergo resection and reanastomosis of trachea or bronchi for the treatment of localized malignancy may develop local recurrence of the tumor. Onset of new cough or other respiratory symptoms of airway disease in such patients should prompt investigation to exclude recurrent bronchogenic carcinoma. Bronchoscopy is one of the diagnostic tools and may reveal the source of pulmonary symptoms (Fig. 15). We stress that not every patient who undergoes surgical treatment for intrathoracic malignancy should be subjected to routine follow-up bronchoscopy. Unless the patient presents with symptoms and clinical and roentgenological signs of recurrent neoplasm, routine periodic bronchoscopy is not indicated. Patients who

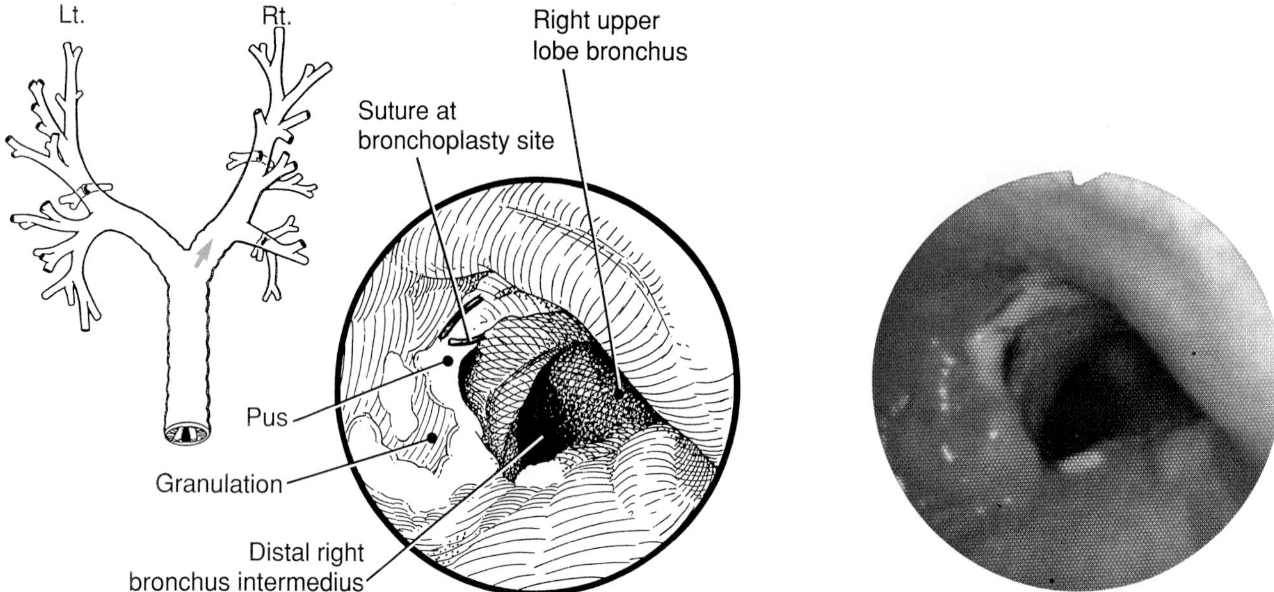

FIG. 14. Granulation tissue formation at anastomotic site caused cough, hemoptysis, and required bronchoscopic biopsy and resection.

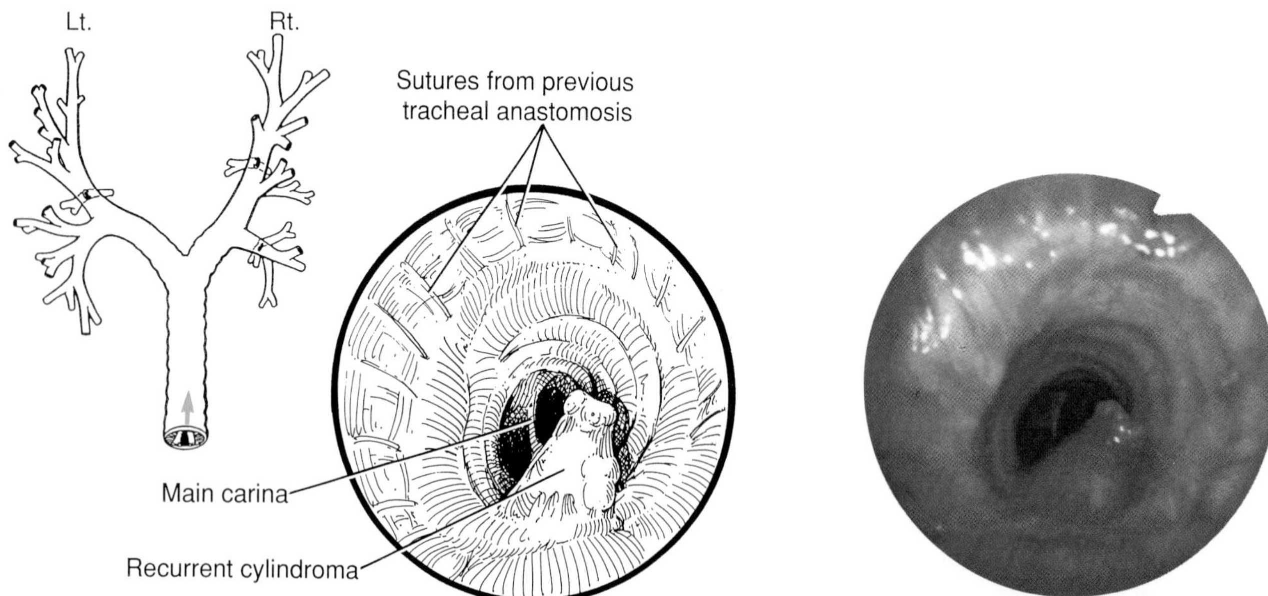

FIG. 15. Recurrent cylindroma of proximal trachea just distal to anastomotic site following resection 4 years earlier; cough and hemoptysis were the presenting symptoms. Sutures from previous anastomosis are visible proximally.

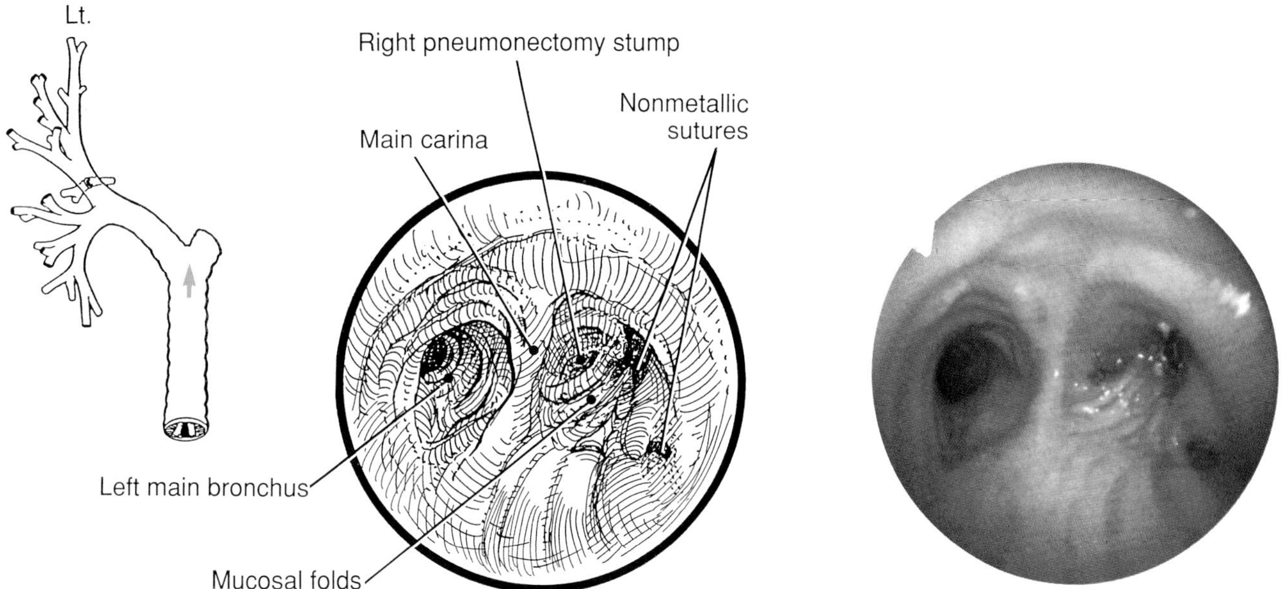

FIG. 16. Loose sutures at right pneumonectomy stump. Cough appearing 2 years after surgery subsided following bronchoscopic removal of sutures.

undergo resection of portions of lung may present with symptoms unrelated to recurrent cancer. The clinical suspicion in such a circumstance is usually biased toward recurrent malignancy and therefore bronchoscopy is indicated. Occasionally, surgical sutures or metallic clips at the site of the lobectomy stump produce cough and hemoptysis and clinically suggest more serious pathology (Fig. 16) (40).

Bronchopleural Fistula and Pneumothorax

Bronchial stump insufficiency following lung resection, with an average incidence of 4 percent, is a serious complication that carries a high mortality. Surgical repairs of these fistulas are technically difficult and carry significant operative risk. Bronchopleural fistulas and persistent pneumothoraces are particularly challenging in the ventilated patient. Alternative treatment methods include bronchoscopic application of fibrin glue sealant to the area of bronchial stump insufficiency. In an experimental animal study, occlusion of infected bronchus stump fistulas was achieved with fibrin sealant (1 ml, 500 units/ml thrombin, 3,500 units/ml aprotinin applied via a flexible bronchoscope). Additional sclerotherapy with 2–3 ml ethoxysclerol was applied around the fistula orifice before fibrin sealing to stimulate fibrosis. Autopsy revealed that all bronchial stump fistulas had healed after the second postoperative week (41). Definitive therapy of the bronchopleural fistula by the bronchoscopic application of a sealing agent to occlude the fistula site has been tried in humans (42). These procedures are normally time consuming and require deep sedation or general anesthesia. Successful application of the technique requires an accurate determination of the segmental location of the air leak in patients with persistent pneumothorax. Balloon tamponade can be accomplished with either the flexible or the rigid bronchoscope. If performed properly, the tamponade will either stop or decrease the air leak through the chest tube. Once the segmental bronchus is identified, further treatment, such as fibrin glue injection or surgery, can be undertaken. The technique of fibrin glue application is described in Chapter 16.

The flexible bronchoscope has been used percutaneously to visualize the track of a bronchopleurocutaneous fistula and to obtain tissue and microbiological specimens for examination (42).

Lung Transplant Patients

In patients undergoing lung transplant, rejection episodes, opportunistic infections, bronchiolitis obliterans, and anastomotic strictures of the tracheobronchial tree are among the most serious complications (43,44). Although currently there are no totally reliable techniques for the diagnosis of lung allograft rejection, bronchoscopic lung biopsy is frequently performed to identify characteristic pulmonary parenchymal changes (44). One study reported that the overall sensitivity and specificity for bronchoscopic lung biopsy were 84 and 100%, respectively (45).

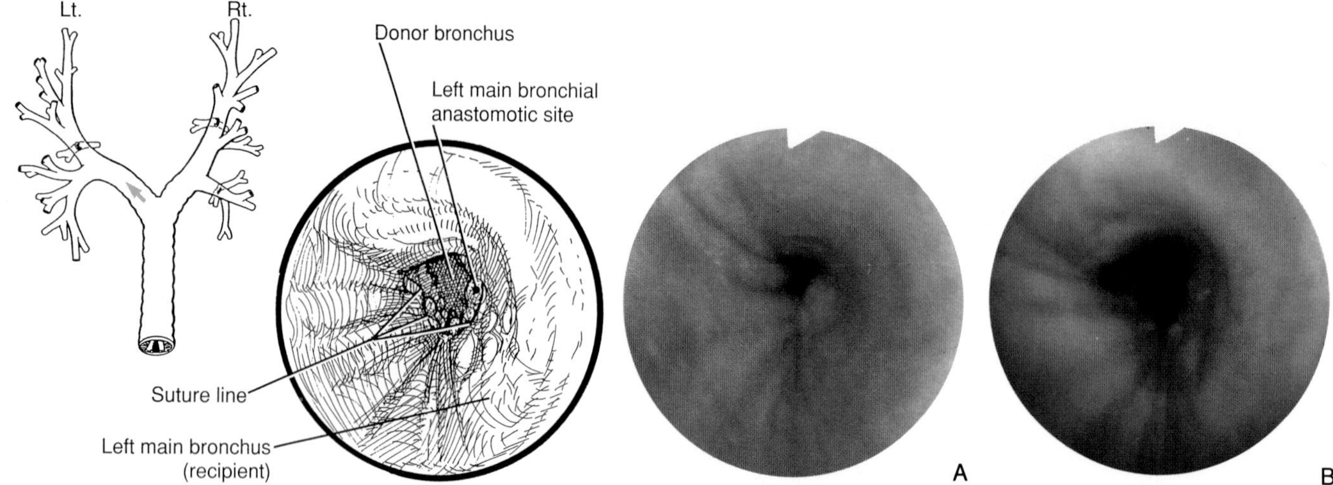

FIG. 17. (A) Left main stem bronchial anastomotic stricture in a lung transplant recipient. **(B)** Increased diameter of the bronchial lumen following bronchoscopic dilatation.

Anastomotic stricture of trachea or main bronchi in lung transplant recipients is a relatively common complication of lung transplantation. This is due to ischemia and recent attempts to revascularize the anastomotic site by wrapping it with omentum have reduced the incidence of this complication. Dilatation or stent placement can be accomplished by bronchoscopy (Fig. 17).

OTHER ISSUES

Bronchoscopic Lung Biopsy vs. Thoracoscopy/Thoracotomy

Bronchoscopic lung biopsy provides adequate lung tissue and thus precludes the need for open lung biopsy in many patients. In recent years, bronchoalveolar lavage has supplanted bronchoscopic lung biopsy in the diagnosis of several diffuse lung diseases, particularly those caused by infections. However, bronchoscopic lung biopsy should be considered when a diffuse or localized interstitial, alveolar, miliary, or fine nodular pattern of disease is present on the chest roentgenogram and when the diagnosis cannot be established by a bronchoalveolar lavage or other less invasive diagnostic technique (46). Lymphangitic carcinomatosis, miliary tuberculosis, diffuse pulmonary mycoses, sarcoidosis, cytotoxic pulmonary disease, and pulmonary eosinophilic granuloma are some of the entities that can be diagnosed in a high proportion of cases (47,48). The diagnosis of idiopathic pulmonary fibrosis by bronchoscopic lung biopsy is somewhat controversial. Tissue diagnosis consistent with idiopathic pulmonary fibrosis is present in various disease processes and hence the diagnosis of idiopathic pulmonary fibrosis established by bronchoscopic lung biopsy tends to be nondiagnostic. Bronchoscopic lung biopsy is useful in diagnosing pulmonary disease in immunocompromised patients. *Pneumocystis carinii* pneumonia may be diagnosed in nearly 100% of cases. The use of touch preparations increases the diagnostic efficacy of bronchoscopic lung biopsy in diagnosing this opportunistic infection. Fungal infections such as aspergillosis and cryptococcosis as well as cytomegalovirus infections may also be diagnosed with bronchoscopic lung biopsy. The advent of bronchoalveolar lavage has added considerably to the diagnostic efficacy of bronchoscopy in the immunocompromised patient, and bronchoscopic lung biopsy is done less frequently than in years past in this group of patients.

In recent years, thoracoscopy (or pleuroscopy) has reemerged as a helpful tool in the diagnosis and treatment of pleural diseases (49–51). However, it is unclear whether this procedure will replace bronchoscopic lung biopsy in the diagnosis of diffuse pulmonary parenchymal disease (52). Obviously, the decision regarding which of the procedures—bronchoalveolar lavage, bronchoscopic lung biopsy, or thoracoscopy—is to be considered in a given patient will depend on the clinical diagnosis and urgency. A clear advantage of thoracoscopy in comparison to bronchoscopic lung biopsy is that much larger pieces of lung tissue can be obtained. It appears that thoracoscopic lung biopsy may obviate the need for standard thoracotomy to obtain tissue diagnosis in patients with diffuse lung disease.

Should All Thoracotomy Patients Undergo Bronchoscopy?

It is not uncommon to proceed directly to thoracotomy in a patient with uncomplicated solitary pulmo-

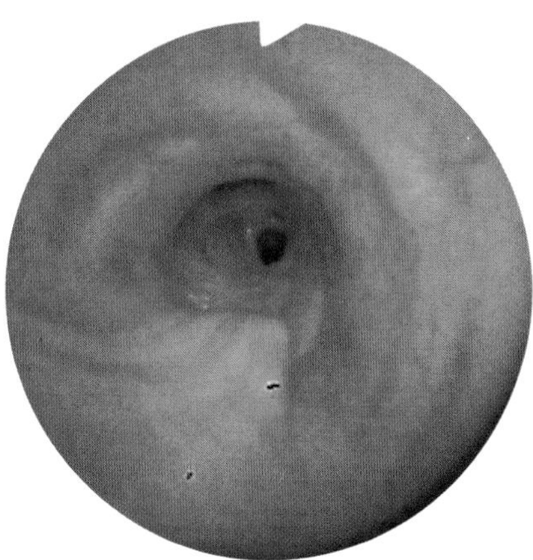

FIG. 18. Bronchoscopy just before thoracotomy for resection of an adenocarcinoma of left lower lobe revealed an unexpected cylindroma in the right bronchus intermedius. Both lesions were resected during separate procedures.

nary nodule. This approach is acceptable in most such situations. However, the possibility of a roentgenologically and clinically occult central airway malignancy with peripheral pulmonary parenchyma metastasis must be considered in all such patients. It has been shown that cancers of the central airways may remain invisible on the chest roentgenograph (53). While we do not recommend or perform routine prethoracotomy bronchoscopy in every patient with peripheral pulonary nodule, we recommend individualizing each patient regarding bronchoscopy. If a patient presents with symptoms and signs suggestive of airway pathology, then a prethoracotomy bronchoscopy is definitely indicated and indeed it may identify the primary tumor in the airway as well as help in establishing the histological type of malignancy (Fig. 18). The results of bronchoscopy may completely change the surgical plan.

Bronchoscopic Needle Biopsy vs. Mediastinoscopy

Certain aspects of bronchoscopic needle aspiration and biopsy were discussed above as well in Chapter 12. The bronchoscopists are utilizing the transbronchial needle aspiration and biopsy to establish the diagnosis of malignant and benign disease in patients with paratracheal, hilar, and mediastinal lymphadenopathy.

REFERENCES

1. Prakash UBS, Offord KP, Stubbs SE. Bronchoscopy in North America: the ACCP survey. *Chest* 1991;100:1668–1675.
2. Prakash UBS, Stubbs SE. The bronchoscopy survey: some reflections. *Chest* 1991;100:1660–1667.
3. American Board of Thoracic Surgery: Booklet of Information; Chicago; 1991:13.
4. Prakash UBS, Abel MD, Hubmayr RD. Mediastinal mass and tracheal obstruction during general anesthesia. *Mayo Clin Proc* 1988;63:1004–1011.
5. Ong GB, Lam KH, Wong J, Lim TK. Factors influencing morbidity and mortality in esophageal carcinoma. *J Thorac Cardiovasc Surg* 1978;76:745–754.
6. Little AG, Ferguson MK, DeMeester TR, Hoffman PC, Skinner DB. Esophageal carcinoma with respiratory tract fistula. *Cancer* 1984;53:1322–1328.
7. Ishihara T, Yamazaki S, Kobayashi K, et al. Resection of the trachea infiltrated by thyroid carcinoma. *Ann Surg* 1982; 195:496–500.
8. Wang KP. Transbronchial needle biopsy for histology specimens. *Chest* 1989;96:226–227.
9. Shure D. Transbronchial biopsy and needle aspiration. *Chest* 1989;95:1130–1138.
10. Shure D. Transbronchial needle aspiration—current status. *Mayo Clin Proc* 1989;64:251–254.
11. Schenk DA, Strollo PJ, Pickard JS, et al. Utility of the Wang 18-gauge transbronchial histology needle in the staging of bronchogenic carcinoma. *Chest* 1989;96:272–274.
12. Mehta AC, Curtis PS, Scalzitti ML, Meeker DP. The high price of bronchoscopy. Maintenance and repair of the flexible fiberoptic bronchoscope. *Chest* 1990;98:448–454.
13. Osinowo O, Harley HRS, Janigan D. Congenital bronchooesophageal fistula in the adult. *Thorax* 1983;38:138–142.
14. Smith BD Jr, Mikaelian DO, Cohn HE. Congenital bronchoesophageal fistula in the adult. *Ann Otol Rhinol Laryngol* 1987; 96:65–67.
15. Cole FH, Cole FH Jr, Khandekar A, Watson DC. Management of broncholithiasis: is thoracotomy necessary? *Ann Thorac Surg* 1986;42:255–257.
16. Dixon GF, Donnerberg RL, Schonfeld SA, Whitcomb ME. Advances in the diagnosis and treatment of broncholithiasis. *Am Rev Resp Dis* 1984;129(6):1028–1030.
17. Bollengier WE, Guernsey JM. Broncholithiasis with aorto-tracheal fistula. *J Thorac Cardiovasc Surg* 1974;68(4):588–592.
18. Arrigoni MG, Bernatz PE, Donoghue FE. Broncholithiasis. *J Thorac Cardiovasc Surg* 1971;62(2):231–237.
19. Lee TS, Wright BD. Tracheobronchial disruption: delayed diagnosis. *Ann Emerg Med* 1980;9:265–267.
20. Payne WS, De Remee RA. Injuries of the trachea and major bronchi. *Postgrad Med* 1971;49:152–158.
21. Travis SPL, Layer GT. Traumatic transection of the thoracic trachea. *Ann R Coll Surg Engl* 1983;65:240–241.
22. Hara KS, Prakash UBS. Fiberoptic bronchoscopy in the evaluation of acute chest and upper airway trauma. *Chest* 1989; 96:627–630.
23. Kirsh MM, Orringer MB, Behrendt DM, et al. Management of tracheobronchial disruption secondary to nonpenetrating trauma. *Ann Thorac Surg* 1976;22:93–101.
24. Flynn AE, Thomas AN, Schecter WP. Acute tracheobronchial injury. *J Trauma* 1989;29:1326–1330.
25. Roxburgh JC. Rupture of the tracheobronchial tree. *Thorax* 1987;42:681–688.
26. Choh JH, Adler RH. Penetrating bullet wound of chest with bronchoscopic removal of bullet. *J Thorac Cardiovasc Surg* 1981;82:150–153.
27. Limper AH, Prakash UBS. Tracheobronchial foreign bodies in adults. *Ann Intern Med* 1990;112:604–609.
28. Weissberg D, Schwartz I. Foreign bodies in the tracheobronchial tree. *Chest* 1987;91:730–733.
29. Stella JP, Kageler WV, Epker BN. Fiberoptic endotracheal intubation in oral and maxillofacial surgery. *J Oral Maxillofac Surg* 1986;44:923–925.
30. Santora AH, Wroe WA. Anesthetic considerations in traumatic tracheobronchial rupture. *South Med J* 1986;79:910–911.
31. Keon TP. Death on induction of anesthesia for cervical node biopsy. *Anesthesiology* 1981;55:471–472.
32. Neuman GG, Weingarten AE, Abramowitz RM, et al. The anesthetic management of the patient with an anterior mediastinal mass. *Anesthesiology* 1984;60:144–147.
33. Piro AJ, Weiss DR, Hellman S. Mediastinal Hodgkin's disease: a possible danger for intubation anesthesia. *Int J Radiat Oncol Biol Phys* 1976;1:415–419.

34. Younker D, Clark R, Coveler L. Fiberoptic endobronchial intubation for resection of an anterior mediastinal mass. *Anesthesiology* 1989;70:144–146.
35. Mustard WT, Bayliss CE, Fearson B, Pelton D, Trusler GA. Tracheal compression by the innominate artery in children. *Ann Thorac Surg* 1969;8:312–319.
36. Dark JH, Sethia B, Pollock JCS. Tracheal resection in an infant with double aortic arch and associated tracheomalacia. *Thorax* 1983;38:798–799.
37. Holman WL, Vaezy A, Postlethwait RW, Bridgman A. Surgical treatment of H-type tracheoesophageal fistula diagnosed in an adult. *Ann Thorac Surg* 1986;41:453–454.
38. Gans SL, Johnson RO. Diagnosis and surgical management of "H-type" tracheoesophageal fistula in infants and children. *J Pediatr Surg* 1977;12:233–236.
39. Payne DK, Anderson WMD, Romero MD, Wissing DR, Fowler M. Tracheoesophageal fistula formation in intubated patients. *Chest* 1990;98:161–164.
40. Shure D: Endobronchial suture. A foreign body causing chronic cough. *Chest* 1991;100:1193–1196.
41. Waclawiczek HW, Chmelizek F, Koller I: Endoscopic sealing of infected bronchus stump fistulae with fibrin following lung resections. Experimental and clinical experience. *Surg Endosc* 1987;1:99–102.
42. Chowdhury JK. Percutaneous use of fiberoptic bronchoscope to investigate bronchopleurocutaneous fistula. *Chest* 1979; 75:203–204.
43. Baldwin JC, Jamieson SW, Oyer PE, et al. Bronchoscopy after cardiopulmonary transplantation. *J Thorac Cardiovasc Surg* 1985;89:1–7.
44. Higenbottam T, Stewart S, Penketh A, Wallwork J. The diagnosis of lung rejection and opportunistic infection by transbronchial lung biopsy. *Transplant Proc* 1987;19:3777–3778.
45. Higenbottam T, Stewart S, Penketh A, Wallwork J. Transbronchial lung biopsy for the diagnosis of rejection in heart–lung transplant patients. *Transplantation* 1988;46:532–539.
46. Stableforth DE, Knight RK, Collins JV, et al. Transbronchial lung biopsy through the fibreoptic bronchoscope. *Br J Dis Chest* 1978;72:108–114.
47. Poe RH, Utell MJ, Israel RH, et al. Sensitivity and specificity of the nonspecific transbronchial lung biopsy. *Am Rev Resp Dis* 1979;119:25–31.
48. Prakash UBS, Stubbs SE. The bronchoscopy survey: some reflections. *Chest* 1991;100:1660–1667.
49. Mathur P, Martin WJ II. Clinical utility of thoracoscopy. *Chest* 1992;102:2–4.
50. Lewis RJ, Caccavale RJ, Sisler GE. Imaged thoracoscopic lung biopsy. *Chest* 1992;102:60–62.
51. Menzies R, Charbonneau M. Thoracoscopy for the diagnosis of pleural disease. *Ann Intern Med* 1991;114:271–276.
52. Mathisen DJ. Don't get run over by the bandwagon. *Chest* 1992; 102:4–5.
53. Shure D. Radiologically occult endobronchial obstruction in bronchogenic carcinoma. *Am J Med* 1991;91:19–22.

Bronchoscopy,
edited by U. B. S. Prakash.
Mayo Foundation © 1994.
Published by Raven Press, Ltd., New York.

CHAPTER 23

Pediatric Rigid Bronchoscopy

Udaya B. S. Prakash and Lauren D. Holinger

Bronchoscopy is performed far less frequently in children than in adults. Airway problems in children that require bronchoscopy are usually congenital or inflammatory or are caused by a tracheobronchial foreign body. The miniature anatomy is more likely to produce acute respiratory distress in children than in adults. The glottis of the newborn has an anteroposterior dimension of 7 mm and posterior transverse dimension of 4 mm. Mucosal edema of 1 mm will reduce the airway lumen to 35% of normal (1–3). The larynx is placed more anteriorly and cephalad, being opposite the third cervical vertebra as opposed to the fourth cervical vertebra in adults. The epiglottis may have a variety of shapes and sizes in normal infants. Additionally, the larynx and thyroid cartilage are more acutely funnel shaped with the cricoid diameter definitely less than the diameter of the glottis. All of these factors make it rather difficult for the bronchoscopist to manipulate the instruments in a confined space.

For the greater part of this past century, bronchoscopies in pediatric patients have utilized the rigid bronchoscope. The diagnostic and therapeutic aspects of the diseases of the tracheobronchial tree in pediatric patients has traditionally depended on the rigid bronchoscope. Even though the introduction, in the mid-1970s, of the smaller diameter flexible bronchoscope to examine the pediatric airways has further contributed to the diagnosis and treatment of diseases in the pediatric population, the pediatric rigid bronchoscope remains an indispensable tool. Prior to the introduction of the pediatric flexible bronchoscope, pediatric bronchoscopy was practiced by surgeons and a few pulmonary specialists. The survey of 871 bronchoscopists, all specializing in adult pulmonary diseases, conducted by the American College of Chest Physicians in 1989 disclosed that pediatric bronchoscopy was practiced by only 13.2% of the respondents. When asked which specialist performed pediatric bronchoscopy in their clinical setting, 14.5% of the survey participants reported that the otolaryngologist performed the procedure, whereas pediatric pulmonary specialist and pediatric surgeon were identified by 12 and 3.1%, respectively (4). The survey suggests that the adult pulmonary specialist has very little exposure to pediatric bronchoscopy.

In view of the widespread use of the flexible bronchoscope in pediatric pulmonology, one is tempted to ask the question, "Is there a role for the rigid bronchoscope in pediatric patients?" A review of 364 rigid bronchoscopies in children (55% were younger than 3 years old) reported that 30–40% of the procedures could have been undertaken with a flexible bronchoscope (5). However, the advantages of the flexible instrument were more evident in children with diseases of the upper airways than in those with parenchymal lung disease.

The superiority of the rigid bronchoscope in the management of tracheobronchial foreign bodies (6–9), dilatation of tracheobronchial strictures, placement of airway stents (10–14), control of massive hemoptysis (15,16), and execution of laser procedures (17–21) is well authenticated. Even though general anesthesia or deep intravenous sedation is required in most cases, rigid bronchoscopy is as safe as flexible bronchoscopy in experienced hands. The current state of bronchoscopy practice reveals that the increasing role of the rigid bronchoscope in the clinical situations outlined above has proven wrong the earlier assertions that the flexible bronchoscope will eventually replace the rigid instrument (22,23). The flexible bronchoscope and the rigid bronchoscope should complement, not compete with, each other (21). In fact, many bronchoscopists who are trained in both techniques prefer to use a com-

U. B. S. Prakash: Division of Thoracic Diseases and Internal Medicine, Rochester, Minnesota 55905.
L. D. Holinger: Department of Pediatric Otorhinolaryngology, Children's Memorial Hospital, Chicago, Illinois 60614.

bination technique of rigid and flexible bronchoscopy. After inspection of the larynx and trachea with the rigid instrument, the flexible bronchoscope can be introduced through the rigid bronchoscope to examine the distal bronchial tree (24).

Because of the structuring of the training programs, the otorhinolaryngologist is more likely to use rigid bronchoscopy whereas the pediatric pulmonary specialist almost exclusively uses the flexible bronchoscope. This reflects the traditional use of the rigid bronchoscope by surgeons (25). A British survey (26) reported that although only 2% of 39,564 bronchoscopies performed between 1974 and 1986 employed the rigid instrument, more than 90% of the rigid bronchoscopies were done by surgeons. With the increasing number of physicians being trained in pediatric pulmonology and flexible bronchoscopy, there exists the possibility of diminishing the exposure of physicians to the rigid bronchoscopic procedures. We emphasize that ideally a pediatric bronchoscopist should be able to use both flexible and rigid bronchoscopes. In spite of the popularity of the pediatric flexible bronchoscope, there are several areas where the rigid bronchoscope has definitive advantages. The role of the flexible bronchoscope and the advantages and disadvantages of the rigid and flexible bronchoscopes in pediatric pulmonary diseases is discussed in Chapter 24. For detailed discussions on the preoperative preparation, medications, and anesthesia for pediatric bronchoscopy, the reader is referred to Chapter 7. In this chapter, we discuss the instrumentation, the indications for rigid bronchoscopy, and the most commonly used techniques.

ADVANTAGES AND DISADVANTAGES

Advantages

The use of the rigid bronchoscope permits excellent control of the airway, the ability to provide general or topical anesthesia, and the use of a wide range of instruments for almost any type of endobronchial manipulation. The most important advantages are that the relatively large internal diameter of the instrument allows the use of auxiliary equipment for extraction of foreign bodies and the fact that the airway is controlled (the rigid bronchoscope is, in essence, a metal endotracheal tube). These are not inconsequential advantages. There is a wide variety of bronchoscopic instrumentation—forceps, baskets, various grasping devices, etc.—available for extraction of foreign bodies and tissue masses. Since such procedures should be undertaken in all but the most unusual circumstances under general anesthesia, control of the airway is an essential part of the technique. The large internal diameter of the rigid bronchoscope allows simultaneous ventilation and manipulation of instruments beyond the distal end of the bronchoscope. However, these instruments (and the glass rod telescope) partially obstruct the airway, and caution is always in order.

Because the airway is controlled, general anesthesia and even complete muscle relaxation are possible. During delicate manipulation of the distal airways (as during biopsy or foreign body extraction), coughing or unexpected movement could have drastic consequences. In the early years of pediatric bronchoscopy, general anesthesia was considerably more risky than with modern agents and techniques, and most procedures were done with sedation and topical anesthesia. Today, there is general agreement that general anesthesia should be employed, as it is safe, effective, and humane, and facilitates rapid completion of the procedure.

Another relative advantage of rigid bronchoscopy is that such procedures are usually performed in the operating room, where every conceivable complication can readily be managed. If bronchoscopy is done in a facility that is not fully staffed and equipped, complications may not be managed as effectively or expeditiously as in the operating room (Fig 1).

The ability to extract foreign bodies from the airways, effect dilatation of tracheobronchial strictures, biopsy endobronchial lesions, and use laser therapy via the bronchoscope is better accomplished with the rigid bronchoscope than with its flexible counterpart. The capacity to suction thick respiratory secretions, mucous plugs, and large amounts of blood from the tracheobronchial tree is also much better with the rigid bronchoscope. Even though the frequency of bronchography has considerably diminished in the recent years, as result of the availability of high-resolution computed tomography of chest, rigid bronchoscopy permits easy instillation of radiocontrast medium and its removal after the bronchograms are obtained. The quality of the optical image obtained with a rigid bronchoscope equipped with a glass rod telescope is unsurpassed and is superior to the image obtained with a flexible bronchoscope.

The cost of rigid instruments is often noted to be lower than that of flexible bronchoscopes. However, this is a slippery issue, since a much greater number of rigid instruments must be purchased in order to have a complete capability. While a flexible bronchoscope costs between $8,000 and $10,000, a rigid bronchoscope costs only a few hundred dollars. However, each glass rod telescope costs several thousand dollars and, like flexible bronchoscopes, is fragile. In order to adequately equip a bronchoscopy facility, one would need a number of telescopes of different lengths, with different viewing angles at the tip. Therefore, the cost may in fact equal if not exceed that for flexible bronchoscopes.

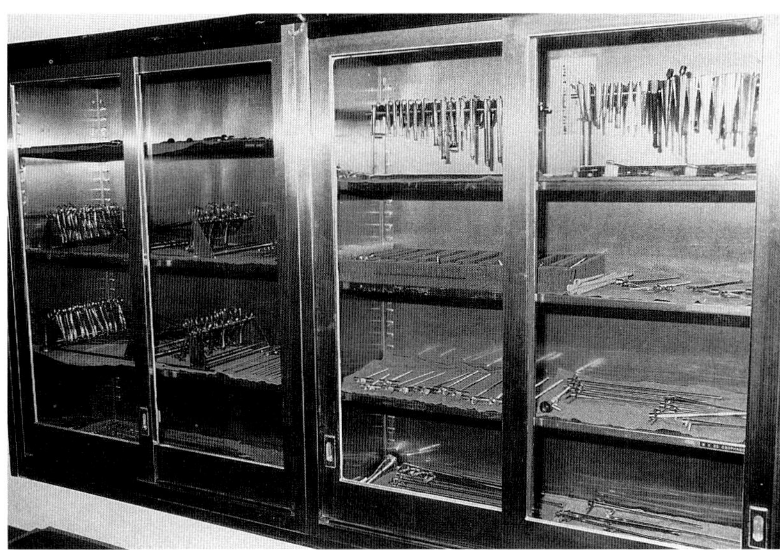

FIG. 1. The well-equipped endoscopic operating room facility is organized so that endoscopic instruments are readily available and easily identified. In the endoscopic suite at the Children's Memorial Hospital in Chicago, instruments are sterilized before being placed in these glass cabinets, where they can be quickly located and retrieved.

Finally, some proponents of rigid bronchoscopy assert that almost anything that can be done with a flexible bronchoscope can be done with a rigid one, thus making flexible instruments an unnecessary part of the bronchoscopist's armamentarium.

Disadvantages

Among the several arguments against the routine use of rigid instruments in pediatric patients, the one most commonly cited is the need for general anesthesia. While the absolute magnitude of the risk of general anesthesia is very small, there is some risk. It clearly adds to the expense of the procedure. The perception of an increased risk associated with general anesthesia undoubtedly contributes to a reluctance on the part of at least some physicians to refer their patients for bronchoscopy, especially if only rigid instrumentation is available in the institution. On the other hand, there are some aspects of general anesthesia for bronchoscopy that are potential pitfalls. Unless care is taken to observe the larynx prior to the introduction of general anesthesia, vocal cord movement cannot be accurately assessed. Likewise, airway dynamics are quite different during anesthesia and positive pressure ventilation (especially if muscular relaxation is used) compared to spontaneous breathing. Since dynamic airway changes of real significance (i.e., bronchomalacia, tracheomalacia) can be missed, most procedures are done with spontaneous respiration. With appropriate training, however, all of these problems can be properly addressed.

Another potential problem with rigid instrumentation is that repeated use of rigid instruments may pose a greater risk of trauma to the airway. While part of this increased risk is associated with the fact that rigid instruments are more likely to be used in high-risk patients (i.e., those with foreign bodies or major airway obstruction), there is also the fact that the larger diameter of the rigid bronchoscope can result in subglottic trauma. Indeed, subglottic edema is usually not a clinical problem and is usually not considered a complication. Selection of an appropriate size bronchoscope and careful manipulation of the upper airway minimizes laryngeal edema.

The rigid bronchoscope, being of relatively large diameter, cannot be passed into the distal airways. Glass rod telescopes (including some devices that utilize the telescope, such as the "optical forceps") can be extended beyond the tip of the bronchoscope and into some of the lower bronchi, but the peripheral range of these instruments is less than that of flexible bronchoscopes. On the other hand, in children, at least, examination of the airways distal to the segmental bronchi is not often necessary, since almost all significant pathology is found in the large airways. Rigid bronchoscopes sometimes cannot be passed beyond an area of stenosis to examine, for example, the airways distal to a congenital tracheal stenosis. The telescope alone may be advanced ahead of a short tracheoscope.

Light normally travels in straight lines, and a 0° rod-lens telescope does not readily allow visualization of the upper lobe bronchi. Telescopes with angled lenses facilitate examination of the upper reaches of the airways. Since most foreign bodies lodge in the central airways or the lower/middle lobe orifices, where they are readily accessible, the inability to reach into the upper lobes is only a minor limitation (5).

Bronchoalveolar lavage has become an increasingly

important part of diagnostic bronchoscopy. This technique mandates the placement of a catheter into a "wedge" position in order to flush the saline into the distal airways (and, more importantly, to get most of it out again). While this can surely be done with a rigid bronchoscope, a flexible bronchoscope is usually used through the rigid tube. Bronchoalveolar lavage is not a specific indication for rigid bronchoscopy under most circumstances.

INSTRUMENTATION

The basic concept of the rigid pediatric bronchoscope has changed little since the turn of the century. The rigid bronchoscope is an open tube (as small as 2.5 mm internal diameter) (Fig. 2) equipped with a wide range of telescopes. To provide excellent optics, the Storz–Hopkins telescopes are available in a variety of sizes with the smallest diameter of 2.5 mm (external diameter), and with a variety of prisms (30°, 70°, etc.) to provide visualization of upper lobe and superior segmental bronchi.

The diameters and the lengths of the tracheobronchial tree are dependent on the age of patients in the pediatric population (Chapter 7). The bronchoscopist has at her or his disposal a wide range of rigid bronchoscopes in various lengths and sizes. The basic design of the instrument is similar except for the decreased diameters and lengths of the bronchoscopes, telescopes, and ancillary instruments such as rod-lenses, forceps, and suction tubes. Standard anesthesia attachments for ventilation are identical to adult rigid bronchoscopes. The bronchoscopist who intends to practice pediatric rigid bronchoscopy is well advised to have available a full range of laryngoscopes, forceps (Fig. 3), and suction catheters (Fig. 4) that can be used in patients of different sizes and ages. In many of the clinical conditions discussed below, the bronchoscopist may use either a rigid laryngoscope, a tracheoscope, or a bronchoscope, depending on the location of the abnormality and the treatment planned.

Bronchoscopes may have proximal illumination as with the Storz system. A prismatic light deflector shines light down the length of the bronchoscope but partially occludes the proximal end. In other systems, such as the bronchoscopes manufactured by Pilling, a light carrier provides distal illumination. This eliminates the distracting reflection of light within the tube itself and the proximal obstruction of the prism.

Either system is commonly used with rod-lens telescopes, which provide excellent illumination, magnification, and depth of field. Visualization far exceeds that obtained by any other means. Rod-lens telescopes are standard for use in pediatric rigid bronchoscopy.

Tracheoscopes are short bronchoscopes without ventilating holes in the side through which longer, small-diameter telescopes can be extended through stenoses and into distal bronchial segments. Using a similar technique with anesthesia by insufflation, telescopes may be used without bronchoscopes through a laryngoscope to examine the larynx, trachea, and bronchi. This technique is particularly effective for examination of the distal airways when a proximal narrowing precludes passage of the bronchoscope itself (Fig. 5).

A wide variety of forceps are available for use through the rigid bronchoscopes. Passive action forceps are of four basic types: (a) forward-grasping forceps, which include peanut forceps; (b) rotation forceps, which allow a sharp object to rotate or tumble so that it can be withdrawn with the point trailing; (c)

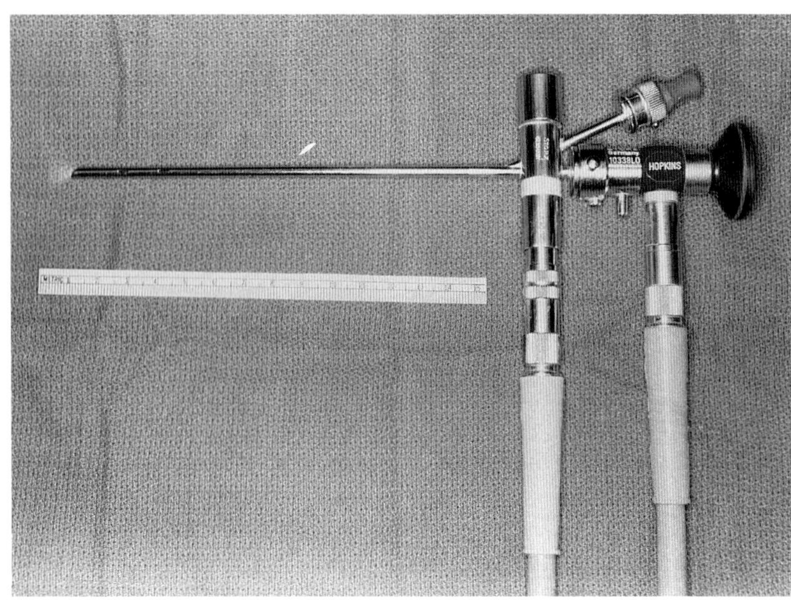

FIG. 2. 2.5 mm × 20 cm rigid bronchoscope with telescope.

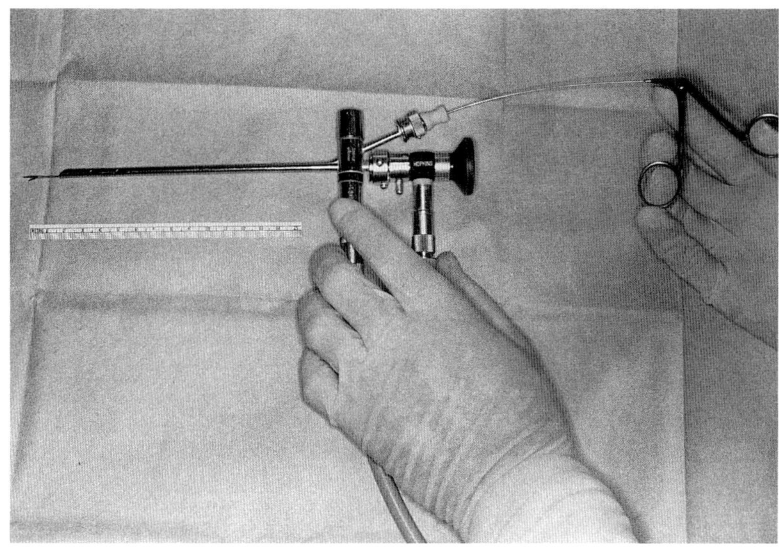

FIG. 3. 3.5 mm × 20 cm rigid bronchoscope with flexible alligator forceps passed through the side channel and into the lumen next to the telescope. This permits close observation of manipulation with the forceps.

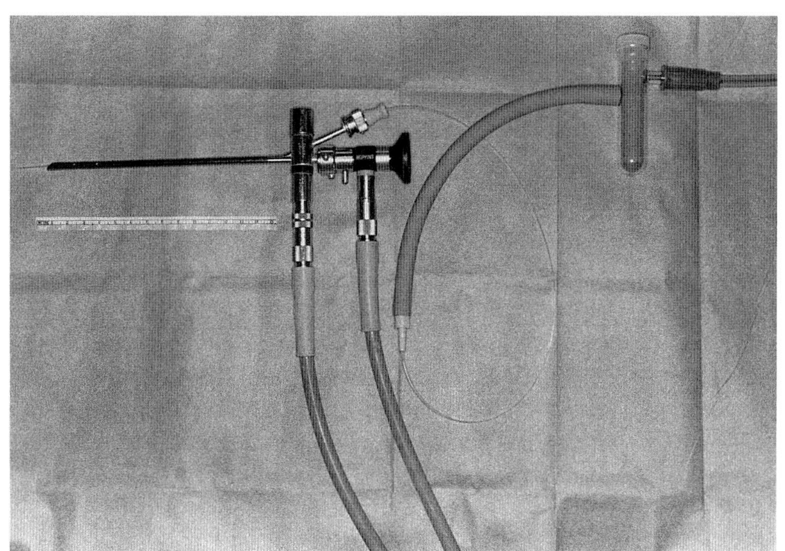

FIG. 4. Flexible suction catheter passed through the side channel of the bronchoscope. The suction catheter can be directed into segmental and subsegmental bronchi for aspiration of secretions, clearing the bronchi and obtaining samples for analysis.

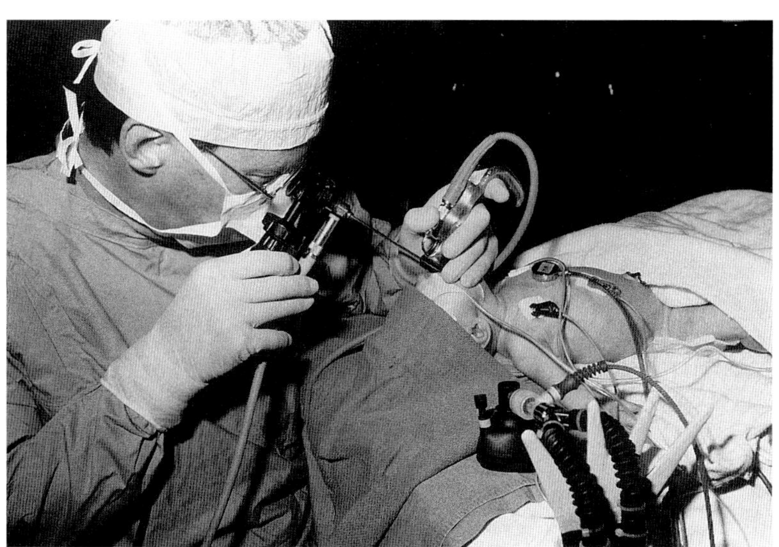

FIG. 5. Bronchoscopy without the bronchoscope! Using this insufflation technique the telescope (with video camera attached) is passed through the laryngoscope and larynx to visualize the tracheobronchial tree. The infant breathes spontaneously during the procedure. Oxygen and halothane is administered through a catheter that passes through the right nostril to the level of the tip of the epiglottis.

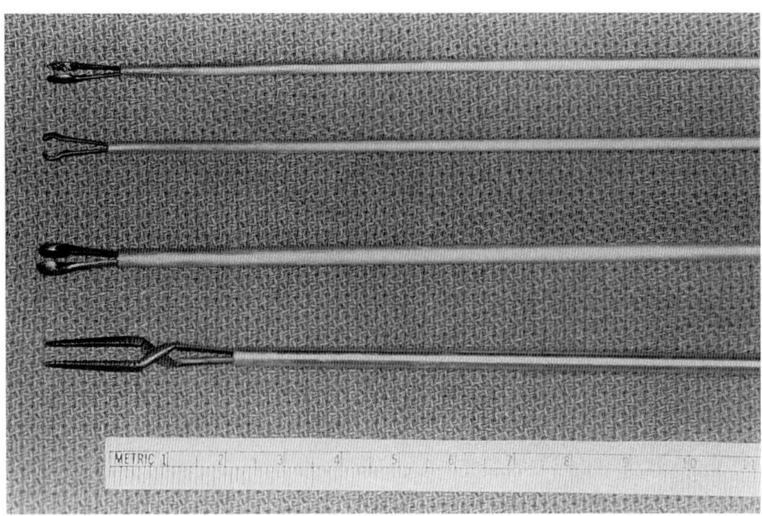

FIG. 6. Four types of passive action forceps, from top to bottom: (1) forward-grasping forceps; (2) rotation forceps; (3) globular object or ball bearing forceps; (4) hollow object forceps.

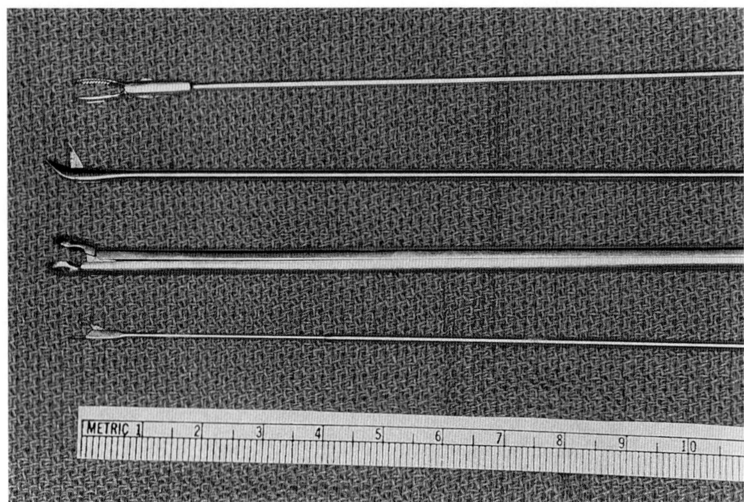

FIG. 7. Positive action forceps from top to bottom: (1) foreign body forceps (peanut type); (2) scissors; (3) medium-sized cupped biopsy forceps; (4) microforceps (biopsy).

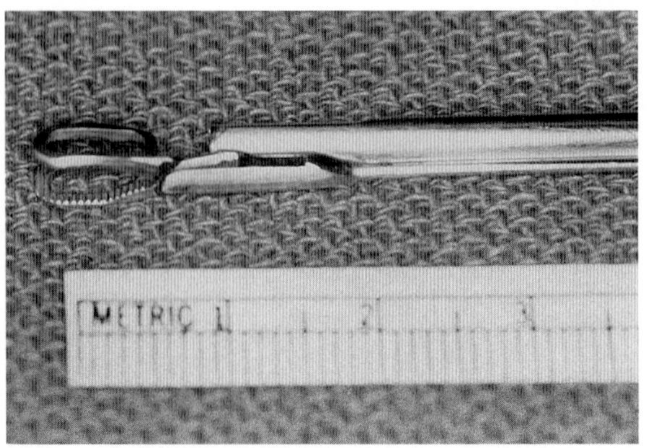

FIG. 8. Tip of the optical forceps (peanut), a center action forceps with the advantages of illumination and vision of the rod-lens telescope.

globular object or ball-bearing forceps, which can also be used for biopsy forceps; and (d) hollow object forceps, used to extract a rivet or .22 shell casing that may lodge in a bronchus so tightly that operating space for forceps cannot be developed between the outside of the object and the bronchial wall (Fig. 6).

Center action forceps (also called positive action forceps because they can be used positively to open the blades to dilate the wall of the bronchus) are manufactured as alligator forceps, scissors, cupped (biopsy) forceps, and microforceps (biopsy) (Fig. 7). Optical forceps combine the rod-lens telescope with a center action forceps for biopsy and foreign body extraction (Fig. 8).

INDICATIONS FOR BRONCHOSCOPY

Since the indications for the flexible and rigid bronchoscopy are similar, this chapter will discuss indications for both instruments. The indications can be broadly classified into diagnostic and therapeutic bronchoscopies (Tables 1 and 2). Frequently, both are simultaneously indicated. For example, in patients with suspected tracheobronchial foreign body, it is common to begin the procedure as a diagnostic bronchoscopy and, if a foreign body is identified, to immediately proceed with therapeutic bronchoscopy. Overall, the number of therapeutic and diagnostic indications for pediatric bronchoscopy are fewer than in adults. The most common indication in a newborn infant is the presence of stridor originating in the upper airways. Respiratory distress of unexplained etiology, suspected laryngomalacia, failure of a lung or a lobe to fully expand and aerate, and suspicion of congenital defects of the tracheobronchial tree, including tracheoesophageal fistula, are some of the commoner indications. In otherwise healthy toddlers and older children, acute onset of upper airway noises, persistent cough, and wheezing suggest the possibility of foreign body in the tracheobronchial tree. While acute infectious processes of the upper respiratory tract such as epiglottitis, tracheobronchitis, and other infections of the upper airway also produce symptoms similar to those elicited by foreign body, the onset of symptoms is rather subacute and most children respond rapidly to appropriate treatment. Causes of airway obstruction in children are listed in Table 3.

TABLE 1. *Indications for diagnostic bronchoscopy*

Persistent unexplained cough or wheeze
Unexplained stridor or dyspnea
Suspected congenital anomalies
Hemoptysis (Chapter 17)
Recurrent infections of airway or lungs (Chapters 13 and 14)
Persistent abnormality of chest roentgenograph
Atelectatic lung, lobe, or segment
Diagnostic bronchoalveolar lavage (Chapters 13 and 14)
Suspected tracheoesophageal or bronchoesophageal fistula (Chapters 16 and 22)
Mediastinal neoplasm (Chapter 22)
Chemical or thermal burns of the tracheobronchial tree
Foreign bodies in the tracheobronchial tree (Chapter 18)
Tracheobronchial strictures and stenoses (Chapter 21)
Lung abscess
Assessment of endotracheal tube placement (Chapter 16)
After airway reconstruction
Prior to bronchography
Thoracic trauma
Miscellaneous

TABLE 2. *Indications for therapeutic bronchoscopy*[a]

Retained secretions, mucous plugs, clots
Necrotic tracheobronchial mucosa
Foreign bodies in the tracheobronchial tree (Chapter 18)
Hemoptysis (Chapter 17)
Obstructing neoplasms (Chapters 19–21)
Strictures and stenoses (Chapter 21)
Bronchogenic cysts (drainage)
Mediastinal lesions
Endotracheal tube placement and replacement
After airway reconstruction (Chapter 22)
Cystic fibrosis
Asthma
Thoracic trauma

[a] Unless specified in parentheses, see Chapters 16 and 24 for other indications for therapeutic bronchoscopy.

TABLE 3. *Causes of airway obstruction in pediatric patients*

Congenital
Congenital subglottic stenosis
Congenital tracheal stenosis
Tracheomalacia, bronchomalacia
Vocal cord paralysis
Extrinsic compression
• Vascular
• Foregut cysts
Acquired
Laryngotracheobronchitis
• Membranous tracheitis
Acute supraglottitis (epiglottitis)
Foreign body
Trauma, internal and external
• Laryngotracheal stenosis

Children who are immunocompromised as a result of congenital or acquired immunodeficiency diseases, malignancies, chemotherapy, malnutrition, or systemic illnesses are prone to develop opportunistic infections, drug toxicity, and other complications peculiar to this group of patients. Bronchoalveolar lavage and/or bronchoscopic lung biopsy can be performed via either flexible or rigid bronchoscope to obtain respiratory secretions and lung tissue.

SPECIAL INDICATIONS FOR RIGID BRONCHOSCOPY

It is obvious from a review of the literature that many bronchoscopists routinely use rigid bronchoscope for all pediatric bronchoscopies. This may be the result of training or of the unavailability of a flexible instrument. In a report on 468 children who required bronchoscopy and in whom all procedures were performed with the rigid instrument and general anesthesia, the age groups of children were as follows: less than 12 months old, 14%; between 1 and 3 years, 39%; over 3 years, 47%; and over 12 years, 4%. In another retrospective report on 1,032 bronchoscopies in 748 children, it was evident that almost all procedures utilized the rigid bronchoscope (26). Among these children, 27.4% were under 6 months of age and the smallest patient weighed 600 g. All the bronchoscopies were performed under general anesthesia, except for a few laryngoscopies performed with a flexible bronchoscope. The most common indications for bronchoscopy were suspected foreign body (16.7%), stridor (14.5%), recurrent respiratory infections (12.3%), and dyspnea (9.6%). Bronchoscopic findings included laryngomalacia (13.8%), subglottic stenosis (7.0%), tracheal compression (10.8%), and tracheal stenosis (2.5%). Bronchoscopy was completely normal in 10.6%.

Tracheobronchial Foreign Body

One of the most common indications for rigid bronchoscopy in pediatric practice is the suspicion of a foreign body in the tracheobronchial tree. Even though other techniques utilizing the flexible bronchoscope, Fogarty catheter, and wire baskets have been used to extract trachebronchial foreign bodies (27,28), we feel that the rigid bronchoscope provides the safest and fastest means to remove the tracheobronchial foreign body (Figs. 9 and 10). There are many ancillary instruments to extract almost any kind of foreign body via the rigid bronchoscope. The diagnosis and treatment of tracheobronchial foreign body is discussed in detail in Chapter 18.

Bronchoscopic Lung Biopsy

The narrow working channel of the flexible bronchoscope allows collection of bronchoalveolar lavage effluent. The same narrow channel, however, makes it impossible to obtain bronchoscopic lung biopsy in smaller children. If a bronchoscopic lung biopsy is required in a small child, the rigid bronchoscope will provide a large channel for the lung biopsy forceps. There are very few papers published on the role of bronchoscopic lung biopsy in pediatric patients (29,30). One report reviewed a 2-year experience in 12 patients (median age, 14.5 years) who underwent bronchoscopic lung biopsy (29). In all 12 patients, the indication for bronchoscopic lung biopsy was a persistently abnormal chest roentgenogram (nine with multiobar infiltrates, two with unilateral infiltrates, and one with a cavitary lesion). Overall, a specific diagnosis was made by bronchoscopic lung biopsy in six patients, including three patients with sarcoidosis, one with lymphoma, and two with eosinophilic granuloma. In three additional patients, nonspecific histological findings on bronchoscopic lung biopsy combined with clinical findings, roentgenographic patterns, and supplemental laboratory data helped support a diagnosis. Fluoroscopic guidance can be used to obtain optimal samples. The technique used is similar to that in adults, as discussed in Chapter 11.

Tracheobronchial Stricture and Stenosis

Congenital webs and stenoses are not uncommon in infants. Acquired laryngotracheal stenosis in children continues to be a problem due to internal laryngeal trauma following the widespread adoption of prolonged endotracheal intubation for respiratory support (31). Less common causes of stenosis secondary to congenital anomalies, external trauma, high tracheot-

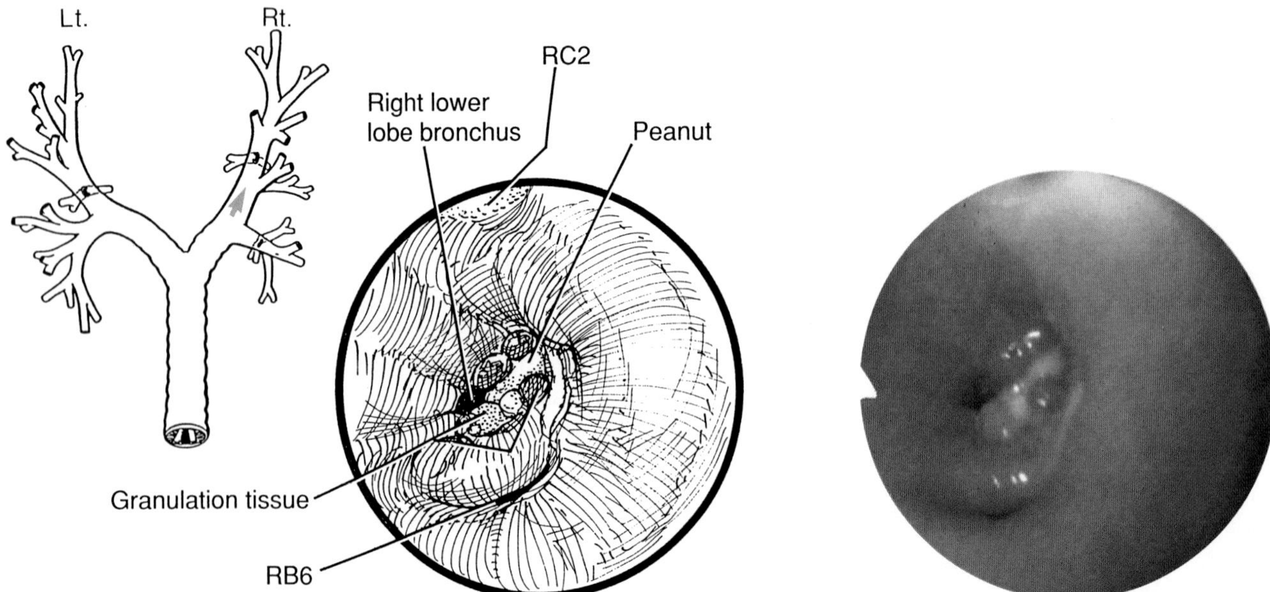

FIG. 9. The effects of subacute retention of foreign body (peanut) in the right lower lobe bronchus of a child. The intense edema and formation of granulation tissue proximal to the foreign body necessitated the use of rigid bronchoscope for successful extraction.

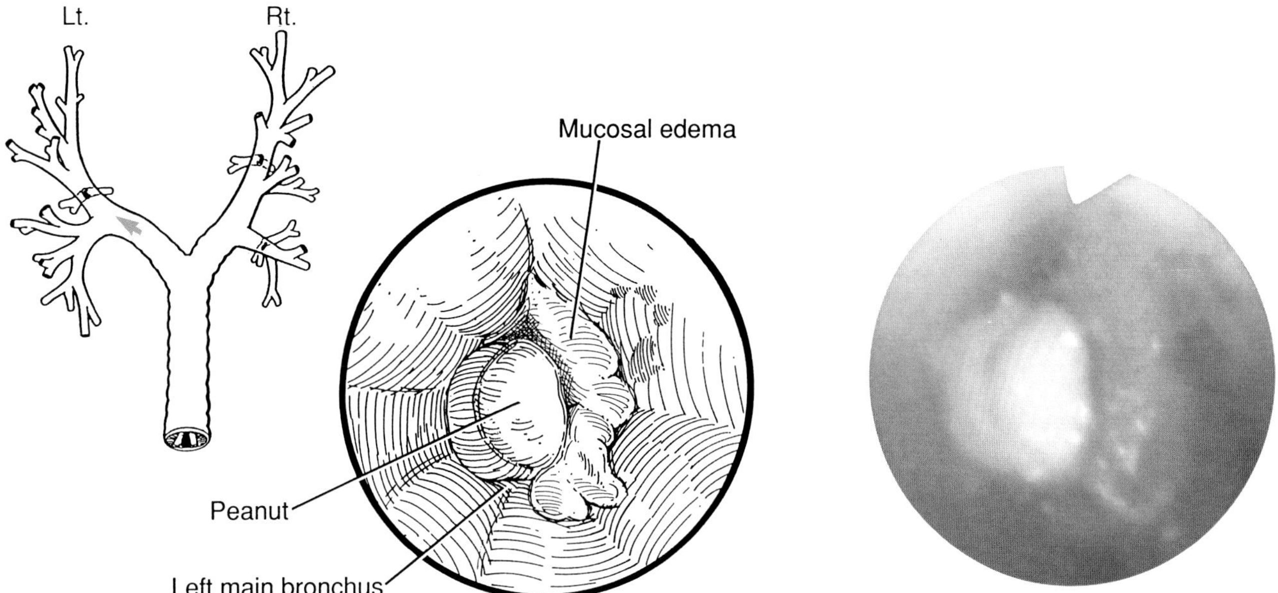

FIG. 10. A foreign body (peanut) in the distal left main stem bronchus. Attempts at flexible bronchoscopic removal using a balloon catheter were unsuccessful. The child was referred for rigid bronchoscopic removal that was accomplished within 5-min.

omy, thermal and chemical burns, and dystrophic cartilage are also seen. Therapy for these difficult problems includes bronchoscopic and surgical treatment. Therapeutic dilatation of tracheobronchial stricture and stenosis can be easily accomplished with a rigid bronchoscope. In one report on 1,607 intubated neonates, low tracheal stenosis was seen in 0.4%. In six cases of acute obstruction, diagnostic bronchoscopy was used to relieve the stenosis by forcefully dilating the trachea (32). The rigid bronchoscope itself can be used as a dilator. Beginning with smaller caliber rigid bronchoscope, the tight stricture can be gradually dilated by using larger caliber instruments. More distal strictures may not be amenable to rigid bronchoscopic dilatation. In such cases, a balloon can be passed through the rigid bronchoscope and inflated at the site of the stenosis to dilate the stricture (33). This type of treatment with a flexible bronchoscope is not possible in pediatric patients.

In addition to dilatation, management of strictures and stenoses may include injection of steroids through the rigid bronchoscope. A fine esophageal varices needle is used to inject triamcinolone 40 mg/ml. This may be used in conjunction with dilatation, laser (discussed below), and/or placement of a stent (discussed below).

Acquired strictures are often associated with granulation tissue. The tip of the bronchoscope may be used to remove these with a coring or shearing technique after which the granuloma is removed with the tip of a suction tube. The CO_2 laser or cupped forceps may also be used to remove granulation tissue.

Occasionally it is necessary to remove sutures that are placed with tracheal resections and sleeve resections. The knot of the suture may rotate into the lumen producing granulation tissue and restenosis. Small scissors, a blade, or forceps may be used through the rigid bronchoscope to remove the sutures.

Laser Bronchoscopy

Most airway tumors in infants and children are benign. Recurrent respiratory papillomatosis is the most common benign tumor of the larynx. Extension to trachea and proximal bronchi occurs in 5–20% of patients (34). The use of a CO_2 laser in the treatment of this disorder is well known (34). Photodynamic therapy using dihematoporphyrin ether in laryngotracheobronchial papillomatosis has been described (35).

Malignant tumors of the tracheobronchial tree are rare in children. When seen, the tumors have been bronchial carcinoid and mucoepidermoid carcinoma of the bronchus (36–39). Presenting symptoms of these rare childhood tumors are chronic cough, hemoptysis, repeated bouts of pulmonary infection, and chest pain. Bronchoscopic examination should be considered in patients with these symptoms and is highly reliable in diagnosing these tumors. The role of rigid bronchoscopy in such instances is to obtain biopsy and, in some cases, to establish an airway in an emergency. Rigid bronchoscopic removal of tracheal cylindromas and similar tumors has been reported. Surgical resection is the treatment of choice. Bronchial carcinoid and mucoepidermoid carcinoma have an excellent prognosis following conservative surgical resection.

The more likely use for the rigid bronchoscopic laser

therapy is the presence of tracheobronchial papillomas. These benign neoplasms are more common in children than in adults. Various types of treatment have been reported in the literature. Favorable results have been achieved by careful, frequent removal of papillomas using forceps, the cryoprobe, or the CO_2 laser (40). The rigid bronchoscope with CO_2 laser permits precise tissue excision and ablation in the treatment of congenital and acquired lesions of the pediatric airway (41).

Tracheobronchial Stents

Another treatment option to treat tracheobronchial stenoses is the long-term insertion and placement of a stent through the narrowed segment of the airway. Insertion and proper placement of tracheal and bronchial stents is best accomplished with the rigid instrument. This therapeutic modality is relatively new, even in adults, and long-term results and complications are not yet discernible.

Mucous Plugs

Expectoration of large, branching bronchial casts, termed *plastic bronchitis,* also known as *fibrinous bronchitis* or *pseudomembranous bronchitis,* is an uncommon condition in children. These extremely thick mucous plugs may produce segmental or lobar atelectasis. Plastic bronchitis has been described in over 40 cases (42). Plastic bronchitis may complicate many diseases including cystic fibrosis, asthma, bronchitis, allergic bronchopulmonary aspergillosis, bronchocentric granulomatosis, congenital tricuspid atresia, and chronic pericardial and pleural effusions (43,44). Idiopathic cases of plastic bronchitis have been described (44). In most cases of bronchial casts, the diagnosis is usually made at bronchoscopy because the clinical picture is not dissimilar from that of tracheobronchial foreign bodies. Chest roentgenographic findings during periods of cast formation may include atelectasis, obstructive emphysema, bronchiectasis, pleural effusion, and pneumomediastinum. Most patients may not be able to expectorate the tenacious casts with medical management alone. In small children, the working channel of the flexible bronchoscope is not capable of removing thick mucous plugs. Removal of such endobronchial matter can be easily achieved with a rigid bronchoscope. Even when the mucous plugs are located in the upper lobe bronchi, special J-shaped catheters can be used through the rigid bronchoscope (45). Postbronchoscopy treatment should include chest physiotherapy with nebulized bronchodilator and acetylcysteine, and an evaluation to determine the underlying etiology.

Management of Severe Upper Airway Obstruction

The rigid bronchoscope is an open tube and therefore most able to establish a temporary airway in an emergency. This may be helpful in laryngospasm, which can occur any time during a laryngoscopic or bronchoscopic procedure, particularly when the patient's anesthesia is too light or the laryngeal topical anesthesia is inadequate.

Acute laryngeal or tracheal infectious processes may require emergent intervention to establish an airway. In cases of acute supraglottitis (acute epiglottitis), severe croup, and bacterial tracheitis, an airway can be initially established with the rigid bronchoscope. Secretions are aspirated and the airway cleared prior to placing a nasotracheal tube that remains in place until the acute inflammation and edema subside and the airway recovers adequate patency. In cases of bacterial tracheitis (membranous croup), aspiration of thick tenacious mucous secretions and crusts may obviate the need for intubation.

Internal laryngeal trauma (as most often occurs following intubation injury) and external laryngeal trauma with laryngeal fracture, edema, and hematoma may produce acute airway obstruction. A temporary airway may be established with the rigid bronchoscope until careful intubation or tracheotomy can be carried out.

Bilateral vocal cord paralysis can produce severe inspiratory obstruction necessitating tracheotomy. Acutely, the airway may be stabilized with the rigid bronchoscope or intubation.

Large obstructing intraluminal tumors may produce acute or subacute obstruction that can best be managed using the rigid bronchoscope. Excision biopsy can be carried out for diagnosis and to establish an airway, especially in small children. These hazardous lesions may be entirely removed with the large forceps while maintaining safe control of the airway. Such lesions may produce any of the hazards that accompany tracheal and bronchial foreign bodies.

The rigid bronchoscope has particular effectiveness in the management of obstructing intraluminal tumors, in the palliation of malignant disease, and in the management of recurrent respiratory papillomatosis involving the trachea and bronchi. A wide variety of techniques may be employed, including forceps, snare, and coring and shearing of tumor tissue with the tip of the bronchoscope. Electrocautery or resectoscope, cryoprobe, and laser may all be effectively employed through the rigid bronchoscope.

Management of Massive Hemmorrhage and Blood Clots

The critical aspect of managing massive hemoptysis is maintaining an adequate airway. Patients will drown in their own blood and die before there is danger from exsanguination. The rigid bronchoscope or an endotracheal tube can be effectively used to maintain the airway. The tip of the rigid bronchoscope or endotracheal tube is directed into the normal lung.

Once the airway has been established, control of the bleeding can be accomplished. Bleeding may be tamponaded using the tip of the bronchoscope, an endotracheal tube cuff, a balloon catheter, or pressure from a sponge carrier placed through the rigid bronchoscope. Electrocautery or laser can be used in some situations to control the bleeding. Vasoconstriction may be employed using cocaine, epinephrine, or 0.05% oxymetazoline (Afrin) on a sponge carrier.

Other Indications

The problem of intubation injuries of the trachea in children is well recognized. In the management of this frequently encountered problem, an aggressive approach combining rigid and flexible bronchoscopic evaluation and tracheal stenting with an endotracheal tube may have to be employed (46).

In the evaluation of tracheoesophageal cleft, fistula, and other unusual congenital anomalies, the rigid bronchoscope provides better visualization, manipulation of anatomic structures, measurements of lengths and diameters of strictures, preoperative evaluation, and photographic documentation (47). Most importantly, the rigid instrument allows excellent control of the airway and assures optimal oxygenation during the procedure. Additionally, the rigid bronchoscope can be utilized as a rigid esophagoscope and accomplish both bronchoscopy and esophagoscopy at one session. Even though some studies claim that computed tomography is superior to bronchoscopy in the evaluation of certain congenital airway diseases (48), we feel that bronchoscopy is invaluable in the assessment of the airway dynamics.

Rigid bronchoscopy is very helpful before, during, and following tracheobronchoplasty procedures to treat congenital or acquired tracheobronchial abnormalities. Such reconstruction can salvage normal bronchial and pulmonary tissue distal to obstructive bronchial lesions. Rigid bronchoscopy is valuable to ensure adequate ventilation during bronchotomy and postoperative bronchoscopic dilatation of anastomotic stricture (49). By means of the new rod-lens telescopic bronchoscopes, the diagnosis of H- or N-type tracheoesophageal fistula in infants and children can now be made definitively. With use of these advanced esophagoscopes and bronchoscopes, the fistula can be demonstrated by bronchoscopy. A small Fogarty catheter is threaded through the opening in the trachea under direct view of the telescope and passed through the fistula into the esophagus (50). The balloon is inflated and the bronchoscope removed, leaving the catheter in place. A proper incision is then made in the neck or chest, depending on the location of the lesion, and the fistulous tract is quickly located by palpation of the balloon and catheter. Then with minimal and accurate dissection, correction is carried out (50).

Bronchography is used less frequently nowadays because of the reliability of high-resolution computed tomography in the diagnosis of bronchiectasis (51). If bronchography has to be obtained in smaller children, the rigid bronchoscope is more versatile in aiding this procedure. In a report on 451 pediatric rigid bronchoscopies, 24% of the procedures, all performed under general anesthesia, preceded bronchography (52). After instilling the bronchographic medium through the long metallic cannula inserted through the rigid instrument, the roentgenograph can be taken and the contrast medium easily suctioned back into the metal cannula.

Large anterior mediastinal masses in children have the propensity to cause tracheal compression, particularly during general anesthesia (53). This complication has resulted in serious respiratory distress and death during induction of anesthesia (54–56). While anticipation of this problem and careful anesthetic management using the routine endotracheal tube can avoid tracheal compression, insertion of the rigid bronchoscope in place of the endotracheal tube to provide ventilation and oxygenation will circumvent the complication.

In the management of long-term sequelae of burn-related tracheobronchial injuries, tracheostomy and frequent bronchoscopy are required to maintain airway patency. Of the 1,092 pediatric admissions over a 5-year period to an institute specializing in the care of burn-related injuries, 9.2% required airway support consisting of endotracheal intubation or tracheostomy for more than 24 hr (57).

Right middle lobe syndrome is characterized by a spectrum of diseases from recurrent atelectasis and pneumonitis to bronchiectasis of the middle lobe (58). The diagnosis in pediatric patients may be delayed or missed because of nonspecific symptoms or findings. An evaluation of 21 children with this problem included bronchoscopy in all to exclude obstruction due to foreign body or tumor. Bronchoscopy was therapeutic in two thirds of the cases, with resolution occurring promptly in one third, and eventually in another third (59).

Pulmonary alveolar proteinosis is a rare disease that usually affects the adult patient (60). Treatment in the adult patient consists of whole-lung lavage utilizing a double-lumen endotracheal tube. For the treatment of pulmonary alveolar proteinosis in small children, however, a double-lumen tube is not available. Nevertheless, whole-lung lavage has been accomplished via a double-lumen Swan–Ganz catheter, introduced bronchoscopically through the side arm of a rigid, 3.5-mm Storz bronchoscope while ventilation to the other lung was maintained through the rigid bronchoscope (61).

The rigid bronchoscope excels as a therapeutic instrument, one through which bronchoscopic surgery may be carried out. The safety of anesthesia and the newer instruments available for use with the rigid bronchoscope have greatly reduced the risk of complications from rigid bronchoscopy (62,63). However, flexible bronchoscopy has revolutionized diagnostic bronchoscopy and allowed more physicians to explore the pediatric airways. Nevertheless, Wood (64) wisely noted that while flexible bronchoscopy is an important diagnostic technique for the study of pediatric patients with pulmonary problems, many pitfalls await the unwary. However, with experience and care, most problems can be overcome or circumvented. The well-trained bronchoscopist who is accomplished in the use of both instruments will not be limited by a prejudice toward either scope. Rather, he or she will select the instrument that is preferable for the specific patient and technical problem at hand. As noted in other chapters in this textbook, the instruments should complement rather than compete with each other.

THE PROCEDURE

The majority of rigid bronchoscopy procedures are better accomplished under general anesthesia. However, deep intravenous sedation can also be used with topical anesthetic (1–4% xylocaine). All pediatric anesthesia demands considerable expertise. Each case should be individualized depending on the patient as well as the length and type of bronchoscopic procedure planned. The communication between the bronchoscopist and the anesthesiologist is critical before and throughout the procedure. Since the bronchoscope and the anesthetic gases and oxygen have to share the same passage during the procedure, it is imperative that the instruments and anesthetic gases perform optimally without posing risks to the patient. The team approach should be stressed as in any surgical procedure. More details regarding premedication and anesthetic management for bronchoscopy are discussed in Chapter 7. Other important data such as case history, chest roentgenograph, results of laboratory tests, and details of previous bronchoscopy procedures and complications should be analyzed prior to the procedure.

The selection of the rigid bronchoscope of the proper size (see Chapter 7) and additional instruments is an important early step. The bronchoscopist should anticipate unsuspected eventualities and be prepared to deal with them. The team approach is an essential part of the procedure and team members should be aware of their respective duties during the procedure. This includes nursing personnel as well as the bronchoscopist and anesthesiologist.

If suspension laryngoscopy is not used, an assistant may have to hold the patient's head freely over the end of the operating table so as to orient the head and the upper airway to help the bronchoscopist. Some leave the patient on the operating table in a supine position and put a rolled up towel between the scapulae to "wing back" the chest and produce extension of the neck.

The introduction of the rigid bronchoscope into the tracheobronchial tree can be accomplished by one of several techniques. Once the infant or child is properly anesthetized and adequate oxygenation assured, the bronchoscopist can use a laryngoscope by placing the tip anterior to the epiglottis in order to get a better visualization before introducing the bronchoscope. Suspension laryngoscopy can also be used to introduce the rigid bronchoscope. Previous training, available facilities, instruments, and paramedical assistance, as well as the patient's underlying disease process and clinical situation dictate the technique of the procedure.

As soon as the rigid bronchoscope has been introduced into the trachea, it is imperative that the bronchoscopist and the anesthesiologist work as a team to assure adequate oxygenation through the bronchoscope by attaching the ventilating apparatus to the side orifice of the rigid bronchoscope. It is important throughout the procedure to assure the lack of trauma from the rigid instrument to teeth and soft tissues of oropharyngeal regions and larynx. If the patient begins to cough in spite of anesthesia, atomizers may be used to instill topical anesthetic through the bronchoscope.

The examination of the tracheobronchial tree should proceed in an orderly manner so that no abnormality is missed. As in adults, it is advisable to first examine the normal side, as determined by chest roentgenograph and clinical examination, and then proceed to the abnormal side. This will depend on the urgency of the situation. Obviously, if a large asphyxiating foreign body is found in the trachea or if serious bleeding is encountered, the first step is to treat these problems before examining the entire tracheobronchial tree. Throughout the procedure, the bronchoscopist should remember to use finesse and not force and unnecessary manipulations that might produce laryngeal edema and trauma to other areas. Application of excessive suction to remove respiratory secretions can easily result in mucosal edema and bleeding, which in turn will produce poor visibility and make the procedure more difficult. Further, excessive use of suction may also result in suctioning of oxygen and anesthetic gases. Because of the small airways and instruments used, particularly in small children, and when working without a telescope, simultaneous visualization and instrumentation are not always possible or optimal. In such circumstances, palpation and a few visual clues may be all the bronchoscopist will have to rely on.

CONTRAINDICATIONS

There are few relative contraindications to both diagnostic and therapeutic rigid bronchoscopy in children. An unstable neck that implies excessive motion of the neck during bronchoscopy, congenital facial anomalies such as micrognathia or microstomia, and technical difficulties due to cervical ankylosis and severe kyphoscoliosis are among the contraindications. Even the severe respiratory dysfunction in immunosuppressed patients with diffuse pulmonary infiltrates is only a relative contraindication to bronchoscopy (65).

Absolute contraindications to bronchoscopy include an unstable cardiovascular status, life-threatening cardiac arrhythmias, extremely severe hypoxemia that is likely to worsen during bronchoscopy, and an inadequately trained bronchoscopist and bronchoscopy team. Thrombocytopenia in not a contraindication to pediatric bronchoscopy unless bronchoscopic lung biopsy or biopsy of a tracheobronchial mucosal lesion is planned.

COMPLICATIONS

A properly performed rigid bronchoscopy is extremely safe and is rarely associated with complications. There were eight minor complications in a series of 386 rigid bronchoscopies and no death or cardiac arrest (66). Minimal edema of the larynx and tracheobronchial tree from instrumentation is usually self-resolving and not dangerous. Diagnostic procedures are not done during acute respiratory tract infections but are deferred until symptoms have resolved for a week or two. However, severe obstruction (as with severe croup) may necessitate emergent therapeutic intervention.

The beneficial effect of intravenous corticosteroids in preventing traumatic laryngeal edema is controversial. A controlled clinical study of 70 children who underwent bronchoscopy for removal of foreign bodies from the tracheobronchial tree administered intravenous dexamethasone to one group and no medication to the second. Intravenous corticosteroids did not reduce the incidence of postbronchoscopy laryngeal edema (67). Trauma to the soft tissues of the oropharyngeal area and damage to teeth and gums can easily be avoided by careful instrumentation and minimal manipulation of the rigid instrument. An unexpected cocaine intoxication following the topical administration of cocaine (30 mg) in a 14-month-old boy undergoing bronchoscopy for removal of a foreign body has been reported; the child recovered completely (68).

An uncommon complication of bronchoscopy reported is the disruption of the posterior tracheal wall. With this mishap, air tracking may present as surgical emphysema, pneumomediastinum, or pneumothoraces, and may be associated with respiratory distress. One report described six children with posterior tracheal wall disruptions; three associated with tracheotomy, one with bronchoscopy, and another with endotracheal intubation (69). Appropriate training and techniques in bronchoscopy should prevent such complications.

A study on the design and aerodynamics of rigid bronchoscope identified two concerns for the bronchoscopist and anesthesiologist. The first concern is selection of an appropriately sized instrument for the pediatric patient because the measurements demonstrated that the stated size of a rigid bronchoscope's internal diameter may differ significantly from its actual size and in many instances the actual diameter may be significantly greater than the stated size. The second problem concerns difficult ventilation of the patient while the bronchoscope is in place. The measurements indicated that major increases in resistance to gas flow through the bronchoscope occurred when smaller caliber instruments with accessory sheaths and/or telescopes were introduced into the bronchoscope (70). The ventilating channel in the 2.5, 3.0, 3.5, and 4.0 rigid bronchoscopes is small, and high inspiratory pressures may be required to deliver a fixed volume of gas. Animal experiments have documented retention of CO_2 when the smaller instruments are used (71). Appropriate knowledge of instruments and preoperative planning should minimize or eliminate these problems.

TRAINING IN RIGID BRONCHOSCOPY

Several aspects of training in bronchoscopy are discussed in Chapter 29. Of all the bronchoscopy procedures, pediatric rigid bronchoscopy is perhaps the most difficult to master. One of the reasons is the small airways and the limited visibility afforded by the very small instruments. Looking through a small-caliber rigid bronchoscope is akin to looking through a drinking straw. Repeated pediatric laryngoscopy and tracheal intubation prior to surgical procedures will provide good basic training in the pediatric anatomy. We have provided bronchoscopic training using cat since its anatomy mimics the pediatric oropharyngolaryngeal anatomy. Large rabbits are used to practice manual skills of foreign body extraction. Mannequins may provide additional help in understanding the tracheobronchial anatomy. Needless to say, repeated performance of pediatric bronchoscopic procedures is essential to attain proficiency. Special training should be sought at major centers specializing in pediatric pulmonology and pediatric bronchoscopy.

ACKNOWLEDGMENT

Input by Robert E. Wood, M.D., to the discussion on advantages and disadvantages is gratefully acknowledged.

REFERENCES

1. Holinger P, Johnston K. Factors responsible for laryngeal obstruction in infants. *JAMA* 1950;143:1229.
2. Tucker G. Infant larynx—direct laryngoscopic observation. *JAMA* 1932;99:1899–1902.
3. Tucker JA. Obstruction of the major pediatric airway. *Otolaryngol Clin North Am* 1979;12:329–341.
4. Prakash UBS, Offord KP, Stubbs SE. Bronchoscopy in North America: the ACCP survey. *Chest* 1991;100:1668–1675.
5. Godfrey S, Springer C, Maayan C, Avital A, Vatashky E, Belin B. Is there a place for rigid bronchoscopy in the management of pediatric lung disease? *Pediatr Pulmonol* 1987;3:179–184.
6. Nunez H, Rodriguez EP, Alvarado C, et al. Foreign body aspiration extraction (letter). *Chest* 1989;96:697.
7. Weissberg D, Schwartz I. Foreign bodies in the tracheobronchial tree. *Chest* 1987;91:730–733.
8. Limper AH, Prakash UBS. Tracheobronchial foreign bodies in adults. *Ann Intern Med* 1990;112:604–609.
9. Holinger PH, Holinger LD. Use of the open tube bronchoscope in the extraction of foreign bodies. *Chest* 1978;73:721–724.
10. Cooper JD, Pearson FG, Patterson GA, et al. Use of silicone stents in the management of airway problems. *Ann Thorac Surg* 1989;47:371–378.
11. Dumon J-F. A dedicated tracheobronchial stent. *Chest* 1990; 97:328–332.
12. Freitag L, Firusian N, Stamatis G, Greschuchna D. The role of bronchoscopy in pulmonary complications due to mustard gas inhalation. *Chest* 1991;100:1436–1441.
13. Prakash UBS. Chemical warfare and bronchoscopy. Editorial. *Chest* 1991;100:1486–1487.
14. Wallace MJ, Charnsangavej C, Ogawa K, et al. Tracheobronchial tree: expandable metallic stents used in experimental and clinical applications. *Radiology* 1986;158:309–311.
15. Wedzicha JA, Pearson MC. Management of massive hemoptysis. *Resp Med* 1990;84:9–12.
16. Editorial. Life-threatening hemoptysis. *Lancet* 1987; 1:1354–1356.
17. Dumon J-F, Shapshay S, Bourcerau J, et al. Principles for safety in application of neodymium-YAG laser in bronchology. Chest 1984;86:163–168.
18. Beamis JF Jr, Shapshay S. More about the YAG. *Chest* 1985; 87:27–28.
19. Hetzel MR, Smith SGT. Endoscopic palliation of tracheobronchial malignancies. *Thorax* 1991;46:325–333.
20. Chan AL, Tharratt RS, Siefkin AD, Albertson TE, Volz WG, Allen RP. Nd:YAG laser bronchoscopy: rigid or fiberoptic mode? *Chest* 1990;98:271–275.
21. Prakash UBS, Stubbs SE. The bronchoscopy survey: some reflections. *Chest* 1991;100:1660–1667.
22. Elliott RC, Smiddy JF. The "territorial domain" of hemoptysis. *Chest* 1964;65:703.
23. Wilson JAS. The flexible fiberoptic bronchoscope. *Ann Thorac Surg* 1972;14:686–88.
24. Becker HD, Kayser K, Schulz V, Tuengerthal S, Vollhaber H-H. Instrumentation and technique. In: *Atlas of bronchoscopy*. Philadelphia: B.C. Decker,Inc; 1991:6.
25. Simpson FG, Arnold AG, Purvis A, Belfield PW, Muers MF, Cooke NJ. Postal survey of bronchoscopic practice by physicians in the United Kingdom. *Thorax* 1986;41:311–317.
26. Puhakka H, Kero P, Erkinjuntti M. Pediatric bronchoscopy during a 17-year period. *Int J Pediatr Otorhinolaryngol* 1987; 13:171–180.
27. Tsueda K, Sjogren S, Debrand M, Pulito AR. Wire basket extraction of foreign bodies from the tracheobronchial tree of small children. *J Ky Med Assoc* 1981;79:13–15.
28. Al-Naaman YD, Al-Ani MS, Al-Ani HR. Non-vegetable foreign bodies in the bronchopulmonary tract in children. *J Laryngol Otol* 1975;89:289–297.
29. Fitzpatrick SB, Stokes DC, Marsh B, Wang KP. Transbronchial lung biopsy in pediatric and adolescent patients. *Am J Dis Child* 1985;139:46–49.
30. Levy M, Glick B, Springer C, et al. Bronchoscopy and bronchography in children. Experience with 110 investigations. *Am J Dis Child* 1983;137:14–16.
31. Cotton RT. Pediatric laryngotracheal stenosis. *J Pediatr Surg* 1984;19:699–704.
32. Louhimo I, Leijala M. The treatment of low retrosternal tracheal stenosis in the neonate and small children. *Thorac Cardiovasc Surg* 1985;33:98–102.
33. Groff DB, Allen JK. Gruentzig balloon catheter dilation for acquired bronchial stenosis in an infant. *Ann Thorac Surg* 1985; 39:379–381.
34. Strong MS, Vaughn CW, Healy GB, Cooperband SR, Clemente MA. Recurrent respiratory papillomatosis: management with the CO_2 laser. *Ann Otol Rhinol Laryngol* 1976;85:508–516.
35. Kavuru MS, Mehta AC, Eliachar I. Effect of photodynamic therapy and external beam radiation therapy on juvenile laryngotracheobronchial papillomatosis. *Am Rev Resp Dis* 1990; 141:509–510.
36. Leiberman A, Bar-Ziv J, Zirkin HJ. Low grade mucoepidermoid tumour of the bronchus in childhood: a therapeutic dilemma. *Eur J Pediatr* 1986;145:130–132.
37. Carr T, Stevens RF, Marsden HB, Morris-Jones P, Kumar S. An unusual presentation of non-Hodgkin's lymphoma (NHL) in a child. *Eur J Surg Oncol* 1986;12:193–195.
38. McDougall JC, Gorenstein A, Unni K, OConnell EJ. Carcinoid and mucoepidermoid carcinoma of bronchus in children. *Ann Otol Rhinol Laryngol* 1980;89:425–427.
39. Verska JJ, Connolly JE. Bronchial adenomas in children. *J Thorac Cardiovasc Surg* 1968;55:411–417.
40. Fearon B, MacRae D. Laryngeal papillomatosis in children. *J Otolaryngol* 1976;5:493–496.
41. Healy GB, McGill T, Simpson GT, Strong MS. The use of the carbon dioxide laser in the pediatric airway. *J Pediatr Surg* 1979; 14:735–740.
42. Muller W, von-der-Hardt H, Rieger CH. Idiopathic and symptomatic plastic bronchitis in childhood. A report of three cases and review of the literature. *Respiration* 1987;52:214–220.
43. Werkhaven J, Holinger LD. Bronchial casts in children. *Ann Otol Rhinol Laryngol* 1987;96:86–92.
44. Bowen A, Oudjhane K, Odagiri K, Liston SL, Cumming WA, Oh KS. Plastic bronchitis: large, branching, mucoid bronchial casts in children. *Am J Roentgenol* 1985;144:371–375.
45. Majid AA. J-Shaped catheter for endobronchial aspiration of right upper lobe bronchus during rigid bronchoscopy in pediatric patients. *Chest* 1991;100:862.
46. Othersen HB Jr. Intubation injuries of the trachea in children. Management and prevention. *Ann Surg* 1979;189:601–606.
47. Stigol LC, Traversaro J, Trigo ER. Carinal trifurcation with congenital tracheobiliary fistula. *Pediatrics* 1966;37:89–91.
48. Hernandez RJ, Tucker GF. Congenital tracheal stenosis: role of CT and high kV films. *Pediatr Radiol* 1987;17:192–196.
49. Black CT, Luck SR, Raffensperger JG. Bronchoplastic techniques for pediatric lung salvage. *J Pediatr Surg* 1988; 23:653–656.
50. Gans SL, Johnson RO. Diagnosis and surgical management of "H-type" tracheoesophageal fistula in infants and children. *J Pediatr Surg* 1977;12:233–236.
51. Wilson JF, Peters GN, Fleshman K. A technique for bronchog-

raphy in children. An experience with 575 patients using topical anesthesia. *Am Rev Resp Dis* 1972;105:564–571.
52. Godfrey S. Bronchoscopy in childhood. *Br J Dis Chest* 1987; 81:225–231.
53. Prakash UBS, Abel MA, Hubmayr RD. Mediastinal mass and tracheal obstruction during general anesthesia. *Mayo Clin Proc* 1988;63:1004–1011.
54. Neuman GG, Wiengarten AE, Abramowitz RM, Kushins LG, Abramson AL, Ladner W. The anesthetic management of the patient with an anterior mediastinal mass. *Anesthesiology* 1984; 60:144.
55. Keon TP. Death on induction of anesthesia for cervical node biopsy. *Anesthesiology* 1981;55:471.
56. Piro AH, Weiss DR, Hellman S. Mediastinal Hodgkin's disease: a possible danger for intubation anesthesia. *Int J Radiat Oncol Biophysiol* 1976;1:415.
57. Calhoun KH, Deskin RW, Garza C, McCracken MM, Nichols RJ Jr, Hokanson JA, Herndon DN. Long-term airway sequelae in a pediatric burn population. *Laryngoscope* 1988;98:721–725.
58. Dees SC, Spock A. Right middle lobe syndrome in children. *JAMA* 1966;197:8–14.
59. Livingston GL, Holinger LD, Luck SR. Right middle lobe syndrome in children. *Int J Pediatr Otorhinolaryngol* 1987; 13:11–23.
60. Prakash UBS, Barham SS, Carpenter HA, Dines DE, Marsh HM. Pulmonary alveolar phospholipoproteinosis: experience with 34 cases and a review. *Mayo Clin Proc* 1987;62:499–518.
61. Moazam F, Schmidt JH, Chesrown SE, et al. Total lung lavage for pulmonary alveolar proteinosis in an infant without the use of cardiopulmonary bypass. *J Pediatr Surg* 1985;20:398–401.
62. Hamilton AH, Carswell F, Wisheart JD. The Bristol Children's Hospital experience of tracheobronchial foreign bodies 1977–87. *Bristol Med Chir J* 1989;104:72–74.
63. Burton EM, Riggs W Jr, Kaufman RA, Houston CS. Pneumomediastinum caused by foreign body aspiration in children. *Pediatr Radiol* 1989;20:45–47.
64. Wood RE. Pitfalls in the use of the flexible bronchoscope in pediatric patients. *Chest* 1990;97:199–203.
65. Olopade CO, Prakash UBS. Bronchoscopy in the intensive care critical care unit. *Mayo Clinic Proc* 1989;64:1255–1263.
66. Puhakka H, Kero P, Valli P, Iisalo E, Erkinjuntti M. Pediatric bronchoscopy. A report of methodology and results. *Clin Pediatr (Phila)*. 1989;28:253–257.
67. Ghorayeb BY, Shikhani AH. The use of dexamethasone in pediatric bronchoscopy. *J Laryngol Otol* 1985;99:1127–1129.
68. Schou H, Krogh B, Knudsen F. Unexpected cocaine intoxication in a fourteen month old child following topical administration. *J Toxicol Clin Toxicol* 1987;25:419–422.
69. Crysdale WS, Forte V. Posterior tracheal wall disruption: a rare complication of pediatric tracheotomy and bronchoscopy. *Laryngoscope* 1986;96:1279–1282.
70. Lockhart CH, Elliot JL. Potential hazards of pediatric rigid bronchoscopy. *J Pediatr Surg* 1984;19:239–242.
71. Rah KH, Salzberg AM, Boyan CP, Greenfield LJ. Respiratory acidosis with the small Storz–Hopkins bronchoscopes: occurrence and management. *Ann Thorac Surg* 1979;27:197–202.

Bronchoscopy,
edited by U. B. S. Prakash.
Mayo Foundation © 1994.
Published by Raven Press, Ltd., New York.

CHAPTER 24

Pediatric Flexible Bronchoscopy

Robert E. Wood and Udaya B. S. Prakash

The first application of bronchoscopy was for the removal of a foreign body from the airway (1). Since foreign body aspiration is a fairly common problem in children, it was quite natural that attention was given early in the development of bronchoscopy to instrumentation and applications in pediatric patients. However, as discussed in Chapter 23, the small size of the pediatric airway imposed severe limitations, as did the problems of anesthetic management. In most centers, pediatric bronchoscopy was primarily limited to foreign body extraction until the development of more advanced instrumentation and anesthetic techniques in the 1960s and 1970s (2).

The Hopkins glass rod telescope enabled bronchoscopists to visualize the airways of infants with amazing detail and clarity, and led to rapid progress in pediatric bronchology. For the first time, it was truly practical to utilize bronchoscopy for diagnostic purposes other than suspected foreign body aspiration or major airway obstruction. The next major revolution in the development of bronchoscopes was the introduction of the flexible bronchoscope in the early 1970s for use in adults, with dramatic impact on medical practice (3). Quite naturally, there was interest in applying this new instrumentation to pediatric patients. However, because of the relatively large size of the instruments, pediatric applications were quite limited. Since 1981, flexible bronchoscopes small enough to be routinely used in infants and children have been commercially available.

R. E. Wood: Department of Pediatric Pulmonary Medicine, University of North Carolina, Chapel Hill, North Carolina 27599.

U. B. S. Prakash: Division of Thoracic Diseases and Internal Medicine, Mayo Clinic, Rochester, Minnesota 55905.

ADVANTAGES AND DISADVANTAGES

Advantages

Flexible bronchoscopes are, as the name implies, flexible. Therefore, they can be passed into and through the airways without themselves introducing (much) mechanical distortion. For an awake patient, they are more comfortable than a rigid instrument. Despite the fact that the image is composed of only several thousand pixels (points of color and light intensity), the image quality is surprisingly good, especially in real time. Still photos taken through a flexible instrument are of generally low quality because each glass fiber (corresponding to one pixel in the composite image) is visible on the image (Fig. 1). However, video or cine films, or direct visualization through the instrument, allow the eye to ignore the pixels and see an image of high quality.

Not only are flexible bronchoscopes capable of traversing the airways relatively atraumatically, they can also go places rigid bronchoscopes cannot, such as the distal branches of the upper lobes. For example, in a 3-month-old infant, one would ordinarily use a 3.2-mm rigid bronchoscope. The tip of this instrument could be expected to reach no further than the lobar orifices, if that far. However, the 3.2-mm flexible bronchoscope could be expected to enter the subsegmental bronchi in all lobes in the same child. With the new 2.2-mm "ultrathin" flexible bronchoscope (Olympus N22), It is quite easy to routinely examine airways as far as 10–14 generations in infants as young as 3 months.

In this context it is appropriate to mention the differences in the nomenclature as regards the size of rigid and flexible bronchoscopes. The size designation of a rigid instrument refers to the minimum internal diame-

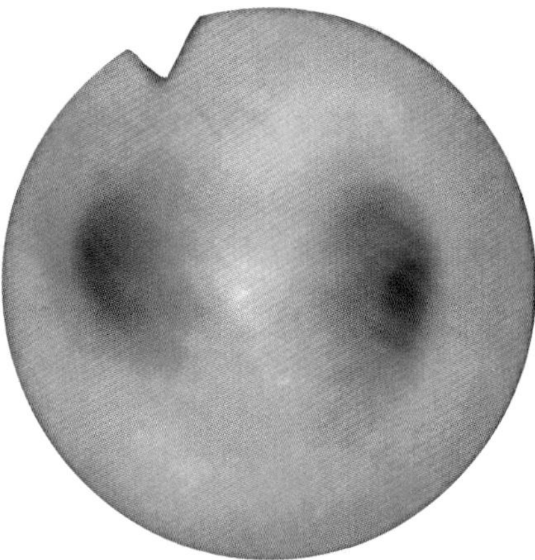

FIG. 1. The bronchoscopic image obtained through the pediatric flexible bronchoscope is not of high quality. The picture is very grainy.

ter, not the outside diameter (4). Thus, a 3.2-mm flexible bronchoscope can easily pass through a 3.5-mm rigid bronchoscope.

A very important aspect of the flexible bronchoscope is that it can be inserted through the nostril or mouth, with the head and neck in a neutral position. Many benefits accrue from nasal insertion. First of all, the entire upper airway is examined as well as the lower airways. Often this is where the pathology is found or where additional pathology is found. Since the neck is not extended, and the mandible does not have to be lifted with a laryngoscope, the natural dynamics of the palate and larynx can be more readily observed. This is of major importance in the evaluation of infants and children with stridor.

General anesthesia is rarely used for flexible bronchoscopy in pediatric patients. Indeed, if general anesthesia is used, bronchoscopy may be more difficult with a flexible instrument than with a rigid one because the airway must be controlled. Since the diameter of the common pediatric flexible bronchoscope is 3.2 mm, it cannot be used through an endotracheal tube smaller than 4.5 mm (Fig. 2). Even then, it will be impossible to ventilate the patient. On the other hand, the flexible bronchoscope can be used through endotracheal tubes, which cannot be done at all with rigid instruments. The ultrathin (2.2-mm) bronchoscope can easily be passed through endotracheal tubes as small as 2.5 mm, and infants intubated with 3.0-mm tubes can be ventilated around the 2.2-mm scope.

If general anesthesia is not used, then pediatric patients generally must be sedated. Spontaneous breathing throughout the examination facilitates the observation of airway dynamics. Topical anesthesia is an absolute necessity and is readily achieved with lidocaine. At the University of North Carolina, about 400 flexible bronchoscopic procedures are performed annually, and general anesthesia is electively utilized only for special situations. These include laser procedures, or procedures on children we know, or have very good reason to suspect, will not do well with sedation. In practice, we use general anesthesia because sedation will be inadequate for a given patient in less than 1% of our patients. This substantially reduces the overall cost of the procedure without increasing risk.

Bronchoalveolar lavage can be performed easily with a flexible bronchoscope. The tip of the scope is gently wedged into a bronchus, and saline is alternately instilled and withdrawn. Although bronchoalveolar lavage is not part of every pediatric procedure, it is a useful and important technique to evaluate the microbiological, cellular, and protein constituents of the lower airways and airway surface fluids.

There are a number of special applications for which the flexible instruments are uniquely suited. These include bronchoscope-assisted intubation, and examination of the airways in patients with mandibular or cervical abnormalities that preclude the use of rigid instruments except through a tracheostomy incision.

Bronchoscopic intubation is a powerful technique that in our experience has often been life saving. In fact, the pediatric flexible bronchoscope is part of the armamentarium of the anesthesiologists at the Mayo Medical Center, and trainees in anesthesia are instructed to intubate patients via pediatric flexible bronchoscope. On average, it should require only about 30 sec for a skilled bronchoscopist to accomplish a nasopharyngoscopy, laryngoscopy, bronchoscopy, and nasotracheal intubation. Once the tube is in position in the trachea, the bronchoscope is withdrawn and the patient ventilated. Then the bronchoscope is reinserted, the optimum position of the tube is verified (thus eliminating the need for a chest radiograph for

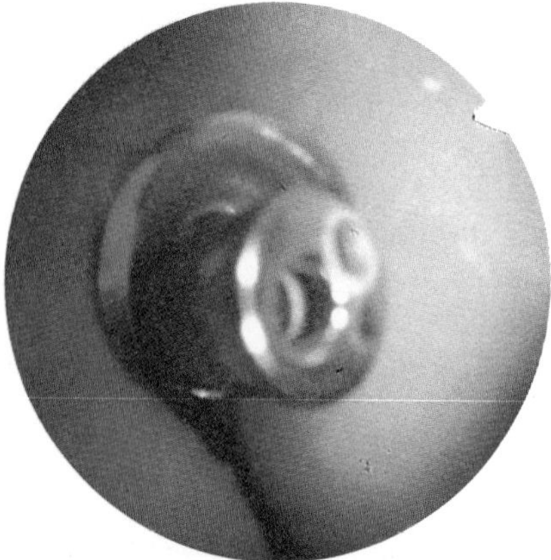

FIG. 2. The most commonly used pediatric bronchoscope (with an outer diameter of 3.2 mm) can pass through a 5.0-mm endotracheal tube as shown in this cephalad view in a model of the tracheobronchial tree.

tube placement), and the lower airways examined more leisurely. There are very few situations in which intubation cannot be achieved using this technique. Patients with cervical or mandibular ankylosis, mandibular hypoplasia, oropharyngeal masses, or other conditions that preclude rigid bronchoscopy usually cannot be intubated for the same reasons. A flexible bronchoscope of appropriate size is thus invaluable in the management of such patients. In patients with tracheostomies, the flexible bronchoscope can be inserted through the stoma and directed retrograde to examine the tracheal surface of the larynx; this is valuable in the evaluation of selected patients with subglottic stenosis. In general, the flexible bronchoscope can be inserted into virtually any orifice and advanced into virtually any anatomic site.

Not only can a flexible bronchoscope be used to insert an endotracheal tube, but the airways can be examined through the tube without having to remove it. As noted earlier, the 2.2-mm ultrathin bronchoscope can easily be passed through a 2.5-mm endotracheal tube, thus allowing the examination of the smallest of intubated infants. At times, however, this procedure can be misleading, if the abnormalities in the airways are proximal to the tip of the endotracheal tube. Such examinations are of great value in many patients with tracheostomies, since the relationship of the tip of the tube to the airway wall can be seen clearly. If the size of the artificial airway is such that the presence of the flexible bronchoscope will preclude ventilation, it is usually possible to complete an examination of the lower airways within 30–40 sec, reinserting the bronchoscope for additional looks if necessary.

In part because of the nature of the flexible bronchoscope and in part because of its relatively small diameter in relation to that of the airways, the incidence of complications is very low (5). It is difficult to make a direct comparison of complication rates since in general higher risk patients are more likely to be studied with a rigid instrument. On the other hand, inappropriate or unskilled use of flexible instruments can surely result in complications (5). In high-risk patients, complications are more likely. To date, only one fatal complication of flexible bronchoscopy in a child has been reported (6).

Because general anesthesia is so rarely used for flexible bronchoscopy, these procedures are usually not performed in an operating room. Indeed, bedside bronchoscopy is not uncommon. While this is cited as a relative advantage, it must be recognized as a potential liability as well. Unless care is taken to provide all necessary equipment, supplies, and trained personnel, bedside bronchoscopy can turn into a disaster. We routinely perform bronchoscopy at the bedside of patients in the pediatric and neonatal intensive care units, but only when they are ventilator-dependent or otherwise cannot be moved. All other procedures are performed in a fully equipped and staffed bronchoscopy suite or operating room.

Disadvantages

The most serious limitations of flexible bronchoscopes are that they at least partially obstruct the airway (the patient must breathe around, rather than through, a flexible scope) and the very limited instrumentation that can be used. Although the flexible bronchoscope is a valuable instrument in the diagnosis of suspected tracheobronchial foreign body aspiration (7), flexible instruments should not be routinely used for foreign body extraction in children except under unusual circumstances (which will be associated with great difficulty and increased risk unless the foreign body is very small). Attempts to perform foreign body extraction with a flexible bronchoscope ignore the advantages of rigid instrumentation (and general anesthesia) and accept the limitations of flexible instrumentation.

The instruments available for extraction of a tracheobronchial foreign body using the flexible bronchoscope are limited but include wire baskets and special forceps (8). The pediatric flexible bronchoscope has been used to extract tracheobronchial foreign bodies in children by using ureteral stone baskets and forceps that can easily traverse the working channel of the pediatric flexible bronchoscope (Figs. 3–5) (9). However, we stress that unless the bronchoscopist is trained in both rigid and flexible bronchoscopy procedures and has all the necessary instruments and facilities to handle the potential complications, flexible bronchoscopes should not be used for extraction of a tracheobronchial foreign body.

Airway obstruction induced by the flexible bronchoscope is a constant concern to the bronchoscopist and mandates continuous patient monitoring (10). On the other hand, virtually all infants 3–3.5 kg and larger can breathe quite adequately around the 3.2-mm flexible bronchoscope, at least for long enough to complete a thorough examination of the lower airways. Supplemental oxygen can be given, but it is not a substitute for careful monitoring and good common sense. Premature infants will not usually be able to ventilate around the 3.2-mm bronchoscope, but infants as small as 540 g can breathe quite readily around an ultrathin (2.2 mm) bronchoscope (5). The airway compromise and inability to oxygenate when the flexible bronchoscope is introduced into tiny airways is a potential problem. The suction channel can be used to deliver supplemental oxygen through the flexible bronchoscope (11). However, this can lead to the development of a pneumothorax if the bronchoscope is wedged into a bronchus (5).

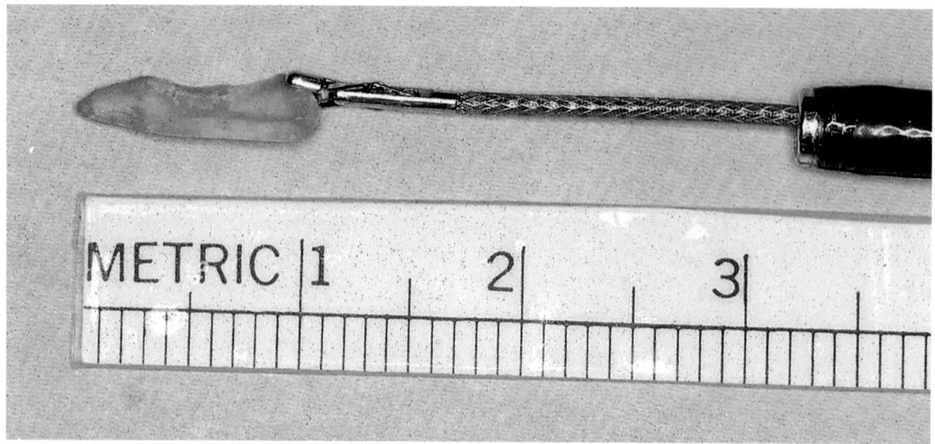

FIG. 3. A ureteral forceps can be easily passed through the working channel of pediatric flexible bronchoscope (outer diameter of 3.2 mm). A sunflower seed was removed using this technique from the left lower lobe of 2-year-old child.

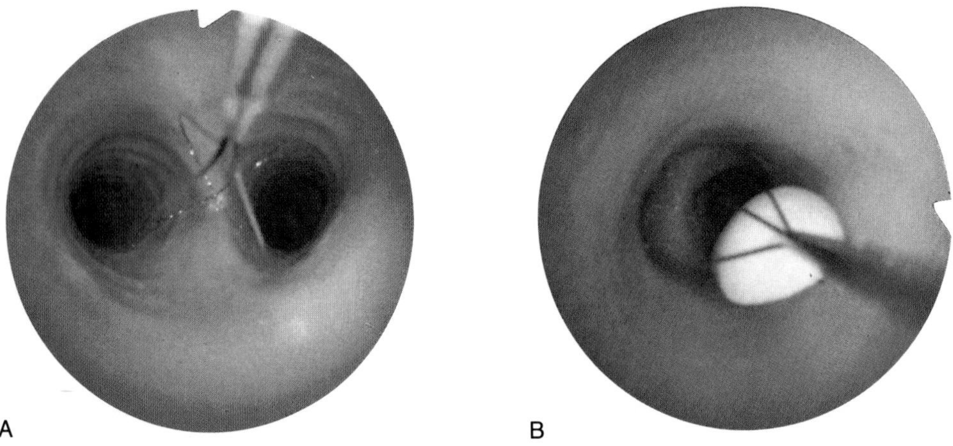

FIG. 4. (A) Ureteral basket in the distal trachea of a model of tracheobronchial tree. This basket can also easily traverse the working channel of pediatric flexible bronchoscope. **(B)** Half a peanut is being grasped and brought out from the distal trachea.

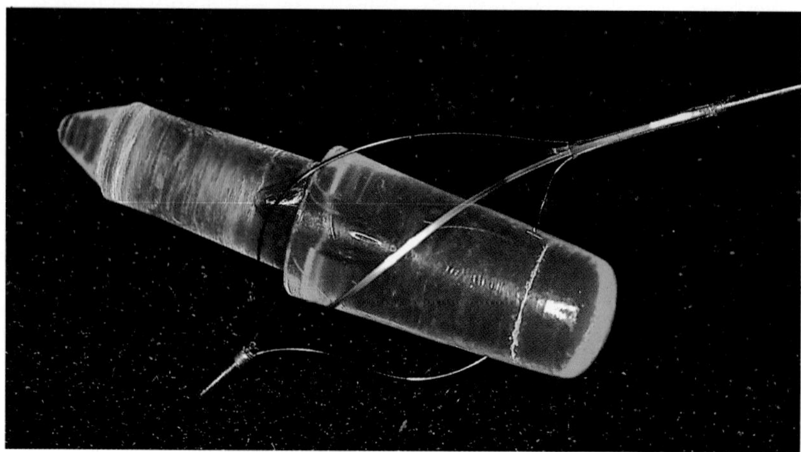

FIG. 5. A small plastic peg was removed from a 3-year-old child's left main bronchus using a pediatric flexible bronchoscope and a ureteral basket.

The necessity to control the airway during general anesthesia may limit the use of flexible bronchoscopes. On the other hand, alternatives are available for selected circumstances. At the University of North Carolina, a nasopharyngeal tube is employed to ventilate infants during general anesthesia with complete muscular relaxation while extended bronchoscopic procedures are performed. This technique was developed to facilitate large-volume bronchopulmonary lavage (12), and we have used it a number of times for laser procedures or with paralyzed infants in the intensive care units.

The quality of the image seen through flexible bronchoscopes has been cited as a drawback (Fig. 1), and it is certainly inferior to that of a glass rod telescope. However, in practice this is not a meaningful limitation. Secretions on the lens can be readily removed by suctioning and lavage with small volumes of saline, or the lens can be gently wiped across the carina.

Since flexible bronchoscopes at least partially obstruct the airway, one must be careful in interpreting observed airway dynamics. Abnormally high pressure gradients induced by the partial obstruction may result in impressive dynamic airway changes. This can be avoided by the careful application of common sense and appropriate instruments (i.e., by switching to an ultrathin instrument when there is a question of too much obstruction by the bronchoscope). On the other hand, even with flexible bronchoscopy, clinically important airway dynamics may not be demonstrable unless the child breathes deeply enough or coughs (13).

Finally, in some situations it may be desirable or necessary to manipulate the airway structures under direct visualization; this is difficult if not impossible with flexible bronchoscopes. For example, with a rigid scope, one can observe the opening of the glottis as the tip of the bronchoscope is passed between the cords, and thus help to differentiate between bilateral abductor paralysis and posterior fixation.

We feel that for the majority of diagnostic procedures the flexible bronchoscope has substantial advantages. On the other hand, for the majority of therapeutic procedures a rigid bronchoscope is superior. It is clear that neither rigid nor flexible bronchoscope is entirely sufficient to accomplish the full range of pediatric bronchoscopy; both instruments (and expertise in their use) are necessary. For example, we have found it very helpful to use the ultrathin flexible bronchoscope through the instrument side port of the rigid bronchoscope to observe and control certain instruments such as balloon catheters (for dilatation of bronchial stenoses) (14). If necessary, the flexible bronchoscope can be passed through the rigid instrument to apply laser therapy or simply to examine the distal bronchial tree (15). This approach combines the airway control of the rigid bronchoscope with the maneuverability of the flexible bronchoscope (7,16–18). Even in pediatric bronchoscopic practice, the flexible and rigid bronchoscopes complement, not compete with, each other (19).

The performance of pediatric flexible bronchoscopy depends on the training of the bronchoscopist and the evolution of practice at each medical center. For instance, at the University of North Carolina, we have evolved a practice model in which the vast majority of diagnostic bronchoscopy is performed by the pediatric pulmonary service, using flexible instruments, while the vast majority of therapeutic bronchoscopy is performed by pediatric surgeons or pediatric otolaryngologists with rigid instruments. In cases where there is uncertainty as to the most appropriate technique, we may be prepared to use either or both. It is not a rare event for us to employ both types of instruments in the same patient, even simultaneously. At the Mayo Medical Center, on the other hand, the pulmonary physicians perform all bronchoscopic procedures, including rigid and flexible procedures in pediatric and adult patients.

Careful documentation of procedures with videotape and review of the tapes with the appropriate surgeon is a time- and cost-effective method, conserving operating room time, reducing cost to the patients, facilitating the detailed planning of surgical procedures, etc. The flexible bronchoscope is also invaluable for intraoperative examinations and for evaluation of postoperative results (20).

THE INSTRUMENTS

The first reports of flexible bronchoscopy in infants and young children were published in 1978, and were descriptions of somewhat crude instruments or adaptations (21,22). In late 1978, Wood and Sherman obtained a prototype of what became the Olympus BF3C4 and used this instrument in patients of all ages, including premature infants (23). Later models of the pediatric flexible bronchoscope (Olympus BF3C10, BF3C20; Pentax FB10X) have had essentially the same physical characteristics (diameter 3.2 mm, suction channel size 1.2 mm, etc.) as the original prototype. Smaller, ultrathin instruments with controlled flexion at the tip (Olympus BF27, BF22, N22) have also become available and have important, though more limited, applications (20,24–26). A major clinical byproduct of the small-caliber flexible bronchoscope has been the ability of the bronchoscopist to use them in adults to reach the distal branches of the bronchial tree to diagnose abnormalities not seen with regular adult flexible bronchoscopes (27). These small-caliber bronchoscopes are also used with increasing frequency in intensive care units to facilitate endotracheal tube changes and to confirm the placement of endotracheal or tracheostomy tubes. However, in older children (median age 10 years), a standard flexible bronchoscope (Olympus BFP20) has been used with topical anesthesia and sedation (28).

Today bronchoscopists have a wide array of choices for instrumentation and technique. Newer imaging techniques such as computed tomography and magnetic resonance imaging have also extended our ability to extract information from the airways of infants and children. The net result of these advances has been to move pediatric bronchology from the dark ages toward enlightenment and to achieve widespread recognition of bronchoscopy as a generally useful diagnostic tool. However, these advances have not been without controversy (23), some of which persists today. The major arguments have centered on the choice of instrumentation (and anesthesia) and the indications for bronchoscopy. Today there is general acceptance of both methodologies as well as the idea of pediatric bronchoscopy as a medical, rather than exclusively a surgical, procedure. More importantly, primary care practitioners are increasingly recognizing the value of diagnostic bronchoscopy and are less reluctant to refer their patients for appropriate evaluation.

INDICATIONS

The indications for diagnostic and therapeutic bronchoscopy are listed in tables 1 and 2 of chapter 23. In this chapter, Table 1 lists indications outlined by the American Thoracic Society (29). Generally, the indications for rigid and flexible bronchoscopy are similar. One of the largest series of flexible bronchoscopy experiences reported (30) included 1,000 procedures (172 laryngoscopies, 828 bronchoscopies) in children less than 10 years of age. A bronchoscopic diagnosis of direct relevance to the primary indication for the procedure was established in 76% of cases; in an additional 15%, abnormalities relevant to a secondary indication were found. Findings were normal in only 9% of cases. The bronchoscope was most useful in the evaluation of patients who had stridor, atelectasis, persistent wheezing, or a suspected foreign body for which there was insufficient evidence to warrant rigid bronchoscopy, as well as for patients who had tracheostomies. In another retrospective study to determine the indications for flexible bronchoscopy in 95 pediatric patients (mean age 6.9 years) who underwent 129 procedures, a specific diagnosis was made in 88% of the cases, of which 48% involved a lower airway disorder (31). The high diagnostic yield and low complication rate strongly support the use of the flexible bronchoscope in the diagnostic evaluation of infants and children who have a variety of pulmonary problems.

TABLE 1. *Indications for flexible bronchoscopy in pediatric patients*[a]

Stridor
Persistent atelectasis
Wheezing
Recurrent/persistent infiltrates
Lung lesions of unknown etiology
Chronic cough
Hemoptysis
Selective bronchography
Equivocal tracheobronchial foreign body
Assessment of position, patency, or airway damage related to endotracheal or tracheostomy tubes
Assessment of injury from toxic inhalation or aspiration
Sampling from lower airway secretions and/or cells by bronchoalveolar lavage
Brush biopsy and bronchoscopic lung biopsy
Aid in difficult intubations
Therapeutic bronchoalveolar lavage
Removal of airway secretions and mucous plugs

[a] Recommended by the American Thoracic Society (29).

The value of bronchoalveolar lavage in the diagnosis of pulmonary infections in adults is well established (32). Bronchoalveolar lavage appears to be a safe, rapid, and reproducible method to diagnose infections in pediatric patients (33,34). In one study of 30 infectious episodes in 20 immunocompromised children, bronchoalveolar lavage provided a specific diagnosis in 56%; the most frequently identified organism was *Candida albicans* (35). In a prospective study (36), the utility of bronchoalveolar lavage with flexible bronchoscopy was assessed in 14 immunocompromised children with pneumonia over a 5-month period; a diagnosis was made by bronchoalveolar lavage in 71% of the children. Flexible bronchoscopy with bronchoalveolar lavage is well tolerated by children with acquired immunodeficiency syndrome complicated by significant tachypnea and hypoxia secondary to infection by *Pneumocystis carinii* (37).

Both partial and total lung lavage using a 3.2-mm flexible bronchoscope has been accomplished in young infants to treat severe pulmonary alveolar proteinosis (38). Bronchial washing for the quantification of lipid-laden macrophages has been suggested as a test for the diagnosis of recurrent aspiration of food substances in children (39).

The flexible bronchoscope has been found to be useful in the diagnosis of suspected tuberculosis. In one study of 121 flexible bronchoscopies in 54 children suspected of having tuberculosis, typical bronchial abnormalities were detected in 31 children. Bronchoscopy was important in the management of these patients, as it indicated a need for resection of granulation tissue by rigid bronchoscopy and guided the surgical decision (40).

In the diagnosis of diffuse infiltrates due to noninfectious diseases, the diagnostic yield tends to be lower.

One study reviewed 60 consecutive flexible bronchoscopies in 48 pediatric cancer patients with undiagnosed pulmonary infiltrates. Diagnostic procedures included 40 brushings, 50 bronchoalveolar lavages, and 6 bronchoscopic lung and mucosal biopsies during a 36-month period (41). The overall diagnostic yield was 27%; the diagnoses included infection, pulmonary leukemia, and lymphoma. Subsequent specific diagnoses had to be obtained by other procedures (open biopsy, needle aspiration, or autopsy) in 10 patients with negative bronchoscopy. The largest proportion of specific diagnoses came from lavage (14/50) and the smallest from brushings (1/40). A positive bronchoscopic result may be useful, but negative bronchoscopic findings do not justify delaying other diagnostic procedures or discontinuing antibiotic and antifungal therapy in children with cancer and pulmonary infiltrates.

Flexible bronchoscopy has proved useful as a safe bedside technique for critically ill pediatric patients in whom evaluation of the airway under general anesthesia is deemed unsafe (30). The flexible instrument can be used effectively and safely in pediatric intensive care units. A study of 87 children in the pediatric intensive care unit utilized four different-sized bronchoscopes to perform 61 diagnostic laryngoscopic procedures, 35 diagnostic bronchoscopic procedures, and 8 therapeutic bronchoscopic procedures (42). Diagnostic information was obtained in 91 of 96 procedures. Of the 8 therapeutic procedures, 7 were considered successful. Small-caliber bronchoscopes have been employed in the bedside evaluation of pediatric patients in the intensive care units (24,43–45).

Bronchoscopic determination of endotracheal tube position has been found to be safe and as accurate as chest roentgenograph (46). Ultrathin flexible bronchoscopes have been used to assist intubation of pediatric patients with difficult airway problems such as mandibular hypoplasia and Pierre–Robin syndrome (5,25,47). New applications possible with the ultrathin instruments include bronchoscopic transnasal intubation with endotracheal tubes as small as 2.5 mm inside diameter, inspection of the upper lobe segments in infants weighing less than 2.5 kg, and evaluation of the lower airways through endotracheal tubes as small as 2.5 mm inside diameter or tracheostomy tubes as small as no. 00 (3.1 mm inside diameter). Although these ultrathin instruments have no suction channel and are thus incapable of removing airway secretions or obtaining specimens, they can be extremely useful for many clinical purposes in infants and young children (5,20,25,48).

Flexible bronchoscopes can be used as therapeutic instruments in a variety of clinical situations. In a report on 46 bronchoscopies completed on 29 infants and 17 small children with persistent unilobar or multilobar atelectasis, the atelectasis resolved in all 29 infants and 10 of 17 (59%) small children after direct visualization, bronchial washing, and removal of mucous plugs and/or secretions (49). The procedure resulted in resolution of respiratory distress and cough within 24 hrs, as well as early hospital discharge in all patients regardless of complete or partial radiographic improvements. Arterial blood gases were improved or normalized in 16 patients. Despite the small (1.2-mm) suction channel, very large mucous plugs can often be removed with a flexible bronchoscope (5,50).

Bronchoscopy in children with bacterial tracheitis helps in confirming the diagnosis, removing adherent secretions, monitoring the course of the disease, and judging the appropriate time for the removal of the endotracheal tube (51).

Bronchopulmonary dysplasia is frequently encountered in pediatric practice. The application of bronchoscopy as a diagnostic tool in this disease has been valuable to the understanding of the clinical problems. A review of 129 flexible bronchoscopies in 47 children with bronchopulmonary dysplasia revealed that the two most common indications for bronchoscopy included evaluation of previously diagnosed subglottic stenosis and airway abnormalities (33 and 32%, respectively) (52). Other indications included persistent or recurrent infiltrates or atelectasis, need for cultures, stridor, failure to extubate, hoarseness, and persistent wheeze. Bronchoscopic diagnoses included adenoidal hypertrophy, laryngotracheobronchomalacia, vocal cord abnormalities, interarytenoid membrane, subglottic stenosis, granulomas including partial or near-total airway occlusion, bronchial stenosis, generalized inflammation, edema, polyps, tracheal bronchi, anomalous bronchial anatomy, and inspissated secretions (52,53).

In neonates, the flexible bronchoscope is valuabe in the examination of the airway and in the management of emergency situations such as suspected tube blockage or malposition and difficult intubations (5,25,54). A high yield of diagnostic information has been obtained especially in both postextubation patients and in patients presenting with upper airway obstruction (55). No major complications have been observed (5,25,56).

Bronchoscopic lung biopsy is performed less commonly in children than in adults (57,58). Therefore, limited data are available on the use of bronchoscopic lung biopsy in pediatric patients (29). The narrow working channel of the pediatric flexible bronchoscope allows for bronchoalveolar lavage, but it is not feasible to obtain bronchoscopic lung biopsy in smaller children. If a bronchoscopic lung biopsy is required in a small child, then a rigid bronchoscope will provide a large channel for the biopsy forceps. In most circumstances, if a lung biopsy is needed in a child, an open biopsy will be more satisfactory. One report (57) reviewed an experience in 12 patients (median age 14.5 years), all of whom had indications for bronchoscopic lung biopsy; a specific diagnosis was made in six patients (sarcoidosis, lymphoma, eosinophilic granuloma). In three additional patients, nonspecific histological findings combined with clinical, roentgenographic, and laboratory data helped support a diagnosis. Bronchoscopic lung biopsy has also been used in children who have undergone lung transplantation (59). Adequate lung tissue can be obtained in more than 84% of procedures (60,61). However, a 12.5% incidence of pneumothorax has been noted (60). Fluoroscopic guidance is advisable to obtain optimal samples (19). The technique used is similar to that in adults, as discussed in Chapter 11. Flexible bronchoscopes have been used to close bronchopleural fistulas with fibrin and tissue glues (62,63).

CONTRAINDICATIONS

There are no absolute contraindications to flexible bronchoscopy in pediatric patients. However, bronchoscopy should only be performed when the relative benefits outweigh the risks. According to the guidelines provided by the American Thoracic Society, situations that present a serious risk of complications during flexible bronchoscopy include coagulopathy or bleeding diathesis that cannot be corrected, massive hemoptysis, severe airway obstruction, severe refractory hypoxemia, and unstable hemodynamics including dysrhythmia (29).

Nevertheless, we believe that these are only relative contraindications and that each patient should be carefully considered as a candidate for bronchoscopy even when one or all of the above-listed factors are present. For example, thrombocytopenia poses minimal risk if no biopsy is performed. Diagnostic bronchoalveolar lavage is safe in severely thrombocytopenic patients (19). If the refractory hypoxemia is the result of a bronchoscopically treatable process, then a therapeutic bronchoscopy should be immediately undertaken after making sure that the patient is given adequate amounts of supplemental oxygen. Likewise, if significant hemoptysis is judged to be amenable to bronchoscopic therapy, one should not withhold the procedure as long as the procedure itself does not aggravate the problem. Obviously, the procedure should not be performed by inexperienced physicians, nor without extensive and comprehensive preparation for any possible complication.

COMPLICATIONS

The incidence of serious complications related to flexible bronchoscopy in pediatric practice is small (9,30,31,64). The complications can be divided into those related to medications used before or during the procedure and those secondary to the bronchoscopy itself. The former account for nearly half of the complications associated with flexible bronchoscopy (29). Minor and reversible complications such as benign arrhythmias and transient hypoxemia are the result of difficulty in ventilation, increased airway resistance, excessive sedation, and disturbances in ventilation-perfusion relationships. These complications can be avoided or minimized by careful execution of the procedure (10,29,64–71). Mechanical complications of flexible bronchoscopy in pediatric patients may include epistaxis, hemoptysis, and pneumothorax (5,56). A review of the results of 129 flexible bronchoscopy procedures performed on 47 children with bronchopulmonary dysplasia revealed that minor complications (epistaxis, transient bradycardia, mild nasopharyngeal bleeding, and mild worsening of upper airway obstruction) occurred in 3.1% of procedures, but no severe complications occurred (52). In the author's own series of 1,095 procedures (5), complications occurred in 2.9%; most of these were minor, and all resolved uneventfully. Bronchoalveolar lavage can be performed safely even in those with significant hypoxemia and immunocompromised status (72).

The flexible bronchoscope can be used safely in a critical care unit. In a study involving 87 children in a pediatric intensive care unit, the morbidity was minimal and no mortalities occurred (42). An ultrathin flexible bronchoscope has been used to remove bronchial secretions without interruption of mechanical ventilation in infants (73). In a report on 46 pediatric flexible bronchoscopies completed on 29 infants and 17 small children between 1 and 2 years of age with persistent unilobar or multilobar atelectasis, atelectasis resolved in all 29 infants and in 10 of 17 (59%) small children. Only one infant experienced minor epistaxis and another had transient minimal stridor. None of the 17 small children developed complications (49). Only one fatality following flexible bronchoscopy has been reported in a pediatric patient (6).

THE PROCEDURE

Children must be safe and comfortable during a bronchoscopic procedure. It is rarely necessary to employ general anesthesia for flexible bronchoscopy in children, but this modality should be used when sedation and other techniques are inadequate or inappropriate.

Children are usually good hypnotic subjects and, if handled properly, can perform amazingly well with minimal chemical sedation. In any event, the way in which a child (and the child's parents) is prepared for a procedure can have a major impact on the conduct of the procedure. Great attention should be paid to hypnotic principles in the preparation of children for bronchoscopy (Chapter 7). Using nonthreatening, positive, reassuring words, the procedure is described to the child and parents, so that the child's anxiety is minimized before the child enters the procedure room. Some form of presedation (oral chloral hydrate, oral midazolam) is generally recommended to attenuate anxiety. In a small percentage of infants, this alone may be sufficient, but in almost all children an intravenous access should be established to administer sedatives (midazolam, 0.05–0.1 mg/kg and meperidine 0.5–2.0 mg/kg). These drugs are given in fractional doses, with careful and continuous monitoring, and titrated to the desired effect. The child should be comfortable and relaxed, yet capable of responding to verbal or at least physical stimulation. Occasionally, an agitated child will fail to respond to the above and may be induced with a small dose of an ultra-short-acting barbiturate (methohexital, 1.0 mg/kg). This will produce light general anesthesia for 60–90 sec, and the bronchoscopist must be prepared to support ventilation and the airway. Following a dose of barbiturate given in this setting, the child almost always reaches the desired state of sedation from the drugs previously given. However, it is useful to pass the bronchoscope through the nose during the minute or two when the effects of the barbiturate are maximal.

Children are further prepared for flexible bronchoscopy by ensuring that their stomachs are empty. Older children are kept fasting for at least 4 hr, while younger children may be allowed to have small amounts of clear liquids until 2 hr prior to the scheduled time for the procedure. However, longer fasting periods (4–6 hr) are required if general anesthesia is to be used. In children younger than about 4–5 years, it is advisable to pass a suction catheter through the nose and into the stomach before beginning the bronchoscopy. This not only ensures that the stomach is empty, but it also gives a useful test of the patient's degree of sedation and topical anesthesia, and clears the nose and pharynx of secretions as well.

Topical anesthesia of the larynx is essential for safe and comfortable flexible bronchoscopy. This is accomplished in pediatric patients by direct instillation of 0.3–1.0 ml of 2% lidocaine (preservative-free) into the nostril with the patient supine, followed by direct application of another 1–2 ml of 2% lidocaine to the larynx and subglottic space directly through the bronchoscopy. If further topical anesthesia is necessary in the lower airways, 1% lidocaine is used.

Pediatric patients undergo flexible bronchoscopy in a supine position. When specimens are to be obtained from the lower airways for culture or cytology, it can be useful to place the patient in a Trendelenburg position prior to administration of topical anesthesia. This minimizes the risk of orotracheal aspiration, although it does not eliminate it.

Because children will almost always require sedation for bronchoscopy, it is also essential to provide for effective monitoring after the procedure is completed. In practice, the child usually remains in the bronchoscopy room for some minutes after the bronchoscope is withdrawn, while the specimens are prepared and paperwork is completed. This is a useful time to observe the patient for physiological stability and to speak with parents about the findings and their interpretation. The patient is then moved to an appropriate recovery area for further monitoring prior to discharge.

Unless the child has an artificial airway, the bronchoscope is inserted through the nose (this is useful even in many patients who do have a tracheostomy or an endotracheal tube). Frequently, pathological findings in the nasopharyngeal airway may be clinically unsuspected, so it is important to look as carefully in this area as in the lower airways.

A 3.2-mm flexible bronchoscope can be used in children of virtually any age and size, down to at least 700 g (5). The smaller the child, the less likely he or she will be to ventilate around the bronchoscope, although most children larger than about 3–3.5 kg will ventilate easily. Careful monitoring is necessary to ensure that the child continues to ventilate and oxygenate well. If this is not the case, then the procedure can be and *must be* completed within 30–45 sec. Fortunately, most skilled bronchoscopists can examine the entire lower airways within this time frame; repeated passes can be made if necessary, with hyperoxygenation between. Alternatively, an ultrathin bronchoscope can be used; infants as small as 540 g have been found to ventilate satisfactorily around this instrument (5).

In virtually every other respect, flexible bronchoscopies in children are conducted as in adults, although there are some subtle differences in techniques many of which are described in Chapter 9. With experience, each bronchoscopist will develop her or his own modifications.

TRAINING IN PEDIATRIC FLEXIBLE BRONCHOSCOPY

A survey of 871 North American bronchoscopists, all specializing in adult pulmonary diseases, conducted by the American College of Chest Physicians (ACCP) revealed that 13.2% of the respondents practiced pediatric bronchoscopy (74). In pediatric practice, surgeons (otolaryngologists and pediatric surgeons) and pediatric pulmonary specialists seem to perform the majority of bronchoscopies. An informal survey revealed that the former group is more likely to use rigid bronchoscopy whereas the latter almost exclusively uses flexible bronchoscopy. The ACCP survey suggests that the adult pulmonary specialist has very little exposure to pediatric bronchoscopy. This is not inappropriate, due to the lack of training in pediatric pulmonology as well as an increasing number of pediatric pulmonologists who are trained to perform bronchoscopy (50,75).

The American Thoracic Society has provided broad guidelines for pediatric flexible bronchoscopy (29). For training and teaching purposes, photographic equipment such as still or video camera and a teaching attachment is highly desirable. Unless specially equipped, hospital treatment rooms and general ward patient rooms are not adequate settings for flexible bronchoscopy. Flexible bronchoscopy should be incorporated into a comprehensive training program where trainees acquire expertise in pediatric airway anatomy, physiology, and pathophysiology as well as the manual skills. Training in bronchoscopy should include manual skills, interpretation of findings and indications, and knowledge of pharmacological agents employed in bronchoscopy (29). Some animal species may serve as valuable sources to learn observation of airway dynamics and nontraumatic manipulation of the bronchoscope (75). Further details regarding bronchoscopy training can be found in Chapter 29.

THE FUTURE OF PEDIATRIC BRONCHOSCOPY

The future lies in the imagination of bronchoscopists and instrument makers, involving new applications and new, possibly smaller, instruments. As this is written, the 2.2-mm flexible bronchoscope with distal angulation has just been marketed for general use. This step alone may increase the clinical use of flexible bronchoscopy in infants and children. New applications will follow, as more physicians apply their skills and imagination to clinical problems. On the other hand, the laws of physics are immutable, and instruments can only be made so small. We do not foresee the development of ultrathin bronchoscopes with working suction channels, for example.

A new generation of pediatric flexible bronchoscopes is on the horizon, with larger suction channels, capable of being used for limited instrumentation such as bronchoscopic lung biopsy. These instruments will bring important new capabilities and will greatly facilitate the care of a new generation of pediatric patients who, for example, have undergone lung transplantation.

In part because of the ease with which flexible bronchoscopes may be used and the low complication rate associated with their use, bronchoscopy has become an important research tool in the investigation of a number of pulmonary disorders. Recently, a working group was convened by the National Institutes of Health to discuss the research use of bronchoscopy and to update the guidelines for investigational procedures. The consensus of the group was that indications for investigative bronchoscopy could be considerably liberalized and that, while there are certainly very special considerations in the use of pediatric patients in clinical research, "age alone is not a contraindication to the use of bronchoscopy as a research tool" (76). The 1990s will see an explosion in the application of bronchoscopy to the problems of pediatric pulmonology.

Flexible bronchoscopy is being used more frequently in research protocols to study a variety of lung diseases. In the study of asthma in children, bronchoalveolar lavage has been used to study the relationship between the number of inflammatory cells in the bronchoalveolar lavage effluent and airway hyperresponsiveness (77). Bronchoscopy has been used to study mucosal structural abnormalities in children with cystic fibrosis (78,79). Tracheal injury is common and may lead to chronic complications in premature infants who are mechanically ventilated. Bronchoscopes have been used in such infants to carefully identify the factors that predispose to chronic airway problems (80).

Bronchoscopy is a very important tool in the diagnosis and management of infants and children with lung diseases. As with any tool, its safe and effective application depends on the skill, training, and judgment of the person operating it. We strongly disagree with statements such as, "flexible fiberoptic endoscopy as a technical procedure requires no specialized training" and "the technique itself is similar to routine endotracheal tube suctioning" (81). It should only be practiced by those who will do a sufficient number of procedures to develop and maintain their skill. There are many specific tools with which to examine and sample the airways of children, and the bronchoscopist must choose the proper tool for the proper situation and indications. Judicious use of the most appropriate tool in the most appropriate fashion at the most appropriate time will result in improved care for our most precious assets: our children.

REFERENCES

1. Patterson EJ. History of bronchoscopy and esophagoscopy for foreign body. *Laryngoscope* 1926;36:157–175.
2. Gans SL, Berci G. Advances in endoscopy of infants and children. *J Pediatr Surg* 1971;6:199–223.
3. Sackner MA. State of the art: bronchofiberscopy. *Am Rev Resp Dis* 1975;111:62.
4. Lockhart CH, Elliot JL. Potential hazards of pediatric rigid bronchoscopy. *J Pediatr Surg* 1984;19:239–242.
5. Wood RE. Spelunking in the pediatric airways: explorations with the flexible fiberoptic bronchoscope. *Pediatr Clin North Am* 1984;31:785–799.
6. Wagener JS. Fatality following fiberoptic bronchoscopy in a two-year-old child. *Pediatr Pulmonol* 1987;3:197–199.

7. Wood RE, Gauderer MW. Flexible fiberoptic bronchoscopy in the management of tracheobronchial foreign bodies in children: the value of a combined approach with open tube bronchoscopy. *J Pediatr Surg* 1984;19:693–698.
8. Tsueda K, Sjogren S, Debrand M, Pulito AR. Wire basket extraction of foreign bodies from the tracheobronchial tree of small children. *J Ky Med Assoc* 1981;79:13–15.
9. Prakash UBS, Midthun DE, Stelck MJ. Removal of large tracheobronchial foreign body in children using flexible bronchoscope. Unpublished data.
10. Schnapf BM. Oxygen desaturation during fiberoptic bronchoscopy in pediatric patients. *Chest* 1991;99:591–594.
11. Monden Y, Nakahara K, Fujii Y, Nanjo S, Ohno K, Kawashima Y. Trans-FBS-channel ventilation during the flexible bronchoscope (FBS) examination in infant. *Endoscopy* 1984; 16:175–178.
12. McKenzie B, Wood RE, Bailey A. Airway management for unilateral lung lavage in children. *Anesthesiology* 1989;70:550–553.
13. Wood RE. Pitfalls in the use of the flexible bronchoscope in pediatric patients. *Chest* 1990;97:199–203.
14. Groff DB, Allen JK. Gruentzig balloon catheter dilation for acquired bronchial stenosis in an infant. *Ann Thorac Surg* 1985; 39:379–381.
15. Brutinel WM, Cortese DA, Edell ES, McDougall JC, Prakash UBS. Complications of Nd:YAG laser therapy (editorial). *Chest* 1988;94:902–903.
16. Hetzel MR, Smith SGT. Endoscopic palliation of tracheobronchial malignancies. *Thorax* 1991;46:325–333.
17. Godfrey S. Bronchoscopy in childhood. *Br J Dis Chest* 1987; 81:225–231.
18. Godfrey S, Springer C, Maayan C, Avital A, Vatashky E, Belin B. Is there a place for rigid bronchoscopy in the management of pediatric lung disease? *Pediatr Pulmonol* 1987;3:179–184.
19. Prakash UBS, Stubbs SE. The bronchoscopy survey: some reflections. *Chest* 1991;100:1660–1667.
20. Wood RE, Azizkhan RG, Lacey SR, Sidman J, Drake A. Surgical applications of ultrathin flexible bronchoscopes in infants. *Ann Otol Rhinol Laryngol* 1991;100:116–119.
21. Wood RE, Fink RJ. Applications of flexible fiberoptic bronchoscopes in infants and children. *Chest* 1978;73:737–740.
22. Tucker JA, Silberman HD. Flexible fiberoptic pediatric bronchoscope. A new instrument. *Ann Otol Rhinol Laryngol* 1978; 87:558–559.
23. Wood RE, Sherman JM. Pediatric flexible bronchoscopy. *Ann Otol Rhinol Laryngol* 1980;89:414–416.
24. Fan LL, Sparks L,M, Dulinski JP. Applications of an ultrathin flexible bronchoscope for neonatal and pediatric airway problems. *Chest* 1986;89:673–676.
25. Wood RE. Clinical applications of ultrathin flexible bronchoscopes. *Pediatr Pulmonol* 1985;1:244–248.
26. Arnold JE. Advances in pediatric flexible bronchoscopy. *Otolaryngol Clin North Am* 1989;22:545–551.
27. Prakash UBS. The use of pediatric fiberoptic bronchoscope in adults. *Am Rev Resp Dis* 1985;132:715–717.
28. Raine J, Warner JO. Fiberoptic bronchoscopy without general anaesthetic. *Arch Dis Child* 1991;66:41–44.
29. Green CG, Eisenberg J, Leong A, Nathanson I, Schnapf BM, Wood RE. Flexible endoscopy of the pediatric airway. *Am Rev Resp Dis* 1992;145:133–235.
30. Wood RE. The diagnostic effectiveness of the flexible bronchoscope in children. *Pediatr Pulmonol* 1985;1:188–192.
31. Fitzpatrick SB, Marsh B, Stokes D, Wang KP. Indications for flexible fiberoptic bronchoscopy in pediatric patients. *Am J Dis Child* 1983;137:595–597.
32. Reynolds HY. State of the art: bronchoalveolar lavage. *Am Rev Resp Dis* 1987;135:250–263.
33. de Blic J, Blanche S, Daniel C, Le-Bourgeois M, Scheinmann P. Bronchoalveolar lavage in HIV infected patients with interstitial pneumonitis. *Arch Dis Child* 1989;64:1246–1250.
34. de Blic J, McKelvie P, Le-Bourgeois M, Blanche S, Benoist MR, Scheinmann P. Value of bronchoalveolar lavage in the management of severe acute pneumonia and interstitial pneumonitis in the immunocompromised child. *Thorax* 1987;42:759–765.
35. Farge A, Bellon G, Bouffet E, et al. Bronchoalveolar lavage by fibroscopy in immunodepressed children. *Pediatrie* 1989; 44:45–51.
36. Pattishall EN, Noyes BE, Orenstein DM. Use of bronchoalveolar lavage in immunocompromised children with pneumonia. *Pediatr Pulmonol* 1988;5:1–5.
37. Birriel JA Jr, Adams JA, Saldana MA, et al. Role of flexible bronchoscopy and bronchoalveolar lavage in the diagnosis of pediatric acquired immunodeficiency syndrome-related pulmonary disease. *Pediatrics* 1991;87:897–899.
38. Mahut B, de-Blic J, Le-Bourgeois M, Beringer A, Chevalier JY, Scheinmann P. Partial and massive lung lavages in an infant with severe pulmonary alveolar proteinosis. *Pediatr Pulmonol* 1992; 13:50–53.
39. Colombo JL, Hallberg TK. Recurrent aspiration in children: lipid laden alveolar macrophage quantitation. *Pediatr Pulmonol* 1987;3:86–89.
40. de Blic JD, Azevedo I, Burren CP, Bourgeois ML, Lallemand D, Scheinmann P. The value of flexible bronchoscopy in childhood pulmonary tuberculosis. *Chest* 1991;100:688–692.
41. Stokes DC, Shenep JL, Parham D, Bozeman PM, Marienchek W, Mackert PW. Role of flexible bronchoscopy in the diagnosis of pulmonary infiltrates in pediatric patients with cancer. *J Pediatr* 1989;115:561–567.
42. Fan LL, Sparks LM, Fix FJ. Flexible fiberoptic endoscopy for airway problems in a pediatric intensive care unit. *Chest* 1988; 93:556–560.
43. Ward RF, Arnold JE, Healy GB. Flexible minibronchoscopy in children. *Ann Otol Rhinol Laryngol* 1987;96:645–649.
44. Ovassapian A, Dykes MH, Yelich SJ. Difficult pediatric intubation—an indication for the fiberoptic bronchoscope (letter). *Anesthesiology* 1982;56:412–413.
45. Rucker RW, Silva WJ, Worcester CC. Fiberoptic bronchoscopic nasotracheal intubation in children. *Chest* 1979;76:56–58.
46. Vigneswaran R, Whitfield JM. The use of a new ultra-thin fiberoptic bronchoscope to determine endotracheal tube position in the sick newborn infant. *Chest* 1981;80:174–177.
47. Kleeman PP, Jantzen JP, Bonfils P. The ultra-thin bronchoscope in management of the difficult paediatric airway. *Can J Anaesth* 1987;34:606–608.
48. de Blic J, Delacourt C, Scheinmann P. Ultrathin flexible bronchoscopy in neonatal intensive care units. *Arch Dis Child* 1991; 66:1383–1385.
49. Nussbaum E. Pediatric bronchoscopy and its application in infantile atelectasis. *Clin Pediatr (Phila)* 1985;24:379–382.
50. Wood RE, Postma D. Endoscopy of the airway in infants and children. *J Pediatr* 1988;112:1–6.
51. Kasian GF, Bingham WT, Steinberg J, et al. Bacterial tracheitis in children. *Can Med Assoc J* 1989;140:46–50.
52. Cohn RC, Kercsmar C, Dearborn D. Safety and efficacy of flexible endoscopy in children with bronchopulmonary dysplasia. *Am J Dis Child* 1988;142:1225–1228.
53. Miller RW, Woo P, Kellman RK, Slagle TS. Tracheobronchial abnormalities in infants with bronchopulmonary dysplasia. *J Pediatr* 1987;111:779–782.
54. Finer NN, Etches PC. Fiberoptic bronchoscopy in the neonate. *Pediatr Pulmonol* 1989;7:116–120.
55. Vauthy PA, Reddy R. Acute upper airway obstruction in infants and children. Evaluation by the fiberoptic bronchoscope. *Ann Otol Rhinol Laryngol* 1980;89:417–418.
56. Fan LL, Flynn JW. Laryngoscopy in neonates and infants: experience with the flexible fiberoptic bronchoscope. *Laryngoscope* 1981;91:451–456.
57. Fitzpatrick SB, Stokes DC, Marsh B, Wang KP. Transbronchial lung biopsy in pediatric and adolescent patients. *Am J Dis Child* 1985;139:46–49.
58. Levy M, Glick B, Springer C, Mogle P, Vatashsky E, Drexler H, Godfrey S. Bronchoscopy and bronchography in children. Experience with 110 investigations. *Am J Dis Child* 1983; 137:14–16.
59. Whitehead B, Scott JP, Helms P, et al. Technique and use of transbronchial biopsy in children and adolescents. *Pediatr Pulmonol* 1992;12:240–246.
60. Muntz HR, Wallace M, Lusk RP. Pediatric transbronchial lung biopsy. *Ann Otol Rhinol Laryngol* 1992;101:135–137.

61. Scott JP, Higenbottam TW, Smyth RL, et al. Transbronchial biopsies in children after heart–lung transplantation. *Pediatrics* 1990;86:698–702.
62. Malfroot A, Van Tussenbroek F, Van Nooten G, Dab I. Endoscopic diagnosis and closure of a bronchopleural fistula. *Pediatr Pulmonol* 1991;11:280–282.
63. Wood RE, Lacey SR, Azizkhan RG. Endoscopic management of large, post-resection bronchopleural fistulas with methacrylate adhesive ("super glue"). *J Pediatr Surg* 1992;27:201–202.
64. Nussbaum E. Flexible fiberoptic bronchoscopy and laryngoscopy in children under 2 years of age: diagnostic and therapeutic applications of a new pediatric flexible fiberoptic bronchoscope. *Crit Care Med* 1982;10:770–772.
65. Albertini RE, Harrell JH, Kurihara N, Moser KM. Arterial hypoxemia induced by fiberoptic bronchoscopy. *JAMA* 1974; 230:1666–1667.
66. Karetzki MS, Garvery JW, Brandsetter RD. Effect of fiberoptic bronchoscopy on arterial oxygen tension. *NY State J Med* 1974; 74:62–63.
67. King EG. Hypoxemia during fiberoptic bronchoscopy (editorial). *Chest* 1984;65:117–118.
68. Matsushima Y, Jones RL, King EG, Moysa G, Alton JD. Alterations in pulmonary mechanics and gas exchange during routine fiberoptic bronchoscopy. *Chest* 1984;86:184–188.
69. Belen J, Neuhaus A, Markowitz D, Rotman HH. Modification of the effect of fiberoptic bronchoscopy on pulmonary mechanics. *Chest* 1981;79:516–519.
70. Peacock AJ, Benson-Mitchell R, Godfrey R. Effect of fibreoptic bronchoscopy on pulmonary function. *Thorax* 1990;45:38–41.
71. de Blic J, Scheinmann P. Fibreoptic bronchoscopy in infants. *Arch Dis Child* 1992;67:159–161.
72. Frankel LR, Smith DW, Lewiston NJ. Bronchoalveolar lavage for diagnosis of pneumonia in the immunocompromised child. *Pediatrics* 1988;81:785–788.
73. Shinwell ES. Ultrathin fiberoptic bronchoscopy for airway toilet in neonatal pulmonary atelectasis. *Pediatr Pulmonol* 1992; 13:48–49.
74. Prakash UBS, Offord KP, Stubbs SE. Bronchoscopy in North America: the ACCP survey. *Chest* 1991;100:1668–1675.
75. Wood RE, Pick JR. Model systems for learning pediatric flexible bronchoscopy. *Pediatr Pulmonol* 1990;8:168–171.
76. Workshop summary and guidelines: investigative use of bronchoscopy, lavage, and bronchial biopsies in asthma and other airway diseases. *J Allergy Clin Immunol* 1991;88:808–814.
77. Ferguson AC, Wong FW. Bronchial hyperresponsiveness in asthmatic children. Correlation with macrophages and eosinophils in broncholavage fluid. *Chest* 1989;96:988–991.
78. Sherman JM. Bronchial lavage in patients with cystic fibrosis: a critical review of current knowledge (review). *Pediatr Pulmonol* 1986;2:244–226.
79. Wunderlich P, Kemmer C, Fischer R, et al. Bronchial secretions and bronchial mucosa in children with cystic fibrosis: comparison of bronchoscopic, biochemical, bacteriological, microscopic and ultrastructural findngs. *Acta Paediatr Hung* 1986; 27:123–131.
80. Schellhase DE, Graham LM, Fix EJ, Sparks LM, Fan LL. Diagnosis of tracheal injury in mechanically ventilated premature infants by flexible bronchoscopy. *Chest* 1990;98:1219–1225.
81. Dietrich KA, Strauss RH, Cabalka AK, Zimmerman JJ, Scanlan KA. Use of flexible fiberoptic endoscopy for determination of endotracheal tube position in the pediatric patient. *Crit Care Med* 1988;16:884–887.

Bronchoscopy,
edited by U. B. S. Prakash.
Mayo Foundation © 1994.
Published by Raven Press, Ltd., New York.

CHAPTER 25

Complications of Bronchoscopy

Samuel E. Stubbs and W. Mark Brutinel

The morbidity and mortality associated with bronchoscopy and its associated procedures are low. The indications for rigid bronchoscopy and flexible bronchoscopy are similar, and contraindications are few. Each instrument has proponents for its preferred uses (1). The rigid bronchoscope is preferred for massive bleeding and certain foreign bodies whereas the flexible bronchoscope is preferred for patients who have structural abnormalities of the neck or require mechanical ventilation. Complications from use of each instrument are similar; however, with the rigid instrument one has the additional risk of damage to dentures, soft tissue trauma leading to airway perforation or subglottic edema, and significant hemorrhage. With larger instruments, severe hemorrhage may occur on obtaining a biopsy that includes the wall of a significant-sized vessel or a very vascular tumor or aneurysm. Unlike the flexible bronchoscope, the rigid bronchoscope permits direct access to the bleeding site for topical application of gauze packing that may be soaked in epinephrine, ventilation of the patient, and application of large suction devices. Bronchoscopy today is largely flexible bronchoscopy (2). Except where indicated, this chapter will deal primarily with flexible bronchoscopy and its complications.

Bronchoscopists should be familiar with factors known to increase a patient's risk for bronchoscopy (Chapter 8) as well as the type of complications that can occur and their management. The goal of the bronchoscopist should be to provide a safe procedure free of complications in an efficient manner with minimal discomfort for the patient. This can only be accomplished by careful preoperative evaluation, an assessment of the indication for the procedure relative to the risk for the patient, careful preparation of the patient, and the use of skillful techniques. Facilities and equipment should be available to deal with emergencies that can occur (Chapter 7).

One can identify several areas from which complications of flexible bronchoscopy arise (3). Premedication and sedatives may lead to respiratory depression, hypotension, syncope, or an agitated state of hyperexcitement. Local anesthesia may be associated with laryngospasm, bronchospasm, seizures, or cardiorespiratory arrest. Most flexible bronchoscopies are performed under local anesthesia; however, general anesthesia may be used when indicated (Chapter 7). Bronchoscopy and its related procedures including brushing and biopsy of localized lung lesions, bronchoscopic lung biopsy, and bronchoalveolar lavage may also be associated with bronchospasm, laryngospasm, hypoxemia, cardiac arrhythmias, fever, pneumonia, pneumothorax, and hemorrhage (Table 1). Some complications deserve special consideration and will be discussed in more detail later in this chapter.

In 1974 Credle and associates reported a review of the complications of flexible bronchoscopy in 24,521 procedures (4). Of 250 questionnaires that were mailed to various centers in the United States, 192 replies were reported. The incidence of minor complications was 0.2%; major complications 0.08%; and mortality 0.01%. Major complications were defined as those which by their nature were serious or required specific resuscitative measures. Approximately half of the life-threatening complications were associated with premedication or topical anesthesia.

PREMEDICATION

There were four major complications and nine minor complications related to premedication reported in the review (4). Excessive premedication resulted in four serious episodes of respiratory depression, one of which required intubation. Three patients who re-

S. E. Stubbs and W. M. Brutinel: Division of Thoracic Diseases and Internal Medicine, Mayo Clinic, Rochester, Minnesota 55905.

TABLE 1. *Complications of bronchoscopy*

Drugs	
Premedication and intraoperative sedation:	Respiratory depression, apnea, hypotension, syncope, hyperexcitable state, allergic reaction
Local anesthesia:	Respiratory arrest, seizures, methemoglobinemia, laryngospasm, bronchospasm, allergic reaction, nausea and vomiting
Bronchoscopy and Associated Procedures	
General:	Laryngeal edema, hypoxia, hypercarbia, bronchospasm
Cardiovascular:	Atrial and ventricular arrhythmias, myocardial ischemia, angina, cardiac arrest
Infectious:	Temperature elevation, bacteremia, pneumonia, metastatic infections, inoculation of infectious agent (bacterial, mycobacterial, fungal, viral [human immunodeficiency virus]), intrabronchial contamination by abscess cavity contents
Therapeutic suctioning:	Hypoxia, bleeding
Bronchial brushing, bronchial biopsy, bronchoscopic lung biopsy:	Hemorrhage, perforation of bronchus/lung, pneumothorax, broken brush, broken forceps
Bronchoscopic needle aspiration:	Hemorrhage, perforation of the great vessels, hemomediastinum, pneumomediastinum, pneumothorax
Endobronchial laser therapy:	Hypoxia, hemorrhage, perforation of esophagus, bronchus or lung, pneumothorax, fire, death
Bronchoalveolar lavage:	Fever, pneumonitis, bronchial bleeding, bronchospasm, pneumothorax
Foreign body removal:	Massive hemoptysis, airway obstruction
Other:	See text

ceived a narcotic premedication experienced apnea; two were managed with narcotic antagonists, but the other developed a ventricular arrhythmia and required vigorous resuscitation. Transient hypotension and syncope occurred in seven patients. Pretreatment with an anticholinergic and performance of the procedure in the supine position should help offset this complication. A hyperexcitable state was reported in one instance; certainly, this can be a problem for patients who become agitated and develop a state of panic leading to a need to abort the procedure. Many patients tolerate flexible bronchoscopy well without sedating premedication and, when needed, the agent and dose used should take into consideration the patient's cardiovascular, hepatic, and mental status (3).

LOCAL ANESTHESIA

In Credle's survey (4) there was one mortality, seven major complications, and three minor complications. Excessive tetracaine was felt responsible for respiratory arrest in three cases, two seizures, methemoglobinemia in one case, and death in a patient who was not seriously ill. An excessive dosage of lidocaine was responsible for two unspecified minor complications and a seizure. The concentration of lidocaine in the blood after topical applications may be 30–50% of that obtained by rapid intravenous administration (3). Xylocaine has a wider margin of safety than tetracaine, and with a total dose of lidocaine of 300 mg there is little risk of clinical toxicity or toxic blood levels. One must use caution in patients with cardiac or hepatic disease when higher doses are occasionally needed to provide adequate local anesthesia. As with adverse reactions to premedications, facilities and drugs must be available to treat seizures and provide cardiorespiratory support in the event of cardiovascular collapse or respiratory arrest (Chapter 7). Laryngospasm with airway obstruction associated with tonic contraction of the laryngeal and pharyngeal structures may occur with application of a local anesthetic or manipulation of the vocal cords and adjacent structures. Minor cases may be treated with hyperoxygenation. Stubborn cases may require ventilation by positive airway pressure with 100% oxygen. Intravenous sedation and small doses of a drug such as succinylcholine may be necessary if these measures are not successful.

MAJOR COMPLICATIONS

In 1976 Suratt and associates reported on a review of 48,000 bronchoscopies reported in 323 responses from 1,041 mailed questionnaires (5). Twelve deaths (0.02%) were reported; 2 of these occurred after administration of tetracaine, 2 had acute myocardial infarctions, and 2 patients with previously bleeding tumors bled massively following biopsy and lavage. Life-threatening cardiovascular complications occurred in 27 patients (0.5%) with 10 cardiac arrests. Life-threatening airway complications occurred in 52 patients including bronchospasm in 17 instances and hemorrhage in 5 patients. Life-threatening reactions to topical anesthesia occurred in 41 instances including the 2 deaths. A previously unreported problem of broken brushes was reported in 4 instances. In this review of complications, all of the patients who died had at least 1 of 4 serious underlying illnesses: myocardial disease, severe chronic obstructive lung disease, serious pneumonia, or cancer.

In 1978 Pereira and associates reported on the frequency of complications in a prospective study of 908 patients from 13 hospitals (6). Major complications including respiratory arrest, pneumonia, pneumothorax, and airway obstruction occurred in 1.7%. One death resulted in a mortality rate of 0.1%. Minor complications (6.5%) included vasovagal reactions, fever, cardiac arrhythmias, bleeding, obstruction of the airways, nausea and vomiting, pneumothorax, psychotic reactions, and aphonia. Bronchoscopic lung biopsy performed in 85 patients resulted in 4 pneumothoraces (5%).

HYPOXIA

Hypoxia has been well recognized as one of the complications of bronchoscopy (7–15) and is known to occur frequently (13,15–17). With the newer flexible bronchoscopes having large suction channels and the procedure being performed in more critically ill patients, the potential for hypoxia is even greater. This complication is more frequently appreciated now that pulse oximetry is readily available, and supplemental oxygen is administered routinely by 88.9% of respondents in a recent survey of bronchoscopic practice in the United States. In this same survey, 84.2% of respondents routinely used oximetry (18). The more severely ill the patient, the more likely that hypoxia will occur and the more severe the hypoxia is likely to become. In acutely ill, ventilated patients, one study documented an average decline in the PaO_2 of 26% at the end of the procedure compared to baseline with a slight rise in $PaCO_2$. Fourteen patients developed clinical hypoxemia defined by a PaO_2 lower than 60 mm Hg. Patients with the adult respiratory distress syndrome and those who frequently exceeded the peak airway pressure settings for their ventilator were at increased risk of developing a PaO_2 of less than 60 mm Hg. A mild but significant reduction in the PaO_2 persisted for up to 2 hr after the procedure (7). Hypoxia can also occur during bronchoalveolar lavage (8,10,11). With proper attention to the patient's oxygenation, hypoxia should infrequently be a problem during bronchoscopy. Depending on the patient's baseline oximetry or arterial blood gas determination, oxygen supplementation may be as simple as use of a nasal cannula, a close-fitting mask with a hole or diaphragm cut in it (14), an open-face tent, or an endotracheal tube with adapter. In those patients already receiving supplemental oxygen by one of these methods, an increase in the fraction of inspired oxygen (FiO_2) prior to starting the procedure should be considered as long as CO_2 retention is not a problem. Also, attention should be given to maintaining an increase in FIO_2 for an adequate time following the patient's procedure to assure return to the baseline arterial oxygen tension.

HYPERCARBIA

The flexible bronchoscope takes up space in the airway, and resistance to breathing is increased. An adult patient with adequate respiratory reserve can easily compensate for a mild increase in resistance to breathing by normal respiratory mechanisms. Significant hypercarbia with respiratory acidosis is rare but can occur in patients who develop acute severe bronchospasm or in those marginal patients whose respiratory reserve is minimal. By increasing airway resistance one can overcome the patient's ability to compensate resulting in an increased arterial CO_2 level, respiratory acidosis, and a decrease in respiratory drive, thereby entering into a vicious cycle toward respiratory failure. The bronchoscopist should be aware of this possibility and be prepared to deal with it. In patients with high alveolar-arterial oxygen gradients, despite oxygen supplementation, and CO_2 retention, placement of an endotracheal tube with a balloon cuff over the bronchoscope should be considered. Oxygen supplementation and ventilatory support can then be provided as needed. Careful observation following the procedure to assure the patient will be able to ventilate adequately prior to extubation is important, particularly when sedation is used.

Patients with diffuse pulmonary disease present a special challenge to the bronchoscopist. These patients can have a large alveolar-arterial oxygen gradient, low arterial oxygen levels despite oxygen supplementation, and low carbon dioxide levels. There is usually an associated tachypnea. They can develop respiratory failure with hypoxia, severe hypercarbia, and respiratory acidosis following the procedure. Immunocompromised patients frequently present with this clinical picture, and bronchoscopy with bronchoalveolar lavage can be a life-saving diagnostic procedure in these patients. Thus, the potential benefits justify the procedure. The bronchoscopist should be prepared to support the patient with intubation and mechanical ventilation if necessary following the procedure while diagnostic material is being analyzed and definitive therapy is being planned.

BRONCHOSPASM

Patients with increased airway reactivity are at high risk for development of complications (19,20). Bronchospasm as a complication of bronchoscopy can be severe and potentially life threatening (19). Especially worrisome are patients with unrecognized bronchial hyperactivity who are examined without pretreatment with bronchodilators or corticosteroids. Although fortunately this is rare, these patients can quickly develop severe respiratory distress and potentially progress to respiratory failure. Patients with asthma undergoing bronchoscopy should be on optimal treatment. If there is any question regarding this aspect of their care, one can premedicate patients with inhaled, intravenous, or oral bronchodilators. Corticosteroids by any of these three routes can also be used as long as adequate time is allowed for them to take effect. Bronchodilators have been shown to reduce the decrease in forced expiratory volume in 1 sec (FEV_1) with bronchoscopy and should greatly reduce the chance of severe bronchospasm occurring (21,22). Large doses of atropine (1–2 mg) administered parenterally or by inhalation may be helpful in reducing the bronchoconstrictive effects of bronchoscopy (19,23). One may also have an infusion containing aminophylline for administration during the procedure (24). The intravenous line would provide a quick access for the administration of a corticosteroid should it be desired. Having available facilities for intubation and respiratory support is imperative.

The exact cause of bronchospasm in patients undergoing bronchoscopy is still debatable. Studies have shown that local anesthesia with lidocaine alone without bronchoscopy can cause a decrease in the FEV_1 (25). Using 25°C saline for bronchoalveolar lavage will decrease the peak expiratory flow rate and the forced expiratory $flow_{25-72}$ in healthy subjects. This response doesn't occur when 37°C saline is used (11). Pre- and postbronchoscopy testing with histamine challenges does not show a change in the airway responsiveness. However, those patients that have a heightened responsiveness to histamine challenge will show a greater decrease in the FEV_1 following bronchoscopy (26,27). The risks and potential benefits of bronchoscopy must be constantly assessed in those patients with bronchial hyperreactivity. If such patients are adequately pretreated with appropriate medication, the risk of bronchoscopy can be greatly reduced. It is reassuring that bronchoscopy and bronchoalveolar lavage have been reported to be safe in asthmatic patients with no or minimal symptoms and an FEV_1 of greater than 60% of predicted (28). Patients with chronic obstructive pulmonary disease also benefit from pretreatment for bronchial hyperreactivity (21).

HEMODYNAMIC EFFECTS OF BRONCHOSCOPY

Bronchoscopy induces significant hemodynamic changes that are maximal during passage through the larynx and during suctioning. The mean arterial pressure can increase by 30%, heart rate by 43%, cardiac index by 28%, and mean pulmonary arterial occlusion pressure by 26% compared with prebronchoscopic control values (29). The changes are of little consequence in patients with normal cardiovascular function and blood supply. In patients with coronary artery ischemia and reduced cardiac function, they may be significant. With the potential for hypoxemia with flexible bronchoscopy there is an increased risk for myocardial infarction and arrhythmias in such patients. Fortunately, myocardial infarction is uncommon in patients undergoing flexible bronchoscopy, but the risks should be carefully weighed in patients with significant coronary artery disease and unstable cardiac function.

CARDIAC ARRHYTHMIAS

Arrhythmias have been noted with bronchoscopy and can lead to asystole and death (30), although this is fortunately extremely rare. Patients with coronary artery disease have the potential to develop ischemia (31) and therefore an increased risk for development of serious cardiac arrhythmias. The most common arrhythmia is a sinus tachycardia, and when all arrhythmias are combined, the incidence can approach 70–80% (32,33). Fortunately, major arrhythmias such as ventricular tachycardia are much less common (approximately 4%). The incidence of major arrhythmias was found to decrease from 8% to 4% when prebronchoscopic and postbronchoscopic electrocardiographic recordings were compared. This was considered to be related to the blood lidocaine concentrations that developed from the topical anesthetic applied to the respiratory mucosa (32). Thus, lidocaine topical anesthesia may have a protective effect in terms of the incidence of cardiac arrhythmias. Atenolol has also been shown to reduce the number of cardiac arrhythmias when used prior to bronchoscopy (34). Prior to bronchoscopy, the patient's cardiovascular status should be carefully assessed, myocardial ischemia should be treated aggressively, and arrhythmias should be adequately treated to reduce the chance of myocardial infarction or life-threatening arrhythmia. In a recent survey of bronchoscopists in the United States, 74.6% routinely use electrocardiographic monitoring during bronchoscopy (18). We strongly endorse this practice, along with the routine use of oximetry, which can allow for early intervention to prevent the dangerous combination of hypoxia, myocardial ischemia, and arrhythmias.

INFECTIOUS COMPLICATIONS

Fever can occur following bronchoscopy; 16% of patients developed fever in one study (6). Parenchymal infiltration was also found in 6% of patients in this study. In a more recent study fever occurred in 27% of cases without evidence of bacteremia (35). The exact cause of the fever elevation is uncertain. Dramatic elevations of tumor necrosis factor have been observed (36). Bacteremia following bronchoscopy has been reported in isolated case reports, sometimes with serious consequences (37–40). Serious bacteremic events appear to be associated with gram-negative organisms, particularly *Pseudomonas,* and can develop dangerous consequences despite prophylactic antimicrobial therapy (41). Pneumonia has been reported following bronchoscopy (42).

Lung abscesses have also occurred and have been reported complicating bronchoscopic lung biopsies (43). Massive intrabronchial aspiration of the contents of pulmonary abscess cavities can also occur (44). Fortunately, these episodes are rare. The possibility of aspirating abscess cavity contents following bronchoscopy has raised questions about the place of bronchoscopy in the evaluation and treatment of lung abscesses. Hammer and associates described massive aspiration of the contents of a large abscess cavity 2 hr following the introduction of a cytology brush into the cavity of the abscess (44). Harber and Terry reported a fatality rate of 9.3% in 440 patients with lung abscesses (45). It was felt that aspiration of abscess cavity contents contributed to a fatal outcome in 7 of 33 patients in their series. A number of these patients had rigid bronchoscopy during the course of their evaluation. They concluded that one should limit bronchoscopy to carefully selected patients in whom it appears likely to be of significant therapeutic or diagnostic benefit. Certainly, one may need to evaluate the patient for an obstructing lesion such as a malignancy or foreign body. Some measures that may be taken to minimize or prevent aspiration of the contents of a lung abscess include (a) minimal use of depressant drugs and local anesthetics in an effort to preserve to some degree the protective defenses such as the gag and cough reflexes, (b) positioning the patient in a lateral or head-down position until all airway reflexes have returned to help prevent aspiration of material to the unaffected side, and (c) careful intraoperative and postoperative observation for the development of sudden aspiration by personnel prepared to treat this complication rapidly. General anesthesia would appear to increase the risk because of a more profound effect on the protective reflexes of the airways. Clearly, one should have adequate suction equipment available and be prepared to intubate the patient if necessary. It is recommended that high airway pressures be avoided during resuscitation of patients with cardiopulmonary arrest since this may promote release and dissemination of additional infected material (45,46).

Currently, due to the low incidence of bacteremia, bacterial endocarditis prophylaxis is not recommended in patients undergoing flexible bronchoscopy (Chapter 8). Physicians can use their discretion in patients with prosthetic heart valves and previous bacterial endocarditis. Bacterial endocarditis prophylaxis is recommended for rigid bronchoscopy (46,47). Multiple pseudo-outbreaks of bacterial, fungal, and tuberculosis infections have been reported due to contaminated bronchoscopes (48–54). A particular concern is transmission of tuberculosis, and a recent article indicated the need to pay close attention to suction valves (55). Transmission of *Mycobacterium tuberculosis* has been documented (56), and the human immunovirus has been cultured from bronchoscopes used in patients who are infected with this virus (57). Thus to prevent transmission of these infectious agents, meticulous care must be taken in the cleaning of the bronchoscope between procedures. Manufacturer's instructions should be followed carefully. Use of appropriate disinfecting and sterilizing agents for adequate amounts of time as well as thorough cleaning of suction channels and valve parts should be undertaken (Chapter 29). Metastatic *Pseudomonas* endophthalmitis (58), extension of pulmonary tuberculosis (59), bacteremic pneumonia (40), and bacteremia with meningitis (39) have been reported following bronchoscopy. Fortunately, these are uncommon and present in the literature as single-case reports. The literature would also suggest that chemoprophylaxis will not prevent these isolated unfortunate incidents, and the treatment will have to be tailored according to the individual patients.

COMPLICATIONS PERTAINING TO SPECIFIC PROCEDURES

Brushings

There have been few studies looking at the complication rate with the use of the cytology brush in bronchoscopy. Fortunately, these complications are rare. They can induce bleeding and have the potential for perforating the pleura causing a pneumothorax. Breaking of the brushes has been reported (60). One study reported four instances of breakage of the tip of a cytology brush. The brushes were reusable, suggesting that repeated use and bending of the tip may be a factor. Three of the four brushes were removed, with one patient requiring thoracotomy, and one brush was left in place for 18 months without complications (5). Current bronchoscopic brushes are well made and if they are used properly this should rarely be a problem. An unusual complication of a brush piercing the bronchus has been described (61). The use of vigorous pressure against resistance was felt to be related to penetration of the bronchus producing a hook deformity of the brush. After several attempts, the brush was successfully removed with no development of complications.

Bronchial Biopsies and Bronchoscopic Lung Biopsies

The risk of bronchoscopy is increased if bronchoscopic biopsy is performed. The main concerns are bleeding and pneumothorax. The bronchoscopic lung complication rate was increased from 0.12% to 2.7% and the mortality rate went from 0.04% to 0.12% if bronchoscopic lung biopsy was included in the procedure (62). Bleeding from bronchial and bronchoscopic lung biopsies was addressed in a large study of 600 patients; 193 patients had biopsies under direct vision, 132 had biopsies under fluoroscopic guidance, and 13 had bronchoscopic lung biopsies for diffuse disease. Brisk hemorrhage was reported to be present in six of the patients. One of the biopsies was taken under direct vision from a bronchogenic carcinoma, and the other five biopsies were by the bronchoscopic technique. Of these five patients, one had usual interstitial pneumonia and patients were on cytotoxic-immunosuppressive and corticosteroid therapy (three renal transplants, one leukemia). In one case, the rigid bronchoscope was needed to manage excessive hemorrhage. No deaths occurred (63). A subsequent study of 438 patients who had bronchoscopic lung biopsy revealed severe hemorrhage in 9% of routine cases, 29% in immunosuppressed patients, and 45% of uremic patients; there was one death (64). Fatal pulmonary hemorrhage has been reported. In one case, a patient died from a massive, fatal pulmonary hemorrhage following a bronchoscopic lung biopsy of the right middle lobe. The patient had a normal prothrombin and partial thromboplastin time and platelets of 93,000/μl. He had been examined through the nasal route without an endotracheal tube and the massive hemorrhage prevented insertion of either an endotracheal tube or a rigid bronchoscope. Tracheostomy was performed but did not succeed in controlling the hemorrhage. Examination of the bronchoscopic lung biopsy showed a leukemic infiltrate and autopsy confirmed the diagnosis. A small (0.5-mm) artery was found to have been biopsied along with the adjacent bronchus and lung (65). Bronchoscopic lung biopsy of 15 patients on mechanical ventilation had a 20% occurrence of self-limited bleeding. All the patients who had bleeding survived and were eventually weaned from mechanical ventilation (66). Patients with thrombocytopenia are at increased risk for bleeding. Twenty-five bronchoscopies were performed in 24 patients with a mean platelet count of 30,000/μl (7,000–60,000/μl). There were three patients who had self-limited endobronchial bleeding and one patient with a fatal pulmonary hemorrhage. All patients who had bleeding complications received platelet transfusions. The patients with self-limited bleeding had prothrombin times that were normal or only very slightly prolonged and one had a slightly elevated partial thromboplastin time. The patient with fatal hemorrhage had a platelet count of 23,000/μl and elevated prothrombin and partial thromboplastin times. This fatal case had received platelet transfusions and fresh frozen plasma before and during the bronchoscopy (67). Wedging the bronchoscope in the bronchus to the area of lung being biopsied has been suggested to control hemorrhage if it occurs. There has been one report of an air embolism related to increased pressure from wedging the bronchoscope (68). The advantage gained in controlling hemorrhage from bronchoscopic biopsies probably outweighs the small risk of this complication. Wedging the flexible bronchoscope into the bronchus in the area being biopsied is not absolutely required as long as the bronchoscopist is able to immediately reach the affected bronchus if bleeding occurs. The bronchoscopist must be prepared to deal with life-threatening bleeding and hemoptysis (Chapter 17).

Bronchoscopic lung biopsy should have a low incidence of pneumothoraces. The incidence of pneumothorax has been reported to be between 1% and 4% (69–72). It has been reported that fluoroscopy is unnecessary in bronchoscopic lung biopsies (72). However, in one mail survey of bronchoscopists in the United Kingdom, the incidence of pneumothorax without fluoroscopy was 2.9% and when fluoroscopy was used the incidence decreased to 1.8% (62). A small study of bronchoscopic lung biopsies during mechanical ventilation (73) revealed a higher incidence of pneumothoraces (13%). A 7% incidence of tension pneumothorax has been reported (66). If a bronchoscopist feels that bronchoscopic lung biopsy is indicated with mechanical ventilation, preparation should be made to control the pleural space with thoracostomy tubes if necessary. Studies have shown that routine chest roentgenogram following bronchoscopic lung biopsy is not cost-effective (71). We favor use of fluoroscopic guidance for bronchoscopic lung biopsies. With fluoroscopy one can more precisely place the biopsy forceps in an area of localized disease or near the pleura for a peripheral bronchoscopic lung biopsy in diffuse disease (74). Acute chest pain or dyspnea following bronchoscopic lung biopsy should make one suspect pneumothorax. A chest X ray or fluoroscopy can confirm the diagnosis and lead to appropriate measures to expand the lung (72).

Consistent with the finite life of many medical instruments, alligator biopsy forceps have also been reported to break during the course of flexible bronchoscopy (75). In this instance, metal fatigue was thought to have been a factor. The forceps had been used for 50, 30, and 10 cases, respectively. One patient was reported to have coughed and expectorated one of the broken forceps. The fate of the other two patients is unknown; however, subsequent chest roentgenogram showed no evidence of a foreign body.

Bronchoscopic Needle Aspiration

Bronchoscopic needle aspiration and biopsy has been found safe and few complications have been reported. Pneumothorax, hemomediastinum, and fever can occur following this type of needle aspiration or biopsy (76–80). Fortunately, these are only case reports and this procedure should be considered safe with rare complications in properly selected patients (Chapter 12).

Endobronchial Laser Therapy

The use of laser technology to treat malignant airway obstruction can lead to significant complications, including airway obstruction, massive hemorrhage, pneumothorax, and esophageal perforation. These problems can be dealt with by the appropriate measures, and the mortality should not exceed 2% (81). The selection of patients, equipment, and technique contributes to reducing the incidence of complications with endobronchial laser therapy. Also the bronchoscopist must be ready to respond to the problem of massive pulmonary hemorrhage and airway obstruction (Chapter 17).

Bronchoalveolar Lavage

Bronchoalveolar lavage is being used increasingly in the evaluation of patients with diffuse lung disease, especially those possibly infectious in etiology. Minor complications requiring only symptomatic treatment occur in less than 5% of procedures and include hypoxia, pneumothorax, fever, pneumonitis, bronchial bleeding, and bronchospasm (8,10,11,82–86). It was reported that PaO_2 fell a mean of 32 mm Hg in 28 patients given supplemental oxygen during bronchoalveolar lavage. The PaO_2 fell to less than 60 mm Hg in 76% of patients (8). The mean time for the oxygen tension to return to baseline was 53 min. Bronchoalveolar lavage is an atraumatic procedure and can be used in patients with abnormal coagulation parameters and low platelet counts (87). Pneumothorax has been reported in a patient who coughed suddenly following wedging of the bronchoscope in the lingula at the beginning of the lavage. Pleuritic chest pain and dyspnea led to the obtaining of a chest X ray showing a left pneumothorax. It was proposed that high intraalveolar tension during cough with no air flow could result in rupture of a bleb and resultant pneumothorax (84).

Other Complications

Flexible bronchoscopy is a low-morbidity procedure, but it can be associated with unusual complications that in themselves may threaten the life of the patient. For example, cerebral air embolism complicating bronchoscopic lung biopsy is an uncommon complication (68). Using the wedge procedure described by Zavala (88) to obtain a bronchoscopic lung biopsy in a patient subsequently found to have miliary tuberculosis, the patient developed a grand mal seizure approximately 10 sec following removal of the forceps and had a respiratory arrest. A clinical diagnosis of air embolism was made, and the patient died 3 days later. The bronchoscopic lung biopsy specimens showed a 3-mm segment of pulmonary vein. The authors were concerned that the wedging of the bronchoscope at the beginning of the exhalation may have played a role in causing the venous air embolism. They recommended that the bronchoscope not be wedged until the lung biopsy had been taken at the end of exhalation.

Historically, the rigid bronchoscope has been the instrument used for removal of foreign bodies from the lungs. Although massive hemoptysis associated with removal of foreign bodies is uncommon, Reiss reported exsanguinating hemoptysis following the removal of a small-caliber cartridge casing from the right main stem bronchus of a 12-year-old child who had "swallowed a bullet seven years previously" (89). The rigid instrument was used in this instance. With the increasing use of the flexible instrument for foreign body work, one must be aware of this potential risk and be prepared to deal with it.

Fatal hemorrhage has also occurred following flexible bronchoscopy on a patient with mycotic aneurysms of the pulmonary artery (90). A young man who used heroin had received treatment for pneumonia that became more extensive and included a large, round opacity in the left upper lobe with a left hilar shadow. Following bronchoscopy in an attempt to brush an extrinsically compressed left lower lobe, the patient suffered an immediate hemoptysis of 2 L. Although he survived the initial episode of bleeding, he died following a second episode of 1.5 L 56 hr later. At postmortem examination he was found to have multiple aneurysms of the pulmonary artery. Organized vegetations were found within the right atrium. Bronchoscopists are often called on to do diagnostic procedures for intravenous drug abusers. They should be aware that these patients are at risk for the development of endocarditis, septic pulmonary emboli, mycotic aneurysms, and massive hemoptysis (90).

Carcinoid tumors may be very vascular and bleed easily following manipulation and biopsy. Acute carcinoid syndrome has also been reported to occur during bronchoscopic biopsy of a solitary nodule in a 39-year-old woman (91). As a specimen was being removed, the patient developed marked facial flushing, diaphoresis, hypertension, and tachycardia. The procedure was aborted; however, the symptoms and findings recurred with a second attempt. The tumor was found to produce serotonin and adrenocorticotropic hormone. Although symptoms subsided following termination of the flexible bronchoscopy, the patient had severe hypotension during surgery that responded to massive doses of corticosteroids. The possibility of acute carcinoid syndrome and other hormonal syndromes should be kept in mind when one obtains a biopsy from a lesion suspected of being a carcinoid tumor.

Bronchoscopists are often asked to do bronchoscopy on patients who have mediastinal masses and superior vena caval obstruction. One should keep in mind that these masses may markedly compromise the airway when patients are supine producing respiratory distress. General anesthesia may magnify this problem, which may become more severe following extubation of the patient in the postoperative period. Superior vena caval obstruction may also become worse with the development of laryngeal edema and stridor. Local anesthesia and careful manipulation are recommended followed by close observation in the immediate postoperative period (92).

The flexible bronchoscope can be a useful instrument in difficult intubations or patients in whom conventional intubation may present risk as with cervical cord lesions. During the course of an awake tracheal intubation requested because of an unstable spinal lesion, a flexible bronchoscope used to aid intubation exited an endotracheal tube through the Murphy eye (93). The endotracheal tube had been placed into the left naris followed by blind insertion of the flexible bronchoscope. At that point, the glottis could be seen; however, the endotracheal tube could not be passed over the bronchoscope because of firm resistance. Direct laryngoscopy confirmed that the bronchoscope had exited the endotracheal tube by the Murphy eye. The bronchoscope and endotracheal tube were removed as a unit, the tip of the bronchoscope was redirected, and intubation was readily accomplished. To avoid this complication and potential damage to the glottic structures, the endotracheal tube can be passed over the bronchoscope prior to its insertion, or the bronchoscope can be advanced through the endotracheal tube under direct vision.

Temporomandibular joint dislocation can occur following flexible bronchoscopy or gastroscopic examination infrequently. It is felt that it more often occurs following trauma, sudden wide-opening movements of the mouth, prolonged wide opening of the mouth during dental procedures, or extreme capsular laxity and chronic subluxation of the temporomandibular joint (94). Age may be a contributing factor. It has also been suggested that one consider using a mouthpiece with a diameter of less than 2 cm for the procedure (95). When patients complain of pain around the jaw or difficulty in swallowing following flexible bronchoscopy, this complication must be considered so that manual reduction of the temporomandibular joint dislocation might be accomplished.

Flexible bronchoscopy can be a cause for the development of a large bronchial cast. Following transbronchial lung biopsy through an oral endotracheal tube, brisk bleeding led to the development of a large clot that adhered to the endotracheal tube and extended into both the right and left main stem bronchi (96). Attempts to remove the clot were unsuccessful. When active bleeding had ceased, a cast of the trachea and main stem bronchi were removed along with the endotracheal tube. Zavala described a similar complication in which a large clot formed obstructing the trachea and endotracheal tube (63). Removal of the endotracheal tube with clot followed by the passing of a rigid bronchoscope were effective in preventing cardiac arrest in this situation. Thereafter, vigorous suction was possible along with the packing of a bronchus with gauze tape in addition to other measures such as placing the patient in the lateral decubitus position with the bleeding lung down.

Bronchoscopists are asked to do examinations on patients with serious infections that can potentially affect personnel performing the examination. Since it is impossible to identify these patients in all circumstances, the potential hazard to the bronchoscopist dictates that he or she be vigilant in protecting all individuals involved in the examination (97–100). Working with the infection control committee of the institution, guidelines should be established for dealing with potential pathogens such as *Mycobacterium tuberculosis,* hepatitis viruses, and the human immunoviruses related to the acquired immunodeficiency syndrome. This requires gloves, appropriate protective attire, masks, and close-fitting eye protection in addition to extreme care to avoid inadvertent injury by a contaminated needle. Adequate procedure room ventilation is essential to reduce the risk of airborne pathogens infecting bronchoscopy personnel. The best measures for protecting surgeons and others exposed to blood and body fluids of infected patients are still being worked out (100).

REFERENCES

1. Landa JF. Bronchoscopy: general considerations. In: Sacker MA, ed. *Diagnostic techniques in pulmonary disease.* New York: Marcel Dekker; 1981:655–695.
2. Prakash UBS, Stubbs SE. Bronchoscopy: indications and technique. *Semin Resp Med* 1981;3:17–24.
3. Fulkerson WJ. Current concepts: fiberoptic bronchoscopy. *N Engl J Med* 1984;311:511–515.
4. Credle WF Jr, Smiddy JF, Elliott RC. Complications of fiberoptic bronchoscopy. *Am Rev Resp Dis* 1974;109:67–72.
5. Suratt PM, Smiddy JF, Gruber B. Deaths and complications associated with fiberoptic bronchoscopy. *Chest* 1976; 69:747–751.

6. Pereira W Jr, Kovnat DM, Snider GL. A prospective cooperative study of complications following flexible fiberoptic bronchoscopy. *Chest* 1978;73:813–816.
7. Trouillet JL, Guiguet M, Gibert C, et al. Fiberoptic bronchoscopy in ventilated patients. Evaluation of cardiopulmonary risk under midazolam sedation. *Chest* 1990;97:927–933.
8. Gibson PG, Breit SN, Bryant DH. Hypoxia during bronchoalveolar lavage. *Aust N Z J Med* 1990;20:39–43.
9. Guerra LF, Baughman RP. Use of bronchoalveolar lavage to diagnose bacterial pneumonia in mechanically ventilated patients. *Crit Care Med* 1990;18:169–173.
10. Hendy MS, Bateman JR, Stableforth DE. The influence of transbronchial lung biopsy and bronchoalveolar lavage on arterial blood gas changes occurring in patients with diffuse interstitial lung disease. *Br J Dis Chest* 1984;78:363–368.
11. Lin C, Wu J, Huang W. Pulmonary function in normal subjects after bronchoalveolar lavage. *Chest* 1988;93:1049–1053.
12. Matsushima Y, Jones RL, King EG, Moysa G, Alton JD. Alterations in pulmonary mechanics and gas exchange during routine fiberoptic bronchoscopy. *Chest* 1984;86:184–188.
13. Dubrawsky C, Awe RJ, Jenkins DE. The effect of bronchofiberscopic examination on oxygenation status. *Chest* 1975; 67:137–140.
14. Albertini RE, Harrell JH, Moser KM. Management of arterial hypoxemia induced by fiberoptic bronchoscopy. *Chest* 1975; 67:134–136.
15. Randazzo GP, Wilson AF. Cardiopulmonary changes during flexible fiberoptic bronchoscopy. *Respiration* 1976; 33:143–149.
16. Karetzky MS, Garvey JW, Brandsetter RD. Effect of fiberoptic bronchoscopy on arterial oxygen tension. *NY State J Med* 1974;74:62–63.
17. Lindholm CE, Ollman B, Synder JV, Miller EG, Grenvik A. Cardiorespiratory effects of flexible fiberoptic bronchoscopy in critically ill patients. *Chest* 1978;74:362–368.
18. Prakash UBS, Offord KP, Stubbs SE. Bronchoscopy in North America: the ACCP survey. *Chest* 1991;100:1668–1675.
19. Sahn SA, Scoggin C. Fiberoptic bronchoscopy in bronchial asthma: a word of caution. *Chest* 1976;69:39–42.
20. Dreisin RB, Albert RK, Talley PA, Kryger MH, Scoggin CH, Zwillich CW. Flexible fiberoptic bronchoscopy in the teaching hospital. *Chest* 1978;74:144–149.
21. Nakhosteen JA. Bronchofiberscopy in asthmatics: a method for minimizing risk of complications. *Respiration* 1978; 36:112–116.
22. Belen J, Neuhaus A, Markowitz D, Rotman HH. Modification of the effect of fiberoptic bronchoscopy on pulmonary mechanics. *Chest* 1981;79:516–519.
23. Zavala DC, Godsey K, Bedell GN. The response to atropine sulfate given by aerosal and intramuscular routes to pateints undergoing fiberoptic bronchoscopy. *Chest* 1981;5:512–515.
24. Rosenow EC III, Andersen HA. Bronchoscopically induced bronchospasm. *Chest* 1976;70:565–566.
25. Peacock AJ, Benson-Mitchell R, Godfrey R. Effect of fibreoptic bronchoscopy on pulmonary function. *Thorax* 1990; 45:38–41.
26. Soderberg M, Lundgren R. Flexible fiberoptic bronchoscopy does not alter airway responsiveness. *Respiration* 1989; 56:182–188.
27. Djukanovic R, Wilson JW, Lai CK, Holgate ST, Howarth PH. The safety aspects of fiberoptic bronchoscopy, bronchoalveolar lavage, and endobronchial biopsy in asthma. *Am Rev Resp Dis* 1991;143:772–777.
28. Summary and recommendations of a workshop on the investigative use of fiberoptic bronchoscopy and bronchoalveolar lavage in asthmatics. *Am Rev Resp Dis* 1985;132:180–182.
29. Lundgren R, Haggmark S, Reiz S. Hemodynamic effects of flexible fiberoptic bronchoscopy performed under topical anesthesia. *Chest* 1982;82:295–299.
30. Riggs JE. Bronchoscopy-induced fatal asystole in tetanus: the result of combined carotid-body chemoreceptor and vasovagal reflexes. *South Med J* 1990;83:955–956.
31. Dombret MC, Juliard JM, Farinotti R. The risks of bronchoscopy in coronary patients. *Rev Mal Resp* 1990;7:313–317.
32. Elguindi AS, Harrison GN, Abdulla AM, et al. Cardiac rhythm disturbances during fiberoptic bronchoscopy: a prospective study. *J Thorac Cardiovasc Surg* 1979;77:557–561.
33. Katz AS, Michelson EL, Stawicki J, Holford FD. Cardiac arrhythmias. Frequency during fiberoptic bronchoscopy and correlation with hypoxemia. *Arch Intern Med* 1981;141:603–606.
34. Fassoulaki A, Kaniaris P, Kotsanis S. Atenolol pretreatment in fiberoptic bronchoscopy. Effect on cardiac arrhythmias, heart rate and arterial blood pressure. *Acta Anaesthesiol Belg* 1980;31:279–284.
35. Pedro Botet ML, Ruiz J, Sabria M, et al. Bacteremia after fibrobronchoscopy. Prospective study. *Enferm Infecc Microbiol Clin* 1991;9:159–161.
36. Standiford TJ, Kunkel SL, Strieter RM. Elevated serum levels of tumor necrosis factor alpha after bronchoscopy and bronchoalveolar lavage. *Chest* 1991;99:1529–1530.
37. Timms RM, Harrell JH. Bacteremia related to fiberoptic bronchoscopy. A case report. *Am Rev Resp Dis* 1975;111:555–557.
38. Beyt BE Jr, King DK, Glew RH. Fatal pneumonitis and septicemia after fiberoptic bronchoscopy. *Chest* 1977;72:105–107.
39. Alexander WJ, Baker GL, Hunker FD. Bacteremia and meningitis following fiberoptic bronchoscopy. *Arch Intern Med* 1979; 139:580–583.
40. Etzkorn ET, McAllister CK. Bacteremic pneumonia after fiberoptic bronchoscopy. *Milit Med* 1987;152:263–264.
41. Robbins H, Goldman AL. Failure of a "prophylactic" antimicrobial drug to prevent sepsis after fiberoptic bronchoscopy. *Am Rev Resp Dis* 1977;116:325–326.
42. Muers M, Lane D. Acute pneumonia and pneumothorax as a complication of transbronchial biopsy. *Endoscopy* 1980; 12:183–187.
43. Hsu JT, Barrett CR Jr. Lung abscess complicating transbronchial biopsy of a mass lesion. *Chest* 1981;80:230–232.
44. Hammer DL, Aranda CP, Galati V, Adams FV. Massive intrabronchial aspiration of contents of pulmonary abscess after fiberoptic bronchoscopy. *Chest* 1978;74:306–307.
45. Harber PH, Terry PB. Fatal lung abscesses: review of 11 years' experience. *South Med J* 1981;74:281–283.
46. Dajani AS, Bisno AL, Chung KJ, et al. Prevention of bacterial endocarditis. Recommendations by the American Heart Association. *JAMA* 1990;264:2919–2922.
47. Vasanthakumar V, Bhan GL, Perera BS, Taft P. A study to assess the efficacy of chemoprophylaxis in the prevention of endoscopy related bacteraemia in patients aged 60 and over. *Q J Med* 1990;75:647–653.
48. Kennedy M. Pseudoepidemic of *Rhodotorula rubra* in patients undergoing fiberoptic bronchoscopy (letter). *Infect Control Hosp Epidemiol* 1990;11:334–336.
49. Richardson AJ, Rothburn MM, Roberts C. Pseudo outbreak of *Bacillus* species: related to fibreoptic bronchoscopy (letter). *J Hosp Infect* 1986;7:208–210.
50. Siegman Igra Y, Inbar G, Campus A. An "outbreak" of pulmonary pseudoinfection by *Serratia marcescens*. *J Hosp Infect* 1985;6:218–220.
51. Bezel R, Salfinger M, Brandli O. The transmission of mycobacteria through the fiberoptic bronchoscope. *Schweiz Med Wochenschr* 1985;115:1360–1365.
52. Goldstein B, Abrutyn E. Pseudo outbreak of *Bacillus* species: related to fibreoptic bronchoscopy. *J Hosp Infect* 1985; 6:194–200.
53. Sammartino MT, Israel RH, Magnussen CR. *Pseudomonas aeruginosa* contamination of fibreoptic bronchoscopes. *J Hosp Infect* 1982;3:65–71.
54. Schleupner CJ, Hamilton JR. A pseudoepidemic of pulmonary fungal infections related to fiberoptic bronchoscopy. Infect Control 1980;1:38–42.
55. Wheeler PW, Lancaster D, Kaiser AB. Bronchopulmonary cross colonization and infection related to mycobacterial contamination of suction valves of bronchoscopes. *J Infect Dis* 1989;159:954–958.
56. Nelson KE, Larson PA, Schraufnagel DE, Jackson J. Transmission of tuberculosis by flexible fiberbronchoscopes. *Am Rev Resp Dis* 1983;127:97–100.

57. Hanson PJ, Collins JV. AIDS and the lung. 1. AIDS, aprons, and elbow grease: preventing the nosocomial spread of human immunodeficiency virus and associated organisms. *Thorax* 1989;44:778–783.
58. Boisjoly HM, Jotterand VH, Bazin R, Bergeron MG. Metastatic *Pseudomonas* endophthalmitis following bronchoscopy. *Tubercle* 1988;69:57–61.
59. Rimmer J, Gibson P, Bryant DH. Extension of pulmonary tuberculosis after fiberoptic bronchoscopy. *Tubercle* 1988; 69:57–61.
60. Olesen LL, Thorshauge H, Nielsen BA. Breakage of the wire cytology brush during fiberoptic bronchoscopy (letter). *Chest* 1987;92:188.
61. Fuentes-Otero F, Garcia-Vinuesa G, Tellez F, Rincon P, Perez-Miranda M. Unusual complication during bronchial brushing through the flexible fiberoptic bronchoscope. *Chest* 1980; 78:901–902.
62. Simpson FG, Arnold AG, Purvis A, Belfield PkW, Muers MF, Cooke NJ. Postal survey of bronchoscopic practice by physicians in the United Kingdom. *Thorax* 1986;41:311–317.
63. Zavala DC. Diagnostic fiberoptic bronchoscopy: techniques and results of biopsy in 600 patients. *Chest* 1975;68:12–19.
64. Zavala DC. Pulmonary hemorrhage in fiberoptic transbronchial biopsy. *Chest* 1976;70:584–588.
65. Flick MR, Wasson K, Dunn LJ, Block AJ. Fatal pulmonary hemorrhage after transbronchial lung biopsy through the fiberoptic bronchoscope. *Am Rev Resp Dis* 1975;111:853–856.
66. Papin TA, Grum CM, Weg JG. Transbronchial biopsy during mechanical ventilation. *Chest* 1986;89:168–170.
67. Papin TA, Lynch JP III, Weg JG. Transbronchial biopsy in the thrombocytopenic patient. *Chest* 1985;88:549–552.
68. Erickson AD, Irwin RS, Teplitz C, Corrao WM, Tarpey JT. Cerebral air embolism complicating transbronchoscopic lung biopsy. *Ann Intern Med* 1979;90:937–938.
69. Hanson RR, Zavala DC, Rhodes ML, Keim LW, Smith JD. Transbronchial biopsy via flexible fiberoptic bronchoscope; results in 164 patients. *Am Rev Resp Dis* 1976;114:67–72.
70. Hernandez Blasco L, Sanchez Hernandez IM, Villena Garrido V, de Miguel Poch E, Nunez Delgado M, Alfaro Abreu J. Safety of the transbronchial biopsy in outpatients. *Chest* 1991; 99:562–565.
71. Frazier WD, Pope TL Jr, Findley LJ. Pneumothorax following transbronchial biopsy. Low diagnostic yield with routine chest roentgenograms. *Chest* 1990;97:539–540.
72. de Fenoyl O, Capron F, Lebeau B, Rochemaure J. Transbronchial biopsy without fluoroscopy: a five year experience in outpatients. *Thorax* 1989;44:956–959.
73. Pincus PS, Kallenbach JM, Hurwitz MD, et al. Transbronchial biopsy during mechanical ventilation. *Crit Care Med* 1987; 15:1136–1139.
74. Prakash UBS, Stubbs SE. The Bronchoscopy Survey; some reflections. *Chest* 1991;100:1660–1667.
75. Malik SK, Behera D. Breakage of alligator biopsy forceps: an unusual complication during fiberoptic bronchoscopy. *Chest* 1984;85:837–838.
76. Harrow EM, Oldenburg FA Jr, Lingenfelter MS, Smith AM Jr. Transbronchial needle aspiration in clinical practice. A five-year experience. *Chest* 1989;96:1268–1272.
77. Gay PC, Brutinel WM. Transbronchial needle aspiration in the practice of bronchoscopy. *Mayo Clin Proc* 1989;64:158–162.
78. Kucera RF, Wolfe GK, Perry ME. Hemomediastinum after transbronchial needle aspiration (letter). *Chest* 1986;90: 466.
79. Schenk DA, Bower JH, Bryan CL, et al. Transbronchial needle aspiration staging of bronchogenic carcinoma. *Am Rev Resp Dis* 1986;134:146–148.
80. Witte MC, Opal SM, Gilbert JG, et al. Incidence of fever and bacteremia following transbronchial needle aspiration. *Chest* 1986;89:85–87.
81. Brutinel WM, Cortese DA, McDougall JC, Gillio RG, Bergstralh EJ. A two-year experience with the neodymium-YAG laser in endobronchial obstruction. *Chest* 1987;91:159–165.
82. Pirozynski M, Sliwinski P, Radwan L, Zielinski J. Bronchoalveolar lavage: comparison of three commonly used procedures. *Respiration* 1991;58:72–76.
83. Jarjour NN, Calhoun WJ. Bronchoalveolar lavage in stable asthmatics does not cause pulmonary inflammation. *Am Rev Resp Dis* 1990;142:100–103.
84. Ruiz F, Casado T, Monso E. Pneumothorax during bronchoalveolar lavage (letter). *Chest* 1989;96:1441–1442.
85. Pirozynski M, Sliwinski P, Zielinski J. Effect of different volumes of BAL fluid on arterial oxygen saturation. *Eur Resp J* 1988;1:943–947.
86. Martin II WJ, Smith TF, Sanderson DR, et al. Role of bronchoalveolar lavage in the assessment of opportunistic pulmonary infections: utility and complications. *Mayo Clin Proc* 1987;62:549–557.
87. Stover DE, White DA, Romano PA, Gellene RA. Diagnosis of pulmonary disease in acquired immune deficiency syndrome (AIDS). Role of bronchoscopy and bronchoalveolar lavage. *Am Rev Resp Dis* 1984;130:659–662.
88. Zavala DC. Transbronchial biopsy in diffuse lung disease. *Chest* 1978;73:727–733.
89. Rees JR. Massive hemoptysis associated with foreign body removal. *Chest* 1985;88:475–476.
90. Morgan JM, Morgan AD, Addis B, Bradley GW, Spiro SG. Fatal haemorrhage from mycotic aneurysms of the pulmonary artery. *Thorax* 1986;41:70–71.
91. Sukumaran M, Wilkinson ZS, Christianson L. Acute carcinoid syndrome: a complication of flexible fiberoptic bronchoscopy. *Ann Thorac Surg* 1982;34:702–705.
92. Quong GG, Brigham BA. Anaesthetic complications of mediastinal masses and superior vena caval obstuction. *Med J Aust* 1980;2:487–488.
93. Nichols KP, Zornow MH. A potential complication of fiberoptic intubation. *Anesthesiology* 1989;70:562–563.
94. Kepron W. Bilateral dislocations of the temporomandibular joint complicating fiberoptic bronchoscopy. *Chest* 1986; 90:465.
95. Kim SK, Kim K. Subluxation of the temperomandibular joint. Unusual complications of transoral bronchoscopy. *Chest* 1983; 83:288–289.
96. Fairshter RD, Riley CA, Hewlett RI. Large bronchial casts. *Arch Intern Med* 1979;139:522–525.
97. Woodcock A, Campbell I, Collins JVC, et al. Bronchoscopy and infection control. *Lancet* 1989;2:270–271.
98. Morice A. Hazard to bronchoscopists. *Lancet* 1989;1:448.
99. Panlilio AL, Foy DR, Edwards JR, et al. Blood contacts during surgical procedures. *JAMA* 1991;265:1533–1537.
100. Gerberding JL, Schecter WP. Surgery and AIDS: reducing the risk. *JAMA* 1991;265:1572–1573.

Bronchoscopy,
edited by U. B. S. Prakash.
Mayo Foundation © 1994.
Published by Raven Press, Ltd., New York.

CHAPTER 26

Processing of Bronchoscopy Specimens

Jeffrey L. Myers and Samuel E. Stubbs

Collection of respiratory secretions, bronchoalveolar lavage, and biopsy of endobronchial and pulmonary parenchymal abnormalities for diagnostic purposes are the most important applications of bronchoscopy. The diagnostic yield from bronchoscopy is directly related to the proper collection and optimal processing of the specimens. Several different types of cytological and histological specimens can be obtained (Table 1). Each type of specimen must be appropriately handled in order to obtain reliable laboratory results (1). This requires careful communication between the bronchoscopist and the pathologist. This chapter summarizes general principles of specimen processing that can be applied in nearly all practice settings.

Principles governing handling of bronchoscopy specimens are generally the same for samples obtained with either the rigid or the flexible bronchoscope. The rigid bronchoscope readily yields larger biopsy and fluid specimens. However, a number of technical advances have improved the variety and quality of specimens available with the flexible bronchoscope, and we will focus on specimens obtained with the flexible instrument.

SPECIMEN TYPES

Bronchial washings, bronchial brushings, bronchoscopic needle aspirates and needle biopsies, and endobronchial as well as bronchoscopic lung tissue biopsies represent the five major types of specimens obtained through the flexible bronchoscope (Table 1). Bronchoalveolar lavage is discussed elsewhere (Chapter 13). Most bronchoscopy specimens are used to evaluate possible malignancies, pulmonary infections, or diffuse roentgenographic abnormalities. To some extent, the clinical setting dictates which of the above specimen types is most appropriate and most useful, but in most circumstances a combination of samples provides the best chance of making a specific diagnosis (1–3). Regardless of the sample type, however, all specimens should be carefully labeled *in the bronchoscopy suite* before being transported to the laboratory. In addition, a brief clinical history including a differential diagnosis and any specific questions or concerns should accompany the specimen to the laboratory.

Bronchial Washings

Bronchial washings are obtained by instilling an isotonic solution, such as 0.9% saline, through the flexible bronchoscope and collecting the material in a suitable sterile trap. Washings usually are collected continuously during the course of the procedure and are therefore "contaminated" by secretions from all examined lobes as well as the oral cavity and upper respiratory tract (4). Washings are mainly used to evaluate malignancies and certain pulmonary infections. We find it useful to submit bronchial washings for fungal and mycobacterial smears and cultures, and for cytological examination. Aliquots for microbiology should be taken from the trap using a sterile technique and placed in appropriate transport containers. The aliquot for cytology need not be collected in a sterile fashion. A minimum of 15 ml of undiluted fluid should immediately be sent to the cytology laboratory for processing. If rapid transport to the cytology laboratory is not possible, the sample should either be refrigerated or be placed in a labeled specimen bottle containing an equal volume of a fixative such as 2% Carbowax solution (50% ethanol with 2% Carbowax 1450, Union Carbide Corp.) (Table 2).

J. L. Myers: Department of Surgical Pathology, Mayo Clinic, Rochester, Minnesota 55905.
S. E. Stubbs: Division of Thoracic Diseases and Internal Medicine, Mayo Clinic, Rochester, Minnesota 55905.

TABLE 1. *Types of bronchoscopy specimens*

Specimen type	Utility
Bronchial washings	Fungal, mycobacterial cultures Cytological diagnosis of malignancy Cytological diagnosis of certain infection (e.g., *Pneumocystis,* CMV)
Bronchial brushings	Bacterial (aerobic/anaerobic) cultures Cytological diagnosis of malignancy Cytological diagnosis of certain infections (e.g., CMV)
Bronchoscopic needle aspirates and needle biopsies	Cytological/histopathological diagnosis of primary carcinomas Staging of mediastinal and tracheobronchial lymph node metastases
Endobronchial biopsies	Histopathological diagnosis of centrally located neoplasms Peribronchiolar granulomas (e.g., sarcoidosis)
Bronchoscopic lung biopsies	Histopathological diagnosis of primary and metastatic neoplasms Infectious disorders Certain diffuse nonneoplastic diseases

TABLE 2. *Appropriate fixatives for bronchoscopy specimens submitted for cytological or histopathological evaluation*

Specimen type	Fixative
Bronchial washings	50% ethanol with 2% Carbowax (Union Carbide Corp.)
Bronchial brushings	95% ethanol (smears); 50% ethanol with 2% Carbowax (Union Carbide) (fluid for agitating brush)
Bronchoscopic needle aspirates	95% ethanol (smears); 50% ethanol with 2% Carbowax (Union Carbide) (flushings from needle)
Bronchoscopic needle biopsies	10% formalin
Endo-, transbronchoscopic biopsies	10% formalin
Electron microscopy	Trump's fixative (4% formaldehyde, 1% glutaraldehyde)

Bronchial Brushings

Bronchial brushings, like bronchial washings, are used to evaluate patients suspected of having pulmonary malignancies or pulmonary infections. Brushings tend to be most useful for evaluating centrally located tumors. The technique for bronchial brushing has been described elsewhere (Chapters 9 and 10). Protected catheter brushes should be used for bacterial cultures as described by Wimberley and associates (5).

Smears for cytological evaluation are prepared directly from the brush by rolling the brush in a circular motion in a region about the size of a quarter dollar on a previously labeled frosted glass slide (Fig. 1). The smears should be done quickly and immediately fixed in 95% ethanol for a minimum of 10 min prior to staining; delays cause excessive air-drying artifact that interferes with cytological interpretation. Multiple smears (e.g., two or three) should be prepared, depending on the amount of material on the brush. After preparing smears the brush can be vigorously agitated in fluid to rinse adherent cells. For cytological preparations the brush should be agitated in a fixative such as 2% Carbowax. The fluid can then be filtered or placed in a cytocentrifuge for preparation of Papanicolaou-stained slides. For cultures the brush should be agitated or submitted intact in a sterile medium such as lactated Ringer's solution.

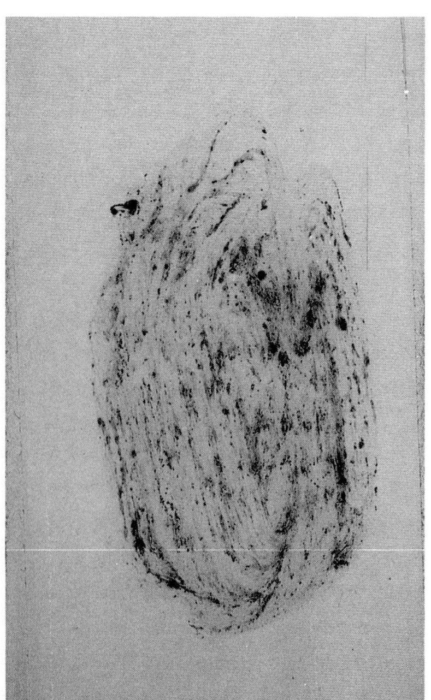

FIG. 1. Photograph of a properly prepared bronchial brushing (2.2× actual size). The material is smeared from the brush onto a circumscribed area approximately 20 mm in diameter on a labeled glass slide.

Bronchoscopic Needle Aspirates and Biopsies

Bronchoscopic needle aspirates and needle biopsies are primarily used to diagnose lung carcinomas and to stage mediastinal and tracheobronchial lymph node metastases (6–10). Properly prepared smears are essential to the successful interpretation of aspirated specimens. Smears can be prepared by personnel from either the bronchoscopy suite or the cytology laboratory, but whomever is responsible should be well versed in the technique. The technique for bronchoscopic needle aspiration and biopsy is described in Chapter 12. It is imperative that pressure be released on the syringe plunger before withdrawing the thin needle containing the aspirated sample. After the needle is withdrawn, the syringe should be removed from the apparatus, the plunger pulled back to introduce air into the syringe, and the syringe reconnected to the apparatus. The tip of the needle is then placed near the frosted edge of a previously labeled slide and a single drop of fluid expressed using gentle pressure from the syringe. The drop of material is then quickly smeared in a manner analogous to preparation of peripheral blood smears, and the slide is immediately fixed in 95% ethanol. After all the material has been smeared, the needle can be rinsed by repeated flushings into a container of 2% Carbowax solution. Alternatively, the entire specimen can be flushed into a container of fixative without direct preparation of smears. Tissue biopsies obtained with larger cutting needles should be placed directly into 10% formalin.

Endobronchial Mucosal- and Bronchoscopic Lung Biopsies

Direct biopsy of bronchial lesions and bronchoscopic lung biopsy of distal pulmonary parenchyma yield tissue samples that are useful for evaluating a variety of lung diseases. The manner in which the biopsy tissue is handled depends to some extent on the differential diagnosis. In general, bronchoscopically obtained biopsies should not be submitted for special procedures such as immunofluorescence and electron microscopy. Routine microscopic examination offers the best opportunity to make a specific diagnosis in these small specimens, and in most cases the tissue should be entirely submitted for light microscopy. In rare circumstances (e.g., occasional patients with diffuse alveolar hemorrhage or suspected immune complex–mediated disorders) additional biopsy fragments can be obtained for immunofluorescence or electron microscopy; however, open lung biopsies are preferable for these sorts of procedures. Biopsy fragments submitted for immunofluorescence should be rapidly transported in saline to the appropriate laboratory. Biopsies submitted for ultrastructural studies should immediately be placed into an appropriate fixative, such as 4% formaldehyde and 1% glutaraldehyde (Trump's fixative). Electron microscopy also can be useful in evaluating bronchial biopsies from patients suspected of having immotile cilia syndrome, but nasal mucosal biopsies are equally useful and are more easily obtained.

Frozen section examination of bronchoscopic biopsies should be avoided except in situations where an immediate diagnosis is needed or when necessary to emergently assess specimen adequacy. The number of bronchoscopists who routinely use frozen section examination of bronchoscopic biopsies is quite low. The mail survey of 871 bronchoscopists in North America reported that only 2.6% of bronchoscopists utilized frozen section techniques on a routine basis, whereas 73% rarely used it; 22% of bronchoscopists indicated that the facility for frozen section examination was not available to them (11). The likelihood of making a specific diagnosis on bronchoscopic biopsies can be maximized if the entire specimen is submitted for routine processing. Frozen tissue is subject to artifactual distortion that interferes with the pathologist's ability to make an accurate diagnosis, and a certain amount of tissue is irretrievably lost for subsequent evaluation.

When the biopsy forceps is withdrawn from the subject, the specimen should be placed on a sterile glass slide with a drop of sterile saline or on a sterile tissue or towel moistened with saline. This avoids unnecessary drying of the tissue. Gauze should be avoided because tissue fragments become entrapped within the fine mesh. The sample can be dislodged from the biopsy device using gentle pressure from the tip of a sterile 25- or 22-gauge needle, or using a small forceps. When the procedure has been concluded and all biopsy specimens collected, the tissue should be quickly transferred to a container filled with an appropriate fixative such as 10% formalin. Alternative fixatives may be preferred in certain circumstances. Because the small biopsy fragments are pale and difficult to see, it may be preferable to have the bronchoscopist fold the fragments into a piece of moistened filter paper and load the filter paper into a labeled tissue cassette before placing the specimen into fixative. Dipping the filter paper into a dilute solution of eosin is helpful in identifying small tissue fragments.

Tissue from bronchoscopic biopsies should be processed in the usual manner for preparation of paraffin-embedded sections. Step-sectioning (Fig. 2) the paraffin block at several levels (i.e., at least two or three) increases the likelihood of making a specific diagnosis in certain conditions, such as sarcoidosis (12). Unstained slides should be prepared from sections cut between the various levels and retained for possible special stains.

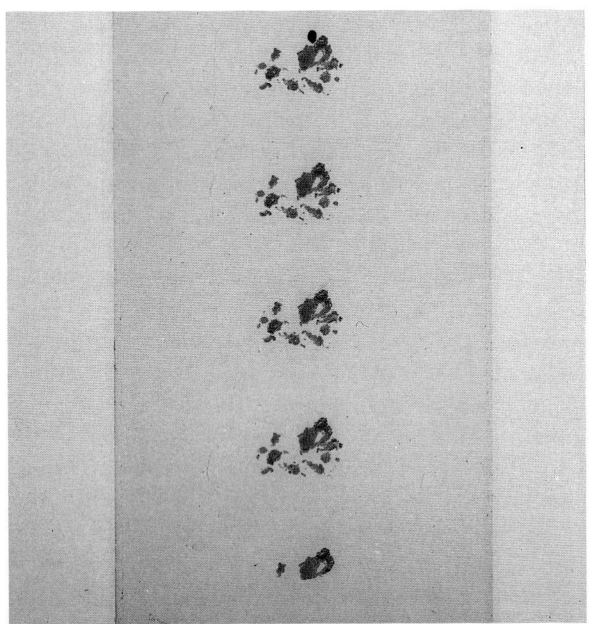

FIG. 2. Photograph illustrating step sections of a bronchial biopsy (2.2 × actual size). A ribbon of tissue sections (i.e., step sections) is fixed to a single slide and stained. Each tissue section includes all of the biopsy fragments, the largest measuring 2.3 mm in its greatest dimension.

MICROBIOLOGY

Fungi can be identified from bronchial washings either directly from smears or from cultures. Smears are prepared by first treating an aliquot with potassium hydroxide to remove cellular debris, smearing a drop of the resulting fluid on a glass slide, and staining with an appropriate fungal stain. Mucous plugs, if present, should be removed from the washings, fixed in 10% formalin, and processed in a routine fashion for paraffin sections that can be examined with a fungal stain, such as silver methenamine. Bronchial washings are also useful in identifying *Pneumocystis carinii* and cytomegalovirus (CMV) infections (13). These organisms can be identified in smears prepared in the manner described below (see "Neoplasms").

Mycobacterial organisms also can be identified in bronchial washings by either smears or cultures. The sample is first decontaminated and concentrated using alkali, acid, and centrifugation. Smears can be prepared directly from the concentrated fluid and stained for organisms. The concentrated fluid can also be plated on appropriate media for cultures. The yield of mycobacterial cultures from bronchial washings tends to be low and may be related to an inhibitory effect of lidocaine (14). Nonetheless Jett et al. showed that bronchial washings are useful in patients suspected of having mycobacterial disease in whom smears from spontaneously expectorated or induced sputum are negative (15). Unfortunately, identification of mycobacteria may require several weeks of culture. Application of specific DNA probes using polymerase chain reaction technology allows rapid identification of mycobacterial organisms in routinely processed bronchial washings and may soon become the procedure of choice (16). A technique of bronchial brushing using a protected catheter brush eliminates or reduces oropharyngeal contamination of lower respiratory tract secretions obtained for bacterial culture (5). This technique, when coupled with quantitative culture estimates, can be used to differentiate between contaminants and true pathogens (5). Once the protected catheter brush specimen has been obtained (Chapter 14), the brush is placed in 1 ml of sterile lactated Ringer's solution. The specimen should be delivered to microbiology without delay to maintain viability of both aerobic and anaerobic bacteria. Bacterial cultures are then performed by streaking 0.1 ml of the sample onto culture media. The number of colonies that grow is used to estimate the number of colony-forming units per milliliter of sample (17).

Tissue biopsies, especially bronchoscopic lung biopsies, can be extremely useful in evaluating pulmonary infections (18), particularly in immunocompromised hosts (19,20). In general, the tissue can be handled in a routine manner and fixed in 10% formalin. The diagnosis of infection is established on the basis of histological examination and special staining procedures that are easily applied to routinely processed tissue. Special stains for organisms should be done in nonimmunocompromised patients only if the histological changes (e.g., bronchopneumonia, granulomas) suggest infection; stains for *Pneumocystis carinii* should be done in all patients with interstitial pneumonia in whom a specific etiology is not known. In contrast, special stains should be done on all biopsies from immunocompromised patients regardless of the histopathological findings. Stains should include acid-fast stains and silver stains for fungi and *Pneumocystis*. Immunoperoxidase stains for CMV and herpes simplex viruses also can be applied to paraffin sections using commercially available antibodies in selected cases.

Touch preps can be used for rapid diagnosis of certain infections in immunocompromised hosts. These are prepared by lightly touching the biopsy specimen onto the surface of a labeled glass slide, immediately fixing the slide in 95% ethanol, and staining the slide with appropriate special stains. This technique is most useful for diagnosing *Pneumocystis carinii* infection, particularly in human immunodeficiency virus–infected patients. In our experience the sensitivity of this technique is limited, however, and it may damage the tissue and interfere with routine light microscopy.

Furthermore, rapid processing of bronchoalveolar lavage specimens has supplanted the need for this special technique in most cases.

NEOPLASMS

All five types of bronchoscopically obtained specimens are used to evaluate pulmonary tumors. Bronchial washings and brushings are least sensitive, particularly in peripherally situated tumors, but both are useful and can increase the sensitivity of mucosal or lung biopsy alone (2,3).

A 15-ml aliquot from the bronchial washings should be sent to the cytology laboratory fresh or in a solution of 2% Carbowax. Purulent secretions are difficult to process and may not be suitable for cytological examination. Nonbloody unfixed specimens are transferred to a 50-ml plastic centrifuge tube and thoroughly mixed with two parts of 2% Carbowax fixative per one part specimen. The specimen should be allowed to remain in fixative for at least 1 hr. We find it useful to then homogenize fixed specimens, including those samples placed in 2% Carbowax at the time they are collected, using the blender technique described by Saccomanno (21). Smears can be prepared directly from the resulting homogenate. Grossly bloody washings are processed differently and are first centrifuged in 50-ml plastic tubes for 5–8 min. After centrifugation, material from the top of the tube is removed with a wooden applicator and placed on a slide. A second slide is used to gently break apart any visible lumps or clots. The slides are then quickly immersed in 95% ethanol for fixation. The sediment remaining in the bottom of the centrifuge tube is removed with the wooden applicator after the supernatant has been decanted and slides are prepared in the manner described above. If the specimen is very bloody, smears should be immersed in Carnoy's solution for 2–3 min to lyse red blood cells prior to fixation in 95% ethanol. The routine Papanicolaou method is the method of choice for staining fixed smears.

Processing of bronchial brushings and bronchoscopic needle aspirates and needle biopsies has been described previously (see "Specimen Types"). These specimens can be extremely helpful in diagnosing and classifying centrally located tumors, but only if appropriately handled. Properly prepared cytological preparations are particularly useful in classifying small cell carcinomas that may appear crushed and uninterpretable in tissue sections.

Endobronchial and bronchoscopic lung biopsies represent the "gold standard" in bronchoscopic diagnosis and classification of lung neoplasms. Diagnosis requires only routine paraffin sections in the vast majority of cases. Immunohistochemistry has largely supplanted the need for electron microscopy in difficult cases and can be performed on routinely processed tissue. Indeed, there are few if any circumstances when tissue should be separately submitted for special procedures, such as electron microscopy. It is extremely difficult to determine on the basis of gross inspection alone whether or not small tissue fragments are representative of tumor, and triaging tissue carries a substantial risk of sending nonneoplastic tissue for light microscopy while sending tumor for special studies and *vice versa*. Frozen sections should also be avoided, except in emergency situations, because of the risk of losing diagnostic material.

DIFFUSE LUNG DISEASE

Bronchoscopic lung biopsies frequently yield helpful information in patients with diffuse lung disease and can be obtained with either the rigid or the flexible bronchoscope. Bronchoalveolar lavage also can be useful in certain circumstances and is discussed elsewhere (Chapter 13). The likelihood of making a specific diagnosis is dependent in part on the number of biopsies obtained. Four to six biopsy specimens should be obtained in most circumstances. More recently, it was suggested that as many as three to four biopsies per lobe of one lung may increase the yield of specific diagnoses (22). As with lung tumors, routine light microscopy offers the best opportunity to make a specific diagnosis in patients with diffuse lung disease. Tissue biopsies should be processed in the manner described previously, with two or three routinely stained sections cut at various levels. Unstained sections should be retained for possible special stains.

Correlation of biopsy results with clinical data is essential to accurate interpretation of bronchoscopic lung biopsies in patients with diffuse lung disease. Lung biopsies are most useful in diagnosing granulomatous disease (i.e., sarcoidosis), acute or subacute infections, and lymphangitic metastases. Entities with unique histological features, including eosinophilic granuloma (histiocytosis X, Langerhans' cell granulomatosis) and lymphangioleiomyomatosis, can be diagnosed with bronchoscopic lung biopsy in a minority of patients. Recognition of less specific tissue reactions, such as bronchiolitis obliterans with organizing pneumonia (BOOP), can lead to a specific diagnosis (i.e., "idiopathic BOOP") if carefully correlated with clinical, physiological, and radiographic information. The presence of mild alveolar septal thickening as well as peribronchial and peribronchiolar inflammation and fibrosis ("interstitial fibrosis") are completely nonspecific findings and should be interpreted with caution.

Although bronchoscopic lung biopsies can be useful in supporting a clinical diagnosis of usual interstitial pneumonia/idiopathic pulmonary fibrosis, the findings are rarely specific and must be interpreted in light of the clinical data.

Bronchoscopic lung biopsy has a limited role in the evaluation of patients suspected of having pneumoconioses. Inherent sampling problems usually preclude specific diagnosis, as with other nonneoplastic diffuse lung disease. Microanalysis (energy-dispersive X-ray spectroscopy) can be useful in selected cases (e.g., hard metal pneumoconiosis), however, and can be performed on routinely processed paraffin-embedded tissue. Metal-containing fixatives, such as B-5 or Zenker's, interfere with analysis and should be avoided in this circumstance.

Frozen sections are rarely indicated for evaluating bronchoscopic lung biopsies in patients with diffuse lung disease. The only potential role is in patients suspected of having immune-mediated illnesses, such as anti–glomerular basement membrane disease, in whom immunofluorescence studies may be helpful. Routine light microscopy still should be the first step in trying to establish a tissue diagnosis (e.g., diffuse alveolar hemorrhage). Immunofluorescence of bronchoscopic lung biopsies is relatively insensitive; for that reason, examination of biopsies from other sites (e.g., kidney) coupled with appropriate serological studies are preferable for making specific clinicopathological diagnoses. Open lung biopsy is the procedure of choice if immunofluorescence is considered essential for diagnosis.

REFERENCES

1. Kvale PA. Collection and preparation of bronchoscopic specimens. *Chest* 1978(Suppl);73:707–12.
2. Saltzstein S, Harell J II, Cameron T. Brushings, washings, or biopsy? Obtaining maximum value from flexible fiberoptic bronchoscopy in the diagnosis of cancer. *Chest* 1977;71:630–632.
3. Kvale P, Bode F, Kini S. Diagnostic accuracy in lung cancer. Comparison of techniques used in association with flexible fiberoptic bronchoscopy. *Chest* 1976;69:752–757.
4. Bartlett JG, Alexander J, Mayhew J, Sullivan-Sigler N, Gorbach SL. Should fiberoptic bronchoscopy aspirates be cultured? *Am Rev Resp Dis* 1976;114:73–78.
5. Wimberley N, Faling LJ, Barlett JG. A fiberoptic bronchoscopy technique to obtain uncontaminated lower airway secretions for bacterial culture. *Am Rev Resp Dis* 1979;119:337–343.
6. Gay P, Brutinel W. Transbronchial needle aspiration in the practice of bronchoscopy. *Mayo Clin Proc* 1989;64:158–162.
7. Harrow E, Oldenburg F Jr, Lingenfelter M, Smith A. Transbronchial needle aspiration in clinical practice. A five-year experience. *Chest* 1989;96:1268–1272.
8. Schenk D, Bryan C, Bower J, Myers D. Transbronchial needle aspiration in the diagnosis of bronchogenic carcinoma. *Chest* 1987;92:83–85.
9. Schenk D, Strolle P, Pickard J, et al. Utility of the Wang 18-gauge transbronchial histology needle in the staging of bronchogenic carcinoma. *Chest* 1989;96:272–274
10. Shure D. Transbronchial biopsy and needle aspiration. *Chest* 1989;95:1130–1138.
11. Prakash UBS, Offord KP, Stubbs SE. Bronchoscopy in North America: the ACCP survey. *Chest* 1991;100:1668–1675.
12. Takayama K, Nagata N, Miyagawa Y, Hirano H, Shigematsu N. The usefulness of step sectioning of trancheobronchial lung biopsy specimen in diagnosing sarcoidosis. *Chest* 1992; 102:1441–1443.
13. Rorat E, Garcia R, Skalom J. Diagnosis of *Pneumocystis carinii* pneumonia by cytologic examination of bronchial washings. *JAMA* 1985;254:1950–1951.
14. Kvale PA, Johnson MC, Wroblewski DA. Diagnosis of tuberculosis: routine cultures of bronchial washings are not indicated. *Chest* 1979;76:140–142.
15. Jett JR, Cortese DA, Dines DE. The value of bronchoscopy in the diagnosis of mycobacterial disease: a five-year experience. *Chest* 1981;80:575–578.
16. American Society for Microbiology. *Manual of clinical microbiology*. Washington DC, 1991.
17. Teague RB, Wallace RJ Jr, Awe RJ. The use of quantitative sterile brush culture and Gram stain analysis in the diagnosis of lower respiratory tract infection. *Chest* 1981;79:157–161.
18. Wallace JM, Deutsch AL, Harrell JH, Moser KM. Bronchoscopy and transbronchial biopsy in evaluation of patients with suspected active tuberculosis. *Am J Med* 1981;70:1189–1194.
19. Feldman N, Pennington J, Ehrie M. Transbronchial lung biopsy in the compromised host. *JAMA* 1977;238:1377–1379.
20. Katzenstein A, Askin F. Interpretation and significance of pathologic findings in transbronchial lung biopsy. *Am J Surg Pathol* 1980;4:223–234.
21. Saccomanno G. Sputum cytology: collection, fixation, and concentration of sputum, bronchial aspirates, and bronchial brushings. *Lab Med* 1979;523–527.
22. Gascoigne A, Ashcroft T, Veale D, Gibson G, Corris P. Use of transbronchial lung biopsy in the diagnosis of diffuse lung disease (abstract). *Am Rev Resp Dis* 1991;143:A57.

Bronchoscopy,
edited by U. B. S. Prakash.
Mayo Foundation © 1994.
Published by Raven Press, Ltd., New York.

CHAPTER 27

Documentation of Bronchoscopic Findings

Udaya B. S. Prakash and Eric S. Edell

It is imperative that the bronchoscopic findings and the procedural details performed in each patient be accurately documented. Properly recorded information not only provides important information to other physicians but also becomes a permanent part of the patient's medical history. In our opinion, preparation of these accurate chronicles and their maintenance is an inherent part of the optimal practice of bronchoscopy. Equally important is the fact that correct recording of bronchoscopy procedures and findings provide essential communication between bronchoscopist and nonbronchoscopist. In certain types of medical practice one group of physicians, e.g., pulmonary physicians, perform all bronchoscopy procedures prior to thoracotomy or other surgical procedures. In such instances, a properly recorded detail of bronchoscopy findings will provide important information that is essential for the thoracic surgeon, oncologist, or others involved in providing medical care to the patient. This allows accurate planning for further evaluation or treatment. Studies of a bronchoscopic practice will be facilitated by accurate record keeping. It is essential that the recording of the procedure be as brief as necessary to convey the findings. Lengthy notes not only confuse the reader by providing unnecessary information but also inadvertently obscure the critical details.

DOCUMENTATION CATEGORIES

The systems to document procedural details and bronchoscopic findings can be classified into the following types: typed or handwritten records, photographic (prints or transparency slides), and video or movie film recordings. Irrespective of the system used, it is good practice to first describe the visual findings and then the details of procedures, followed by the details of complications related to the bronchoscopy. In this chapter, we will describe each of these systems and comment on the merit of each system.

U. B. S. Prakash and E. S. Edell: Division of Thoracic Diseases and Internal Medicine, Mayo Clinic, Rochester, Minnesota 55905.

Paper Record

Typewritten or handwritten notes are most commonly used by the majority of bronchoscopists. Visual findings of each bronchoscopy and details of the procedure performed should be succinctly documented. Many bronchoscopists use a rubber stamp or a preprinted diagram of the bronchial tree to mark the abnormalities observed and locations from where the biopsies are obtained. The type of recording on paper is also dependent on the policies of individual medical institutions. In our practice, for instance, details of all surgical procedures including bronchoscopy are typed on special surgical sheets. The written or typed record of a bronchoscopy procedure as well as the results of bronchoscopically obtained cultures and biopsies should be stored with the rest of the patient's medical history.

Photographic Record

Newer cameras and attachments are available for both flexible and rigid bronchoscopes. It is now easy to obtain fine-quality still photographic prints and 35-mm transparency slides of bronchoscopic findings. Special processing is not necessary for the photographic prints and slides since standard film can be used and processed by commercial vendors. However, photographic laboratories specializing in endoscopic photography are located in many cities and are willing to assist the bronchoscopist if necessary. Since the images obtained by 35-mm transparencies are small, special film or processing may be needed to obtain larger images (1,2). Instantly processed bronchoscopic images can be obtained by using a Polaroid system.

The clinical role of the photographic prints and 35-mm transparency slides is somewhat limited. Generally, official records of bronchoscopy procedures do not include bronchoscopic photographs or slides. Follow-up photographs are helpful in assessing the results of treatment. Storage and deterioration of image quality with time are among the disadvantages. The bronchoscopist should also consider the cost of photographic equipment and processing expenses in relation to its role in clinical practice. The photographic documentation, however, is extremely helpful for the purposes of teaching, lecturing and publication of scientific papers and atlases (3–8).

Video Record

An increasing number of bronchoscopists are now using video imaging (video flexible bronchoscopy) in lieu of still photography (9–11). A mail survey of 871 bronchoscopists in North America in 1990 observed that 14% of the bronchoscopists were routinely using videobronchoscopy (12). The major advantages encompass the ability to record the dynamic bronchoscopy, edit the image, insert alphanumeric characters into the bronchoscopic image, and incorporate sound (commentary on the bronchoscopic procedure). Videobronchoscopy is superbly suited to teach bronchoscopic techniques to large numbers of students (13). The newer systems allow recording of dynamic images as well as still photographs from the video screen. Video recordings are far more helpful in clinical practice since the images are live. In our view, the exchange of recordings among bronchoscopists, thoracic surgeons, and other physicians may have contributed to a decrease in the number of unnecessary repeat bronchoscopies.

The disadvantages of videobronchoscopy include the high cost of the equipment, the need for extra storage space for the video equipment and video cassettes, and the lack of a good method to incorporate the recording into the patient's other medical records. It is also difficult to employ the equipment in limited spaces such as patient rooms and critical care units. Permanent video recording of normal bronchoscopic findings in all patients is clinically unproductive and unwarranted. Special procedures, rare and difficult problems, and follow-up of tracheobronchial tumors treated by laser or brachytherapy, stent placements, tracheobronchoplasty procedures, and research applications are some examples where permanent video recordings can be helpful (14–19).

Movie Record

Prior to the advent of the video camera, 16-mm movie cameras were used to record bronchoscopic images (20). The cameras were bulky and hence cumbersome to use. At present, the videobronchoscopy has virtually replaced the movie cameras.

WHAT TO RECORD

Irrespective of the recording method used, the description of bronchoscopic findings and the details of the procedure performed, specimens obtained, and intraoperative and immediate postoperative complications should be recorded. In our large referral practice, we frequently come across bronchoscopy records of patients who have undergone the procedure at other medical institutions. It is not uncommon to find extremely verbose dictations. It is unnecessary to record at length the clinically irrelevant normal findings. For example, detailed recording of normal finding in each bronchus and its branches is not indicated. The following is an example of the recording of bronchoscopy in an immunocompromised patient with diffuse pulmonary process. The procedure was performed to obtain diagnostic bronchoalveolar lavage for identification of pathogenic organisms:

> The patient was brought to the bronchoscopy suite and placed in the chair for nebulization of the topical anesthetic. . . . There was no gagging or other complications during the application of the topical anesthetic agent. Then the patient was placed in a supine position, provided supplemental oxygen, and an attempt was made to administer intravenous sedative. . . . the intravenous line was found to be clotted and therefore, a new line was inserted over the dorsum of the left hand. . . . The bronchoscope [name of the manufacturer and model number mentioned] was inserted through the right nostril. . . . Both the vocal cords moved normally during phonation and a careful examination of the vocal apparatus and surrounding structures revealed no anomalies. . . . The subglottic and upper third of the trachea was normal as were the middle and distal thirds of the trachea. The shape of the tracheal lumen was normal. . . . The bronchoscope was then introduced into the left main bronchus. The mucosa was normal and there was no obvious evidence of mucosal pathology. . . . The bronchoscope was then introduced into the left upper lobe. . . .

The report went on to describe each and every bronchus, the method of wedging the bronchoscope to obtain bronchoalveolar lavage, and the lack of hypoxemia, bleeding, pneumothorax, and other complications in the patient. Obviously, this is an extreme example of redundant and irrelevant details in this patient. A simple note, shown below, should have sufficed:

A transoral bronchoscopy using topical anesthesia, intravenous sedation, and endotracheal tube revealed no visible abnormalities of the larynx or the tracheobronchial tree. Normal saline, 100 ml, was used for bronchoalveolar lavage and about 70 ml of pinkish lavage effluent was aspirated from the lateral segment of right middle lobe and sent for analysis according to immunosuppressed patient protocol. There were no complications.

On the other hand, if a bronchoscopy is performed for the evaluation of hemoptysis, it is important to mention that all the bronchi (that could be visualized) were examined and that there was no evidence of old or new blood in the tracheobronchial tree. Only the pertinent positive and negative findings should be recorded, based on the clinical information and the indication for bronchoscopy.

Each bronchoscopy record should contain the following information: patient's name, identification number, age, date of the procedure, and indication for bronchoscopy. The type and dose of topical anesthetic, intravenous sedation, general anesthesia, and other pharmacological agents used should be included. The route of insertion of the bronchoscope should be mentioned. It is useful to develop a routine to first describe the bronchoscopy findings and then the procedural details followed by the details of complications. Ideally, the description should mention if the larynx is normal or not. If the rest of the bronchoscopic examination is visually normal, a simple statement to that effect is adequate, and if the procedure is performed to the satisfaction of the bronchoscopist, a clear narrative of abnormal findings should suffice. Technical difficulties and complications should be mentioned at the end of the report. The reason for not doing a planned procedure (e.g., a bronchoscopic lung biopsy that cannot be performed because of excessive cough or noncooperation by patient) should be mentioned. Preliminary results from frozen section analysis should not form part of the permanent bronchoscopic diagnosis because the final analysis may provide a different diagnosis.

In the photographic documentation, whether it is a print or slide format, it is time consuming and inconvenient to label the names of bronchi and the findings. If the photographic images are to be incorporated into the permanent medical record, all pertinent information mentioned above should be included. The bronchoscopist should mark the photographic images so that any physician can easily understand the anatomic orientation of the image.

Video documentation of the bronchoscopic findings can include text if the video equipment can generate text characters. Sound (commentary) recording of the findings is helpful to other physicians who may wish to view the recording.

BRONCHOSCOPIC PHOTOGRAPHY

Photographic Equipment

Since newer cameras and video machines are constantly introduced into the market, it is impossible to list all the available bronchoscopic photography equipment. The basic essentials, however, include the bronchoscope, light source, camera, camera adapter, and appropriate film. The bronchoscopist should evaluate several brands and use them on a trial basis before purchase. The requirements for bronchoscopic photography and videobronchoscopy have been published (21–24). Most of the cameras currently availablc for still photography have the capability to automatically adjust for the light, the light source, and the bronchoscope. Bronchoscopic light sources are classified as simple or automatic. The former has a lamp and brightness control, whereas the latter is equipped with a complex photographic exposure system for both still and video photography. Proper installation of either a halogen or a xenon bulb is critical for providing maximum brightness.

Bronchoscopic cameras for still photography are available in 35-mm, 110-mm, or Polaroid formats. Most cameras in use at present are 35-mm single-shutter-speed manual cameras; the correct exposure is determined by the automatic light source. Camera adapters, available in different focal lengths or magnification ratios, are necessary to connect the bronchoscope to the light source (25). Unfortunately, the bronchoscopic and photographic equipment made for one brand is incompatible with other brands.

The single most important part of the photographic equipment for use with the flexible bronchoscope is the bronchoscope itself. The quality of image obtained with standard flexible bronchoscope is not as sharp and clear as that with the flexible bronchoscopes specially made for photography. The quality of the photographs captured through the rigid bronchoscope will depend on the telescope system used. For still photography, standard 35-mm color transparency film for slides and color negative film with ASA 200/400 are recommended. Tungsten film must be used for halogen light sources. Color negative or print film produces color negatives from which color prints can be developed; slides may be also made from the negatives. This is the film type recommended for those who wish both a print for publication or record keeping and a slide for lecture (25). Photographic laboratories that specialize in endoscopic photography can provide films for larger images or enlarge images obtained using standard film.

Generally, the photographs obtained with a rigid bronchoscope and Hopkins rod telescope system provide the best images. The panel of bronchoscopic images shown in Fig. 1 show the variations in the quality of images obtained with different bronchoscopes. The least satisfactory still images are those directly captured from a video monitor. The quality of the picture captured through the pediatric (ultrathin) flexible bronchoscopes are also very grainy and hazy (Fig. 2).

Currently, the bronchoscopic images obtained using the Hopkins rod telescope system through the rigid bronchoscope are far superior to those obtained with even the best pictures captured through the latest model of flexible bronchoscope. The panel of rigid bronchoscopic images shown in Fig. 3 demonstrate the differences in the quality of images.

The quality of the video image is also dependent on the type of bronchoscope used as well as the camera and resolution of the video monitor. Newer high-resolution monitors provide sharper and more true-to-life images. The quality of images can be improved by using bronchoscopes with the highest density of fiberoptics. Obviously, the best video image is obtained with a rigid telescope system. Video images have been improved immensely since the days of 16-mm cameras. Currently, several vendors provide add-on video cameras that utilize charged couple device (CCD) technology. These cameras have been used for standard home video recording and have revolutionized the quality of the images obtained. More recently, Ikeda and colleagues applied this technology to the tip of the flexible bronchoscope (26). The CCD bronchoscope provides the highest resolution of both video and still imaging (Fig. 4).

Handling the Photographic Equipment

The bronchoscopist who plans to employ the photographic equipment should be familiar with the technical details and operational procedure. Although the newer bronchoscopic cameras for still photography automatically adjust for light exposure, the bronchoscopist should check and make sure that the adjustments in the light source are appropriate. Experimentation with different exposures will ultimately provide the bronchoscopist with correct settings. The photographic

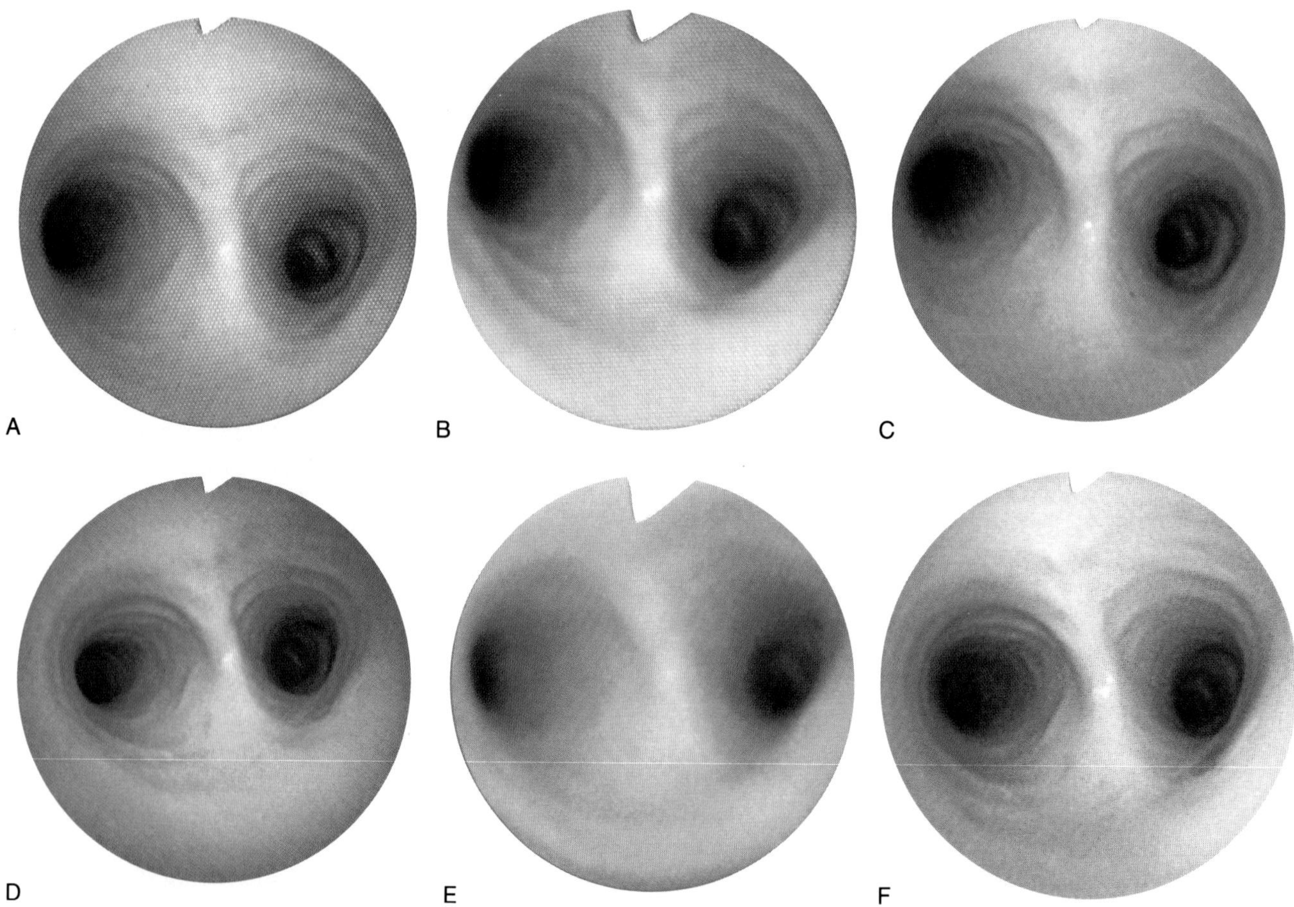

FIG. 1. Bronchoscopic photographs of distal trachea of a model tracheobronchial tree. All images were obtained using same camera, film, and light settings. Different models of Olympus bronchoscopes used were **(A)** 1T10, **(B)** P10, **(C)** P20, **(D)** C620, **(E)** M27, and **(F)** 6C10. Differences in the granularity of images are the result of variations in the arrangement of fiberoptic bundles.

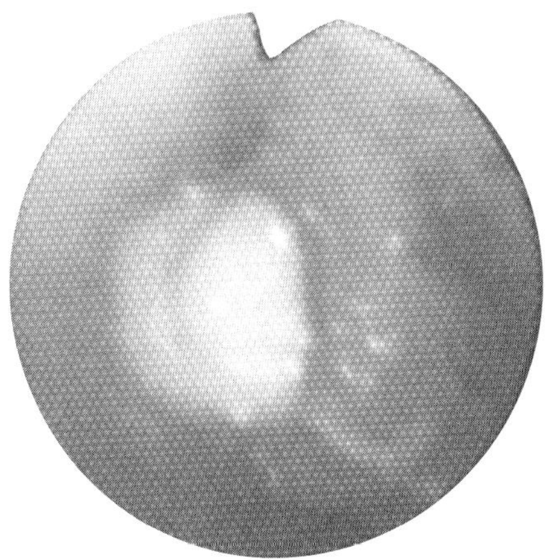

FIG. 2. Bronchoscopic image of a foreign body captured with an earlier model of a pediatric flexible bronchoscope.

equipment should be protected from water and chemicals used during bronchoscopy as well as secretions from the patient.

Preparation of the Patient

Since bronchoscopic photography and videobronchoscopy are simple extensions of standard bronchoscopy, the preparation of the patient for bronchoscopic photography does not merit special consideration. However, it should be noted that addition of photography or video recording for the purposes of publication or teaching will invariably lengthen the duration of the procedure (27). If special or time-consuming procedures are planned along with photographic documenta-

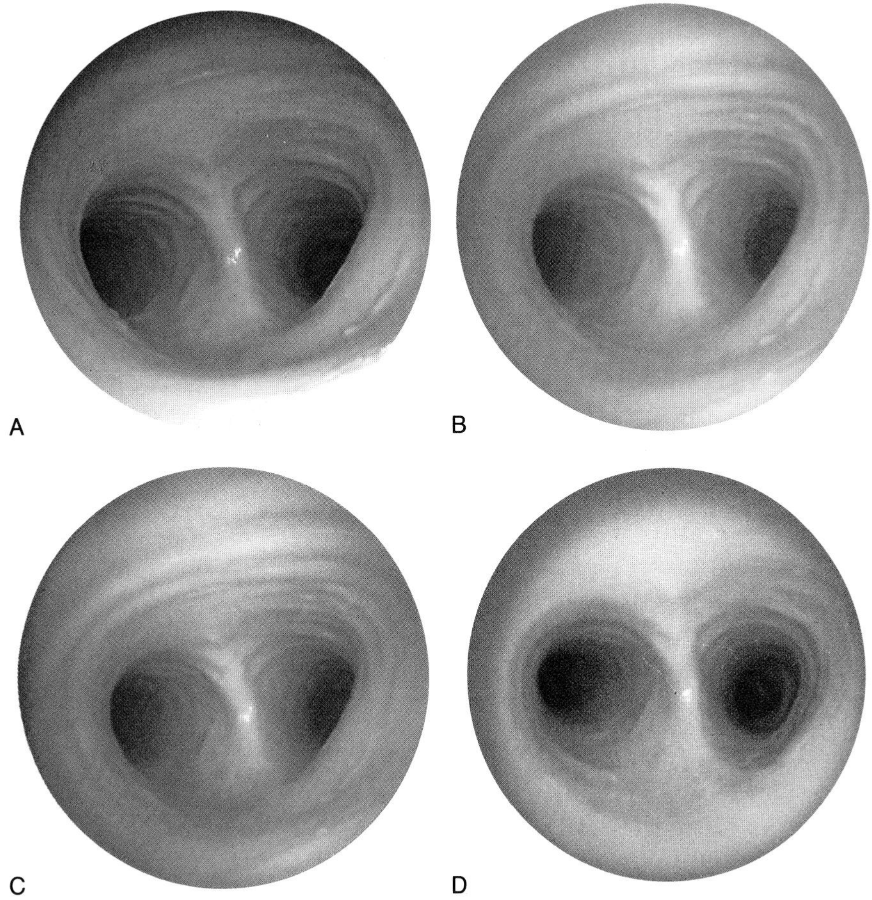

FIG. 3. Bronchoscopic photographs of distal trachea of a model tracheobronchial tree. All images were obtained using same rigid bronchoscope, camera, film, and light settings. The only difference was the model of Hopkins rod telescope used: **(A)** Storz telescope, **(B)** Wolff laser telescope, **(C)** Storz telescope made for rigid esophagoscopy, and **(D)** Storz telescope for pediatric rigid bronchoscopy. The last image shows a faint rim of darkness because of the slightly reduced field of view.

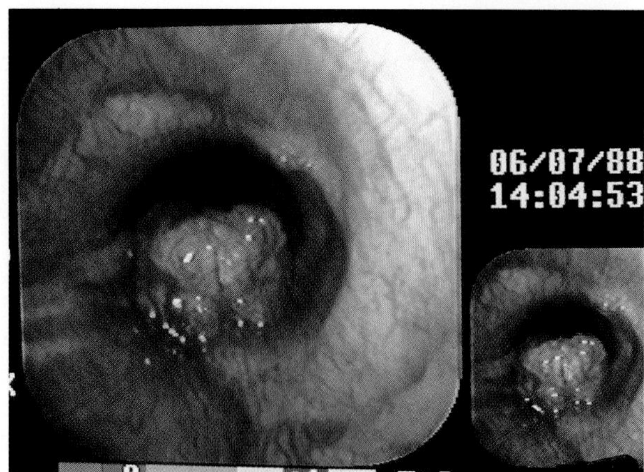

FIG. 4. Bronchoscopic image obtained through a charged couple device (CCD) bronchoscope (also known as video bronchoscope). The quality of images is superior to that captured with regular flexible bronchoscopes.

tion, then general anesthesia may be required (27,28). For most flexible bronchoscopic photography in adults, mild to moderate intravenous sedation with excellent topical anesthesia should suffice. Almost all rigid bronchoscopy procedures will require general anesthesia or deep intravenous sedation.

Photographic Techniques

Before commencing bronchoscopic photography, the focusing of the camera and the bronchoscope should be completed. The distal (objective) lens of the bronchoscope or the telescope should be cleaned with a defogging agent. If coughing by the patient is a problem, extra topical anesthetic may be required. For the videobronchoscopy with permanent recording, an assistant should be instructed to start and stop the recording upon signal from the bronchoscopist. An alternative method is to record the entire procedure and then edit the tape. However, this is time consuming.

For still photography, once the site to be photographed is selected, either the bronchoscopist or an assistant can release the shutter. Excessive blood or liquid in the photographic site will produce bright reflections and adversely affect the photographic image. Similar problems are encountered when an attempt is made to secure a close-up of a glistening endobronchial lesion such as a tumor. To avert this problem, the photographic angle of approach should be changed or the secretions removed, or the bronchoscope should be pulled away from the lesion. Another problem is the rapid breathing by the patient. A solution to this is to reassure and instruct the patient to breathe slowly. If this measure does not succeed, the patient should be asked to hold a breath during which time the camera shutter should be released.

Proper anatomic orientation is important to make sense of the photographs at a later date. A close-up of an endobronchial lesion will provide the proximate picture of the lesion but not its relation to adjacent structures. To obtain a proper perspective, the photograph of a lesion should also include an identifiable tracheobronchial landmark if possible. For instance, if a picture of a tumor in the right main stem bronchus also shows the main carina and a portion of the left main bronchus, then the viewer will be able to assess the size of the tumor and plan appropriate treatment. An option is to take photographs of the lesion close up as well as from a distance (Fig. 5). When a very close view is planned, the objective lens of the bronchoscope or telescope may touch the lesion; mucus or blood may cover the lens. Bronchoscopically removed specimens can be photographed through the bronchoscope even though the image obtained is somewhat distorted due to "fish's eye view" of the optics (Fig. 6). Since bronchoscopic photography is a high-magnification process, minute changes in the distance from the bronchoscope's objective lens to the lesion can result in large excursions in exposure. A change of 2 mm in distance results in a two–f-stop change in exposure (25). Sharp photographic images can be obtained when the distance between the objective lens and the object is 5–15 mm. Since the top of the 35-mm transparency slides are always oriented to the pointer in the flexible bronchoscope, pictures may not always show the anatomic anterior at the top of the slide. To get a consistently correct orientation, the bronchoscopist should try to flex the tip of the bronchoscope in such a way that the patient's anatomic anterior is always at the top of the photographic image. This is particularly important if a large number of 35-mm transparency slides are to be collected for teaching purposes.

Storage

The videocassette should be properly cataloged and stored in a proper location; the video equipment to study the images should be located close to the video library. The video tapes should have labels with patient identification, diagnosis, and date. Similarly, 35-mm transparency slides should be catalogued and stored appropriately (29).

Troubleshooting

When the photographs are consistently poor in quality, the light source, the flash contact between the bronchoscope and the light source, and the camera should be inspected. Most problems encountered in bronchoscopic photography are related to the automatic light source system. There are several electrical contacts that must be made between the camera and

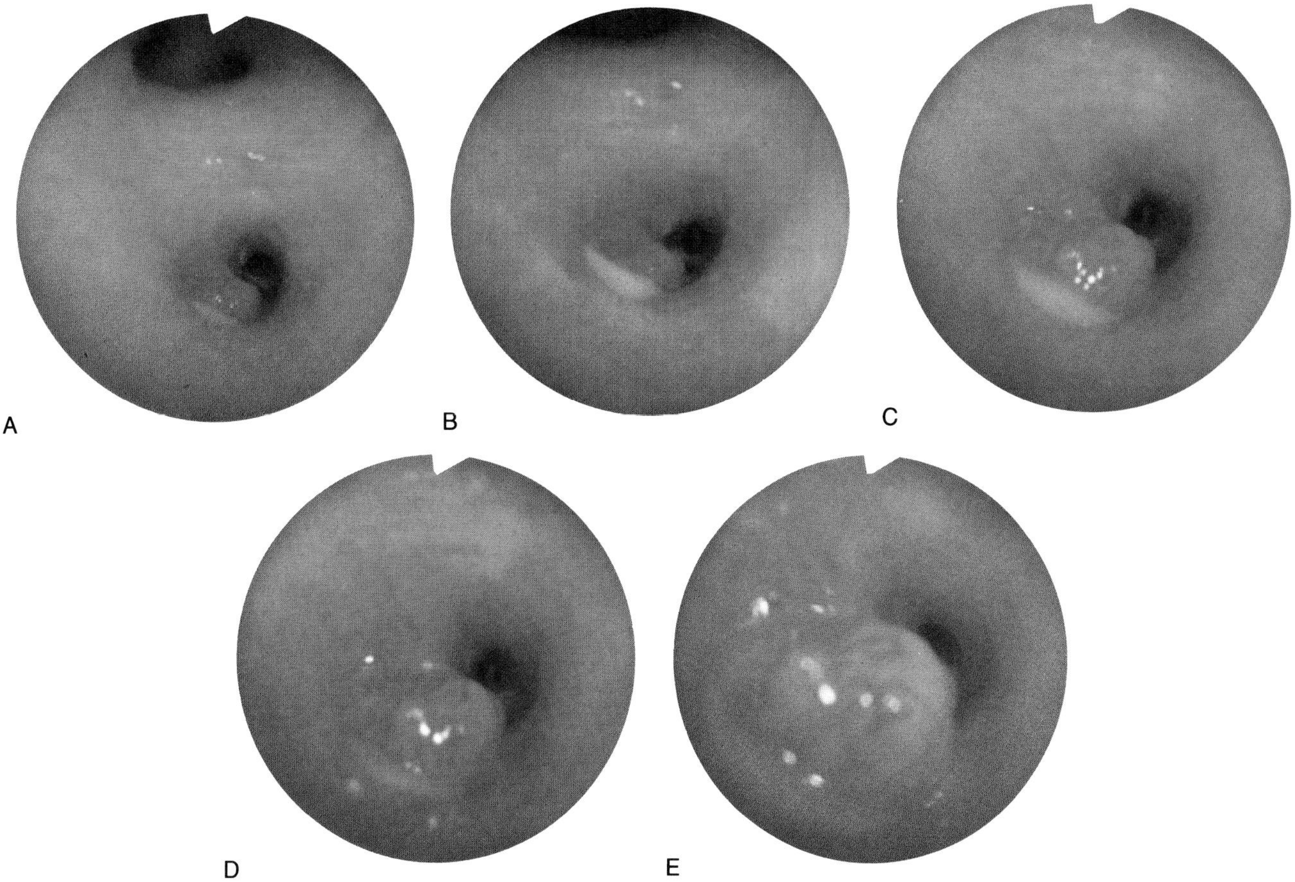

FIG. 5. Lesion located at the entrance to right lower lobe lesion photographed from different distances. **(A)** This distant image provides an identifiable landmark, namely, the right middle lobe bronchus. **(B–D)** Progressively closer images provide further details of the lesion itself. **(E)** Very close exposure provides macroscopic details of the lesion, such as its vascularity, possible site of attachment to bronchial wall, and relation to distal bronchial tree, etc.

the adapter, the adapter and the bronchoscope, and the bronchoscope and the light source. Dirt, moisture, or dry residue from cleaning or disinfecting solutions will cause a failure of the photographic system (25). The electrical contacts must be kept clean and dry and the connector pins on the light source should be properly aligned. Different exposure settings and film should be tested. The service departments of the bronchoscope and camera manufacturers should be contacted for further assistance.

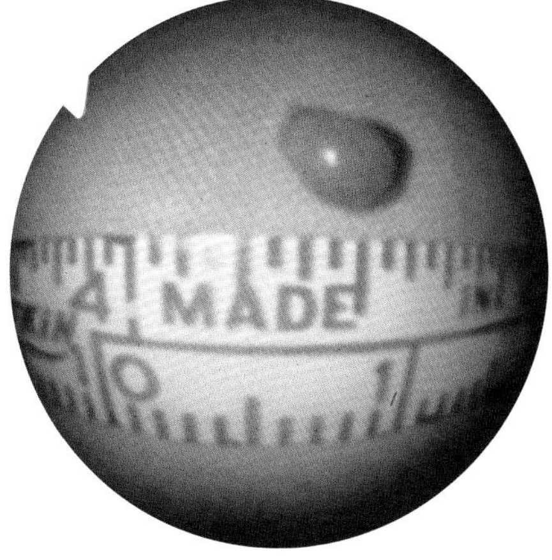

FIG. 6. Bronchoscopic photograph of a bronchoscopically removed specimen.

REFERENCES

1. Ollman B, Lindholm CE, Barkman PE. Making enlargements from small fibre-optic transparencies. *Med Biol Illus* 1975; 25:231–234.
2. Morgan E. Personal communication.
3. Ikeda S. *Altas of flexible bronchofiberscopy*. Baltimore: University Park Press; 1974.
4. Kitamura S. *Color atlas of clinical application of fiberoptic bronchoscopy*. Chicago: Year Book; 1990.
5. Becker HD, Kayser K, Schulz V, Tuengerthal S, Vollhaber H-H. *Atlas of bronchoscopy*. Philadelphia: BC Decker; 1991.
6. Cavaliere S, Beamis J. *Atlas of therapeutic bronchoscopy: laser stents*. Brescia, Italy: Sergio Cavaliere; 1991.
7. Stradling P, Stradling JR. *Diagnostic bronchoscopy: a teaching manual*. Edinburgh: Churchill Livingstone; 1991.
8. Kato H, Horai T. *A colour atlas of endoscopic diagnosis in early stage lung cancer*. London: Wolf; 1992.
9. Ikeda S. Bronchial television endoscopy. *Chest* 1989;96:(1 Suppl)41S–42S.

10. Rayl JE, Hall CJ Jr, Rourke D, Spindler LJ. Requirements for television-bronchoscopy. *Chest* 1978:73(5 Suppl)764–767.
11. Cunanan OS, Mazza JE. Integrated electronic display model for teaching bronchoscopy. *Chest* 1977;72:364–365.
12. Prakash UBS, Offord KP, Stubbs SE. Bronchoscopy in North America: the ACCP survey. *Chest* 1991;100:1668–1675.
13. Rayl JE, Pittman JM, Shuster JJ. Preclinical training in bronchoscopic diagnosis of cancer. *Chest* 1988;93:824–827.
14. Finer NN, Etches PC. Fiberoptic bronchoscopy in the neonate. *Pediatr Pulmonol* 1989;7:116–120.
15. Pingleton SK. Bronchoscopic photography of a bronchial carcinoid tumor associated with unilateral hypoperfusion of the lung. *Endoscopy* 1983;15:31–33.
16. Nakhosteen JA, Niederle N. Small cell lung cancer. Serial bronchofiberscopy and photographic documentation—the bridge sign. *Chest* 1983;83:12–16.
17. Ihde DC, Cohen MH, Simms EB, Matthews MJ, Bunn PA, Minna JD. Evaluation of response to chemotherapy with fiberoptic bronchoscopy in non–small cell lung cancer. *Cancer* 1980;45:1693–1696.
18. Marsh BR, Frost JK, Erozan YS, Carter D. Occult bronchogenic carcinoma. Endoscopic localization and television documentation. *Cancer* 1972;30:1348–1352.
19. Toomes H, Vogt-Moykopf I, Heller WD, Ostertag H. Measurement of mucociliary clearance in smokers and nonsmokers using a bronchoscopic video-technical method. *Lung* 1981;159:27–34.
20. Yoshida S. The Yoshida new bronchoscope and photo-cine-*Laryngoscope* 1966;76:1582–1590.
21. Stradling P. Photography within the human bronchial tree. *J Audiovis Media Med* 1978;1:192–193.
22. Berci G. Flexible fiber and rigid (pediatric) bronchoscopic instrumentation and documentation. Quo Vadis? *Chest* 1978; 73:(Suppl)768–775.
23. Rayl JE, Hall CJ Jr, Rourke D, Spindler LJ. Requirements for television-bronchoscopy. *Chest* 1978;73(Suppl):764–767.
24. Holinger PH. Open tube endoscopic photography in otorhinolaryngology and bronchoesophagology. *Acta Otorhinolaryngol Belg* 1975;29:1074–1077.
25. Morgan SJ. Endoscopic photography. In: Tams TR, ed, *Small animal endoscopy*. St. Louis: CV Mosby; 1990:25–30.
26. Ono R, Edell ES, Ikeda S. Recent advances in bronchoesophagology. Amsterdam: Elsevier; 1990:49–53.
27. Fuller WR, Davies DM, Stradling P. Anaesthesia for bronchoscopy prolonged by teaching and photography. *Anaesthesia* 1972; 27:292–300.
28. Morgan M, Lumley J, McCormick PW, Stradling P. Anaesthesia for bronchoscopic photography. *Anaesthesia* 1969;24:343–354.
29. Prakash UBS. A simplified system to filing and retrieval of 35-mm teaching slides in medicine. *Arch Intern Med* 1985; 145:1680–1682.

Bronchoscopy,
edited by U. B. S. Prakash.
Mayo Foundation © 1994.
Published by Raven Press, Ltd., New York.

CHAPTER 28

Maintenance of the Bronchoscope and Bronchoscopy Equipment

Mickie J. Stelck, Marsha J. Kulas, and Atul C. Mehta

The bronchoscope and other equipment employed in bronchoscopic procedures are surgical instruments and should be treated with the utmost care. There are two major distinctions between the bronchoscope and other surgical instruments. First, bronchoscopy is not a sterile procedure and therefore, the need to maintain absolute sterility is not imperative. Second, while most surgical instruments, including the rigid bronchoscope, are made of stainless steel and durable materials and therefore can withstand harsh usage and the steam autoclave, the flexible bronchoscope is a very delicate and easily damaged instrument and requires special handling. The majority of the instruments used in rigid bronchoscopy can be disinfected or sterilized in the standard manner used for the sterilization of other surgical equipments or in the same manner described below for the cleaning of the flexible bronchoscope.

THE FLEXIBLE BRONCHOSCOPE

The flexible bronchoscope has become a workhorse of modern pulmonary practice (1). The instrument is now routinely used for both diagnostic and therapeutic procedures such as Nd:YAG laser photoresection, brachytherapy, and photodynamic therapy (2–4). The flexible bronchoscope is a delicate, sophisticated, and expensive instrument and proper maintenance is mandatory for its durability and to avoid expensive repairs (5). Besides, in the era of acquired immunodeficiency syndrome (AIDS), proper cleaning of the instrument is of the utmost importance for the prevention of both the spread of communicable diseases and false-positive results (6). The fact that the base price of this instrument varies from $8,000 to $12,000 is reason enough to take special care of this delicate instrument.

There are two aspects of proper maintenance of the flexible bronchoscope: (a) its routine care and (b) prevention of damage. The key aspects of routine care involve the cleaning, disinfection, sterilization, storage, and transportation of the instrument, which are routinely carried out by paramedical personnel such as nurses, physicians' assistants, or respiratory therapists by following a well-rehearsed schedule. However, the responsibility of preventing damage to the instrument during its use belongs to the bronchoscopist. Joint efforts are required on the part of both teams in proper care of the instrument.

Routine Care

Cleaning

Following each use, the instrument should be cleaned and disinfected or sterilized prior to its storage for the next procedure. Before subjecting the instrument to either disinfection or sterilization, it is cleaned in the following fashion. The exterior of the instrument is wiped off with a dry gauze. The working channel of the instrument is cleaned using providone (Betadine) solution suction for approximately 10 sec. Then the suction valve is removed and the instrument is immersed in the cleaning solution. The cleaning solution could be simple tap water and an enzymatic neutral detergent (6). The majority of flexible bronchoscopes marketed currently are submersible instruments. However, the bronchoscopists who are using the older non-

M. J. Stelck and M. J. Kulas: Bronchoscopy Section, Mayo Clinic, Rochester, Minnesota 55905.
A. C. Mehta: Department of Pulmonary and Critical Care Medicine, Cleveland Clinic Foundation, Cleveland, Ohio 44195.

immersible models should follow the manufacturer's recommendations. The proximal control unit and the umbilical cord of the *non*submersible bronchoscopes should never be allowed to dip into the cleaning solution. It is recommended by most manufacturers that after each use of the flexible bronchoscope a "leak test" be performed for early detection of damage either to the working channel or to the outer sheath of the flexible bronchoscope (7). In a busy bronchoscopy practice, this could be a cumbersome undertaking; however, it is our recommendation that the leak test must be performed following each bronchoscopic needle aspiration and Nd:YAG laser photoresection performed through the flexible bronchoscope. The method of performing the leak test is described in the instruction manual for each flexible bronchoscope (7). An air leak through either side of the working channel indicates perforation of the plastic tubing lining the working channel, which usually occurs as a result of improper bronchoscopic needle aspiration or biopsy, repeated excessive bending of the instrument, or use of damaged flexible accessories (5). The repair cost of such a damage is around $3,500. An air leak occurring from the surface of the instrument indicates damage to the rubber sheath located at the distal end or polyurethane tubing covering the proximal flexible portion of the bronchoscope. Such damage is usually the result of rubbing the exterior of the instrument against sharp objects or a part of routine wear and tear (Fig. 1). The repair of such damage is around $350. A positive leak test requires immediate repair of the instrument to prevent further damage to the inner mechanism of the instrument. Once any type of fluid enters into the flexible bundle, the visual field appears foggy and proper endobronchial examination becomes impossible.

Following completion of the leak test, the instrument is scrubbed softly with the gauze and then removed from the cleaning solution. The working channel of the flexible bronchoscope is then brushed with the cleaning brush and once again Betadine suction is used for approximately 10 sec, followed by water rising. Once cleaned in this fashion, the instrument is then ready for either disinfection or sterilization.

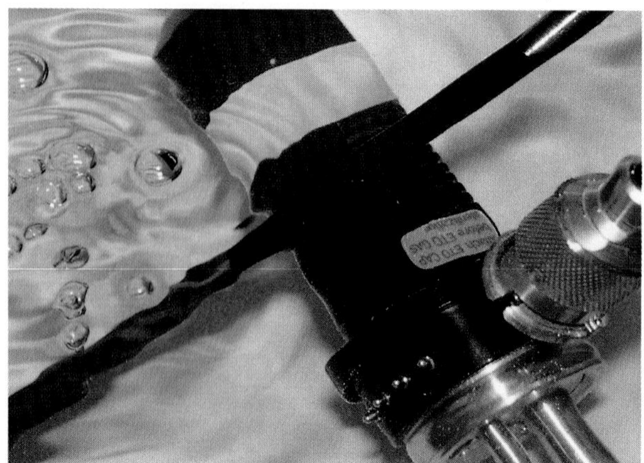

FIG. 1. Positive "leak test." Note air leak from the external surface of the flexible bronchoscope (see text).

Beside cleaning the instrument, it is extremely important to decontaminate the instrument after using it in patients suffering from infectious diseases. A recent study by Hanson and colleagues documented contamination of the flexible bronchoscope by a variety of organisms including *Pneumocystis carinii* following its use in patients with AIDS. Proper cleaning of instruments with Keymed autodisinfector in 5% neutral detergent prior to disinfection of the instrument using glutaraldehyde was found to be useful in removing all detectable contaminants to an acceptable level (6).

Disinfection

There are three levels of disinfection. High-level disinfection denotes elimination of all vegetative organisms and viruses and most but not necessarily all bacteria or fungal spores. Intermediate disinfection calls for elimination of all vegetative pathogenic bacteria and mycobacteria (including *Mycobacterium tuberculosis*) but not necessarily all viruses (smaller and nonenveloped viruses are more resistant to disinfection). Low-level disinfection is nearly comparable to sanitization and implies elimination of most pathogenic bacteria. Prior to its introduction into the patient's tracheobronchial tree, the flexible bronchoscope should be either disinfected or sterilized (see below) to prevent the spread of communicable diseases. For the purpose of disinfection, any of the chemicals such as isopropyl alcohol, glutaraldehyde, or phenol can be used. Glutaraldehyde 2% (Cidex) is the most popular chemical used for this purpose. Submersion of the flexible bronchoscope in glutaraldehyde for more than 10 min destroys all vegetative pathogens such as *Pseudomonas aeruginosa,* viruses (polio virus type I, adenovirus type II, herpes simplex type I and II, influenza type A, vaccinia, coronavirus, cytomegalovirus, rhinovirus type XIV), and 99.8% of *Mycobacterium tuberculosis* organisms. To remove 100% of *M. tuberculosis* organisms, one needs to submerse the instrument in glutaraldehyde solution for 45 min at 25°C. Davis and colleagues found that a 15-min disinfection procedure with either aqueous glutaraldehyde or an iodophor, coupled with initial vigorous mechanical cleaning of the bronchoscope and its accessories, is a quick and reliable method for preventing the contamination of the bronchoscope with mycobacteria (8). A common practice of submersing the flexible bronchoscope for 20 min in 2% glutaraldehyde solution for disinfection following routine procedures is acceptable. It should be pointed out that certain state laws in the United States ban the pouring of used glutaraldehyde solution into the sink. This measure is aimed at the protection of the environment and certain species of fish in the lakes and rivers. If this policy becomes nationwide then use of other less toxic disinfectant solutions such as peracetic acid would become popular. Another disadvantage of glutaraldehyde is that it corrodes steel parts of the instrument following more than 24 hr after exposure. Other disinfecting agents such as isopropyl alcohol and phenol are not as effective sporicidals as glutaraldehyde.

Following submersion of the instrument into the disinfectant solution for the recommended period of time, the exterior of the instrument is rinsed with distilled water and the working channel of the instrument with sterile water followed by air suction drying. A large pan should be used to submerse the flexible bronchoscope in a disinfectant solution to prevent excessive coiling of its flexible portion. Repeated excessive coiling can lead to damage to the working channel of the instrument. In recent years, mechanical devices used for washing and disinfecting of the bronchoscope have been removed from the market because of the possibility of colonization of the filters used in these devices by gram-negative organisms and eventual contamination of the instrument.

Sterilization

Sterilization means the complete elimination of all viable microorganisms including all spores. It can be performed by submersing the instrument in formaldehyde or using ethylene oxide (ETO) gas. The latter is the most practical and popular method of sterilizing the instrument. ETO is effective against all types of microorganisms; it is easily available, noncorrosive, and penetrates through a mass of dry materials. High pressures are not required for its effectiveness. However, ETO is somewhat toxic and instruments should not be used for at least 12 hr after completion of ETO gas sterilization.

Submersible flexible bronchoscopes are completely sealed to make them air-tight. A pressure difference that develops between the interior and exterior of the body of the scope can lead to severe damage. Prior to ETO gas sterilization, and ETO venting cap must be placed at the proximal end of the umbilical cord of the instrument to equalize pressure between the exterior and interior of the instrument and thus to prevent rupture of the rubber or polyurethane sheath of the flexible bronchoscope (Fig. 2) (5). Once again, the instrument should not be excessively coiled during the sterilization. A hard-walled sterilization pan with a lockable lid provides a protective way of storing the instrument.

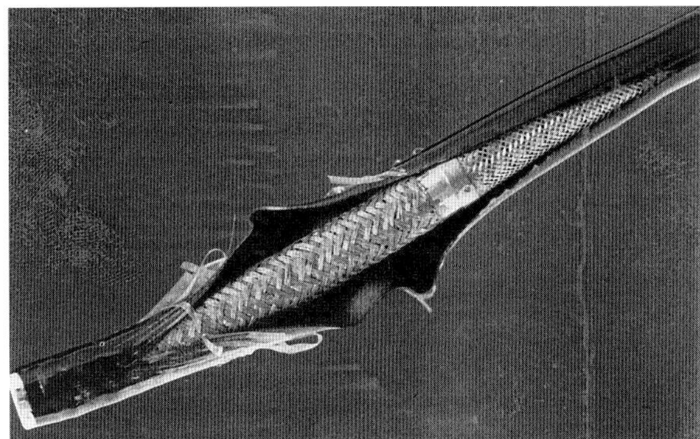

FIG. 2. Failure to place ETO venting cap prior to gas sterilization leading to rupture of the outer sheath of the flexible bronchoscope. From ref. 5, with permission.

Clamps or ties should be used to prevent excessive movement of the instrument during sterilization. Care must be taken not to exceed the recommended pressure, temperature, humidity, exposure time, and gas concentration guidelines during ETO gas sterilization. These guidelines are easily obtainable from the instruction manual supplied by the manufacturer. The flexible bronchoscope should never be autoclaved, boiled, or cleaned using ultrasonic devices.

Both sterilization as well as disinfection described above are adequate means of cleaning the instrument, even after its use in patients with hepatitis or human immunodeficiency virus infection (6). However, one must follow institution-specific guidelines in this regard. The role of the bronchoscope as a vector in the spread of infection from one patient to another and as a cause of pseudoepidemics (cross-contamination) is a potential risk of improper disinfection and sterilization procedures (9). This topic is discussed at length in Chapter 14.

Storage

Following disinfection or sterilization, the flexible bronchoscope should be stored properly between uses. Prior to its storage, the instrument should be dried with special attention paid to its distal tip, lenses, and electrical contacts. The control lock should be released and the instrument stored in a straight, vertical position. The storage area should be dry, well ventilated, devoid of extreme temperatures, away from direct sunlight and high humidity. Storage of bronchoscopes is best when the insertion tube can be maintained straight to avoid the development of a curve. The storage cabinet should be tall enough to accommodate the entire length of the working portion of the flexible bronchoscope in the vertical position. A wall cabinet in which the bronchoscope can be hung is probably a better option (see Chapter 3, this volume). This will prevent curved-fixed configuration of the flexible portion of the instrument (memory curve). If a drawer is used for storage, the tip of the instrument should be protected from getting caught when the drawer closes. Instruments should not be stored in the carrying case. The carrying case should be used only for the purpose of transportation of the instrument. Bacterial colonization of the carrying case is quite frequent and can lead to contamination of the instrument. Excessive exposure of the flexible bronchoscope to radiation may result in yellowish discoloration and darkening of both the fiber bundles and the visual image (see below) (10). Therefore, it should never be stored in the X-ray department where fluoroscopy or roentgenograhic studies are routinely performed. Storing of the flexible bronchoscope with the ETO venting cap in place may allow evaporation of moisture that develops over time from the leak test.

Transportation

At times it may be necessary to transport the flexible bronchoscope away from the bronchoscopy suite for a variety of purposes including demonstration or repair. Long-distance transportation of the instrument may be carried out in the carrying case provided by the manufacturer to avoid external damage or excessive coiling of the instrument. Extreme care should be taken while closing the lid of the carrying case as severe damage to the bronchoscope can occur if its body is accidentally pinched between the lids (5). This damage would be similar to that caused by the patient biting the instrument. This scenario would lead to damage to the delicate quartz filament resulting in the appearance of black spots in the field of vision reducing the quality of the image. Once again, during transportation the ETO venting cap must be placed at the proximal end of the instrument to equalize pressure between the exterior and the interior of the instrument. This protocol is mandatory to prevent damage to the instrument during air transport.

Prevention of Damage to Flexible Bronchoscope

Areas of potential damage to the instrument are listed in Table 1. The physician performing the procedure is solely responsible for prevention of such damage to the instrument.

Improper Handling

The objective and ocular lenses and the quartz filaments of the instrument are vulnerable to trauma during its routine use. Accidental striking of the distal end

TABLE 1. *Maintenance of flexible fiberoptic bronchoscope*

(A) Routine care:	1) Bedside cleaning
	2) Disinfection
	3) Sterilization
	4) Storage
	5) Transportation
(B) Prevention of damage from:	1) Improper handling
	2) Fluoroscopy
	3) Transbronchial needle aspiration
	4) Nd:YAG laser photoresection
	5) Electrosurgery
	6) Improper lubrication
	7) Uncooperative patient

of the instrument on a hard surface can fracture the objective lens. To prevent damage to the flexible bronchoscope, the novice bronchoscopist should recognize the damaging moves. Due care should be taken to prevent excessive angulation of the instrument, which most commonly occurs at the most proximal portion of the flexible insertion tube (Fig. 3) and can be minimized by allowing adequate distance between the patient's face and the instrument control unit. One can use a step stool to increase this distance or lower the height of the bronchoscopy table. If the procedure is performed while the patient is in a sitting position, the distance can easily be adjusted by the bronchoscopist's stepping backward. Excessive twisting of the distal flexible portion of the instrument can damage the quartz filaments, once again resulting in the appearance of black spots in the field of vision. If the rotation of the flexible insertion tube is required, it should be performed by flexing or extending the wrist rather than twisting the flexible portion of the scope, thus limiting the torque applied to the instrument (5).

The working channel of the instrument is lined by a delicate plastic tubing. A paradox that needs to be understood is the fact that the fancier and more expen-

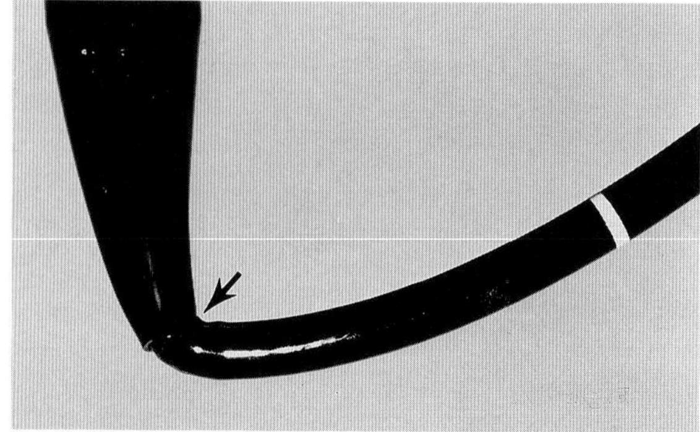

FIG. 3. Forced, repeated, excessive angulation causing damage to proximal most flexible portion of the flexible bronchoscope.

sive flexible bronchoscopes, which provide a high degree of angulation and maneuverability, are lined by a much thinner (vulnerable) plastic tubing to increase the flexibility. If this tubing is perforated, fractured, or lacerated, liquids can seep into the fiberoptic quartz filaments fogging the field of vision and making further examination impossible. This tubing is vulnerable to damage from the use of flexible bronchoscopic instruments (Fig. 4). In our experience this is a major drawback of the submersible bronchoscopes as its immersion into the cleaning solution increases the likelihood of fluids seeping into the inner mechanism of the instrument including the quartz filaments. Repair of such damage to thc plastic tubing requires dismantling the entire instrument to replace the tubing and costs more than $3,500.

The most proximal flexible portion of the instrument is highly vulnerable to such damage because the instruments inserted through the working channel impact on this portion of the tubing while negotiating the angulation. To prevent such damage, the proximal most flexible portion of the instrument should be kept as straight as possible during insertion of any instrument through the working channel. In our experience, a recently introduced flexible bronchoscope with a separate distal port for instrument insertion reduces the angulation between the port and the working channel and is less vulnerable to such damage.

One should be aware of the diameter of the working channel of the flexible bronchoscope. Flexible instruments with diameters equal to or larger than that of the working channel of the instrument should not be forcefully inserted into the channel. For example, an 18-gauge bronchoscopic needle aspiration used to obtain a histology specimen cannot be passed through the working channel of the Olympus BF-1T20 flexible bronchoscope because its 15-mm-long metal needle will not negotiate the acute angle between the insertion port and the working channel of the flexible bronchoscope (11,12). Fortunately, both the needle and the flexible bronchoscope are replaced by their modified versions.

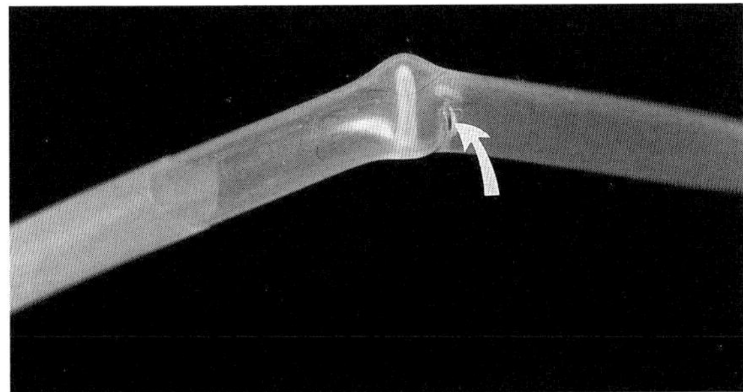

FIG. 4. Perforation **(arrow)** of the working channel of the flexible bronchoscope caused during bronchoscopic needle aspiration or biopsy. The kink in the tubing represents proximal most flexible portion of the flexible bronchoscope. From ref. 5, with permission.

Fluoroscopy

Fluoroscopic guidance is often used during bronchoscopic lung biopsy, thus exposing the fiberoptic bundles within the flexible bronchoscope to radiation. Kato and colleagues study the relationship between X irradiation and changes in the functional properties of flexible bronchoscopes by utilizing scanning electron microscopy, electron spin resonance, and thermoluminescent dosimetry techniques to determine the nature of the changes and their possible reversibility (10). Decreases in light transmission were observed at exposures above 5 roentgens (R), color changes were observed above 25 R, and electron spin resonance absorption changes occurred above 100 R. These changes were proportional to the X-ray doses. The results showed that to prevent X irradiation to the fiberoptic bundles, the flexible bronchoscope should not be subjected to more than 15 min of fluoroscopy per week.

Bronchoscopic Needle Aspiration

Improperly performed bronchoscopic needle aspiration or biopsy is the single most cause for producing perforation of the plastic tubing of the flexible bronchoscope (5,14). Due to the availability of retractable versions, nonretractable metallic needles used to obtain either histology or cytology specimens should not be inserted through the working channel of the instrument (15,16). Such needles can easily lacerate the plastic tubing during its insertion, especially while negotiating the curves of the instrument. During the use of retractable needles, it should be ascertained that its beveled end is fully protected inside the metal hub, which is located at the distal end of its plastic catheter. Care should also be taken not to place the sharp end of the needle proximal to the hub, where it may easily perforate its own plastic tubing during forward thrust and subsequently damage the channel of the flexible bronchoscope (Fig. 5). The proximal most flexible portion of the flexible bronchoscope should be kept as straight as possible and the distal tip kept in a neutral forward-viewing position during insertion of the needle through the working channel. The metal needle should not be pushed out of its catheter unless the catheter is adequately visualized outside the flexible bronchoscope in the endobronchial tree. After obtaining the specimen, the flexible bronchoscope should be optimally straightened for smooth withdrawal of the needle with its catheter. As mentioned previously, the leak test should be

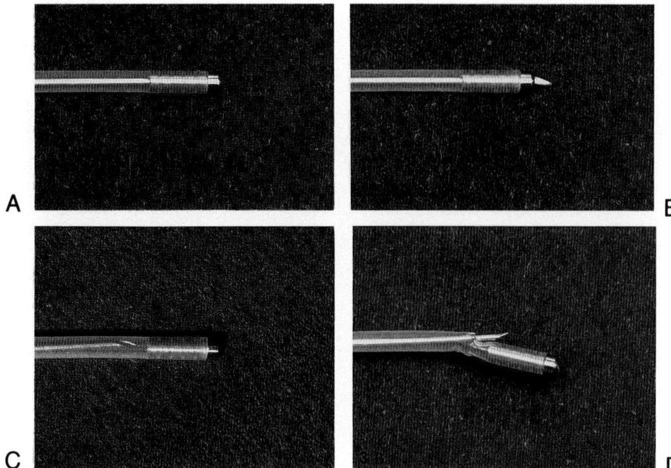

FIG. 5. (A) Correct position of the metal needle prior to bronchoscopic needle aspiration. Note that entire beveled end is placed inside the metal hub. **(B)** Incorrect position of the metal needle. Note that sharp end of the needle is jutting out of the metal hub, which can lacerate the working channel of the flexible bronchoscope. **(C, D)** Incorrect position of the metal needle. Placement of the metal needle proximal to the metal hub can perforate its own plastic catheter during forward thrust and consequently damage the working channel of the flexible bronchoscope.

performed after each bronchoscopic needle aspiration to rule out damage to the working channel. This will allow early identification of damage to the instrument and help identify flaws in the technique. In our opinion, bronchoscopic needle aspiration should be performed only by experienced bronchoscopists or under their direct supervision.

Laser Bronchoscopy

Symptomatic malignant as well as benign endobronchial lesions are now being palliated with various laser bronchoscopy procedures (17). Many bronchoscopists use the flexible bronchoscope for such procedures (2,18). Whether flexible or rigid bronchoscopy is used, safe instrumentation in laser surgery involves the following three basic principles: first, the armamentarium used in conjunction with the operative procedure should be nonflammable; second, the surfaces of instruments should be nonreflective; and third, there must be a provision for adequately evacuating smoke and steam from the operative field (19–21). With the powerful capabilities of laser therapy comes an inherent danger of endobronchial ignition (22). The flexible bronchoscope is made up of combustible materials that make it vulnerable to endobronchial fire. Concomitant use of a highly combustible polyvinylchloride (PVC) endotracheal tube to facilitate insertion of the flexible bronchoscope further increases the risk. Extreme care should be taken to avoid the possibility of endobronchial ignition while performing this procedure through the instrument (23). The laser beam should never be fired unless the tip of the laser fiber is adequately visualized inside the endobronchial tree and is at least 5 mm away from the end of the instrument. It should be ascertained that coaxial coolant, either gas or normal saline, is constantly flowing by the side of the laser fiber during the use of laser energy; otherwise the metal casing located at the distal end of the noncontact fiber can get warmed up and damage the working channel during its withdrawal (Fig. 6). In our opinion, safety of the use of "bare fiber" through the flexible bronchoscope has not been proven as yet and should be avoided as far as possible. Unprotected bare fiber appears to be more vulnerable to the damage and if the damaged portion of the bare fiber is positioned inside the working channel of the flexible bronchoscope severe damage to the instrument can occur (Fig. 7) (24). Both the tip of the laser fiber and the flexible bronchoscope should be kept free of any carbon particles because these charred black particles absorb a significantly higher amount of energy than the surrounding tissue and start the ignition. Alcohol or alcohol-based solutions should not be used to clean the laser fiber tip to avoid the possibility of combustion. One important caution that needs to be exercised during Nd:YAG laser photoresection is that the concentration of supplemental oxygen should not exceed 40% and no combustible anesthetic agent should be used during the procedure. If the procedure is being performed through a PVC endotracheal tube, optimal distance (>4 cm) should be maintained between its tip and the treatment site. If midtracheal or upper tracheal lesions are being treated, the procedure should be performed using a metal jet injection cannula or rigid bronchoscope (25). A low-power density and short-duration pulses minimize the chances of endobronchial ignition.

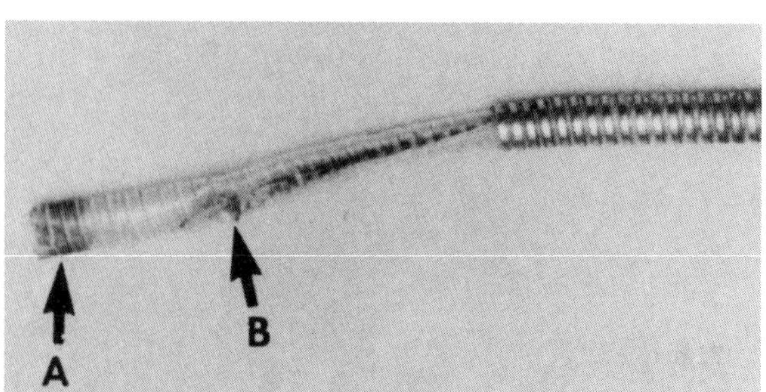

FIG. 6. Damaged distal end of the working channel of the flexible bronchoscope. Note charring **(A)** and perforation **(B)**, caused by heated metal casing of the noncontact laser fiber when the coaxial gas flow was accidentally shut off. From ref. 5, with permission.

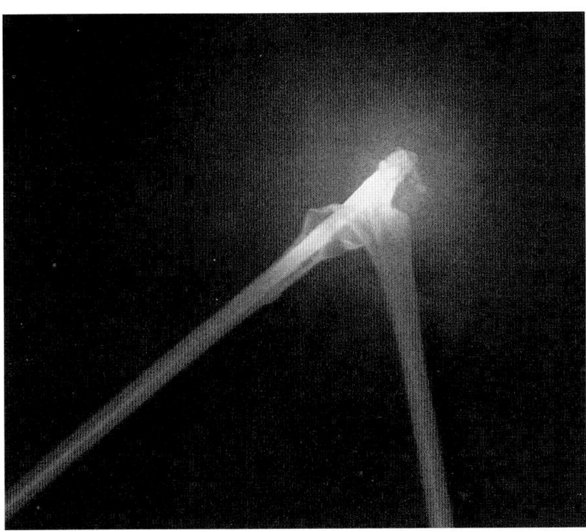

FIG. 7. Application of laser energy through a cracked filament leading to its fracture and burning of the protective plastic tubing.

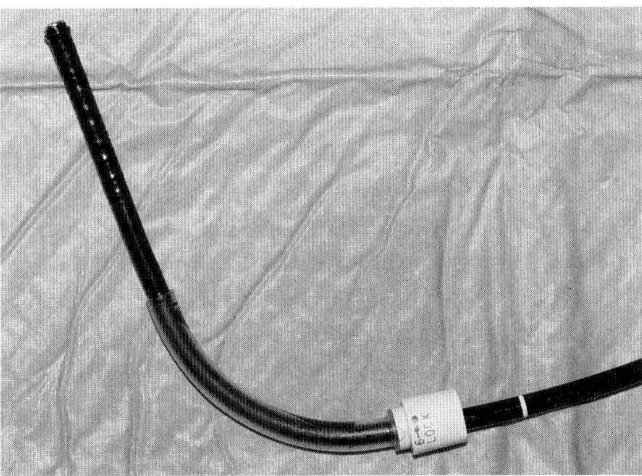

FIG. 8. Selection of an improper size of flexible bronchoscope for a procedure through the tracheostomy tube can lead to patient distress and/or getting the instrument stranded inside the tube and requiring immediate and simultaneous removal of both gadgets.

Electrosurgery

Electrocauterization through the flexible gastrointestinal endoscopes is an accepted treatment for gastrointestinal bleeding. In recent years, there has been increasing interest in the application of this modality in the management of endobronchial lesions; however, unlike endoscopes used for gastrointestinal procedures, flexible bronchoscopes are not electrically grounded (26–28). If the wire electrocautery loop inadvertently touches the tip of the flexible bronchoscope, the current could ground through the instrument and the bronchoscopist, generating sparks at either end of the instrument, leading to severe damage to the flexible bronchoscope and injury to the patient as well as the bronchoscopist. In the presence of high concentrations of oxygen, this could start an endobronchial fire as well. A firm understanding of the basic principles of electrocautery and familiarization with the equipment and accessories being used as well as maintaining low concentrations of inspired oxygen will decrease the risk of this type of damage. Because of its special design, bipolar cautery might be safer than wire-loop cautery in this regard (28). Use of endobronchial electrocauterization, however, is still considered experimental.

Lubrication

The flexible bronchoscope should be well lubricated when it is to be inserted through the tracheostomy or endotracheal tube. One should be aware of the size of the endotracheal tube as well as the diameter of the flexible bronchoscope to avoid damage to the instrument or respiratory distress to the patient (Fig. 8). Performing a flexible bronchoscopy through an endotracheal tube using an adult flexible bronchoscope requires a 8.5 size tube, although the bronchoscope can be passed with some difficulty through a 7.0 endotracheal tube. Otherwise the procedure should be performed using a pediatric flexible bronchoscope. Use of a bronchoscope through a small-size endotracheal tube can also lead to tearing of the distal rubber sheath of the flexible bronchoscope. Petroleum-based lubricants should never be used as these may cause premature wear and deterioration of the rubber sheath of the flexible bronchoscope. Only water-soluble lubricants should be used for this purpose. It is a good practice to note the size of an endotracheal tube necessary for the easy passage and proper ventilation for each bronchoscope in the institution. This can save valuable time in an emergency.

Damage Caused by the Patient

The patient's cooperation is essential to avoid possible injury to the instrument. Although the examination can be performed while the patient is in the sitting position, the supine position provides greater patient relaxation and lessens the likelihood of vasovagal attack, which could lead to inadvertent grabbing or pulling of the instrument by the patient. When the procedure needs to be performed either through an endotracheal tube or transoral route, a mouthpiece (bite guard) must be used to protect the instrument from accidental compression by the patient's teeth leading to severe damage to the fiber bundles (Fig. 9). This mouthpiece should be made of a firm plastic material and be securely fastened to the patient's face. If the specially designed bite block is not available, an oral airway or

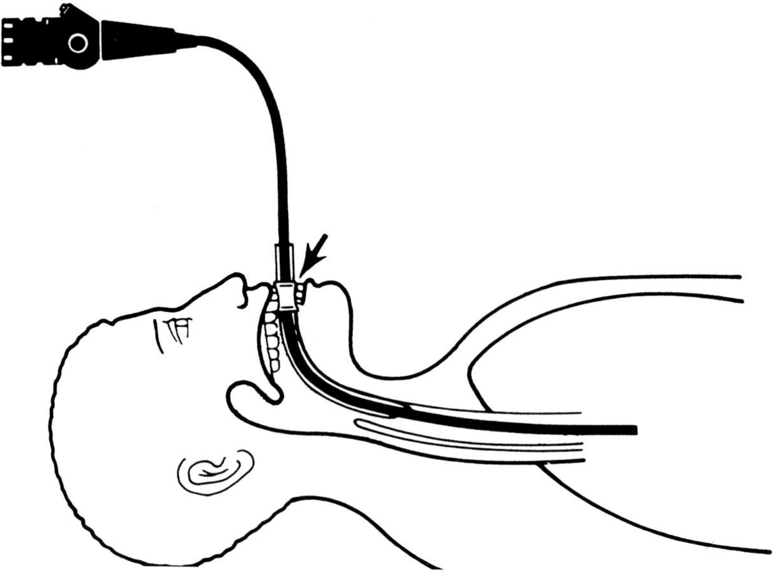

FIG. 9. A bite block to protect the delicate flexible bronchoscope is essential if the oral route is employed to insert the bronchoscope. Reproduced with permission from Zavala, DC: Flexible fiberoptic bronchoscopy. A handbook. University of Iowa Press, 1978.

a dental bite block should be placed between the upper and lower molar teeth. Even if a patient is under general anesthesia, similar precautions are necessary. In the absence of a bite block or other protective device, a patient can bite through an endotracheal tube and damage the flexible bronchoscope (Fig. 10).

Financial Impact of the Damage to Flexible Bronchoscopes

Damage to the flexible bronchoscope may lead to expensive repairs or require replacement of the instrument. Strict adherence to proper maintenance procedure can minimize the damage and related repair cost as well as maximize the life span of the instrument. At the Cleveland Clinic Foundation between 1985 and 1990, 5,652 bronchoscopy procedures, including 212 Nd:YAG laser procedures, were performed by six pulmonary fellows under the direct supervision of one of the seven staff physicians. Procedures were assisted by either registered nurses or respiratory therapists. Eighteen- and 22-gauge bronchoscopic needle aspirations were performed when indicated. Until 1988, no special efforts had been made for the maintenance of the flexible bronchoscope. In 1987 alone, $34,260 ($39.80/procedure) was spent to repair damaged flexible bronchoscopes (Fig. 11). Interestingly, close atten-

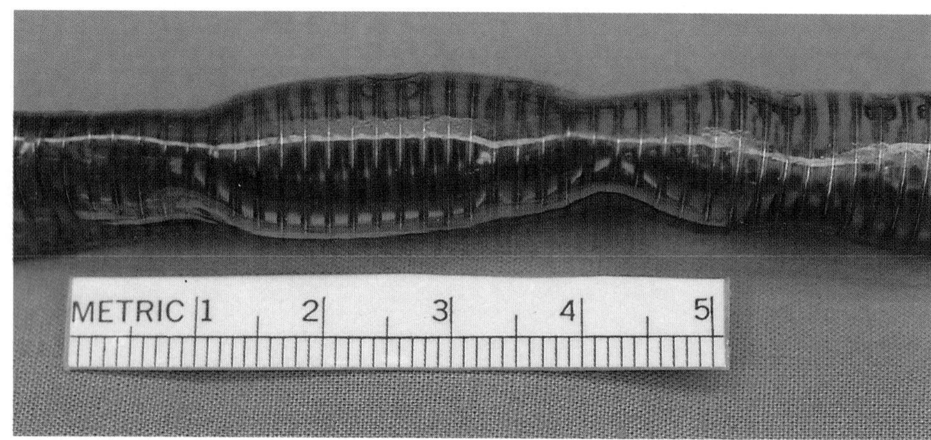

FIG. 10. Endotracheal tube chewed and permanently damaged by a patient who underwent bronchoscopy without a bite block.

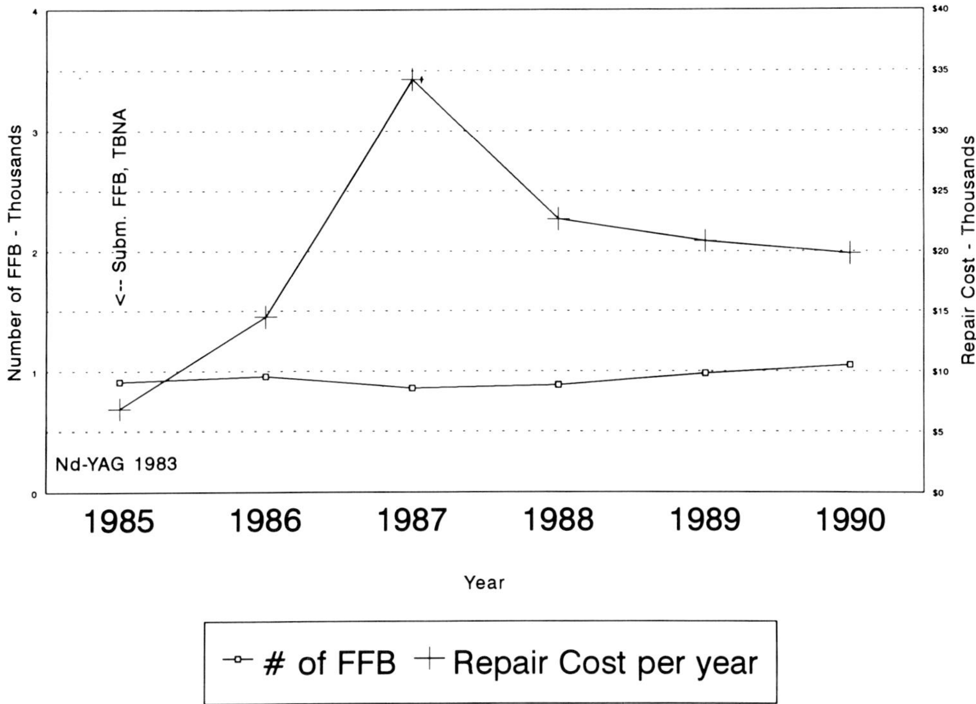

FIG. 11. Introduction of submersible flexible bronchoscope (FFB) and bronchoscopic needle aspiration (TBNA) or biopsy in 1985 increased repair cost to $39.80 per procedure (total $34,260) for year 1987. Nd:YAG laser therapy program started in 1983 didn't contribute significantly to the repair cost. Proper maintenance procedure reduced the repair cost to $18.80 per procedure (total $19,810) for the year 1990.

tion to the repair cost revealed that 87% of the total cost was spent on repairs caused by human error (bronchoscopic needle aspiration Nd:YAG laser therapy, sterilization and transportation of the flexible bronchoscope, and patient-related damage) and could have been prevented. Routine wear and tear, such as impaired angle control, frozen distal tip, broken control arm wire, and worn-out outer sheath, were some of the unpreventable but minor damages. Uniform, extra effort to minimize damage to the flexible bronchoscope in the areas of both routine care as well as prevention of the damage, as described previously, reduced the repair cost to $18.80/procedure; total cost to $19,810 for year 1990. Besides, over the last 3 years and even after 3,300 bronchoscopic procedures, none of the routinely used 10 flexible bronchoscopes required replacement.

Instruction Manual

Manufacturers of the flexible bronchoscope provide instruction manuals containing explicit directions to avoid many of the above-mentioned complications. Unfortunately, only a small number of individuals involved with the procedure familiarize themselves with the information. In a survey conducted at the Cleveland Clinic Foundation involving pulmonary fellows, staff physicians, referring pulmonary physicians, and previously trained fellows, only 11% reported ever having used this information. We believe that this manual is an underutilized resource and should be recommended at the beginning of the training. This information should be readily available at the area where the procedure is usually performed; it should be updated as new techniques are developed with procedures that differ from those described in the original manual.

In summary, flexible bronchoscopes are sophisticated yet delicate instruments that are vulnerable to various types of damage. Even minor damage may require extensive repair. The institution of a proper care program can minimize the repair cost while maximizing the life span. The instruction manuals are very valuable resources for this purpose and should be read by all involved.

THE RIGID BRONCHOSCOPE

The majority of the rigid bronchoscopes are made of steel, even though some bronchoscopists continue to use earlier brass instruments. The newer applications such as laser bronchoscopy, stent placement, and balloon dilatation have resulted in the resurgence of rigid bronchoscopy. To accommodate these procedures, many accessory instruments are necessary; many are made of plastic, rubber, and other easily damageable materials. Some rigid bronchoscopes have rubber nipples on them to provide a seal at a point of insertion and these must be replaced if they rip. All instruments used in rigid bronchoscopy are washed and then disinfected in glutaraldehyde solution for 45 min, rinsed, and dried.

The rigid bronchoscope itself can be subjected to standard techniques of cleaning, disinfection, and sterilization. The accessories, however, are treated in the same fashion as described above for the cleaning of the flexible bronchoscope. The older rigid bronchoscopes contain a narrow channel in the wall of the instrument itself to carry the light source. After each use, the light carrier and the bulb should be thoroughly cleaned. The channel should be cleaned with a brush.

The glass rod telescopes used in rigid bronchoscopy are delicate instruments. The rigid glass rods are easily broken if the steel encasing is subjected to undue bending. The rigid telescopes should be constantly checked for clarity in the optics. The ideal time to do this is after disinfection, especially after gas sterilization. Special defogging agents are available for maintaining the clear sight through the distal end of the glass rod. The telescopes should be stored in foam padding. The distal end of the glass rod should be checked periodically for evidence of chipping or cracking. Among the delicate instruments used in rigid bronchoscopy are the light cords. The cords should be coiled gently and not pinched. The light cords should be checked for excessive bundle breakage. This is accomplished by holding one end of the cord up to a light and looking at the other end; broken bundles will appear as dark spots.

The rigid bronchoscopy forceps used for biopsy and removal of the foreign bodies require preoperative evaluation to ascertain the ease of operation, tight closure, and alignment of the cups or jaws. Periodic lubrication of joints and hinges will maintain proper function.

Other Bronchoscopy Equipment

Occasionally it is necessary to do a bronchoscopy at the bedside of a patient or in the intensive care unit when the patient is already intubated. A portable bronchoscopy unit (bronchoscopy cart) is used for this purpose. After the procedure, all the equipment used for the procedure should be separated from unused instruments and taken for cleaning as described above. The cart itself needs to be kept clean by wiping with a germicide solution, particularly in grooves and edges of the drawers.

Bronchoscopic accessories for both the flexible and rigid bronchoscopes come in many styles and sizes. The forceps used for biopsies and removal of debris and foreign bodies become slower in opening after multiple uses and may need fresh application of a lubricating agent. The flexible forceps can be stored either by hanging or in a drawer. Bending and kinking of the instrument should be avoided. When cleaning the forceps, each cup should be cleaned with a brush to thoroughly remove debris. The forceps with an impaler needle between the cups should be handled carefully to avoid accidental puncture injury and breakage of the needle.

Instruments employed in the extraction of foreign bodies from the tracheobronchial tree include baskets, grasping forceps, claws, and balloon catheters. Some of these appliances are made with delicate wires and easily become misshapen and unusable. Before insertion through the working channel of the flexible bronchoscope, they should be examined for damage and to assure that they move easily in and out of their sheaths and function properly. The baskets, claws, balloon catheters, and similar delicate equipment should be stored inside their sheaths.

Two types of brushes are commonly used through the flexible bronchoscope to collect the specimens for cytology and culture. A sheathed microbiology brush comes packaged sterile from the manufacturer and is for single-use only. The cytology brush tip should be handled in such a way that the brush tip does not get bent frequently. Multiple uses cause metal fatigue and result in the breakage and loss of the brush tip in the tracheobronchial tree. One-time use of the cytology brush prevents such mishaps and cross-contamination. The manufacturer's recommendations should be followed to avoid these mishaps.

Disposable instruments such as transbronchial needles should be used only once. Damaged reusable accessories such as biopsy forceps and cleaning brushes should be replaced rather than repaired due to the delicate nature of the parts involved. This will help prevent trauma to the flexible bronchoscope and provide patient safety as well (13).

Light sources, video equipment, cameras, fluoroscopes, and other instruments used in bronchoscopy should be subjected to regular periodic maintenance according to manufacturer guidelines. Adequate inventory of spare parts such as fuses and bulbs for the light source, film rolls, and batteries for the camera should be maintained. When buying spare parts, the purchaser should ascertain that the parts are compatible with the existing system.

Some cameras are sealed and can be immersed in liquid disinfectant after the plug end of the camera cord is sealed with its cap; the attachments cannot be immersed. Normally, wiping the camera with a germicide solution is sufficient. Excessive talc particles from the bronchoscopist's gloves tend to collect in the camera unless the talc is washed off after donning of the glove.

After bronchoscopy is completed in a patient known to have a highly contagious disease, the cleaning of the bronchoscopy suite itself is first done with a 0.5% sodium hypochlorite solution for all surfaces and the floor. The floor is soaked for 15 min, then everything is cleaned again with a germicidal solution. All tables, the bed surface, and the bronchoscopy cart are wiped with a general cleaner that is a germicide, fungicide, virucide, deodorizer, and mildew-stat all in one. Routine cleaning includes the use of only the germicidal soution.

REFERENCES

1. Ikeda S. Flexible bronchofiberscope. *Ann Otol Rhinol Laryngol* 1970;79:916–917.
2. Unger M. Neodymium:YAG laser therapy for malignant and benign endobronchial obstruction. *Clin Chest Med* 1985; 6:277–290.
3. Schray MF, McDougall JC, Martinez A, Cortese DA, Brutinel MW. Management of malignant airway compromise with laser and low dose rate brachytherapy. *Mayo Clin Exp Chest* 1988; 93(2):264–269.
4. Edell E, Cortese DA. Bronchoscopic phototherapy with hemato-porphyrin derivative for treatment of localized bronchogenic carcinoma: a 5-year experience. *Mayo Clin Proc* 1987;62:8–14.
5. Mehta AC, Curtis PS, Scalzitti M, Meeker DP. The high price of bronchoscopy: maintenance and repair of the flexible fiberoptic bronchoscope. *Chest* 1990;98:448–454.
6. Hanson PJV, Gor D, Clarke JR, et al. Recovery of the human immunodeficiency virus from the fiberoptic bronchoscope. *Thorax* 1991;46:410–412.
7. Olympus BF-1T10 (OES bronchofiberscope instruction manual) section maintenance, 6–20.
8. Davis D, Bonekat HW, Andrews D, Shigeoka JW. Disinfection of the flexible fiberoptic bronchoscope against *Mycobacterium tuberculosis* and *M gordonae*. *Thorax* 1984;39:785–788.
9. Prakash UBS. Does the bronchoscope propagate infection? *Chest* 1993;104:552–559.
10. Kato H, Suzuki T, Ito A, Tanaka M, Urahashi S. Changes in optic glass-fibers due to X-ray irradiation. *Chest* 1979; 76:672–677.
11. Curtis P, Mehta AC, Kavuru MS. Olympus BF-1T20 fiberoptic bronchoscope and a flexible 18 gauge transbronchial aspiration needle. *Chest* 1989;95:1172.
12. Dillon DJ. Response to the editor regarding Olympus BF-1T20 fiberoptic bronchoscope and 18 gauge transbronchial needle aspiration. *Chest* 1989;95:1172.
13. Khalil HY, Mehta AC. Bronchoscopy begets bronchoscopy. *Chest* 1992;101:884–885.
14. Kelley SJ, Wang KP. Transbronchial needle aspiration. *J Thorac Imag* 1987;2:330–344.
15. Wang KP. Flexible transbronchial needle aspiration or biopsy for histological specimen. *Chest* 1985;86:860–863.
16. Mehta AC, Kavuru MS, Meeker DP, Gephardt GN, Nunez C. Transbronchial needle aspiration for histology specimens. *Chest* 1989;96:1228–1232.
17. Cavaliere S, Focedi P, Farina PL. Nd-YAG laser bronchoscopy: a five year experience with 1396 applications in 1000 patients. *Chest* 1988;94:15–21.
18. Livingston DR, Mehta AC, Golish JA, Ahmand M, DeBoer G, Tomaszewski MZ. Palliation of malignant transbronchial obstruction by Nd-YAG laser: an update of experience at the Cleveland Clinic Foundation. *J Am Osteopath Assoc* 1987; 87:226–234.
19. Ossoff RH, Karlan MS. Safe instrumentation in laser surgery. *Otolaryngol Head Neck Surg* 1984;92:644–648.
20. Dumon JF, Shapshay S, Bourcereau J, et al. Principles for safety in application of neodymium-YAG laser in bronchology. *Chest* 1984;86:163–168.
21. Davis RK, Simpson GT II. Safety with the carbon dioxide laser. *Otolaryngol Clin North Am* 1983;16:801–813.
22. Krawtz S, Mehta AC, Wiedemann HP, DeBoer G, Schoeff KD, Tomaszewski MZ. Nd-YAG laser induced endobronchial burn: management and long term follow-up. *Chest* 1989;95:916–918.
23. Mehta AC. Lasers application in respiratory care. In: Stoller JK, Kacmarek RM, eds. *Current respiratory care techniques and therapy*. Ontario: BC Decker; 1988;101–106.
24. Casey KR, Fairfax WR, Smith SJ, Dixon JA. Intratracheal fire ignited by the Nd-YAG laser during treatment of tracheal stenosis. *Chest* 1983;84:295–296.
25. Mehta AC, Livingston DR, Levine H, et al. Ventilatory management during Nd-YAG photoresection of subglottic or higher tracheal lesions. *Trans Am Bronchoesoph Assoc* 1986;148–153.
26. Barlow DE. Endoscopic applications of electrosurgery: a review of basic principles. *Gastrointest Endosc* 1982;28:73–76.
27. Hooper RH, Jackson FN. Endobronchial electrocautery. *Chest* 1989;87:712–713.
28. Marsh BR. Bipolar cautery for the fiberoptic bronchoscope. *Ann Otol Rhinol Laryngol* 1987;96:120–121.

Bronchoscopy,
edited by U. B. S. Prakash.
Mayo Foundation © 1994.
Published by Raven Press, Ltd., New York.

CHAPTER 29

Teaching Bronchoscopy

Paul A. Kvale and Udaya B. S. Prakash

Teaching and learning bronchoscopy are interdependent phenomena. It seems intuitively obvious that a student of bronchoscopy must have teachers, or else the learning of bronchoscopy would not be possible. While there are many fine atlases on bronchoscopy, very little has been written about how bronchoscopy is best taught. The professional organizations specializing in pulmonary diseases have not provided specific guidelines regarding the training of physicians in bronchoscopy. However, many organizations have published guidelines regarding bronchoscopy and related procedures (1–9). But these guidelines have been broad and loosely structured, and hence the training of new pulmonary physicians in bronchoscopy has to a large extent depended on the teachers' training in the procedure and postgraduate courses. This has led to wide variations in the application of bronchoscopy techniques in clinical practice (10,11). Even among bronchoscopists, there is considerable disagreement as to the training methods and the number of procedures needed to become proficient and remain competent in the procedure (10). In this chapter we will attempt to define the process of how to teach bronchoscopy, calling on our own experiences and thoughts, as well as the techniques for teaching that have been described or learned from many other instructors in the field of bronchoscopy practice.

Every medical student or postdoctoral trainee has heard the phrase, "See one, do one, teach one." This trite little saying applies to procedural practices more than the cognitive aspects of medicine. Students who desire to learn bronchoscopy can (and perhaps often do) acquire their skills by watching others and then repeating the same techniques that are observed. Initially this is done under supervision and then with increasing independence. Learning to perform bronchoscopy necessarily involves repetition of the procedure in sufficient numbers to develop proficiency. Intuitively, one might think that a minimum number of procedures might be specified so as to predict that any reasonably dexterous person could become proficient should that goal be met. However, there is great variability in manual dexterity among people attempting to learn how to perform bronchoscopy. While the approach of repetition is likely eventually to produce a qualified practitioner of bronchoscopy, a better plan includes the identification of specific educational objectives followed by a process of implementation over a period of years with checkpoints as the process evolves.

There are four or five groups of physicians who do almost all bronchoscopic procedures worldwide: (a) pulmonary/critical care physicians (both adult and pediatric); (b) otorhinolaryngologists; (c) thoracic surgeons; (d) anesthesiologists; and (e) general surgeons (10,12). Anesthesiologists who perform bronchoscopy usually do so for two specific applications: to facilitate placement of endotracheal tubes or to check the position of a tube that has already been inserted. General surgeons who perform bronchoscopy usually do so because they practice in a geographic locale where pulmonary physicians, otolaryngologists, or thoracic surgeons are not readily available. The vast majority of physicians performing diagnostic and therapeutic bronchoscopy belong to the first three groups, with more bronchoscopy done by pulmonary physicians than any other group. This was not always the case, however. In the era when the only type of bronchoscope available was the rigid bronchoscope, a relatively small cadre of bronchoscopists or bronchoesophagologists performed most such procedures. These individuals would train additional persons via the preceptor

P. A. Kvale: Department of Pulmonary and Critical Care Medicine, University of Michigan School of Medicine, Detroit, Michigan 48202.

U. B. S. Prakash: Division of Thoracic Diseases and Internal Medicine, Mayo Clinic, Rochester, Minnesota 55905.

method. In the current era, when most bronchoscopy is done with the flexible type of instrument, far more physicians from all of these disciplines perform bronchoscopy. Although the absolute number of bronchoscopy procedures is greater now than was true in the midportion of the twentieth century, the greater number of bronchoscopists and the need to train them systematically virtually demands that a structured approach to teaching be adopted. Regardless of which training program is involved, the methods for teaching bronchoscopy can be adapted readily to training programs in any of the specialties mentioned.

SETTING GOALS AND DEVELOPING THE CURRICULUM

The five essentials of bronchoscopy training include (a) theoretical knowledge of pulmonary anatomy, pathophysiology, and clinical pulmonology, (b) development of manual skills, (c) interpretation of bronchoscopic findings, (d) knowledge of indications, contraindications, and complications, and (e) understanding of pharmacological agents used in bronchoscopy. Ideally, a bronchoscopist should be well versed in all aspects of pulmonary diseases (both adult and pediatric) and both rigid and flexible bronchoscopy techniques. This goal may not be achievable because of the lack of training facilities and the ever-increasing "superspecialization" in certain clinical areas. For instance, a survey of 871 bronchoscopists in North America conducted by the American College of Chest Physicians revealed that the physicians specializing in adult pulmonary diseases had very little exposure to or training in pediatric bronchoscopy (10). Our own experience suggests that there are very few programs, particularly in North America, that provide comprehensive training programs in both adult and pediatric bronchoscopy.

Larger training programs typically introduce their students to the practice of bronchoscopy by simply assigning the student to the bronchoscopy rotation during some months of the training program. Smaller programs, or programs in which the total volume of bronchoscopy is only a minor part of many other procedures that must be learned, integrate time for bronchoscopy with other parts of the curriculum or learning program. While either approach is a satisfactory operational style to train students of bronchoscopy, the same programs usually develop a core curriculum for all aspects of the training program.

The core curriculum is a standard teaching tool, applied to medical practice and also to educational programs in any other walk of life, including elementary and secondary education. A similar approach is desirable for teachers of bronchoscopy. Much less will be left to chance by a careful, written development of the core curriculum and teaching goals. This set of educational goals should be given and explained to the student of bronchoscopy sometime near the beginning of the training program. All too often the volume of written material distributed on the first few days of a training program overwhelms the students to whom it is given, so the faculty member must intermittently review this set of written goals and the curriculum with the student to emphasize how and why it contains the information within it.

The most logical end point is to train the student in the proficient manipulation of the bronchoscope so that the patient is managed safely with the optimal diagnostic and therapeutic efficacy. As with any tool, its safe and effective application depends on the skill, training, and judgment of the person operating it. We do not agree with statements such as, "flexible fiberoptic endoscopy as a technical procedure requires no specialized training" and "the technique itself is similar to routine endotracheal tube suctioning" (13). It should only be practiced by those who will do a sufficient number of procedures to develop and maintain their skill. To accomplish this goal, the faculty members must promote a scholarly approach to this procedural skill, not just the manipulative skills. Students of bronchoscopy require guidance for reading selected literature relevant to bronchoscopy and specific structure to develop the patient care aspects of bronchoscopy. This includes a thorough knowledge of pulmonary anatomy, pathophysiology, clinical aspects of pulmonary disorders, indications and contraindications for the procedure, complications and their management, organizing the procedure, preparation of the patient for the procedure, the procedure itself, and the postprocedure care of the patient. The curriculum for bronchoscopy should contain cognitive as well as practical objectives (manual dexterity, recognition, and management skills).

DIDACTIC PRESENTATIONS

We begin our discussion here with the assumption that the physician who wishes to learn bronchoscopy skills has adequate knowledge of pulmonary anatomy, pathophysiology, and clinical aspects as well as the indications, contraindications, and complications of bronchoscopy. One of the best ways to orient the student to bronchoscopy is by utilizing standard audiovisual techniques in a lecture format. Typically 1 or 2 hr of lecture with slides is adequate for the beginning student. The content of such lectures should be broad in scope, beginning with an explanation of the indications and contraindications for bronchoscopy. The lectures can include an overview of the equipment, beginning with the bronchoscope itself, with regard to both various design features and the perceived advantages and disadvantages of each type of instrument. Auxiliary equipment, such as light sources, monitoring devices, sampling instruments, and photographic capabilities, should be described. The potential for diagnostic yield in each disease category should be outlined. Complications of bronchoscopy and their prevention/management must be stressed. Although other issues such as anesthetic and sedation techniques can be described, these are points that might better be reserved for the time when patients are managed in the bronchoscopy suite itself.

BRONCHOSCOPY ROOM

Time can be set aside when no patients are present in order to orient the student bronchoscopist to the physical structure of the bronchoscopy arena. All of the equipment and its purposes are reviewed. Support personnel are introduced along with a description of their roles. In fact, it is often useful to have the support personnel explain the layout of the area, assisting in demonstrating how the equipment operates and where all of the materials are stored. Especially important is the identification of the location of emergency drugs, instruments, and other devices for managing emergencies. The various devices for physiological monitoring of the patient during and after the procedure should be demonstrated during these orientation sessions.

It is highly desirable in a teaching program to have a variety of bronchoscopes available, preferably from more than one manufacturer. The faculty member may have strong preferences for one company's product, but the student is helped by an opportunity to see and eventually use as many different bronchoscopes as can reasonably be made available.

During these sessions without patients, the bronchoscopes should be removed from their storage areas, and the student should review all the different parts of the equipment and what purpose each part serves. The bronchoscope should be disassembled and reassembled, noting the alignment of removable pieces such as the inserts for the suction/biopsy channel. All bundles within flexible bronchoscopes should be explained, including the fact that the bundles are composed of thousands of filaments that can and do break. The need to avoid trauma to the bronchoscope and its parts must be emphasized. This includes passage of sampling instruments through the hollow channel of the flexible bronchoscope. The linkage at the distal tip can be broken by forcing a sampling instrument when the bronchoscope is in a fully flexed position. Likewise, avulsing tissue with too much force can result in a disruption of the linkage of the flexion control. Special emphasis is needed for the proper position of the shaft of the bronchoscope when transbronchial needles are passed through its channel.

Cleaning and caring for the bronchoscope when it is not in use deserves emphasis, including all aspects of the manufacturer's recommendations for preventing inadvertent damage if the instrument is immersed. Although sterilization of rigid bronchoscopes is done in autoclaves, flexible bronchoscopes must be cleaned and disinfected quite differently to avoid damage. The potential cost of mistakes in handling instruments improperly must be stressed.

Light sources for the bronchoscopes should be analyzed and explained, including a demonstration of the controls to adjust light intensity. Proper connections between bronchoscope and light source can be demonstrated. The initial discussion should be limited to the major aspects necessary with this component, reserving finer details like changes in the settings for various types of photography until the student has more experience with the basics.

Sampling instruments should be displayed and discussed in detail. A variety of cytology brushes can be used, and the student needs to understand the potential from long or short bristles with regard to cell recovery and trauma to tissues. Similar aspects for microbiology sampling devices and forceps of different designs should be discussed and carefully inspected by faculty and student together. Availability of other sampling devices, such as curettes, together with their advantages and disadvantages as well as how they are used should be discussed. Disposable (single-use) and reusable sampling instruments deserve review.

The next item for review is infection control measures. This includes proper disposal of sharps, cleaning of spills of blood or other body fluids, and disinfection of the bronchoscope to prevent cross-contamination. The student must be told of the need for protective garments, personal eye protection to avoid splash injuries/infection potential, and masks. All bronchoscopists should be tested for hepatitis antibody titers, and those who do not have native immunity must be vaccinated. Tuberculin reactivity should be known at the beginning of bronchoscopy training, and retesting must be done at least on an annual basis. Tuberculin converters should be treated in the standard fashion.

Additional equipment, such as fluoroscopy units, should be explained. Location of on/off switches, changes in exposure settings, collimator devices, and the like must be reviewed. The importance of protective shields for all personnel together with radiation safety measures and dosimeter monitoring badges/rings can be emphasized. The location of cutoff switches and fire extinguishers should be identified.

It is imperative that the bronchoscopy student be taught to recognize that the performance of bronchoscopy is a team effort and that absolute cooperation is essential to the successful completion of the procedure. It is important for the student to know that in many centers the care and maintenance of bronchoscopy equipment is handled by nursing personnel who can provide more information on the technical details of the instruments.

THE BRONCHOSCOPE

The student should be taught the proper way to hold a flexible bronchoscope during these sessions. For example, although most people are right-handed and the natural tendency may be to place the right hand at the top of a flexible bronchoscope, the instrument was originally designed with the intent to have the left hand at the top where the manipulation controls are located (Shigeto Ikeda, MD, personal communication). The light source bundle and suction port are connected to the left side of the proximal end of the bronchoscope. When the left hand is used in the upper position, the weight of the bronchoscope is balanced across the second metacarpal with excellent balance and very little stress on the muscles and tendons of the operator who is manipulating the instrument (Fig. 1). Doing it the opposite way, with the right hand at the proximal end of the bronchoscope, may increase the risk for chronic overuse problems such as tendinitis. However, this has not been a reported problem. In fact, ambidexterity in bronchoscopy is an advantage, particularly in dealing with difficult-to-reach anatomic areas. The student should also be taught how to push or pull the control lever to get the desired amount of flexion or extension of the distal tip of the bronchoscope, with emphasis on the ability to flex forward into a desired location, or reverse flex (extend) the distal tip of the bronchoscope without the need to spin the bronchoscope about its long axis in order to cannulate bronchi that are located more posterior or anterior. There should be emphasis on keeping the shaft of the bronchoscope straight between the two hands of the operator, so that any spin motion of the instrument is reflected in the distal end without the resultant torque, which attenuates the rotation of the entire shaft if the shaft of the bronchoscope is not held straight between the operator's hands (Fig. 2). We have observed many bronchoscopy students trying to twist the shaft of the bronchoscope in order to turn the tip to the desired position. This maneuver does not accomplish what the student seeks and moreover is likely to damage the fibers within. The student should be shown the proper way to switch hand positions with a rotatory motion from index fingertip control of the lever to thumb control of the lever, without losing up/down (axial location) position of the tip of the bronchoscope. It should be emphasized that this should be done when the point of discomfort for pronation/supination of the wrist has been reached.

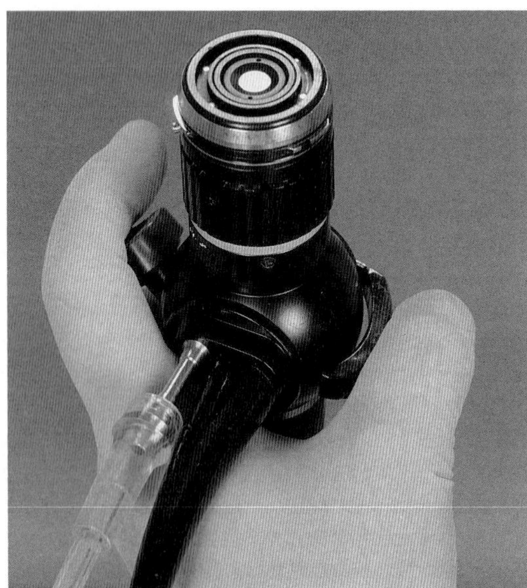

FIG. 1. When the operator's left hand is uppermost, the light source bundle and suction port are supported by the second metacarpal, which balances the instrument far better than when the operator has the right-hand uppermost. This position produces less stress on the muscles and tendons.

SELECTED READING

The faculty has an obligation to guide the student's reading about bronchoscopy. Certain books about bronchoscopy should be available to the student in the medical library, and the student should be expected to read them. Our review of the available literature suggests that most of the books on bronchoscopy are color atlases on bronchoscopic findings in various diseases but didactic review of the literature and techniques are discussed in only a few of the volumes (14–32). Therefore, we have resorted to developing a "bronchoscopy syllabus" by compiling pertinent review articles of importance on all bronchoscopy and related topics. Current review articles ought to be kept on file and distributed to the students early in the bronchoscopy experience. Other articles of importance about selected aspects should be organized by section, and the student should read and become familiar with each facet of bronchoscopy practice as described in the literature. An expanded bibliography should also be developed for additional reading on issues of concern as they are identified during the years of training. Obviously, such bibliographies must be updated by the faculty as new developments and changes in approaches take place.

A
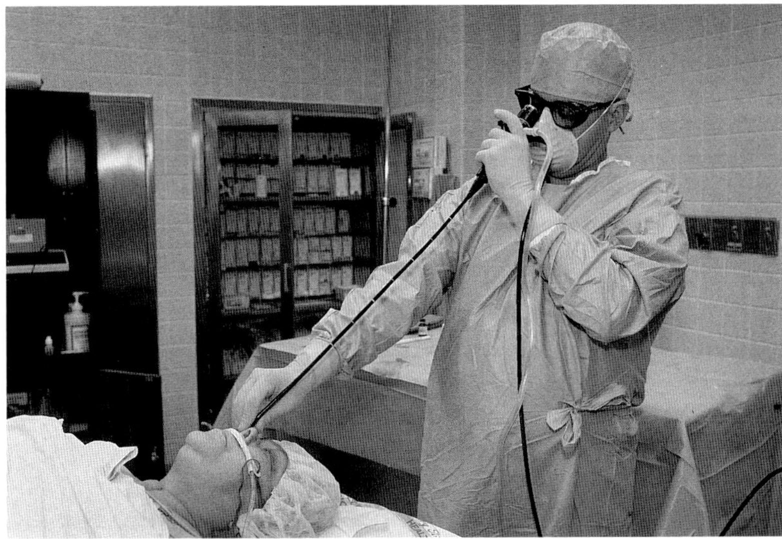

B
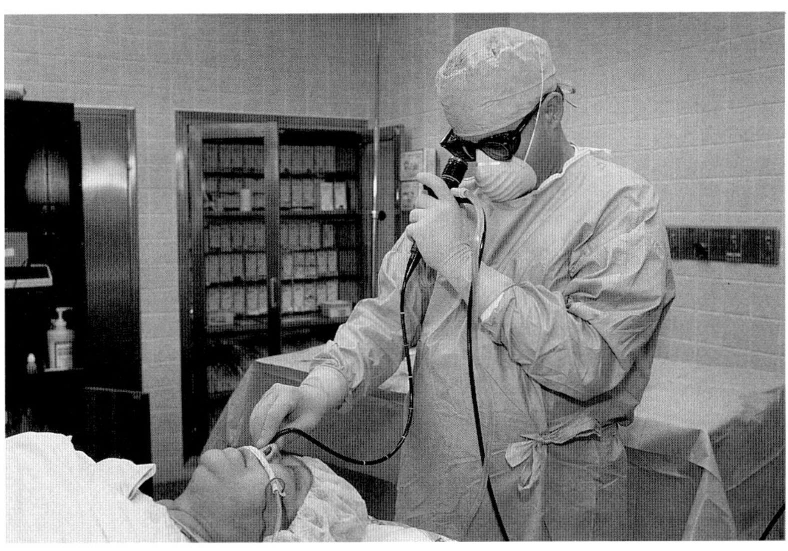

FIG. 2. (A) Proper position of the hands on the shaft of the flexible bronchoscope: the hands are sufficiently far apart so that the shaft of the instrument is kept straight. **(B)** Incorrect position of the hands on the shaft. Note that there is an exaggerated S shape in the shaft. If the operator attempts to rotate the proximal end of the bronchoscope, there will be torque in the shaft, so that the distal end of the bronchoscope does not rotate through the same arc that occurs with the rotation applied at the proximal end of the instrument.

VIDEOTAPES AND 35-mm TRANSPARENCY SLIDES

Each teaching institution should be stocked with tapes that can be purchased commercially to facilitate the beginning student of bronchoscopy. Alternatively, videotaping equipment is readily available to make one's own tapes for teaching purposes. Rayl and colleagues (33) developed an outstanding compendium of teaching videotapes that greatly facilitate the preclinical training for bronchoscopy practice. The five videotape programs with a paraphrasing of the description by Rayl and colleagues follows.

Bronchoscopic Checkpoints

This is a 19-min videotape that is a demonstration of a systematic method for airway examination with the flexible bronchoscope. The discussion on bronchopulmonary segments are detailed. with a description of 8 anatomic checkpoints that can be used to maintain constant orientation or be rapidly reoriented during a bronchoscopic procedure.

Endoscopic Examination of the Upper Airway Using the Flexible Bronchoscope

This 11-min tape is a description of how to systematically examine the upper airway, checking up to 49 anatomic structures to rule out malignancy. Again, the tape emphasizes how the operator can use certain landmarks within the upper airway to maintain orientation during this phase of a bronchoscopic examination.

Bronchoscopic Features of Acute Inflammation

This is a 16-min tape that discusses and displays the four features of acute airway inflammation: purulent exudate, erythema, edema, and intermittent longitudinal ridges. The speakers emphasize when to perform biopsies to differentiate benign airway inflammation from a similar abnormality that might be interpreted as malignant.

Bronchoscopic Features of Chronic Inflammation

This is a 15-min tape on which are displayed 20 sequences from bronchoscopic examinations that show the four features of chronic inflammation, including mucus, longitudinal light bands, transverse mucosal ridges, and dilated ducts of mucus glands. Again, the speakers outline those features of chronic inflammation that indicate the need for biopsy to exclude carcinoma.

Bronchoscopic Features of Carcinoma

On this 30-min tape the speakers present 44 bronchoscopic clips illustrating 18 pathological features that can be associated with carcinoma in the lumen, wall, or extraluminal in location. There is emphasis on the indications for biopsy to establish a precise diagnosis.

Other Sources

An additional tape that, at a minimum, should be part of the required viewing of any bronchoscopy student relates to use of the transbronchial needle. There is much potential for expensive damage to a flexible bronchoscope when this sampling instrument is used, especially by the novice bronchoscopist who is not taught properly. Such a tape should be reviewed very early during the bronchoscopy learning time, and again several more times during the course of the continuing experience with this device.

There are several sources where a compendium of videotapes can be purchased or rented by institutions involved in bronchoscopy training. They include (a) National Audiovisual Center (NAC), Customer Service Section, 8700 Edgeworth Drive, Capitol Heights, MD 20743-3701 (telephone: 301-763-1896); (b) Health Sciences Consortium (HSC), 103 Laurel Avenue, Carrboro, NC 27510 (telephone: 919-942-8731); (c) Veterans Administration Library Network (VALNET), in any VA Medical Center through their library service (telephone: 202-389-5130); (d) National Library of Medicine (NLM), Collection Access Section, Public Services Division, 8600 Rockville Pike, Bethesda, MD 20894 (telephone: 301-496-5511); (e) American College of Chest Physicians (ACCP), 3300 Dundee Road, Northbrook, IL 60062-2348 (telephone: 708-498-1400); and (e) Health Sciences Consortium (HSC), 201 Silver Cedar Court, Chapel Hill, NC 27514 (telephone: 919-942-8731).

Personal collection of 35-mm transparency slides by the faculty should be used during didactic teaching sessions. The slides and the color atlases as well as the videotapes should provide ample examples of normal and abnormal bronchoscopic findings. At present we are unaware of any commercially available slide sets that can be purchased for personal use.

PRACTICE SESSIONS IN NONHUMAN MODELS

There are several ways to help the student gain manipulation skills before attempting to perform bronchoscopy in human patients: use of inanimate models, live nonhuman animals, and airways or arteries obtained from slaughterhouses. The former are readily available for commercial purchase. Not all training programs have access to an animal laboratory that can be made available for bronchoscopy training. Airways or arteries are not difficult to obtain for training purposes, but their usefulness is greatest for the teaching of laser bronchoscopy rather than to help the beginning student of diagnostic bronchoscopy and standard therapeutic bronchoscopy (foreign bodies and retained secretion removal).

Several different inanimate models are currently available for purchase. The most widely used is a silastic model of the tracheobronchial tree that was developed by Zavala (Zavala bronchoscopic lung model, Medi-Tech Inc., 150 Coolidge Avenue, Watertown, MA (02172) (Fig. 3). Other models include a latex tracheobronchial model (Richard Wolf Medical Instruments Corp., 7046 Lyndon Avenue, Rosemont, IL 60018); an ALM II model (Fig. 4A) which, like the Zavala model, is based on a casting of the adult human tracheobronchial tree but which is said to be more detailed and realistic (Fig. 4B) (APM, Inc., Research Triangle Park, NC); the Laerdal adult intubation model (Fig. 5) and the Laerdal infant intubation model (both are available from Armstrong Industries, Inc., 3660 Commercial Avenue, P.O. Box 7, Northbrook, IL 60062). The Nakhosteen model also uses plastic cast and provides both normal and abnormal bronchoscopic findings. Only one of the models should suffice and should be a requisite for every training program in bronchoscopy, and the student bronchoscopist should spend several hours at the outset, practicing manipulation of the bronchoscope within the model to learn spatial relationships and to hone skills. The faculty member can coach the student as he or she begins to work with the model, but it is equally appropriate to have a more senior resident or fellow work with the junior resident or fellow with the model. The student should be expected to return to the model from time to time as the training years continue, particularly to practice

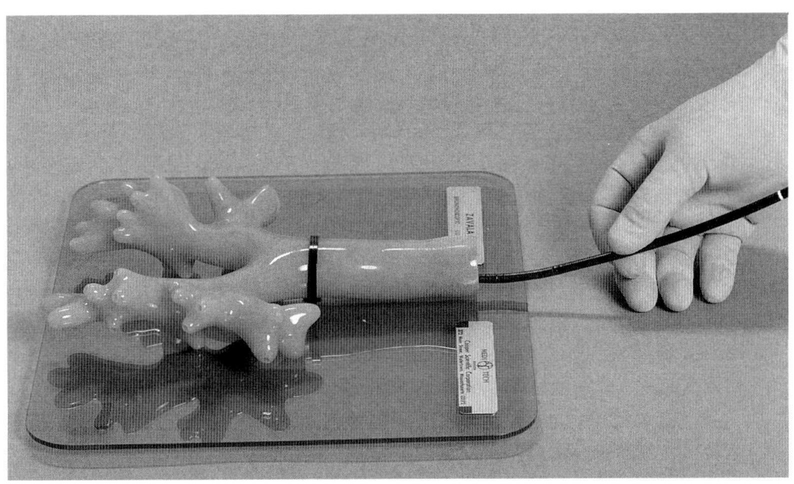

FIG. 3. The Zavala bronchoscopic lung model.

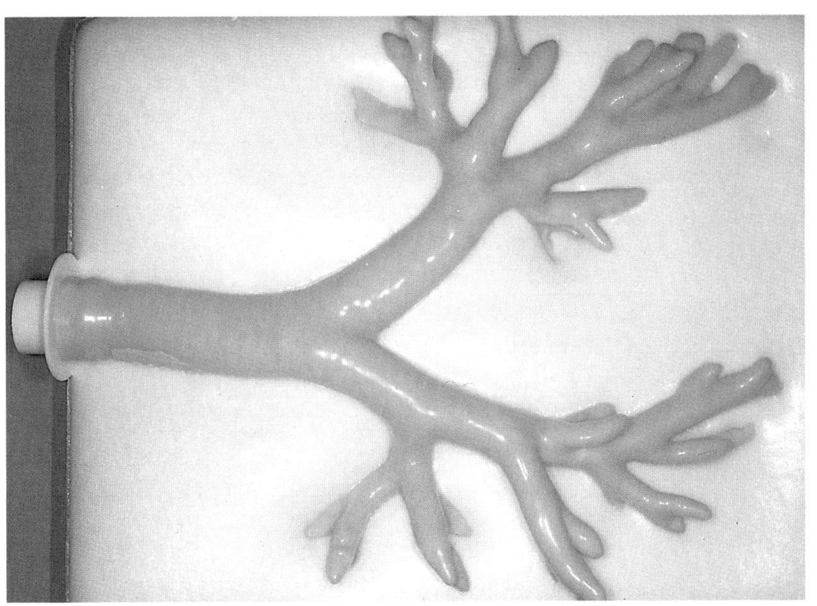

A

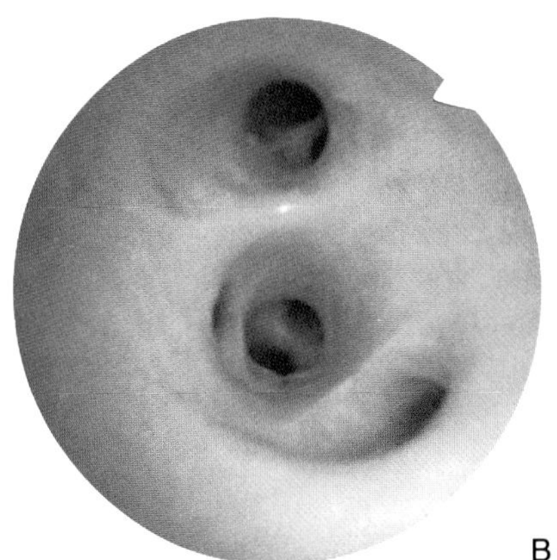

B

FIG. 4. (A) The ALM model of tracheobronchial tree. **(B)** The bronchial tree in this model.

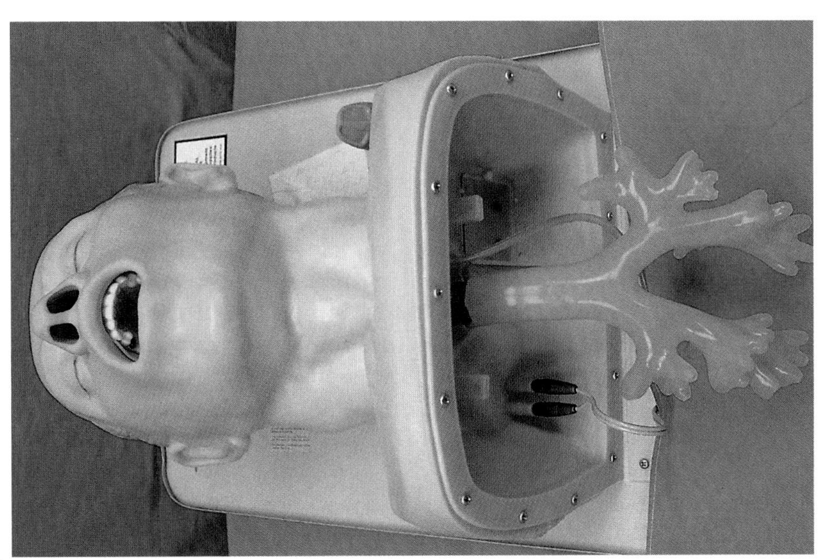

A

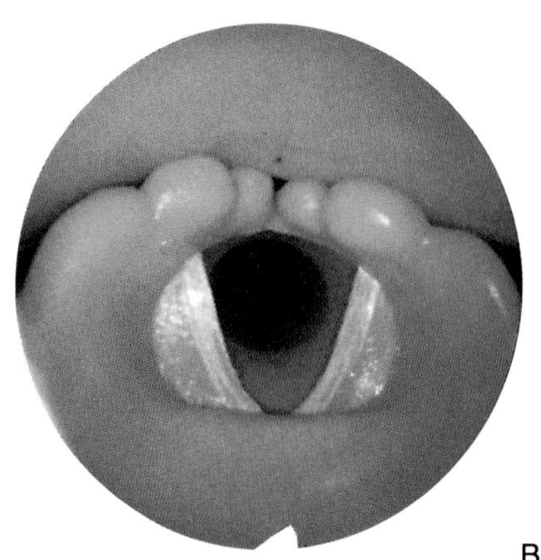

B

FIG. 5. (A) Laerdal adult intubation model used with Zavala model of tracheobronchial tree. **(B)** Bronchoscopic image of the larynx in the Laerdal model.

use of various sampling instruments. This is especially valuable in learning to use the transbronchial needle and retrieval instruments for foreign bodies.

The Laerdal intubation models can be fitted to one of the models of the tracheobronchial tree, as was described by King et al. (34). These authors removed the trachea and main stem bronchi from the Laerdal model and substituted the Zavala model (Fig. 5A). They were able to use the combined model for practice and teaching of both flexible and rigid bronchoscopy intubation, which is particularly important if the training program has the additional goal of helping the student to gain skills with a rigid bronchoscope. Each of these models must be lubricated with silicone spray in order to prevent problems with friction as the student practices with them.

Living animal models can also be used for the practice of rigid or flexible bronchoscopy. The most widely used animal model is the dog, but its long neck and trachea make it difficult to explore much beyond the main stem bronchi. Moreover, transnasal insertion is not usually possible because the dog's nares are easily traumatized and bleed readily. Other animal models include the cat, rabbit, and rhesus monkey. Cats and rabbits are particularly useful for the early phase of learning to bronchoscope infants and children, but each has its limitations because of differences in the anatomy when compared to humans (9,35). The rhesus monkey's airways most closely resemble those of humans, but such an animal model is expensive and not available for most training programs. Wood and Pick (35) provide a more detailed discussion of the advantages and disadvantages of all four animal models. Many of the models mentioned above can be used to train rigid bronchoscopy techniques. However, a better training model for rigid bronchoscopy is the use of animal models. Insertion and removal of a tracheobronchial foreign body can be easily taught with dogs, cats, or rabbits.

When animals are used by students for their education, such work should be under the direct supervision of an experienced teacher. The rules for the care of such animals must be the same as for animals used for research. Animals used for bronchoscopy training must receive every consideration for their comfort; they must be properly housed, fed, and their surroundings kept in a sanitary condition. The postbronchoscopy care of animals should be such as to minimize discomfort and pain, and in any case should be equivalent to accepted practices in schools of veterinary medicine (36).

OTHER FORMS OF TRAINING

The clinical usefulness of bronchoscopy and bronchoscopy skills can be disseminated by regular workshops and postgraduate courses (37–39). Following four workshops on flexible bronchoscopy for anesthesiologists in Britain, a survey observed that 35% of the attendees were able to introduce flexible bronchoscopy in their practice (38). We believe that for a new student of bronchoscopy, an individualized, intensive, and well-focused training is important.

CLINICAL TRAINING WITH HUMANS

Ideally, the first few procedures might be done with patients who have general anesthesia. This is not a difficult requirement for training programs in the surgical disciplines and anesthesiology. However, for training programs in pulmonary and critical care medicine, the suggestion that a general anesthetic be administered is neither possible nor appropriate. The next best substitute is to start with procedures that are done on patients who are intubated and mechanically ventilated in the critical care unit, as most such patients are paralyzed and highly sedated. The disadvantage of such an approach is that there may be major problems with hypoxemia from the primary disease process, and a lengthy bronchoscopic examination for the beginning student of bronchoscopy has its own set of hazards.

Familiarity with the History and Physical

The student should be expected to learn as much about the patient as possible before the bronchoscopy is started. The history and physical examination can be performed directly with the patient, but this is not always practical in a training program where multiple physicians request procedures to be done by colleagues including the student bronchoscopist. An understanding must exist that there is a dual responsibility for communicating the details of all relevant history and physical findings between the physician who has decided that a bronchoscopy is to be done and the team of physicians, including the student bronchoscopist, who will actually perform the procedure. This communication must include the various diagnostic possibilities, which will greatly influence the choice of sampling methods and the laboratory specimens needed to optimize the diagnostic yield. Likewise, if the bronchoscopy is scheduled for therapeutic purposes, similar precise communication is needed; an example is the type and suspected location of a foreign body that must be removed. Only through such communication can the student and faculty choose the correct array of instruments that might be needed for a successful procedure.

Checkpoints Before Bronchoscopy

The student of bronchoscopy also needs to be taught to check for potential problems that might lead to complications during or after the procedure. Patients must be asked about intake of drugs that might alter the approach to the procedure or give rise to a delay in the timing of the procedure. A simple history for bleeding diatheses together with questions about intake of drugs known to interfere with platelet function (salicylate, dipyridamole, nonsteroidal antiinflammatory agents) is satisfactory for the prevention of a bleeding complication. However, many bronchoscopists will routinely check a coagulation profile or a bleeding time before going ahead with the procedure. The student should be taught that this "routine" practice is primarily a medical-legal defensive maneuver, as the performance of such tests on a *routine* basis does not lead to fewer bleeding complications (10,11,40).

Some patients who require bronchoscopy may be taking anticoagulants; timing the interruption of these drugs and performing the bronchoscopy requires precision, if the anticoagulants are mandatory, as may be the case with a prosthetic cardiac valve. Diabetes mellitus that requires insulin for control may necessitate changes in dose and timing of insulin on the day of the procedure, plus the administration of glucose solutions for a few hours before, during, and after the bronchoscopy. Chronic intake of narcotic analgesics or alcohol may alter the dose of sedative medications that the student will prescribe as a part of awake sedation. Prior or current use of systemic corticosteroids will be important in that parenteral supplementation with cortisone may be needed intraoperatively.

Reviewing Roentgenographic Studies

The student should be taught to independently review all available chest roentgenographic images, including current and old chest roentgenographs and computed tomographic images. Before the procedure is started, the faculty member can listen to the student's description of the images and assist the student to understand the abnormalities that are present. This is an excellent time for the student and faculty member to integrate the history, physical findings, and laboratory data already available with the findings present on the plain chest roentgenograph and computed tomographic images. It also presents a challenge for understanding the anatomy of the lungs and planning the approach to a specific location with the bronchoscope.

Some procedures are best deferred if all the needed images have not been done. For example, lesions that are located near the apex of the lung may not be readily seen on the lateral chest roentgenogram. This is an opportunity for the faculty member to teach the student how to anticipate better diagnostic yield by postponing the procedure until computed tomographic images are available, since knowledge of the precise anteroposterior position of the abnormality in question will facilitate proper placement of the sampling instruments. Another example is the presence of enlarged mediastinal lymph nodes, where precise localization with computed tomography greatly enhances diagnostic yield from bronchoscopic needle aspirates.

Anesthetic Techniques

Faculty members need to have familiarity with a variety of techniques to anesthetize the airways. One method may be greatly preferred because of its simplicity or its efficacy. Alternative approaches require discussion and occasional demonstration. If there are multiple faculty members, particularly where the faculty has had its training in different institutions, the student will have a greater opportunity to see, compare, and try several ways to accomplish effective anesthesia for bronchoscopy. The techniques chosen for transnasal intubation will be different from those used for transoral intubation. Likewise, when an endotracheal tube is inserted, the approach to use of local anesthetics may be different. Proper use of sedating drugs, including the potential adverse consequences, must be emphasized. The need to keep reversing agents readily available in case of excessive respiratory depression must be stressed by the faculty member. Adjunctive approaches, such as the use of intravenous lidocaine to suppress cough, require demonstration. The various anesthetic approaches are discussed in Chapter 7, so that no attempt will be made at this point to describe them other than to emphasize the role of the faculty member to teach the student one good way for most procedures, but with a variety of alternatives.

Although rigid bronchoscopy can be done with awake sedation, passing a rigid bronchoscope into the airway typically causes the patient enough discomfort that a general anesthetic is preferred. Moreover, with the proper choice of muscle-paralyzing agents in conjunction with a general anesthetic, the student will have less difficulty in mastering the technique of inserting this instrument into the patient's trachea and bronchi. However, use of a paralyzing agent makes it important that the anesthesiologist and/or the faculty member keep careful watch of the time the student spends in an efforts to insert the rigid bronchoscope while the patient is apneic, lest hypoxemia become a problem.

Setting Time Limits for the Student

If the student has spent time with the model, it is usually possible to set time limits for the student under direct faculty supervision so that the patient has no problems because of the length of the procedure. Setting time limits for the student of bronchoscopy is an often overlooked issue for faculty members. As most flexible bronchoscopy is done with awake sedation and a local anesthetic, the faculty member must always remember the dual responsibility to the patient and to the student. It is reasonable to expect patients in a teaching program to allow bronchoscopy students to gain experience while the patients undergo bronchoscopy, but not at the expense of a procedure that is prolonged to the point of major discomfort for the patient or the risk of complications that can be avoided by a procedure done expediently (41). As the student gains more experience with humans, it will be possible to do the entire procedure quickly and efficiently. At the beginning, it is more reasonable to have the student perform only a part of the procedure and then relinquish control of the bronchoscope to the faculty member in the interest of patient safety and comfort.

Use of the Teaching Sidearm (Lecturescope)

One of the great advances in the art of teaching a student to perform flexible endoscopic procedures was the development of the teaching sidearm or lecturescope. This device can be fitted onto the proximal end of the bronchoscope, so that the faculty member can directly visualize what the student is seeing at exactly the same time.

Among the disadvantages of the teaching sidearm is its extra weight at the proximal end, which stresses the muscles, ligaments, and tendons of the operator. Also, the light transmitted through the optical bundles of the bronchoscope is split so that some of the light enters the eye of the primary operator, while another portion of the total light energy is diverted into the teaching sidearm for the faculty member. This is only a minor problem, as a rule; however, it is the faculty member's responsibility to assure that the power output of the light source is sufficient to provide ample light for student and faculty at the same time. The newer models of teaching sidearms are lighter and provide better illumination.

During use of the teaching sidearm, the faculty member can coach the student on each aspect of manipulating the bronchoscope for maximum efficiency. This includes instructions to flex or extend the tip of the bronchoscope with the control lever, rotate the bronchoscope in a clockwise or counterclockwise motion about its long axis, or push or pull backward on the bronchoscope for axial movement into or out of the airways. At the beginning, each of these motions will be asynchronous. The faculty member must coach the student until all three basic motions begin to flow as one integrated motion while the bronchoscope is passed from one position to the next.

Use of Videobronchoscopy

More and medical centers are using videobronchoscopy on a routine basis, not only to train bronchoscopy students but also in the routine clinical bronchoscopy (42–44). The newer video bronchoscopes have a chip camera mounted in the tip of the bronchoscope itself, and the image is digitized and transmitted by cable up the shaft of the bronchoscope into a processor. The image is then reconstructed and displayed on the video monitor. With the newer video bronchoscopes, the only image that can be viewed is from the video monitor, rather than from the proximal end of the bronchoscope itself. The major advantages of videobronchoscopy include the magnification of images on the screen, the ability to simultaneously teach several students, and the ability to record the findings for future use, either as a teaching tool or for discussion with other physicians involved in the patient's care. The obvious disadvantages are the cost of purchasing the equipment and the need for extra space for storage. One of the least appreciated but clinically significant disadvantages of letting the student train exclusively using the videobronchoscopy equipment is related to the type of camera used to transmit the bronchoscopic image to the video monitor. Many newer cameras attached to the bronchoscope do not allow the bronchoscopist to directly view the tracheobronchial tree through the bronchoscope. We have had experience with several bronchoscopists who were entirely trained by a videobronchoscopy system and when required to perform bronchoscopy without the video system were unable to show adequate hand–eye coordination and expressed their inability to perform bronchoscopy without the video system. Since videobronchoscopy is not available in all medical centers and cannot be used in limited spaces such as patient rooms and critical care units, it is highly desirable to train the student without the use of videobronchoscopy. Once the student has mastered the bronchoscopy techniques, then switching to video system should not pose a problem.

Intubation

During the first week the student might concentrate solely on the process of intubating patients transnasally and transorally with the flexible bronchoscope until it has been passed through the glottis into the subglottic larynx/proximal trachea. This, too, must be limited by time (e.g., not greater than 5 min of effort) as well as by the need to avoid laryngospasm from excessive stimulus to the vocal cords. The faculty member must instruct the student bronchoscopist on how to traverse the naris and the oral cavity with the least discomfort to the patient; such an approach also lessens the likelihood of epistaxis. Typically, the space between the floor of the nose and the inferior turbinate is larger than any other part of the naris. In many patients, the posterior part of the naris and the nasopharynx has enough redundant tissue that visualization of the lumen is lost momentarily. The student must be coached to gently push through this area without manipulating the lever that controls flexion/extension of the tip of the bronchoscope, since it will usually follow the natural curvature into the oropharynx and the hypopharynx. Upon entering the hypopharynx, the faculty member must emphasize those landmarks that assist the student in maintaining control of the patient and facilitate the further introduction of topical anesthetics in the correct locations.

Most patients who are awake but sedated will sense the stimulus from the bronchoscope as the glottis is approached. Rate and depth of respiration are likely to change, and the student should be taught to talk gently but with firmness and reassurance, so that the patient can avoid repeated efforts to swallow, cough, or otherwise breathe in a way that makes the intubation more difficult. The student must be reminded to tell the patient to anticipate each new stimulus that is likely to occur, such as the instillation of additional topical anesthetic, or the actual insertion of the bronchoscope through the glottis and into the proximal trachea.

Manipulation of the Flexible Bronchoscope

One of the more difficult things for the student to learn, and that is perhaps most pronounced at the beginning phases of acquiring the manipulative skills, is to integrate three separate motor skills into a single fluid motion. The three separate movements are axial motion of the shaft of the bronchoscope, rotatory motion of its tip, and flexion or extension of the tip, which is controlled by the lever at the proximal end near the eyepiece. Moving from the hypopharynx into the trachea requires the student to align the bronchoscope in the midline above and slightly posterior to the arytenoid cartilages, then flex the tip of the bronchoscope anteriorly as the arytenoids are passed, and then posteriorly once again in order to stay near the posterior commissure of the true vocal cords, which are much wider than the anterior commissure. This motion, when viewed in the sagittal plane, is like a gently sloping "S." The faculty member can explain and diagram the motion for the student as well as demonstrate the integrated motion during the procedure and with an inanimate model.

Transoral intubation with the flexible bronchoscope is often more difficult for the student to master. This is because the tongue is so muscular and the flexible bronchoscope is easily pushed out of the midline. The faculty member must instruct the student on the proper use of a bite block, as an uncooperative patient can bite the shaft of the bronchoscope causing damage that is expensive to repair. The faculty must also stress the absolute requirement to keep the bronchoscope in the midline with the shaft of the instrument held straight between the operator's two hands, lest torquing of the shaft interfere with the ability to find the landmarks in the hypopharynx and larynx. In most training programs, the faculty will perform flexible bronchoscopy with the patient supine on a procedure table, or upright in a chair such as those used by otolaryngologists for indirect laryngoscopy. The student should be encouraged to learn both approaches to the patient, as there are likely to be some patients who cannot comfortably be approached in one position or the other. Since the orientation is exactly the opposite in these two positions, the student must learn to anticipate whether a downward deflection of the control lever will move the tip of the bronchoscope anterior or posterior, depending on which patient body position is being used.

It is the preference of some bronchoscopists to perform the majority of flexible bronchoscopies through a previously placed endotracheal tube. Whether this is the case or not, there are clearly some patients who are better managed with an endotracheal tube in place before the flexible bronchoscope is inserted. The faculty member must review these situations with the student and ensure that the student gains the needed experience in placing an endotracheal tube for these individuals.

Manipulation of the Rigid Bronchoscope

The opportunities for training in rigid bronchoscopy have significantly diminished as a result of the widespread use of the flexible bronchoscope. However, there are many indications for the use of rigid bronchoscopy and the details as well as the techniques are discussed in Chapter 4. One instructional point is that the bronchoscopy student should make use of every opportunity to perform rigid bronchoscopy. The first step is to practice endotracheal intubation on both adult and pediatric patients scheduled for surgery under general anesthesia. This provides ample experience in traversing the upper airways with the help of various laryngoscopes and endotracheal tubes. The student should develop expertise with monocular vision by looking through a drinking straw. As a rule, intubation with a rigid bronchoscope is more difficult for the student bronchoscopist to learn. No standard teaching sidearm is available for moment-to-moment verbal coaching of the student as use of the rigid bronchoscope is begun. However, a special adapter can be attached to the rigid telescope eyepiece and the video camera used with the flexible bronchoscope can be used to let student and teacher view the student's performance on the video monitor simultaneously. The faculty member must demonstrate the peroral passage of a rigid bronchoscope, emphasizing the greater potential for inadvertent damage to teeth, soft tissues, and the larynx itself. The student should be given the opportunity to look through the hollow illuminated shaft of the rigid bronchoscope at each important point along the way to a successful intubation. When the student is the person manipulating the rigid bronchoscope through the mouth and into the trachea, the faculty member must be immediately to the side of the student, looking into the bronchoscope and the rod telescope (if a special video camera attachment is unavailable), coaching the student on the precise position of the tip at each point along the way. In addition, the student must be taught how to assume the most comfortable posture for himself or herself. Furthermore, rigid bronchoscopy requires that the student be taught to take the time to properly position the patient's body on the table, perhaps with a rolled-up towel or blanket between the scapulae, in order to improve the extension of the patient's head and neck to make the insertion of the rigid bronchoscope easier with less potential for trauma.

Immediately After the Intubation

The student must be taught that a paramount part of the procedure, in terms of comfort for the patient, is to keep the tip of the bronchoscope in the center of the airway lumen, off the wall as much as possible. This applies to the trachea as well as all the more distal airways. By doing so, the cough receptors within the mucosa will be stimulated less often and the patient will be kept under better control. By avoiding contact with the airway wall by the tip of the bronchoscope, there is less trauma to the tissues and the examination will proceed in a quicker fashion.

Immediately after passing the bronchoscope through the glottis in an awake-sedated patient, the maximum stimulus to cough will occur, and the patient will usually experience some breathing difficulty because of the increased resistance from having the bronchoscope within the airway lumen. The student should be taught to push the bronchoscope caudad approximately 2–3 cm below the glottis on the first thrust, since the coughing that the patient will normally experience at this moment often will expel the tip of the bronchoscope cephalad. This can cause inadvertent extubation if the bronchoscope has not been pushed downward for this distance. The student must be coached to push or pull the control lever and rotate the bronchoscope about its long axis, preferably as an integrated motion, in order to position the tip of the bronchoscope directly in the middle of the airway lumen and off the airway walls. At this point, the student should be taught to pause while a small amount of additional lidocaine is instilled through the channel of the bronchoscope to facilitate suppression of the cough reflex.

The bronchoscopy assistant is typically the person who will instill the lidocaine or other fluids into the bronchoscope when requested by the operator. The student should be taught to present the opening for insertion of the end of the syringe to the bronchoscopy assistant, so that a connection can be made quickly and easily. Frequently the student becomes so involved in manipulating the bronchoscope or looking through the viewing lens that the assistant has difficulty in making the connection and instilling the desired solution. Since the patient is most likely to be experiencing some difficulty holding still at this point, the instructor must repeatedly and calmly lead the student through each phase of this particular sequence.

BRONCHOSCOPIC PROCEDURES

Systematic Examination of the Airways

When the patient has resumed a more relaxed posture and coughing has been controlled, the faculty member can concentrate on coaching the student while the student holds and manipulates the primary bronchoscope and the faculty member views the same image through the teaching sidearm. The student should be taught to return to the few centimeters of airway that he or she quickly passed through (the subglottic larynx and the proximal part of the trachea), as the mucosa in this area is often not carefully inspected for abnormalities if such a "pull-back" maneuver is not done. Examination of this region of the airway can be deferred until the rest of the procedure has been completed, but it is usually better to inspect the proximal trachea and subglottic larynx at this point in order to avoid the inadvertent omission of this part of the examination. The faculty member needs to emphasize this part of the examination in two specific situations: (a) with cigarette smokers, who are at risk of carcinoma of the larynx as well as bronchogenic carcinoma, and (b) among patients who have been intubated previously. In the latter circumstance, when stenosis of the subglottic larynx or proximal trachea is suspected, the student will need additional supervision and coaching to avoid inadvertent obstruction of the airway by the bronchoscope at the stenotic segment of the airway. The usual thrust of the bronchoscope for 2–3 cm must be modified in this circumstance.

After the initial coughing has been controlled and the subglottic larynx and proximal trachea have been examined, the student requires coaching by the faculty as the student moves the bronchoscope caudad to the distal trachea. Additional lidocaine is instilled at this point, and then into each main stem bronchus. The usual approach is then to proceed down the right main bronchus, as it descends from the trachea at a less acute angle than the left main bronchus. The faculty coaches the student through rotatory motions, flexion and extension of the tip of the bronchoscope with the control lever, and the gentle forward motion of the tip as each lobe and segment is inspected. The faculty member must continue to emphasize and coach the student to keep the tip of the bronchoscope in the middle of each airway lumen to minimize trauma and the stimulus that will lead to more coughing by the patient. Then the faculty member can help the student as the bronchoscope is withdrawn from the right side, and a similar approach with coaching of each manipulation skill is developed while the left side is inspected.

Typically, it is easier to proceed past the right upper lobe and directly down the intermediate bronchus at first. Less manipulation of the tip of the bronchoscope is required to cannulate and inspect the middle lobe and right lower lobe than the right upper lobe. The faculty member needs to emphasize the careful naming of each lobar and segmental bronchus, helping the student to remain oriented by the notch at the periphery of the viewing image by reference to the hours on a clock face. That way, the student can respond to suggestions for clockwise or counterclockwise rotation, and to flex or reverse-flex (extend) commands on manipulation of the control lever.

On the left side, it is usually easier to proceed directly into the lingula initially, as this bronchus is straight ahead when the tip of the bronchoscope is passed down the left main bronchus. After examining the lingula, the student should be coached to complete the examination of the remaining part of the upper lobe before proceeding to the lower lobe on the left side. Another system to develop as routine habit is to examine each side by bronchial nomenclature, i.e., begin sequentially by examining B1–B10. There are situations when this sequence can or should be altered, such as when the airways encountered are distorted and following this sequence would be more difficult.

One additional manipulation skill deserves special emphasis by the faculty: the method for cannulating the superior segment of the lower lobe bronchus. Two possible ways to cannulate the lower lobe superior segment should be learned. The first is to make a mental note of the position of the superior segment orifice as an hour on the clockface, but bypass the superior segment and cannulate the trunk of the lower lobe first. Then the basal segments are inspected, followed by a pull-back maneuver, with the notch of the viewing image positioned 180° opposite the place where the student has noted the position of the superior segmental orifice. As the tip of the bronchoscope is slowly withdrawn cephalad, a gentle reverse flex of the tip is advised, and the tip of the bronchoscope will "fall into" the superior segmental bronchus as the tip reaches its orifice (Fig. 6). This maneuver is typically easier to master, since there is less stress on the student's wrist as he or she accomplishes it. The other way to cannulate the superior segmental bronchus is to spin the bronchoscope around on its long axis, changing hand position in the process, so that the notch in the perimeter of the viewing image is at the same position on the clockface as the position of the superior segmental bronchial orifice, followed by a flexion maneuver of the tip of the bronchoscope into the orifice as it is cannulated (Fig. 7). Both methods should be taught to the

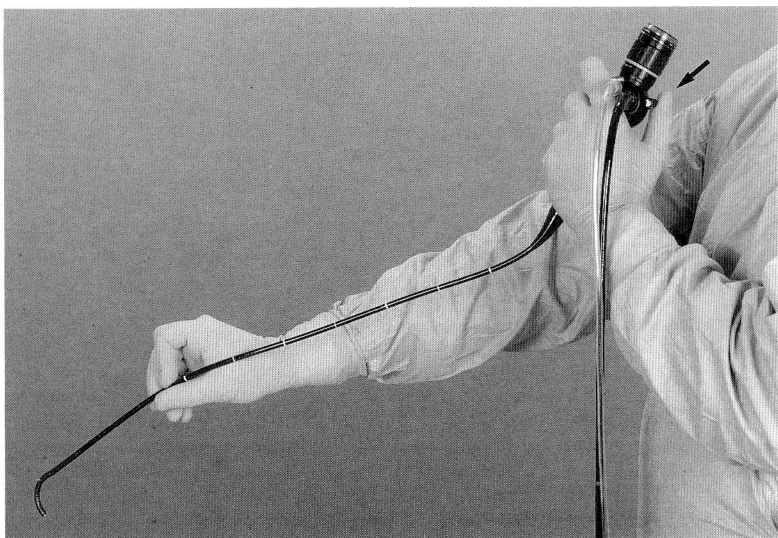

FIG. 6. Cannulation of the superior segment of a lower lobe bronchus: the easier way to perform this maneuver is to not rotate the instrument all the way around 180°, maintaining control of the flexion–extension lever with the thumb of the left hand. As the thumb pushes the lever upward **(arrow)**, the distal tip of the bronchoscope will be "reverse-flexed" downward into the superior segment as the bronchoscope is pulled slightly cephalad from a beginning position just beyond this segmental orifice.

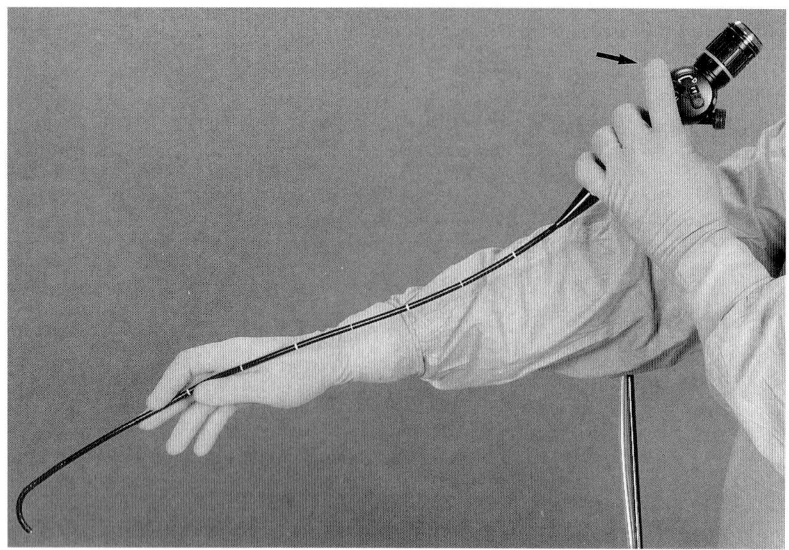

FIG. 7. Alternative approach to cannulation of the superior segment of a lower lobe bronchus: the bronchoscope has been rotated through an arc of 180°. Now the control lever is pulled down by the index finger **(arrow)**, so that the distal tip of the bronchoscope is flexed forward (down) into the superior segmental orifice.

student, as a particular method will sometimes be needed because of distortion or simply because of a mechanical advantage to the operator.

Tailoring the Inspection

There must be some flexibility in the method of examining the airways with a bronchoscope. For example, when bronchoscopy is done to identify the place from which brisk hemoptysis is occurring, the student must appreciate that the examination is very much different from when the procedure is being done to search for an occult carcinoma with a positive sputum cytology and a normal chest roentgenograph. In the paragraphs that follow, we have categorized the various approaches in different clinical settings, with recommendations about how to instruct the student to fine-tune the procedure to the specific objectives that must be accomplished.

Central Endoscopically Visible Lung Cancer

After reviewing the clinical presentation, plain chest roentgenographs, and computed tomograms (if the latter study was done prior to the bronchoscopy), it is often possible to predict that a tumor is likely to be seen within the visual reach of the bronchoscope and to decide that the only real objective of the bronchoscopy is to make a cytological and/or histological diagnosis. When this is the case, we suggest that the student be taught to proceed directly to the bronchus where the tumor is located, obtain the requisite specimens to facilitate the diagnosis, and not prolong the procedure more than is required to reach these objectives. This is especially true when it has already been determined that curative therapy is not a consideration.

When the tumor is thought to be resectable based on the clinicoroentgenographic assessment, the student must learn that additional time should be spent to look for endoscopic findings that indicate resectability or nonresectability, such as submucosal spread proximally or involvement of the main carina of the trachea. Likewise, if an operative procedure is likely, the student must learn the features that indicate the proximal extent for transection of the bronchus in order to predict that the margin will be clear or free of tumor. The student should be taught which findings would be consistent with lung-sparing resections such as a sleeve right upper lobectomy as well as how to identify the distal as well as the proximal margins in such a case. We also suggest, in this situation where a unilateral tumor is identified and thought to be resectable, that the student learn to carefully inspect the contralateral side for an occult simultaneous second primary, as this would alter the therapeutic approach drastically.

Bronchoscopically Invisible Peripheral Masses/Infiltrates

The initial phase of the examination may differ little from the approach outlined for central, visible tumors. However, once it has been determined that the abnormality evident on the roentgenographic studies is not within the visual reach of the bronchoscope, the student must be taught that sampling instruments can be placed in or near the lesion only by ceasing to observe the image through the bronchoscope, and transfer attention to the image on the video monitor which displays the fluoroscopic image (Fig. 8). Initially, this is

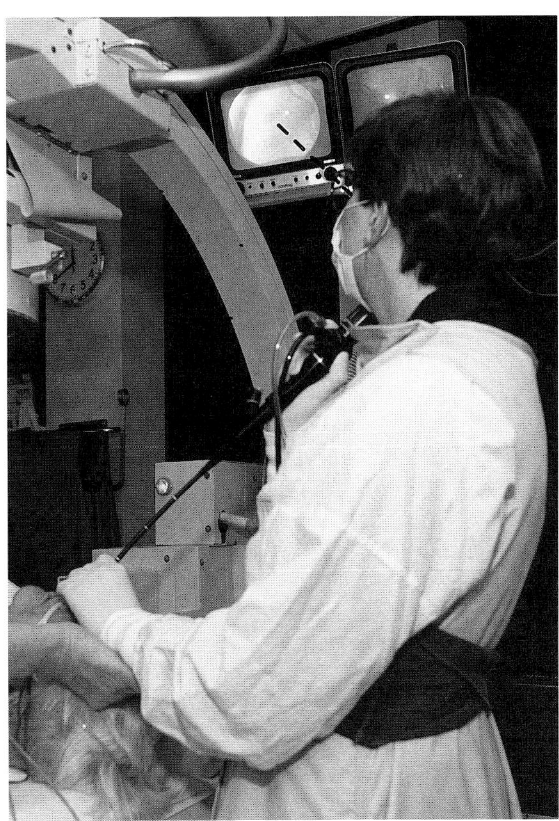

FIG. 8. When samples are taken from a mass in the periphery of the lung (which cannot be visualized through the bronchoscope), the student must be taught to look at the video monitor for the fluoroscopic image while manipulating the tip of the bronchoscope as the lesion is approached with sampling instruments. Note the line of sight **(dotted line)** toward the video monitor instead of looking into the bronchoscope.

a difficult concept to impart to the student of bronchoscopy, as the natural tendency in manipulating the tip of the bronchoscope up or down, or in a rotatory fashion, is to watch the deflection through the viewing image of the bronchoscope itself.

When a sample is desired from a localized peripheral lesion, the student must adopt the discipline to imagine the change in direction of the tip of the bronchoscope from the motions imparted and observed on the video monitor. We suggest that this can be done initially by the faculty member demonstrating the various motions of the bronchoscope tip while the faculty and student both watch the video monitor. As the initial trials by the student are likely to be slower and more cumbersome, such a demonstration will minimize the fluoroscopy time to which the patient is subjected. Then, when the student performs her or his initial efforts and watches the video monitor, we find that the faculty can facilitate the learning experience by placing the faculty member's hands directly over the hands of the student on the proximal end of the bronchoscope, to guide the rotatory motions as the tip and sampling instruments are directed a little more anterior or posterior, or with flexion and extension of the tip which allows the tip to be deflected upward or downward as the peripheral lesion is approached with the sampling instruments. Once this concept has been demonstrated and the student is helped by simultaneous manipulation with the faculty, the student can improve her or his skills if the faculty coaches the student verbally in rotatory motions and flexion/extension of the tip for subsequent cases. This is best accomplished by both faculty and student observing the video monitor simultaneously as the student performs the manipulations and obtains the samples.

Searching for an Endoscopically Occult Malignancy

In any individual training program, there are not likely to be many patients who present with a radiographically occult lesion (but with a sputum cytology specimen from which malignant cells clearly have been identified). Nevertheless, the student must be taught to anticipate this situation, as it may be encountered sometime during a practice lifetime.

The greatest difference in approach to a patient like this, as compared with a radiographically obvious tumor, is that more time is required to inspect each and every part of the tracheobronchial tree that is accessible to the flexible bronchoscope. Almost all patients who have a positive sputum cytology for malignant cells and a normal chest roentgenograph will have tumors that can be found within the central airways that are accessible to a flexible bronchoscope. Approximately 15% of such patients may have a tumor that is obvious endoscopically, and the tumor may even occlude the involved bronchus completely (45). Most of these tumors will be located at a segmental bronchus rather than at a larger bronchus such as a lobar or main stem bronchus (45). Many radiographically occult tumors will be much more subtle, however. The faculty member must emphasize the abnormalities that are much more easily overlooked, such as minor irregularity of the mucosa, localized erythema or pallor of the mucosa, and loss of the normal longitudinal striations. These findings are especially well described and displayed in one of the videotapes that was recommended as part of the preclinical training (''Bronchoscopic Features of Carcinoma''). The faculty must also emphasize the need to spend more time on parts of the airways that are often bypassed quickly, such as the subglottic portions of the larynx immediately beneath the true vocal cords.

Hemoptysis

There are several important points which the faculty must emphasize to the student that differentiate the bronchoscopic approach to the patient who is to undergo this procedure because of hemoptysis. The potential value of rigid or open tube bronchoscopes must be discussed, especially if hemoptysis is massive and there is potential for asphyxiation when blood in the airways is not removed quickly.

Nevertheless, most patients who present with hemoptysis will be examined with a flexible bronchoscope. The faculty member can emphasize the times when the patient should be intubated with a standard oral or nasal endotracheal tube to protect the airway. The faculty should stress that an approach through an endotracheal tube will facilitate removal and cleaning of the lens of the flexible bronchoscope, in contrast to other situations where a flexible bronchoscope can be used safely without the need to have previously intubated the patient.

We suggest that the faculty member discuss the probability that the site of bleeding will be identified in relation to the timing that the bronchoscopic examination is done (at the time the hemoptysis occurs, as opposed to an examination that is delayed for 48 hr or more).

So far as the actual procedure itself is concerned, the faculty should emphasize that one key point to be determined is the site from which bleeding is occurring, particularly if hemoptysis is of such volume that intervention might be needed (surgical resection, bronchial artery embolization, etc.). We suggest that under these circumstances the student be taught to approach the examination at the level of bronchi on both sides rather than to completely examine one side before going to the other side. That way, it is far more likely that the location from which the bleeding is occurring can be identified with confidence, without the interference from trauma to the mucosa from suctioning, or making incorrect inferences because of blood that might have been aspirated into the contralateral side. The nose, naso/oro/hypopharynx, and larynx are examined first to exclude these sites as the source of bleeding. An attempt is made to assure that blood is present below the true vocal cords so as to assure that the problem is really hemoptysis rather than another bleeding source that the patient may have confused with hemoptysis. Then the trachea is examined, followed by the two main stem bronchi. The next level to examine is all five lobes at their orifices, before attempting a more detailed examination of the segmental bronchi, which receive attention near the conclusion of the procedure.

In addition to trying to localize the site from which the bleeding is occurring, the student should be taught to determine whether the blood is old and clotted, or whether active bleeding (at least oozing) is present. Only in the latter circumstance can the bronchoscopist make confident statements to the interventional physician (thoracic surgeon or interventional radiologist) and guide therapeutic decisions. The cause of the bleeding may be determined by the bronchoscopist from what is seen visually, but often he or she must settle for identification of the site from which the bleeding is occurring.

Obtaining Microbiology Samples

The faculty should instruct the student about the potential yield from different sampling techniques such as use of a protected telescoping brush, protected catheter, and bronchoalveolar lavage. The need to minimize the use of local anesthetics through the channel of the bronchoscope must be emphasized by the faculty, as these agents will interfere with the growth of almost all types of bacteria from bronchoscopy specimens. Since the bronchoscope will always be contaminated by normal flora that reside in the upper aerodigestive tract, the student must learn the importance of quantitative processing of specimens to differentiate contaminants from true lower respiratory tract pathogens.

Bronchoscopy in the Management of Endotracheal Tubes

There are several key points where the bronchoscope is used for managing endotracheal tubes that we suggest the faculty member emphasize and demonstrate to the bronchoscopy student during the course of her or his training. The first is that the bronchoscope can be used to facilitate placement of an endotracheal tube under direct visualization. We suggest that the faculty member emphasize its utility for difficult intubations, particularly when there is a deformity of the upper aerodigestive tract. The prior placement of the endotracheal tube over the shaft of the flexible bronchoscope can be demonstrated, with proper lubrication of the endotracheal tube to facilitate its insertion by sliding the tube over the bronchoscope after the latter has been passed through the glottis. The usual need to have an assistant for this maneuver should be emphasized.

Next the student can be taught to use a flexible bronchoscope to check the position of the tip of an endotracheal tube so as to prevent improper insertion into a main stem bronchus (usually on the right side because of its less acute angle as it arises from the trachea). The student can learn to use the bronchoscope as the balloon of the endotracheal tube is first deflated, then reposition the endotracheal tube the proper distance above the carina, and finally reinflate the balloon as the tube is secured in the desired location.

Changing endotracheal tubes with the aid of a bronchoscope, particularly for intubated and mechanically ventilated patients, should be taught in the intensive care unit with close support and supervision by the faculty member. This is a particularly good time to make use of the teaching sidearm, as the side-by-side removal of the old endotracheal tube and reinsertion of the new one can be difficult when there is much edema of the vocal cords and the supraglottic tissues in the larynx. We suggest that a third person, typically a nurse or respiratory therapist, time the effort by the student while this technique is learned and that the faculty member take the bronchoscope and new endotracheal tube to complete the reintubation when the student requires more than 60–90 sec of effort on her or his own with the faculty member coaching the process as the effort is viewed through the teaching sidearm.

Finally, the use of a small-diameter flexible bronchoscope to facilitate and check for proper placement of double-lumen endotracheal tubes can be taught to the student of bronchoscopy who expects to use double-lumen tubes. This is especially important for trainees in thoracic surgery and anesthesiology, as single-lung ventilation is a requisite for the proper conduct of thoracic surgical procedures. For the nonsurgeon pulmonary physician who envisions high-volume lung lavage (as for pulmonary alveolar lipoproteinosis), mastery of placement of double-lumen endotracheal tubes with ultrathin flexible bronchoscopes is also mandatory (46).

Aspirating Secretions

We suggest that the student be taught to selectively apply bronchoscopy for secretions that the patient cannot clear through ordinary coughing and/or respiratory therapy methods. Selective cannulation of the bronchi with the flexible bronchoscope can be far more effective than blind suctioning transnasally or through an endotracheal tube. However, the faculty should emphasize that a flexible bronchoscope increases the airway resistance, particularly if the internal diameter of the endotracheal tube is smaller than 8.5 mm. Since secretions can be aspirated more efficiently with a bronchoscope with a large suction channel, the student should be taught to change the endotracheal tube to prevent undue difficulty in ventilating the patient during the procedure itself. We also suggest that the student be taught not to overuse bronchoscopy to aspirate secretions, as simpler techniques are less expensive and work very well in most patients (47).

The Immunocompromised Host

The utility of bronchoscopy to define specific causes of pulmonary complications in immunocompromised hosts has been repeatedly emphasized during the past two decades, particularly since organ transplantation and the human immunodeficiency virus (HIV) epidemic have become much more common. We suggest that the faculty teach the different probabilities for specific diagnoses, depending on the reason the patient is immunocompromised and the type of clinical or radiographic presentation.

The student must be taught to recognize specific abnormalities that are best handled by observation without tissue or microbiological confirmation, e.g., endobronchial Kaposi's lesions in HIV-infected patients. The need to maximize the safety of the procedure, since many patients who are immunocompromised are more likely to have coagulopathies, must be emphasized. Toward this goal, the high yield from simple high-volume bronchoalveolar lavage when the suspected diagnosis is *Pneumocystis* pneumonia, should be emphasized so that additional sampling procedures are not done when they are not clearly indicated or would increase the probability of a complication such as bleeding.

Retrieval of Foreign Bodies

Not all bronchoscopists will gain a great deal of expertise in removing foreign bodies from the airways. On the other hand, few bronchoscopists will practice without occasionally encountering a foreign body. The two key points that the faculty should emphasize are how to suspect and then to recognize a foreign body in the airway, and the possible ways foreign bodies can be removed endoscopically. We suggest that the student be taught that a newly aspirated foreign body may appear as an easily recognized object, such as a pin or a peanut, but that a foreign body that has been in the airways for more than a few hours (especially when there is a delay of several days or more in performing the bronchoscopy) may not appear as a foreign body at all. The masking of such a situation by secretions, granulation tissue, and edema deserves emphasis.

The techniques for retrieval of foreign bodies from airways are best taught with an inanimate model, followed by a nonhuman animal model. The student who desires to learn these techniques should do so not just with a flexible bronchoscope but with a rigid bronchoscope as well (48). In fact, the greater utility of a rigid bronchoscope with its wider variety of retrieval instruments for various kinds of foreign bodies must be emphasized to the student. Unless there is a commitment to learn rigid bronchoscopy well, the student should be taught that prompt referral of patients with foreign bodies to other bronchoscopists with these skills is preferable to lengthy efforts at retrieving the foreign body with a flexible bronchoscope.

Laser Bronchoscopy and Brachytherapy

In the majority of training programs it is not necessary to attempt routine teaching of the specialized techniques of laser bronchoscopy and brachytherapy. As a critical volume of activity with laser bronchoscopy and brachytherapy is needed to gain and maintain skills, we believe that not all students of bronchoscopy should attempt to learn these procedures. Like standard bronchoscopy practice, a minimal volume of procedures is needed to learn either skill and constant repetition of these procedures is also required to maintain proficiency (49). Several teaching models for laser bronchoscopy have been successfully employed to teach laser bronchoscopy techniques (50,51). Using these models, bronchoscopists can become familiar with laser bronchoscopic equipment and appreciate the interaction of laser and soft tissue in a controlled setting in the laboratory before applying this therapy to patients.

Various Biopsy Procedures

We suggest that the student acquire solid skills in manipulating the bronchoscope itself before beginning to master the use of various sampling instruments through the operating channel of the bronchoscope. The faculty member can demonstrate ex vivo how to use each of the sampling instruments and then proceed with a similar demonstration of their use with patients undergoing the procedure. Again, at some point the student should manipulate the sampling instruments, initially by viewing through the teaching sidearm while the faculty member positions the bronchoscope onto the lesion or locus within the lung that sampling is planned. Eventually, the student should be challenged to place the sampling instrument onto the desired locus while at the same time manipulating the bronchoscope, while the faculty member observes through the teaching sidearm and operates the movable parts of the sampling instrument. It is important to emphasize that all sampling should be done gently so as to avoid excessive trauma to the tissues with a greater potential for bleeding as the primary complication of concern. Proper positioning of biopsy forceps, using fluoroscopic guidance, should include instruction on how to reduce the probability of pneumothorax and the wedge technique (52) to control any bleeding that might occur. Also deserving of emphasis is that avulsing tissue with the forceps has the potential to damage the distal end of the bronchoscope if done forcefully, causing the bronchoscope to telescope over the forceps with breakage of the linkage inside the bronchoscope when the tissue suddenly releases the applied force.

Among the more difficult techniques of sampling to teach is the method for performing transcarinal or transbronchial needle aspiration. The actual techniques are discussed in detail in Chapter 12. We suggest that the faculty member defer teaching of this skill until the student has become proficient in virtually all other aspects of diagnostic bronchoscopy, particularly since there is increased risk of damaging the bronchoscope with the needle if there are errors in the manipulation of both bronchoscope and needle (53).

Selective Sampling

The student should be taught to selectively process samples that are retrieved at bronchoscopy in accord with the diagnostic problems under consideration rather than take a "shotgun" approach to the laboratory processing, which has a low yield and increases the overall costs of the procedure. The faculty member should emphasize that, whereas the student may initially think that one or two extra methods of processing the material is relatively inexpensive for a single patient, perpetuation of this approach generally in the practice of bronchoscopy becomes extremely expensive to patients and their insurance carriers when viewed collectively.

We also suggest that the student be taught that the methods of obtaining samples are constantly refined and changed as additional clinical and basic research studies are conducted worldwide. For example, gene probes for the identification of various mycobacterial species are likely to be applied to samples obtained at bronchoscopy and will replace standard culture methods in the future.

Managing Complications

The faculty must constantly help the student to prevent complications by appropriate and careful planning. Despite this effort, complications will occur from time to time. The most frequent complication related to intubation is laryngospasm, and the student should be taught that this usually can be managed expectantly and/or by instilling epinephrine or lidocaine directly onto the cords while the bronchoscope is held just above them. The faculty should be prepared to intervene quickly should laryngospasm persist and the patient require reintubation with an endotracheal tube. Other problems related to intubation with a rigid bronchoscope, such as broken teeth or trauma to the soft tissues of the pharynx, are again best taught by emphasizing prevention. Cardiac rhythm disturbances and myocardial events during the procedure are infrequent, but managing them can be taught as a team approach when they are recognized.

The two primary complications that deserve emphasis are pneumothorax and bleeding. Pneumothorax is infrequent, if there has been emphasis on proper technique in obtaining samples, particularly bronchoscopic lung biopsies. A postprocedure assessment with the fluoroscope is usually all that is required, provided the patient has not complained of pleuritic chest pain or shortness of breath at the time of bronchoscopic lung biopsy. Rarely is a postprocedure chest roentgenograph of value to assess for pneumothorax in the absence of new symptoms of pain or dyspnea (54,55). Management of bleeding is the primary concern for the faculty member, and is again best taught by demonstration after discussing the key features of suctioning blood to clear the airway, tamponading the site that bleeds after biopsy, and topically applying epinephrine. More advanced ways to control bleeding should be discussed, such as packing the bronchus with gauze, using a Fogarty balloon-tipped catheter, or using a laser to photocoagulate the bleeding site.

Record Keeping

The importance of clear and concise record keeping for the operative procedure is best taught by showing examples of reports and use of a template that the student can follow. The faculty member can demonstrate the components for reports as they are prepared and then challenge the student to do likewise with direct supervision and assistance as the skills in preparing reports are developed. The reports should be reviewed carefully by the faculty member and then changed as necessary after a discussion of the changes and the reasons for them with the student.

Postoperative Care

This discussion is divided into immediate and late care of the patient after completion of bronchoscopy.

Immediate Care

The importance of continued monitoring of the patient in a recovery suite should be emphasized. A systematic plan to check vital signs and adequacy of oxygenation deserves emphasis. The importance of allowing time for the metabolism/excretion of sedating drugs and of testing the patient regarding the ability to ambulate before he or she is discharged should be discussed and demonstrated, with involvement of support personnel such as nurses. Record keeping and precise tagging and bagging of specimens should be demonstrated.

Later Care

The student should be taught to check the results of all specimens as they are processed in the laboratory. An important part of this exercise is to encourage the student to review specimens with the pathologist, so that a mental correlation can be made with the gross findings as seen at the time of the bronchoscopy and the microscopic picture of the specimens that were retrieved. The student should be taught to arrange a follow-up visit for the patient and to effectively communicate test results and bronchoscopic findings to the patient as well as any referring physicians. Finally, the student should be taught to develop contingency plans for further investigation in cases where the bronchoscopy did not achieve the desired goals, such as providing a definitive diagnosis.

Billing

Billing is a part of the teaching process that faculty members often overlook. It is surprising how quickly a student who did not learn proper billing learns how to do it on her or his own when the training days are over! Nevertheless it is appropriate for the faculty member to review proper coding of the procedure with the student and then supervise the student as bills for the procedure are prepared.

Allowing the Student to "Solo"

At some point in the training of a student of bronchoscopy it is important for the faculty to allow the student to perform all aspects of intubating the patient and manipulating the bronchoscope without direct assistance. Obviously, the timing will vary from student to student, but it is important for the faculty member to challenge the student when there is sufficient confidence in the student's skills that such challenge is reasonable. The student must develop the skills to recognize abnormalities and be able to describe them in words so that all who might need to have this information communicated hear it in a relatively standard or uniform fashion. Use of the teaching sidearm serves as a hindrance to the student's developing confidence and may actually increase the total time spent in performing a given bronchoscopy. We suggest that the student be given a defined period of time to operate the bronchoscope in solo fashion, then verbally describe all abnormalities to the faculty member, who can take the bronchoscope and quickly repeat the inspection to assure that the student's description is accurate and complete. If errors in recognition of abnormalities are evident, it becomes appropriate to attach the teaching sidearm to the bronchoscope and discuss the differences of opinion with the student so that the overall learning process is enhanced.

BECOMING PROFICIENT AND REMAINING COMPETENT

In the mail survey of 871 bronchoscopists in North America conducted by the American College of Chest Physicians (10), more than 60% of respondents observed that at least 50 procedures were necessary to become competent, and more than 50% estimated that to remain competent at than 50 procedures per year were required (Table 1). This issue, namely, the number of bronchoscopy procedures to become proficient and remain competent, is controversial and somewhat threatening to bronchoscopists because of its implications regarding credentials and related matters. The eligibility requirements to appear for the pulmonary certification of the American Board of Internal Medicine do not specify that a specific number of bronchoscopies must have been performed by the candidates during the training (56). The American Board of Thoracic Surgery, on the other hand, requires its candidates to have performed at least 25 bronchoscopy and esophagoscopy procedures (57). To become proficient in the procedure, performance of 50–100 bronchoscopies (flexible and rigid) has been suggested (58). An individual who completed a training program in pulmonary diseases reported that at least 100 bronchoscopies were needed to achieve proficiency (59). We infer that at least 50 bronchoscopy procedures may be necessary to become competent in routine flexible bronchoscopy. This should include biopsy of visible tracheobronchial lesions, BAL, and therapeutic bronchoscopy. In addition, the performance of at least 10 bronchoscopic lung biopsy, 10 laser procedures, and 10 rigid bronchoscopies may be necessary to achieve competence in these specialized procedures. Incontrovertibly, some physicians, in spite of "performing" many more than 50 bronchoscopies, may remain incompetent and lack confidence in achieving expertise in the procedure. Therefore, the decision as to whether someone is competent to perform bronchoscopy should not be made solely on the basis of the number of bronchoscopies "performed." The program director or the director of bronchoscopy at the training institution should judge and certify the competence of each candidate and recommend and provide remedial training if necessary (11). Several studies have reported on various techniques of training to strengthen bronchoscopy skills (33,37,38,58). At least 50 bronchoscopies per year may be necessary to maintain expertise in the procedure. We stress that the performance of the procedure on a regular basis is far more important than the numbers alone. Frequent attendance at postgraduate meetings and workshops dealing with bronchoscopy should be part of the plan to preserve the expertise.

TABLE 1. *Number of bronchoscopies required to become and remain competent*

Number of bronchoscopies required	Respondents %	Respondents *n*
To become competent		
≥50	61.1	532
26–50	28.6	249
≤25	9.0	78
No response	1.4	12
	100.0	*871*
To remain competent		
≥50	8.5	74
26–50	33.4	291
≤25	50.9	443
No response	7.2	63
	100.0	*871*

From Prakash et al. (10), with permission.

REFERENCES

1. Committee on Bronchoesophagology of the American College of Chest Physicians. Standards for training in endoscopy. *Chest* 1976;69:665–666.
2. Guidelines for competency and training in fiberoptic bronchoscopy. Section on Bronchoscopy, American College of Chest Physicians. *Chest* 1982;81:739.
3. Greve JJ, Adamson J, Caldwell EJ III, Edsall JR, Sugg WC, Zavala DC. Guidelines for Bronchoscopy. *ATS News* 1983 (Winter).
4. Sokolowsky JW, Burgher LW, Jones FL. Guidelines for fiberoptic bronchoscopy. *ATS News* 1986 (Spring).
5. Guidelines for fiberoptic bronchoscopy in adults. American Thoracic Society. Medical Section of the American Lung Association. *Am Rev Resp Dis* 1987;136:1066.
6. National Institutes of Health workshop summary. Summary and recommendations of a workshop on the investigative use of fiberoptic bronchoscopy and bronchoalveolar lavage in individuals with asthma. *J Allergy Clin Immunol* 1985;76:145–147.
7. Summary and recommendations of a workshop on the investigative use of fiberoptic bronchoscopy and bronchoalveolar lavage in asthmatics. *Am Rev Resp Dis* 1985;132:180–182.
8. Summary and recommendations of a workshop on the investigative use of fiberoptic bronchoscopy and bronchoalveolar lavage in asthmatic patients. *Chest* 1985;88:136–138.
9. Green CG, Eisenberg J, Leong A, Nathanson I, Schnapf BM, Wood RE. Flexible endoscopy of the pediatric airway. *Am Rev Resp Dis* 1992;145:233–235.
10. Prakash UBS, Offord KP, Stubbs SE. Bronchoscopy in North America: the ACCP survey. *Chest* 1991;100:1668–1675.
11. Prakash UBS, Stubbs SE. The bronchoscopy survey: some reflections. *Chest* 1991;100:1660–1667.
12. Simpson FG, Arnold AG, Purvis A, Belfield PW, Muers MF, Cooke NJ. Postal survey of bronchoscopic practice by physicians in the United Kingdom. *Thorax* 1986;41:311–317.

13. Dietrich KA, Strauss RH, Cabalka AK, Zimmerman JJ, Scanlan KA. Use of flexible fiberoptic endoscopy for determination of endotracheal tube position in the pediatric patient. *Crit Care Med* 1988;16:884–887.
14. Jackson C: *Bronchoscopy and esophagoscopy; a manual of peroral endoscopy and laryngeal surgery*. Philadelphia: WB Saunders; 1927.
15. Jackson C. *Bronchoscopy, esophagoscopy and gastroscopy; a manual of peroral endoscopy and laryngeal surgery*. Philadelphia: WB Saunders; 1934.
16. Jackson C, Jackson CL. *Bronchoesophagology*. Philadelphia: WB Saunders; 1950.
17. Huzly A. *An atlas of bronchoscopy*. New York: Grune and Stratton; 1960.
18. Kassay D. *Clinical applications of bronchology*. New York: Blakiston; 1960.
19. Ikeda S. *Atlas of flexible bronchofiberscopy*. Baltimore: University Park Press; 1974.
20. De Kock MA. *Dynamic bronchoscopy*. Berlin: Springer-Verlag; 1977.
21. Faber LP, Andersen HA. American College of Chest Physicians; American Broncho-Esophagological Association, World Congress on Bronchoscopy, San Francisco. *Chest* 1977; 73:(5)(Suppl)1977.
22. Zavala DC. *Flexible fiberoptic bronchoscopy: a training handbook*. Iowa City: Univ. of Iowa Press; 1978.
23. Nakhosteen JA, Zavala DC. *Atlas und lehrbuch der flexiben bronchoskopie*. Berlin: Springer-Verlag; 1983.
24. Oho K, Amemiya R. *Practical fiberoptic bronchoscopy*. Tokyo: Igaku-Shoin; 1984.
25. Dumon J-F. *YAG laser bronchoscopy*. New York: Praeger; 1985. (*Surgical science series*; vol 5).
26. Collins J, Goldstraw P, Dhillon P. *Practical bronchoscopy*. Oxford: Blackwell Scientific; 1987.
27. Du Bois RM, Clarke SW. *Fiberoptic bronchoscopy in diagnosis and management*. Orlando: Grune and Stratton; 1987.
28. Kitamura S. *Color atlas of clinical application of fiberoptic bronchoscopy*. Chicago: Year Book; 1990.
29. Becker HD, Kayser K, Schulz V, Tuengerthal S, Vollhaber H-H. *Atlas of bronchoscopy*. Philadelphia: BC Decker; 1991.
30. Cavaliere S, Beamis J. *Atlas of therapeutic bronchoscopy*: Laser–stents. Brescia, Italy: Cavaliere; 1991.
31. Stradling P, Stradling JR. *Diagnostic bronchoscopy: a teaching manual*. Edinburgh: Churchill Livingstone; 1991.
32. Kato H, Horai T. *A colour atlas of endoscopic diagnosis in early stage lung cancer*. London: Wolf; 1992.
33. Rayl JE, Pittman JM, Shuster JJ. Preclinical training in bronchoscopic diagnosis of cancer. *Chest* 1988;93:824–827.
34. King EG, Sproule BJ, Yamamoto I. A teaching model for bronchoscopy. *Chest* 1976;70:72–73.
35. Wood RE, Pick JR. Model systems for learning pediatric flexible bronchoscopy. *Pediatr Pulmonol* 1990;8:168–171.
36. Federation Board. Guiding principles in the care and use of animals. *Fed Proc*, January 1986.
37. Ovassapian A, Yelich SJ, Dykes MH, Golman ME. Learning fibreoptic intubation: use of simulators v. traditional teaching. *Br J Anaesth* 1988;61:217–220.
38. Dykes MH, Ovassapian A. Dissemination of fibreoptic airway endoscopy skills by means of a workshop utilizing models. *Br J Anaesth* 1989;63:595–597.
39. Puterman M, Gorodischer R, Leiberman A. Tracheobronchial foreign bodies: the impact of a postgraduate educational program on diagnosis, morbidity, and treatment. *Pediatrics* 1982; 70:96–98.
40. Lind SE. The bleeding time does not predict surgical bleeding. *Blood* 1991;77:2547–2552.
41. Fuller WR, Davies DM, Stradling P. Anaesthesia for bronchoscopy prolonged by teaching and photography. *Anaesthesia* 1972; 27:292–300.
42. Ikeda S. Bronchial television endoscopy. *Chest* 1989;96:(1; Suppl)41S–42S.
43. Rayl JE, Hall CJ Jr, Rourke D, Spindler LJ. Requirements for television-bronchoscopy. *Chest* 1978;73(5;Suppl)764–767.
44. Cunanan OS, Mazza JE. Integrated electronic display model for teaching bronchoscopy. *Chest* 1977;72:364–365.
45. Shure D. Radiologically occult endobronchial obstruction in bronchogenic carcinoma. *Am J Med* 1991;91:19–22.
46. Prakash UBS, Barham SS, Carpenter HA, Dines DE, Marsh HM. Pulmonary phospholipoproteinosis. Experience with 34 cases and a review. *Mayo Clin Proc* 1987;62:499–518.
47. Olopade CO, Prakash UBS. Bronchoscopy in the intensive care critical care unit. *Mayo Clin Proc* 1989;64:1255–1263.
48. Limper AH, Prakash UBS. Tracheobronchial foreign bodies in adults. *Ann Intern Med* 1990;112:604–609.
49. Kvale PA. Training in laser bronchoscopy and proposal for credentialing. *Chest* 1990;97:983–996.
50. Beamis JF Jr, Shapshay SM, Setzer S, Dumon J-F. Teaching models for Nd:YAG laser bronchoscopy. *Chest* 1989; 95:1316–1318.
51. Lanzafame RJ, Rogers DW, Hinshaw JR. Teaching laser bronchoscopy with laboratory models. *Surg Gynecol Obstet* 1989; 168:65–66.
52. Zavala DC: Zavala DC. Transbronchial biopsy in diffuse lung disease. *Chest* 1978;73:727–733.
53. Mehta AC, Curtis PS, Scalzitti ML, Meeker DP. The high price of bronchoscopy. Maintenance and repair of the flexible fiberoptic bronchoscope. *Chest* 1990;98:448–454.
54. Milam MG, Evins AE, Sahn SA. Immediate chest roentgenography following fiberoptic bronchoscopy. *Chest* 1989;96:477–479.
55. Frazier WD, Pope TL Jr, Findley LJ. Pneumothorax following transbronchial lung biopsy. Low diagnostic yield with routine chest roentgenograms. *Chest* 1990;97:539–540.
56. Hudson LD, Benson JA Jr. Evaluation of clinical competence in pulmonary disease. *Am Rev Resp Dis* 1988;138:1034–1035.
57. American Board of Thoracic Surgery. Booklet of information, Chicago: January 1991;13.
58. Faber LP. Bronchoscopy training. *Chest* 1978;73:776–778.
59. Dull WL. Flexible fiberoptic bronchoscopy. An analysis of proficiency. *Chest* 1980;77:65–67.

Bronchoscopy,
edited by U. B. S. Prakash.
Mayo Foundation © 1994.
Published by Raven Press, Ltd., New York.

CHAPTER 30

Optimal Bronchoscopy

Udaya B. S. Prakash and Samuel E. Stubbs

The word *optimism* is derived from Leibnitz's doctrine that the world is the best of all possible worlds. Optimal bronchoscopy, to position the word in a narrow focus, represents performance of ideal bronchoscopy from the bronchoscopist's as well as the patient's view. The concept of optimal bronchoscopy also encompasses a cost-effective approach to bronchoscopy. The latter is no longer an inconsequential concern because of the limited economic resources available for health care in the 1990s. Even though there are no rigidly established standards regarding the practice of bronchoscopy, broad guidelines have been published by specialty organizations (1–5). Clearly, bronchoscopy practice has been one of evolution over the past century during which there has been a continuum of changes in the disease processes that require bronchoscopy. The changes in the indications, instrumentation, and techniques for bronchoscopy have contributed to the difficulty in establishing rigid guidelines. Therefore the recommendations we provide here may become invalid in the future as new technologies develop. Certain aspects of optimal bronchoscopy techniques discussed in Chapter 9 are aimed mainly at the novice bronchoscopist. The other chapters in this textbook also deal with the technical details and the diagnostic and therapeutic yield from various bronchoscopy procedures. Much of the discussion here is based on our reflections on the results of a mail survey we conducted for the American College of Chest Physicians (ACCP) (6,7).

THE OPTIMAL BRONCHOSCOPIST

An "optimal bronchoscopist" should be able to perform both flexible and rigid bronchoscopy in adult as well as pediatric patients. To be able to accomplish this, a bronchoscopist should be well versed in the clinical aspects of pulmonary medicine as well as the anatomy of upper and lower airways in children and adults, proficient in identification and utilization of appropriate instruments for use in both flexible and rigid bronchoscopy, and trained in all types of bronchoscopy-related procedures. This definition of an ideal bronchoscopist obviously begets the question, "does an optimal bronchoscopist exist in the 1990s?" The "endoscopists" in the first 70 years of this century were worthy of this definition because they performed bronchoscopies and esophagoscopies in children as well as adults and developed great expertise in the procedures. However, the training of physicians in many subspecialties, the development of gastroenterology and pediatric pulmonology as distinct subspecialties, and the refinement of fiberoptic instruments in the 1960s has greatly thwarted the development of adequate numbers of such specialists. Another unfortunate trend in the recent years has been the emergence of "interventional bronchoscopy" and "interventional bronchoscopists." These phrases denote a two-tier system in which one group of bronchoscopists performs "routine bronchoscopy" and the other performs special bronchoscopy procedures such as laser bronchoscopy and placement of tracheobronchial prosthesis.

The continued emphasis on "superspecialization" and the results of the ACCP survey suggest that the number of "ideal bronchoscopists" will gradually diminish. This is more of a problem in the Western countries. As a result of the above influences, the terms *endoscopy* and *endoscopist* have largely become nontenable and likewise the terms *bronchoesophagology* and *bronchoesophagologist* are perilously close to becoming oxymorons. A plausible plan to increase the number of ideal bronchoscopists embraces the idea that all well-qualified bronchoscopists attempt as much

U. B. S. Prakash and S. E. Stubbs: Division of Thoracic Diseases and Internal Medicine, Mayo Clinic, Rochester, Minnesota 55905.

as possible to take advantage of every opportunity to participate in pediatric and adult bronchoscopy as well as to utilize flexible and rigid bronchoscopy skills.

In the North American and most Western European countries, adult bronchoscopy is performed by pulmonologists, thoracic surgeons, and otorhinolaryngologists. Specialists in critical care medicine and anesthesia who manage critical care units sometimes provide limited therapeutic bronchoscopy services such as bronchoscopic aspiration of secretions and endotracheal tube placements. In other countries, the abovementioned specialists as well as general surgeons and specialists in endoscopy provide bronchoscopy as well as other endoscopic procedures. Irrespective of the primary medical specialty training, every bronchoscopist must be adequately trained in anatomy, physiology, and the disorders of the upper and lower airways. It is also important to emphasize that the bronchoscopy should be performed by physicians and not by nonphysicians. We totally disagree with publications that have stated that "flexible fiberoptic endoscopy as technical procedure requires no specialized training" and that "the technique itself is similar to routine endotracheal tube suctioning" (8). While bronchoscopy is a safe procedure when performed by well-trained physicians, its inadvertent use by nonphysicians or inadequately trained physicians could lead to life-threatening complications.

THE OPTIMAL BRONCHOSCOPE

The introduction of the flexible bronchoscope in the late 1960s sparked lively discussions between the stern proponents of flexible and rigid bronchoscopy (9–13) with each group criticizing the problems associated with the bronchoscope favored by the opposing group and forecasting the end of that particular bronchoscope. The significant numbers of disapproving comments in the more recent literature on the role of the rigid bronchoscope are reminiscent of analogous reproach of the flexible bronchoscope when it was first introduced into clinical practice more than two decades ago (9–11). Contrary to earlier assertions that the flexible bronchoscope will eventually replace the rigid bronchoscope (12,13), recent years have seen an increase in the clinical role played by the rigid bronchoscope (7).

Historically, the rigid bronchoscope has been utilized by surgeons. A postal survey of British bronchoscopists observed that although only 2% of 39,564 bronchoscopies performed between 1974 and 1986 employed the rigid bronchoscope, more than 90% of the rigid bronchoscopies were done by surgeons (14). That report also noted that the flexible fiberoptic bronchoscope was used by 81% of bronchoscopists, both flexible and rigid instruments by 9%, and the flexible bronchoscope through the rigid bronchoscope by 8%. In the ACCP survey (6), only 8% of the survey respondents used the rigid bronchoscope. Nevertheless, the superiority of the rigid bronchoscope in the treatment of massive hemoptysis (15,16), laser procedures (17–20), cryotherapy (21,22), removal of tracheobronchial foreign bodies (23–26), dilatation of tracheobronchial strictures, and placement of airway stents (27–31) is well established (also see Chapter 17). However, there are those who have questioned the need for rigid instrument in the current practice of bronchoscopy (32–36).

Introduction of bronchoscopic laser therapy was largely responsible for the revival of rigid bronchoscopy. During the early days of laser bronchoscopy, the bronchoscopists would ablate the entire tumor with laser energy. It is now evident that the "laser ablation" of large tumors in major airways to a large extent involves physical removal of tumor tissue with rigid bronchoscopic forceps or use of the rigid bronchoscope itself as a "coring" and "dilating" instrument. While most of the tumor is resected in this manner, the laser is used either initially and/or terminally to coagulate and/or cauterize vascular lesions and vascular stalks of pedunculated tumors. A significant advantage of this technique is the shorter time needed to treat the lesions via the rigid bronchoscope (19). Bronchoscopists who use only the flexible bronchoscope for laser therapy of large airway lesions schedule several sessions because of the long duration involved. Indeed, studies have documented that there is a statistically significant difference in the number of laser therapy sessions utilized by flexible and rigid bronchoscopies to palliate airway lesions, with the rigid instrument requiring only one session and the procedure employing the flexible bronchoscope requiring a mean of two sessions (19,37).

The bronchoscopy section at the Mayo Clinic has carried out more than 500 laser bronchoscopies and, except for the initial 20% of the procedures in which the flexible instrument was employed, we and our associates have been using the rigid bronchoscope as the primary instrument in almost all the laser bronchoscopies and feel that the rigid bronchoscope is preferable to the flexible instrument for laser applications. The contention that the flexible instrument is ideal for treatment of lesions in the distal or peripheral airway is rather unconvincing because such cases are infrequent and the indications for palliative therapy debatable (7). Even in such uncommon situations, we believe that the rigid bronchoscope is better because a flexible bronchoscope can be passed, if required, through the lumen of the rigid bronchoscope to apply laser therapy (38). This approach combines the safety of the rigid instrument with the maneuverability of the flexible bronchoscope (19). In our opinion, bronchoscopists who wish to use laser should be competent in both flexible and rigid bronchoscopic techniques (20,38). Furthermore, the bronchoscopists who perform laser therapy should ideally have the facilities to provide other bronchoscopic treatments such as brachytherapy and stent placement. Recent studies have shown that brachytherapy following Nd:YAG laser therapy may significantly potentiate the duration of survival in patients with malignant airway disease compared to palliation with the Nd:YAG laser alone (39).

Even though the flexible bronchoscope has been used to insert airway stents for palliation of obstructed major airways, the advantage provided by the rigid bronchoscope in the placement, manipulation, and removal of such stents is unsurpassed. A major advantage is the ability to provide adequate ventilation during airway manipulation. Parallel to this is the ease with which the rigid bronchoscope can be implemented to dilate major airway strictures and stenoses. The larger dilator balloons are at times unable to traverse the working channel of the flexible bronchoscope and frequently, particularly when force is used, the balloons rupture. The size of the balloon is not a major consideration when the rigid bronchoscope is used. Lastly, the rigid bronchoscope itself can be used as an airway dilator.

The bronchoscope of choice for removal of a tracheobronchial foreign body in children is the rigid bronchoscope (40,41). Success rates exceeding 98% can be achieved with a rigid bronchoscope (42,43). Optically guided extraction instruments permit precise localization and removal. However, the flexible bronchoscope has been employed to extract pediatric foreign bodies. Used in conjunction with the Fogarty balloon in children who were 2 years of age or younger, a success rate of 82% was reported in one series (44). Even though the diagnostic use of the pediatric flexible bronchoscope is a safe, definitive, and cost-effective method for the identification of tracheobronchial foreign bodies in pediatric patients (45), the bronchoscopist who wishes to use the flexible instrument for this purpose should be aware of the risk of losing the foreign body in the narrow subglottic space and have the means to prevent the potential asphyxia. Detection of a tracheobronchial foreign body should ideally be followed by immediate removal of it at the same bronchoscopy session. It is neither cost-effective nor safe to diagnose the foreign body by flexible bronchoscopy and then postpone the rigid bronchoscopic extraction or transfer the patient to another area for rigid bronchoscopy.

Management of tracheobronchial foreign bodies in adults has gradually undergone considerable evolution mostly because of wider application of flexible bronchoscopy in clinical practice. Traditionally, rigid bronchoscopy has been the preferred treatment for adults (46). Many reports have indicated that flexible bronchoscopy may be a valuable therapeutic option for adults (41,47–52). Some bronchoscopists have proposed that flexible bronchoscopy is preferable to rigid bronchoscopy both in the initial evaluation and for removal of tracheobronchial foreign bodies in adults (41,53). We disagree that the flexible instrument is superior to the rigid bronchoscope for extracting the foreign bodies. In our own experience, flexible bronchoscopy has been successful in 60% of patients in contrast to a 98% success rate associated with rigid bronchoscopy (25). We admit that flexible bronchoscopy is superior in specific cases where the foreign body is impacted too far distally to be reached with the rigid bronchoscope or in cases where instability of the cervical spine prevents the use of the rigid bronchoscope. Other explicit indications for flexible bronchoscopy include foreign bodies in patients who are mechanically ventilated and patients with trauma or fractures of the jaw, cervical spine, or skull. Even though there are many types of baskets, grasping claws, electromagnets, balloon catheters, suction tubes, and other instruments available for use through the flexible bronchoscope (54–62), we feel that most of these instruments are somewhat flimsy in construction, awkward to use, and ill suited to grasp or extract all foreign bodies. Bronchoscopists planning to use the flexible bronchoscope in foreign body removal should be aware of the problems and hazards that may develop if improperly managed (63).

Finally, we believe that both flexible and rigid bronchoscopes are "optimal" instruments in the hands of a bronchoscopist trained in bronchoscopic procedures using both instruments. Rigid adherence to use of either the rigid or flexible bronchoscope for all bronchoscopic procedures due to lack of training in one or the other constitutes suboptimal practice of bronchoscopy. The flexible and rigid bronchoscopes should complement, and not compete with, each other (7).

INDICATIONS

Are too many bronchoscopies being performed in current clinical practice? The traditional and newer indications for diagnostic and therapeutic bronchoscopies permit greater latitude in the application of this procedure. The safety of flexible bronchoscopy and ease with which a well-trained bronchoscopist can perform bronchoscopic procedures has probably contributed to the "overuse" of bronchoscopy. Additionally, other "enticements" are also involved (64,65). It is our bias that many bronchoscopic procedures are unnecessary. It is increasingly important for bronchoscopists to consider the indications for the procedure carefully with attention regarding the diagnostic information that the procedure can provide. The scheduling of bronchoscopy to obtain specimens from the respiratory tract should be tempered with the knowledge that each additional test increases the cost of the procedure.

The major indications for bronchoscopy reported by the participants in the ACCP survey are shown in Table 1. As expected, suspicion of pulmonary malignancy, lung nodules and masses, hemoptysis, and unexplained pulmonary parenchymal and interstitial processes were the most common indications for bronchoscopy. The timing and the role of bronchoscopy in the evaluation of hemoptysis is discussed in detail in Chapter 17 and the usefulness of bronchoscopy in the diagnosis, staging, and follow-up of patients with lung cancer is discussed in Chapter 22, this volume. Routine periodic bronchoscopy following surgical treatment of lung cancer has been recommended and the procedure inappropriately considered analogous to colonoscopic follow-up of malignancy of the large intestine (66). Performance of such "routine" bronchoscopy following surgical resection of lung cancer in the absence of clinical indications for bronchoscopy is inappropriate and constitutes "unnecessary" bronchoscopy (67). The bronchoscopic restaging of patients with lung cancer responding to therapy is not cost effective because the subsequent management is not affected by the results. In a study of 139 patients with small cell lung cancer who achieved complete response to therapy and underwent repeat bronchoscopy for restaging, 87.7% were negative, 5.8% were inconclusive, and, despite other evidence suggesting that there was complete response, 6.5% of patients showed persistence of cancer and this group of patients survived for a shorter period than the other two groups of patients. However, the survival difference was not significant (68). The telling finding was that the cost of rebronchoscopy per patient restaged was Can. $14,960. The authors' concluded that restaging bronchoscopy should not be done in responding patients with limited small cell lung cancer, thus potentially saving health care dollars as well as reducing patient inconvenience with no detrimental effect on survival.

TABLE 1. *The five most common indications for bronchoscopy[a]*

Indications	Respondents, % (*n*)
Mass/nodule/suspicious lesion/cancer	96.4 (840)
Hemoptysis/bleeding	81.1 (706)
Pneumonia/infection	65.1 (567)
Diffuse/interstitial disease in nonimmunocompromised patient	62.1 (541)
Therapeutic bronchoscopy for lobar or segmental atelectasis	56.4 (491)
Cough/wheeze	23.4 (204)
Immunocompromised patient	15.4 (134)
AIDS/HIV positive	14.7 (128)
Trachea/stridor	2.2 (19)
ICU/ventilator	1.5 (13)
Other[b]	4.7 (41)

From Prakash et al. (6), with permission.

[a] Each respondent was asked to list the five most common indications for bronchoscopy in his/her practice. AIDS = acquired immunodeficiency syndrome, HIV = human immunodeficiency virus, ICU = intensive care unit.

[b] Aspiration, 10; brachytherapy, 8; asthma, 4; effusion, 5; weight loss, 4; research, 3; surgical, 3; protected brushing, 2; failure to wean, 1; vasculitis, 1.

One of the most common indications for bronchoscopy in the current practice is persistent or chronic cough. Even though bronchoscopy carries a low diagnostic yield in the evaluation (69–73), nearly a quarter of the ACCP survey participants listed cough as one of the five most common indications for the procedure (Table 1). Granted that bronchoscopy is presumably directed at "excluding tracheobronchial etiology" of cough in the absence of apparent abnormality of the chest roentgenograph, we postulate that bronchoscopy is overused in this group of patients. However, in meticulously chosen patients with chronic cough and a nonlocalizing chest roentgenogram, bronchoscopy can be useful (74,75). Careful clinical examination and correlation with the chest roentgenogram may exclude many bronchoscopic procedures. However, it is likely that cough will remain a common indication for bronchoscopy (7).

Interestingly, about 15% of bronchoscopists consider respiratory complications in patients with acquired immunodeficiency syndrome (AIDS) and other immunocompromised states among the five most common indications for bronchoscopy (6). This reflects the increasing frequency with which these two groups of patients are encountered in current clinical practice as well as the well-authenticated role of bronchoscopy in the diagnosis of respiratory problems in these two groups. The most important role of bronchoscopy in these patients is its ability to obtain specimens to identify the etiological agents of pulmonary infections. Nevertheless, repetition of bronchoscopy within a short time after the initial procedure for identification of respiratory infection is unwarranted (76). Bronchoalveolar lavage is a well-tolerated procedure in critically ill, mechanically ventilated patients, provided that risk factors for complications are corrected before the procedure and one adheres to procedural guidelines focused on patient safety (77–81). Clinically important complications are uncommon.

Chest roentgenographic abnormalities are among the most common indications for bronchoscopy. If bronchoscopy is planned solely on the basis of chest roentgenographic abnormalities, then a careful clinical evaluation should be undertaken before hastily proceeding with bronchoscopy. The chest roentgenographic abnormalities that are more likely to be diagnosed by bronchoscopy include lobar collapse, mass lesions (>4 cm), and diffuse pulmonary parenchymal process (82). Pleural effusion is often used as an indication for bronchoscopy despite the documentation that bronchoscopy has a limited role in the investigation of pleural effusion. In patients with pleural effusion, bronchoscopy is more likely to be diagnostic in those presenting with a cough and in those with other chest roentgenographic abnormalities (83).

Many of the repeat bronchoscopic procedures can be averted by excellent documentation of bronchoscopic findings and procedures and by communication with the patient and primary physician. Details of the documentation techniques are discussed in detail in Chapter 27.

PREBRONCHOSCOPY TESTS

Among the cost-cutting measures should be included elimination of many prebronchoscopy tests obtained on a routine basis. The number of prebronchoscopy tests and the number of bronchoscopists who routinely obtain many unwarranted tests is astounding (Table 2) (6). It is imperative that the bronchoscopist consider each patient individually and order tests preoperatively on the basis of the patient's clinical status and the potential risks of the procedure planned (7). In our view, procuring a meticulous and relevant history with specific attention to the presence of underlying likely risk factors, an accurate cardiopulmonary examination, and a chest roentgenogram are three of the most important prebronchoscopy requirements. A posteroanterior and lateral chest roentgenogram is essential to plan optimal specimen collection from focal abnormalities.

TABLE 2. *Tests required before bronchoscopy*

Test	Respondents who require test, % (*n*)
Chest radiograph	89.4 (779)
Platelet count	70.3 (612)
Prothrombin time	70.3 (612)
Complete blood cell count	61.5 (536)
Electrocardiogram	42.4 (369)
Arterial blood gas analysis	38.7 (337)
Potassium	27.9 (243)
Pulmonary function tests	26.8 (233)
Creatinine	24.8 (216)
Glucose	19.7 (172)
Others[a]	13.9 (121)

From Prakash et al. (6), with permission.

[a] Other tests used by respondents: activated partial thromboplastin time, 6.8% (59); oximetry, 4.0% (35); blood urea nitrogen, 1.0% (9); history and physical examination, 0.3% (3); blood type and cross-match, 0.1% (1).

Smaller lesion may need to be better defined by simple tomography. Computed tomography of chest on a routine basis is not necessary prior to bronchoscopy. However, if computed tomography and other imaging procedures are already planned for other reasons, it is better to schedule them before bronchoscopy so that the bronchoscopist will have the additional advantage of using the information in planning biopsy and other bronchoscopic procedures. Some bronchoscopists obtain bronchography prior to brushing and biopsy of nodular lesions (36), with the reason for the bronchography being the ability to identify the bronchus leading to the nodular lesion. This, in our opinion, is an unnecessary test and only adds to the time taken to evaluate the lesion and to the patient's discomfort.

We have previously advocated that an otherwise healthy individual scheduled to undergo bronchoscopy does not require a complete blood count, a hemostatic survey, blood chemistry, and urinalysis (7). Of all the tests in the blood chemistry, estimation of serum creatinine is probably the most important because platelet dysfunction secondary to renal failure is associated with a clinical hemorrhagic tendency that can be quite severe (84). Further, a 45% incidence of bleeding following bronchoscopic lung biopsy has been reported in uremic patients (85,86). Nevertheless, only 25% of the ACCP survey participants routinely required a creatinine level before bronchoscopy (Table 2). It should be noted that the relationship between abnormal platelet function and the risk of hemorrhage in patients with renal dysfunction is unclear. Zavala is of the opinion that "any biopsy procedure is avoided, if at all possible, on a uremic patient because of hemorrhage" (86). If bronchoscopic lung biopsy is absolutely needed, the clotting mechanism should be normalized by the administration of fresh-frozen plasma or deamino-8$_{D}$-arginine-vasopressin (see Chapter 17, this volume). Patients with platelet counts of less than 50,000/mm^3 should receive six to ten packs of platelet transfusion before bronchoscopic lung biopsy (85,86). In our practice, a serum creatinine level of ≥3 mg/dl is considered a relative contraindication to bronchoscopic lung biopsy (7).

We stress that no single test designed to examine the integrity of the coagulation system can predict hemorrhage during surgery. Measurement of bleeding time, while inexpensive, is not warranted as a routine screening test because of the inability of this test to predict the risk of hemorrhage in individual patients (87,88). Similarly, routine estimation of prothrombin time and the activated partial thromboplastin time should be avoided. It is far more important to obtain a clinical history of bleeding diathesis and related information from the patient than routinely schedule tests to identify abnormalities of coagulation. Spontaneous bleeding from the tracheobronchial tree or pulmonary parenchyma is unusual even in congenital coagulopathies such as hemophilia (89), and tests to ascertain hemorrhagic disposition should be individualized. Prebronchoscopy coagulation screening should be limited to patients with active bleeding, known or clinically suspected bleeding disorders, liver disease, renal dysfunction, malabsorption, malnutrition, or other conditions associated with acquired coagulopathies (7,90). The British postal survey reported that 66–75% of bronchoscopists included evaluation of platelet count, prothrombin time, or clotting time prior to bronchoscopic lung biopsy (14). The incidence of significant blood loss as a result of bronchoscopic procedures is so low that grouping of blood type and cross-matching, obtained by 22% of British bronchoscopists prior to bronchoscopy (14), is unnecessary.

Two tests obtained commonly and routinely by many bronchoscopists are pulmonary function tests and arterial blood gas analysis. Among the British bronchoscopists, 66% routinely obtain pulmonary function tests before bronchoscopic lung biopsy (14). Considering that even the severe respiratory dysfunction encountered in immunosuppressed patients with diffuse pulmonary infiltrates is only a relative contraindication to bronchoscopy (77,81), routine evaluation of pulmonary functions before bronchoscopy is unnecessary. However, if a patient is scheduled to undergo both bronchoscopy and pulmonary function testing within a period of 72 hr, we suggest that the pulmonary function tests be performed first because bronchoscopy itself can provoke bronchial mucosal edema which in turn results in spuriously abnormal pulmonary function test results (91–93). Prebronchoscopy evaluation of arterial blood gases has been endorsed by some bronchoscopists (94). We feel that routine measurement of arterial blood gases before bronchoscopy is not indicated in all patients scheduled to undergo bronchoscopy. Noninvasive tests such as pulse oximetry, sphygmomanometry, and electrocardiographic monitoring should be used to obtain adequate information during the procedure in most cases.

TABLE 3. *Other premedications used*[a]

Premedication	Respondents reporting use, % (*n*)
Codeine	13.9 (121)
Midazolam (Versed)	10.2 (89)
Hydroxyzine (Vistaril)	7.9 (69)
Diazepam (Valium)	7.2 (63)
Morphine	7.1 (62)
Promethazine (Phenergan)	5.1 (44)
Hydromorphone (Dilaudid)	2.1 (18)
Pentobarbital (Nembutal)	1.4 (12)
Fentanyl (Sublimaze)	1.3 (11)
Lidocaine (Xylocaine)	1.1 (10)
Lorazepam (Ativan)	0.8 (7)
Albuterol	0.3 (3)
Other[b]	3.6 (19)
	60.6 (528)

From Prakash et al. (6), with permission.

[a] Premedications other than atropine, meperidine, and glycopyrrolate.

[b] Diphenhydramine hydrochloride (Benadryl), butorphanol (Stadol), prochlorperazine (Compazine), and phenobarbital were used by two respondents each. Hydrocortisone, magnesium sulfate, droperidol (Inapsine), alprazolam (Xanax), benzonatate (Tessalon), tetracaine (Pontocaine), hydrochlorothiazide, steroid aerosol, chlordiazepoxide hydrochloride (Librium), nalbuphine (Nubain), and isoetharine were used by one each. The drugs named are those mentioned by survey respondents.

PREMEDICATION

The routine administration of premedication prior to bronchoscopy varies among bronchoscopists and patient groups. Some bronchoscopists use medications before bronchoscopy while others use anticholinergic agents and sedatives during the procedure. Other bronchoscopists have promoted bronchoscopy without any premedications (95). Indeed, a small number of ACCP survey participants and 6% of bronchoscopists in a British survey used no premedication (6,14). Granted that both flexible and rigid bronchoscopic procedures can be performed without premedication and intraoperative sedation, routine avoidance of premedication is unjustified, unless there are compelling reasons to do so. Patient surveys have documented that prior to bronchoscopy many patients are more fearful of the potential diagnosis of malignancy than of dyspnea and asphyxiation (96). Prebronchoscopy medication to diminish anxiety should be contemplated for most patients with the stipulation that the medication and dosage be individualized for each patient. Routine administration of an antisialagogue such as atropine or glycopyrrolate is generally recommended to reduce secretions, prevent bradycardia, and inhibit other vasovagal responses (14,97–102). Among the North American bronchoscopists, 83.2% used atropine as a premedication (6), whereas among the British bronchoscopists, 71% used atropine and 16% scopolamine (14). Because of the lower incidence of undesirable side effects, glycopyrrolate is currently recommended as the anticholinergic agent of choice for bronchoscopy (103). Additionally, a drug capable of producing sedation or anxiolysis (e.g., codeine, meperidine, morphine, or barbiturate) should be administered approximately 30–45 min before the procedure. The wide variety of premedications used by the bronchoscopists in the ACCP survey is indeed startling (Table 3).

SEDATION

As in the case of premedications, there is wide variation among bronchoscopists regarding the routine use of intraoperative sedatives (97). With newer and safer sedatives being available in the current practice, the routine use of sedatives during bronchoscopy has increased. Sedation is not synonymous with topical anesthesia and one does not replace the other, even though together they provide optimal operating conditions for the bronchoscopist. Antegrade amnesia, relaxation, and patient cooperation are the clinical end points when using intravenous sedatives for bronchoscopy (96). A controlled double-blind study reported that patients prefer intravenous benzodiazepine to placebo (101). In the absence of contraindications, the majority of patients should be provided the advantage of an intraoperative sedative. However, the bronchoscopist should cautiously choose the agent and dosage of sedation individually for each patient.

The wide diversity of intravenous sedative drugs and the drug combinations used by the ACCP survey bronchoscopists was surprising (Table 4). It is irrational on a pharmacological basis to use two or more opiates or more than one benzodiazepine. Since no single agent produces amnesia, anxiolysis, and analgesia, a combination of two drugs (a benzodiazepine and an opiate) may be required in many patients. However, combination of three or more sedatives is not only unnecessary but also escalates the danger of respiratory depression.

The overwhelming superiority of midazolam over diazepam in endoscopy procedures is well documented (104–113). Currently, midazolam is the drug of choice for almost all bronchoscopy procedures (7,108,112). In the ACCP survey, only 48% of the survey participants categorized midazolam as the sedative of choice. In contrast to diazepam, midazolam has a shorter half-life, a larger volume of distribution, a faster total body clearance, and achieves significant antegrade amnesia in twice as many patients and at lighter levels of sedation (99,105–107,114–117). The suggested dose of midazolam for conscious sedation is 0.07 mg/kg, but cautious titration is needed. The dose specification for midazolam is sex-dependent; males require about 1.0 mg more than females (118). Since elderly patients are especially susceptible to midazolam, extreme caution is advised for its employment in this group of patients (98,118,119). Bronchoscopists should be aware of the availability of a benzodiazepine antagonist, flumazenil, which can reverse the sedative effects of midazolam.

While cautious use of sedatives permits performance of smoother bronchoscopy, it should be observed that up to half of the life-threatening complications have been ascribed to sedative administration (114). A drawback of sedative use from the bronchoscopist's perspective is the suppression of the patient's ability to participate and react to commands such as those to make a special attempt to suppress coughing and signal the perception of chest pain during bronchoscopic lung biopsy, the latter signifying proximity of the biopsy forceps to the visceral pleura. Hypoventilation with secondary hypercarbia is a potential complication in patients with severe chronic obstructive pulmonary disease who are administered sedation.

TABLE 4. *Intravenous sedatives used*[a]

Sedative	Respondents, % (*n*)
Midazolam (Versed)	48.1 (419)
Diazepam (Valium)	24.5 (213)
Meperidine (Demerol)	5.7 (50)
Fentanyl (Sublimaze)	3.6 (31)
Morphine	3.6 (31)
Lorazepam (Ativan)	0.7 (6)
Other[b]	1.7 (15)
	87.3 (761)

From Prakash et al. (6), with permission.

[a] Intravenous sedation was used routinely by 51%, sometimes by 23%, and rarely by 24%; only 2% did not respond to this question.

[b] Hydromorphone (Dilaudid), droperidol (Inapsine), and pentobarbital (Nembutal) were used by two respondents each. Promethazine (Phenergan), butorphanol (Stadol), magnesium sulfate, prochlorperazine (Compazine), hydroxyzine (Vistaril), and oxymorphone (Numorphan) were used by one each. Three physicians wrote that they "never use intravenous sedation." The drugs named are those mentioned by survey respondents.

TOPICAL ANESTHESIA

Judicious use of topical anesthetic agents is essential for the uneventful completion of bronchoscopic procedures. Complications of excessive use of anesthetic agents are discussed in Chapter 7, this volume. However, most adults who undergo bronchoscopy do not usually require the maximal dose that can be administered without encountering toxicity. An overwhelming majority of bronchoscopists employ lidocaine as the main topical anesthetic agent whereas many use other agents (such as benzocaine or cocaine) for the initial application (120). One study reported little difference in effectiveness between cocaine and lidocaine (121). However, because the cardiovascular and allergic side effects are more common with cocaine, lidocaine may be the preferred anesthetic for bronchoscopy (122). The majority of publications on this topic have concentrated their discussions on the mode of administration. One study evaluated nasal anesthetic regimens using different medications and found that sprayed anesthetics contribute little to nasal anesthesia and any regimen appeared acceptable when viscous lidocaine was used (123). Another study compared the three different methods of local anesthesia (4 ml of 2.5% cocaine by tracheal injection (cricoid), by bronchoscopic injection of cocaine, or 4 ml of 4% lidocaine delivered by nebulizer 20 min before the procedure) and reported that both the patients and the bronchoscopists preferred the tracheal method to either bronchoscopically injected cocaine or nebulized lidocaine (124). Others have also shown that a single injection of lidocaine, 100 mg, via cricothyroid puncture is safe and is associated with less cough (125). Individual training and practice will most likely determine the preferred method of topical anesthetic application. As discussed in Chapter 9, there is no one optimal method of application of topical anesthetic. Suffice it to say that every bronchoscopist should be ready to utilize an alternative method if a favorite technique cannot be used in a given patient. Many publications have discussed the types of topical anesthetic agents available, although the majority of the bronchoscopists use lidocaine (14,126–128).

GENERAL ANESTHESIA

General anesthesia is unnecessary for most adult flexible bronchoscopies. Even rigid bronchoscopy can be safely performed with deep intravenous sedation (129). Complicated or technically difficult procedures, most rigid bronchoscopies, most time-consuming laser bronchoscopies, and extreme patient apprehension are circumstances in which general anesthesia may be desirable. Almost all rigid bronchoscopies in pediatric patients will require general anesthesia. It is surprising to note that 16.5% of North American bronchoscopists and 12% of British bronchoscopists routinely use general anesthesia for bronchoscopic procedures (6,14). This is an exceedingly high number and it is hoped that more and more bronchoscopists will avoid general anesthesia on a routine basis.

SUPPLEMENTAL OXYGEN

Bronchoscopy in patients with underlying pulmonary disorders is well known to produce iatrogenic hypoxemia (130–134). This fact is important since a majority of patients who undergo bronchoscopy have underlying pulmonary dysfunction and bronchoscopic procedures can further aggravate the pulmonary dysfunction and contribute to hypoxemia. As noted above, an increasing number of immunosuppressed patients with diffuse lung disease have severe hypoxemia that can be aggravated by bronchoscopy. Further, the newer flexible bronchoscopes with larger suction channels have the ability to aspirate large volumes of gas from the lungs. For these reasons, administration of supplemental oxygen during bronchoscopy is indicated in most patients (135,136). This recommendation should be tempered with the advice that each patient be carefully evaluated before bronchoscopy. This practice was reported by 89% of North American bronchoscopists but only 18% of British bronchoscopists use supplemental oxygen on a routine basis (6,14). Pulse oximetry, can be very valuable to estimate the adequacy of oxygenation whether or not additional oxygen is given. In patients with severe chronic obstructive pulmonary disease and hypoxia-driven ventilation, excessive supplemental oxygen may suppress the hypoxic drive and produce hypoventilation and exacerbate preexisting hypercarbia.

ORAL VERSUS NASAL INSERTION

The oral versus the nasal insertion of the bronchoscope, applicable only with the flexible bronchoscope, is to a large extent dependent on one's initial training and one's subsequent proficiency in the utilization of either route (137–143). One third of the ACCP survey participants used only the nasal route and 6% used only the oral route (Table 5). Even though only 43% of the bronchoscopists in the ACCP survey reported using both routes, we emphasize that every bronchoscopist should be able to perform bronchoscopy by both routes, since each method has its own distinct advantages. Our observations of bronchoscopists suggest that they continue to employ the route of insertion learned during their bronchoscopy training and more or less adhere to it during their career.

The oral route of insertion of the flexible bronchoscope permits insertion of a large orotracheal tube through which the bronchoscope can be readily inserted or removed for cleaning or removal of a biopsy specimen. Oral insertion is quicker and, even without an orotracheal tube, it can be inserted and removed easily. The risk of epistaxis is eliminated by the use of the oral route of insertion. The disadvantages include the interference of the tongue during insertion and slightly increased gag reflex.

The nasal route is easy to learn since the nasal passage performs as a stent for the passage of the flexible bronchoscope. This allows excellent inspection of the upper airways and examination of the glottis and trachea under dynamic or static conditions. The nasal approach is ideal for a brief examination when excessive manipulation of the airway is not contemplated, as in postoperative inspection after a bronchoplasty procedure, placement of brachytherapy catheters, and assessment of results of treatment for major airway obstruction.

TABLE 5. *Responses pertaining to bronchoscopic technique*[a]

Question	Routinely	Sometimes	Rarely	No response
Do you use an endotracheal (oral or nasal) tube?[b]	6.7 (58)	13.7 (119)	78.2 (681)	1.5 (13)
Do you use BAL in a nonimmunocompromised patient?	24.0 (209)	16.9 (147)	57.6 (502)	1.5 (13)
Do you use BAL in an immunocompromised patient?	76.8 (669)	5.5 (48)	15.8 (138)	1.8 (16)
Do you use TBNA in malignant disease?[c]	11.8 (103)	29.2 (254)	49.4 (430)	9.6 (84)
Do you use TBNA in nonmalignant disease?[d]	2.3 (20)	3.7 (32)	82.5 (719)	11.5 (100)
Do you use fluoroscopy for TBLB?	75.3 (656)	6.4 (56)	11.0 (96)	7.2 (63)
Do you perform TBLB in a nonimmunocompromised patient?	68.8 (599)	20.3 (177)	8.8 (77)	2.1 (18)
Do you obtain a chest radiograph after TBLB?	79.0 (688)	3.6 (31)	9.9 (86)	7.6 (66)
Do you hospitalize a patient after TBLB?	12.1 (105)	6.7 (58)	72.8 (634)	8.5 (74)
Do you use frozen-section examination of biopsy specimens?[e]	2.6 (23)	1.5 (13)	72.9 (635)	1.5 (13)
Do you use videobronchoscopy?	13.8 (120)	0.0 (0)	73.8 (643)	12.4 (108)

From Prakash et al. (6), with permission.

[a] Values are the percentage of the group of 871 respondents who made a response, with the number shown in parentheses. "Routinely" = ≥85% of cases; "sometimes" = 6% to 84% of cases; "rarely" = ≤5% of cases; BAL = bronchoalveolar lavage; TBNA = transtracheal/transbronchial needle aspiration; TBLB = transbronchoscopic lung biopsy.

[b] Thirty-one respondents commented that they used an endotracheal tube in the following settings: TBLB, high-risk patients, respiratory failure, intensive care unit, general anesthesia, laser bronchoscopy, serious hemorrhage and patients receiving supplemental oxygen.

[c] Comments from respondents included the following: damage to scope, 31; poor results, 27; use only in paratracheal disease, 10; need better training, 7; needle does not work, 7; always positive, 2; pathologist does not like samples, 2; radiology department will not allow use of fluoroscopy machine, 2.

[d] Comments from survey respondents included the following: use in suspected sarcoid, 2; use in infections, 2; not indicated in any condition, 8; not trained in TBNA; looks dangerous, 2.

[e] One hundred eighty seven (21.5%) respondents reported that the facility for frozen-section examination was not available to them.

ENDOTRACHEAL TUBE

A vast majority of flexible bronchoscopic procedures can be performed without using an endotracheal tube for the insertion of the bronchoscope. Indeed, only 6.7% of ACCP survey participants routinely used endotracheal tubes for bronchoscopy (Table 5). However, the use of an endotracheal tube, either orally or nasally, permits easy and quick removal and reinsertion of the flexible bronchoscope to clean the lens and remove mucous plugs from the channel. The proper insertion of an endotracheal tube is not associated with complications and can be easily accomplished following application of topical anesthesia and lubrication. Another advantage to the use of an endotracheal tube is the ease of administration of supplemental oxygen. Furthermore, the flexible bronchoscope can be removed and reintroduced swiftly if hemorrhage and clots become a problem; with bleeding, one has control of the airway from the outset if an endotracheal tube is employed.

BRONCHOALVEOLAR LAVAGE

The safety and important role of bronchoalveolar lavage in identifying infectious agents is well established. Nevertheless, we believe the technique is being employed inappropriately in many clinical situations. Repeat bronchoalveolar lavage within a short period is unlikely to provide additional useful information. It is inappropriate to perform bronchoalveolar lavage for identification of bacteria in a patient who is already receiving multiple antibiotics (144). An appropriate clinical role has not been defined for bronchoalveolar lavage to study the alveolar cells in nonimmunosuppressed patients with diffuse lung disease. Yet we frequently encounter patients who have been subjected to repeated bronchoalveolar lavage for the monitoring of diffuse diseases such as idiopathic pulmonary fibrosis, hypersensitivity pneumonitis, and sarcoidosis. Until further studies prove the value of bronchoalveolar lavage in the diagnosis and treatment of diffuse inflammatory (noninfectious and nonmalignant) diseases, bronchoscopists should refrain from routinely using bronchoalveolar lavage in all nonimmunosuppressed patients. In our opinion, the finding that nearly one fourth of bronchoscopists in the ACCP survey perform bronchoalveolar lavage on a routine basis is an obvious example of the inappropriate use of this bronchoscopic technique (Table 5) (6).

We hasten to emphasize that bronchoalveolar lavage is of diagnostic utility in certain diffuse pulmonary parenchymal disorders such as pulmonary eosinophilic granuloma (histiocytosis X), eosinophilic pneumonia, pulmonary alveolar proteinosis, and primary or secondary pulmonary malignancies (145–154). Bronchoalveolar lavage is very valuable in the diagnosis of lymphangitic carcinomatosis involving the lungs (155–157).

BRONCHOSCOPIC LUNG BIOPSY

It is evident that the number of bronchoscopic lung biopsies has decreased because of the increasing application of bronchoalveolar lavage and the recent popularity of thoracoscopic lung biopsy in immunosuppressed patients with diffuse lung diseases. The ACCP survey participants reported that nearly 70% of the bronchoscopists perform bronchoscopic lung biopsy routinely in diffuse lung disease in nonimmunosuppressed patients (Table 5). Until further studies are performed to better define the clinical role of bronchoalveolar lavage in these disorders, this approach is proper (7). However, the need for a biopsy has to be assessed after a thorough evaluation of the clinical features of each patient. Bronchoscopic lung biopsy is not an indication for routine hospitalization of patients after the procedure, even though a longer period of observation after biopsy may be required (158).

PROTECTED CATHETER BRUSH

Protected catheter brush technique is a valuable procedure to obtain bacterial cultures from the lower respiratory tract (see Chapter 14). Our review of the techniques used suggests wide variation in the utilization of the technique, indications, and application of the results in the management of patients. Since the results obtained from protected catheter brush technique correlate with the those obtained from bronchoalveolar lavage, it is not necessary to perform both procedures to identify bacteria in the same patient (77,78,159–162). Bronchoalveolar lavage technique has some advantages over protected brush catheter since it does not require sophisticated equipment and permits sampling from larger areas of the distal bronchial tree.

CULTURES AND CYTOLOGY

Routine culture of bronchoscopically obtained secretions for bacteria, fungi, and mycobacteria and for cytological studies is inappropriate. Unless there are clear indications in the clinical data to suggest an infectious or neoplastic etiology for the pulmonary process, the practice of routinely submitting the respiratory secretions for culture and cytology should be avoided. We have encountered many examples of unnecessary tests. For instance, repeated therapeutic bronchoscopies for retained secretions or atelectasis do not call for culture each time the patient is submitted to bronchoscopy. Bronchoscopy to exclude tracheobronchial involvement in a patient with esophageal cancer should not routinely include cytological analysis of respiratory secretions because such patients routinely aspirate esophageal secretions along with malignant cells from the esophagus into their respiratory tract. Therefore a positive cytology of the respiratory secretions will be meaningless.

BRONCHOSCOPIC NEEDLE ASPIRATION/BIOPSY

Despite several publications that have reported on the clinical utility of bronchoscopic needle aspiration/biopsy (163–166), many bronchoscopists too often find the technique to be unconvincing (Table 5) (6). First, the needles, irrespective of which manufacturer produces the needles, possess several technical difficulties. The majority of the needles available today are rather flimsy and bend easily or damage the outer sheath. In our experience, it is quite common to use two or more needles in one patient because of the improper function of the needle. Second, the well-documented high rate of needle-induced damage to the inner lining of the flexible bronchoscope is a serious consideration for the bronchoscopists who possess a limited number of flexible bronchoscopes (167). Third, the very low frequency of use of the transtracheal/bronchial needle aspiration in malignant and nonmalignant diseases and the large number of negative comments regarding this procedure suggest that bronchoscopic needle aspiration/biopsy has not gained popularity among bronchoscopists (6). As noted in an editorial (168), the role of this technique in the diagnosis of respiratory diseases seems equivocal to many.

Unquestionably, one can sample malignant nodules, masses, or lymph nodes employing this technique. This can be exceedingly valuable in preoperative staging of a patient with lung cancer who is a poor surgical risk. The diagnosis of small cell cancer by this technique may obviate a more invasive surgical procedure. In our opinion, however, in an otherwise healthy individual without evidence for metastatic disease, one must weigh the experience of the bronchoscopist, pathologist, and surgeon acting as a team in their desire to offer the patient the best chance for good results (7). In many cases, a direct surgical approach seems appropriate. See Chapter 12 for a detailed discussion on this topic.

THERAPEUTIC BRONCHOSCOPY

The indications and techniques for therapeutic bronchoscopy are discussed in Chapters 6 and 16. We believe that therapeutic bronchoscopy is somewhat overused for the aspiration of respiratory secretions in patients with chronic obstructive pulmonary disease, cystic fibrosis, asthma, and postoperative atelectasis (169). Many of these conditions can be medically managed with conservative therapy including chest percussion, aerosol therapy, and encouragement of the patient to cough effectively. Routine bronchoscopy following lung resection, exacerbation of asthma, cystic fibrosis, bronchiectasis, and similar disorders should be avoided.

The management of airway emergencies such as can occur with stent placement for neoplastic obstruction or foreign bodies require close cooperation of a skilled team. Facilities, equipment, and drug supplies should be maintained in a constant state of readiness. Personnel should maintain an acceptable level of proficiency; this may require an ongoing continuing education program.

FLUOROSCOPY

The use of fluoroscopy to obtain biopsy specimens from localized and diffuse pulmonary lesions has been debated in the literature. More than 75% of ACCP survey participants routinely use fluoroscopy for bronchoscopic lung biopsy (Table 5). There are many who feel that fluoroscopy is not necessary (170–172). While we partly concur with this tenet and believe that adequate bronchoscopic lung biopsy specimens can be obtained without fluoroscopic guidance in a patient with a diffuse pulmonary parenchymal process, we emphasize that the use of fluoroscopy permits the bronchoscopist to select the maximally abnormal areas for biopsies. Furthermore, fluoroscopic guidance enables accurate positioning of the forceps in the periphery of the lung for bronchoscopic lung biopsy near the pleura. A mail survey of 231 British bronchoscopists observed that the incidence of pneumothorax following bronchoscopic lung biopsy was 1.8% when fluoroscopy was used and the incidence significantly increased to 2.9% when fluoroscopy was not used (14). Fluoroscopy is not absolutely essential to perform bronchoscopic needle aspiration and biopsy. However, if a small paratracheal or hilar lymph node or lesion is the target of needle aspiration, then fluoroscopic guidance may assist the bronchoscopist in the accurate placement of the needle. It appears that the cost of fluoroscopy equipment and/or the "control" of the fluoroscopy unit (bronchoscopist versus roentgenologist) are the main impediments to the optimal use of fluoroscopy (6). If a fluoroscopy unit is readily available, the bronchoscopist should use it to obtain maximal diagnostic yield.

An advantage provided by the fluoroscope is its ability to assess the possibility of pneumothorax immediately after the bronchoscopic lung biopsy. Except in unusual cases the use of fluoroscopy should obviate the need to routinely obtain a chest roentgenogram after bronchoscopic lung biopsy (173–175). Routine chest roentgenography following bronchoscopy and/or bronchoscopic lung biopsy is not indicated (176). Chest roentgenography following bronchoscopy should be reserved for patients who exhibit symptoms and signs of pneumothorax, atelectasis, or unexplained respiratory distress following bronchoscopy.

The employment of fluoroscopy requires use of appropriate measures to protect the personnel from radiation hazards by limiting exposure time and use of protective shields.

BRONCHOSCOPY SUITE

As noted in Chapter 3, while it is convenient to have a dedicated operating room or other facility for performing bronchoscopy, the procedure can be safely performed in other areas, provided trained personnel and implements are accessible to handle and treat complications. The safety of bronchoscopy has been well authenticated by earlier studies involving multiple medical centers (177–179). However, recent years have seen the introduction of many new bronchoscopic applications and wide variations in the methods. Despite the potential for new complications as a result of these techniques, the rates for both minor and major complications have remained low (6). Nonetheless, we feel that the proven safety of bronchoscopy should not lead to complacency and indiscriminate use of the procedure (7).

Routine hospitalization for bronchoscopy is unnecessary. Even bronchoscopic lung biopsy, laser bronchoscopy, or other difficult bronchoscopic procedures do not automatically require overnight observation in the hospital. Careful postbronchoscopy observation, for several hours if appropriate, may be all that is required in such situations. Bronchoscopy is primarily an outpatient procedure. Routine hospitalization following bronchoscopic lung biopsy, recorded by 12% of ACCP survey participants, seems unjustified (Table 5). Complications such as significant bleeding, pneumothorax, respiratory distress, and other complications may require hospitalization for further evaluation and management (170,172,173,180,181).

COMPLICATIONS

Prevention and minimization of complications is part of optimal bronchoscopy. Life-threatening complications can be horrifying experiences for both the patient and the bronchoscopist. The low incidence of complications from bronchoscopic procedures is well established. However, the established safety of bronchoscopy should not induce complacency in its application. One topic that deserves special emphasis here concerns the risk of infection caused by bronchoscopy itself. Theoretically, bronchoscopy has the potential to transmit infection from the tracheobronchial tree to distant organs. It may intuitively seem that bronchoscopic procedures pose a greater risk of producing this complication because the instrument traverses the oropharyngeal area and carries with it the indigenous microorganisms to the distal tracheobronchial tree and pulmonary parenchyma. Nevertheless, postbronchoscopy infections, bacteremia, and sepsis are very uncommon (182–184). Therefore, routine culture of blood and other nonpulmonary specimens following bronchoscopy is not warranted.

ENDOCARDITIS PROPHYLAXIS

Is bronchoscopy a risk factor for infective endocarditis in susceptible individuals? We believe that the risk is very low and antibiotic prophylaxis is somewhat overused. The number of patients reported to have developed infective endocarditis following bronchoscopy has been extremely low. Prospective studies have recorded the exceedingly low risk of bacteremia following bronchoscopy (182,185). The American Heart Association (186) has recommended endocarditis prophylaxis for "rigid bronchoscopy" but not for "flexible bronchoscopy with or without biopsy." However, the recommendations include the following statement: "In patients who have prosthetic heart valves, a previous history of endocarditis, or surgically constructed systemic-pulmonary shunts or conduits, physicians may choose to administer prophylactic antibiotics even for low-risk procedures that involve the lower respiratory tract" (186). According to the Working Party of the British Society for Antimicrobial Chemotherapy (187), prophylactic antibiotics are not indicated prior to bronchoscopy. We generally concur with that suggestion even though some have argued that the benefits of routine antibiotic prophylaxis far outweigh the risk of endocarditis (188).

In our opinion, each patient should be individualized and treated accordingly. In susceptible individuals, as defined by the American Heart Association (186), either flexible or rigid bronchoscopy with bronchoalveolar lavage, biopsy of mucosa or lung, or other invasive procedures involving significant mucosal or pulmonary parenchymal trauma (laser bronchoscopy, stent placement, tracheobronchial dilatation, etc.) should be given endocarditis prophylaxis. Another indication for endocarditis prophylaxis in a susceptible individual is the presence of documented and active pulmonary or tracheobronchial infections such as lung abscess, bronchiectasis, or pneumonia in an immunocompromised patient. Bronchoscopy, either flexible or rigid, for endobronchial visualization, suction of tracheobronchial secretions or mucous plugs, or extraction of tracheobronchial foreign body does not require endocarditis prophylaxis (183).

PROTECTION OF BRONCHOSCOPY PERSONNEL

A review of the literature suggests that the risk of transmitting infection from patient to patient or from patient to bronchoscopist or bronchoscopy personnel through the bronchoscope is minimal (183). Nonetheless, infection control policies in bronchoscopy practice should comply with the following: (a) infection control precautions should apply to all patients, whether a patient is deemed infectious or not; (b) all equipment used should be dismantled (suction valve, etc.) and thoroughly washed in an appropriate neutral detergent immediately after use to remove respiratory secretions and to reduce contamination; an ultrasonic cleaner may be used prior to the disinfecting process so that the debris can be removed from the bronchoscopic accessories if manual cleaning fails; (c) strict maintenance of "clean" and "infected" areas in the bronchoscopy suite so that contaminated instruments are separated from sterile and clean equipment, (d) medical personnel in contact with each patient should wear simple barrier clothing, masks, gloves, and goggles routinely; (e) heavily contaminated bronchoscopes should be disinfected for at least 20 min (30–40 min for *M. tuberculosis*, 40 min for all unknown cases, and 4–6 hr for *M. avium-intracellulare*) in alkaline glutaraldehyde (2%) after cleaning; (f) bronchoscopy specimens for studies should be handled appropriately; (g) used disposable material should be discarded properly; (h) bronchoscopists and paramedical personnel actively involved in bronchoscopy should be vaccinated against hepatitis B virus; (i) as it is difficult to thoroughly clean nonimmersible flexible bronchoscopes, they should be phased out as soon as possible; and (j) each flexible bronchoscope should be regularly tested for leaks. If a leak is detected, the instrument should not be submersed until the leak is repaired; ethylene oxide sterilization should be considered in this situation (183).

COMPETENCY AND PROFICIENCY

Performance of 50–100 bronchoscopies (flexible bronchoscopy and rigid bronchoscopy) has been recommended to attain proficiency (189). A pulmonary specialist who completed a training program in respiratory diseases reported that a minimum of 100 bronchoscopies were necessary to acquire proficiency (190). The American Board of Thoracic Surgery requires its candidates to have performed at least "25 bronchoscopy and esophagoscopy" procedures (191). On the other hand, the eligibility requirements to appear for the pulmonary certification of the American Board of Internal Medicine do not stipulate that a definite number of bronchoscopies must have been performed by candidates during training (192). We believe that a minimum of 50 bronchoscopy procedures may be essential to achieve competency in routine flexible bronchoscopy. This should include biopsy of visible tracheobronchial lesions, bronchoalveolar lavage, and therapeutic bronchoscopy. Additionally, the completion of at least 10 bronchoscopic lung biopsies, 10 laser procedures, and 10 rigid bronchoscopy may be needed to develop proficiency in these specialized techniques (7). Undeniably, some physicians, despite the "performance" of many more than 50 bronchoscopic procedures, may remain incompetent and lack confidence in acquiring competence in the bronchoscopy. In such situations, the program director or the director of bronchoscopy at the training institution should judge and certify the competence of each candidate and recommend and provide remedial training if necessary. A minimum of 50 bronchoscopies per year may be required to maintain competence in the procedure. We and others emphasize that the performance of the procedure on a regular basis is vastly more consequential than the numbers alone (7,193).

TRAINING AND TEACHING

To produce optimal bronchoscopists, training programs in bronchoscopy should provide excellent training opportunities to students of bronchoscopy. Simple observation by a student is an insufficient method of training. Performance of bronchoscopy in both animals and humans should be included in the training program. Competency in special procedures such as laser bronchoscopy and stent placement will require additional training. The details of training and teaching are discussed in Chapter 29.

NEWER PROCEDURES

Description of newer diagnostic or therapeutic techniques invariably attracts a significant number of physicians to institute these in their practices. All too often, before the technique is validated by a sufficient number of well-designed studies, the clinicians begin routinely employing them in their clinical practice. Once this "entrenchment" occurs, the procedures attain undeserved clinical validity and it becomes almost impossible to discourage physicians from utilizing the unproven techniques. In the field of bronchoscopy, bronchoalveolar lavage, laser therapy, and stent placement are some examples. Bronchoalveolar lavage, as discussed above, is being used routinely by many bronchoscopists for the diagnosis of noninfectious and nonmalignant diffuse lung diseases such as sarcoidosis and idiopathic pulmonary fibrosis even though the test's clinical role is questionable. When laser therapy via bronchoscope was introduced, there was a rush to perform this procedure for both benign and malignant lesions by many bronchoscopists. Currently, the trend is to introduce airway stents for questionable disorders of the airways. Ideally, bronchoscopists should conduct multicenter studies to establish the clinical role of newer or questionable practices.

GUIDELINES

Bronchoscopists are divided on whether or not strict guidelines for bronchoscopy should be instituted (6). Certain basic guidelines, e.g., what type of training is required to perform bronchoscopy, can be established. However, even this may vary from country to country because of the variations in medical training. Well-defined guidelines for bronchoscopy may help avert improper and conceivably superfluous bronchoscopic procedures. When guidelines for a procedure are broad or nonexistent, the frequency of inappropriate use escalates. One study observed the inappropriate use of upper gastrointestinal endoscopy among 17% of gastroenterologists (194).

BRONCHOSCOPY FEES

In the opening paragraph of this chapter, we wrote that cost is an important aspect of optimal bronchoscopy. In the United States, the physician's charges for performing bronchoscopy are separate from charges for the processing of specimens, the use of the operating room, and the use of anesthesia personnel. Our informal survey of bronchoscopists from several countries reveals that there is a vast difference in the bronchoscopists' fees for the procedure and the governmental regulations, financial status of each country, and type of bronchoscopy practices. Therefore, it is impossible to relate the cost of bronchoscopy in different countries. Even in a single country, the United States for instance, there is a wide variation in the fee structure. In 1990, the average prevailing weighted reimbursement (professional fee) from the third-party payers for bronchoscopy in the USA was U.S. $333 and the average allowable fee U.S. $287. In the same year, the prevailing low and high fees among 10 states in the USA were U.S. $234 and U.S. $500, respectively (195). We believe that although more consistent structuring of the professional fee for bronchoscopy seems desirable on the surface, it may be inappropriate due to the complexity of economic influences in different regions of the United States. This observation perhaps applies to other nations and various regions of each country.

Cost containment in bronchoscopy includes proper care and maintenance of bronchoscopy equipment and training of bronchoscopy personnel. These aspects are addressed in Chapters 3 and 28.

REFERENCES

1. Committee on Bronchoesophagology of the American College of Chest Physicians: Standards for training in endoscopy. *Chest* 1976;69:665.
2. Guidelines for competency and training in fiberoptic bronchoscopy. Section on Bronchoscopy, American College of Chest Physicians. *Chest* 1982;81:739.
3. Greve JJ, Adamson J, Caldwell EJ III, Edsall JR, Sugg WC, Zavala DC. Guidelines for Bronchoscopy. *ATS News* 1983 (Winter).
4. Sokolowsky JW, Burgher LW, Jones FL. Guidelines for fiberoptic bronchoscopy. *ATS News* 1986 (Spring).
5. Guidelines for fiberoptic bronchoscopy in adults. American Thoracic Society. Medical Section of the American Lung Association. *Am Rev Resp Dis* 1987;136:1066.
6. Prakash UBS, Offord KP, Stubbs SE. Bronchoscopy in North America: the ACCP survey. *Chest* 1991;100:1668–1675.
7. Prakash UBS, Stubbs SE. The bronchoscopy survey: some reflections. *Chest* 1991;100:1660.
8. Dietrich KA, Strauss RH, Cabalka AK, Zimmerman JJ, Scanlan KA. Use of flexible fiberoptic endoscopy for determination of endotracheal tube position in the pediatric patient. *Crit Care Med* 1988;16:884.
9. Tucker GF, Olsen AM, Andrews AH Jr, Pool JL. The flexible fiberscope in bronchoscopic perspective. *Chest* 1973;64:149.
10. Grant IWB. Safety and fibreoptic bronchoscopy. *Br Med J* 1974;4:464.
11. Stradling P, Poole G. Safety and fibreoptic bronchoscopy. *Br Med J* 1974;4:717.
12. Elliott RC, Smiddy JF. The "territorial domain" of hemoptysis. *Chest* 1964;65:703.
13. Wilson JAS. The flexible fiberoptic bronchoscope. *Ann Thorac Surg* 1972;14:686.
14. Simpson FG, Arnold AG, Purvis A, Belfield PW, Muers MF, Cooke NJ. Postal survey of bronchoscopic practice by physicians in the United Kingdom. *Thorax* 1986;41:311.
15. Wedzicha JA, Pearson MC. Management of massive hemoptysis. *Resp Med* 1990;84:9.
16. Editorial. Life-threatening hemoptysis. *Lancet* 1987;1:1354.
17. Dumon J-F, Shapshay S, Bourcerau J, et al. Principles for safety in application of neodymium-YAG laser in bronchoscopy. *Chest* 1984;86:163.
18. Beamis JF Jr, Shapshay S. More about the YAG. *Chest* 1985; 87:27.
19. Hetzel MR, Smith SGT. Endoscopic palliation of tracheobronchial malignancies. *Thorax* 1991;46:325.
20. Chan AL, Tharratt RS, Siefkin AD, Albertson TE, Volz WG, Allen RP. Nd:YAG laser bronchoscopy. Rigid or fiberoptic mode? *Chest* 1990;98:271.
21. Marasso A, Gallo E, Massaglia GM, Onoscuri M, Bernardi V. Cryosurgery in bronchoscopic treatment of tracheobronchial stenosis. *Chest* 1993;103:472.
22. Vergnon J-M, Schmitt T, Alamartine E, Barthelemy J-C, Fournel P, Emonot A. Initial combined cryotherapy and irradiation for unresectable non-small cell lung cancer. *Chest* 1992; 102:1436.
23. Nunez H, Rodriguez EP, Alvarado C, et al. Foreign body aspiration extraction. *Chest* 1989;96:697.
24. Weissberg D, Schwartz I. Foreign bodies in the tracheobronchial tree. *Chest* 1987;91:730.
25. Limper AH, Prakash UBS. Tracheobroncial foreign bodies in adults. *Ann Intern Med* 1990;112:604.
26. Holinger PH, Holinger LD. Use of the open tube bronchoscope in the extraction of foreign bodies. *Chest* 1978;73:721.
27. Cooper JD, Pearson FG, Patterson GA, et al. Use of silicone stents in the management of airway problems. *Ann Thorac Surg* 1989;47:371.
28. Dumon J-F. A dedicated tracheobronchial stent. *Chest* 1990; 97:328.
29. Freitag L, Firusian N, Stamatis G, Greschuchna D. The role of bronchoscopy in pulmonary complications due to mustard gas inhalation. *Chest* 1991;100:1436–1441.
30. Prakash UBS. Chemical warfare and bronchoscopy. Editorial. *Chest* 1991;100:1486.
31. Wallace MJ, Charnsangavej C, Ogawa K, et al. Tracheobronchial tree: expandable metallic stents used in experimental and clinical applications. *Radiology* 1986;158:309.
32. Dedhia HV, Lapp NL. Nd:YAG laser bronchoscopy: rigid or fiberoptic mode? *Chest* 1991;100:587.
33. Whitlock WL, Brown CR, Young MB. Tracheobronchial foreign bodies. *Ann Intern Med* 1990;113:482.
34. de Castro FR, Lopez L, Varel A, Freixinet J. Tracheobronchial stents and fiberoptic bronchoscopy. *Chest* 1991;99:792.
35. Lan RS, Lee CH, Chiang YC, Wang WJ. Use of fiberoptic bronchoscopy to retrieve bronchial foreign bodies in adults. *Am Rev Resp Dis* 1989;140:1734.
36. Oho K, Amemiya R. Open tube bronchoscope or flexible fiberoptic bronchoscope? In: Oho K, Amemiya K, eds. *Practical fiberoptic bronchoscopy*. Tokyo: Igaku-Shoin; 1984:1.
37. George PJM, Garrett CPO, Nixon C, Netzel MR, Nanason EM, Millard FJC. Laser treatment for tracheobronchial tumours: local or general anesthesia? *Thorax* 1987;42:656.
38. Brutinel WM, Cortese DA, Edell ES, McDougall JC, Prakash UBS. Complications of Nd:YAG laser therapy. Editorial. *Chest* 1988;94:902.
39. Shea JM, Allen RP, Tharrat RS, Chan AL, Siefkin AD. Survival of patients undergoing Nd:YAG laser therapy compared with Nd:YAG laser therapy and brachytherapy for malignant airway disease. *Chest* 1993;103:1028.
40. Mantel K, Butenandt I. Tracheobronchial foreign body aspiration in childhood. A report on 224 cases. *Eur J Pediatr* 1986; 145:211.
41. Case 48, 1983. Case records of the Massachusetts General Hospital. *N Engl J Med* 198;309:1374.
42. Black RE, Choi KJ, Syme WC, Johnson DG, Matlak ME. Bronchoscopic removal of aspirated foreign bodies in children. *Am J Surg* 1984;148:778.
43. Kosloske AM. Bronchoscopic extraction of aspirated foreign bodies in children. *Am J Dis Child* 1982;136:924.
44. Monden Y, Morimoto T, Taniki T, Uyama T, Kimura S. Flexible bronchoscopy for foreign body in airway. *Tokushima J Exp Med* 1989;36:35.
45. Wood RE, Gauderer MW. Flexible fiberoptic bronchoscopy in the management of tracheobronchial foreign bodies in children: the value of a combined approach with open tube bronchoscopy. *J Pediatr Surg* 1984;19:693.
46. Jackson C, Jackson CL. *Diseases of the air and food passages of foreign body origin*. Philadelphia: WB Saunders; 1936.
47. Zavala DC, Rhodes ML. Experimental removal of foreign bod-

ies by fiberoptic bronchoscopy. *Am Rev Resp Dis* 1974; 110:357.
48. Lillington GA, Ruhl RA, Peirce TH, Gorin AB. Removal of endobronchial foreign body by fiberoptic bronchoscopy. *Am Rev Resp Dis* 1976;113:387.
49. Ikeda S. *Atlas of flexible bronchoscopy*. Baltimore: University Park Press; 1974.
50. Barrett CR Jr, Vecchione JJ, Bell AL Jr. Flexible fiberoptic bronchoscopy for airway management during acute respiratory failure. *Am Rev Resp Dis* 1974;109:429.
51. Wanner A, Landa JF, Nieman RE Jr, Vevaina J, Delgado I. Bedside bronchofiberscopy for atelectasis and lung abscess. *JAMA* 1973;224:1281.
52. Lan R-S, Lee C-H, Chiang Y-C, Wang WJ. Use of fiberoptic bronchoscopy to retrieve bronchial foreign bodies in adults. *Am Rev Resp Dis* 1989;140:1734.
53. Whitlock WL, Brown CR, Young MB. Tracheobronchial foreign Bodies. *Ann Intern Med* 1990;113:482–483.
54. Moss R, Kanchanapoon V. Stone basket extraction of a bronchial foreign body (letter). *Arch Surg*. 1986;121:975.
55. Inhaled foreign bodies. Editorial. *Br Med J* 1980;282:1649.
56. Dajani AM. Bronchial foreign body removed with a Dormia basket. *Lancet* 1971;1:1076.
57. Kosloske AM. The Fogarty balloon technique for the removal of foreign bodies from the tracheobronchial tree. *Surg Gynecol Obstet* 1982;155:72.
58. Zavala DC, Rhodes ML. Foreign body removal: a new role for the fiberoptic bronchoscope. *Ann Otol Rhinol Laryngol* 1975; 84:650.
59. Heinz GJ III, Richardson RH, Zavala DC. Endobronchial foreign body removal using the bronchofiberscope. *Ann Otol Rhinol Laryngol* 1978;87:50.
60. Fieselmann JF, Zavala DC, Keim LW. Removal of foreign bodies (two teeth) by fiberoptic bronchoscopy. *Chest* 1977;72:241.
61. Zavala DC, Rhodes ML, Richardson RH, Bedell GN. Fiberoptic and rigid bronchoscopy: the state of the art. Editorial. *Chest* 1974;65:605.
62. McCullough P. Wire basket removal of a large endobronchial foreign body. *Chest* 1985;87:270.
63. Hiller C, Lerner S, Varnum R, et al. Foreign body removal with the flexible fiberoptic bronchoscope. *Endoscopy* 1977;9:216.
64. Sen RP, Walsh TE. Bronchoscopy. Enough or too much? *Chest* 1989;96:710.
65. Rohwedder JJ. Enticements for fruitless bronchoscopy. *Chest* 1989;96:708.
66. McCaughan JS. Bronchoscopy in North America: the ACCP survey. (letter). *Chest* 1992;102:1639.
67. Prakash UBS, Stubbs, SE. Bronchoscopy in North America: the ACCP survey. (letter). *Chest* 1992;102:1640.
68. Feld R, Pater J, Goodwin PJ, Grossman R, Coy P, Murray N. The restaging of responding patients with limited small cell lung cancer. *Chest* 1993;103:1010.
69. Irwin S, Curley FJ, French CL. Chronic cough. The spectrum and frequency of causes, key components of the diagnostic evaluation, and outcome of specific therapy. *Am Rev Resp Dis* 1990;141:640–647.
70. Poe RH, Israel RH, Utell MJ, Hall WJ. Chronic cough: bronchoscopy or pulmonary function testing. *Am Rev Resp Dis* 1982;126:160–162.
71. Poe RH, Harder RV, Israel RH, Kallay MC. Chronic persistent cough: experience in diagnosis and outcome using an anatomic diagnostic protocol. *Chest* 1989;95:723–728.
72. Irwin RS, Curley FJ. Is the anatomic, diagnostic work-up of chronic cough not all that it is hacked up to be? (editorial). *Chest* 1989;95:711.
73. Irwin RS, Corrao WM, Pratter MR. Chronic persistent cough in the adult: the spectrum and frequency of causes and successful outcome of specific therapy. *Am Rev Resp Dis* 1981;123:413.
74. Sen RP, Walsh TE. Fiberoptic bronchoscopy for refractory cough. *Chest* 1991;99:33–35.
75. Shure D. Radiologically occult endobronchial obstruction in bronchogenic carcinoma. *Am J Med* 1991;91:19.
76. Barrio JL, Harcup C, Baier HJ, Pitchenik AE. Value of repeat fiberoptic bronchoscopies and significance of nondiagnostic bronchoscopic results in patients with the acquired immunodeficiency syndrome. *Am Rev Resp Dis* 1987;135:422.
77. Olopade CO, Prakash UBS. Bronchoscopy in the critical care unit. *Mayo Clin Proc* 1989;64:1255.
78. Jimenez P, Saldias F, Meneses M, Silva ME, Wilson MG, Otth L. Diagnostic fiberoptic bronchoscopy in patients with community-acquired pneumonia. Comparison between bronchoalveolar lavage and telescoping plugged catheter cultures. *Chest* 1993;103:1023.
79. Stover DE, Zaman MB, Hajdu SI, Lange M, Gold J, Armstrong D. Bronchoalveolar lavage in the diagnosis of diffuse pulmonary infiltrates in the immunosuppressed host. *Ann Intern Med* 1984;101:1.
80. Chastre J, Viau F, Brun P, et al. Prospective evaluation of the protected specimen brush for the diagnosis of pulmonary infections in ventilated patient. *Am Rev Resp Dis* 1984;130:924.
81. Hertz MI, Woodward ME, Gross CR, Swart M, Marcy TW, Bitterman PB. Safety of bronchoalveolar lavage in the critically ill, mechanically ventilated patient. *Crit Care Med* 1991; 19:1526.
82. Su W-J, Lee P-Y, Perng R-P. Chest roentgenographic guidelines in the selection of patients for fiberoptic bronchoscopy. *Chest* 1993;103:1198.
83. Upham JW, Mitchell CA, Armstrong JG, Kelly WT. Investigation of pleural effusion: the role of bronchoscopy. *Aust N Z J Med* 1992;22:41.
84. George JN, Shattil SJ. The clinical importance of acquired abnormalities of platelet function. *N Engl J Med* 1991;324:27–39.
85. Zavala DC. Pulmonary hemorrhage in fiberoptic bronchoscopy. *Chest* 1976;70:584–588.
86. Zavala DC. Transbronchial biopsy in diffuse lung disease. *Chest* 1978;73:727–733.
87. Rodgers RPC, Levin J. A critical appraisal of the bleeding time. *Semin Thromb Hemost* 1990;16:1–20.
88. Lind SE. The bleeding time does not predict surgical bleeding. *Blood* 1991;77:2547–2552.
89. Connolly JP. Hemoptysis as a presentation of mild hemophilia A in an adult. *Chest* 1993;103:1281.
90. Suchman AL, Mushlin AI. How well does the activated partial thromboplastin time predict postoperative hemorrhage? *JAMA* 1986;256:750–753.
91. Matsushima Y, Jones RL, King EG, Moysa G, Alton JD. Alterations in pulmonary mechanics and gas exchange during routine fiberoptic bronchoscopy. *Chest* 1984;86:184.
92. Belen J, Neuhaus A, Markowitz D, Rotman HH. Modification of the effect of fiberoptic bronchoscopy on pulmonary mechanics. *Chest* 1981;79:516.
93. Peacock AJ, Benson-Mitchell R, Godfrey R. Effect of fibreoptic bronchoscopy on pulmonary function. *Thorax* 1990; 45:38–41.
94. Albertini RE, Harrell JH, Kurihara N, Moser KM. Arterial hypoxemia induced by fiberoptic bronchoscopy. *JAMA* 1974; 230:1666–1667.
95. Colt HG, Morris JF. Fiberoptic bronchoscopy without premedication. A retrospective study. *Chest* 1990;98:1327–1330.
96. Mendes-de-Leon C, Bezel R, Karrer W, Brandli O. Premedication in fiberoptic bronchoscopy from the patient's and the physician's viewpoint—a randomized study for the comparison of midazolam and hydrocodone. *Schweiz Med Wochenschr* 1986; 116:1267–1272.
97. Pearce SJ. Fibreoptic bronchoscopy: is sedation really necessary? *Br Med J* 1980;281:779–780.
98. Goroszeniuk T. Premedication for fibreoptic bronchoscopy: fentanyl, diazepam, and atropine compared with papaveretum and hyoscine. *Br Med J* 1980;281:486.
99. Zavala DC. Complications following fiberoptic bronchoscopy. The "good news" and the "bad news." *Chest* 1978; 73:783–785.
100. Prakash UBS, Stubbs SE. Bronchoscopy: indications and technique. *Semin Resp Med* 1981;3:17–24.
101. Rees PJ, Hay JG, Webb JR. Premedication for fiberoptic bronchoscopy. *Thorax* 1983;38:624–627.

102. Goroszeniuk T, Nicholas IH, Marchant P, Turner JAM, Johnson NM. Premedication for fiberoptic bronchoscopy: fentanyl, diazepam, and atropine compared with papaveretum and lignocaine. *Br Med J* 1980;281:486.
103. Thorburn JR, James MF, Feldman C, Moyes DG, Du-Toit PS. Comparison of the effects of atropine and glycopyrrolate on pulmonary mechanics in patients undergoing fiberoptic bronchoscopy. *Anesth Analg* 1986;65:1285.
104. Driessen JJ, Smets MJ, Goey LS, Booij LH. Comparison of diazepam and midazolam as oral premedicants for bronchoscopy under local anesthesia. *Acta Anaesthesiol Belg* 1982; 33:99.
105. McCloy RF, Pearson RC. Which agent and how to deliver it? A review of benzodiazepine sedation and its reversal in endoscopy. *Scand J Gastroenterol* (Suppl)1990;179:7.
106. Tolia V, Fleming SL, Kauffman RE. Randomized, double-blind trial of midazolam and diazepam for endoscopic sedation in children. *Dev Pharmacol Ther* 1990;14:141.
107. Halim B, Schneider I, Claeys MA, Camu F. The use of midazolam and flumazenil in locoregional anaesthesia: an overview. *Acta Anaesthesiol Scand* (Suppl)1990;92:42.
108. Brouillette DE, Leventhal R, Kumar S, et al. Midazolam versus diazepam for combined esophogastroduodenoscopy and colonoscopy. *Dig Dis Sci* 1989;34:1265.
109. Lee MG, Hanna W, Harding H. Sedation for upper gastrointestinal endoscopy: a comparative study of midazolam and diazepam (comments). *Gastrointest Endosc* 1989;35:82.
110. Sutherland LR, Goldenberg E, Hershfield N, Price L, MacCannell K, Shaffer E. Midazolam in upper gastrointestinal endoscopy: a single-blind dose-finding study. *Clin Invest Med* 1989; 12:99.
111. Boldy DA, Lever LR, Unwin PR, Spencer PA, Hoare AM. Sedation for endoscopy: midazolam or diazepam and pethidine? (comments). *Br J Anaesth* 1988;61:698.
112. Bianchi-Porro G, Baroni S, Parente F, Lazzaroni M. Midazolam versus diazepam as premedication for upper gastrointestinal endoscopy: a randomized, double-blind, crossover study. *Gastrointest Endosc* 1988;34:252.
113. Clyburn P, Kay NH, McKenzie PJ. Effects of diazepam and midazolam on recovery from anaesthesia in outpatients. *Br J Anaesth* 1986;58:872.
114. Shelley MP, Wilson P, Norman J. Sedation for fibreoptic bronchoscopy. *Thorax* 1989;44:769–775.
115. Hennessy MJ, Kirkby KC, Montgomery IM. Comparison of the amnesic effects of midazolam and diazepam. *Psychopharmacology (Berl).* 1991;103:545.
116. Chung F, Cheng DC, Seyone C, Dyck BJ. A randomized comparison of midazolam and diazepam injectable emulsion in cataract surgery. *Can J Anaesth* 1990;37:528.
117. Sanders LD, Davies-Evans J, Rosen M, Robinson JO. Comparison of diazepam with midazolam as i.v. sedation for outpatient gastroscopy. *Br J Anaesth* 1989;63:726.
118. Bell GD, Spickett GP, Reeve PA, Morden A, Logan RFA. Intravenous midazolam for upper gastrointestinal endoscopy: a study of 800 consecutive cases relating dose to age and sex of patient. *Br J Clin Pharmacol* 1987;23:241–243.
119. Smith MT, Heazlewood V, Eadie TO, Tyrer JH. Pharmacokinetics of midazolam in the aged. *Eur J Clin Pharmacol* 1984; 26:381–388.
120. Reed AP. Preparation of the patient for awake flexible fiberoptic bronchoscopy. *Chest* 1992;101:244.
121. Teale C, Gomes PJ, Muers MF, Pearson SB. Local anaesthesia for fibreoptic bronchoscopy: comparison between intratracheal cocaine and lignocaine. *Resp Med* 1990;84:407.
122. Webb J. Local anaesthesia for fibreoptic bronchoscopy—where are we now? *Resp Med* 1990;84:349.
123. Middleton RM, Shah A, Kirkpatrick MB. Topical anesthesia for flexible bronchoscopy. A comparison of our methods in normal subjects and in patients undergoing transnasal bronchoscopy. *Chest* 1991;99:1093.
124. Graham DR, Hay JG, Clague J, Nisar M, Earis JE. Comparison of three different methods used to achieve local anesthesia for fiberoptic bronchoscopy. *Chest* 1992;102:704.
125. Webb AR, Fernando SSD, Dalton HR, Arrowsmith JE, Woodhead MA, Cummin ARC. Local anaesthesia for fibreoptic bronchoscopy: transcricoid injection or the "spray as you go" technique? *Thorax* 1990;45:474.
126. Patterson JR, Balschke TF, Hunt KK, Meffin PJ. Lidocaine blood concentrations during fiberoptic bronchoscopy. *Am Rev Resp Dis* 1975;112:53–57.
127. Jones DA, McBurney A, Stanley PJ, Tovey C, Ward KW. Plasma concentrations of lignocaine and its metabolites during fibreoptic bronchoscopy. *Br J Anaesth* 1982;54:853–877.
128. Fry WA. Techniques of topical anesthesia for bronchoscopy. *Chest* 1978;73:694–696.
129. Perrin G, Colt HG, Martin C, Mak M-A, Dumon J-F, Gouin F. Safety of interventional rigid bronchoscopy using intravenous anesthesia and spontaneous associated ventilation. *Chest* 1992; 102:1526.
130. Editorial. Safety and fiberoptic bronchoscopy. *Br Med J* 1974; 3:542–543.
131. Karetzky MS, Garvey JW, Brandsetter RD. Effect of fiberoptic bronchoscopy on arterial oxygen tension. *NY State J Med* 1974;74:62–63.
132. Dubrawsky C, Awe RJ, Jenkins DG. The effect of bronchofibrescopic examination on oxygenation status. *Chest* 1975; 67:137–140.
133. Randazzo GP, Wilson AF. Cardiopulmonary changes during flexible fiberoptic bronchoscopy. *Respiration* 1976; 33:143–149.
134. Lindholm CE, Ollman B, Snyder JV, Miller EG, Grenvik A. Cardiorespiratory effects of flexible fibreoptic bronchoscopy in critically ill patients. *Chest* 1978;74:362–368.
135. Albertini RE, Harrell JH, Moser KM. Management of arterial hypoxemia induced by fiberoptic bronchoscopy. *Chest* 1975; 67:134–136.
136. Fulkerson WJ. Fiberoptic bronchoscopy. *N Engl J Med* 1984; 311:511–515.
137. Richardson RH. Endotracheal tube bronchoscopy. *Ann Intern Med* 1972;76:512.
138. Sackner MA, Landa JF. Bronchofiberscopy: to intubate or not intubate (editorial). *Chest* 1973;63:302.
139. Smiddy JF, Ruth WE, Kerby GR, et al. Flexible fiberoptic bronchoscope. *Ann Intern Med* 1971;75:971–972.
140. Hodgkin JE, Rosenow EC III, Stubbs SE. Oral introduction of the flexible bronchoscope. *Chest* 1975;68:88–90.
141. Sanderson DR, McDougall JC. Transoral bronchofiberoscopy. *Chest* 1978;73(suppl):701–703.
142. Amikam B, Landa J, West J, et al. Bronchofiberscopic observations of the tracheobronchial tree during intubation. *Am Rev Resp Dis* 1972;105:747–755.
143. Zavala DC, Rhodes ML, Richardson RH, et al. Fiberoptic and rigid bronchoscopy: the state of the art (editorial). *Chest* 1974; 65:605–606.
144. Dotson RG, Pingleton SK. The effect of antibiotic therapy on recovery of intracellular bacteria from bronchoalveolar lavage in suspected ventilator-associated nosocomial pneumonia. *Chest* 1993;103:541.
145. Chollet S, Soler P, Dournova P, Richard MS, Ferrans VJ, Basset F. Diagnosis of pulmonary histiocytosis-X by immunodetection of Langerhans' cells in bronchoalveolar lavage fluid. *Am J Pathol* 1984;115:225–229.
146. American Thoracic Society. Clinical role of bronchoalveolar lavage in adults with pulmonary disease. *Am Rev Resp Dis* 1990;142:481–486.
147. Prakash UBS, Barham SS, Carpenter HA, Dines DE, Marsh HM. Pulmonary phospholipoproteinosis. Experience with 34 cases and a review. *Mayo Clin Proc* 1987;62:499–518.
148. Daniele RP, Elias JA, Epstein PE, Rossman MD. Bronchoalveolar lavage: role in the pathogenesis, diagnosis, and management of interstitial lung disease. *Ann Intern Med* 1985; 102:93–108.
149. Dejaegher P, Demendts M. Bronchoalveolar lavage in eosinophilic pneumonia before and during corticosteroid therapy. *Am Rev Resp Dis* 1984;129:631–632.
150. Linder J, Radio SJ, Robbins RA, Ghafouri M, Rennard I. Bron-

choalveolar lavage in the cytologic diagnosis of carcinoma of the lung. *Acta Cytol* 1987;31:796–797.
151. Bellmont J, DeGracia J, Morales S, Orriols R, Tallado S. Cytologic diagnosis in bronchoalveolar lavage specimens. *Chest* 1990;98:513–514.
152. Prakash UBS. Pulmonary eosinophilic granuloma. In: Lynch JP III, DeRemee RA, eds. *Immunologically mediated pulmonary diseases*. Philadelphia: JB Lippincott; 1991;432–448.
153. Levy H, Horak DA, Leurs MI. The value of bronchial washings and bronchoalveolar lavage in the diagnosis of lymphangitic carcinomatosis. *Chest* 1988;94:1028–1030.
154. Prakash UBS. Pulmonary eosinophilic granuloma. In: Lynch JP III, De Remee RA, eds. *Immunologic pulmonary diseases*. Philadelphia: JB Lippincott; 1991:432.
155. Rennard SI. Bronchoalveolar lavage in the diagnosis of lung cancer. *Lung* 1990;168(suppl):1035.
156. Rennard SI. Bronchoalveolar lavage in the diagnosis of lung cancer. *Chest* 1992;102:331.
157. Gracia JD, Bravo C, Miravittles M, et al. Diagnostic value of bronchoalveolar lavage in peripheral lung cancer. *Am Rev Resp Dis* 1993;147:649.
158. Hernandez-Blasco L, Sanchez-Hernandez IM, Villena-Garrido V, de-Miguel-Poch E, Nunez-Delgado M, Alfaro-Abreu J. Safety of the transbronchial biopsy in outpatients. *Chest* 1991; 99:562.
159. Örtqvist A, Kalin M, Lejdeborn L, Lundberg B. Diagnostic fiberoptic bronchoscopy and protected brush culture in patients with community-acquired pneumonia. *Chest* 1990;97:576.
160. Thorpe J, Baugham R, Frame PT, Wesseler AT, Staneck JL. Bronchoalveolar lavage for diagnosing acute bacterial pneumonia. *J Infect Dis* 1987;155:862.
161. Kahn FW, Jones JM. Diagnosing bacterial respiratory infections by bronchoalveolar lavage. *J Infect Dis* 1987;155:862.
162. Violan JS, de Castro FR, Luna JC, Benitez AB, Alonzo JLM. Comparative efficacy of bronchoalveolar lavage and telescoping plugged catheter in the diagnosis of pneumonia in mechanically ventilated patients. *Chest* 1993;103:386.
163. Wang KP. Transbronchial needle biopsy for histology specimens. *Chest* 1989;96:226.
164. Shure D. Transbronchial biopsy and needle aspiration. *Chest* 1989;95:1130.
165. Shure D. Transbronchial needle aspiration—current status. *Mayo Clin Proc* 1989;64:251.
166. Schenk DA, Strollo PJ, Pickard JS, et al. Utility of the Wang 18-gauge transbronchial histology needle in the staging of bronchogenic carcinoma. *Chest* 1989;96:272.
167. Mehta AC, Curtis PS, Scalzitti ML, Meeker DP. The high price of bronchoscopy. Maintenance and repair of the flexible fiberoptic bronchoscope. *Chest* 1990;98:448–454.
168. Kvale PA. Transbronchial needle aspiration. Is it coming of age? *Chest* 1985;88:161.
169. Stangel P. Bronchoscopy: enough or not enough (letter). *Chest* 1990;89:774.
170. De Fenoyl O, Capron F, Lebeau B, Rochmaure J. Transbronchial lung biopsy: a five year experience in outpatients. *Thorax* 1989;44:956–959.
171. Puar HS, Young RC, Armstrong EM. Bronchial and transbronchial lung biopsy without fluoroscopy in sarcoidosis. *Chest* 1985;87:303–306.
172. Anders GT, Johnson JE, Bush BA, Matthews JI. Transbronchial lung biopsy without fluoroscopy. A seven year perspective. *Chest* 1988;94:557–560.
173. Ahmad M, Livingston DR, Golish JA, Mehta AC, Wiedemann HP. The safety of outpatient transbronchial lung biopsy. *Chest* 1986;90:403–405.
174. Frazier WD, Pope TL Jr, Findley LJ. Pneumothorax following transbronchial lung biopsy. Low diagnostic yield with routine chest roentgenograms. *Chest* 1990;97:539–540.
175. Milam MG, Evins AE, Sahn SA. Routine chest radiography following fiberoptic bronchoscopy. *Am Rev Resp Dis* 1988; 137:401.
176. Milam MG, Evins AE, Sahn SA. Immediate chest roentgenography following fiberoptic bronchoscopy. *Chest* 1989;96:477.
177. Pereira W Jr, Kovnat DM, Snider GL. A prospective cooperative study of complications following flexible fiberoptic bronchoscopy. *Chest* 1978;73:813–816.
178. Credle JF Jr, Smiddy JF, Elliot RC. Complications of fiberoptic bronchoscopy. *Am Rev Resp Dis* 1974;109:67–72.
179. Suratt PM, Smiddy JF, Bruber B. Deaths and complications associated with fiberoptic bronchoscopy. *Chest* 1976; 69:747–751.
180. Aelony Y. Outpatient fiberoptic bronchoscopies (letter). *Arch Intern Med* 1983;143:1837.
181. Ackart RS, Foreman DR, Klayton RJ, Donlan CJ, Munzel TL, Schuler MA. Fiberoptic bronchoscopy in outpatient facilities. *Arch Intern Med* 1983;143:30–31.
182. Djedaini K, Cohen Y, Mier L, et al. Prospective evaluation of the incidence of bacteremia after protected specimen brushing in ICU patients with and without pneumonia. *Chest* 1993; 103:383.
183. Prakash UBS. Does the bronchoscope propagate infection? *Chest* 1993;104:552–559.
184. Spach DH, Silverstein FE, Stamm WE. Transmission of infection by gastrointestinal endoscopy and bronchoscopy. *Ann Intern Med* 1993;118:117.
185. Kane RC, Cohen MH, Fossieck BE Jr, Tvardzik AV. Absence of bacteremia after fiberoptic bronchoscopy. *Am Rev Resp Dis* 1975;111:102.
186. Dajani AS, Bisno AL, Chung KJ, et al. Prevention of bacterial endocarditis. Recommendations by the American Heart Association. *JAMA* 1990;264:2919.
187. Working Party of the British Society for Antimicrobial Chemotherapy. *Lancet* 1983;2:1323.
188. Lewis LD, Cochrane GM. Bronchoscopy, a risk factor for infective endocarditis. *Lancet* 1984;2:1353.
189. Faber LP. Bronchoscopy training. *Chest* 1978;73:776–778.
190. Dull WL. Flexible fiberoptic bronchoscopy. An analysis of proficiency. *Chest* 1980;77:65.
191. The American Board of Thoracic Surgery, Inc. Booklet of Information, Chicago: January 1991:13.
192. Hudson LD, Benson JA Jr. Evaluation of clinical competence in pulmonary disease. *Am Rev Resp Dis* 1988;138:1034.
193. Rocco G, Rizzi A, Robustellini M, Massera F, Pona CD, Rossi G. Training and competence in bronchoscopy. The thoracic surgeon's viewpoint. *Chest* 1993;103:1305.
194. Kahn KL, Kosecoff J, Chassin MR, Solomon DH, Brook RH. The use and misuse of upper gastrointestinal endoscopy. *Ann Intern Med* 1988;109:664–670.
195. Personal communication from Phillip Porte, Health Division, Ryan-McGinn Inc, Washington DC, through the Office of Payment Policy, Health Care Financing Administration.

Bronchoscopy,
edited by U. B. S. Prakash.
Mayo Foundation © 1994.
Published by Raven Press, Ltd., New York.

CHAPTER 31

Newer and Miscellaneous Applications of Bronchoscopy

Udaya B. S. Prakash and Atul C. Mehta

The understanding of the tracheobronchial pathology was greatly enhanced by the introduction of bronchoscopy into clinical practice nearly a century ago. The advent of specialized telescopes for use with the rigid bronchoscope and the flexible bronchoscope in the late 1960s further advanced the capability of the bronchoscopist to examine the distal tracheobronchial tree. Currently, the field of bronchology has evolved into a major branch of pulmonary and bronchoscopy is perhaps the most commonly employed invasive diagnostic procedure in pulmonary diseases. As the quality of instrumentation is improved, newer applications will invariably follow. For example, the development of ultrathin bronchoscopes has permitted the examination of the tracheobronchial tree in the neonates. Preceding chapters have dealt with the traditional as well as newer and currently applied techniques in bronchoscopy. Many recent developments are still in their infancy and their future in the field of bronchoscopy remains to be seen. In this chapter we discuss some of these recent advances in bronchoscopy, particularly in clinical research, and their potential for future application in clinical practice.

THE BRONCHOSCOPE

The manufacturers of flexible bronchoscopes have consistently improved the attributes and performance of these instruments. The quality of the flexible bronchoscopic image is very near to that of the rigid bronchoscope-telescope system. The ability to flex the distal tip of the flexible bronchoscope has increased, thereby allowing the bronchoscopist to easily introduce the instrument into almost all segmental bronchi. Further, the ultrathin flexible bronchoscope now enables bronchoscopists to directly visualize eighth through twelfth branchings of the bronchial tree. Larger working channels and better accessory instruments should allow the bronchoscopist to obtain larger biopsies and higher quality specimens, thereby increasing the diagnostic yield.

The ultra-ultrathin flexible bronchoscope (with an outer diameter of 1.8 mm, a visual angle of 75°, a range of observation of 3–30 mm, an effective length of 950 mm, and a total length of 1,120 mm) has been used to examine the very peripheral airways. The researchers were able to introduce this instrument through the 2.6-mm channel of the conventional flexible bronchoscope to perform alveolobronchography (1). The clinical application for such an instrument in adults is unclear.

The ultrathin flexible bronchoscope is useful in the placement and assessment of endotracheal tubes. Endotracheal intubation may be difficult in situations such as trauma, hemorrhage, or deformity. The availability of an ultrathin bronchoscope facilitates intubation. These small-diameter bronchoscopes are also helpful in visualizing distal endobronchial lesions not seen with the standard flexible bronchoscope (2).

Recently, a new "needle brush" (a cytology brush with a needle at the distal tip) was developed for procuring pathologic specimens from peripheral lesions. It is reported to have a higher diagnostic yield in malignant lung masses or nodules than the regular brush and forceps biopsy (3).

Accessory instruments designed for use with the flexible bronchoscope have been used for nonbroncho-

U. B. S. Prakash: Division of Thoracic Diseases and Internal Medicine, Mayo Clinic, Rochester, Minnesota 55905.

A. C. Mehta: Department of Pulmonary and Critical Care Medicine, Cleveland Clinic Foundation, Cleveland, Ohio 44195.

scopic purposes. In one report, the authors described their experience with a flexible biopsy forceps that was used percutaneously to rapidly retrieve intravascular foreign bodies in six cases (4).

The rigid bronchoscope, while maintaining the basic structural format, has also undergone serial changes to accommodate specialized procedures such as laser bronchoscopy, stent placement, and dilatation of tracheobronchial stenosis. The newer rigid bronchoscopes allow the passage of flexible bronchoscopes, thereby enabling the bronchoscopist to take advantage of the capabilities of both instruments simultaneously.

VIDEOCHIP BRONCHOSCOPE

In order to capture a far better resolution of bronchoscopic image without the interference of the fiber net pattern of the conventional flexible bronchoscopes, a new bronchoscope with a charge-couple device (CCD) has been developed (5). The integrated circuit image-sensing device, which in essence is a tiny television camera, is incorporated into the tip of the flexible bronchoscope. The image captured is transmitted to a video processor for display on a television monitor. This camera is sometimes referred to as a videochip camera because its basic element is a silicon wafer or a chip. A disadvantage of the prototype videochip bronchoscope is its inability to accommodate a biopsy forceps through its 1.8-mm working channel.

Preliminary clinical studies using the videochip bronchoscope have demonstrated that the image quality is far superior and allows for a more accurate and detailed evaluation of mucosal surface, vascular patterns of tracheobronchial mucosa, mucosal folds, and tumor (5). The main clinical applications of this technology will be in the early detection of mucosal neoplastic changes and photographic documentation of bronchoscopic findings. It is likely that the videochip bronchoscopes will become commonplace in the near future, provided the working channel of sufficient diameter can be accommodated without increasing the outer diameter of the instrument.

BRONCHOSCOPIC ULTRASONOGRAPHY (ENDOBRONCHIAL SONOGRAPHY)

The principle underlying the use of ultrasonography in the tracheobronchial tree is the technique's theoretical ability to identify submucosal changes and lesions adjacent (extrabronchial) to the airways. Early diagnosis of mucosal cancer and identification of paratracheal, hilar, or mediastinal lymph nodes by bronchoscopic ultrasonography may alter the current modes of therapeutic approach to bronchogenic carcinoma. The device consists of an echographic camera, a transbronchoscopic ultrasonic probe, a video monitor to visualize the echographic image, and the facility to develop ultrasonographic histograms and echo enhancement. Ono and colleagues (6) described the following specifications for the prototype equipment: maximum diameters of the probe head and the probe transducer (convex type, curvilinear) are 6.3 mm and 5.0 mm, respectively, with a frequency of 7.5 MHz and an effective image field of 34°, and a scanning direction parallel to the axis.

Ono et al. (6) used the bronchoscopic ultrasonography in 25 patients and described that the thoracic aorta, pulmonary artery, esophagus, and peribronchial tissues could be clearly delineated. The probe head's diameter of 6.3 mm limited its insertion into lobar bronchi. In patients with bronchial malignancy, ultrasonography detected invasion of vessel wall and paratracheal lymph nodes. In malignancies involving the upper gastrointestinal tract, the endoscopic ultrasonography is reported to predict lymph node involvement with an 80% probability (7). One prospective study examined the diagnostic role of bronchoscopic ultrasonography in detecting the presence of mediastinal lymph nodes in 32 patients with bronchogenic carcinoma. An Olympus-Aloka EU-M2 or EU-M3 (frequency 7.5 and 12 MHz) was used, and the graded cross-sections of lymph node dissections obtained during subsequent surgery provided the correct diagnosis. Bronchoscopic ultrasonography identified the presence and estimated the size of subcarinal, tracheobronchial, paraaortic, and periesophageal lymph nodes better than computed tomography, with a diagnostic rate of malignancy in 72%. However, lymph nodes behind air-containing organs (paratracheal lymph nodes) could not be identified by ultrasonography. The overall sensitivity was 67% (because the ultrasonographic pattern of malignant lymph nodes was indistinguishable from that of lymphadenopathy secondary to anthracosilicosis) and the specificity was 86% (7). Another study (8) applied bronchoscopic ultrasonography in 100 patients with bronchogenic carcinoma and reported that the bronchial wall is highly echogenic and laminated and the lung parenchyma is echo-rich and patchy. The technique was able to differentiate the echo-poor bronchogenic carcinoma from the highly echogenic normal bronchial wall or lung parenchyma. Endobronchial sonography was also used to measure the length and diameter of bronchial stenoses, which could not be assessed by bronchoscopic visualization or roentgenography, and thus facilitated the correct implantation of stents (8).

The major obstacle to the use of bronchoscopic ultrasonography is the inability to maintain fluid–bronchial mucosal interphase during the procedure. Therefore, the tumors within the lung parenchyma are difficult to identify. Nevertheless, bronchoscopic ultrasonography holds much promise not only in the diagnosis of tracheobronchial mucosal and extrabronchial malignancy but also perhaps in the diagnosis of pulmonary thromboembolism.

DRUGS IN BRONCHOSCOPY

Cough has been a nemesis of the bronchoscopist despite the availability of lidocaine and other topical anesthetics. The presently available antitussives are partially effective in suppressing the cough. A new orally administered drug, levodropropizine, known to inhibit peripheral cough reflexes, has been tried in patients undergoing bronchoscopy. Accurate measurement of the number of coughs during and after bronchoscopy, registered on a magnetic tape and read by a blinded observer, showed that the drug significantly reduced the cough and exhibited excellent tolerability and safety (9).

Pulmonary hemorrhage is a symptom of several pulmonary diseases and a complication of certain bronchoscopic procedures. In an attempt to stop pulmonary hemorrhage, bronchoscopic instillation of glypressin, a vasopressin derivative, has shown that the chemical is as effective as it is when administered intravenously. However, the glypressin plasma level was 251-fold higher after the intravenous than after the endobronchial administration (10).

DIAGNOSTIC BRONCHOSCOPY

The bronchoscope and the bronchoscopic techniques have been applied in newer clinical disorders as well as in well-known diseases. We review several recent papers that describe newer applications of bronchoscopy.

Lung Cancer

The poor prognosis associated with advanced stage lung cancer has prompted clinicians to use newer methods for the early diagnosis of lung cancer. Kato and Horai (11) described the various methods available. Kato and associates (12) developed an excimer dye laser for the early stage diagnosis and treatment of cancer. The excimer laser beam, developed by exciting XeCl, is used for tumor localization and a 630-nm beam obtained with a rhodamine B dye is used for treatment. Fluorescence was recognized in all lesions among 11 patients and the equipment was reported to be effective for localization.

The bronchoscope will remain an invaluable tool in the research studies on lung cancer. In addition to the use of bronchoalveolar lavage, bronchoscopically obtained biopsies can be used for numerous studies. Using the polymerase chain reaction for lung tumor biopsies obtained by flexible bronchoscopy, researchers have been able to map the position of the tumor suppressor genes (13). Similarly, bronchoscopic biopsies have been used to detect and quantitate genetic damage in lung cancer (14).

In one report, the authors described a bronchoscope fitted with a brush to collect cells from patients with lung cancer. The cytological smears were examined with a fluorescent probe for the cell surface enzyme guanidinobenzoatase; abnormal cells were readily distinguished from normal cells, which were deficient in this enzyme (15).

Models of the sequential process of lung carcinomas have been developed in dogs and hamsters. Pulmonary carcinogensis has been studied in animals by using bronchoscopic techniques to deposit specific carcinogens on selected sites in the tracheobronchial mucosa (16). Bronchoscopically obtained specimens have been used to successfully establish new cell lines of small cell lung cancer to assess in vitro sensitivity to chemotherapeutic drugs and irradiation (17). The ability to establish a continually growing tumor cell line from fresh tumor specimens obtained by bronchoscopic techniques has been shown to be associated with decreased survival times in patients with small cell lung cancer. One study demonstrated that in vitro tumor cell growth is an adverse predominant prognostic factor in patients with small cell lung cancer (18).

Attempt has also been made to diagnose early superficial endobronchial tumors by nuclear scanning using a prototype endobronchial scintillation detector (19). Following intravenous administration of the tumor cell–specific radiotracer, ^{57}co-labeled bleomycin, a small thallium-activated sodium iodide (NaI) crystal is inserted through the working channel of the bronchoscope and the suspicious areas of the tracheobronchial tree are scanned. The nuclear count is gathered and the tumor site localized. The diagnosis is confirmed by usual biopsy procedures. The method lacks specificity as well as sensitivity; however, with technical advancements and more tumor cell–specific radiotracer, it seems to hold potential for the early diagnosis of the endobronchial malignancy.

The utility of bronchoalveolar lavage in the diagnosis of peripheral primary lung cancer has been studied. Among 145 patients studied (20), bronchoalveolar lavage was diagnostic of malignancy in 64.8%, although in only 35.9% the cytological diagnosis agreed with the final pathological diagnosis of the resected tumor. Highest yields were obtained in adenocarcinoma (59.2%) and alveolar cell lung cancer (80%).

Bronchioalveolar lavage has been used to obtain alveolar macrophages to study their in vitro tumoricidal activity against lung cancer and renal cell carcinoma cells in several recently published studies (21–23). This experience may form the basis for immunomodulatory treatment in patients with bronchogenic carcinoma.

Bronchoalveolar Lavage

The current clinical usefulness of bronchoalveolar lavage (BAL) in understanding immunological diseases is questionable. Nevertheless, BAL remains a powerful investigative tool. To realize its full potential in the diagnosis and management of diseases involving the lower respiratory tract, there is a great need for standardization of the technical aspects of BAL as well as processing and analysis of the BAL cellular and fluid phase components (24–28). Direct immunological investigation of the human lung has advanced greatly by the use of flexible bronchoscopy, and values for immune components in BAL have been established for normals and used to contrast abnormal findings in certain lung diseases such as sarcoidosis and hypersensitivity pneumonitis (29).

The quantification of intraalveolar phagocytes (dust scavenger cells) in the BAL effluent has been suggested as a method to assess the inhaled particle burden in subjects with pneumoconiosis. The studies to date have shown that the presence of ferruginous bodies is an indication of past occupational exposure and that the quantification of asbestos bodies by BAL is reliable (30,31). It is expected that with future research, in particular long-term prospective epidemiological and clinical studies in pneumoconioses and other interstitial lung diseases, BAL may prove more valuable in the diagnosis and management of such diseases (24,32,33).

The technique of BAL is safe even in immunocompromised patients with hypoxemia (34). BAL has been shown to be useful in the diagnosis of peripheral as well as lymphangitic lung cancer (35).

A number of modifications in BAL have been suggested in order to obtain samples relatively enriched for bronchial material. By fractional processing of BAL effluent returning after injection of each aliquot, it is possible to compare the protein concentrations in bronchial and alveolar lavages (36).

BAL has been studied extensively in the diagnosis of various lung diseases. Its role in noninfectious and nonmalignant diseases remains unclear. A prospective study measured the concentrations of secretory immunoglobulin A (slgA) in bronchial washings obtained from cancerous lungs and concluded that measurement of secretory IgA was clinically useful in the diagnosis of pulmonary malignant neoplasms (37).

BAL studies in dogs following the intravenous administration of phorbol myristate acetate to produce acute, diffuse lung inflammation have shown that there is a direct correlation between BAL percentages and neutrophils present in histological sections, thereby suggesting that BAL accurately reflects changes in the lung parenchyma in acute lung disease (38).

Many severely traumatized patients develop acute respiratory distress syndrome. In a prospective study of severely traumatized patients, Seeger and associates (39) used bronchoscopy to determine the procoagulant activity of BAL effluent. The results showed a several-fold increase in procoagulant activity in all trauma victims within the first 24 hr after injury. They concluded that a marked increase in procoagulant activity occurring in severely injured patients may favor alveolar fibrin deposition and is related to the development of acute respiratory distress syndrome.

BAL has been used to analyze the concentrations of iron, manganese, lead, and chromium in human subjects without occupational or abnormal environmental exposure to metals. The iron concentrations were higher than those of other elements, probably due partly to higher environmental exposure and partly to its essential role in humans. The diagnostic significance of element determination in BAL is unclear (40).

BAL has been measured for levels of phosphatidylcholine in smokers, who had significantly lower levels than nonsmokers (41). Bronchial biopsies have been used to study smoke-related damage to DNA (42). Similar studies may assist in the understanding of pulmonary pathology caused by tobacco smoking.

Pneumonia is a leading cause of morbidity and death in older patients, and immunodeficiency is believed to contribute to their susceptibility. BAL in geriatric subjects has shown significantly elevated numbers of neutrophils, and increased IgG, but not IgA or albumin (43). Further studies are needed to assess the clinical importance of these findings.

Asthma

The recent resurgence in the incidence of asthma and the purported increase in asthma-related mortality has prompted clinicians to study the disease in greater depth by employing bronchoscopy and BAL (44–52). One study examined the bronchoscopically obtained mucosal biopsies from the airways to evaluate the effect of long-term inhaled corticosteroid therapy. Visual inspection of the tracheobronchial tree showed no signs of atrophy, ulcerations, or thrush patches; the only abnormality noted was the epithelial desquamation (53).

Bronchoscopy, bronchial mucosal biopsy, and BAL have been used to obtain further information regarding occupational asthma. For example, detailed studies of bronchoscopically obtained specimens from subjects with asthma caused by toluene diisocyanate (TDI) have shown pathological features, such as inflammatory cell infiltrate and thickening of subepithelial collagen, similar to those described in atopic asthma, and that the avoidance of exposure to the sensitizing agent for 6 months can reverse the reticular basement membrane thickening in the bronchial mucosa but not in the inflammatory cell infiltrate (54–55).

The assay of IgM in the BAL effluent of asthmatics has shown that the increased local IgM concentrations and its increased local production may play a role in the local IgM-mediated reactions in the inflammatory events associated with asthma (56).

Others have shown that in some asthmatic subjects, transient bronchoconstriction and a lowering of oxygen tension can be induced by bronchoscopy and BAL (57).

Ciliary Function

One area in which bronchoscopy has been helpful is in the study of tracheobronchial mucus clearance rate and ciliary function in the airways. The relationship between the pulmonary mechanics and mucus clearance has been studied. King and associates (58), by using direct bronchoscopic visualization of charcoal particle transport, documented that the high-frequency oscillation of the chest wall enhances the tracheal mucus clearance rate in dogs.

Tracheobronchial ciliary dysfunction is responsible for many airway diseases. Continued studies aimed at measurement of ciliary beat frequency, movement of mucous layer, and electron microscopy on biopsies obtained with the bronchoscope will further our understanding of these diseases (59,60).

Other Diagnostic Uses

Inhalation injury to the airways, observed in approximately one third of burn patients treated at burn centers, increases the mortality (61). The development of animal models of inhalation injury using bronchoscopy and other diagnostic tests has made possible the identification of both airway and vascular responses evoked by smoke inhalation. Pruitt et al. (61) reported that early diagnosis, best achieved by bronchoscopy and xenon-133 ventilation perfusion scan, permitted timely application of high-frequency ventilation. This treatment appeared to reduce the incidence of pneumonia and decrease mortality.

Recent advances in the understanding of the genetic basis for cystic fibrosis hold promise for genetic manipulatary therapy. Bronchoscopy and BAL may provide the necessary material for future studies. Evaluation of bronchial epithelial cells obtained by bronchoscopy has been used to study gene abnormalities in patients with cystic fibrosis (62).

The flexible bronchoscope has been used to study the mechanical properties of lung. By wedging the tip of the bronchoscope in subsegmental bronchus, Wagner and colleagues (63) were able to measure peripheral airway resistance in asymptomatic smokers and nonsmoking volunteers. They used a double-lumen catheter through the working channel of the bronchoscope and infused CO_2 (5%) through one lumen and measured pressure through the second lumen.

In recent years lung transplantation has become an accepted treatment for a variety of terminal lung diseases. Successful outcome from the lung transplantation depends heavily on early diagnosis of rejection or infection, which is routinely established through the flexible bronchoscope and bronchoscopic lung biopsy (64–66). In our initial experience at the Cleveland Clinic Foundation in 22 lung transplant patients undergoing 96 flexible fiberoptic bronchoscopy procedures for a variety of indications, we found its positive predictive value at 100% and negative predictive value at 84%, especially in relation to rejection and infection (67). Flexible bronchoscopy will continue to play a major role in management and research in the area of lung transplantation.

THERAPEUTIC BRONCHOSCOPY

Tracheobronchial Stenosis

With the availability of newer modes of therapy including balloon dilatation, stent placement, and laser therapy, bronchoscopic treatment of tracheal stenosis is being applied frequently. With severe tracheal stenosis, maintenance of ventilation during bronchoscopic treatment is crucial. High-frequency jet ventilation techniques may allow the bronchoscopist to provide adequate oxygenation with general anesthesia and proceed with the treatment. In a report, six patients with airway stenosis underwent bronchoscopy under general anesthesia; each was ventilated with a gas mixture of 50% oxygen and nitrogen using manual jet insufflation. Assessment of the effects on alveolar ventilation by blood gas analysis and the transcutaneous monitoring of carbon dioxide tension showed that high-frequency jet ventilation achieves satisfactory operating conditions and provides adequate gas exchanges up to a rate of 300 breaths/min (68).

Stenosis at the anastomotic site is a complication of lung or heart–lung transplantation (66,67). Lack of blood supply at the anastomotic site is thought to be the causative factor. Knowledge of the blood flow in the airway wall may aid in understanding the pathogenesis. Godden and colleagues (69) used flexible bronchoscopy-guided laser–Doppler flowmetry, a technique that detects movement of erythrocytes, to measure tracheal and bronchial wall blood flow in anesthetized sheep. The observations showed that in addition to detecting blood flow from the bronchial artery, the technique also detected collateral circulation. The clinical role of this technique is inapparent now but may become useful in lung transplant patients.

Bronchopleural Fistula

Several types of bronchoscopy-guided treatments for disorders of the tracheobronchial tree have been tried. One area of interest has been the bronchoscopic closure of bronchopleural fistula and persistent pneumothorax. Insufficiency of the bronchial stump following lung resection, with an average incidence of 4%, is a serious complication that carries a mortality of up to 90% (70). Effective application of the bronchoscopic technique of occlusion of a persistent bronchopleural fistula requires a precise identification of the segmental location of the air leak. This has been accomplished by injections of small boluses of $^{Xe}133$ into a number of segmental bronchi through a flexible bronchoscope. Marked increase in radioactivity in the intercostal drainage tube after instillation of the $^{Xe}133$ into the segmental bronchus leading to the fistula can identify the bronchus in question (71). In an experimental study on 18 pigs, flexible bronchoscopic occlusion of infected bronchus stump fistulas was achieved with fibrin sealant (1 ml, 500 units/ml thrombin, 3,500 units/ml aprotinin). At autopsy, all bronchial stump fistulas had healed after the second postoperative week (70). With more clinical experience (72,73), bronchoscopic treatment of bronchopleural fistula in selected cases is likely to become a standard technique.

The bronchoscope has been used to detect a fistula between the pancreas and the bronchial tree. The diagnosis was made by bronchoscopy and biochemical analysis of respiratory secretions (74). Connection between the tracheobronchial tree and gastrointestinal tract through a fistula is sometimes difficult to diagnose. A case has been described in which the bronchoscopically obtained secretion was measured for its low pH, thereby establishing the diagnosis of gastrobronchial fistula (75).

Retained Secretions and Mucous Plugs

One reason for the exacerbation of asthma is the mucoid impaction in the bronchi. Lang et al. (76) performed 51 therapeutic flexible bronchoscopies in 19 patients during 20 episodes of refractory asthma and reported no significant complications. Following bronchoscopy, spirometric measurements increased significantly and correlated with relief of dyspnea and mobilization of secretions with cough. Others have also demonstrated the safety of bronchoscopy in patients suffering from asthma (77). Nevertheless we believe that therapeutic bronchoscopy for removal of respiratory secretion has a limited role in patients with asthma and cystic fibrosis.

Other Therapeutic Uses

The placement of an endobronchial catheter for purposes of bronchoscopic brachytherapy and other diagnostic reasons can be tricky and occasionally difficult. Using a flexible bronchoscope, a "bronchoscopic shuttle" has been used to circumvent some of the limitations (78).

Endobronchial administration of antineoplastic, antifungal, or antituberculous drugs through the bronchoscope is being evaluated. Bronchoscopic administration of radiolabeled monoclonal antibodies with specific targeting of bronchial tumors has been reported to be a feasible technique (79).

PEDIATRIC BRONCHOSCOPY

Newer pediatric bronchoscopes may enter the market and increase the ability of the pediatric bronchoscopist to reach the distal reaches of neonatal airways (80). The ultrathin bronchoscope may further the understanding of neonatal lung diseases. The ultrathin flexible bronchoscope with a single lumen and an outer diameter of 2.7 mm at the distal tip has been utilized to assist intubation of pediatric patients with difficult airways (81). The flexible bronchoscope, however small its outer diameter, interferes with normal breathing by partially obstructing the trachea. The ultrathin bronchoscope, if it has a suction channel, can be used to deliver supplemental oxygen through the suction channel. Ventilation can also be provided through the suction channel of the flexible bronchoscope. Monden and colleagues (82) used a flexible bronchoscope with a channel of more than 1.2 mm in diameter that was directly inserted into the trachea under general anesthesia without an orotracheal tube. The first step was the flushing of pure oxygen into the lung through the channel during inspiration. The next step was the aspiration of expired gases through the channel. Repetition of these two steps adequately maintained optimal ventilation. The physicians were able to perform bronchoscopy continuously for 5 min in most cases.

Bronchoscopy and BAL in children with the acquired immunodeficiency syndrome and acute lower respiratory tract disease has been shown to be a safe and effective diagnostic procedure with a diagnostic yield of 80% in identifications of infectious agents (83).

Major vascular lesions in pediatric patients occasionally produce extrinsic compression of the tracheobronchial tree. In such patients, bronchoscopic examination along with magnetic resonance imaging are the two most important diagnostic tests (84).

Modifications in rigid bronchoscopy for application in pediatric patients continue to be made. Newer instruments allow the use of a rigid bronchoscope along with fiberoptic telescopes. Other accessories described include a J-shaped suction catheter tailored to facilitate aspiration of the right upper lobe bronchus during rigid bronchoscopy in pediatric patients. This suction catheter was used successfully in three patients (85).

OTHER USES

The flexible bronchoscope has been used to measure collateral airway resistance in normal humans. The flexible bronchoscope was introduced under local anesthesia and wedged into a subsegmental bronchus of the right lower lobe; a Swan–Ganz catheter was tightly fitted into the suction port of the bronchoscope and one lumen of the catheter served to deliver a constant flow of 5% CO_2 in air. The pressure in the wedged segment was measured by the other channel. Airway pressure was determined with a flow catheter taped to the side of the bronchoscope (86).

An airway pressure sensor that can be introduced through the flexible bronchoscope has been developed. The airway pressure sensor catheter was introduced to the right lower lobe bronchus through a flexible bronchoscope until the tip is wedged, at which point the bronchoscope is removed. Simultaneous measurements of the mouth flow, mouth pressure, and transpulmonary pressure by the esophageal balloon technique during tidal breathing was accomplished. By this method, researchers were able to obtain central airway resistance and peripheral airway resistance (87).

One approach to the study of the pharmacokinetics of drugs in the lung is to measure their concentrations in bronchial mucosa. Studies by Baldwin and associates (88) indicate that the tracheobronchial mucosal biopsies obtained by bronchoscopy can be utilized for this purpose.

REFERENCES

1. Tanaka M, Satoh M, Kawanami O, Aihara K. A new bronchofiberscope for the study of diseases of very peripheral airways. *Chest* 1984;85:590–594.
2. Prakash UBS. The use of pediatric fiberoptic bronchoscope in adults. *Am Rev Resp Dis* 1985;132:715–717.
3. Wang KP, Britt EJ. Needle brush in the diagnosis of lung mass or nodule through flexible bronchoscopy. *Chest* 1991; 100:1148–1150.
4. Millan VG. Retrieval of intravascular foreign bodies using a modified bronchoscopic forceps. *Radiology* 1978;129:587–589.
5. Ono R, Edell ES, Ikeda S. Newly developed bronchoscope. In: Inoue T, ed. Recent advances in bronchoesophagology. Proceedings of the 6th World Congress of Bronchoesophagology. Amsterdam: Excerpta Medica; 1990:49–53.
6. Ono R, Suemasu K, Matsunaka T. Bronchoscopic ultrasonography in the diagnosis of lung cancer. *Jpn J Clin Oncol* 1993;23: 34–40.
7. Schuder G, Isringhaus H, Kubale B, Seitz G, Sybrecht GW. Endoscopic ultrasonography of the mediastinum in the diagnosis of bronchial carcinoma. *Thorac Cardiovasc Surg* 1991; 39:299–303.
8. Hurter T, Hanrath P. Endobronchial sonography: feasibility and preliminary results. *Thorax* 1992;47:565–567.
9. Guarino C, Cautiero V, Cordaro C, Catena E. Levodropropizine in the premedication to fibrebronchoscopy. *Drugs Exp Clin Res* 1991;17:237–241.
10. Breuer HW, Charchut S, Worth H, Trampisch HJ, Glanzer K. Endobronchial versus intravenous application of the vasopressin derivative glypressin during diagnostic bronchoscopy. *Eur Respir J* 1989;2:225–228.
11. Kato H, Horai T. *Color atlas of endoscopic diagnosis of early stage lung cancer.* St. Louis: Mosby; 1992.
12. Kato H, Imaizumi T, Aizawa K, et al. Photodynamic diagnosis in respiratory tract malignancy using an excimer dye laser system. *J Photochem Photobiol B* 1990;6:189–196.
13. Ganly PS, Jarad N, Rudd RM, Rabbitts PH. PCR-based RFLP analysis allows genotyping of the short arm of chromosome 3 in small biopsies from patients with lung cancer. *Genomics* 1992; 12:221–228.
14. Dunn BP, Vedal S, San RH, et al. DNA adducts in bronchial biopsies. *Int J Cancer* 1991;48:485–492.
15. Steven FS, Lam S, Macaulay C, Palcic B. Fluorescent location of abnormal cells in cell smears obtained from the lungs of patients with lung cancer. *Anticancer Res* 1992;12:625–629.
16. Benfield JR, Hammond WG. Bronchial and pulmonary carcinogenesis at focal sites in dogs and hamsters. *Cancer Res* 1992; 52(Suppl):2687s–2693s.
17. Tanio Y, Watanabe M, Inoue T, et al. Chemo-radioresistance of small cell lung cancer cell lines derived from untreated primary tumors obtained by diagnostic bronchofiberscopy. *Jap J Cancer Res* 1990;81:289–297.
18. Masuda N, Fukuoka M, Matsui K, et al. Establishment of tumor cell lines as an independent prognostic factor for survival time in patients with small-cell lung cancer. *JNCI* 1991;83:1743–1748.
19. Woolfenden JM, Nevin WS, Bradford Barber HB, Donahue DJ. Lung cancer detection using a miniature sodium iodide detector and cobalt-57 bleomycin. *Chest* 1984;85:84–88.
20. Pirozynski M. Bronchoalveolar lavage in the diagnosis of peripheral, primary lung cancer (comments). *Chest* 1992;102:372–374.
21. Thomassen MJ, Wiedemann HP, Barna BP, Farmer M, Ahmad M. Induction of in vitro tumoricidal activity in alveolar macrophages and monocytes from patients with lung cancer. *Cancer Res* 1988;48:3949–3953.
22. Thomassen MJ, Barna BP, Wiedemann HP, Bukowski RM, Farmer M, Ahamd M. Immunologic studies of alveolar macrophages from patients with metatstatic renal cell carcinoma. *Am Rev Resp Dis* 1990;141:1256–1258.
23. Thomassen MJ, Ahmad M, Barna BP, et al. Induction of cytokine messenger RNA and secretions in alveolar macrophages and blood monocytes from patients with lung cancer receiving granulocyte-macrophage colony-stimulating factor therapy. *Cancer Res* 1991;51:857–862.
24. Goldstein RA, Rohatgi PK, Bergofsky EH, et al. Clinical role of bronchoalveolar lavage in adults with pulmonary disease (comments). *Am Rev Resp Dis* 1990;142:481–486.
25. Schumacher U, Mausolf A, Barth J, Welsch U, Petermann W. Recovery of proteins from the broncho-alveolar lavage fluid proposal for a standardisation. *Eur J Clin Chem Clin Biochem* 1992; 30:11–14.
26. Low RB, Giancola MS, King TE Jr, Chapitis J, Vacek P, Davis

GS. Serum and bronchoalveolar lavage of N-terminal type III procollagen peptides in idiopathic pulmonary fibrosis. *Am Rev Resp Dis* 1992;146:701–706.
27. King TE Jr, Mortenson RL. Bronchoalveolar lavage in patients with connective tissue disease. *J Thorac Imag* 1992;7:26–48.
28. Walters EH, Gardiner PV. Bronchoalveolar lavage as reaserch tool. *Thorax* 1991;46:613–618.
29. Reynolds HY, Huck JL. Immunologic responses in the lung. *Respiration* 1990;57:221–228.
30. Dodson RF, Garcia JG, OSullivan M, et al. The usefulness of bronchoalveolar lavage in identifying past occupational exposure to asbestos: a light and electron microscopy study. *Am J Ind Med* 1991;19:619–628.
31. Schwartz DA, Galvin JR, Burmeister LF, et al. The clinical utility and reliability of asbestos bodies in bronchoalveolar fluid. *Am Rev Resp Dis* 1991;144:684–688.
32. Nair P, Rupawate RU, Prabhakaran LC, Bijur S, Kamat SR. Evaluating computed tomography and bronchoalveolar lavage in early diagnosis of pulmonary asbestosis. *Sarcoidosis* 1991; 8:115–119.
33. Newman LS, Orton R, Kreiss K. Serum angiotensin converting enzyme activity in chronic beryllium disease. *Am Rev Resp Dis* 1992;146:39–42.
34. Verra F, Hmouda H, Rauss A, et al. Bronchoalveolar lavage in immunocompromised patients: clinical and functional consequences. *Chest* 1992;101:1215–1220.
35. Rennard SI, Spurzem JR. Bronchoalveolar lavage in the diagnosis of lung cancer (editorial; comment). *Chest* 1992;102:331–332.
36. Rennard SI, Ghafouri M, Thompson AB, et al. Fractional processing of sequential bronchoalveolar lavage to separate bronchial and alveolar samples. *Am Rev Resp Dis* 1990;141:208–217.
37. Pisani RJ, Cortese DA, Homburger HA, Grambsch PM. A prospective pilot study evaluating the effectiveness of secretory IgA measurements in bronchoalveolar lavage to detect non-small cell lung cancer. *Chest* 1990;97:586–589.
38. Weiland JE, Dorinsky PM, Davis WB, Lucas JG, Gadek JE. Validity of bronchoalveolar lavage in acute lung injury: recovered cells accurately reflect changes in the lung parenchyma. *Pathology* 1989;21:59–62.
39. Seeger W, Hubel J, Klapettek K, et al. Procoagulant activity in bronchoalveolar lavage of severely traumatized patients—relation to the development of acute respiratory distress. *Thromb Res* 1991;61:53–64.
40. Romeo L, Maranelli G, Malesani F, Tommasi I, Cazzadori A, Graziani MS. Tentative reference values for some elements in broncho-alveolar lavage fluid. *Sci Total Environ* 1992; 120:103–110.
41. Schmekel B, Khan AR, Linden M, Wollmer P. Recoveries of phosphatidylcholine and alveolar macrophages in lung lavage from healthy light smokers. *Clin Physiol* 1991;11:431–438.
42. Benner SE, Lippman SM, Wargovich MJ, et al. Micronuclei in bronchial biopsy specimens from heavy smokers: characterization of an intermediate marker of lung carcinogenesis. *Int J Cancer* 1992;52:44–47.
43. Thompson AB, Scholer SG, Daughton DM, Potter JF, Rennard SI. Altered epithelial lining fluid parameters in old normal individuals. *J Gerontol* 1992;47:171–176.
44. Bleecker ER, McFadden ER Jr. Hurd SS, Goldstein RA, Ram JS. Investigative bronchoscopy in subjects with asthma and other obstructive pulmonary diseases: whether and when (editorial). *Chest* 1992;101:297–298.
45. Fabbri LM, Ciaccia A. Investigative bronchoscopy in asthma and other airways diseases (editorial; comment). *Eur Resp J* 1992;5:8–11.
46. Bleecker ER, McFadden ER Jr. Hurd SS, Goldstein RA, Ram JS. Investigative bronchoscopy in subjects with asthma and other obstructive pulmonary diseases, Whether and when (editorial). *Chest* 1992;101:297–298.
47. Holgate ST, Wilson JR, Howarth PH. New insights into airway inflammation by endobronchial biopsy. *Am Rev Resp Dis* 1992; 145:2–6.
48. Howarth PH, Djukanovic R, Wilson JW, Holgate ST, Springall DR, Polak JM. Mucosal nerves in endobronchial biopsies in asthma and non-asthma. *Int Arch Allergy Appl Immunol* 1991; 94:330–333.
49. Howarth PH, Wilson J, Djukanovic R, et al. Airway inflammation and atopic asthma: a comparative bronchoscopic investigation. *Int Arch Allergy Appl Immunol* 1991;94:266–269.
50. Bousquet J, Chanez P, Campbell AM, et al. Inflammatory processes in asthma. *Int Arch Allergy Appl Immunol* 1991; 94:227–232.
51. Bentley AM, Menz G, Storz C, et al. Identification of T lymphocytes, macrophages, and activated eosinophils in the bronchial mucosa in intrinsic asthma. *Am Rev Resp Dis* 1992;146:500–506.
52. Berman JS, Weller PF. Airway eosinophils and lymphocytes in asthma. *Am Rev Resp Dis* 1992;145:1246–1248.
53. Laursen LC, Taudorf E, Borgeskov S, Kobayasi T, Jensen H, Weeke B. Fiberoptic bronchoscopy and bronchial mucosal biopsies in asthmatics undergoing long-term high-dose budesonide aerosol treatment. *Allergy* 1988;43:284–288.
54. Saetta M, Maestrelli P, Di-Stefano A, et al. Effect of cessation of exposure to toluene diisocyanate (TDI) on bronchial mucosa of subjects with TDI-induced asthma. *Am Rev Resp Dis* 1992; 145:169–174.
55. Saetta M, Di-Stefano A, Maestrelli P, et al. Airway mucosal inflammation in occupational asthma induced by toluene diisocyanate. *Am Rev Resp Dis* 1992;145:160–168.
56. Hol BE, van-de-Graaf EA, Out TA, Hische EA, Jansen HM. IgM in the airways of asthma patients. *Int Arch Allergy Appl Immunol* 1991;96:12–18.
57. Chetta A, Foresi A, Bertorelli G, Pesci A, Olivieri D. Lung function and bronchial responsiveness after bronchoalveolar lavage and bronchial biopsy performed without premedication in stable asthmatic subjects. *Chest* 1992;101:1563–1568.
58. King M, Zidulka A, Phillips DM, Wight D, Gross D, Chang HK. Tracheal mucus clearance in high-frequency oscillation: effect of peak flow rate bias. *Eur Resp J* 1990;3:6–13.
59. Roth Y, Aharonson EF, Teichtahl H, Baum GL, Priel Z, Modan M. Human in vitro nasal and tracheal ciliary beat frequencies: comparison of sampling sites, combined effect of medication, and demographic relationships. *Ann Otol Rhinol Laryngol* 1991; 100:378–384.
60. Roth Y, Aharonson EF, Teichtahl H, Baum GL, Priel Z, Modan M. Human in vitro nasal and tracheal ciliary beat frequencies: comparison of sampling sites, combined effect of medication, and demographic relationships. *Ann Otol Rhinol Laryngol* 1991; 100:378–384.
61. Pruitt BA Jr, Cioffi WG, Shimazu T, Ikeuchi H, Mason AD Jr. Evaluation and management of patients with inhalation injury. *J Trauma* 1990;30(Suppl):S63–68.
62. Chu CS, Trapnell BC, Curristin SM, Cutting GR, Crystal RG. Extensive posttranscriptional deletion of the coding sequences for part of nucleotide-binding fold 1 in respiratory epithelial mRNA transcripts of the cystic fibrosis transmembrane conductance regulator gene is not associated with the clinical manifestations of cystic fibrosis. *J Clin Invest* 1992;90:785–790.
63. Wagner EM, Bleecker ER, Permutt S, Liu MC. Peripheral airways resistance in smokers. *Am Rev Resp Dis* 1992;146:92–95.
64. Starnes VA, Theodore J, Oyer PE, et al. Pulmonary infiltrates after heart-lung transplantation: evaluation by serial transbronchial biopsies. *J Thorac Cardiovasc Surg* 1989;98:945–950.
65. Clelland CA, Higenbottam TW, Stewart S, Scott JP, Wallwork J. The histological changes in transbronchial biopsy after treatment of acute lung rejection in heart-lung transplants. *J Pathol* 1990;161:105–112.
66. Clelland C, Higenbottam T, Otulana B, et al. Histologic prognostic indicators for the lung allografts of heart–lung transplants. *J Heart Transplant* 1990;9:177–186.
67. Lee F, Kirby T, McCarthy P, et al. Role of flexible fiberoptic bronchoscopy following lung transplantation (abstract). *Chest* 1992;102:198S.
68. Vourch G, Fischler M, Michon F, Melchior JC, Seigneur F. High frequency jet ventilation v. manual jet ventilation during bronchoscopy in patients with tracheo-bronchial stenosis. *Br J Anaesth* 1983;55:969–972.
69. Godden DJ, Wagner EM, Pare PD, Mitzner W, Baile EM. Mea-

surement of airway wall blood flow in sheep by laser-Doppler flowmetry: interpretation and problems. *J Appl Physiol* 1991; 70:641–649.
70. Waclawiczek HW, Chmelizek F, Koller I. Endoscopic sealing of infected bronchus stump fistulae with fibrin following lung resections: experimental and clinical experience. *Surg Endosc* 1987;1:99–102.
71. Lillington GA, Stevens RP, DeNardo GL. Bronchoscopic location of bronchopleural fistula with xenon-133. *J Nucl Med* 1982; 23:322–323.
72. Torre M, Chiesa G, Ravini M, Vercelloni M, Belloni PA. Endoscopic gluing of bronchopleural fistula (published erratum appears in *Ann Thorac Surg* 1987;43:691). *Ann Thorac Surg*, 1987; 43:295–297.
73. Glover W, Chavis TV, Daniel TM, Kron IL, Spotnitz WD. Fibrin glue application through the flexible fiberoptic bronchoscope: closure of bronchopleural fistulas. *J Thorac Cardiovasc Surg* 1987;93:470–472.
74. Iglehart JD, Mansback C, Postlethwait R, Roberts L Jr, Ruth W. Pancreaticobronchial fistula: case report and review of the literature. *Gastroenterology* 1986;90:759–763.
75. Joseph JT, Krumpe PE. Diagnosis of gastrobronchial fistula by measurement of bronchial secretion pH. *Chest* 1989; 96:935–936.
76. Lang DM, Simon RA, Mathison DA, Timms RM, Stevenson DD. Safety and possible efficacy of fiberoptic bronchoscopy with lavage in the management of refractory asthma with mucous impaction. *Ann Allergy* 1991;67:324–330.
77. Van-Vyve T, Chanez P, Bousquet J, Lacoste JY, Michel FB. Godard P. Safety of bronchoalveolar lavage and bronchial biopsies in patients with asthma of variable severity. *Am Rev Resp Dis* 1992;146:116–121.
78. Haruno MM, Williams JH Jr. The flexible fiberoptic bronchoscopic shuttle. *Chest* 1992;102:944–945.
79. Del-Vecchio S, Mansi L, Petrillo A, et al. Endobronchial administration of iodine-131 B72.3 monoclonal antibody in patients with lung cancer. *Eur J Nucl Med* 1991;18:129–132.
80. Stokes DC. Is there room for another pediatric bronchoscope? (editorial). *Pediatr Pulmonol* 1992;12:201–202.
81. Kleeman PP, Jantzen JP, Bonfils P. The ultra-thin bronchoscope in management of the difficult paediatric airway. *Can J Anaesth* 1987;34:606–608.
82. Monden Y, Nakahara K, Fujii Y, Nanjo S, Ohno K, Kawashima Y. Trans-FBS-channel ventilation during the flexible bronchoscope (FBS) examination in infant. *Endoscopy* 1984; 16:175–178.
83. Abadco DL, Amaro-Galvez R, Rao M, Steiner P. Experience with flexible fiberoptic bronchoscopy with bronchoalveolar lavage as a diagnostic tool in children with AIDS. *Am J Dis Child* 1992;146:1056–1059.
84. Hofmann U, Hofmann D, Vogl T, Wilimzig C, Mantel K. Magnetic resonance imaging as a new diagnostic criterion in paediatric airway obstruction. *Prog Pediatr Surg* 1991;27:221–230.
85. Majid AA. J-shaped catheter for endobronchial aspiration of right upper lobe bronchus during rigid bronchoscopy in pediatric patients. *Chest* 1991;100:862.
86. Cormier Y, Laviolette M, Atton L, Series F. Influence of lung volume on collateral resistance in normal man. *Resp Physiol* 1991;83:179–187.
87. Ozawa H, Sugiyama Y, Yanai M, et al. A small airway pressure sensor for humans. *Front Med Biol Eng* 1991;3:177–184.
88. Baldwin DR, Wise R, Andrews JM, Honeybourne D. Quantitative morphology and water distribution of bronchial biopsy samples. *Thorax* 1992;47:504–507.

Bronchoscopy,
edited by U. B. S. Prakash.
Mayo Foundation © 1994.
Published by Raven Press, Ltd., New York.

CHAPTER 32

Atlas of Bronchoscopy

Udaya B. S. Prakash and Sergio Cavaliere

The ability of the bronchoscopist to identify obvious as well as subtle abnormalities in the tracheobronchial tree often determines the subsequent steps in the management of a given patient. Clearly, with experience comes the proficiency to discern variations and nuances in the bronchoscopic appearances in diverse airway disorders. Even in the same pathological process (i.e., bronchogenic carcinoma), the bronchoscopic appearances vary from patient to patient. Not infrequently, even the experienced bronchoscopist cannot make the diagnosis purely on the basis of bronchoscopic appearance of a lesion.

This chapter will demonstrate the bronchoscopic appearances of various disorders photographed by the authors of this book. Figure 1 provides the anatomic orientation to the tracheobronchial tree. The disease

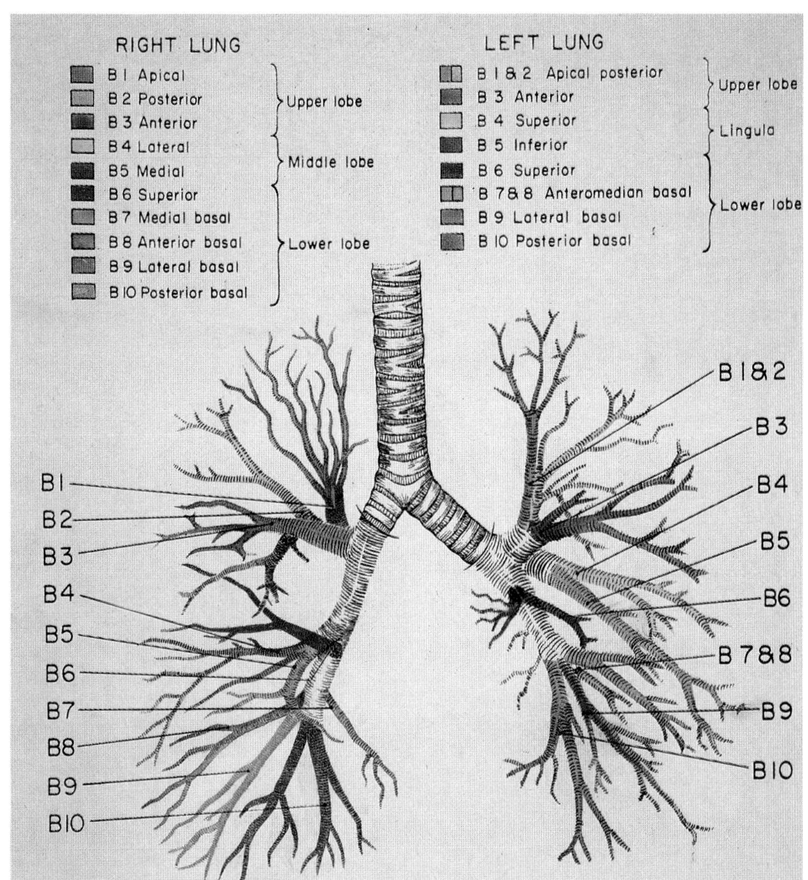

FIG. 1. Tracheobronchial tree and bronchial nomenclature; anteroposterior view shown.

U. B. S. Prakash: Division of Thoracic Diseases and Internal Medicine, Mayo Clinic, Rochester, Minnesota 55905.
S. Cavaliere: Center for Respiratory Endoscopy and Laser Therapy, Spedali Civili 25125, Brescia, Italy.

entities are arranged in alphabetical order. Almost all of the photographs obtained through the flexible bronchoscope were filmed by the members of the section of bronchoscopy at the Mayo Medical Center, Rochester, Minnesota. The majority of the bronchoscopic images obtained through the rigid bronchoscopic system were filmed by one of us (S.C.). Photographs provided by others are acknowledged under the respective figures. We thank all who contributed the bronchoscopic images.

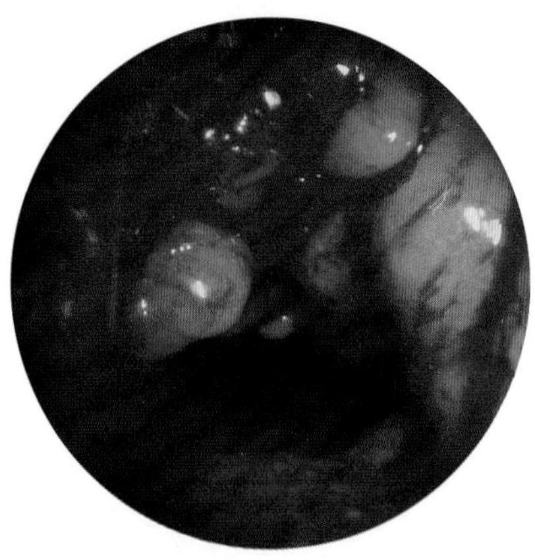

FIG. 3. Tracheal amyloidosis with pseudotumor formation. Tendency to bleed easily can be seen. The latter is not a contraindication to bronchoscopic biopsy. Only available palliative therapy for this disorder is bronchoscopic laser therapy.

AMYLOIDOSIS (Figs. 2–6)

Amyloidosis is a form of plasma cell dyscrasia of unknown etiology characterized pathologically by the extracellular deposition of fibrils derived from the light chain of a monoclonal immunoglobulin. Pulmonary involvement is more common in primary amyloidosis. Pulmonary involvement is broadly classified into tracheobronchial, discrete parenchymal amyloidoma, and diffuse parenchymal amyloidosis. Submucosal depositions of amyloid produce gradual narrowing of the major airways and cause respiratory distress (1,2). Biopsy of mucosal and submucosal lesions usually provides diagnosis.

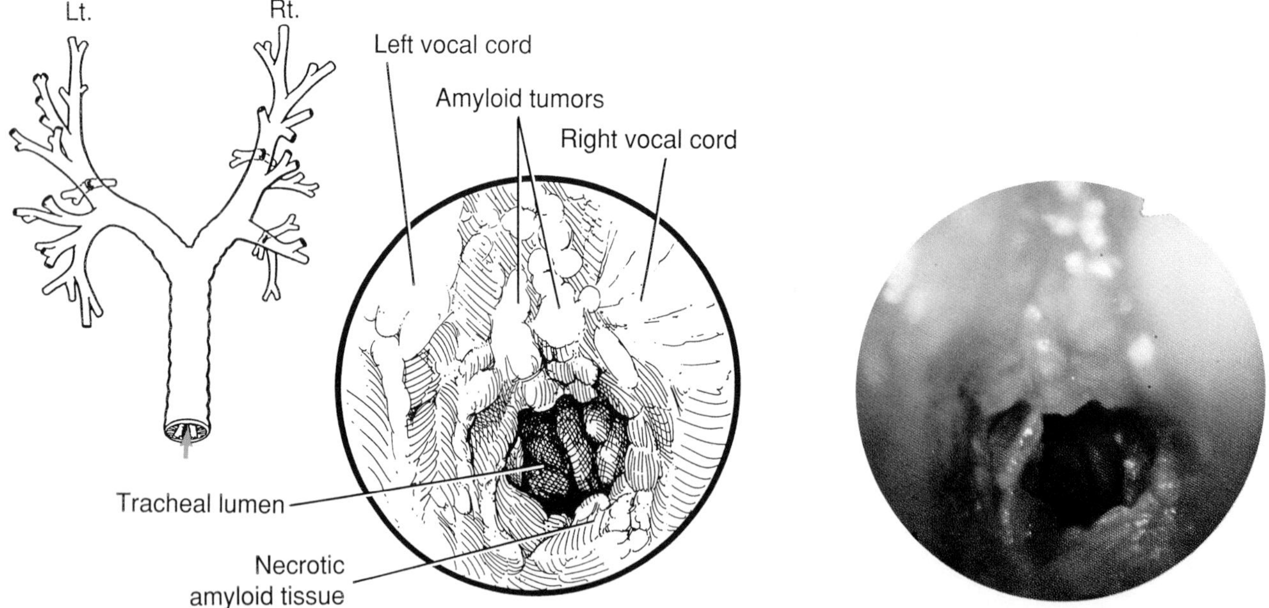

FIG. 2. Laryngeal and subglottic amyloidosis with severe airway obstruction. This patient required tracheostomy followed by Nd:YAG laser therapy. Laser therapy has been described in the treatment of tracheobronchial amyloidosis (3,4).

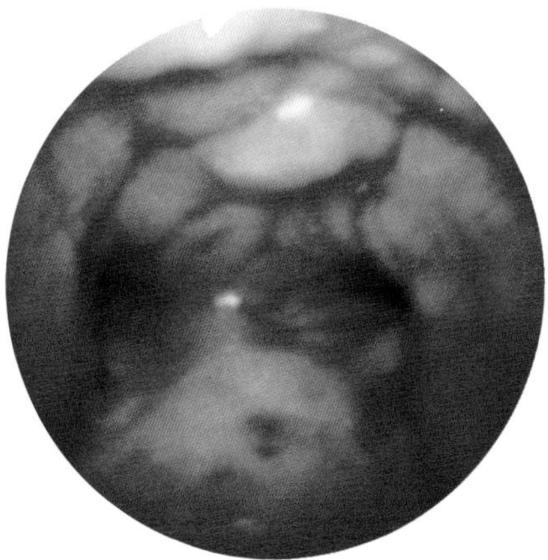

FIG. 4. Diffuse tracheobronchial amyloidosis with multiple mucosal nodules. The differential diagnoses of this bronchoscopic appearance include tracheobronchial amyloidosis, primary or metastatic carcinoma, and tracheopathia osteoplastica.

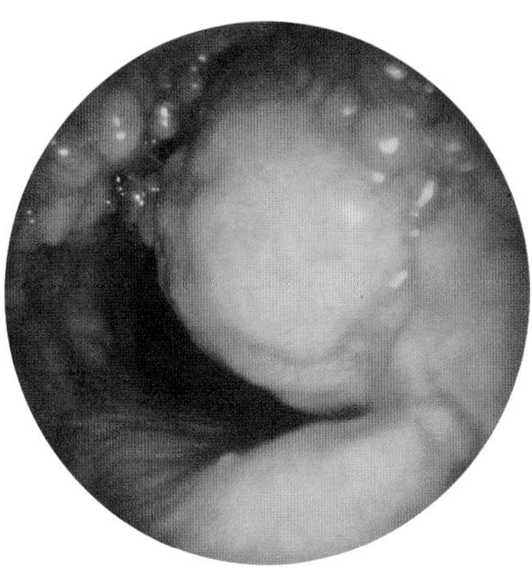

FIG. 5. Amyloid pseudotumors of tracheobronchial tree may occur in various sizes and may block lobar or segmental bronchi.

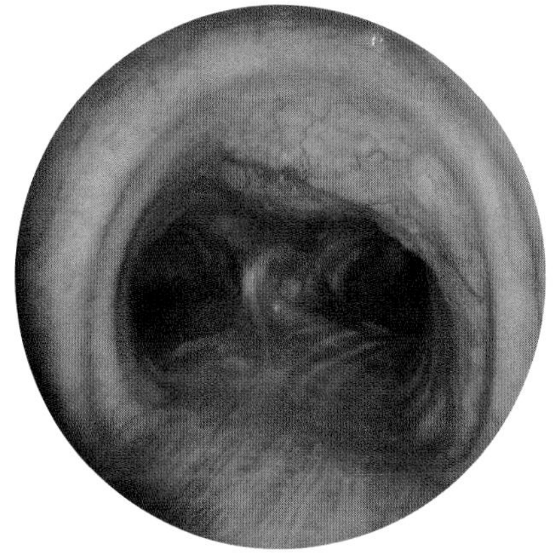

A

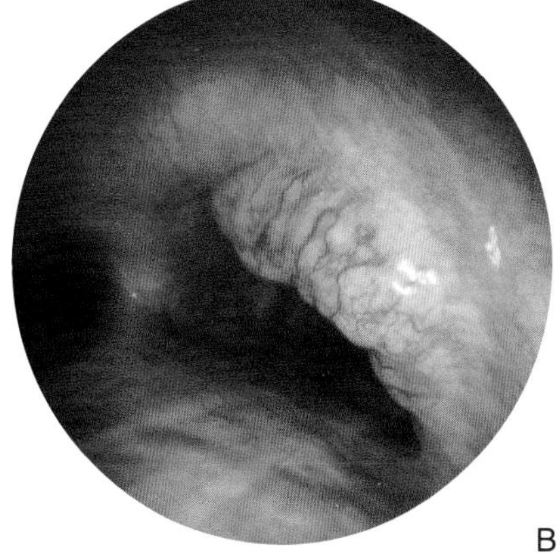

B

FIG. 6. Amyloidosis involving distal trachea (in two different patients) shows mucosal elevation and nodularity **(A)**, and a close-up of the lesion reveals diffuse submucosal capillary proliferation **(B)**.

ANATOMIC VARIATIONS (Figs. 7–16)

Tracheobronchial anomalies can be congenital or acquired. Not all such aberrations cause symptoms or disease. Many of the anatomic variations are incidentally detected during bronchoscopic examination. Congenital tracheobronchial anomalies are more likely to be seen in infants and young children than in adults. The following are some examples.

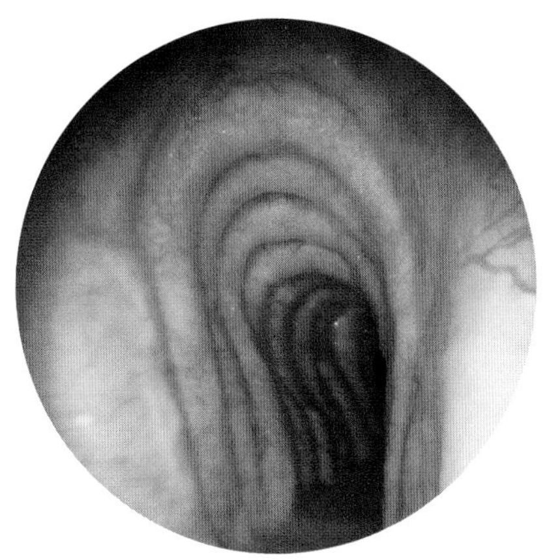

FIG. 7. An inverted U-shaped tracheal lumen. This is not an uncommon finding in bronchoscopy practice. Most patients are asymptomatic. A more severe narrowing of the transverse (coronal) diameter of the trachea is sometimes referred to as "saber sheath" or "scabbard" trachea (5,6). It is more common in men and may be caused by extrinsic compression.

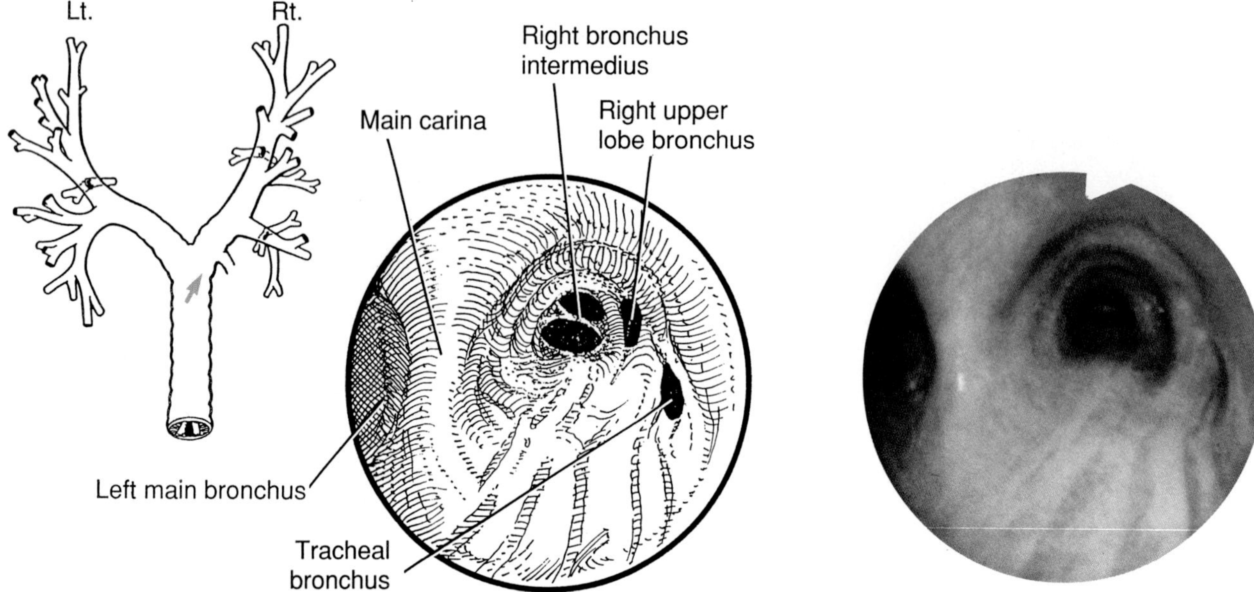

FIG. 8. Accessory tracheal bronchus. The accessory bronchus is almost always right-sided and leads to RB-1. The incidence of accessory tracheal bronchus ranges between 0.1% and 5%, and this anomaly may be associated with other bronchopulmonary abnormalities, tracheal stenosis, or Down's syndrome (7,8).

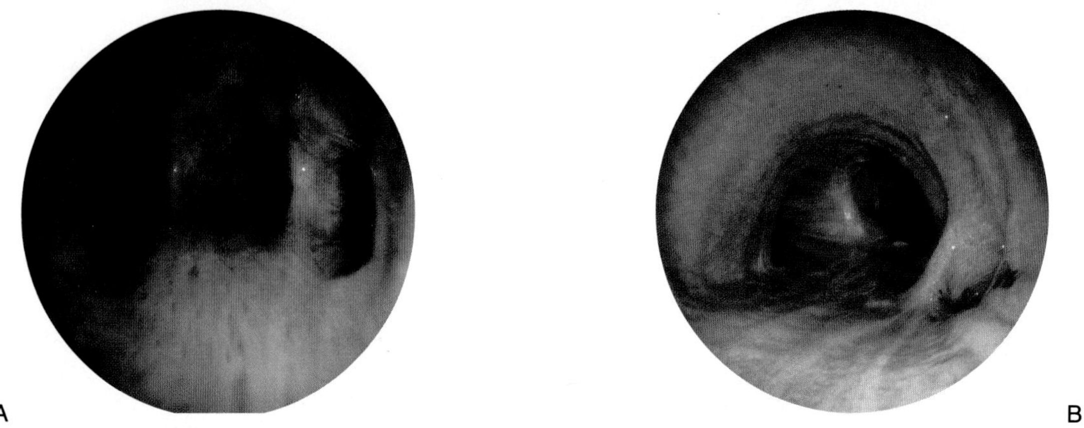

FIG. 9. A large accessory tracheal bronchus on the right; the main carina is seen on the left **(A)**. **B** shows a smaller and more proximal accessory tracheal bronchus on the right. We have observed atelectasis of RB-1 segment when the accessory bronchus was the only airway leading to it (no collateral ventilation) and the cuff of an endotracheal tube was kept inflated over the ostium of the bronchus. A more posterior position of the "accessory bronchus" should alert the bronchoscopist to the possibility of a tracheoesophageal fistula.

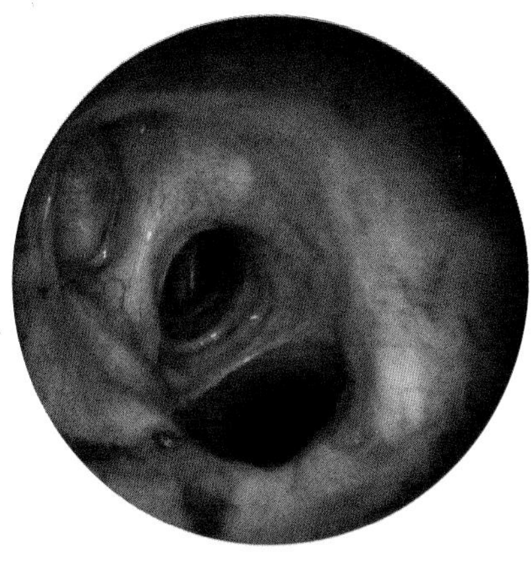

FIG. 10. Trifurcation of left main stem bronchus into left upper lobe, lingula, and left lower lobe. A mirror image of right bronchial tree occurs rarely. Transposition of bronchial tree (right bronchial tree mimicking left bronchial anatomy and vice versa) may be seen in true situs inversus.

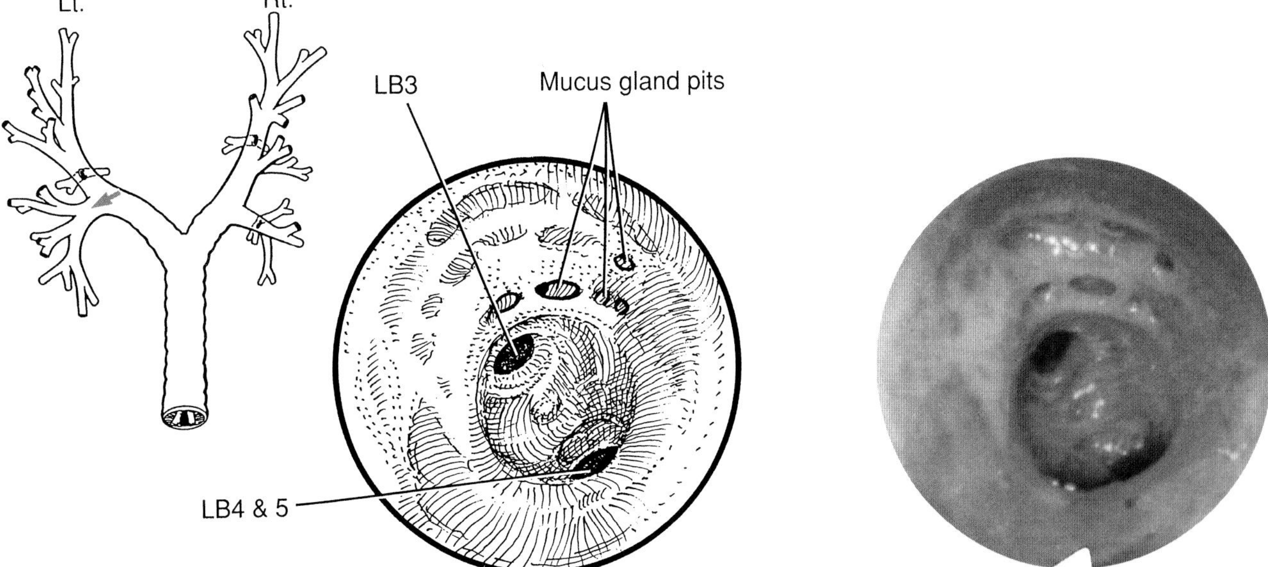

FIG. 11. Dilated mucous ducts (sometimes called mucous gland pits). Although they are thought to be more commonly seen in patients with chronic bronchitis, the clinical significance of these pits is unclear. Some are large enough to look like bronchial openings.

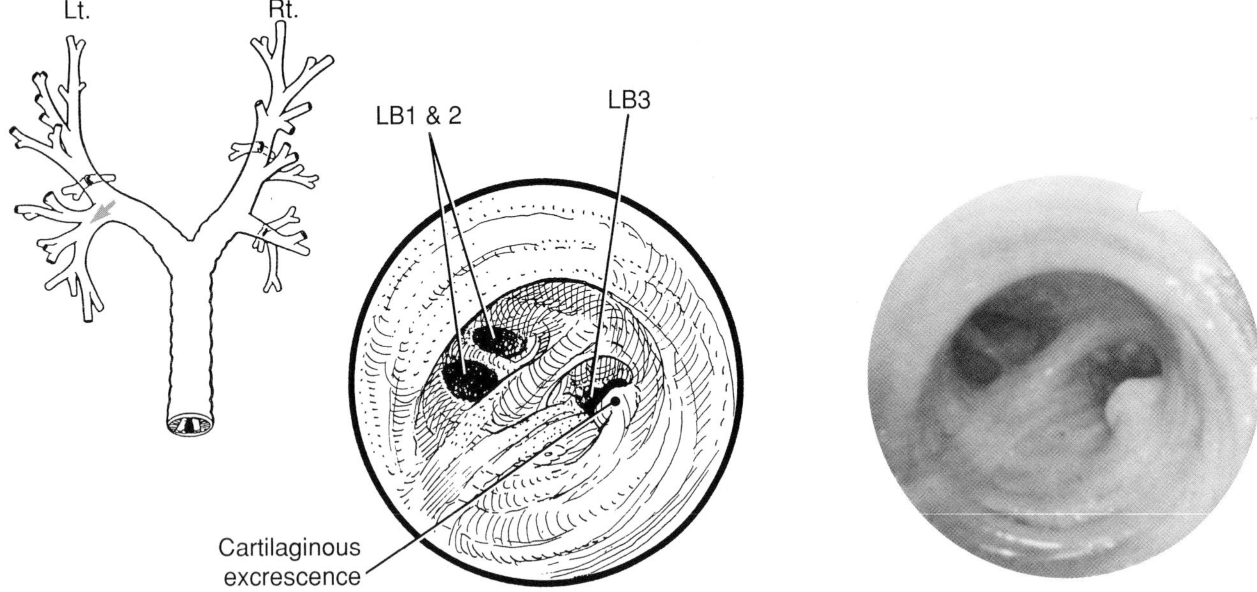

FIG. 12. Cartilaginous excrescence (spur or projection). This is an incidental finding and almost all patients are asymptomatic. Mucosa over such spurs is normal and biopsy is rarely indicated. This benign anomaly is fairly common in elderly subjects. Occasionally, the mucosa overlying the cartilage becomes denuded, thereby exposing the cartilage.

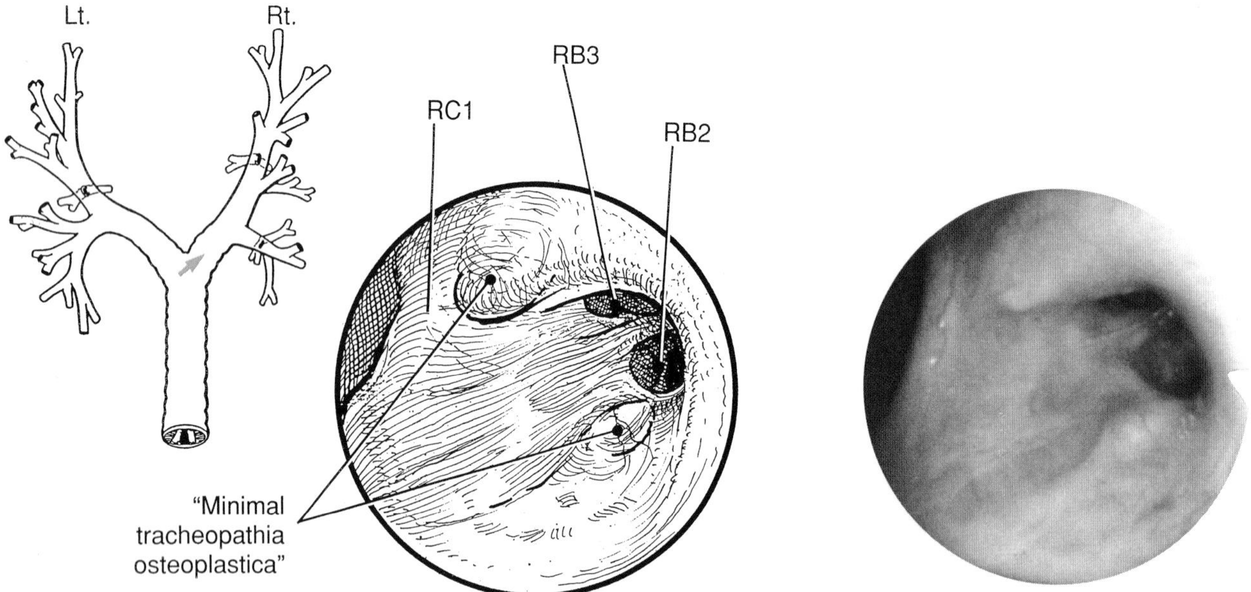

FIG. 13. Cartilaginous distortion in a segmental bronchus. Such deformities are more common in older subjects and following thoracic surgery. These are incidental findings and patients are usually asymptomatic. These projections have been called "minimal tracheopathia" (9).

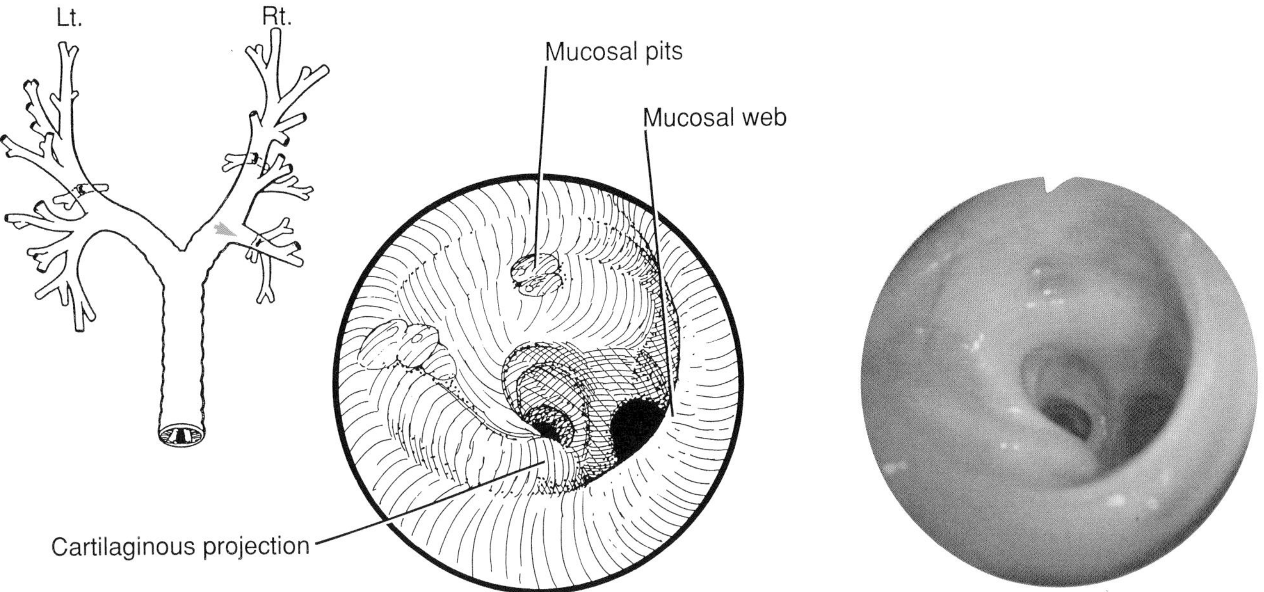

FIG. 14. Slight anatomic distortion of the cartilages, mucous pits, and web-like mucosal reflection. Such variations are not uncommon and are usually incidental and asymptomatic. Chronic bronchitis is reported to predispose to prominent mucous pits (10).

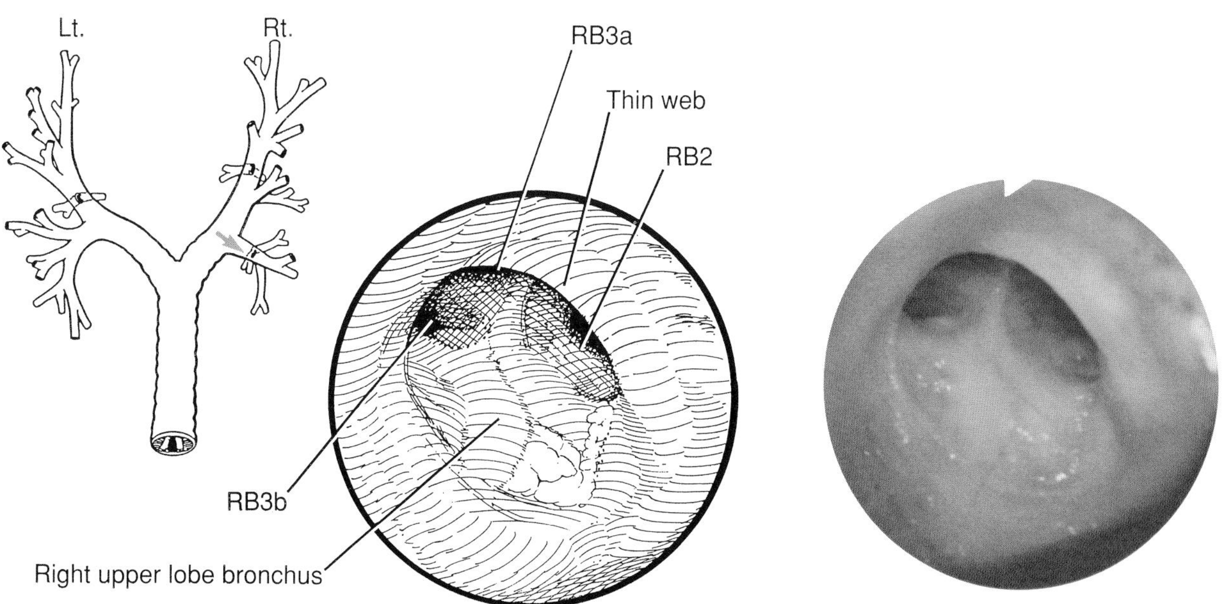

FIG. 15. A more pronounced (almost circular) web-like mucosal abnormality. This is different from the transluminal synechial bands (see under iatrogenic abnormalities).

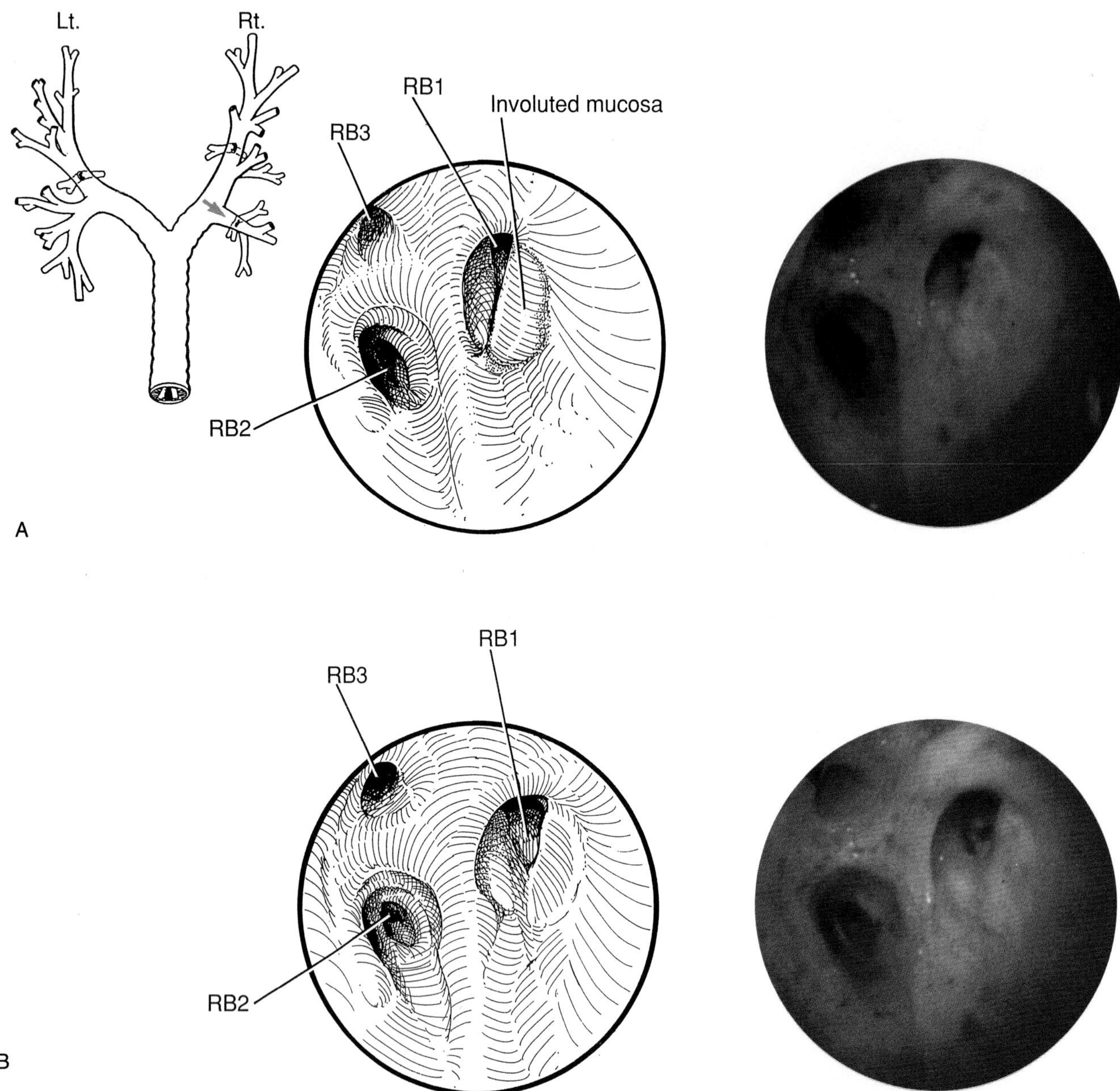

FIG. 16. Mucosal involution (invagination) in RB-1 was wrongly diagnosed as a mucosal tumor and biopsied by an inexperienced bronchoscopist. During forced expiration, a portion of the mucosa involutes to produce a "tumor-like" appearance **(A)**, but on inspiration the mucosal involution disappears **(B)**. The mechanism is unclear but localized abnormality or deficiency of the cartilage may be responsible. Practice of "dynamic" bronchoscopy (see Chapter 9) is helpful in solving such bronchoscopic problems.

ASTHMA (Figs. 17–20)

Uncomplicated asthma rarely produces endobronchial abnormalities. Occasionally, we have observed bronchospasm during bronchoscopy. This manifests itself as sudden narrowing of the bronchial lumen and difficulty in maneuvering the bronchoscope. In asthmatic patients who develop complications such as allergic bronchopulmonary aspergillosis, mucoid impaction syndrome, or plastic bronchitis, bronchoscopy is helpful in the diagnosis and treatment. Plastic bronchitis is an exaggerated form of mucoid impaction in which large mucous casts of an entire bronchial tree are formed. Tight impaction of these casts may require rigid bronchoscopic removal.

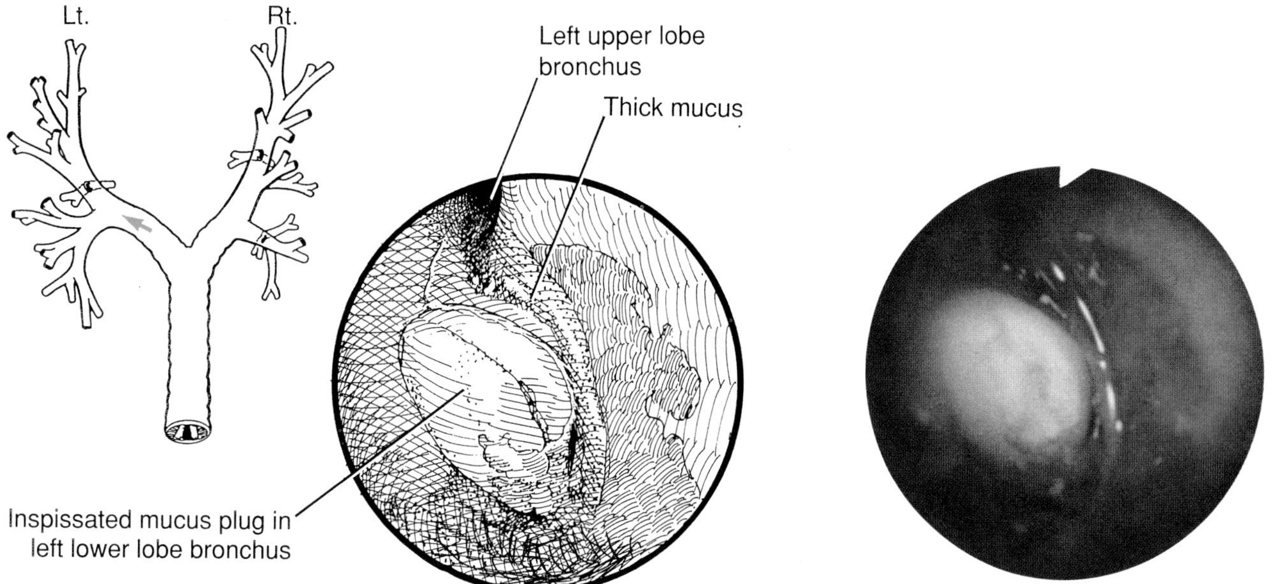

FIG. 17. Asthma with mucoid impaction. Severely inspissated mucous plug had to be removed with a rigid bronchoscope. A piecemeal removal with a flexible bronchoscope can also be attempted but may consume inordinate time in a patient with significant asthmatic symptoms. Mucoid impaction is more common in patients with allergic bronchopulmonary aspergillosis (11).

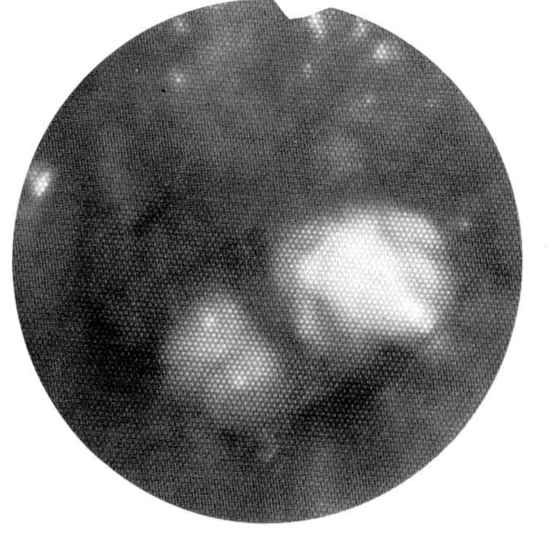

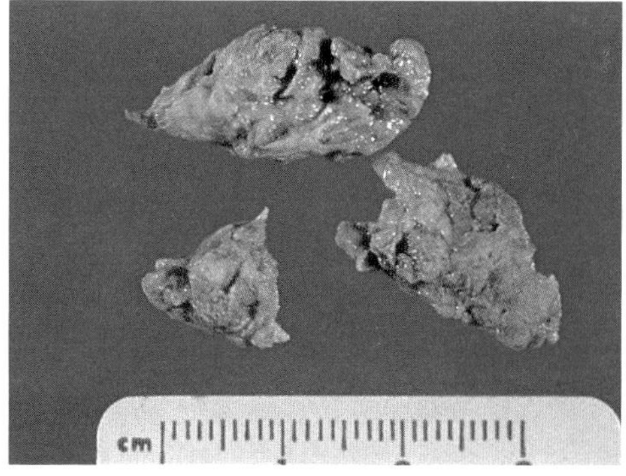

FIG. 18. Large endobronchial mucous plugs in an asthmatic patient **(left)**. Thick inspissated material **(right)**. Courtesy of Atul C, Mehta, M.D.

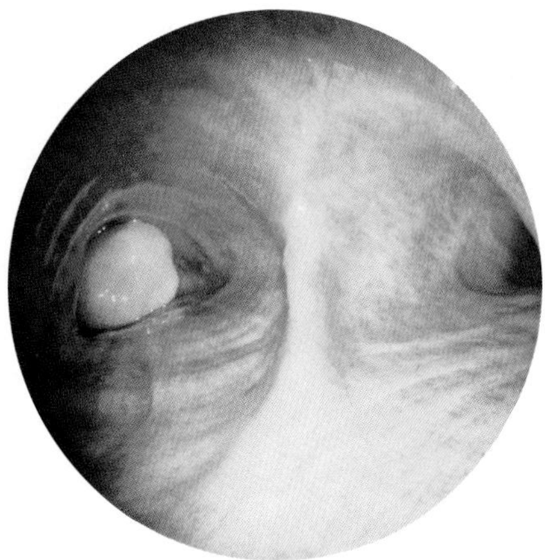

FIG. 19. Left main bronchus obstruction in a patient with allergic bronchopulmonary aspergillosis. Therapeutic bronchoscopy was required to clear the obstructing mucus plug.

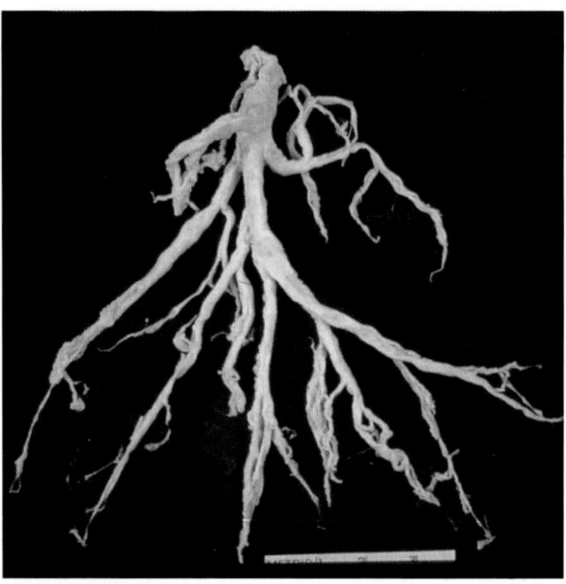

FIG. 20. Plastic bronchitis in a patient without asthma. A large inspissated mucous cast of an entire bronchial tree was removed using flexible bronchoscope and biopsy forceps. Plastic bronchitis has been described in patients with asthma, allergic bronchopulmonary aspergillosis, bronchiectasis, and cystic fibrosis (12–14). Courtesy of James R. Jett, M.D.

BRONCHOLITHIASIS (Figs. 21–28)

Pulmolith or pneumolith denotes a well-defined calcified or ossified nodule within the pulmonary parenchyma. Almost all pneumoliths are asymptomatic and are usually discovered incidentally on chest roentgenograms. When such a calcified nodule erodes into the wall of a bronchus or enters the tracheobronchial lumen, then it becomes a broncholith. Broncholithiasis therefore represents a "stone" in the wall or lumen of the bronchus. Broncholith can also originate from calcification of an intraluminal granulation tissue, as occasionally seen in a chronic tracheobronchial foreign body. The most common etiologies of broncholithiasis include infections by *Mycobacterium tuberculosis*, *Histoplasma capsulatum*, and *Coccidioides immitis*. Symptoms include cough, hemoptysis (in 50%), and localized wheezing.

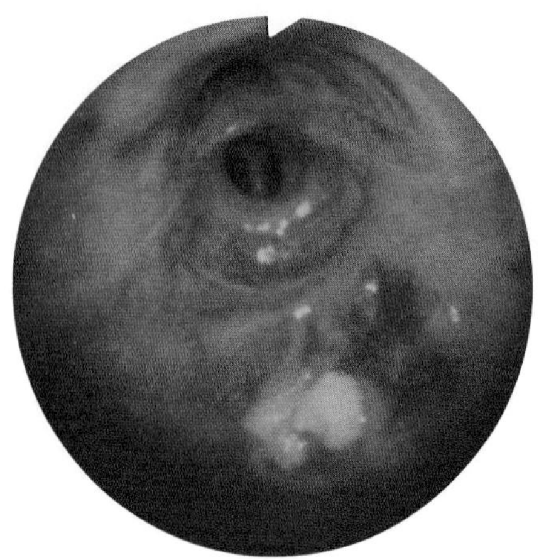

FIG. 21. Broncholithiasis involving the lingular bronchus (LB-4–5). The patient presented with hemoptysis and roentgenological signs of lingular atelectasis. The broncholith occluding the bronchus was removed piecemeal using a flexible bronchoscope.

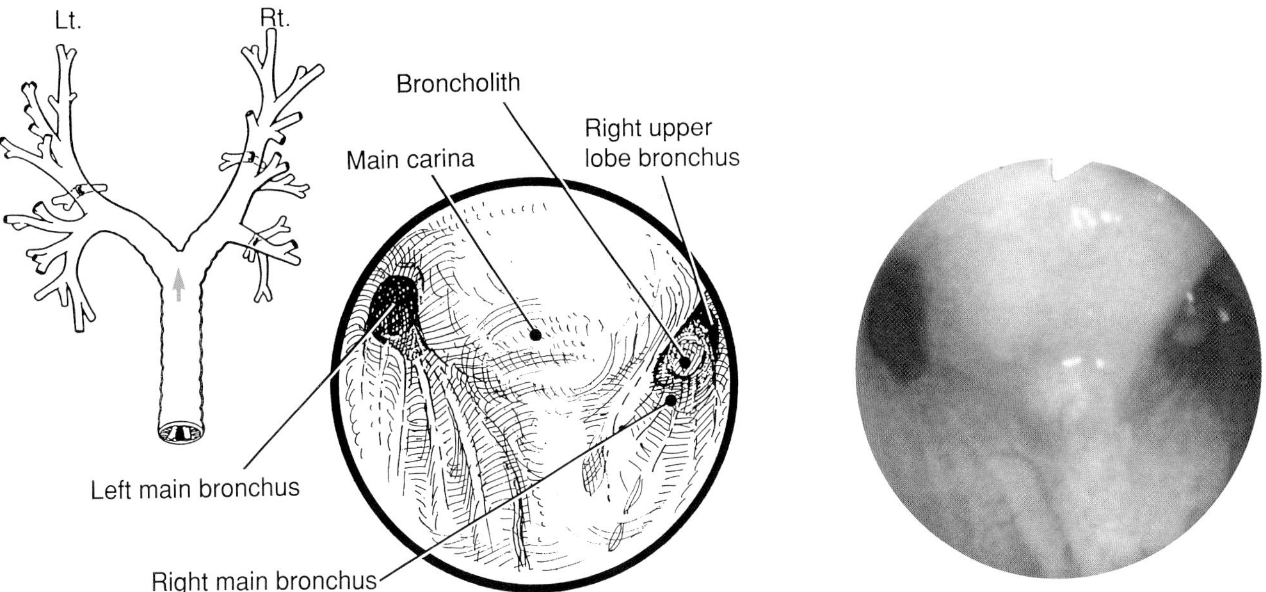

FIG. 22. Broncholithiasis involving right main bronchus. The marked widening of the main carina is due to subcarinal lymphadenopathy caused by histoplasmosis (see Fig. 23).

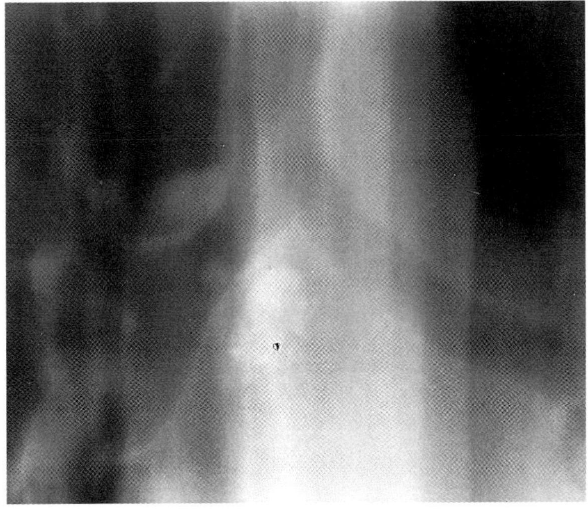

FIG. 23. Broncholithiasis (same patient as shown in Fig. 22) depicted by anteroposterior tomography of main stem bronchi. Calcified mass of subcarinal lymph nodes with intraluminal projection of a broncholith through the medial wall of the right main stem bronchus is seen.

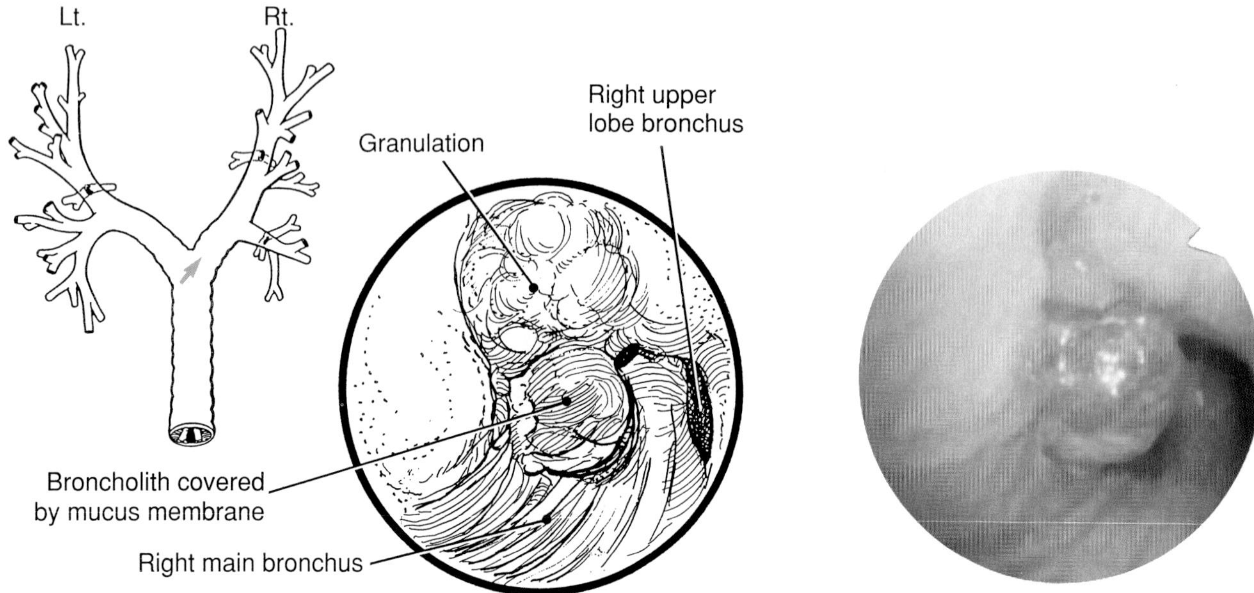

FIG. 24. Broncholith covered by exuberant granulation tissue was erroneously diagnosed as a malignant neoplasm until a biopsy forceps uncovered the broncholith. Bleeding leading to hemoptysis is more common in the presence of granulation tissue. (See Chapter 16 for more details on broncholithiasis.)

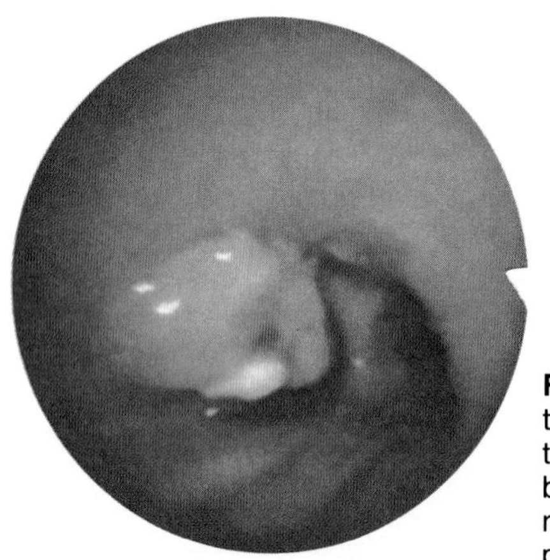

FIG. 25. Broncholith protruding through the granulation tissue (same patient as shown in Fig. 22). The granulation tissue and the broncholith were removed with a flexible bronchoscope. Bleeding was minimal. Bronchoscopic removal of broncholiths has been successful in 19–67% of patients (15,16).

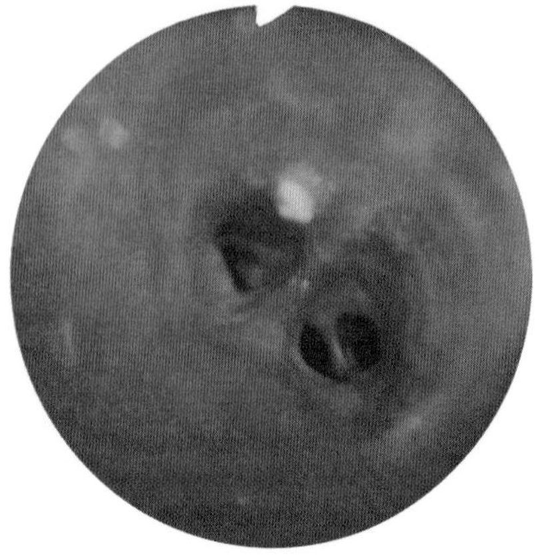

FIG. 26. Broncholithiasis involving RB-5. The patient presented with the chief complaint of cough and hemoptysis soon after sexual intercourse. Postcoital hemoptysis secondary to broncholithiasis has been described.

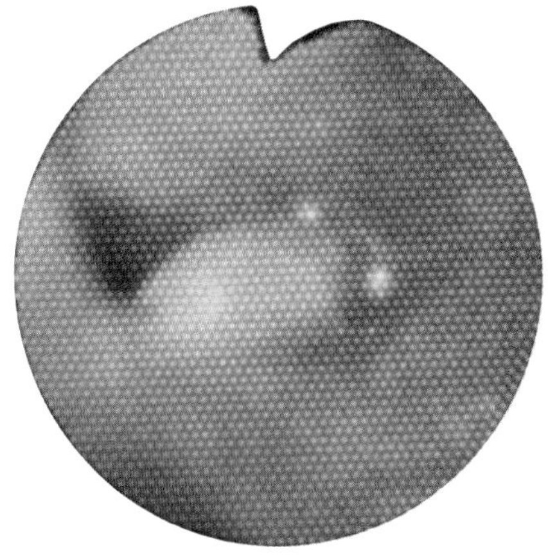

FIG. 27. Broncholith in distal bronchus in the right upper lobe. Significant hemoptysis led to bronchoscopy with a standard flexible bronchoscope that revealed blood streaking. Only with an ultrathin bronchoscope was the broncholith observed.

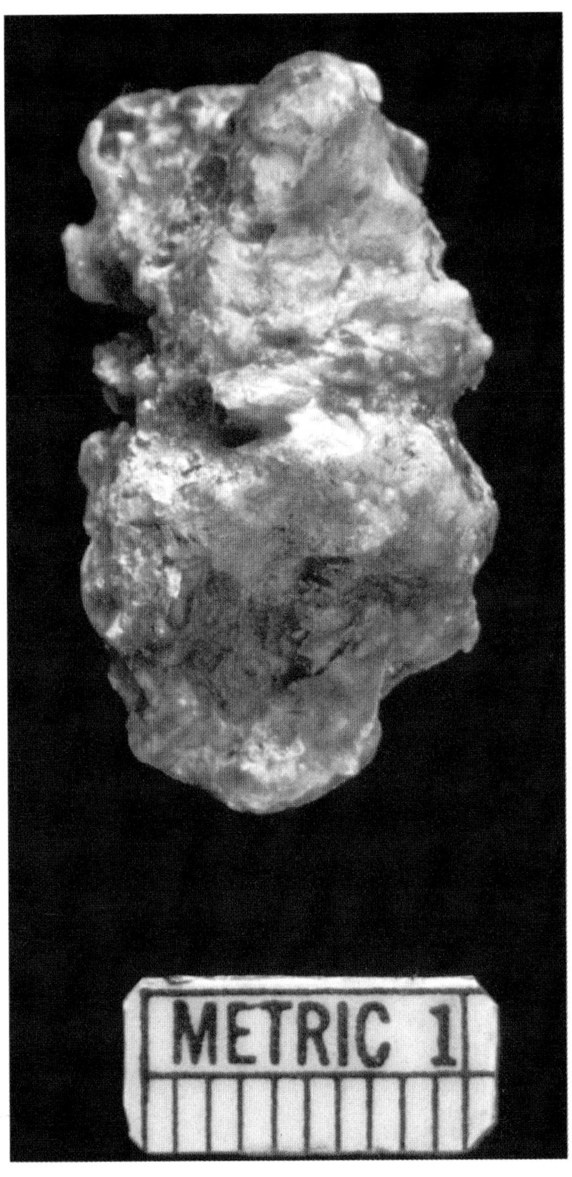

FIG. 28. Broncholith removed with a rigid bronchoscope. Elemental analysis showed that the stone was made of calcium phosphate.

EXTRINSIC COMPRESSION OF AIRWAY (Figs. 29–37)

Extrinsic causes of airway compression include extra-airway disorders such as large mediastinal masses, cysts, tumors, vascular anomalies, esophageal diseases, and skeletal abnormalities. Extrinsic compression by tumors do not necessarily indicate neoplastic extension into the wall or lumen of the airways. Excessive intrathoracic pressure during expiratory maneuver as observed in patients with severe chronic obstructive pulmonary disease and during cough result in the expiratory collapse of airways. Patients with primary tracheal disorders such as tracheobronchomalacia, relapsing polychondritis, and tracheobronchomegaly (Mounier–Kuhn syndrome) also frequently exhibit expiratory collapse of airways during expiratory maneuver.

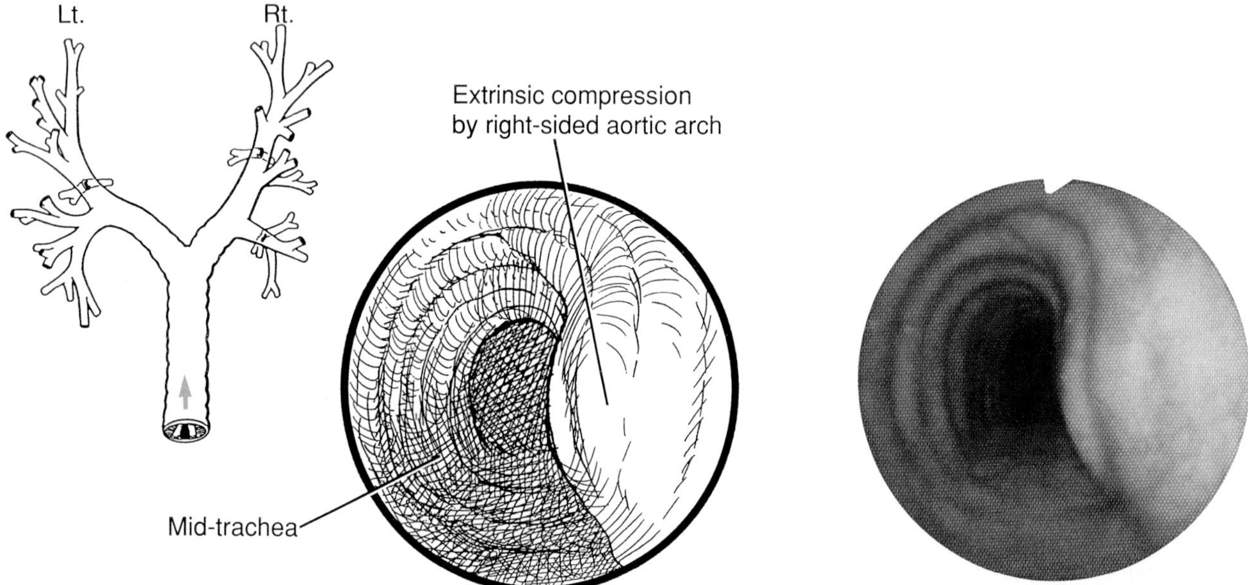

FIG. 29. Extrinsic tracheal compression caused by a right-sided aortic arch. The patient's asthma was exacerbated by this and an aortopexy procedure eliminated tracheal compression. Tracheal compression by right-sided aortic arch has been described (17,18). Pulmonary vascular sling is another well-recognized cause of tracheal compression (19).

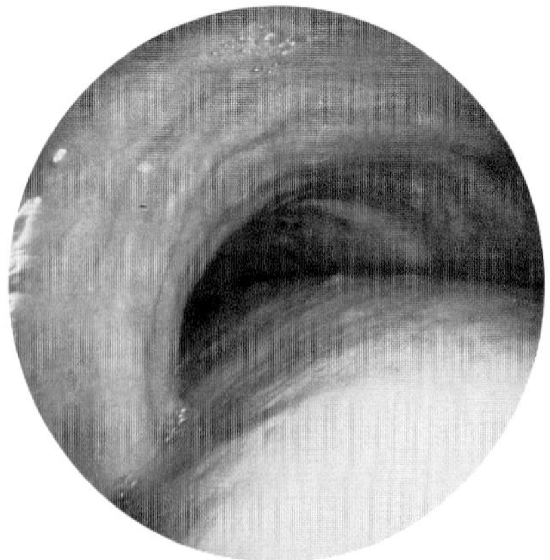

FIG. 30. Collapse of posterior membranous portion of trachea during expiration in chronic obstructive pulmonary disease. Loss of retractive forces is responsible for this finding. The collapse of membranous portion usually extends down to segmental bronchi.

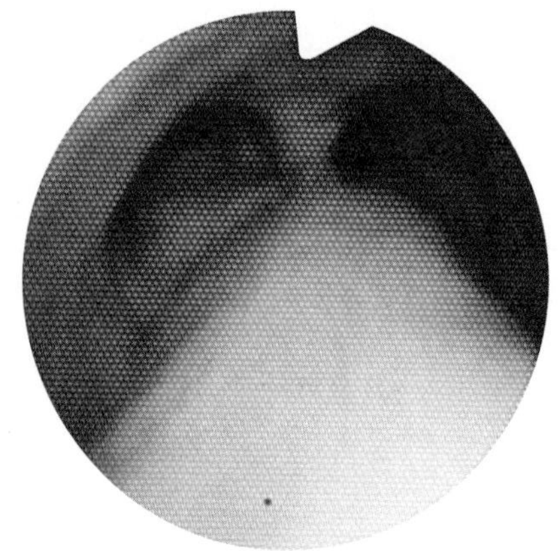

FIG. 31. Extrinsic compression of posterior wall of trachea caused by a large leiomyoma of the esophagus. Usually there is minimal variation in this phenomenon during inspiration and expiration.

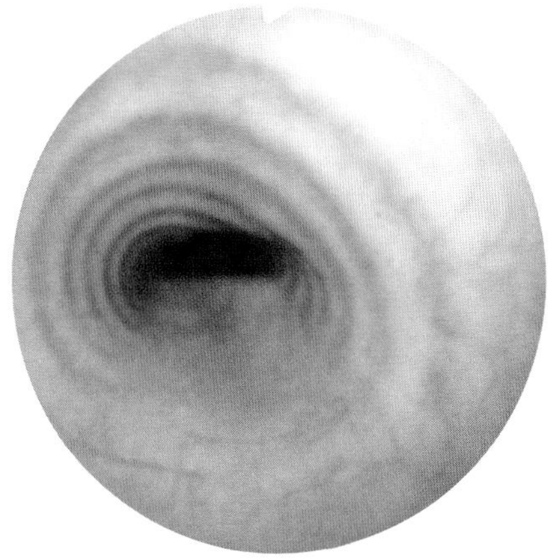

FIG. 32. Aberrant subclavian artery producing a narrow band of extrinsic compression of midposterior trachea.

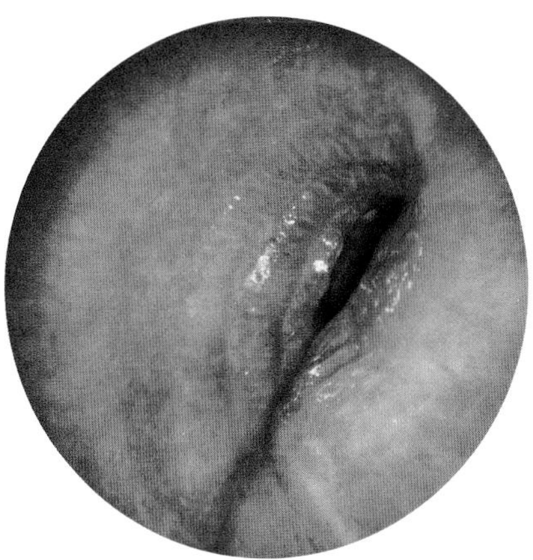

FIG. 33. Extrinsic compression of trachea caused by extraluminal squamous cell carcinoma. Symptomatic relief was obtained by stent placement.

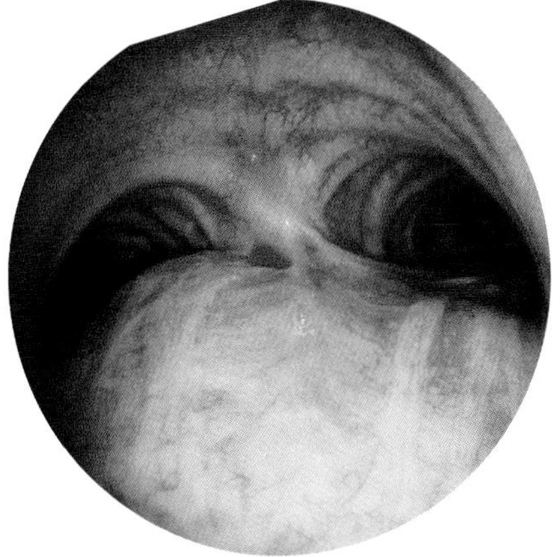

FIG. 34. Extrinsic compression of the distal trachea and left main bronchus caused by squamous cell carcinoma involving mediastinal lymph nodes. A similar case has been reported (20).

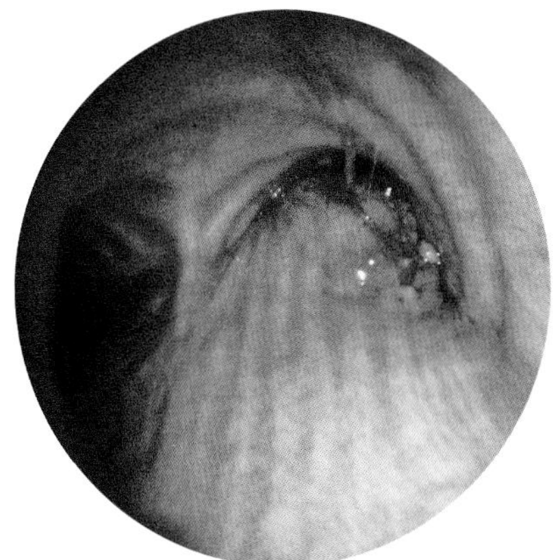

FIG. 35. Extrinsic compression of right main bronchus by adenocarcinoma. Mucosal involvement is also seen. Laser therapy is not indicated in such cases.

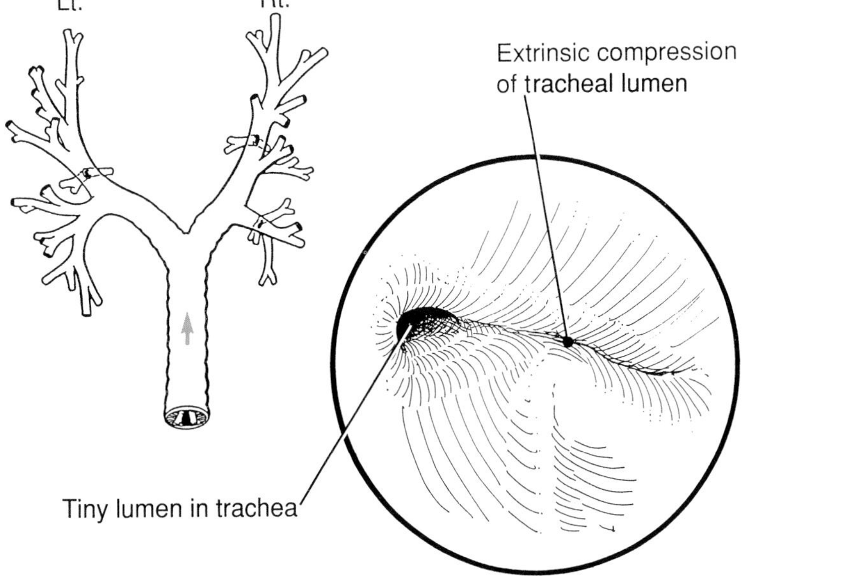

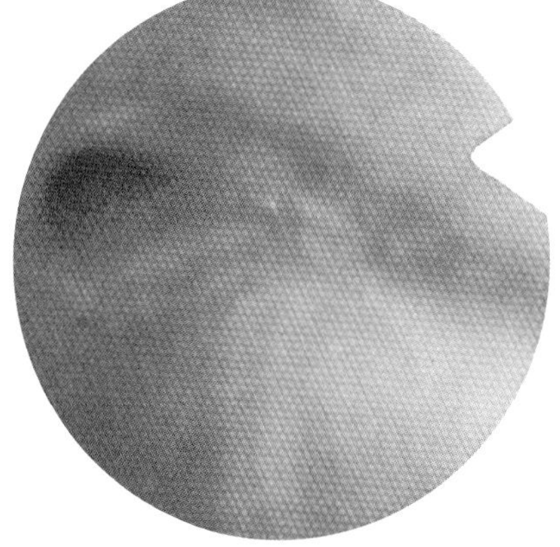

FIG. 36. Severe extrinsic compression of the trachea by truncus arteriosus in a child. Only a tiny slit-like lumen is seen. Surgical correction resulted in relief of the compression. Tracheal compression is a relatively common occurrence in children with truncus arteriosus and anomalous innominate artery (21–25).

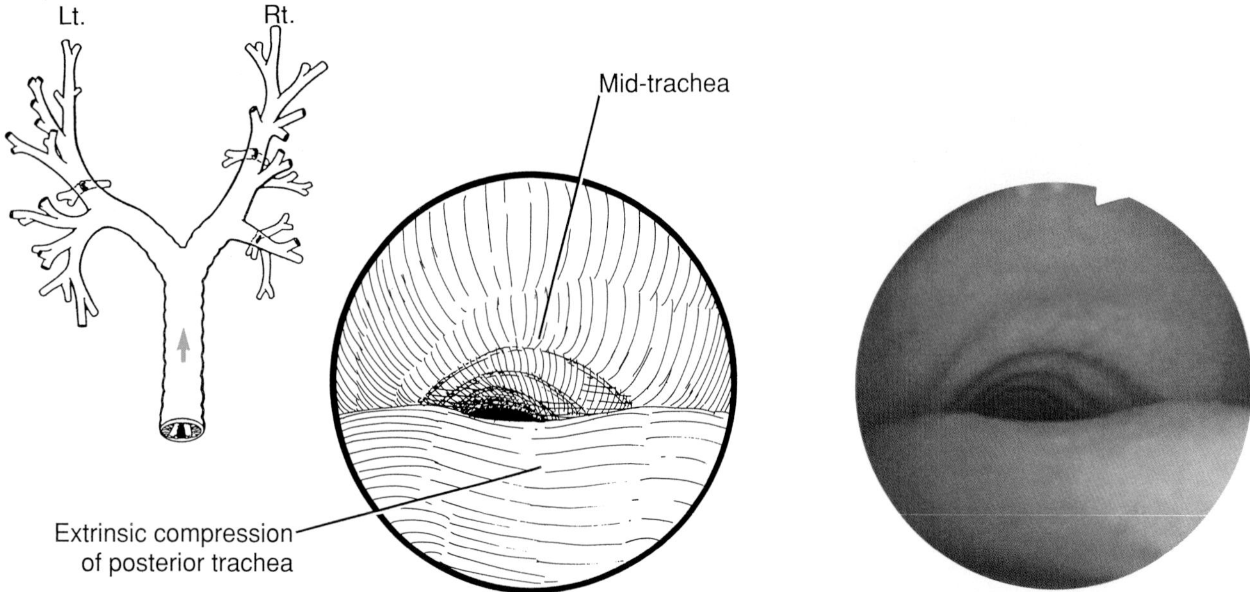

FIG. 37. Extrinsic compression of trachea caused by a large neurogenic tumor in the tracheoesophageal groove. Anterior mediastinal masses can exacerbate tracheal compression during general anesthesia (26–28).

FISTULA (Figs. 38–43)

Fistulous communication between the tracheobronchial tree and nonpulmonary organs is either congenital or acquired. Developmental or congenital fistula results from the failure of embryonic organs to fully form. Acquired fistula is usually encountered in adults and is secondary to neoplasms, trauma, instrumentation, or radiotherapy. The abnormal communications can exist as tracheoesophageal, bronchoesophageal, bronchopleural, bronchovascular, or bronchoperitoneal fistulas.

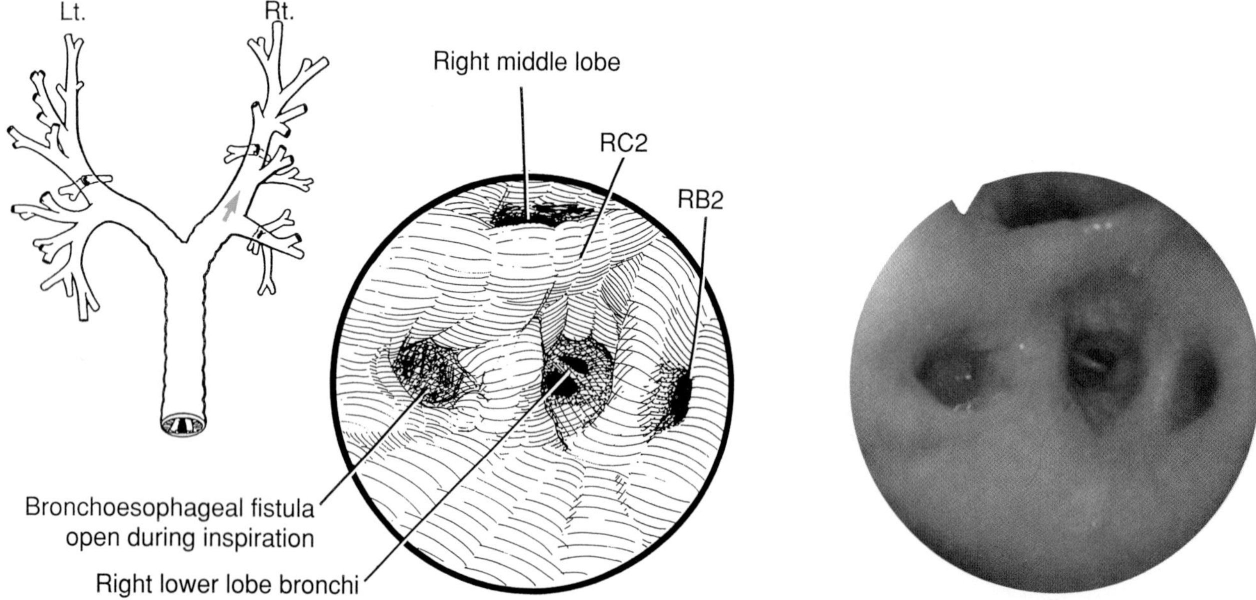

FIG. 38. Bronchoesophageal fistula open during inspiration only. In highly suspicious cases, careful bronchoscopic examination during deep inspiration and expiration should be employed (see Chapter 9). Congenital bronchoesophageal fistula is occasionally encountered in adults (29–31).

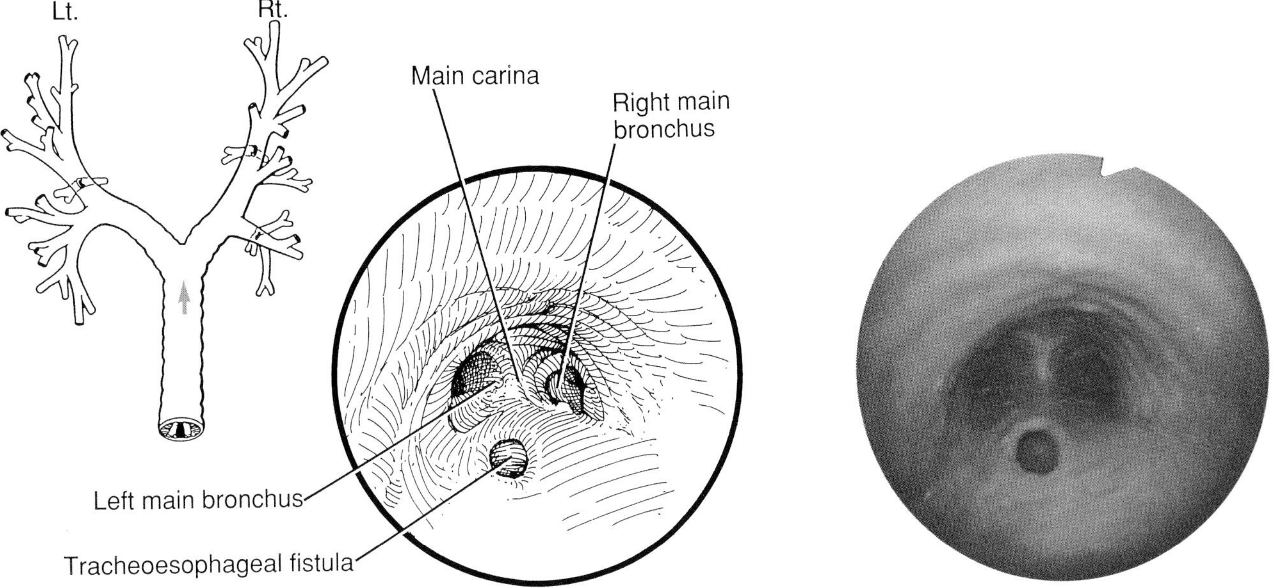

FIG. 39. Tracheoesophageal fistula following radiation therapy of a mediastinal tumor several months earlier. The smooth edges of the fistulous opening suggest the absence of active malignancy. Bronchoscopy helped in the planning of appropriate surgical procedure.

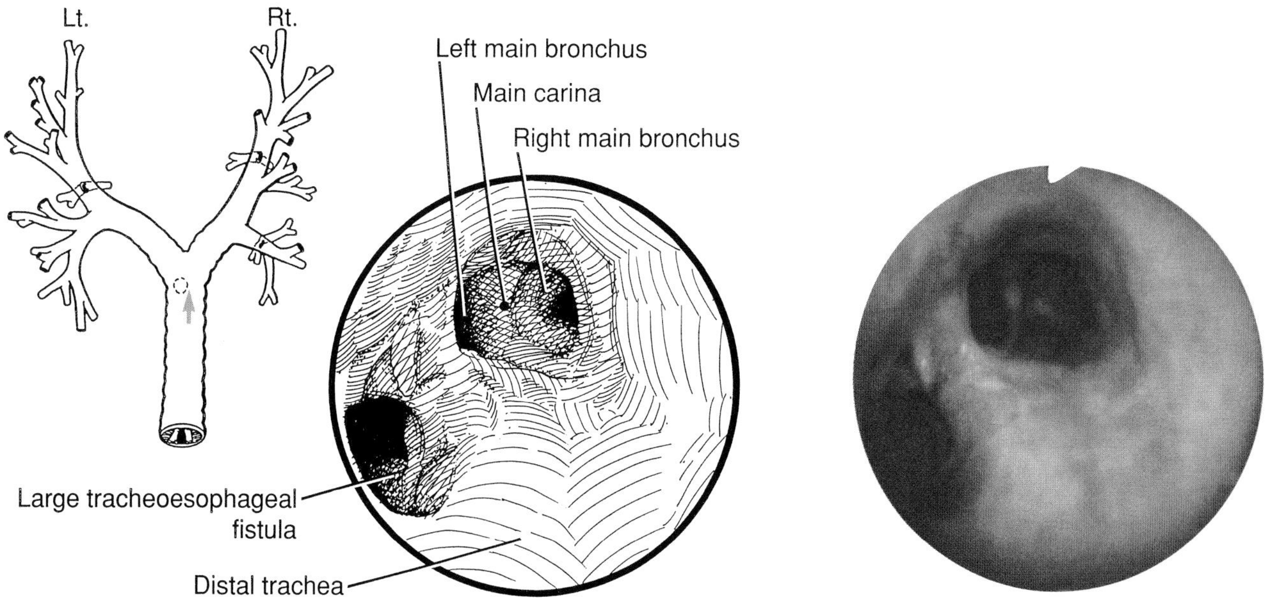

FIG. 40. A large tracheoesophageal fistula caused by carcinoma of the esophagus. An esophageal stent partially prevented episodes of massive esophagotracheal aspiration.

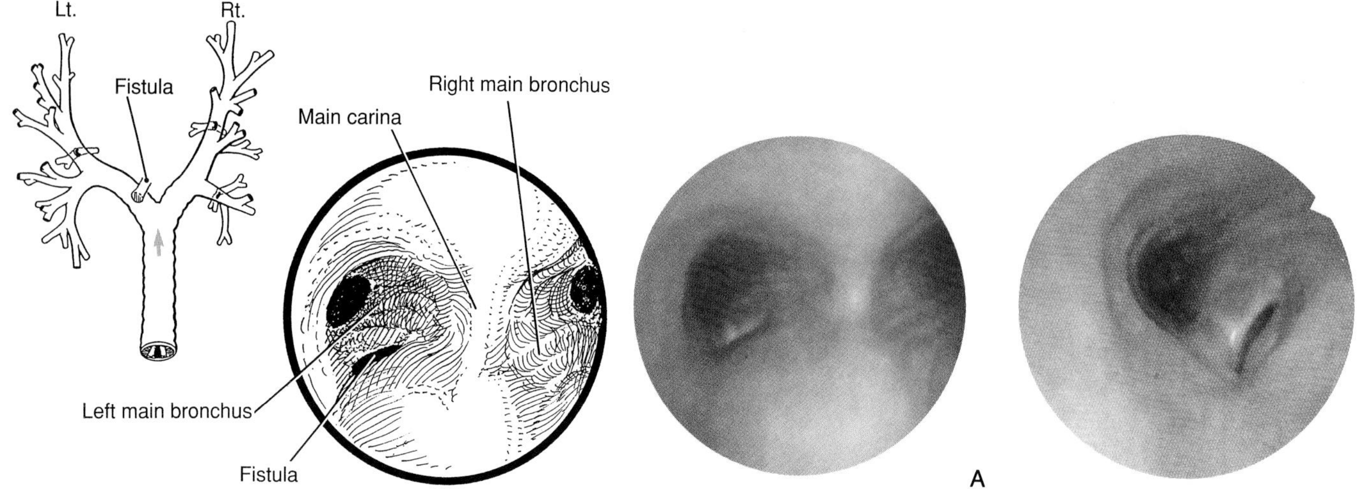

FIG. 41. Fistula between left main bronchus and esophagus caused by previous trauma **(A)** and a close-up view **(B)**.

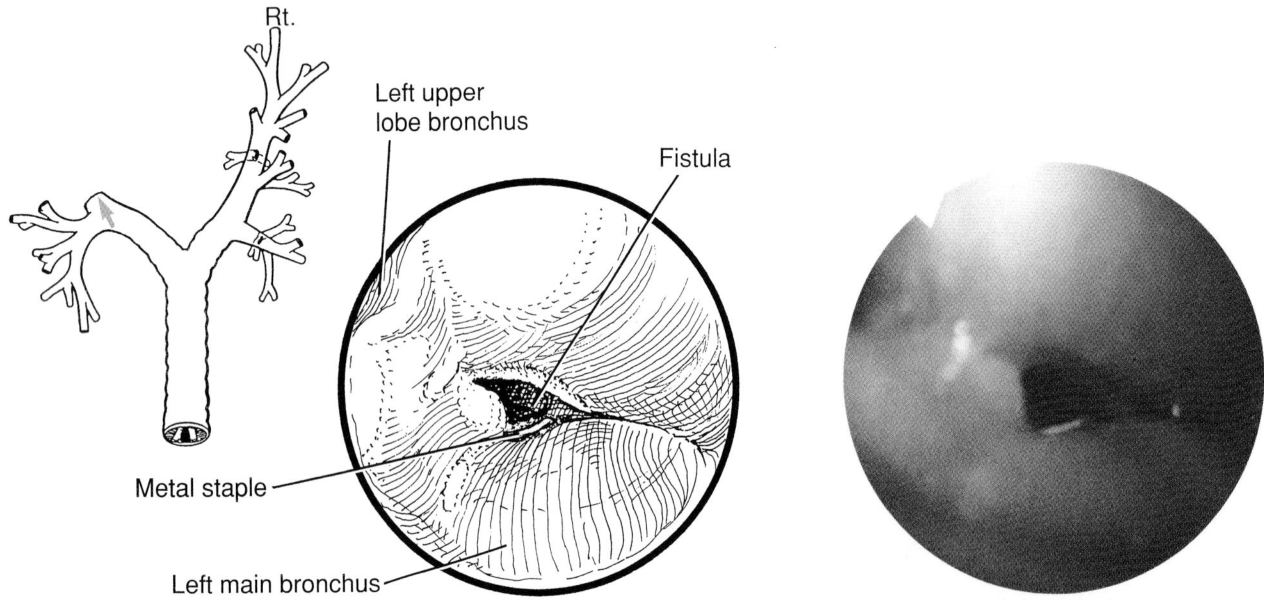

FIG. 42. Bronchopleural fistula following left lower lobectomy. Dehiscence of left lower lobectomy stump and a loose metal staple can be seen. Smaller bronchopleural fistulas have been treated with bronchoscopic fibrin glue therapy (32,33).

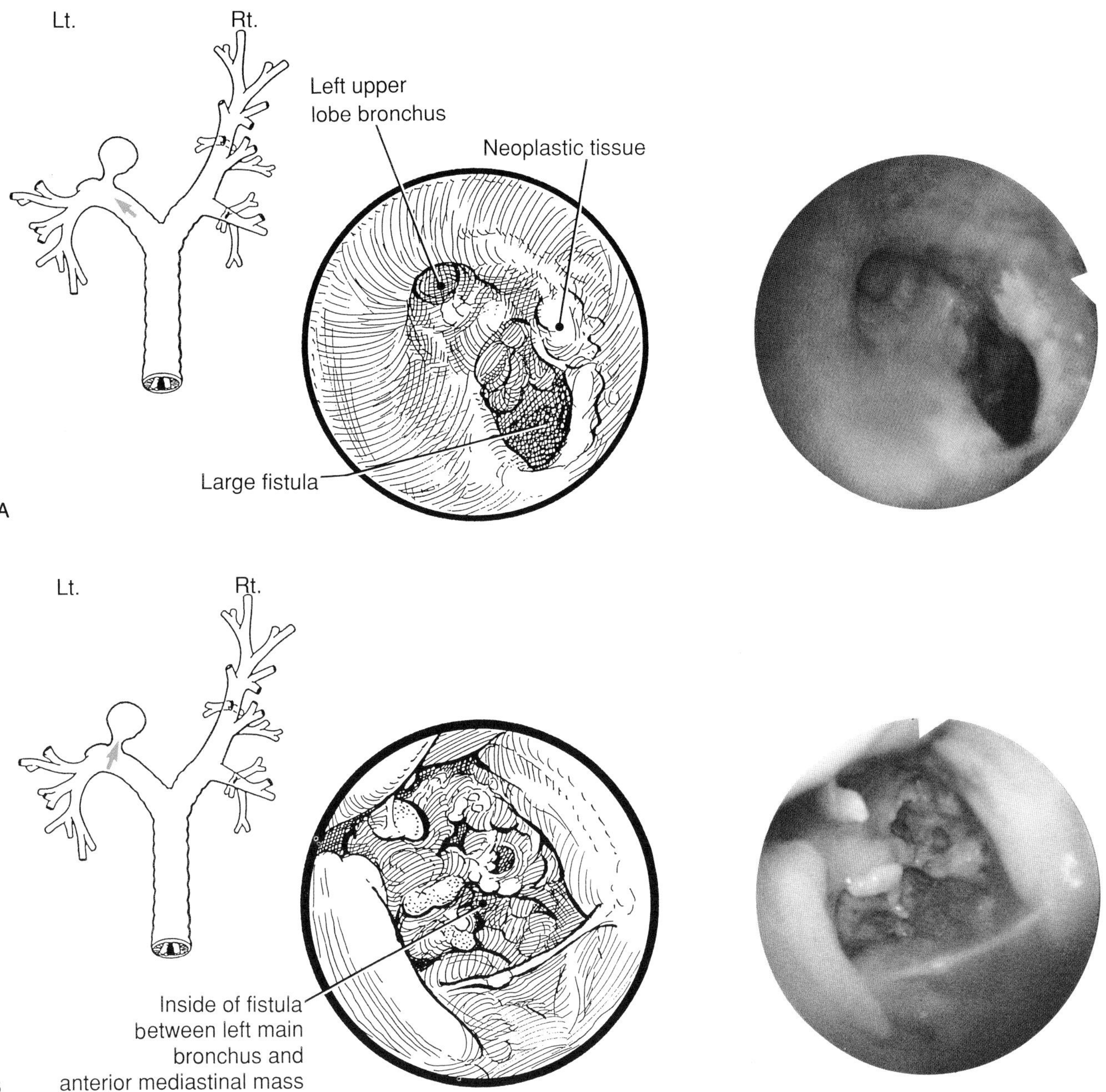

FIG. 43. A large bronchomediastinal fistula following radiation therapy to the mass **(A)**, and an inside view of the fistula and cavity in the mass **(B)**. Similar fistula has been described in a patient whose bronchial anastomotic stump (following lung transplantation) underwent dehiscence (34).

FOREIGN BODIES (Figs. 44–48)

The reader is referred to Chapter 18 for detailed discussions on the diagnosis and treatment of tracheobronchial foreign body in children as well as adults. A tracheobronchial foreign body results from accidental inhalation or iatrogenic causes, and it migrates into the tracheobronchial lumen from an extrabronchial location (35).

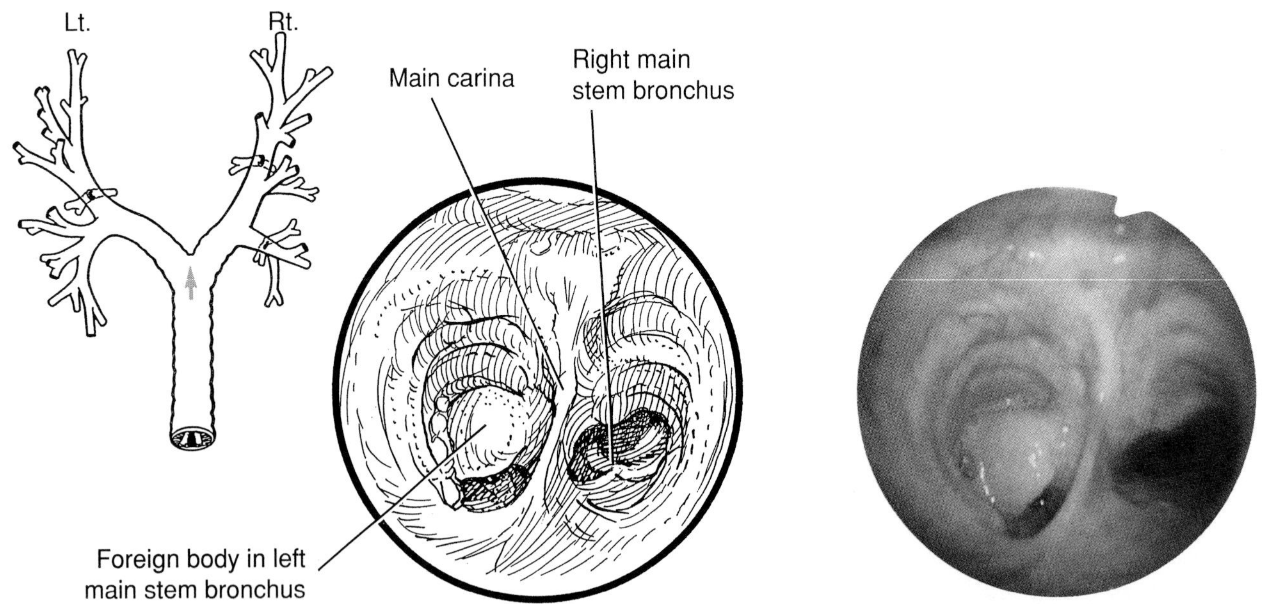

FIG. 44. Foreign body (a large segment of a peach) in an elderly edentulous patient. Flexible bronchoscopic removal was not possible despite repeated attempts. The entire foreign body was removed in a short time using a rigid bronchoscope.

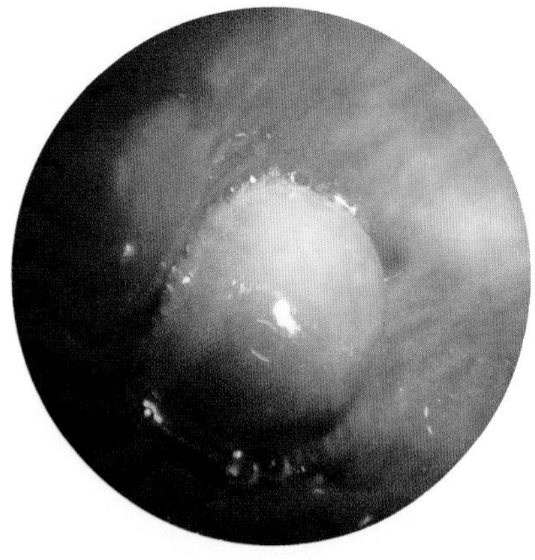

FIG. 45. Foreign body (cherry pit) in the left upper lobe bronchus.

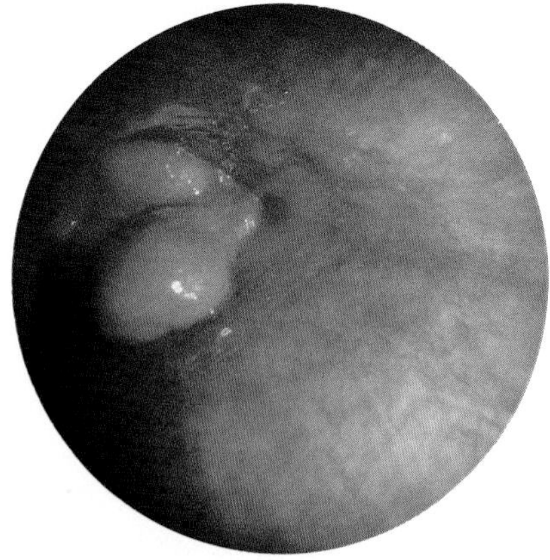

FIG. 46. Foreign body (chicken bone) impaction in the mid–left main bronchus leading to excessive formation of granulation tissue.

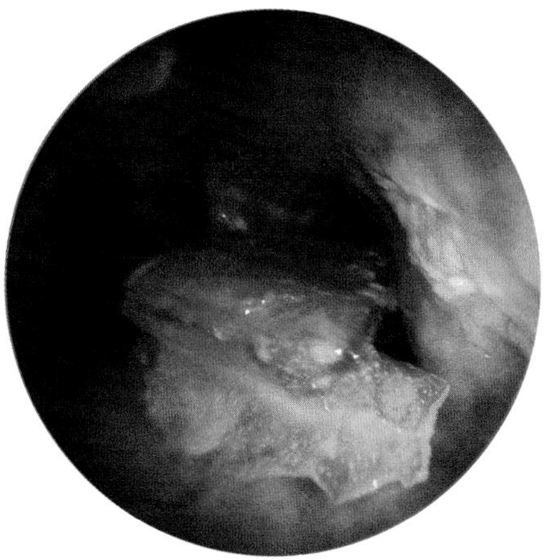

FIG. 47. Foreign body (dental prosthesis) impacted in the distal trachea and right main bronchus.

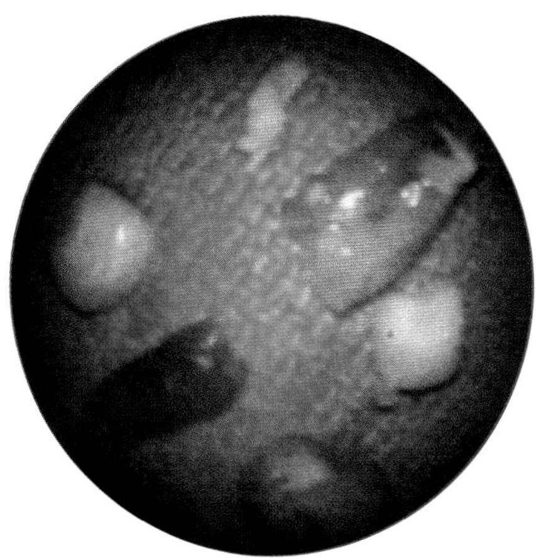

FIG. 48. Foreign bodies (multiple vegetable pieces—beans, corn, and peas) from both bronchial trees in a patient with severe neurological disease. These foreign bodies, photographed through a flexible bronchoscope, were removed using a flexible bronchoscope.

HEMORRHAGIC DISORDERS (Fig. 49)

Hemorrhagic diatheses or disorders pose special problems for the bronchoscopist because of the risk of inducing hemorrhage by bronchoscopic procedures. However, simple bronchoscopy (without biopsies), diagnostic bronchoalveolar lavage, and therapeutic bronchoscopy (aspiration of mucus and plugs) can be accomplished without increasing the risk of bleeding from the tracheobronchial tree.

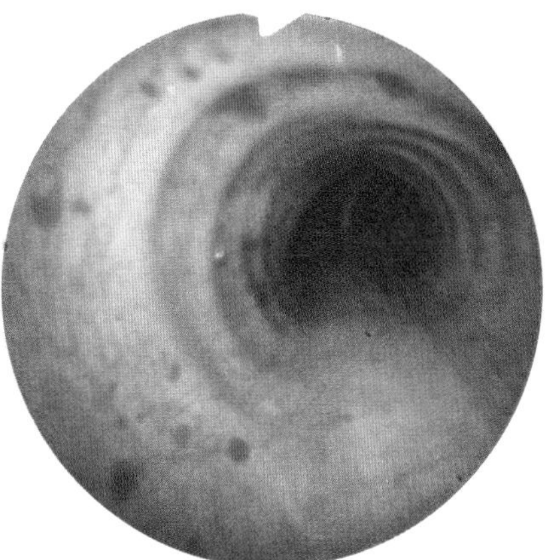

FIG. 49. Tracheal purpura in a patient with thrombocytopenia (platelet count $<200/mm^3$) caused by chemotherapy for leukemia. Note the petechiae are in the intercartilaginous sulci. If the mucosal bleeding was due to bronchoscopy itself, then the petechiae would be located along the cartilaginous ridges. A diagnostic bronchoalveolar lavage was obtained without provoking serious hemorrhage.

IATROGENIC CHANGES (Figs. 50–71)

Foremost among the iatrogenic endobronchial abnormalities are those caused by the bronchoscope itself. These changes can vary from simple mucosal edema to serious bronchoscopy-induced hemorrhage (Chapter 17) (36). Such abnormalities, however, are transient and cause no chronic complications in the majority of patients. Iatrogenic foreign bodies are discussed in Chapter 18. Alterations in the tracheobronchial tree brought on by surgical procedures, radiation therapy, and certain forms of endobronchial therapy can be long-lasting or permanent.

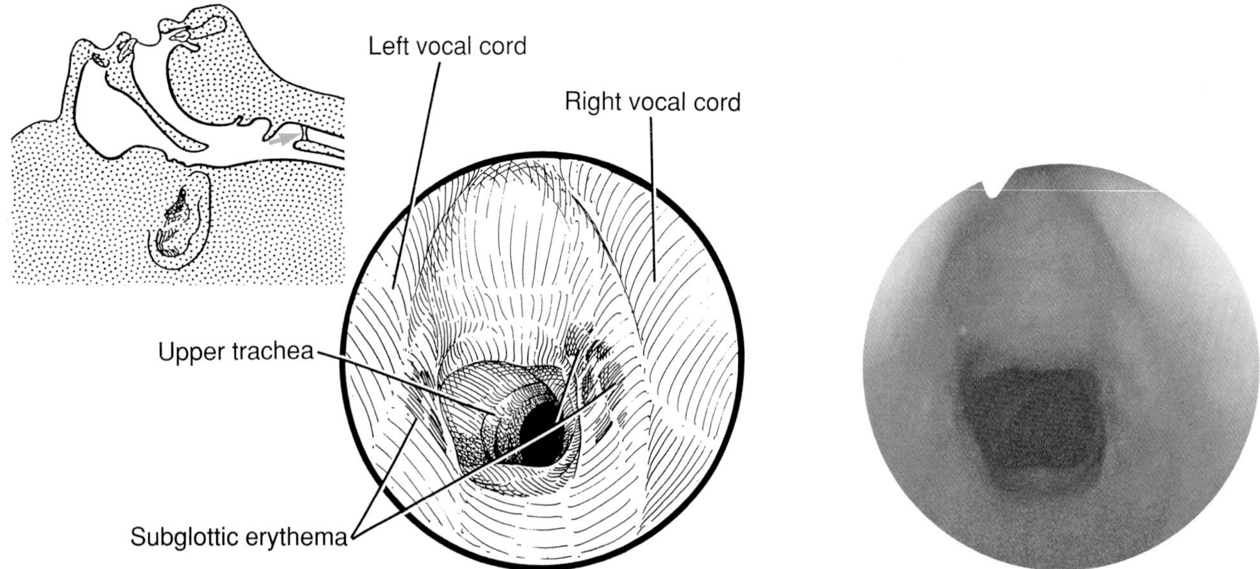

FIG. 50. Subglottic edema and erythema caused by endotracheal intubation. Such minimal changes usually resolve without sequelae.

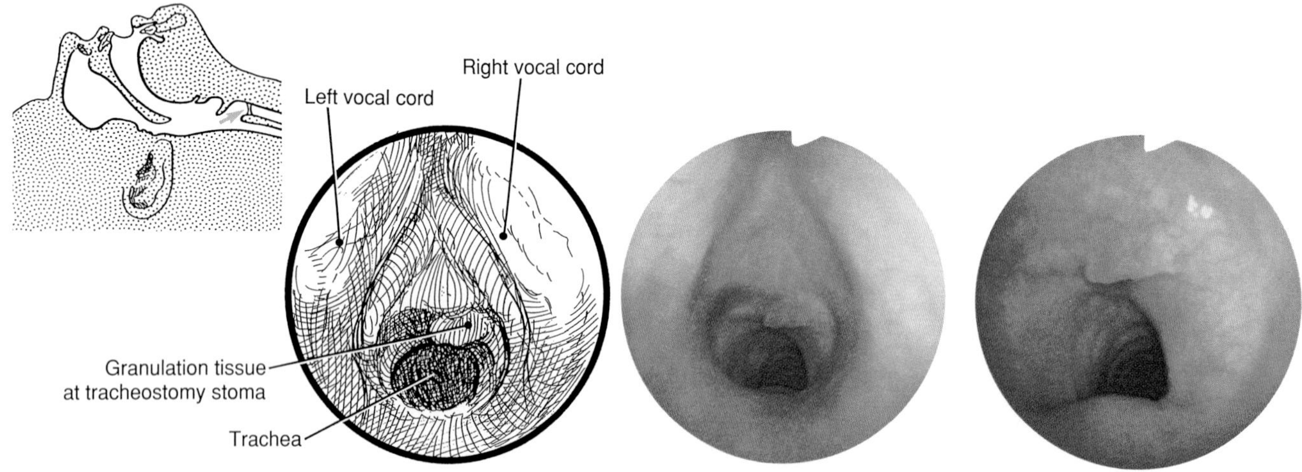

FIG. 51. Mucosal granulation arising in healed tracheostomy stoma **(left)** and a close-up **(right)**. Such granulomas or mucosal tags are usually asymptomatic although larger (and loose) tags may cause cough.

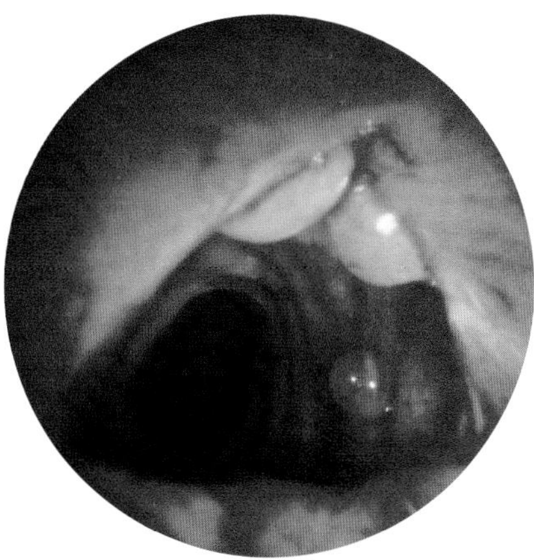

FIG. 52. Multiple tracheal granulomas in a previously tracheotomized patient. Such granulomas may arise from the mucosa coming in repeated contact with the tracheostomy tube. Bronchoscopic (with or without laser) removal may be necessary.

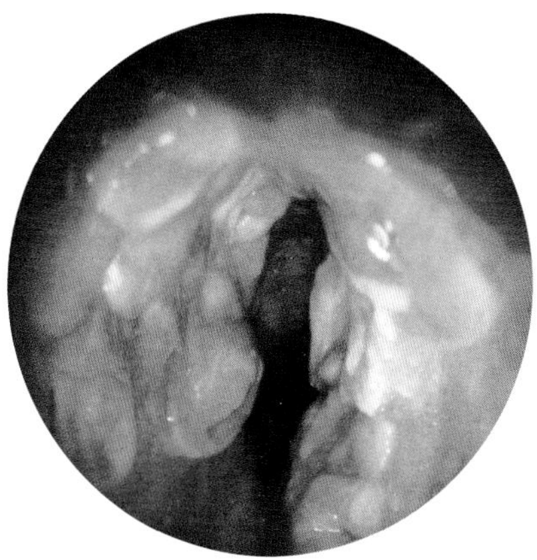

FIG. 53. Exuberant growth of granulomatous tissue in the trachea of a patient with endotracheal tube. Removal of tube is an important aspect of therapy.

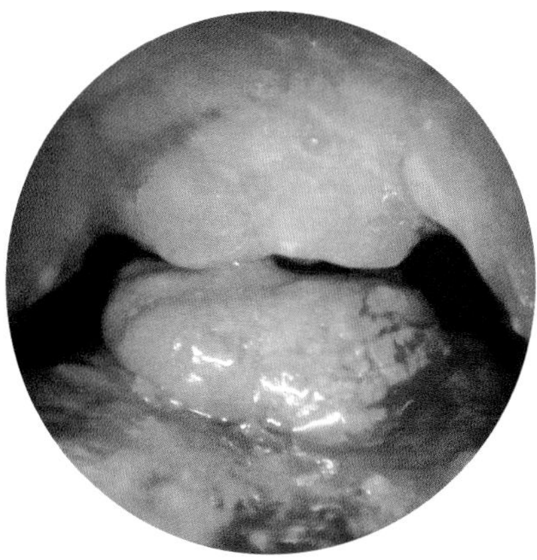

FIG. 54. Extensive anterior and posterior granulation tissue resulting from an endotracheal tube placed after total laryngectomy. Rigid bronchoscopy and Nd:YAG laser therapy resulted in absence of recurrence 9 years later.

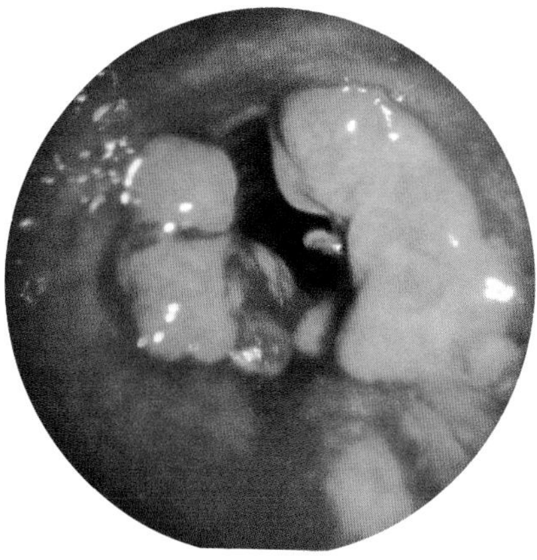

FIG. 55. Extensive granulation tissue formation following tracheal resection and end-to-end anastomosis. Suture material can be seen within the granulation on the right side. No recurrence noted for 7 years after Nd:YAG laser resection.

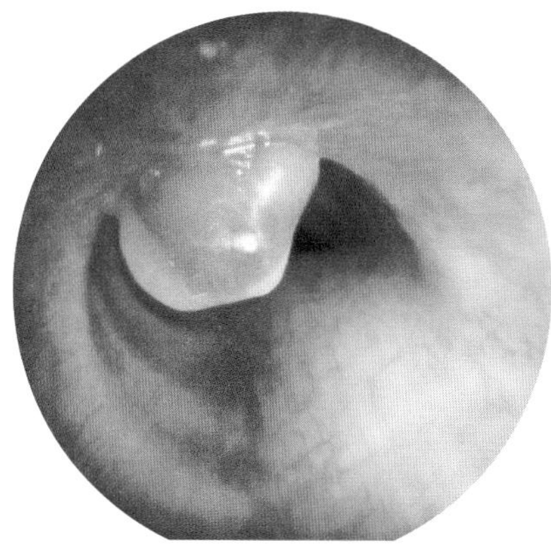

FIG. 56. Suture granuloma at the site of previous tracheostomy. Resected via a rigid bronchoscope and the base treated with Nd:YAG laser.

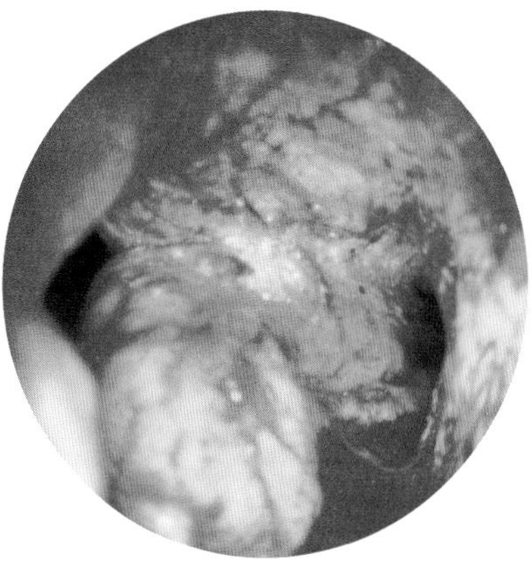

FIG. 57. Trauma induced by repeated suction/aspiration leading to severe inflammation and formation of granulation tissue in distal trachea and main stem bronchi.

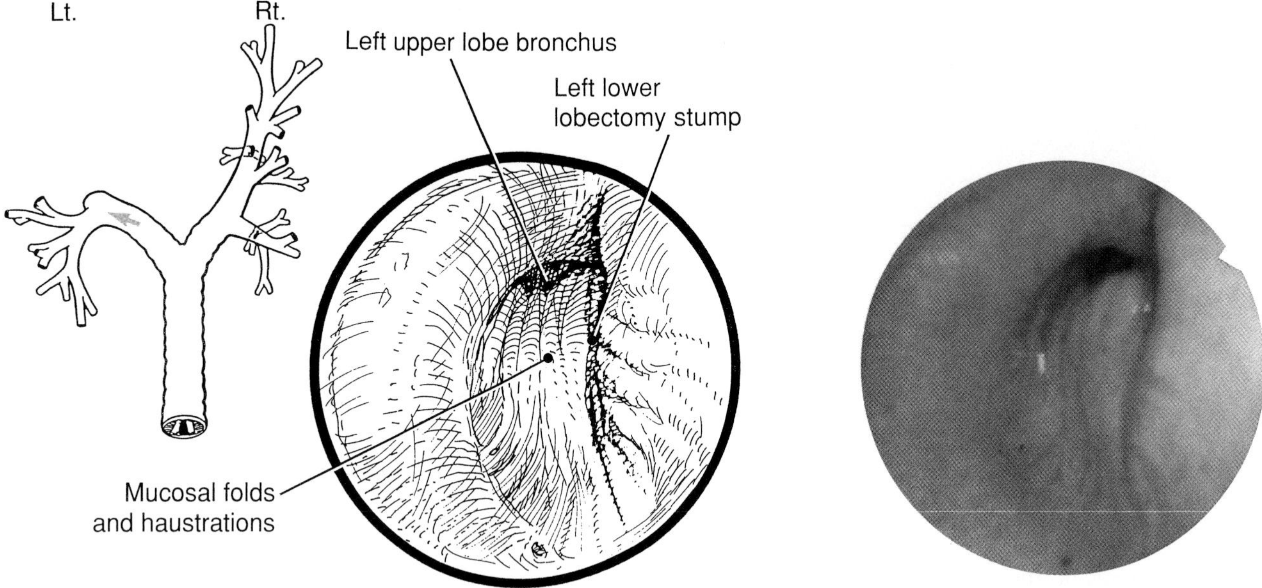

FIG. 58. Postlobectomy distortion of bronchus. Following resection of a lobe or segment, the remaining bronchi may undergo anatomic distortion and produce varying degrees of airway narrowing. This is more common after left lower lobectomy.

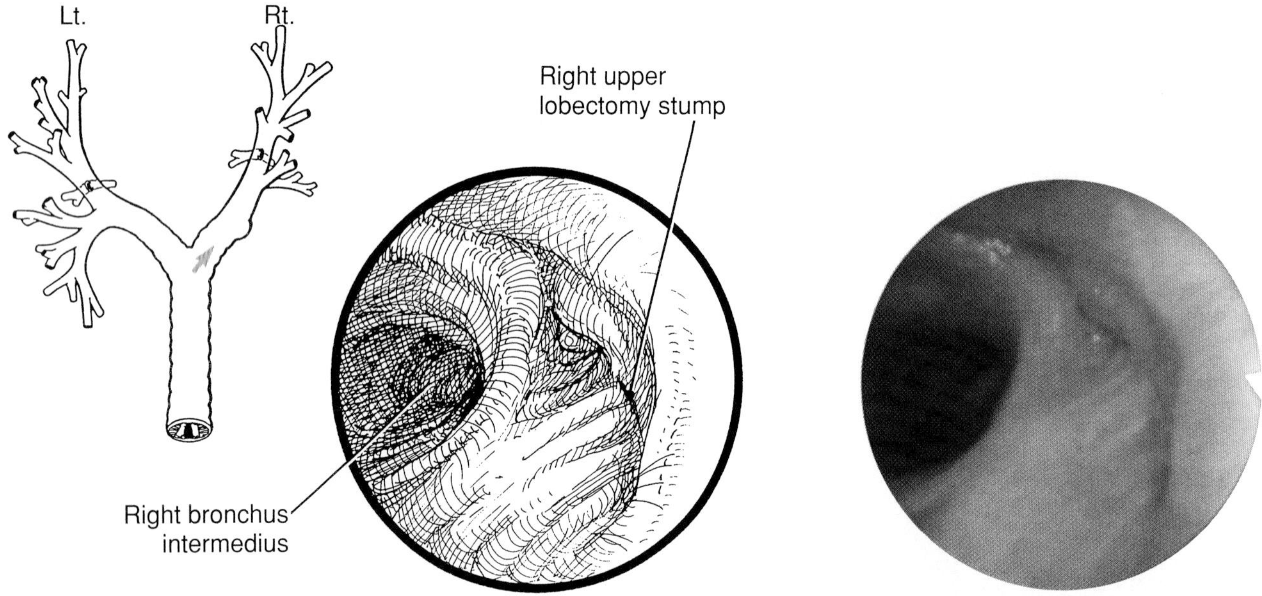

FIG. 59. Right upper lobectomy stump appears healthy. There is no evidence of loose sutures, obvious fistula, or stump recurrence of previously resected carcinoma.

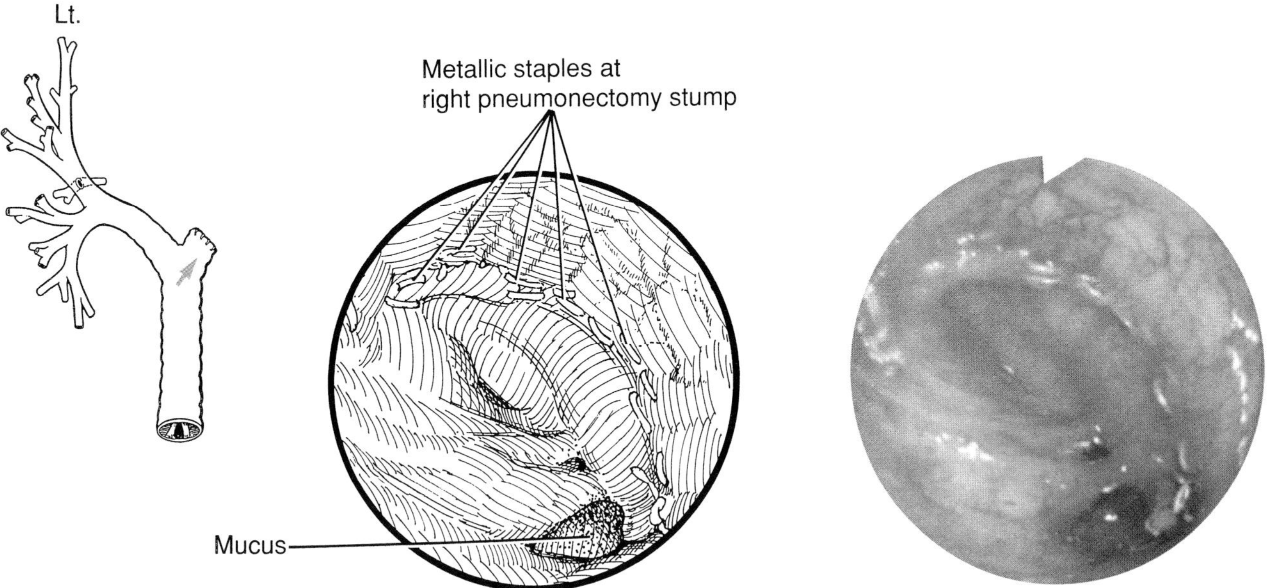

FIG. 60. Right pneumonectomy stump appears healthy. A row of metallic sutures is seen. Small amounts of mucus usually collect in the pits caused by the surgical procedure.

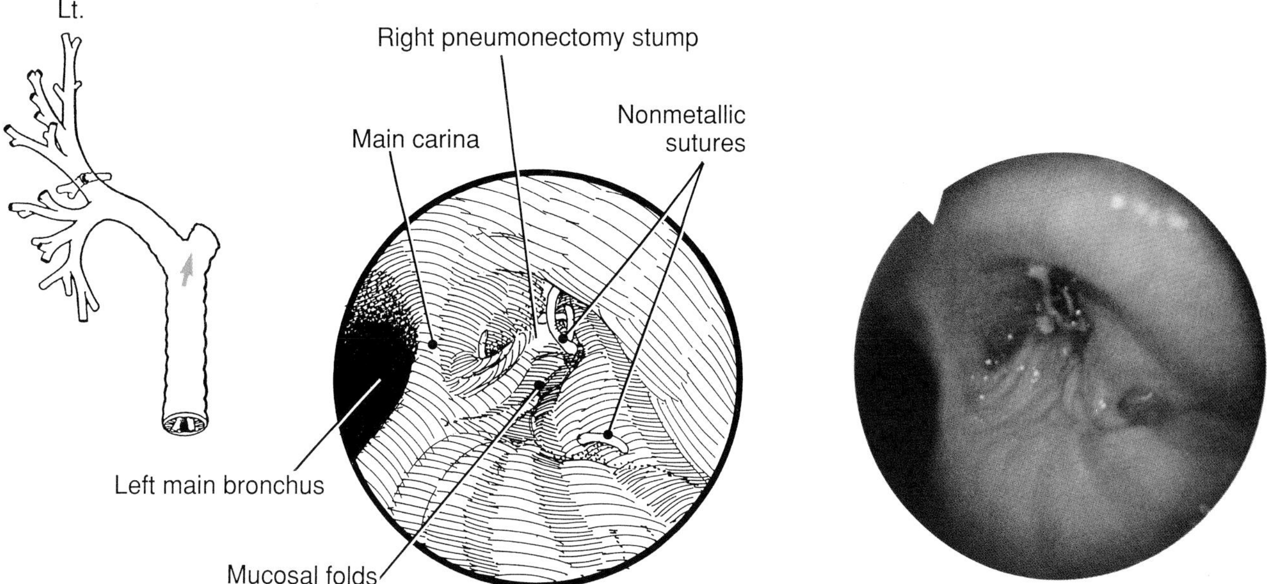

FIG. 61. Sutures at the site of right pneumonectomy. Unless these are very loose or cause cough, removal is not necessary. Endobronchial sutures can cause chronic persistent cough and bronchoscopic removal of suture may be necessary (37).

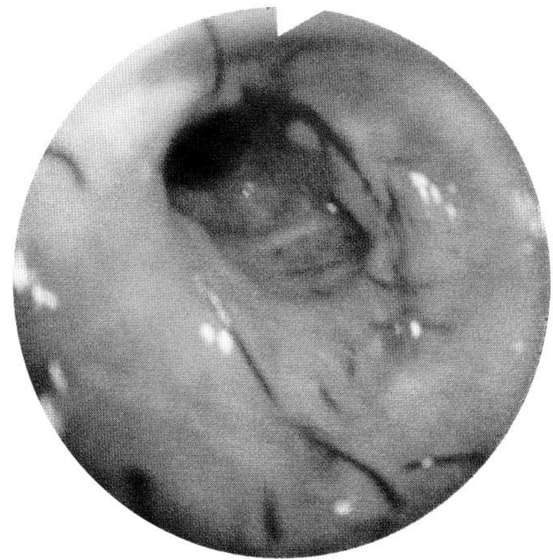

FIG. 62. Nonmetallic sutures at the site of bronchoplasty.

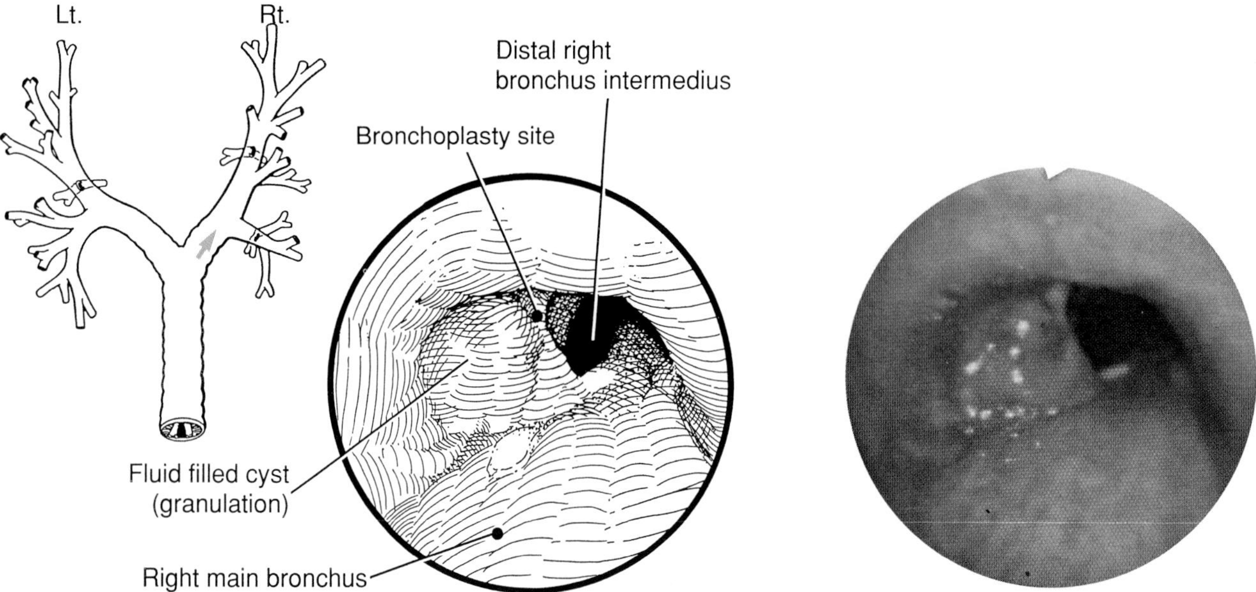

FIG. 63. Granuloma at site of bronchoplasty. Tracheobronchial anastomoses may produce granulation tissue at the anastomotic site. Cough and hemoptysis are the most common symptoms. Removal of granulation tissue can be accomplished with bronchoscopic biopsy removal or Nd:YAG laser therapy.

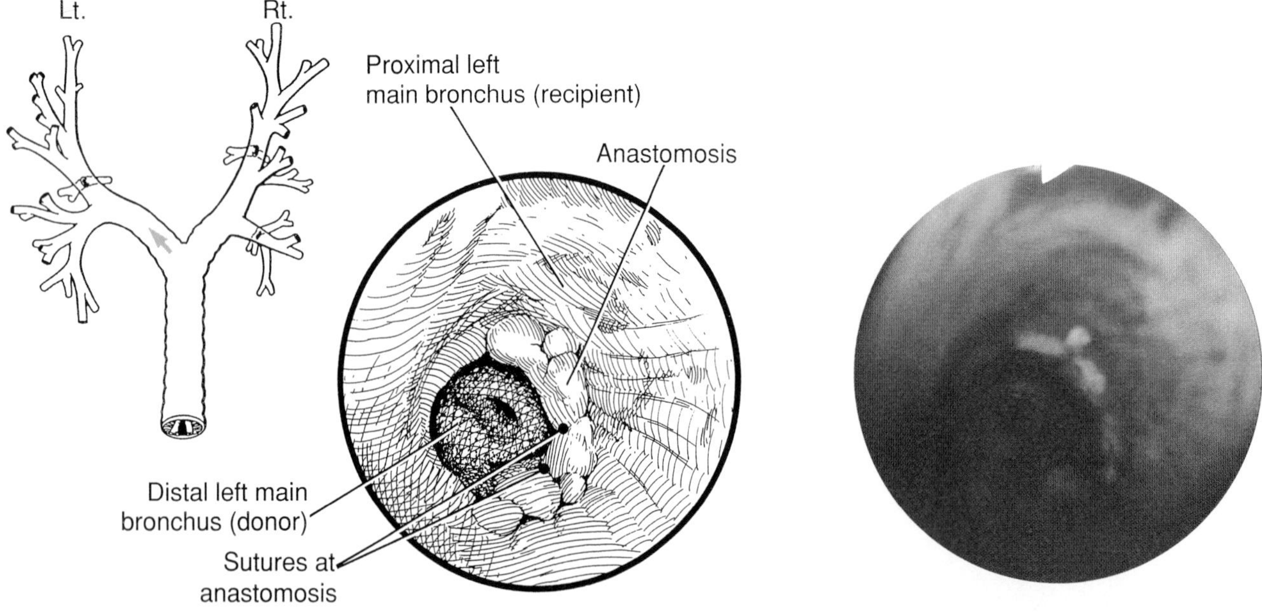

FIG. 64. Left main bronchial anastomosis in a patient with a transplanted lung. Flexible bronchoscopic balloon dilatation and/or bronchial stent therapy have been utilized to treat bronchial strictures that follow lung transplantation (38,39).

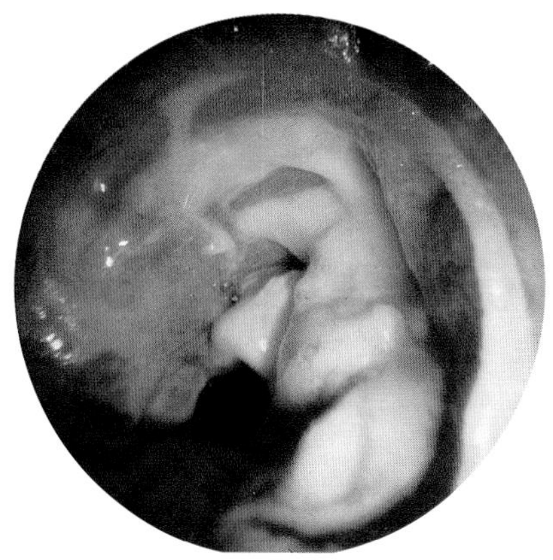

FIG. 65. Radiation-induced necrosis of trachea. Large amount of necrotic material and partially treated tracheal tumor can be seen.

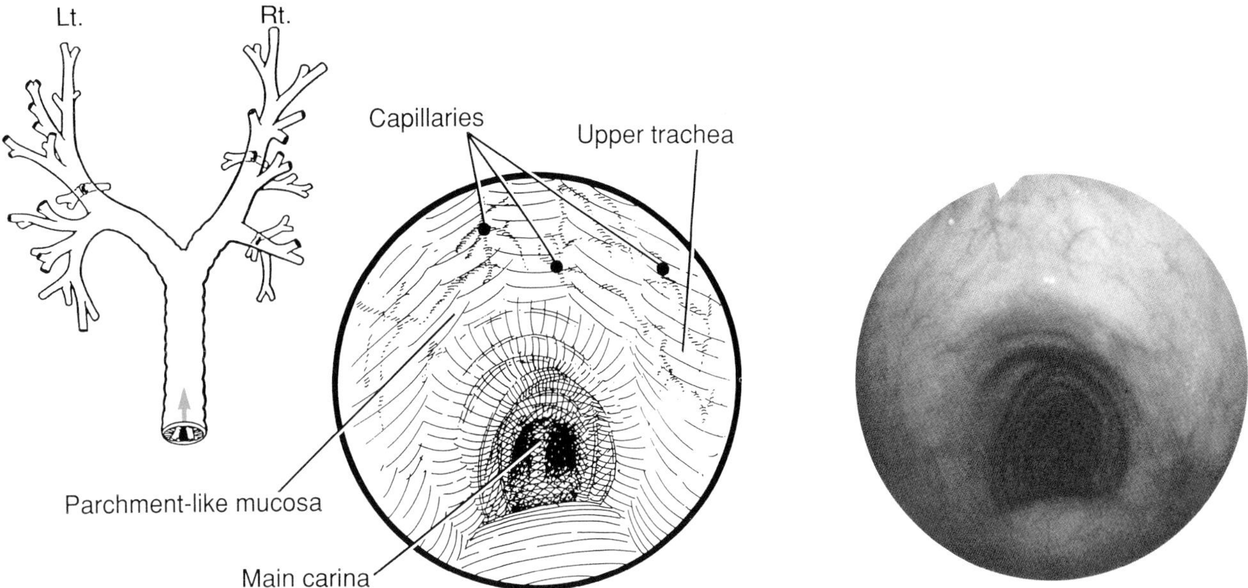

FIG. 66. Radiation-induced mucosal changes in subglottic area. Mucosa looks pale, dry, and exhibits submucosal capillary proliferation. There are no characteristic bronchoscopic findings in radiation-induced airway injury.

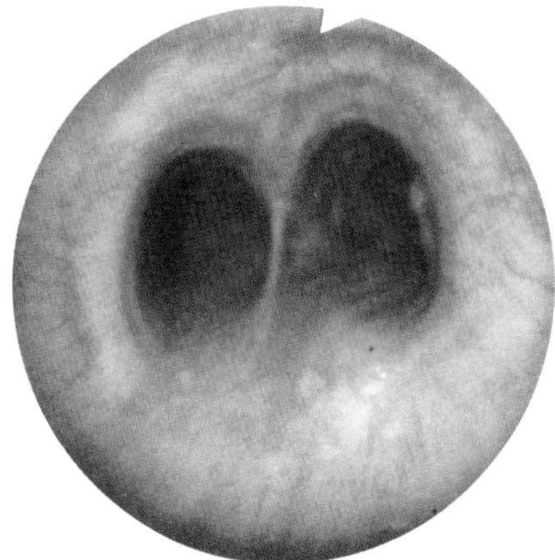

FIG. 67. Radiation-induced bronchitis showing submucosal erythema and prominent capillary network.

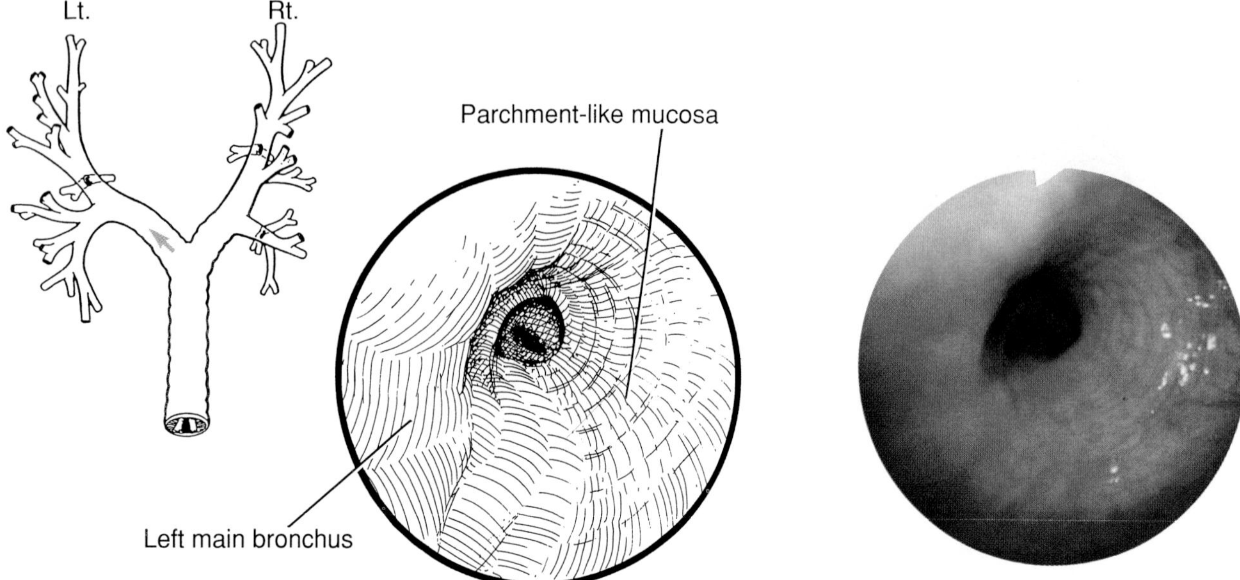

FIG. 68. Radiation-induced mucosal changes in left main bronchus. Submucosal capillary network appears prominent. Mucosa has a "tight" and parchment-like appearance.

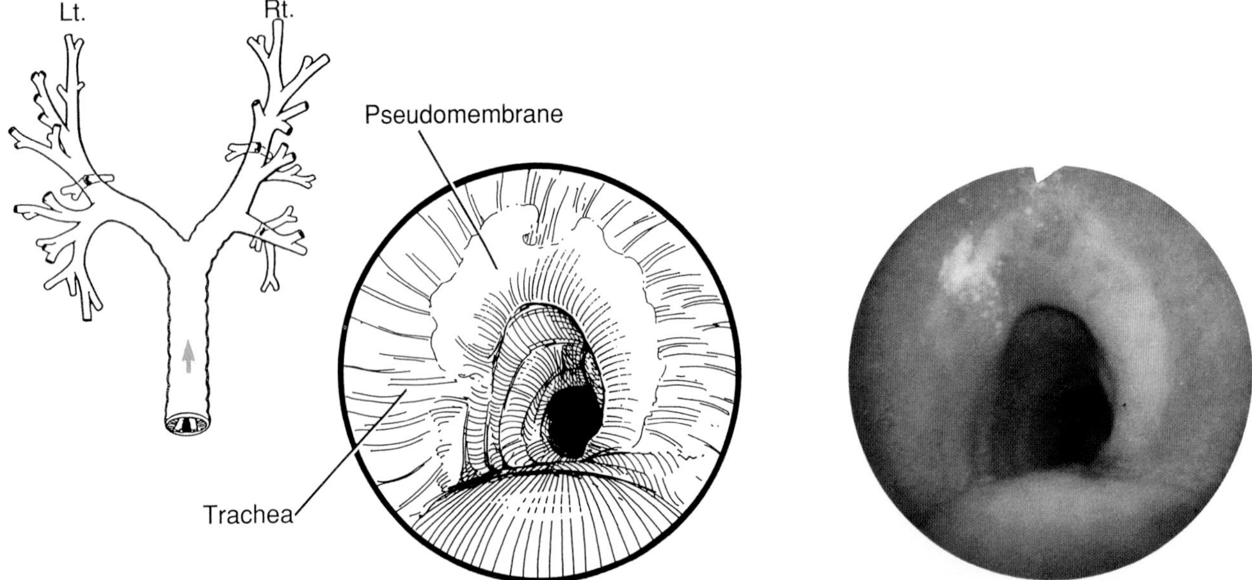

FIG. 69. Photodynamic therapy-induced pseudomembrane formation. This may occur anywhere from 24 hr to several days after the treatment and can cause respiratory distress (40,41). Bronchoscopic removal may be necessary. Pseudomembrane formation also can be seen in tracheobronchial necrotizing aspergillosis and candidiasis.

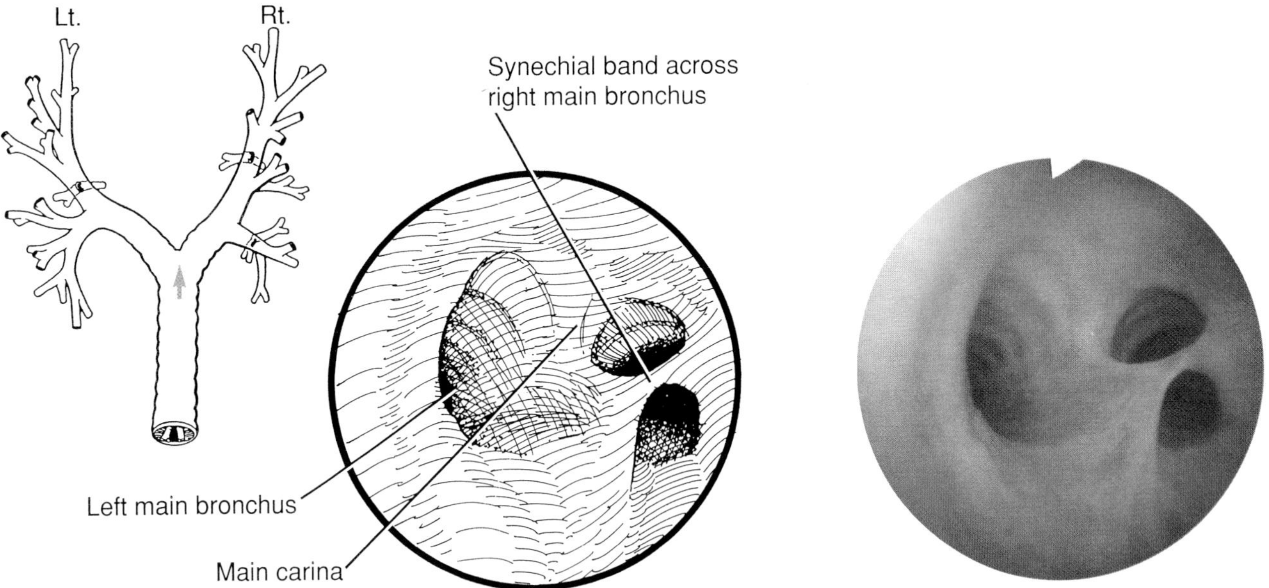

FIG. 70. Synechial band across right main bronchus following radiation therapy to an obstructing tumor. Others have described such endobronchial bands or strings following radiotherapy and also as an incidental finding (42,43).

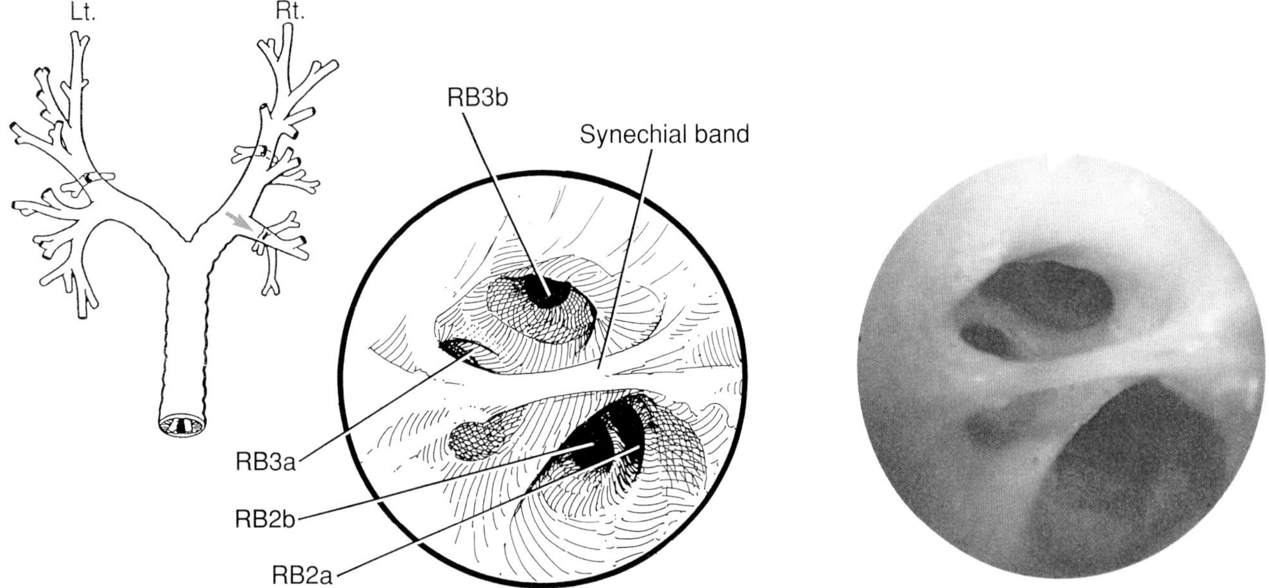

FIG. 71. Synechial band across right upper lobe bronchus following Nd:YAG laser therapy. Patients are usually asymptomatic and resection of synechial bands is not necessary. Severely obstructing bands have been treated with laser ablation (42).

INFECTIONS (Figs. 72–93)

The tracheobronchial tree can be affected by all classes of infectious agents. Indeed, the common cold or "flu" initially affects the tracheobronchial mucosa from which it spreads distally. Very few people undergo bronchoscopy for evaluation of common upper respiratory infections caused by viruses and bacteria. Acute bacterial tracheitis is generally a disease of children and is characterized by a severe infraglottic infection manifested by toxicity, brassy cough, stridor, subglottic edema, and the presence of copious mucopurulent secretions in the trachea (44). The following examples illustrate the bronchoscopic findings in several infectious diseases.

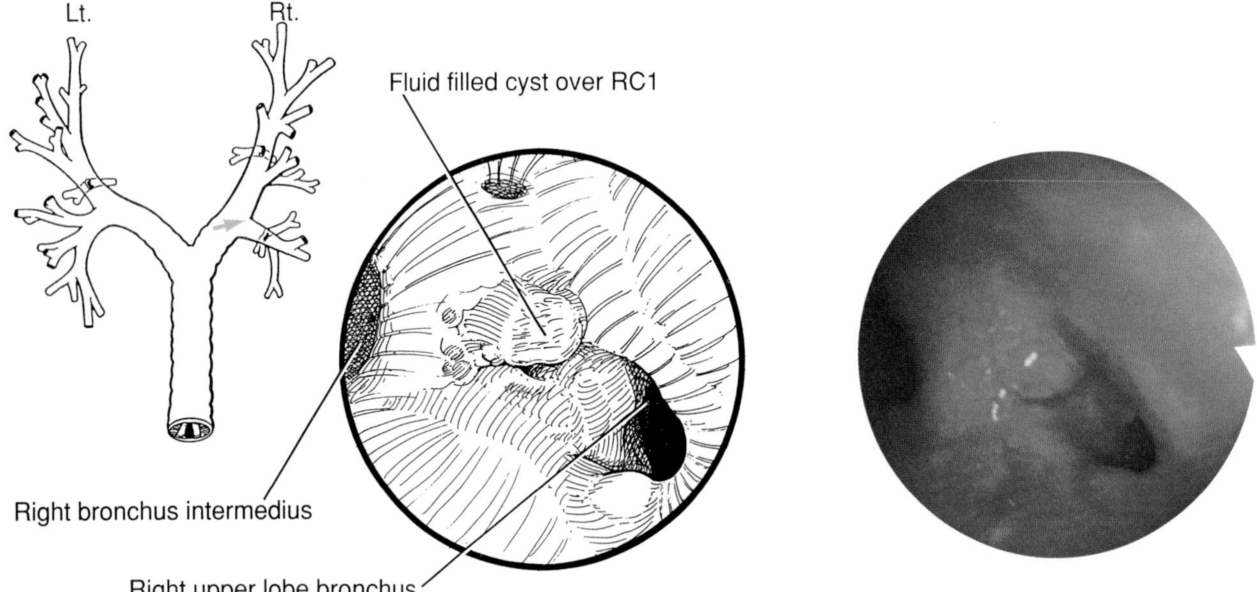

FIG. 72. Herpes vesicle in a patient with acquired immunodeficiency syndrome (AIDS). The patient had extensive esophageal lesions from herpes. Herpetic infection of the tracheobronchial tree may produce mucosal edema, erythema, ulceration, and airway obstruction (45–47).

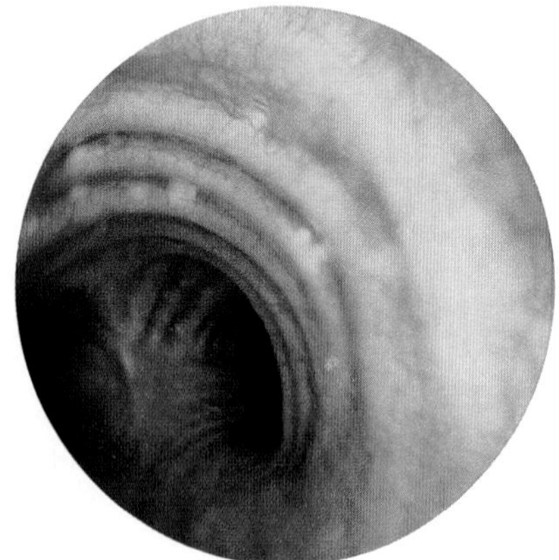

FIG. 73. Multiple viral lesions in the trachea secondary to viral infection.

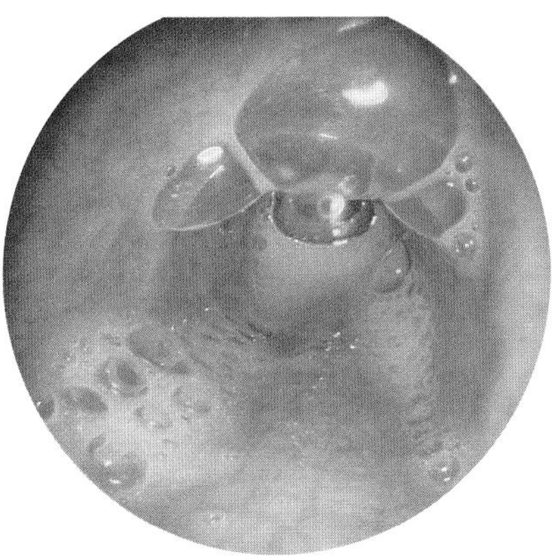

FIG. 74. Purulent secretions caused by bacterial infection of the airways. The secretions can be thin, thick, or inspissated.

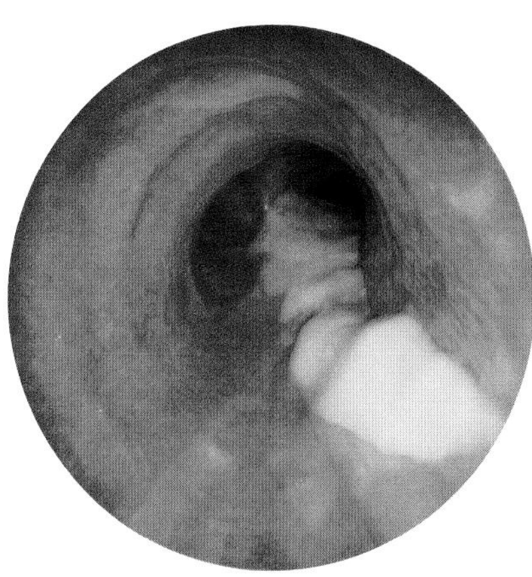

FIG. 75. Thick purulent secretions streaking from right main bronchus in a patient with necrotizing pneumonia.

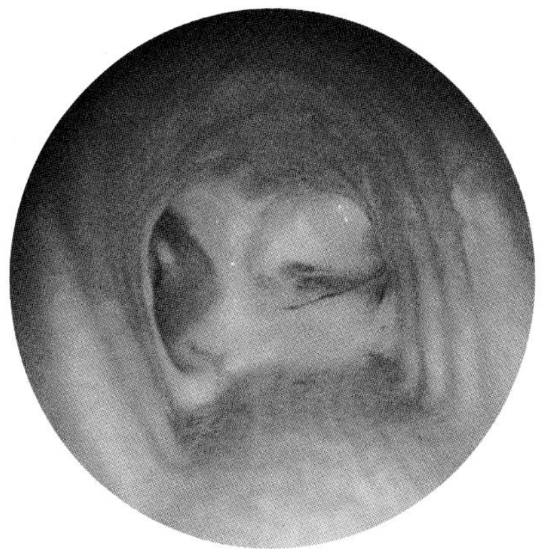

FIG. 76. Thick purulent secretions from both main bronchi. Caused by severe bacterial infection. Bacterial tracheitis is more common in children and the organisms involved include *Staphylococcus aureus, Hemophilus influenzae, Moraxella catarrhalis,* and *Streptococcus pneumoniae* (48).

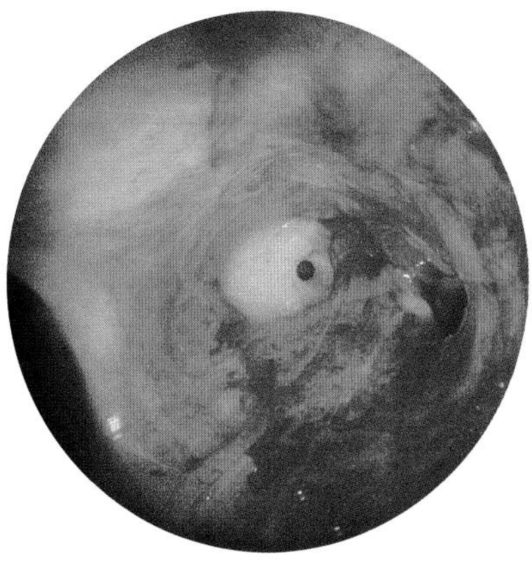

FIG. 77. Purulent secretion oozing from a pinhole stenosis of right bronchus intermedius. Courtesy of Lutz Freitag, M.D.

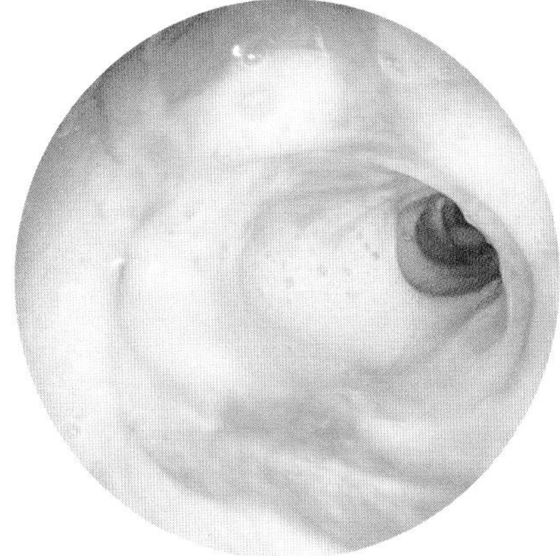

FIG. 78. Pus coming out of right bronchus intermedius in a patient with severe bronchiectasis. Courtesy of Lutz Freitag, M.D.

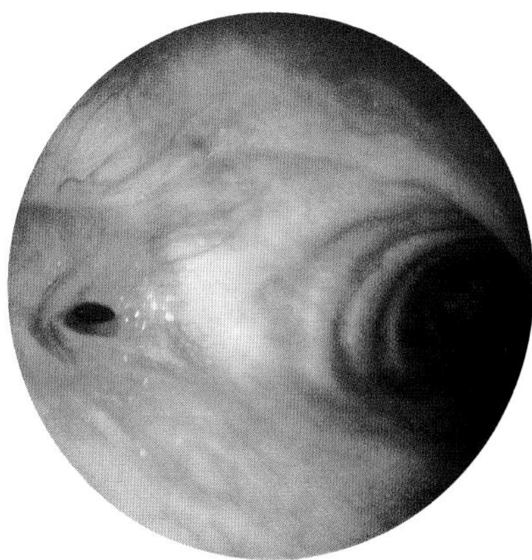

FIG. 79. Tuberculosis-induced stenosis of proximal left main bronchus. Such postinfectious strictures follow endobronchial tuberculosis (49–52).

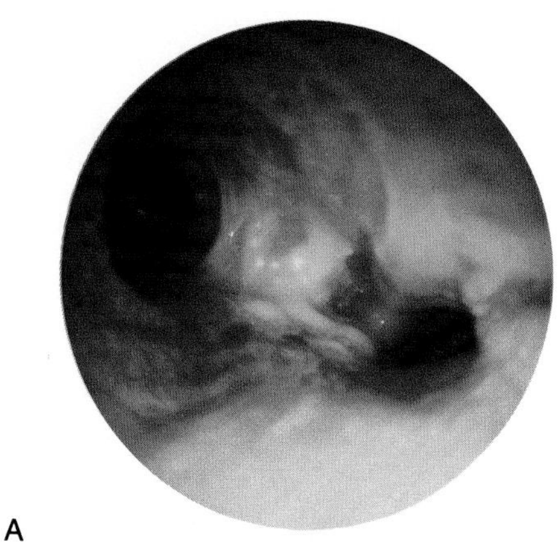

A

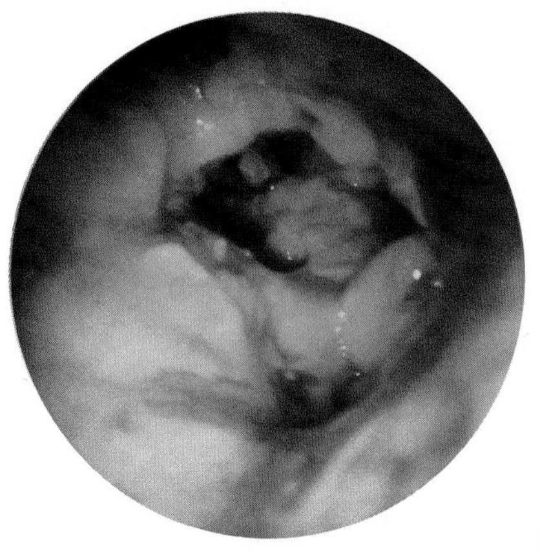

B

FIG. 80. Tuberculosis (active) of distal left main bronchus **(left)** and close-up view of left lower lobe bronchus **(right)**. Mucosal biopsy in such cases will reveal caseous granulomas containing tubercle bacilli. Active endobronchial tuberculosis can mimic bronchogenic carcinoma (51).

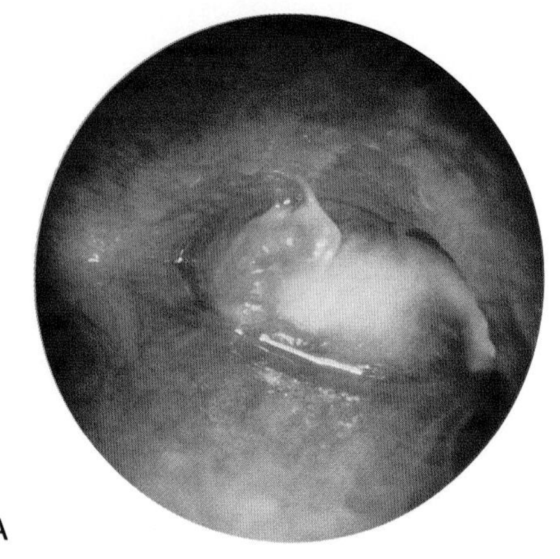

A

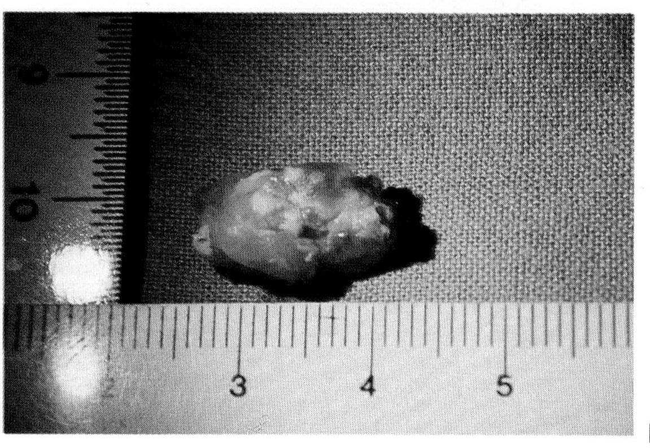

B

FIG. 81. Tuberculous lymphadenopathy eroding into right main bronchus **(left)** and a view of the bronchoscopically resected lymph node **(right)**.

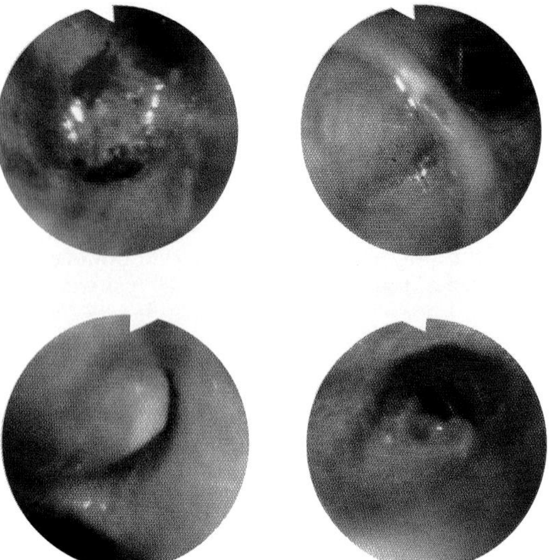

FIG. 82. *Mycobacterium avium* complex infection causing endobronchial lesions in patients with AIDS. These lesions can mimic bronchial carcinoma (53–55). From Mehle et al. (55), with permission.

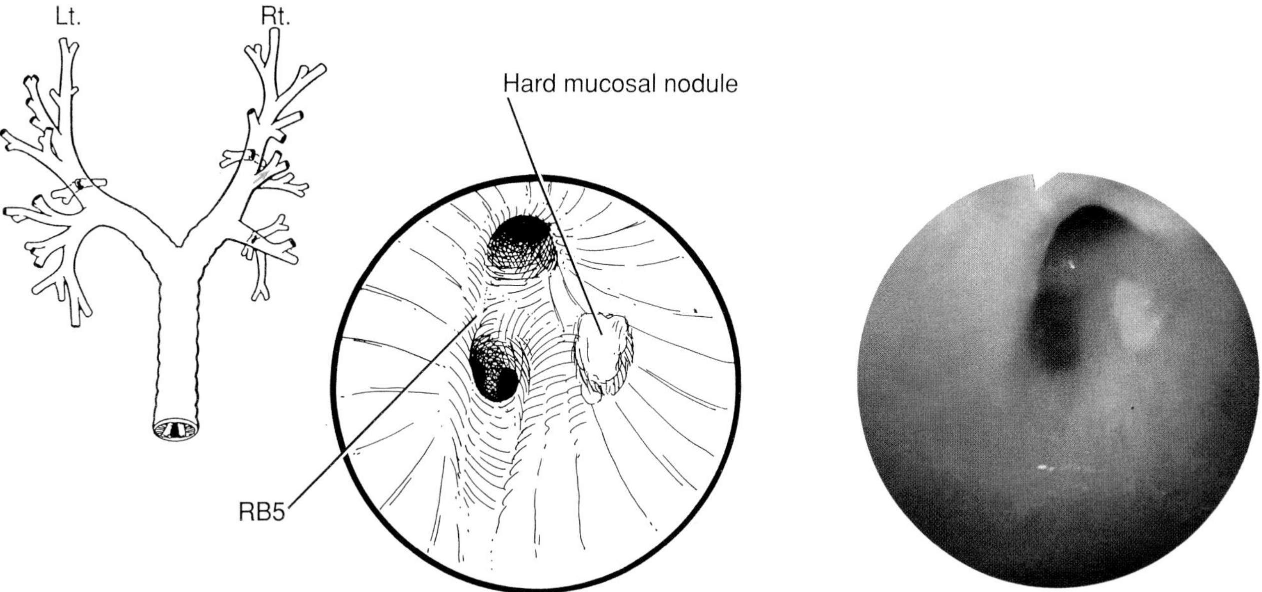

FIG. 83. *Mycobacterium avium* complex infection causing endobronchial nodule in a patient with AIDS. Biopsy revealed caseous granulomas containing acid-fast bacilli.

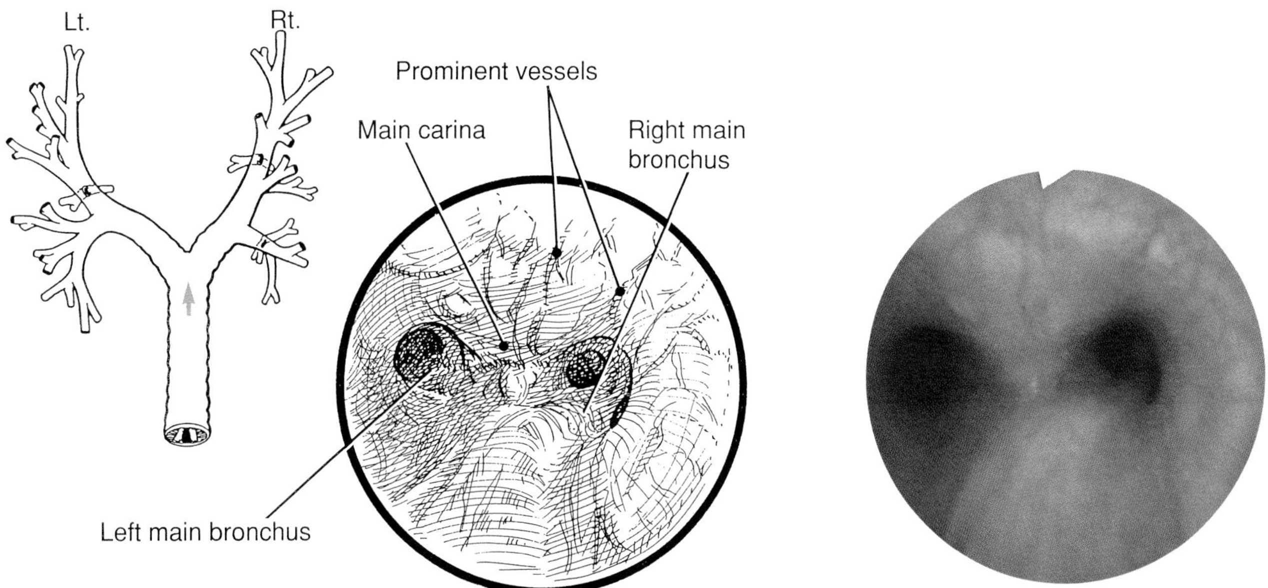

FIG. 84. Histoplasmosis-induced mediastinal granuloma (fibrosing mediastinitis) with secondary tracheobronchial narrowing and hyperemia. Diffuse narrowing of major airways is usually caused by extrinsic compression. Stenosis of major airways has been noted in 45% of patients with mediastinal fibrosis (56). Mucosal biopsy does not show fungal granulomas unless endobronchial infection is present. Most patients with mediastinal granuloma do not have active histoplasmosis.

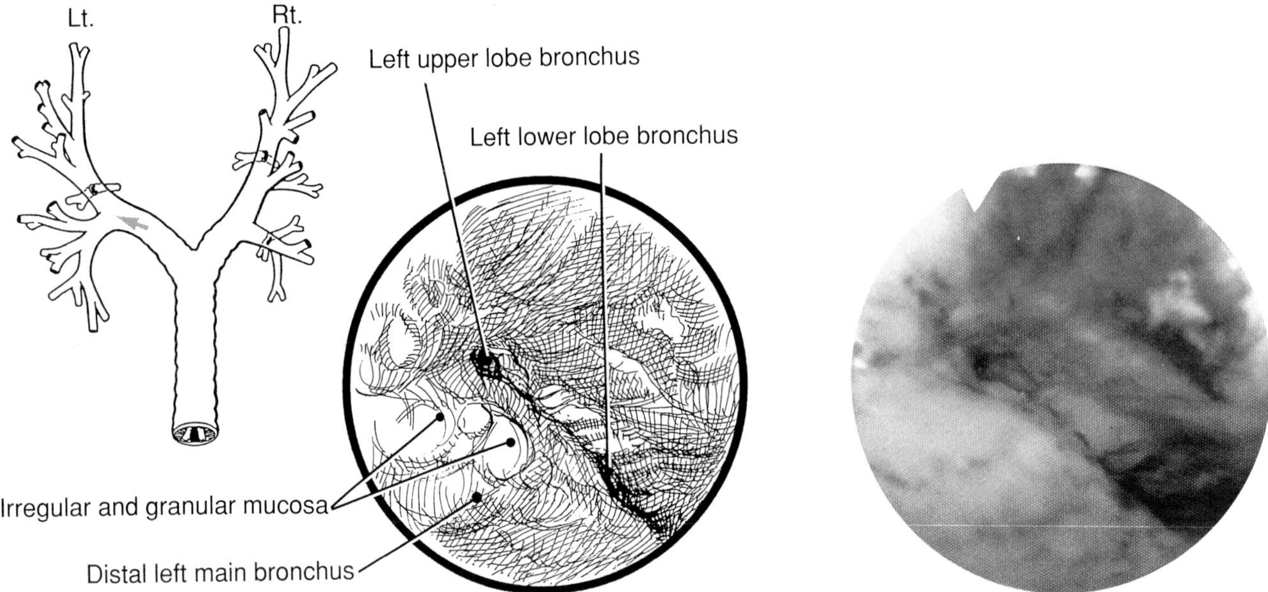

FIG. 85. Histoplasmosis-induced endobronchial narrowing and mucosal abnormality. Mucosal biopsies showed noncaseous granulomas but cultures and special stains were negative for histoplasmosis. Bronchoscopy is the only test of diagnostic importance in one third of patients with pulmonary histoplasmosis (57).

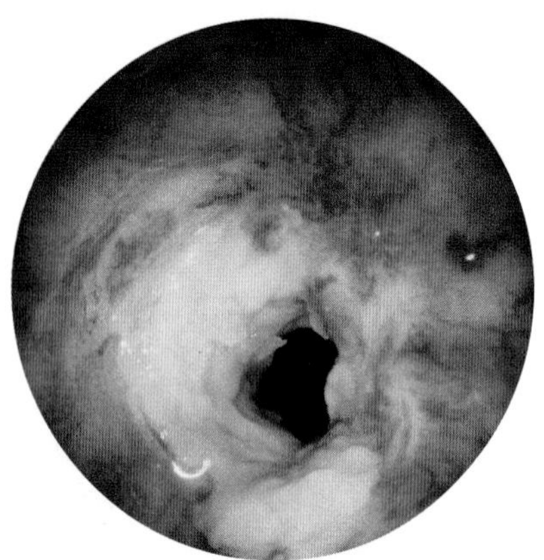

FIG. 86. Necrotizing aspergillosis of the trachea with formation of thick pseudomembrane. Laser vaporization and mechanical dilatation with the rigid bronchoscope was performed. Necrotizing aspergillosis of the tracheobronchial tree is being recognized more frequently in immunosuppressed patients. It is more common in patients undergoing intense chemotherapy for hematological malignancies, following heart–lung or lung transplantation, and AIDS (58–61).

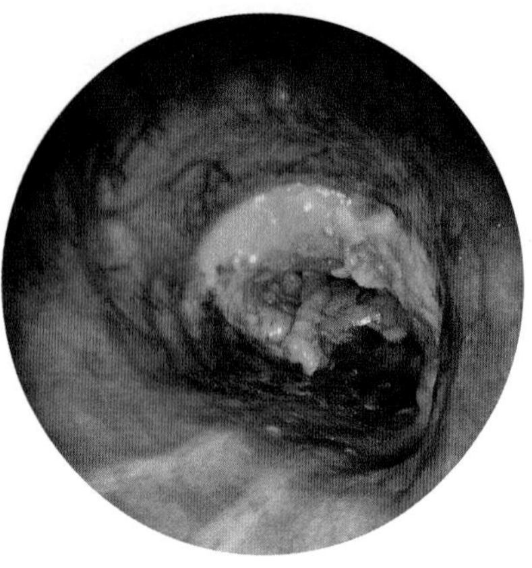

FIG. 87. Necrotizing aspergillosis of the right main bronchus in a patient with chronic myeloid leukemia.

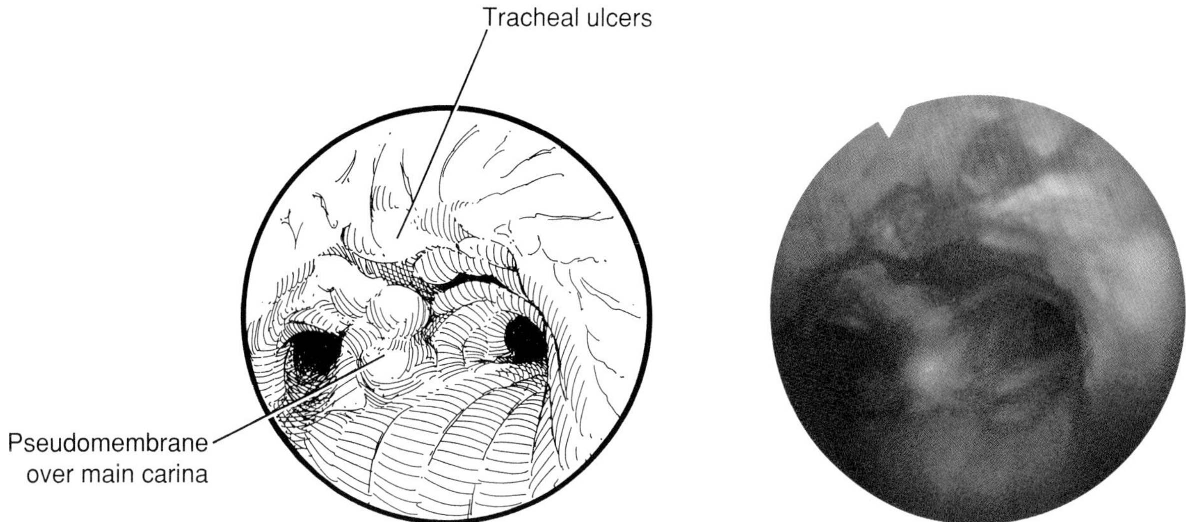

FIG. 88. Necrotizing aspergillosis of distal trachea in a neutropenic patient with non-Hodgkin's lymphoma. Removal of pseudomembrane revealed shallow ulcers.

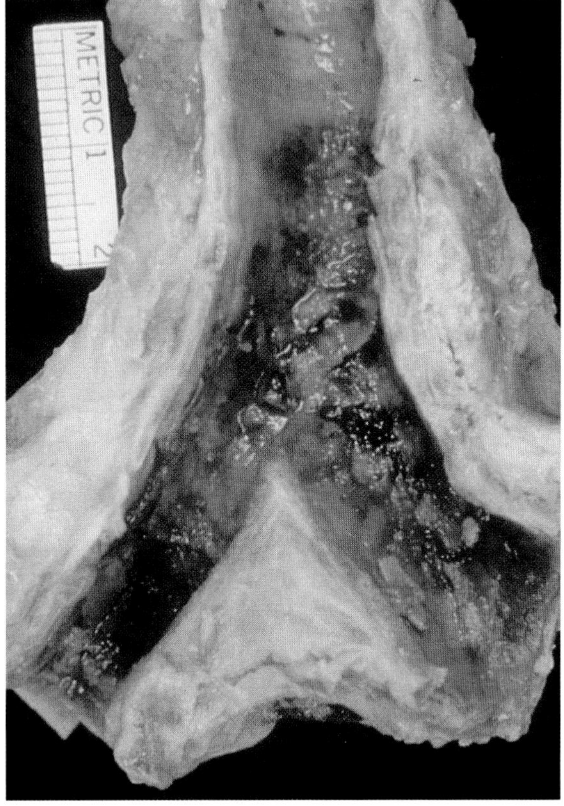

FIG. 89. Trachea and main bronchi removed at autopsy in the patient shown in Fig. 88. Necrotic pseudomembrane can be seen. From ref. 61, with permission.

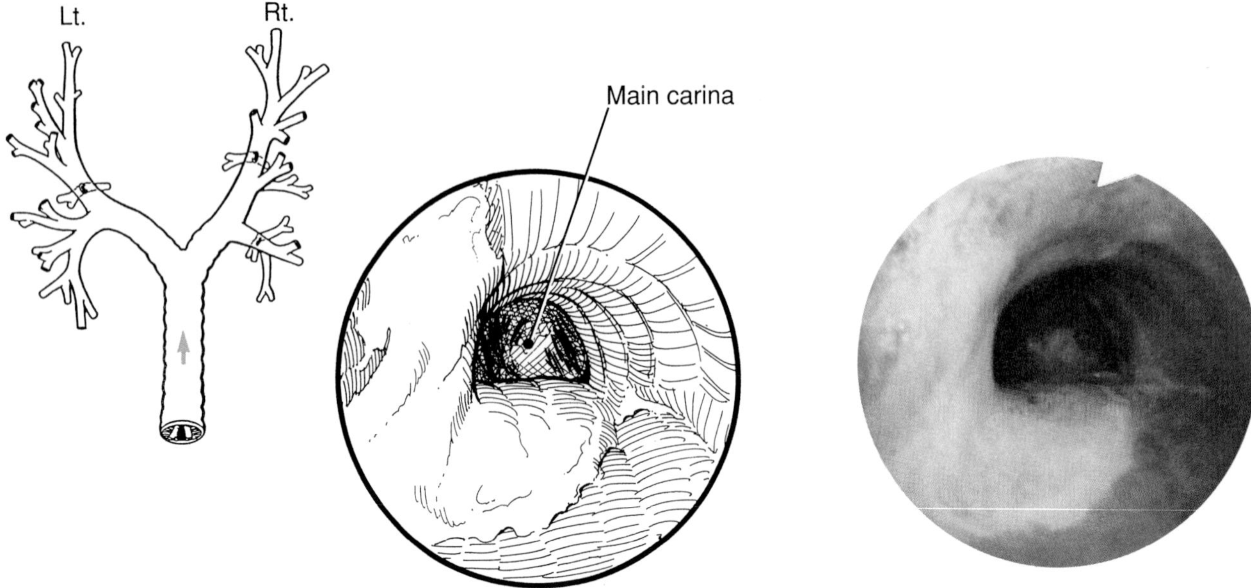

FIG. 90. Invasive candidiasis in a neutropenic patient with leukemia.

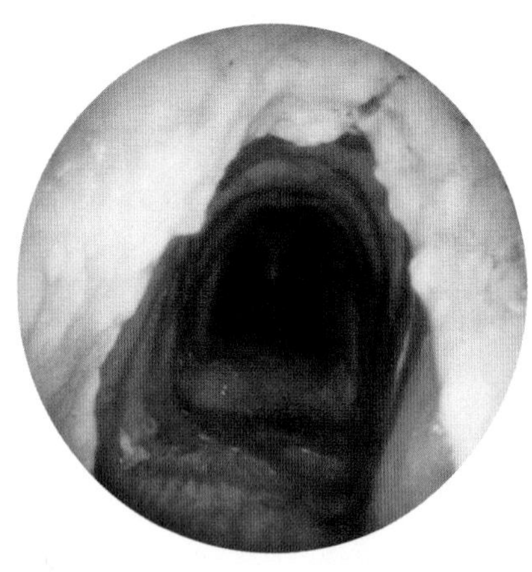

FIG. 91. Necrotizing candidiasis with formation of pseudomembrane in the proximal trachea. Airway obstruction caused by *Candida* has been described (62).

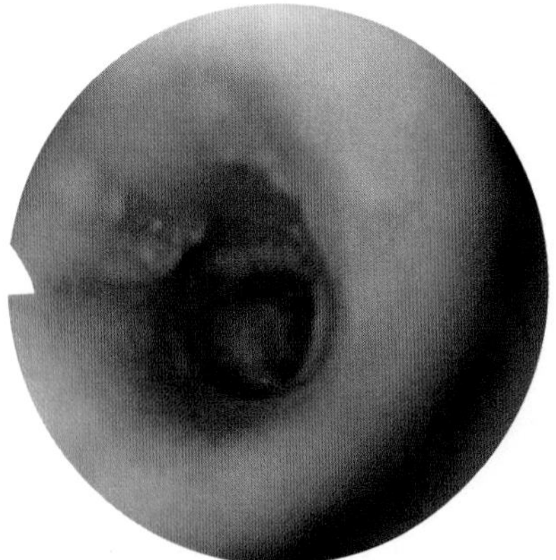

FIG. 92. Zygomycosis (mucormycosis) causing obstructive lesions at the entrance to left upper lobe bronchus. The orifice to the left upper lobe bronchus is completely blocked by granulation tissue and the distal bronchus leads to left lower lobe. Patients with poorly controlled diabetes mellitus are more likely to develop endobronchial zygomycosis (63–66).

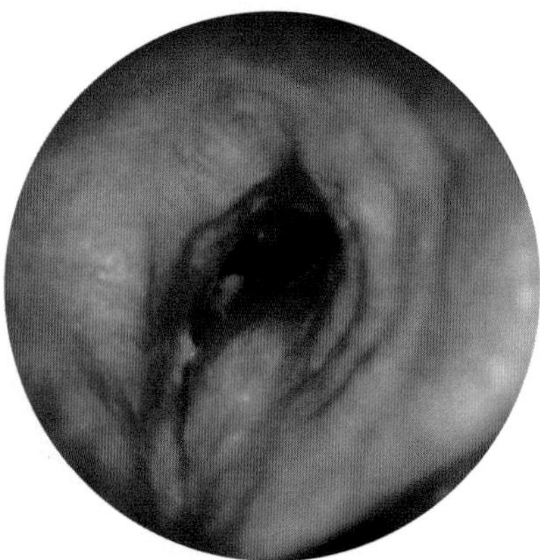

FIG. 93. Syphilis of trachea producing airway inflammation and narrowing. Noncaseous granulomas identical to sarcoid granulomas can be seen in syphilitic pulmonary disease (67).

LARYNX (Figs. 94–107)

Laryngeal examination is an important aspect of the bronchoscopic examination. Unexpected findings may provide clue to the underlying clinical problems. Proximal stationing of the bronchoscope and instructing the patient to engage in different forms of phonation may reveal clinically inapparent vocal cord paralysis, laryngeal abnormalities, or disorders of the epiglottis or the hypopharyngeal structures.

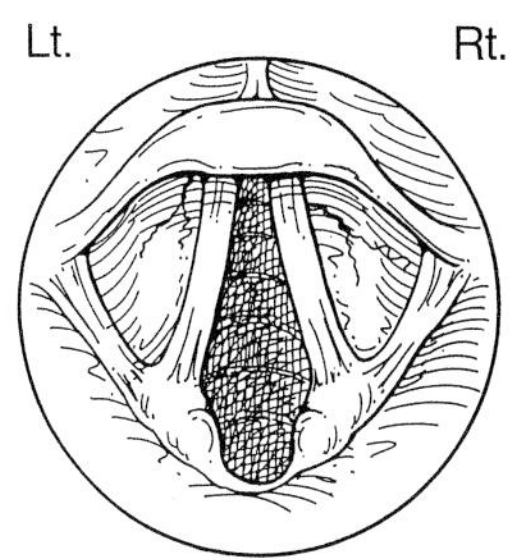

Normal cords.
Quiet breathing.

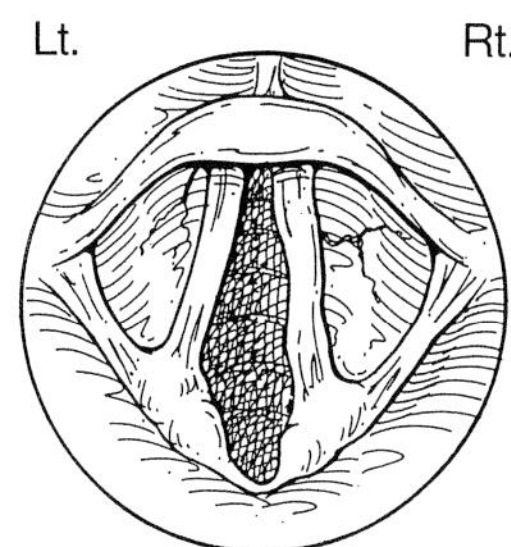

Right recurrent laryngeal nerve paralysis. Quiet breathing. (failure to abduct)

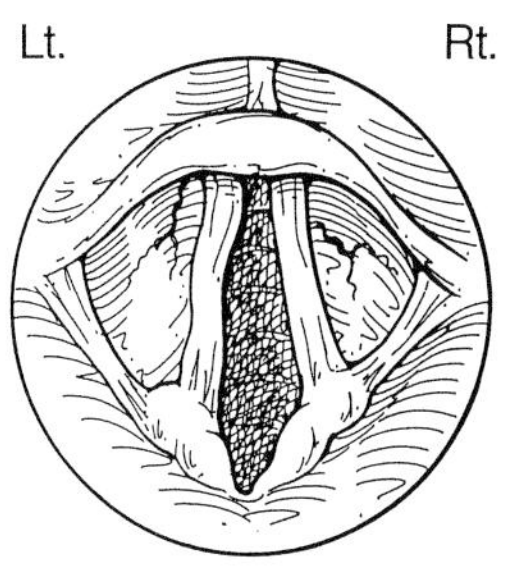

Uncompensated right recurrent laryngeal nerve paralysis during phonation. (failure to adduct)

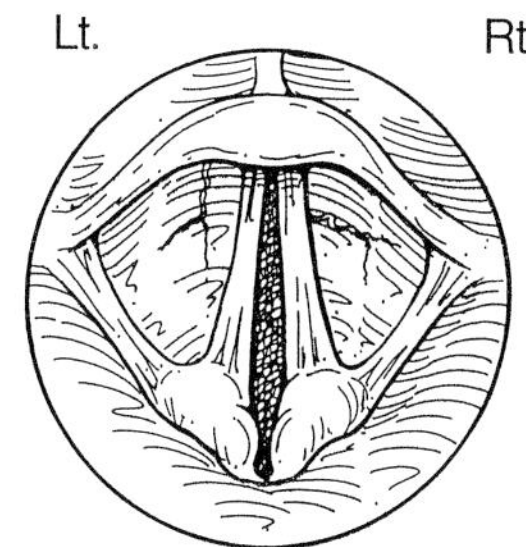

Bilateral recurrent laryngeal nerve paralysis during quiet breathing. (failure to abduct)

FIG. 94. Diagrammatic representation of different types of vocal cord paralysis.

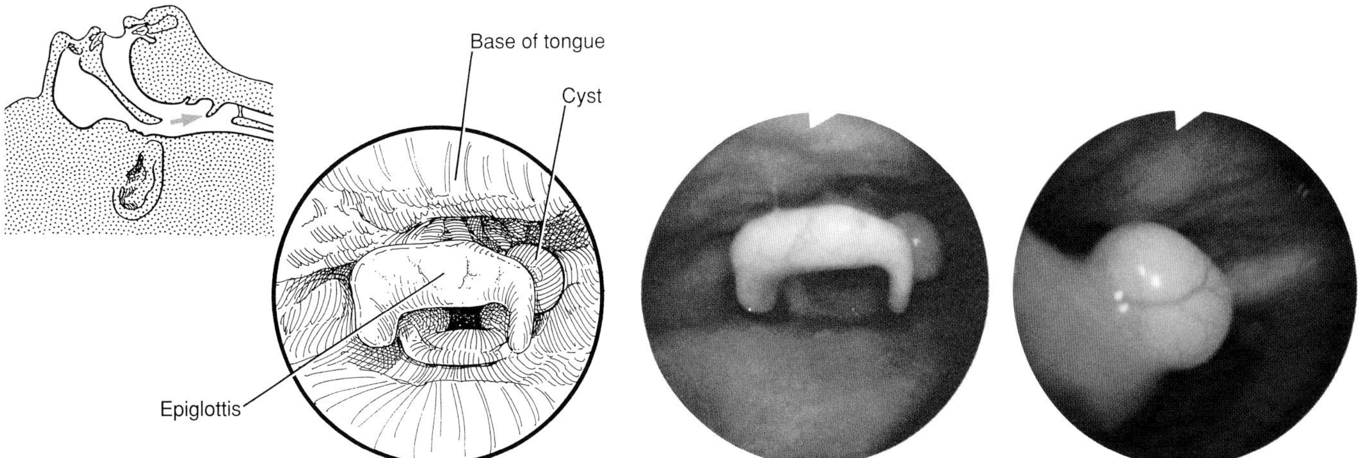

FIG. 95. Epiglottic cyst discovered during bronchoscopy for a suspected bronchial lesion. The patients had no symptoms related the cyst **(left)** and a close-up view **(right)**. Epiglottic cysts can be removed by direct laryngoscopy (68).

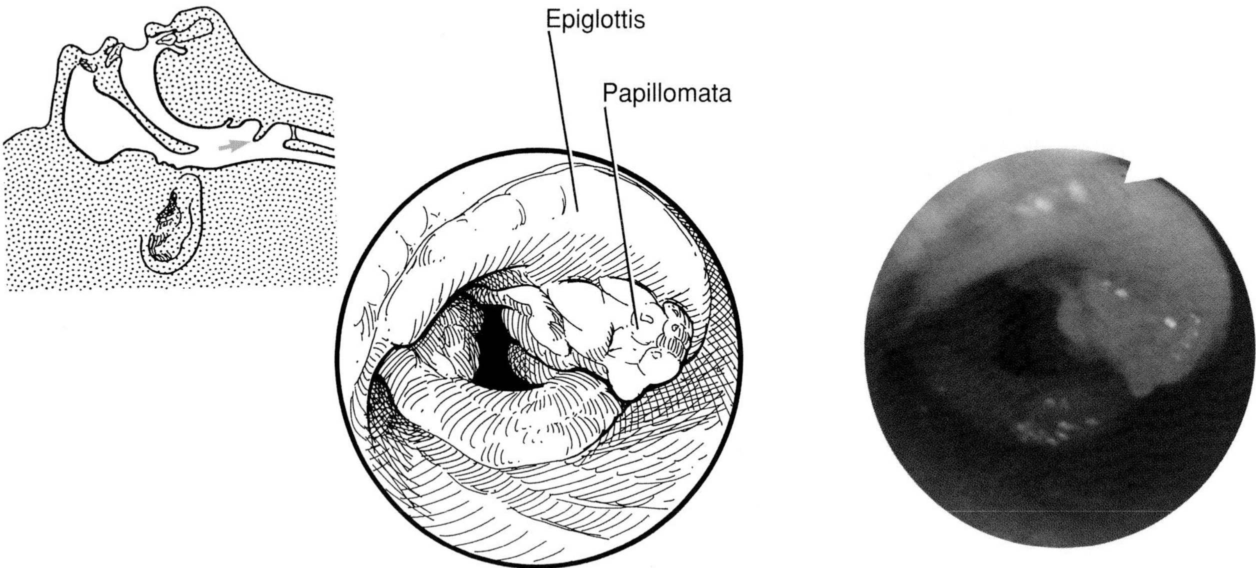

FIG. 96. Papillomatosis involving epiglottis.

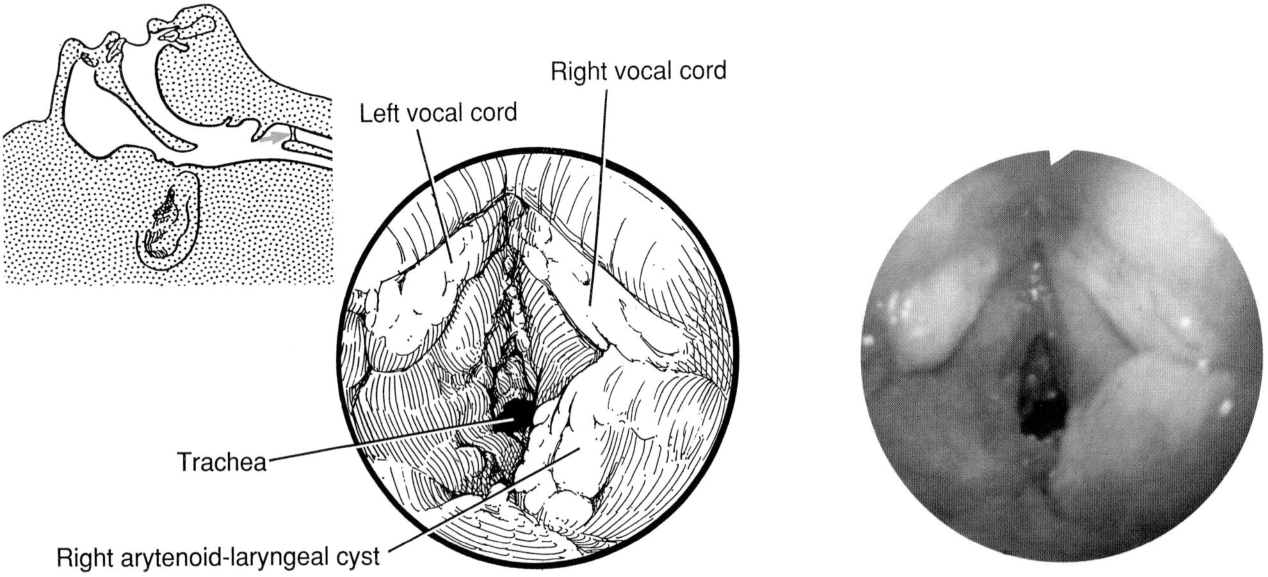

FIG. 97. Arytenoid cyst discovered during bronchoscopy. The patient was asymptomatic. The majority of such cysts are epithelial cysts (69).

FIG. 99. Spastic (adductor) dysphonia. Adduction of anterior two thirds of vocal cords during inspiration **(Top)** and normal appearance during expiration **(Bottom)**. Spasm of laryngeal adductors may result in inspiratory stridor-type breathing abnormality. During inspiratory maneuver, the anterior two thirds of the vocal apparatus remains in apposition causing stridor. In this patient, as in other patients described in the literature, laryngoscopic injection of botulism toxin (botox) relieved the inspiratory stridor (70–72).

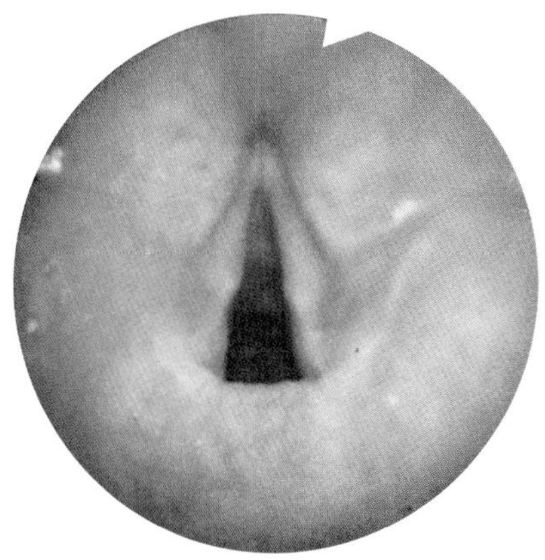

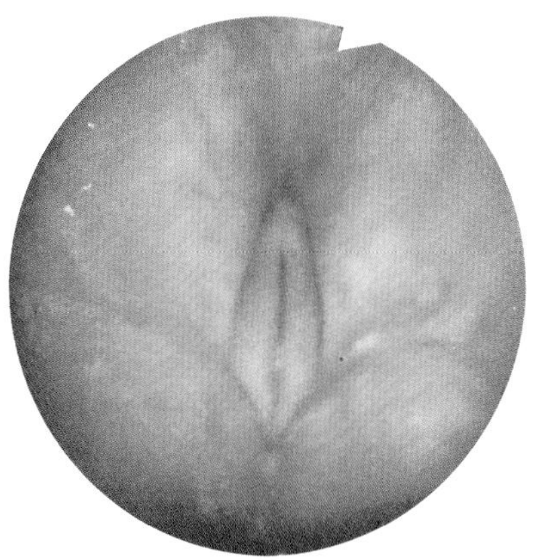

FIG. 98. Normal vocal cord abduction **(left)** and full adduction **(right)**. Phonation during bronchoscopic (or laryngoscopic) visualization will normally reveal the function of the vocal cords. Asking the patient to say "eee" or "hee" will help in assessing the motion of vocal cords.

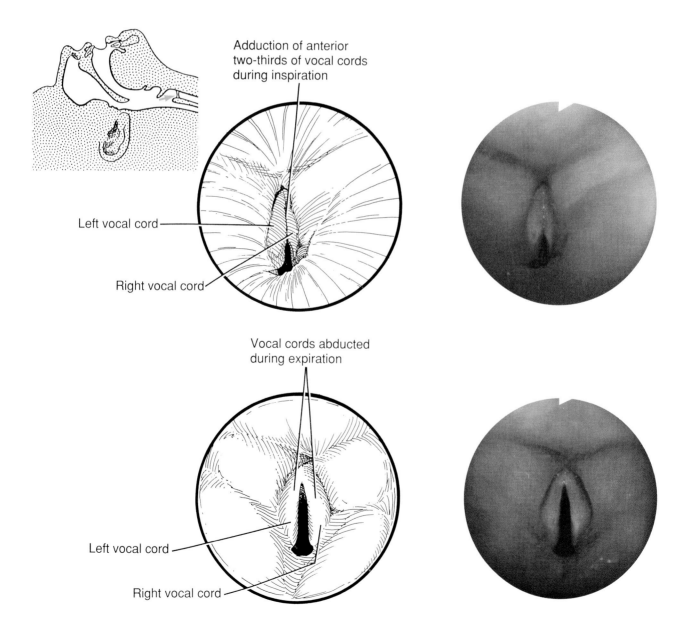

Adduction of anterior two-thirds of vocal cords during inspiration

Left vocal cord

Right vocal cord

Vocal cords abducted during expiration

Left vocal cord

Right vocal cord

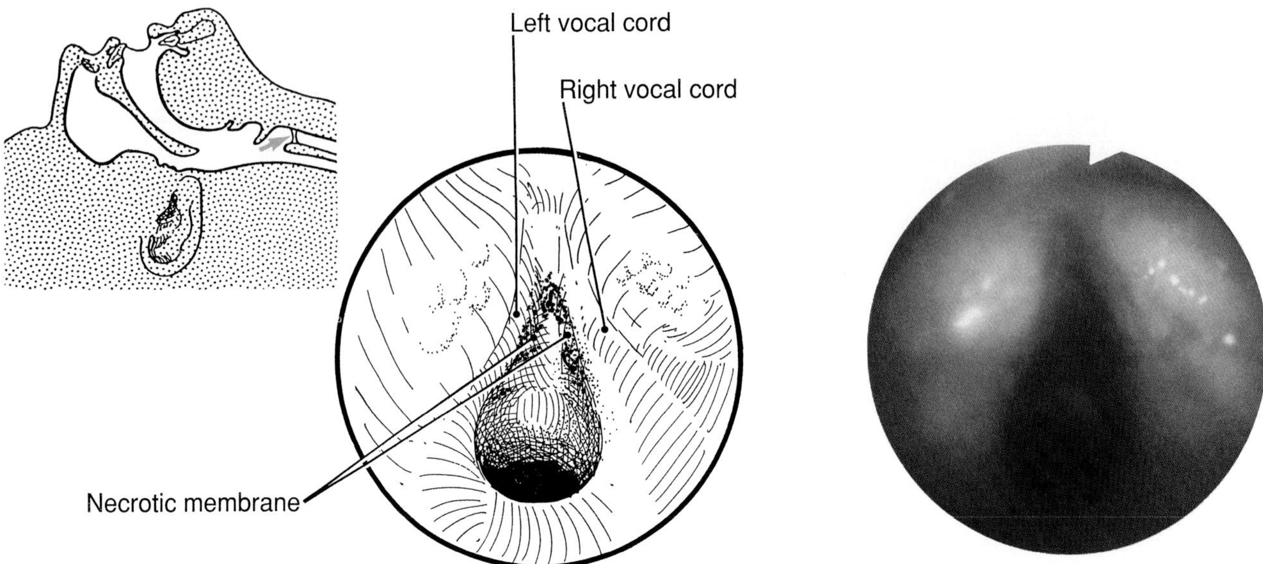

FIG. 100. Necrotizing aspergillosis of the larynx in a neutropenic patient with lymphoma. Dark brown–black pseudomembrane can be seen lining anterior aspects of both vocal cords.

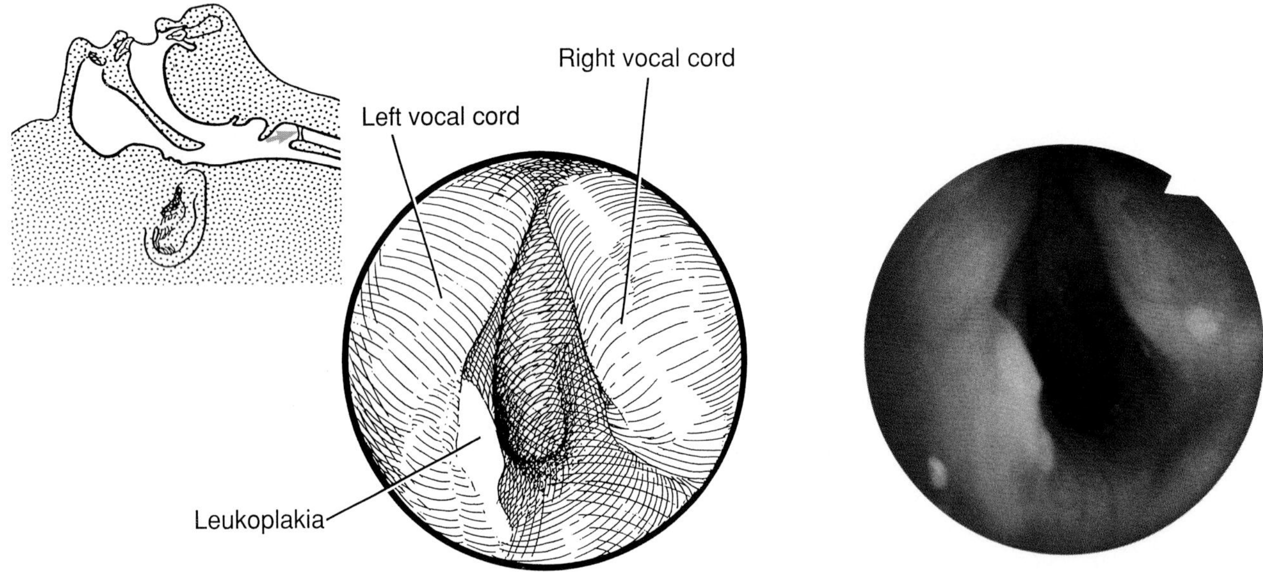

FIG. 101. Early leukoplakia of vocal left cord observed during bronchoscopy. Patient was asymptomatic.

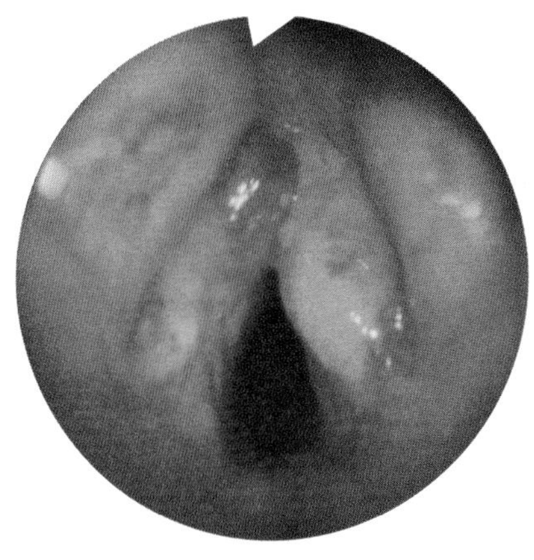

FIG. 102. Advanced leukoplakia recorded during bronchoscopy. Mild hoarseness was the only laryngeal symptom. Biopsy revealed abnormal cells. The patient eventually developed laryngeal cancer.

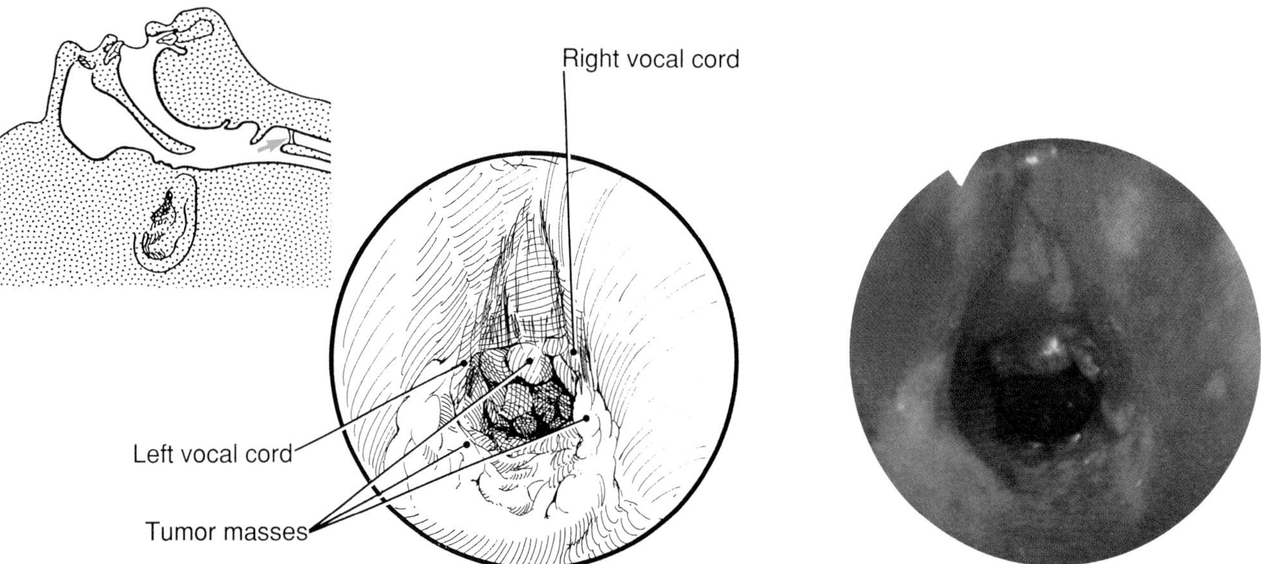

FIG. 103. Squamous cell carcinoma of subglottic area. Patient required a tracheal stent for the symptomatic relief of dyspnea.

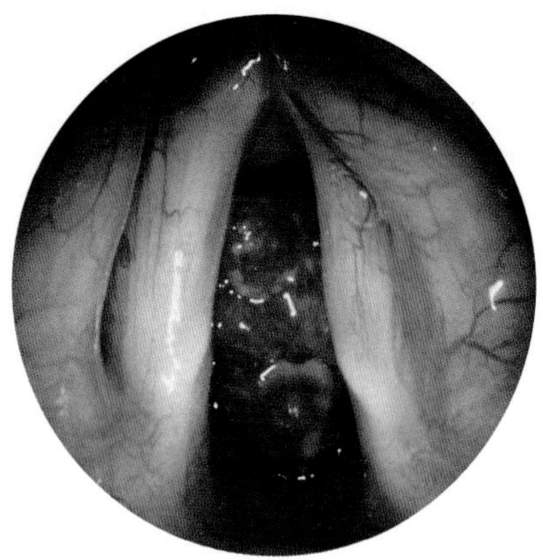

FIG. 104. Colon cancer with subglottic metastasis.

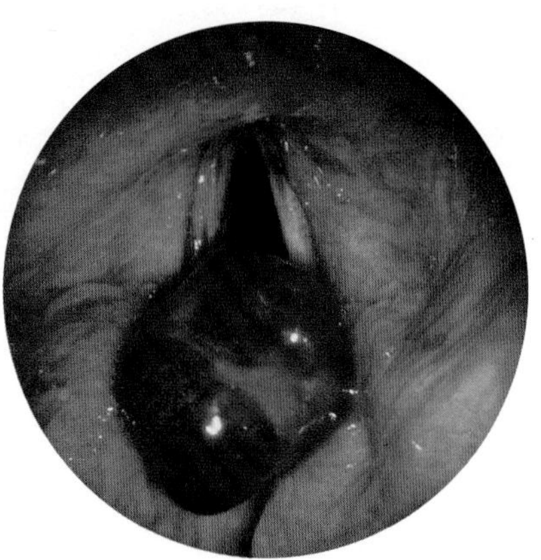

FIG. 105. Postintubation granuloma in subglottic space.

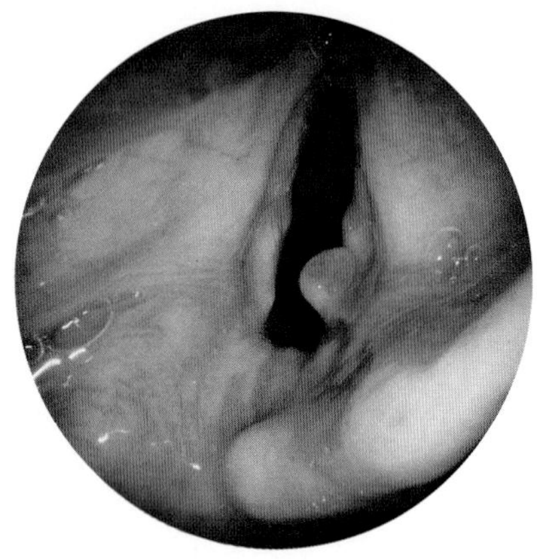

FIG. 106. Postintubation granuloma of vocal cords.

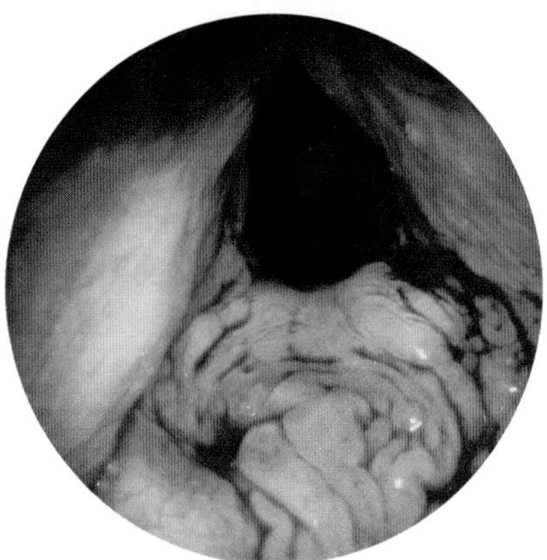

FIG. 107. Amyloidosis of the larynx. This represented a new lesion in a patient who had tracheal amyloidosis treated by Nd:YAG laser 6 years earlier.

LYMPH NODE (Figs. 108–111)

Subcarinal lymphadenopathy can result in loss of the sharp keel-like profile of main carina and diminish respiratory excursions of the carina. It is uncommon to see tracheal distortion from paratracheal lymphadenopathy. Large lymph nodes in the hilar regions may encroach on bronchial tree and produce extrinsic compression. An unusual presentation is the erosion of the tracheobronchial tree by a lymph node.

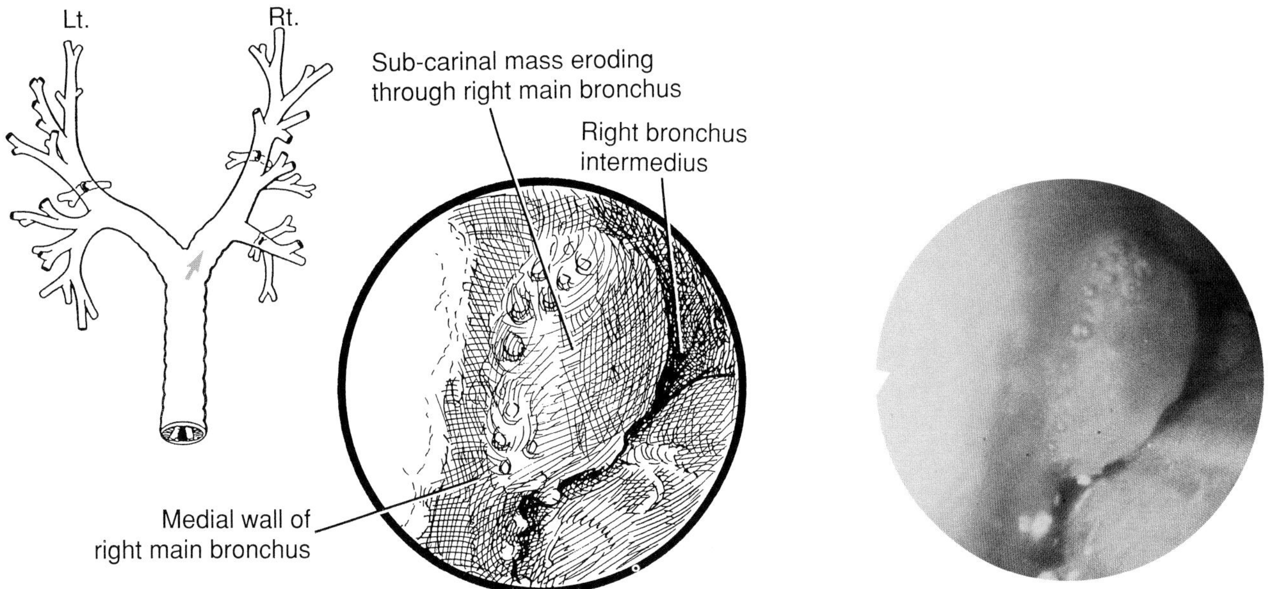

FIG. 108. Lymph node erosion into right main bronchus. Subcarinal mass of lymph nodes were observed on the computed tomography. Biopsy of the lymph node revealed caseous granulomas and cultures were positive for *Mycobacterium tuberculosis.*

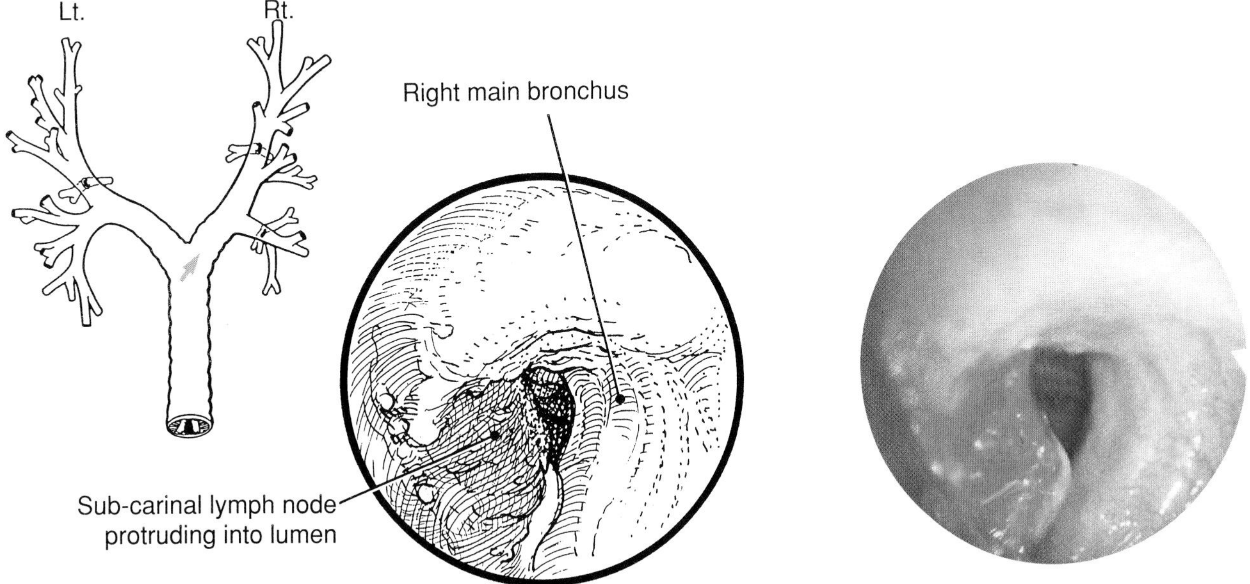

FIG. 109. Lymph node erosion into right main bronchus. Biopsy of the lesion was nondiagnostic but special stains showed a small number of organisms compatible with *Histoplasma capsulatum.*

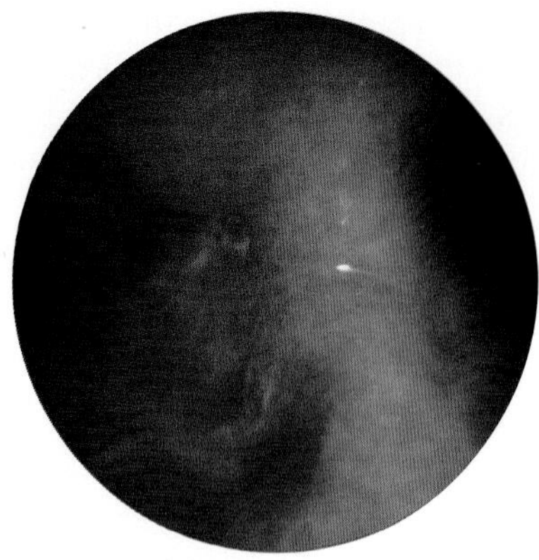

FIG. 110. Tuberculous subcarinal lymph nodes eroding into proximal left main bronchus and causing a secondary fistula.

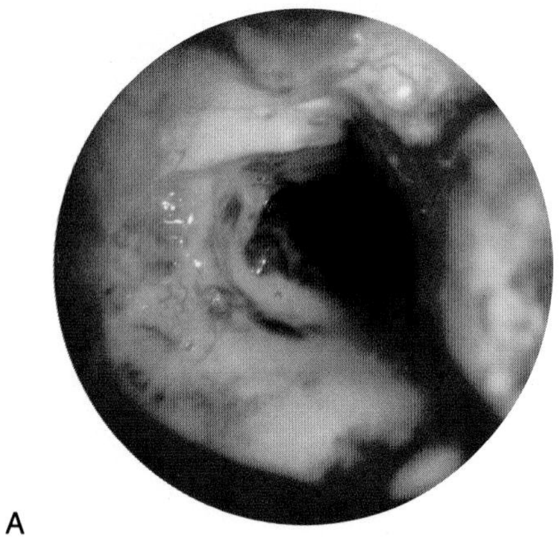

A

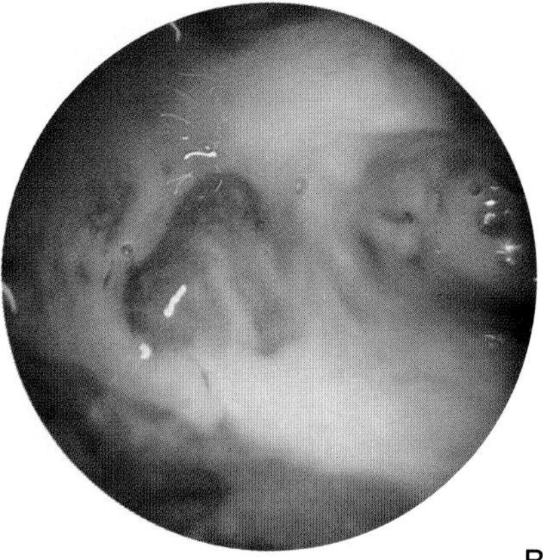

B

FIG. 111. Anthracotic lymph node eroding into medial wall of right main bronchus **(A)** and a close-up view of the bulging node **(B)**.

LYMPHOMA (Figs. 112–115)

Lymphomas are well known to cause pulmonary complications. Hodgkin's lymphoma in particular can manifest as an endobronchial lesion and cause segmental or lobar collapse. Mucosal involvement by lymphoma is also common and may lead to bronchial stenosis (73).

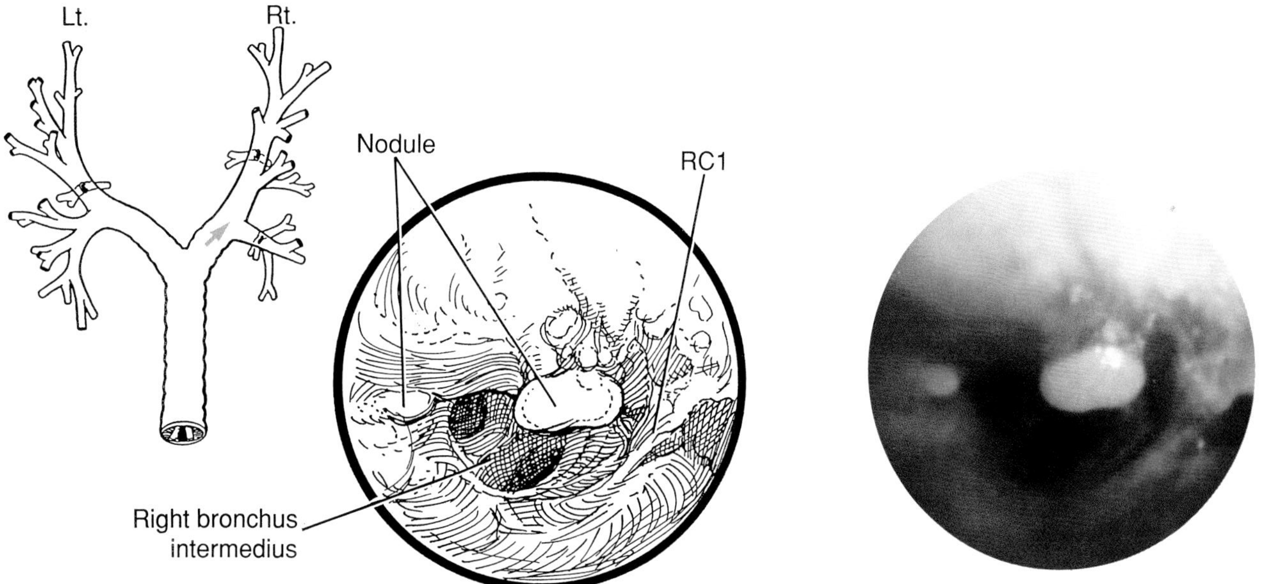

FIG. 112. Hodgkin's lymphoma causing endobronchial polyps. Biopsy of the large whitish nodule showed typical Hodgkin's lymphoma. Orifice to the right upper lobe was blocked by lymphomatous polyp.

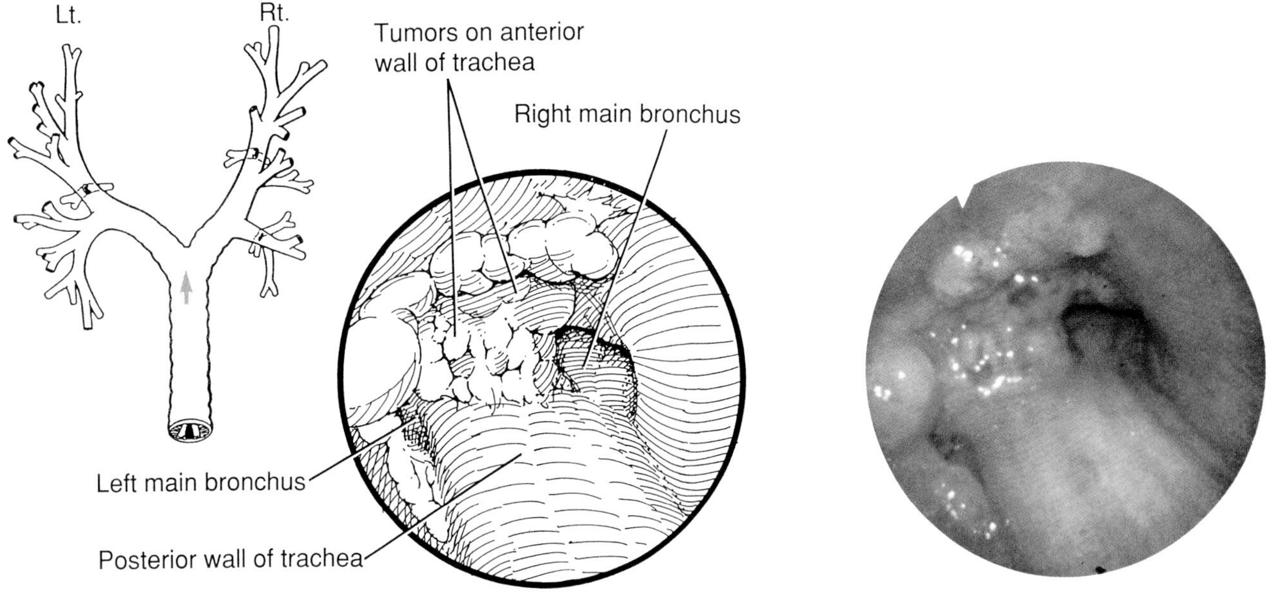

FIG. 113. Lymphosarcoma involving distal trachea and both main bronchi. The left main bronchus is almost totally occluded by tumor mass.

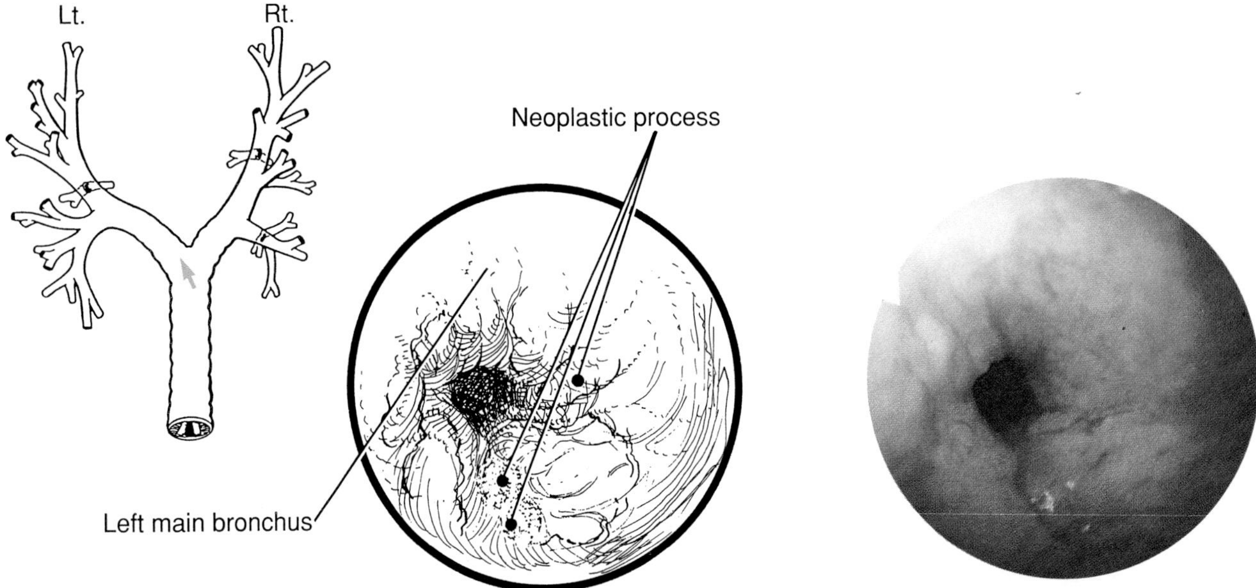

FIG. 114. Non-Hodgkin's histiocytic lymphoma partially obstructing left main bronchus. Biopsy yielded large pieces of soft tumor tissue. Multiple endobronchial tumors and lobar collapse caused by non-Hodgkin's lymphoma have been described (74).

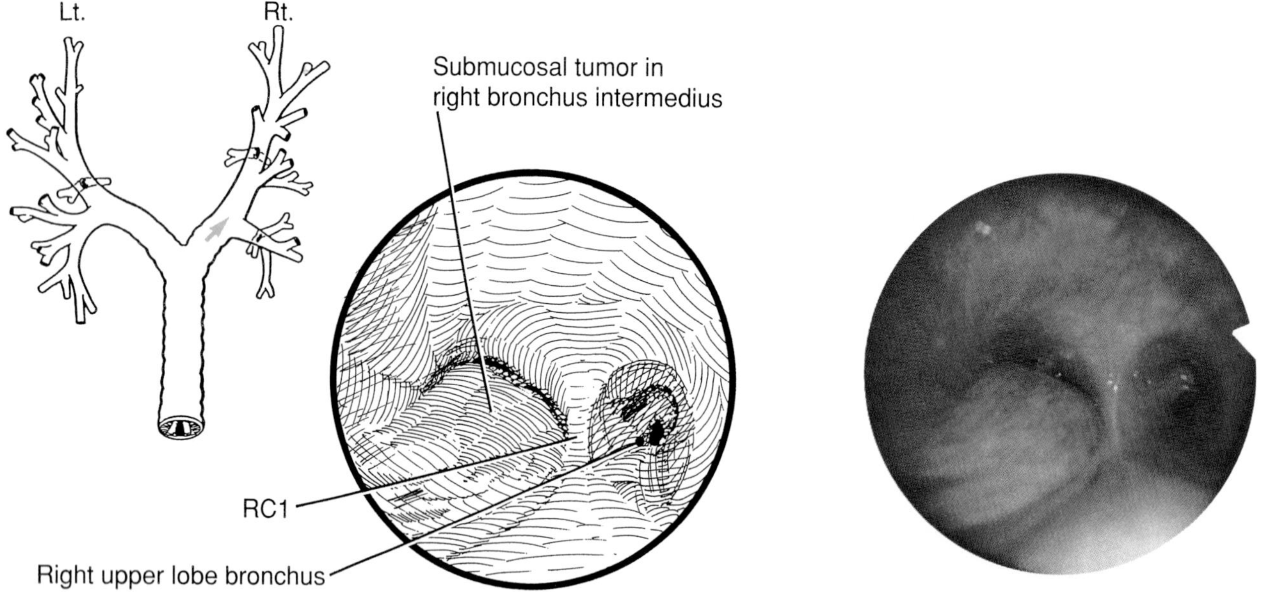

FIG. 115. Lymphoma involving mediastinal lymph nodes causing severe extrinsic compression of right bronchus intermedius. Mucosal biopsies were nondiagnostic; needle aspiration of the mass revealed high-grade lymphoma.

NEOPLASMS, BENIGN (Figs. 116–131)

Several benign neoplasms affect the tracheobronchial tree. Papillomas are more common in children than in adults and they tend to recur despite repeated therapy. Treatment modalities include laser therapy, phototherapy, and bronchoscopic resection. Since 1982 we have treated 157 benign tracheobronchial tumors with mechanical resection and Nd:YAG laser (S.C.). When the base of the lesion was treated as in more than 100 of these cases, nonrecurrence was the rule, except in some cases of extensive papillomatosis.

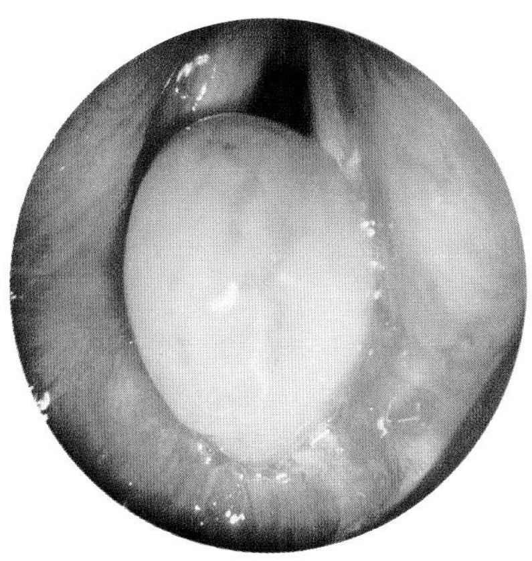

FIG. 116. Inflammatory pseudotumor of subglottic region. Nd:YAG laser resection of the thin pedicle below the right vocal cord allowed removal of the pseudotumor with biopsy forceps.

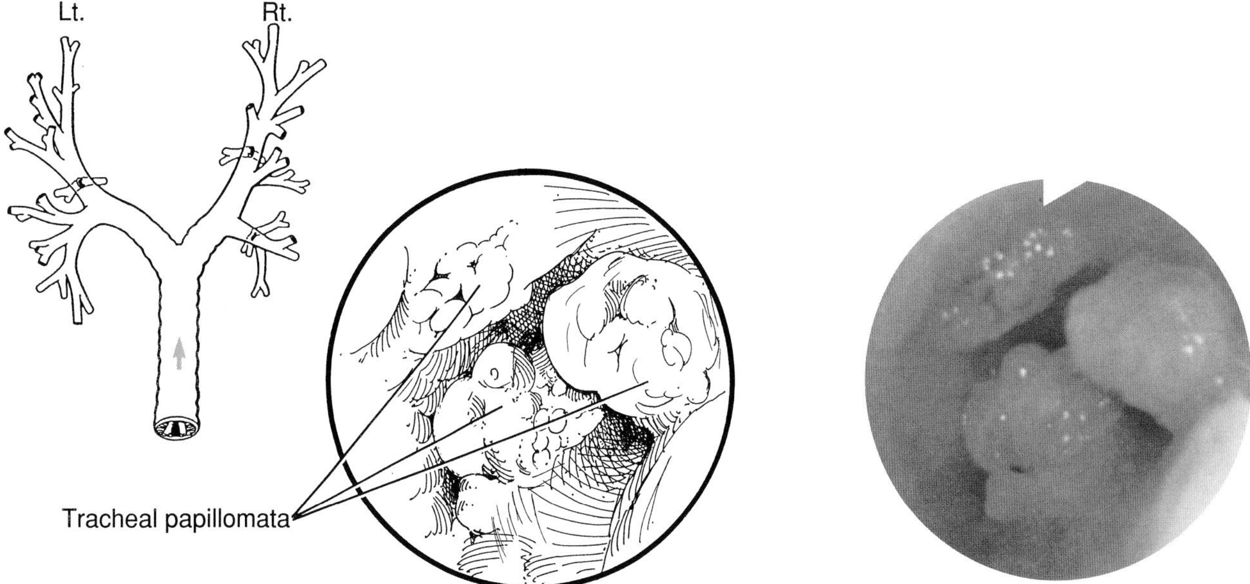

FIG. 117. Papillomas of the upper trachea. Bronchoscopic removal, laser therapy, and bronchoscopic photodynamic therapy have been utilized (75,76).

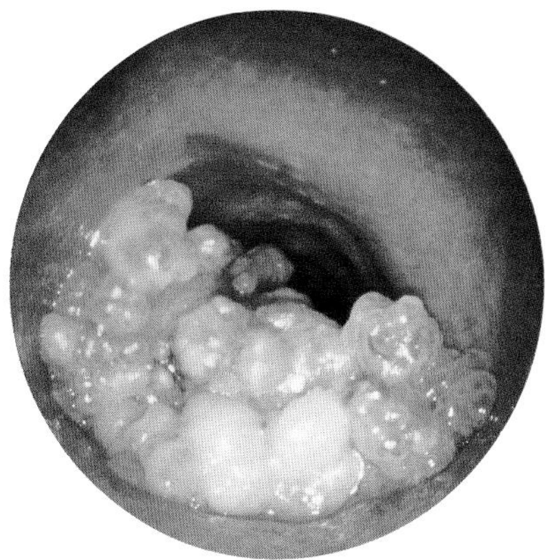

FIG. 118. Papillomatosis of midtrachea.

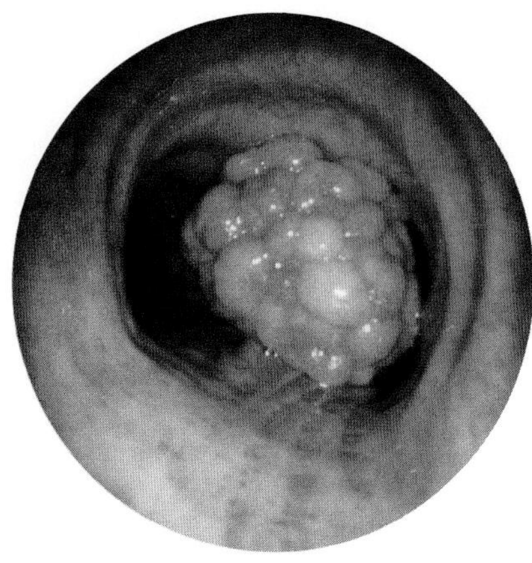

FIG. 119. Papillomatosis of the main carina. A narrow pedicle attached to the main carina was easily resected with a forceps.

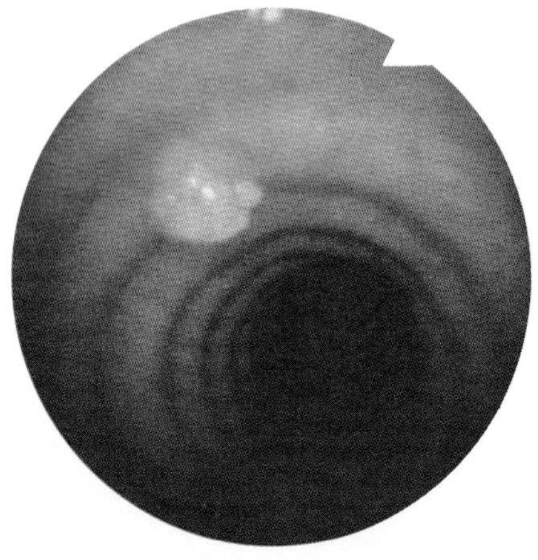

FIG. 120. Benign polyp of the trachea. Patient presented with cough. Biopsy-excision was performed with a flexible bronchoscope.

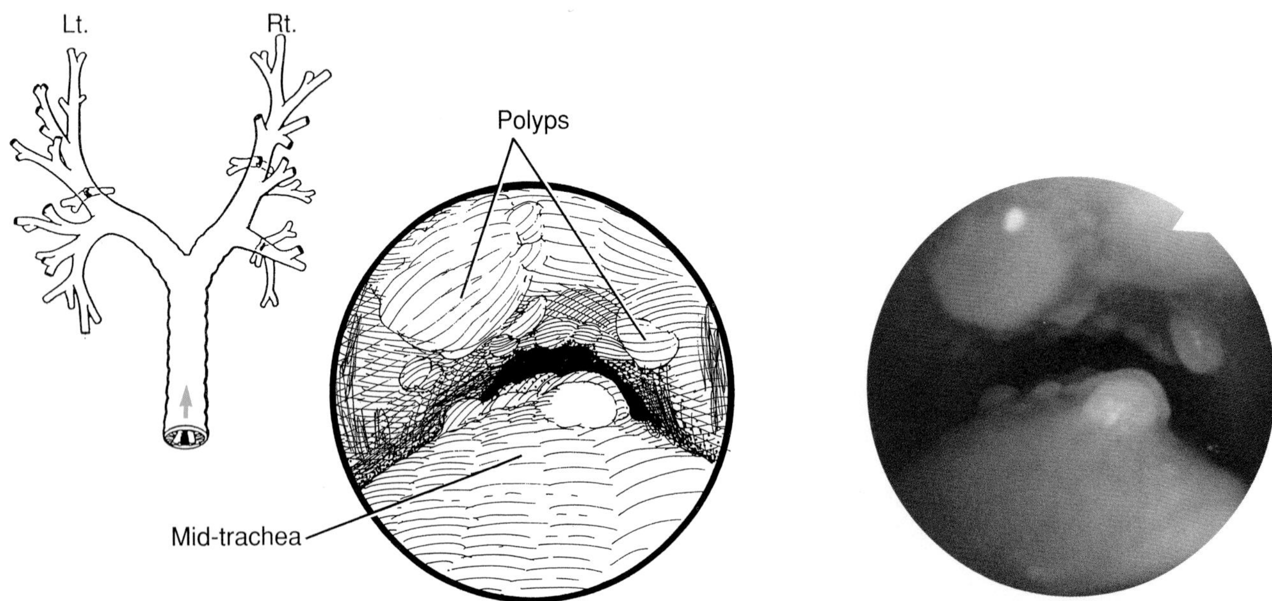

FIG. 121. Multiple benign polyps of the trachea. The etiology of this entity is unclear.

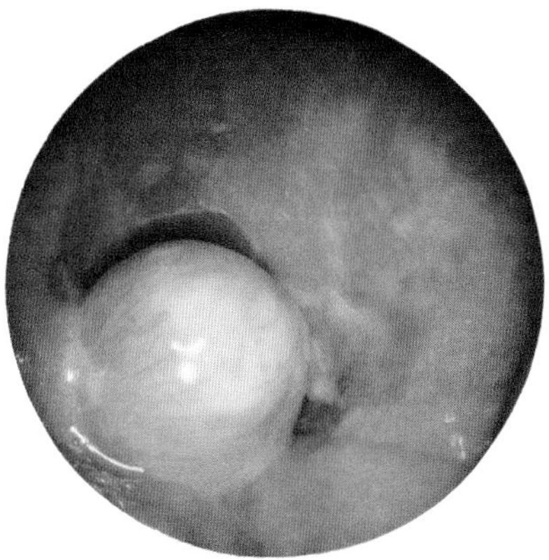

FIG. 122. Inflammatory pseudotumor of trachea.

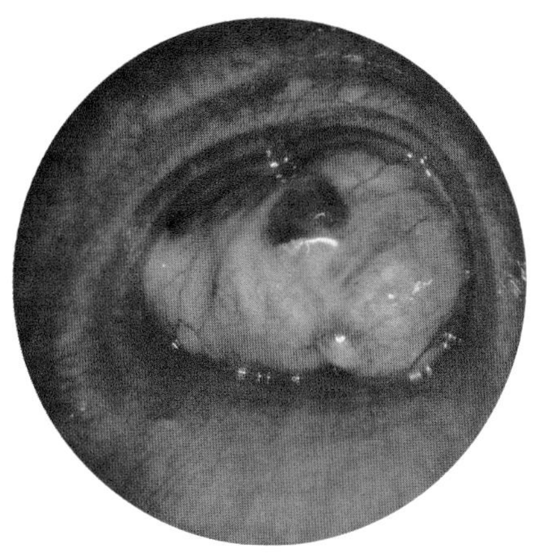

FIG. 123. Benign leiomyoma of trachea. Only 15 cases were reported in the English literature by 1989 (77). Bronchoscopic removal, resection, and reanastomosis of such lesions have resulted in absence of recurrence (77–79). Endobronchial leiomyoma has been described in a patient with uterine leiomyoma (sometimes described as metastasizing benign leiomyoma) (80).

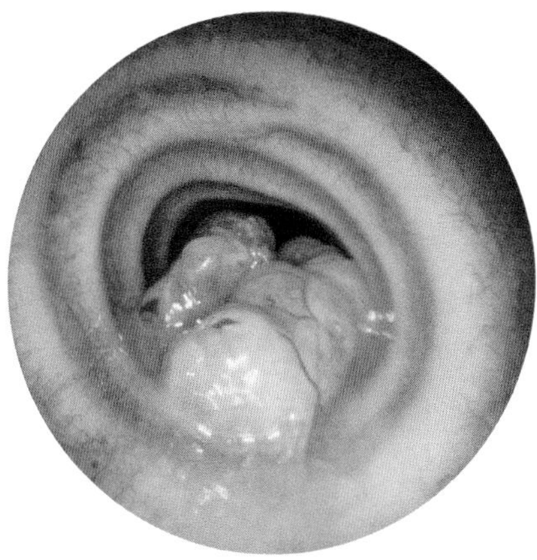

FIG. 124. Neurofibroma of trachea. It can occur singly or as a manifestation of von Recklinghausen's neurofibromatosis (81,82).

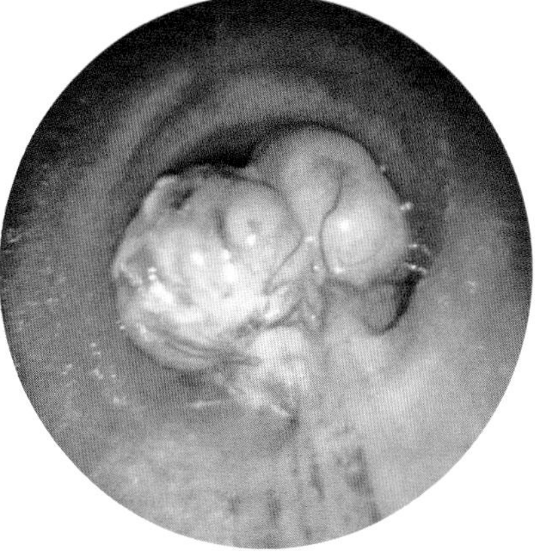

FIG. 125. Schwannoma of trachea with the pedicle of the mass located in the right posterolateral wall. Rigid bronchoscopic Nd:YAG laser therapy resulted in no recurrence after 4.5 years. Schwannoma (neurilemmoma) of the trachea is extremely rare (83).

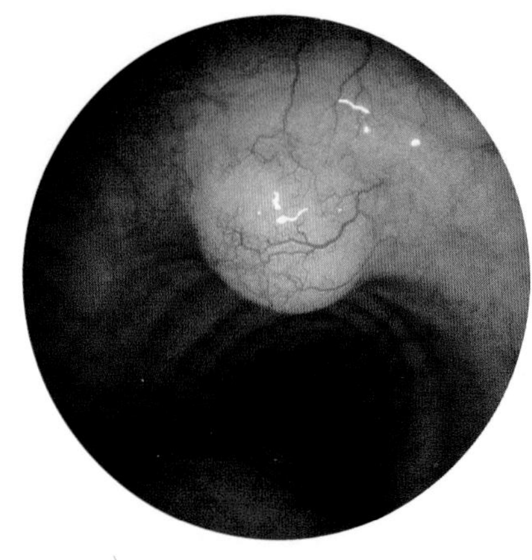

FIG. 126. Chondroma of the anterior tracheal wall. Among 250 cartilaginous tumors of the larynx, 72% were benign chondromas and only eight were tracheal in location (82). Another publication has reviewed the topic of benign cartilaginous tumors of trachea (84).

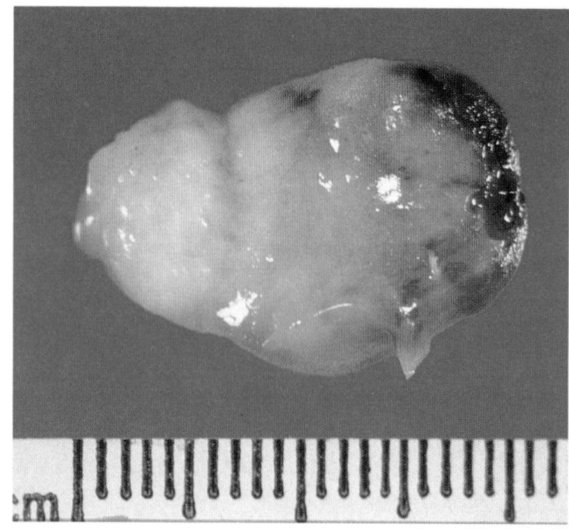

FIG. 127. Lipomatous hamartoma of the trachea-resected specimen. Among 128 benign tumors of the tracheobronchial tree, 38 (30%) were hamartomas (85). Courtesy of Atul C. Mehta, M.D.

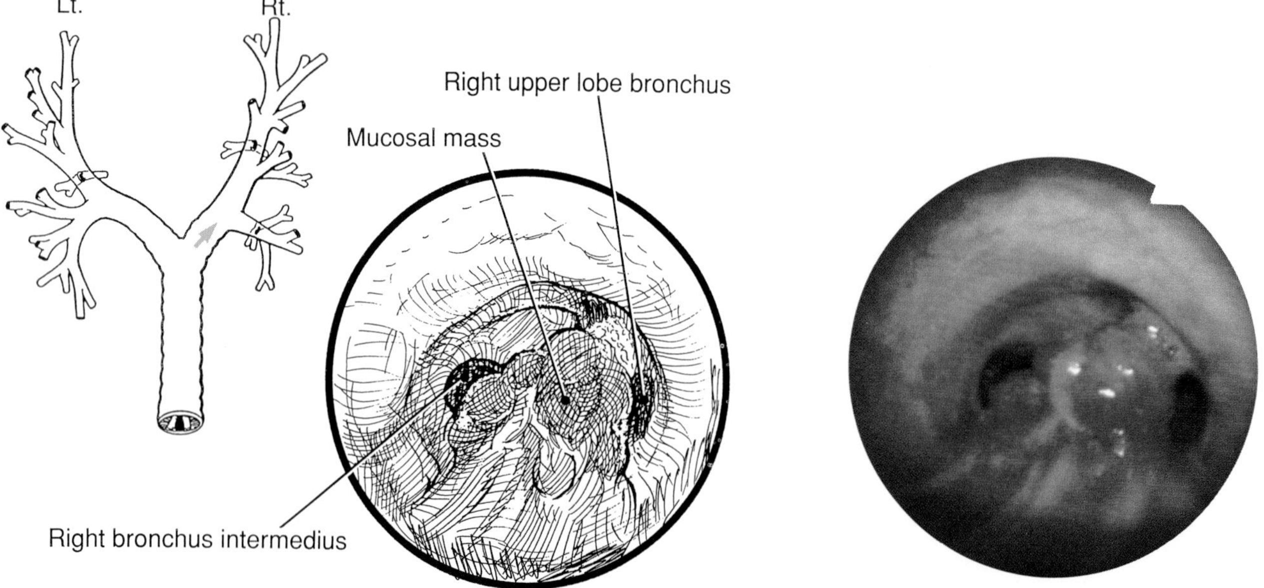

FIG. 128. Benign granuloma of distal right main bronchus presented with chronic cough and hemoptysis. Etiology was unclear. Rigid bronchoscopic resection was carried out with no recurrence after 9 years.

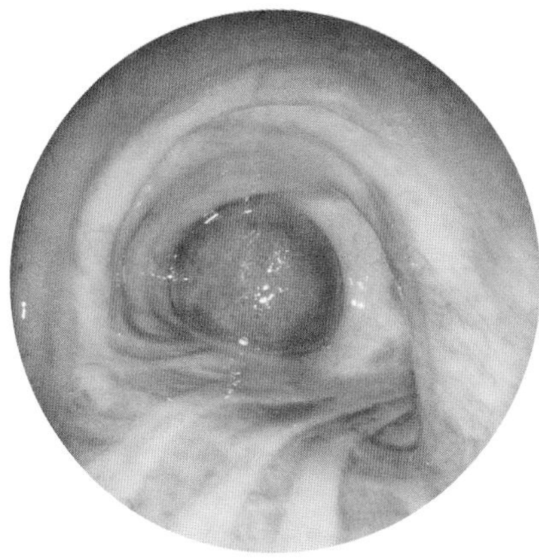

FIG. 129. Benign polyp obstructing proximal bronchus intermedius.

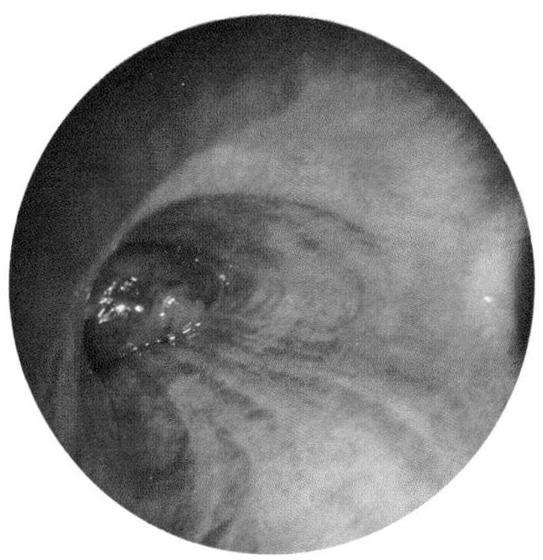

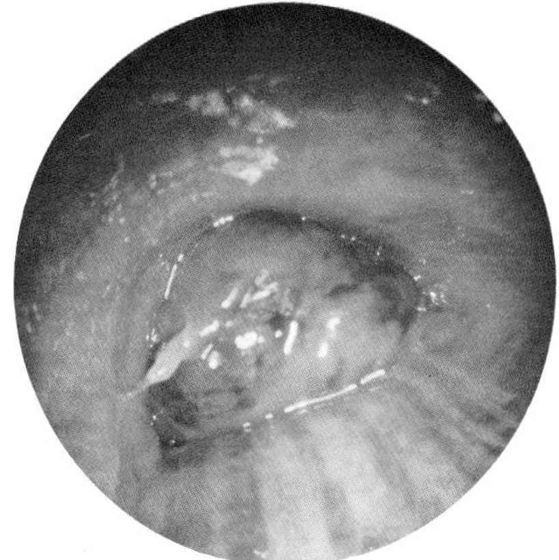

FIG. 130. Chondroma of mid–left main bronchus **(left)** and a close-up view of the lesion **(right)**.

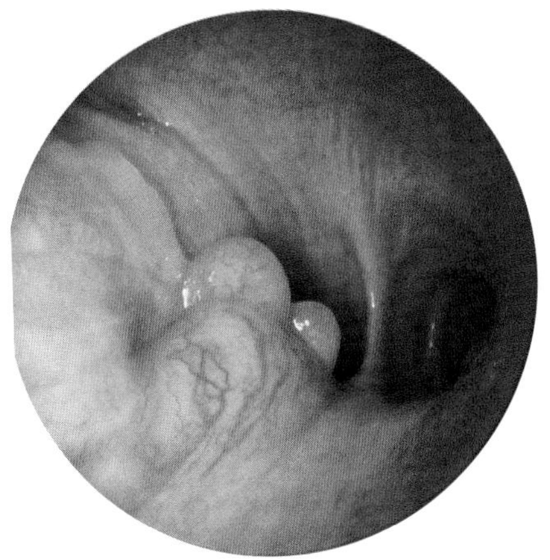

FIG. 131. Lipoma of distal bronchus intermedius. Lipoma of tracheobronchial tree usually arises from the membranous portion of the airway (86).

NEOPLASMS, MALIGNANT PRIMARY (Figs. 132–159)

Both primary and metastatic malignancies affect the tracheobronchial tree. There are no characteristic bronchoscopic features because the bronchoscopic appearance varies depending on the manner in which the tracheobronchial mucosa is affected. The spectrum of bronchoscopic abnormalities vary from subtle mucosal edema, erythema, and irregularity to overtly obvious mucosal masses, polyps, and obstruction of airway lumen. Extrinsic compression of the tracheobronchial tree can occur if the extrabronchial tumors compress it. Direct extension of nonpulmonary tumor, e.g., thyroid and esophageal malignancies, is another form of airway involvement. Occasionally, formation of fistula between the airways and other structures can be visualized at bronchoscopy. The bronchoscopic appearance itself cannot differentiate a primary from a metastatic tumor. Even the bronchoscopically visible increased vascularity of certain lesions, e.g., carcinoid, cannot be relied on to make the histological diagnosis of an endobronchial neoplasm.

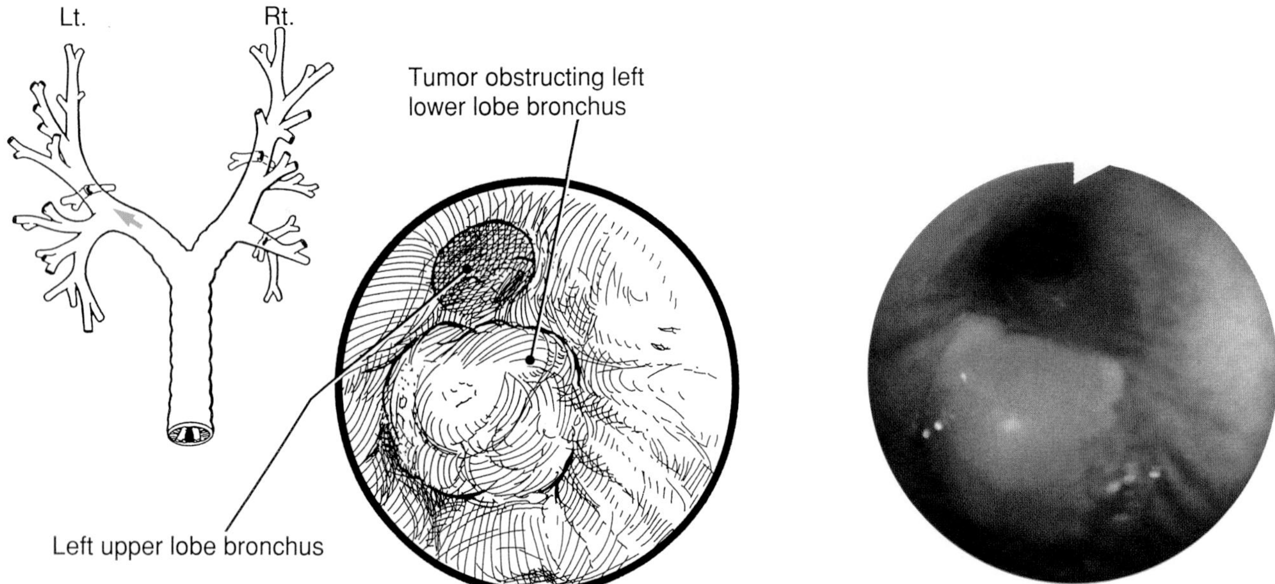

FIG. 132. Squamous cell carcinoma partially obstructing the bronchus to left lower lobe. Necrotic (yellow) material covers the surface of the tumor.

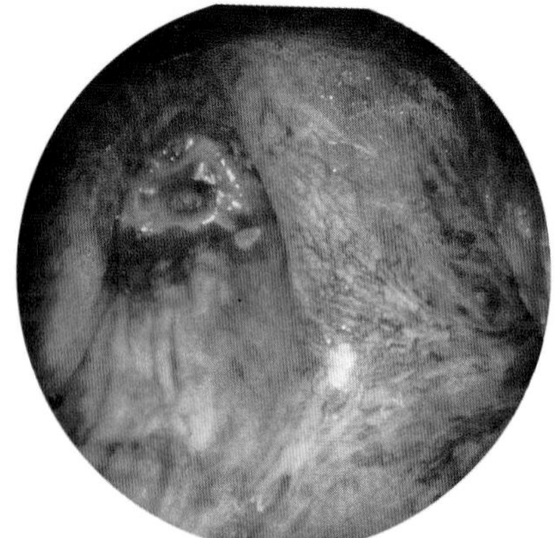

FIG. 133. Squamous cell carcinoma obstructing right bronchus intermedius. Submucosal lymphangitic spread was present.

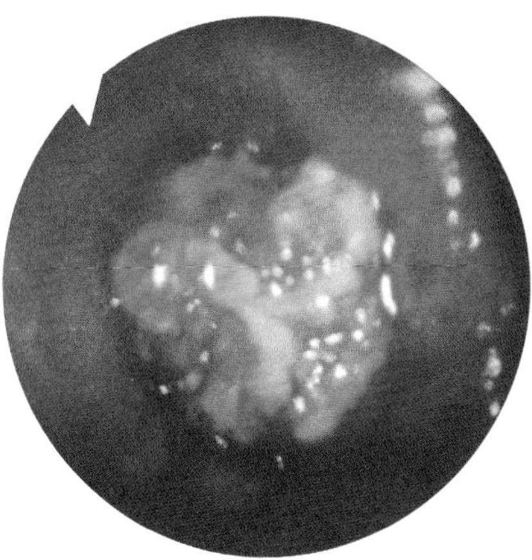

FIG. 134. Squamous cell carcinoma obstructing left main bronchus. Necrotic (whitish) nodules can be seen on the surface of the tumor.

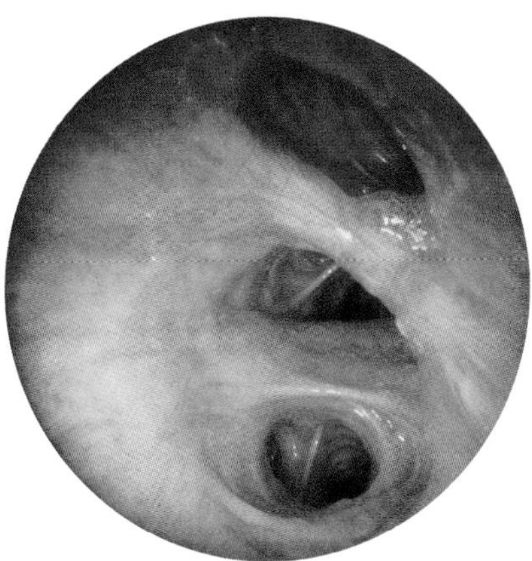

FIG. 135. Squamous cell carcinoma (*in situ*) involving entrance to right middle lobe bronchus.

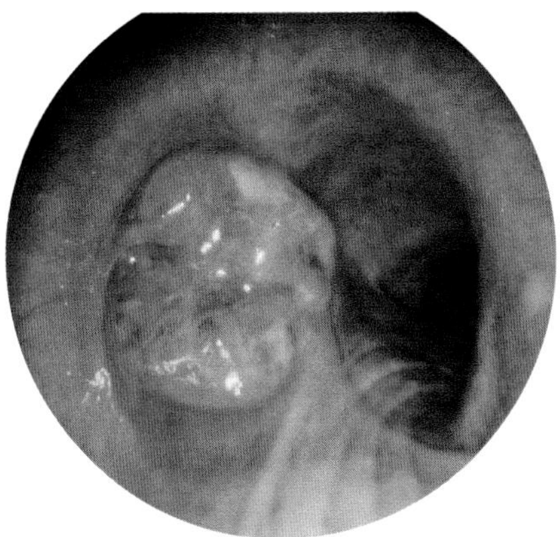

FIG. 136. Squamous cell carcinoma recurring in the stump of previous left pneumonectomy.

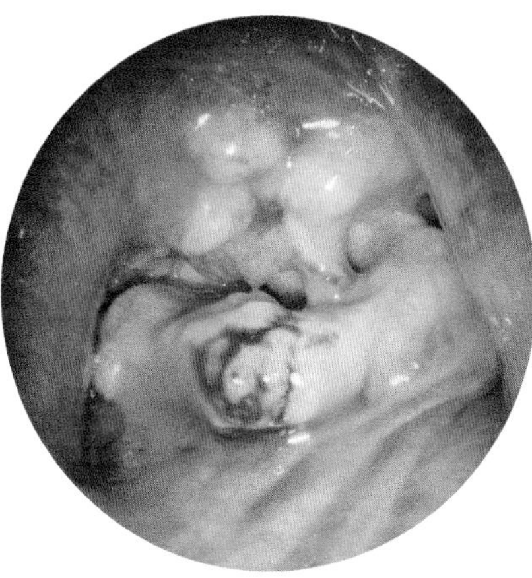

FIG. 137. Squamous cell carcinoma of distal trachea and both main bronchi. Extensive necrosis can be seen.

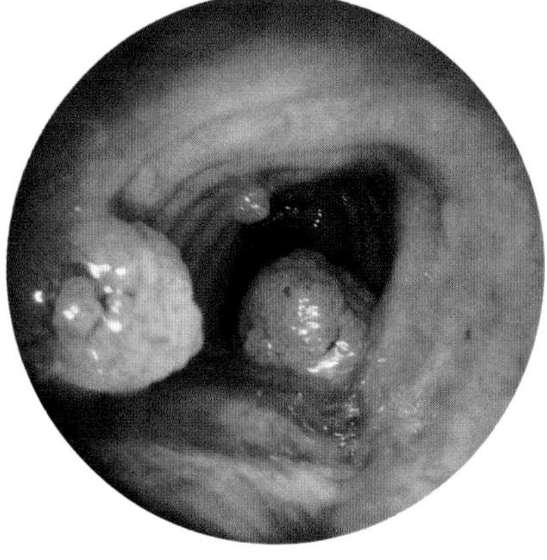

FIG. 138. Tracheal metastases from previously resected (right upper lobectomy) squamous cell carcinoma.

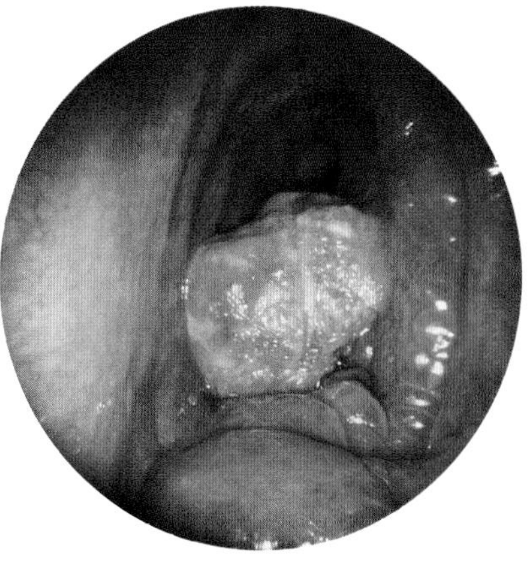

FIG. 139. Squamous cell carcinoma of trachea. Squamous cell carcinoma is the most common malignancy involving the trachea.

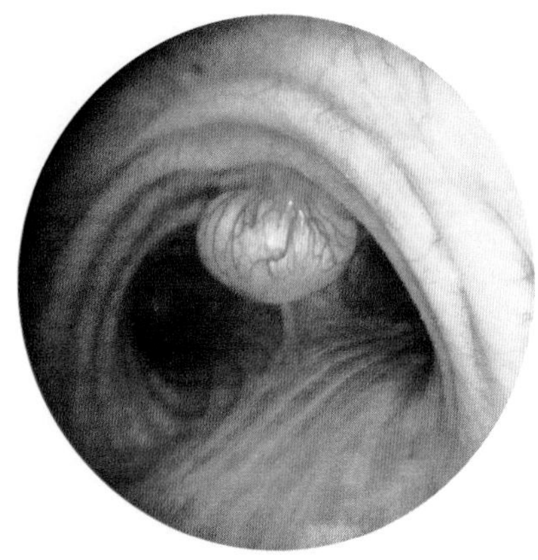

FIG. 140. Metastatic squamous cell carcinoma involving distal trachea. Primary tumor, located in the left upper lobe bronchus, was treated by left upper lobectomy and the tracheal tumor was treated by Nd:YAG laser therapy. No recurrence noted after 4 years.

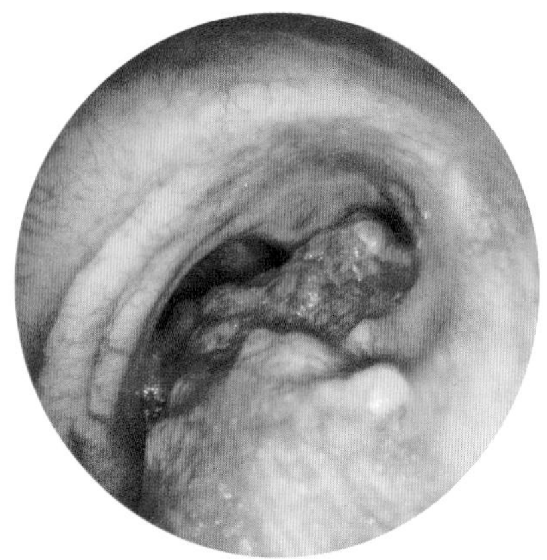

FIG. 141. Adenocarcinoma of distal trachea.

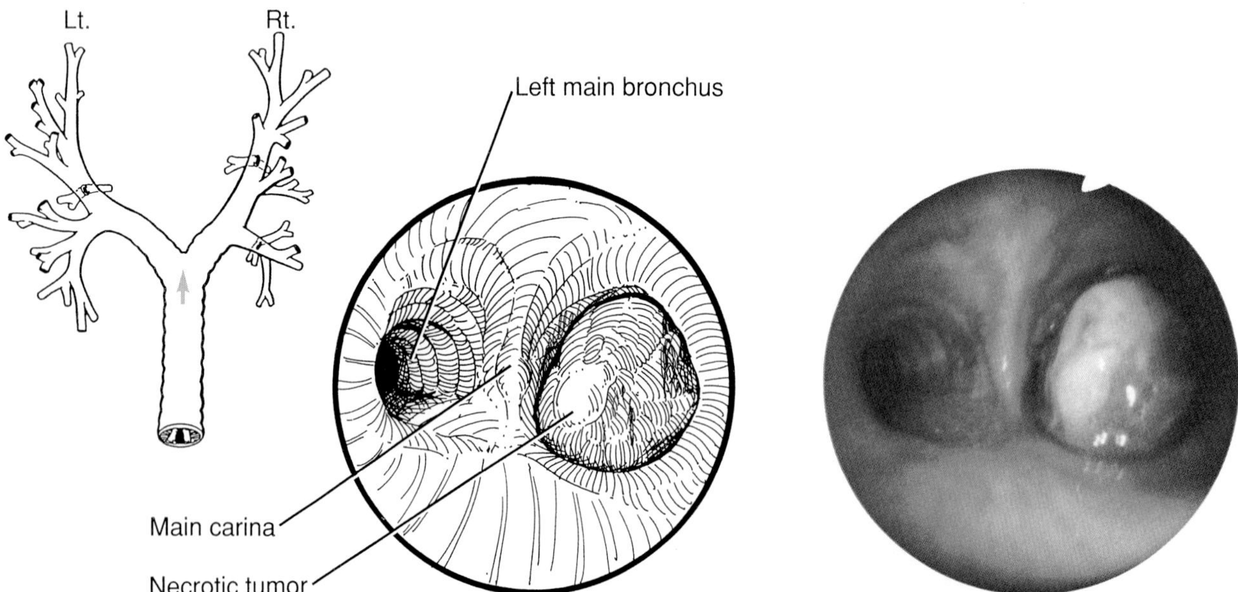

FIG. 142. Adenocarcinoma obstructing right main bronchus. Grayish black discoloration is due to necrosis. Tumor originated in the right upper lobe bronchus.

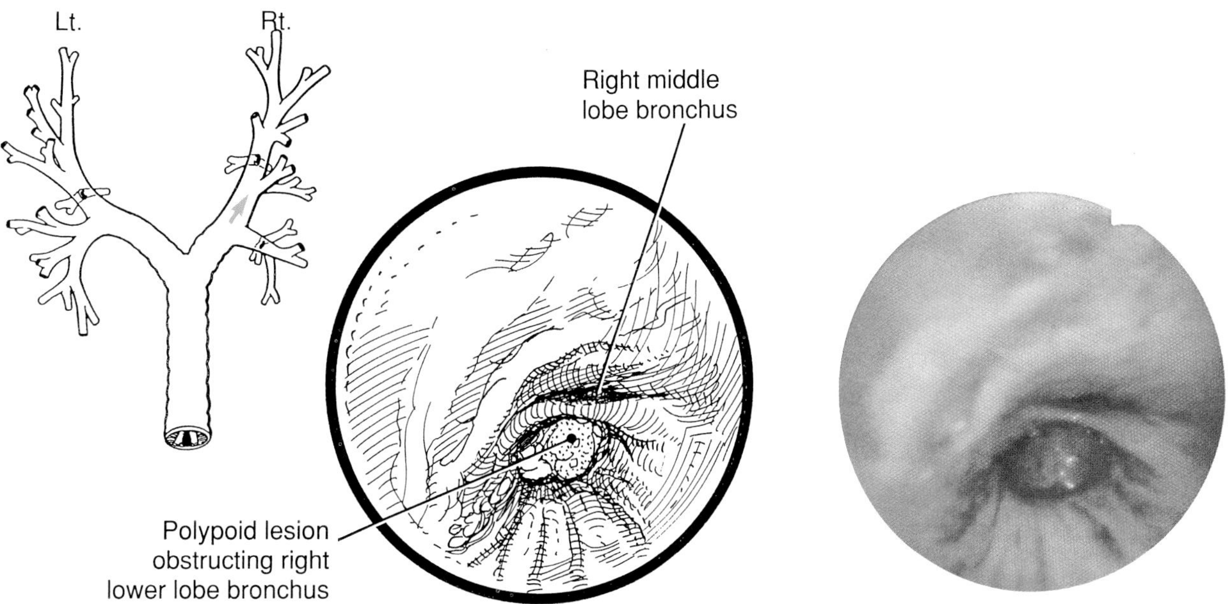

FIG. 143. Large cell carcinoma presenting as an enlarging mass in parenchyma of the lung eventually protruding through right lower lobe bronchus and compressing the right middle lobe bronchus.

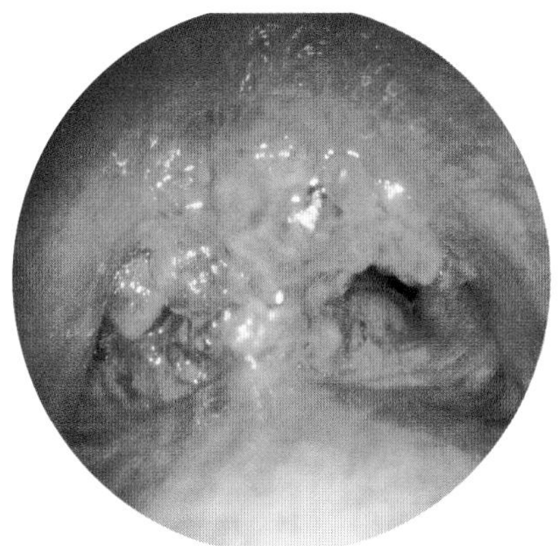

FIG. 144. Adenosquamous carcinoma involving distal trachea and both main bronchi.

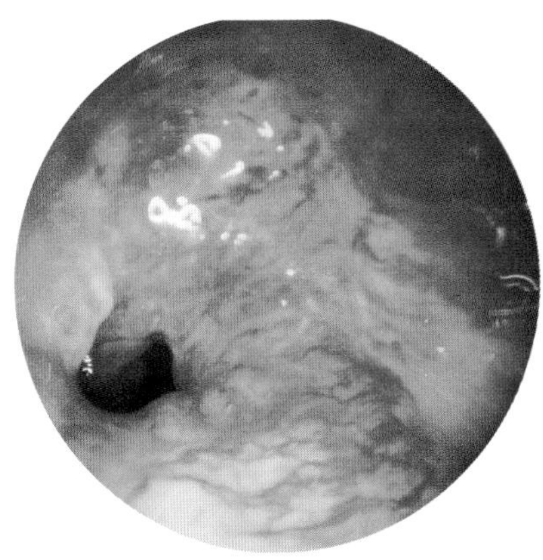

FIG. 145. Small cell carcinoma involving the proximal left main bronchus. Extensive mucosal infiltration by tumor is evident.

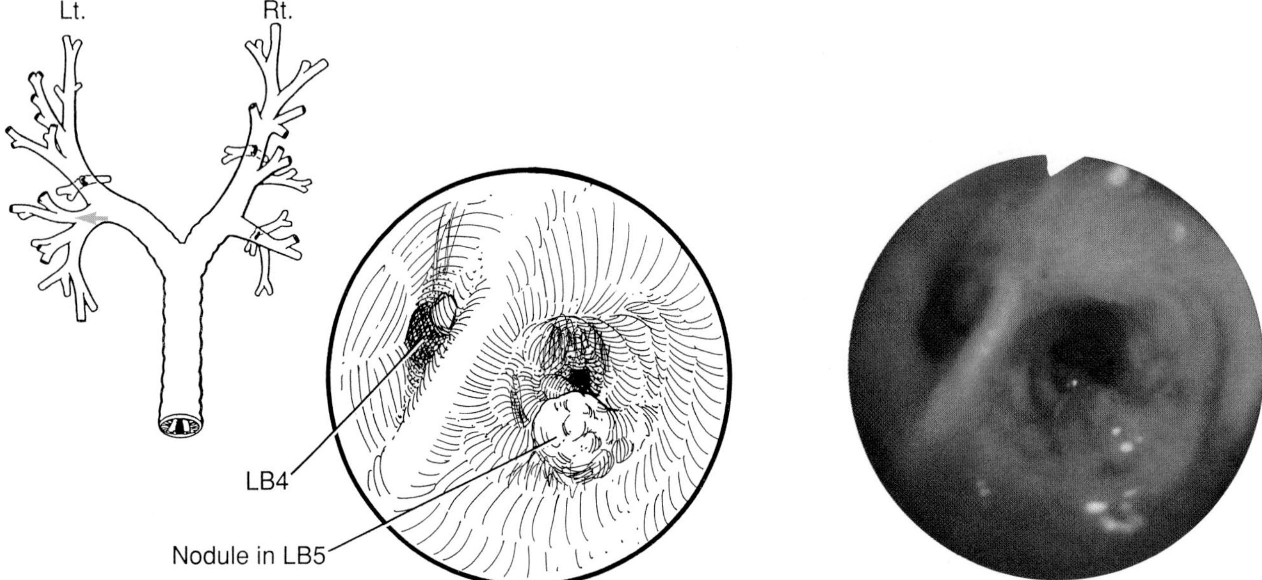

FIG. 146. Alveolar cell carcinoma with endobronchial nodules. This is an unusual presentation because alveolar cell carcinoma usually involves lung parenchyma and not the tracheobronchial tree.

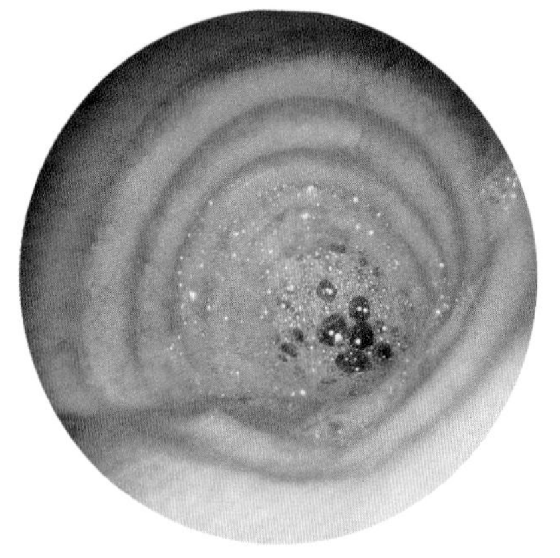

FIG. 147. Alveolar cell carcinoma with severe bronchorrhea. Bronchorrhea is defined as expectoration of more than 100 ml of thin mucous secretion in 24 hr. This manifestation is seen in approximately 20% of patients with diffuse alveolar cell carcinoma.

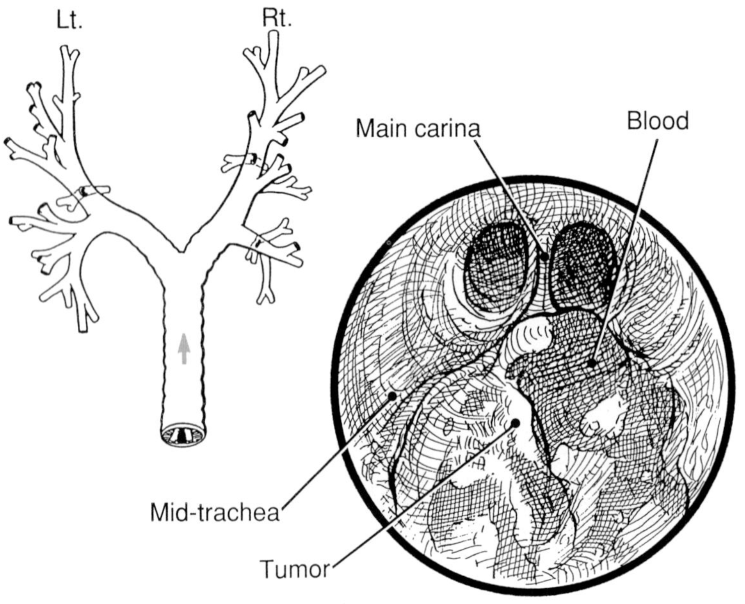

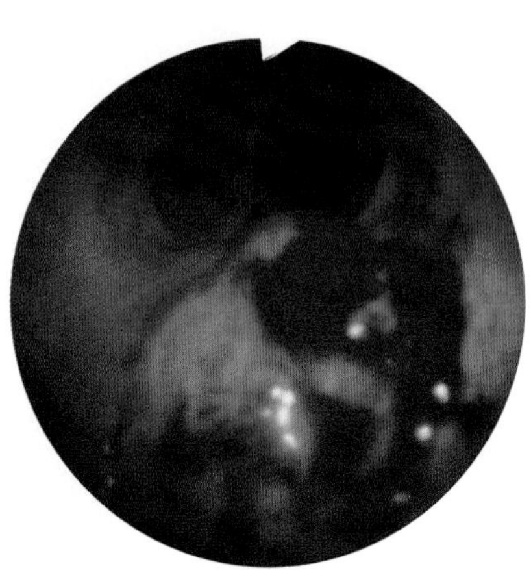

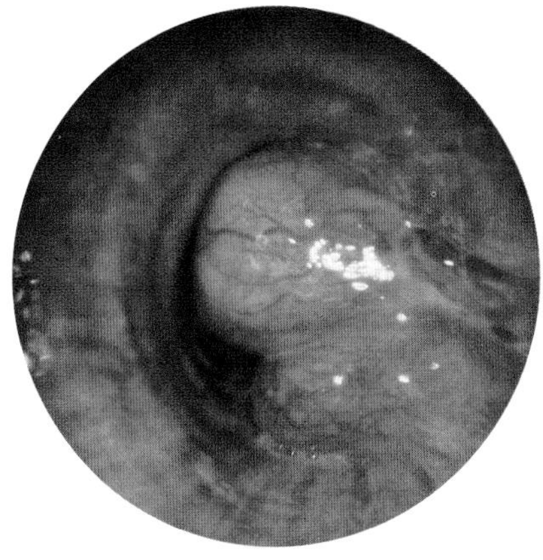

FIG. 149. A large cylindroma of distal trachea. Cylindromas constitute 40% of the malignant tumors of trachea and two thirds of these are surgically resectable (87).

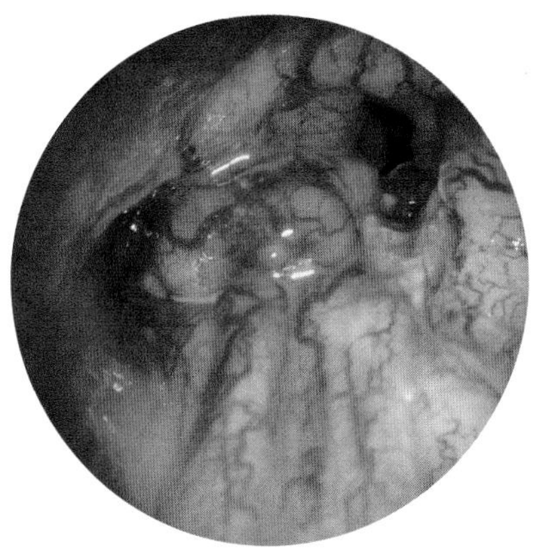

FIG. 150. Cylindroma involving distal trachea and both main bronchi. With repeated laser and stent therapy, patient survived for 3 years.

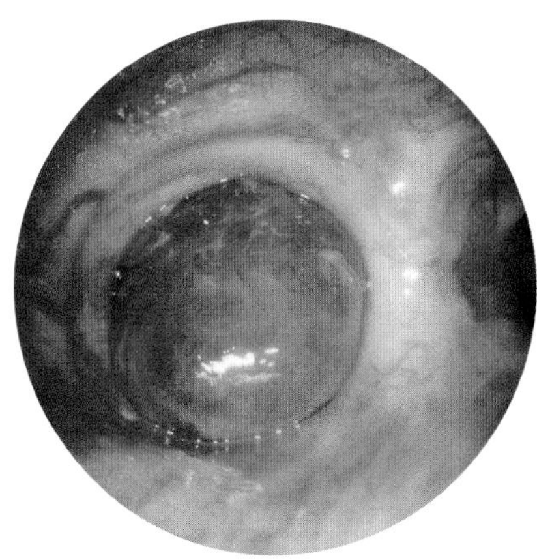

FIG. 151. Carcinoid tumor partially obstructing right bronchus intermedius. The tumor is vascular and smooth—a typical description of carcinoid. However, this appearance is not exclusive to carcinoid. Of the 126 bronchial carcinoid tumors, the diagnostic tests were bronchoscopy (81), bronchoscopic brushing and washing (50), and bronchoscopic biopsy (40) (88).

←

FIG. 148. Cylindroma of midtrachea. Cough and hemoptysis were the main symptoms. Despite tracheal resection and end-to-end anastomosis, the tumor recurred at the anastomotic site. Intraluminal radiation therapy was used with no evidence of progression after 3 years.

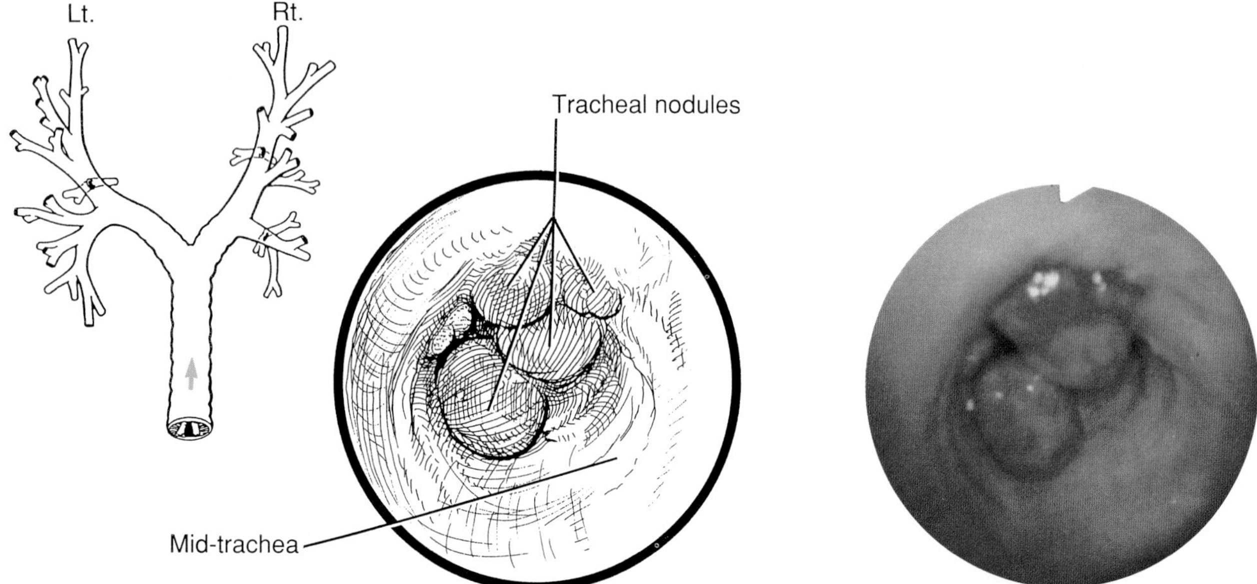

FIG. 152. Carcinoid tumor involving midtrachea. Patient had previously undergone left upper lobectomy for treatment of adenocarcinoma. A review of resected lung tissue suggested atypical carcinoid. The tracheal tumor required multiple Nd:YAG laser treatments. The patient eventually died from hepatic metastases.

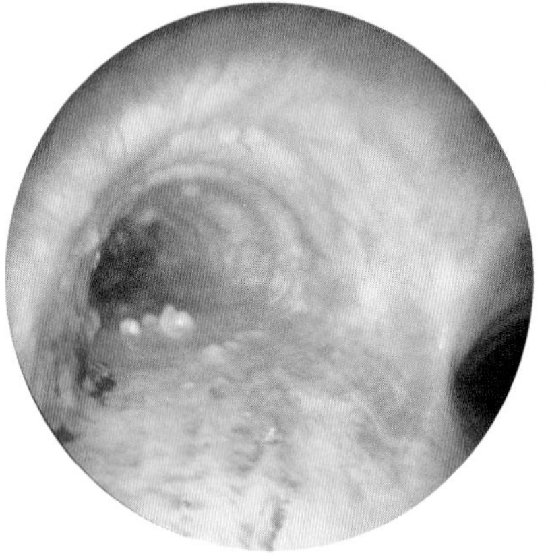

FIG. 153. Carcinoid tumor involving the posterior wall of proximal left main bronchus. These tiny lesions were thought to represent micrometastases.

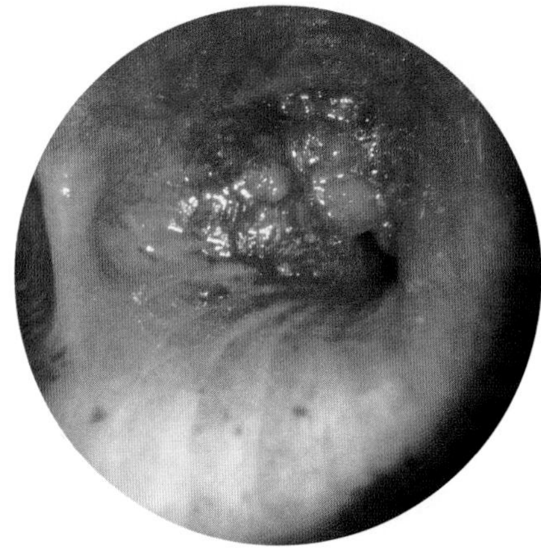

FIG. 154. Carcinoid (atypical) tumor involving right bronchus intermedius.

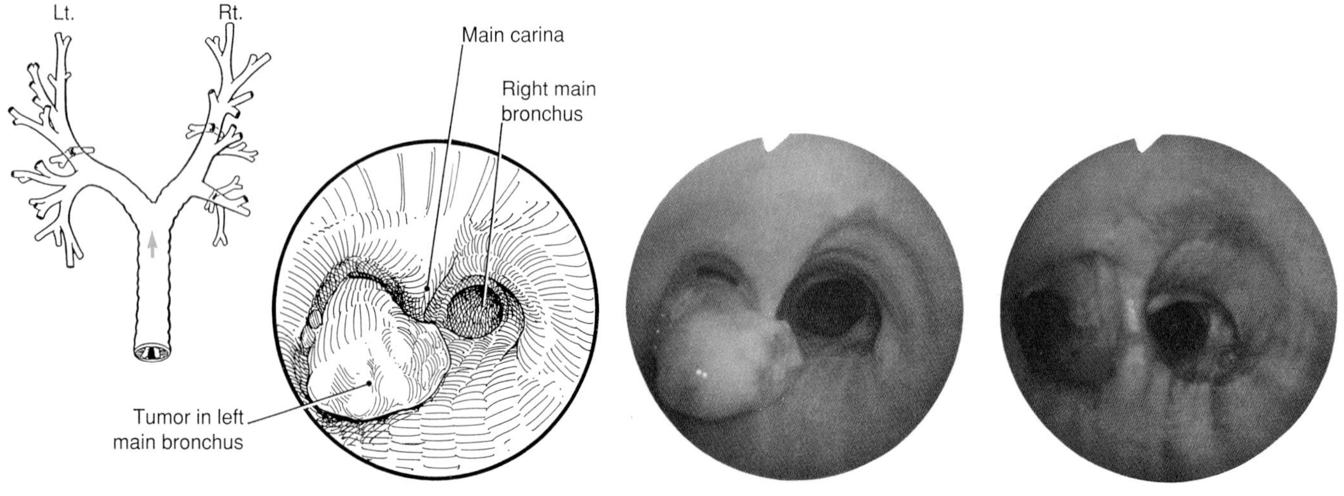

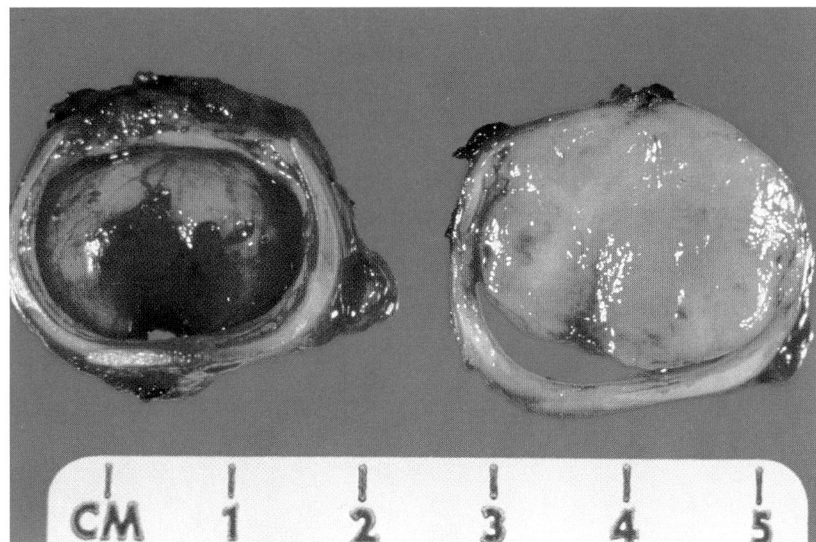

FIG. 156. Plasma cell granuloma of trachea-resected specimen. Plasma cell granulomas of the tracheobronchial tree are very rare. Laser therapy has shown good response (90,91). Courtesy of Atul C. Mehta, M.D.

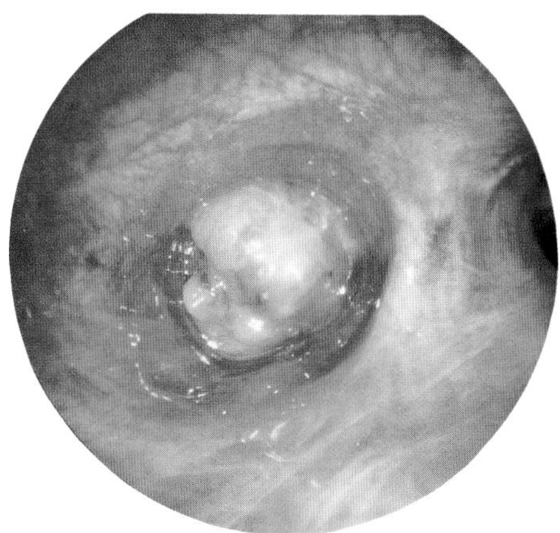

FIG. 157. Myoblastoma of right bronchus intermedius. Endobronchial myoblastoma is rare in the trachea (92). Bronchoscopic bipolar cautery has been used to treat obstructing endobronchial myoblastoma (93).

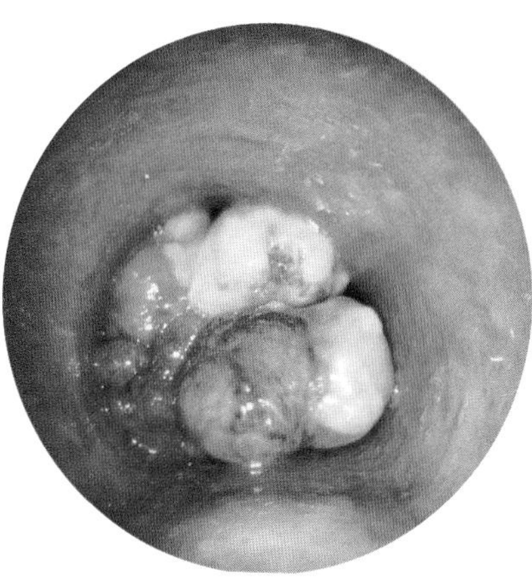

FIG. 158. Glomus tumor of trachea. Bronchoscopic biopsies have been used in the diagnosis and planning of therapy for this rare neoplasm (94,95). Slow growth of this tumor may cause symptoms suggestive of asthma.

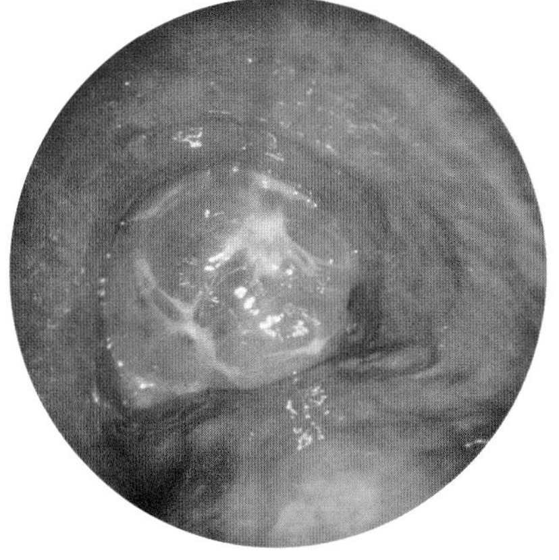

FIG. 159. Paraganglionoma of left main bronchus.

FIG. 155. Carcinoid tumor protruding from left main bronchus **(left)**; and the bronchoscopic appearance immediately after resection of the tumor and reanastomosis **(right)**. Such conservative (lung-sparing) treatment has shown excellent long-term prognosis (89).

NEOPLASMS, METASTATIC (Figs. 160–193)

Tracheobronchial endoluminal metastasis is common in patients with nonpulmonary malignancies. Renal, breast, thyroid, and colon cancers are the most common malignancies associated with tracheobronchial metastases (96). Among 2,388 bronchoscopic examinations in patients with cancer, endobronchial metastases was observed in only 2%. The primary tumors, in order of decreasing frequency, were breast, colon, melanoma, neuroblastoma, leiomyosarcoma, and endometrial tumors (97). In another series of patients with nonpulmonary malignancies and pulmonary metastases, bronchoscopy was most likely to be diagnostic in patients with primary colorectal cancer (79%) and breast cancer (57%), and least likely to be diagnostic in patients with genitourinary tract cancer (33%) (98). However, we have found a significant number of patients with primary prostate cancer with endobronchial metastases. The following are some examples of tracheobronchial metastases from nonpulmonary malignancies.

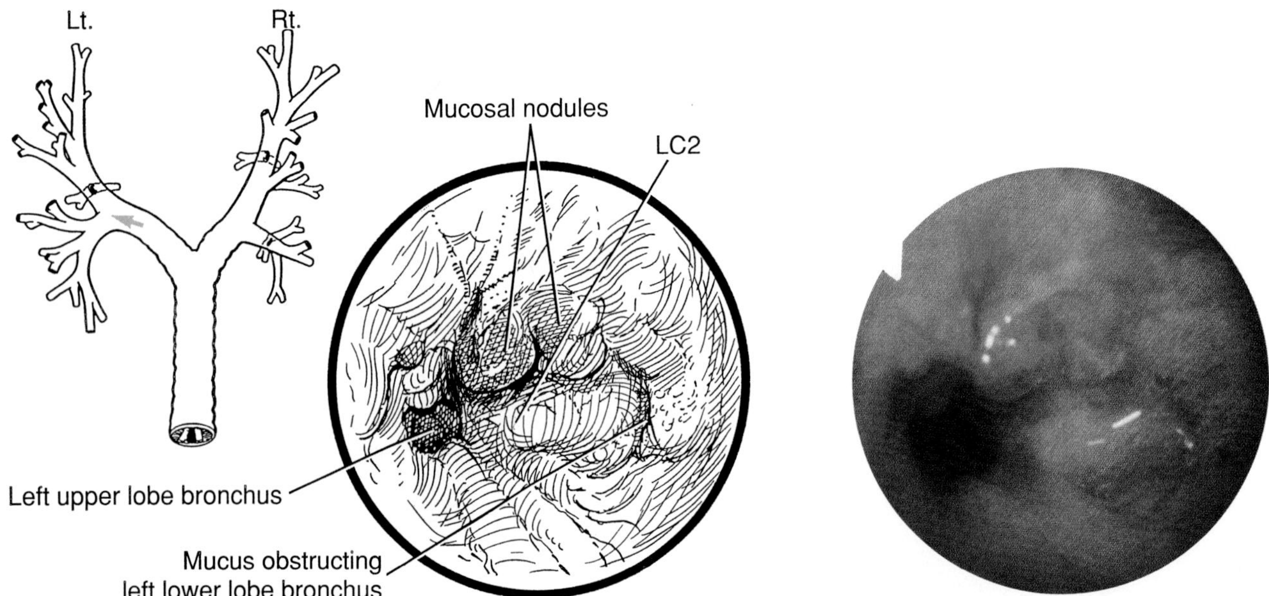

FIG. 160. Breast carcinoma metastatic to left distal main bronchus. Biopsy revealed mucus-producing adenocarcinoma consistent with breast tumor. Among 42 patients with endobronchial metastases from primary carcinoma of breast, clinical features included cough (71%), hemoptysis (25%), and segmental atelectasis (57%) (99).

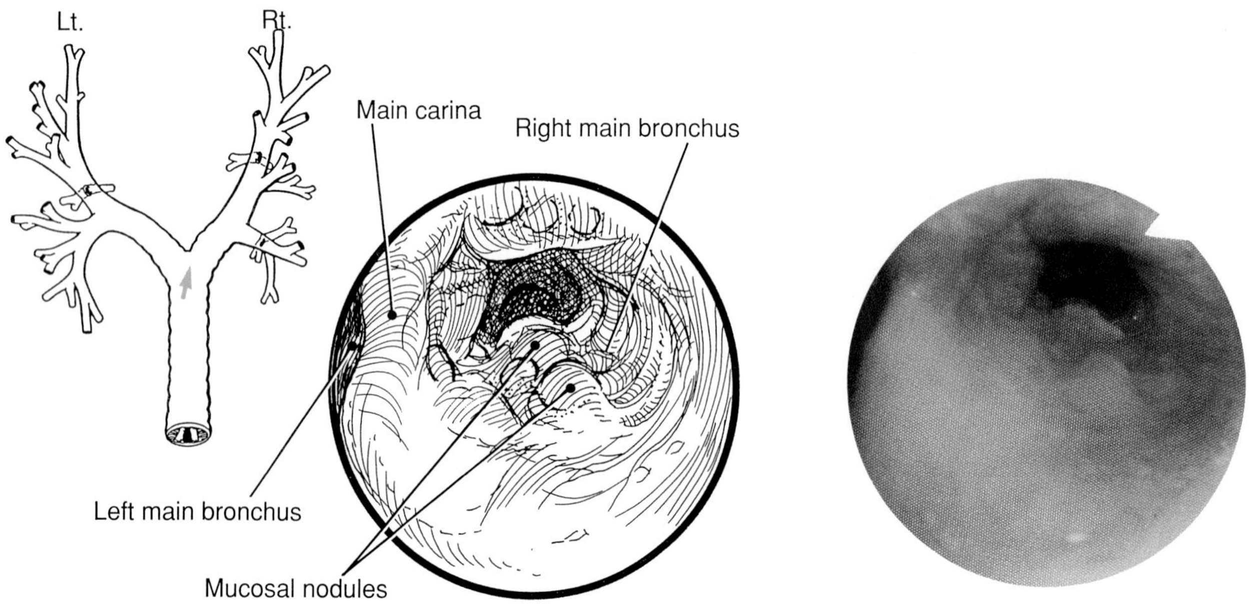

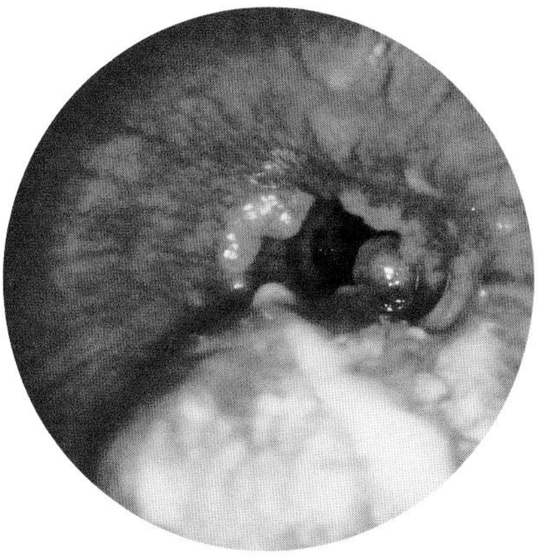

FIG. 162. Breast carcinoma with tracheal metastasis.

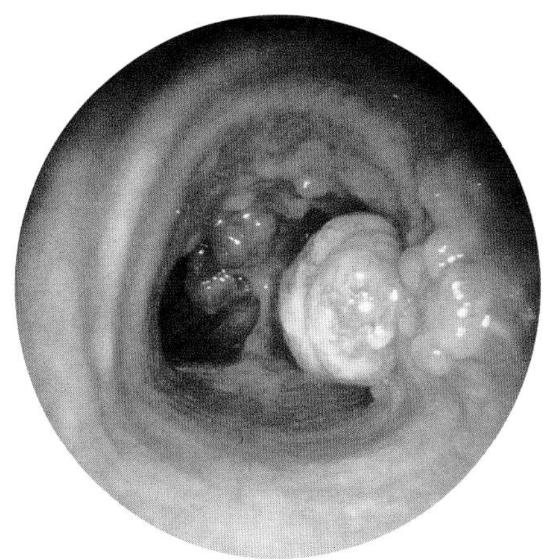

FIG. 163. Breast carcinoma with multiple tracheal metastases.

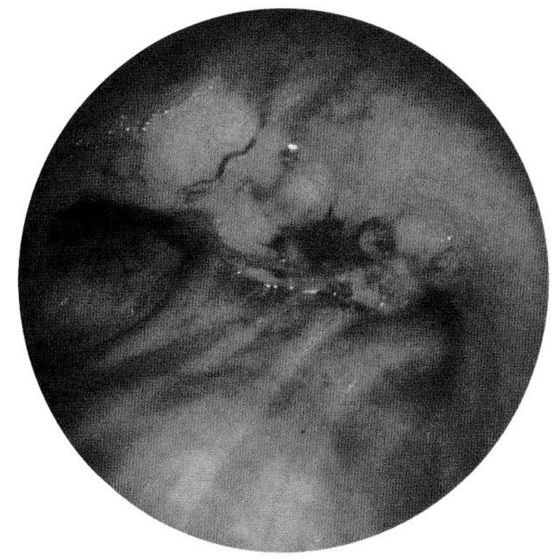

FIG. 164. Breast carcinoma with submucosal lymphangitic metastases.

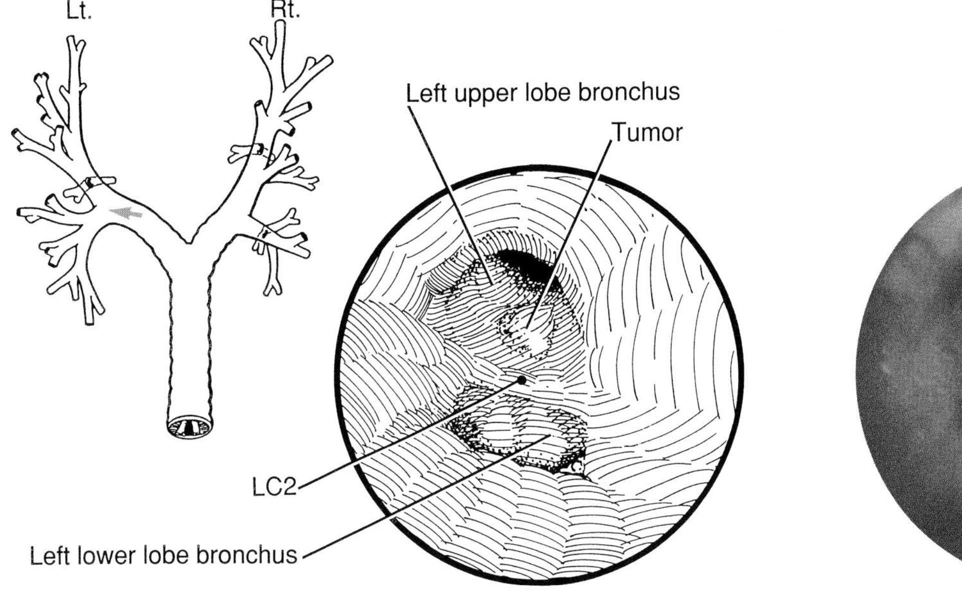

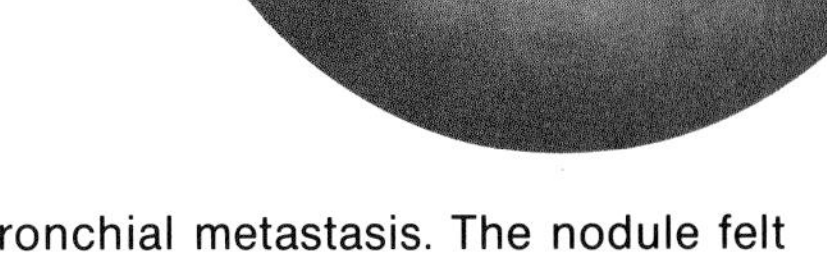

FIG. 165. Chondrosarcoma of left lower femur with endobronchial metastasis. The nodule felt "hard" to the biopsy forceps.

←

FIG. 161. Breast carcinoma with submucosal lymphangitic metastases. Among 660 patients with primary breast cancer, 119 had thoracic metastases but endobronchial metastases were observed in only 7 patients (100). In another study of 1,200 flexible bronchoscopies, only 10 patients had endobronchial metastases from primary breast cancer (101).

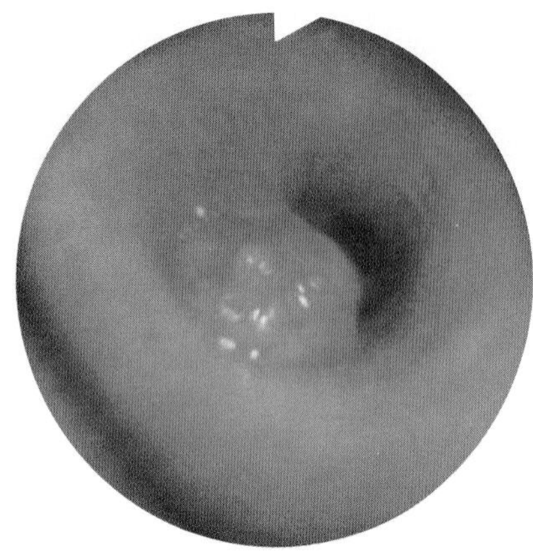

FIG. 166. Chondrosarcoma of pelvic bones with endobronchial metastasis involving left upper lobe bronchus.

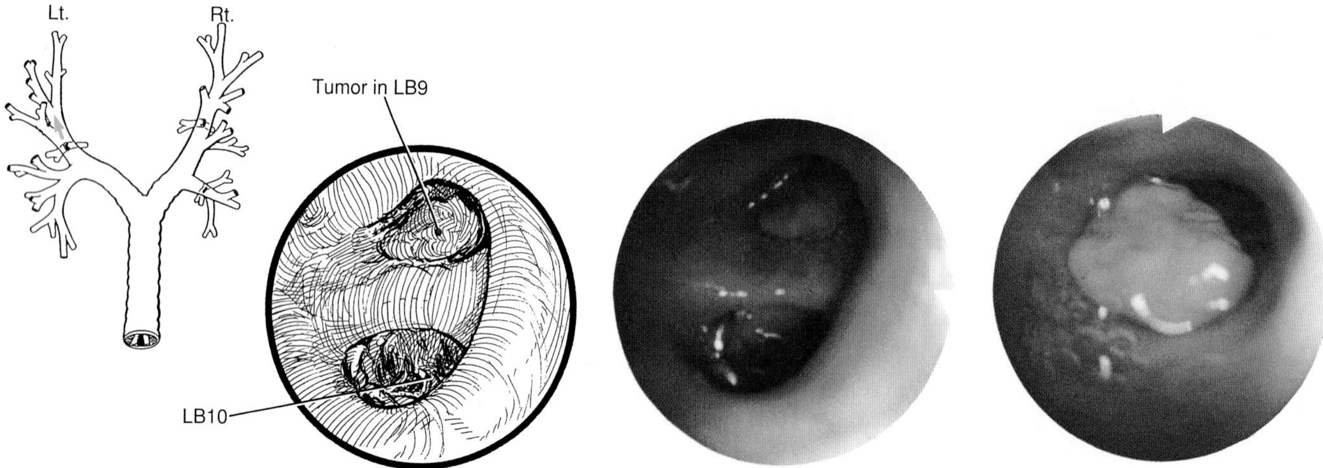

FIG. 167. Colon carcinoma with endobronchial metastasis **(left)**, and a close-up view of the lesion **(right)**. A considerable amount of thin mucus production was noted during bronchoscopy. Biopsy showed mucus-producing adenocarcinoma identical to previously resected colon tumor. A study in 1989 observed that there were only 24 reported cases of endobronchial metastases from colorectal carcinoma (102).

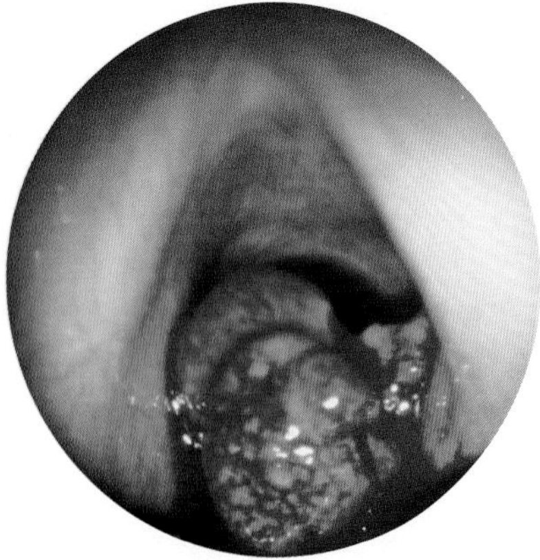

FIG. 168. Colon carcinoma with subglottic tracheal metastasis.

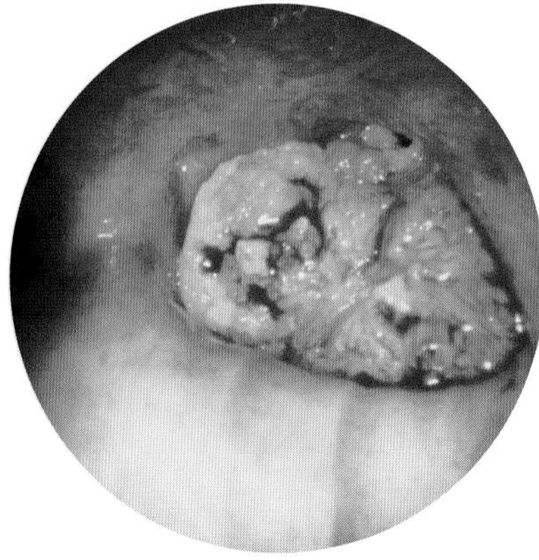

FIG. 169. Colon carcinoma with right main bronchial metastasis.

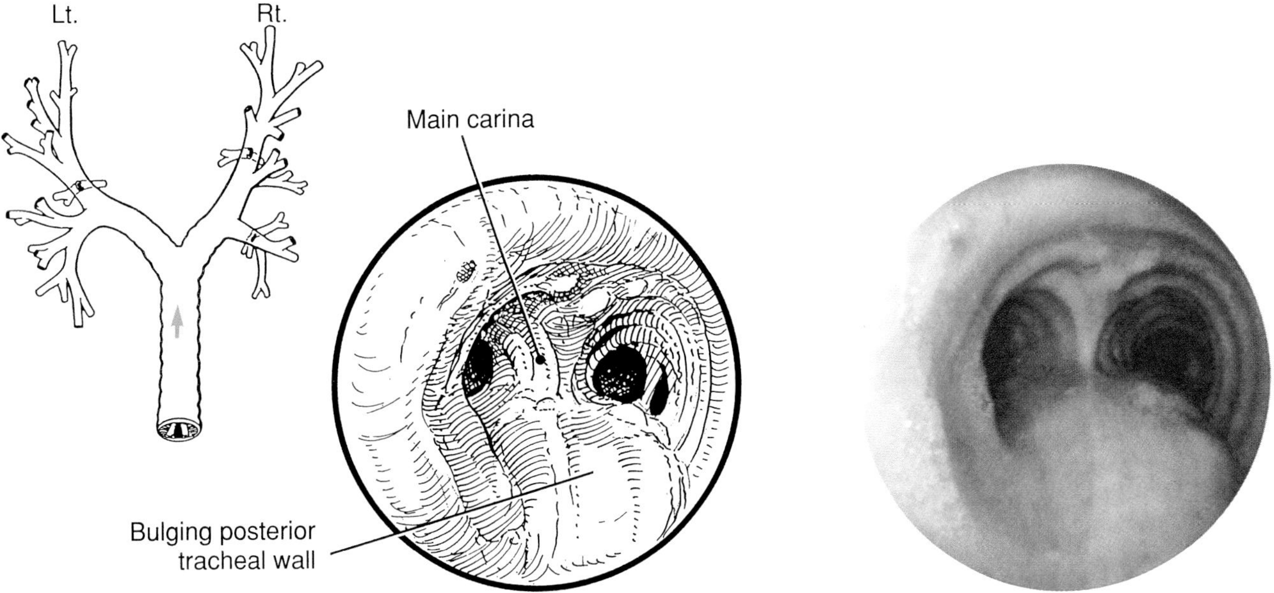

FIG. 170. Esophageal carcinoma causing bulging of posterior tracheal wall. Mucosa itself is uninvolved.

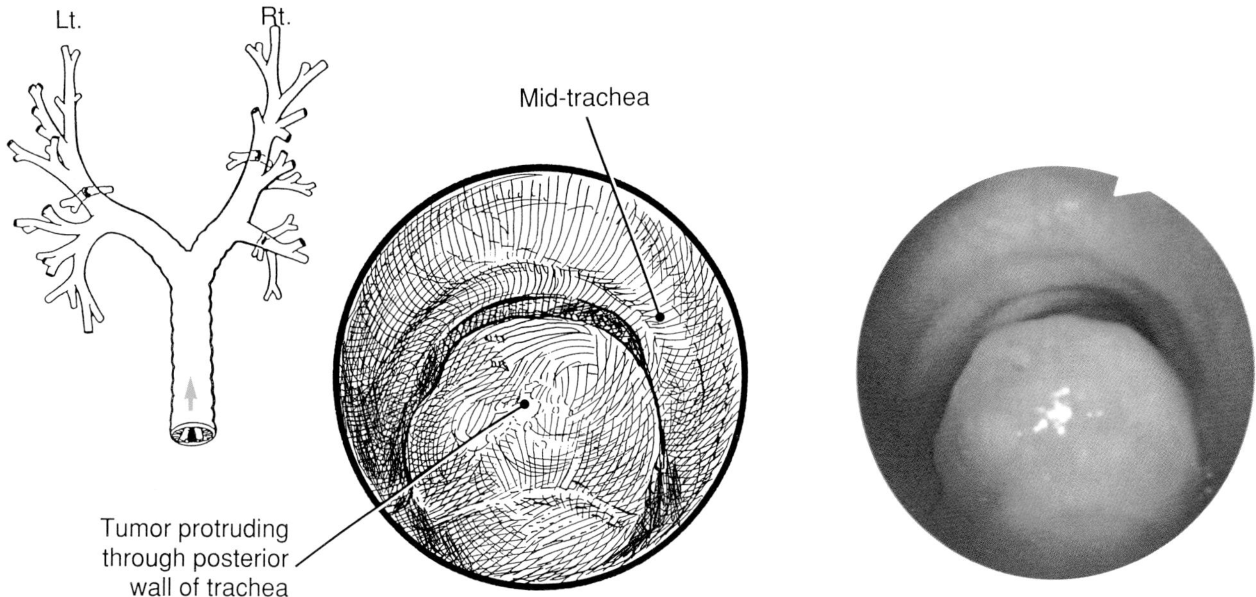

FIG. 171. Esophageal carcinoma with direct extension through the posterior tracheal wall.

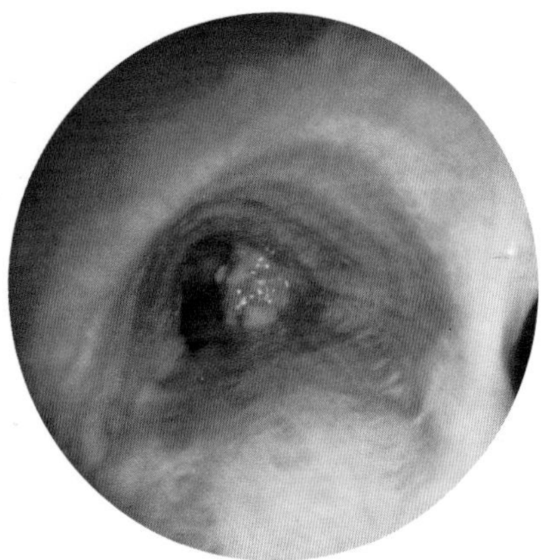

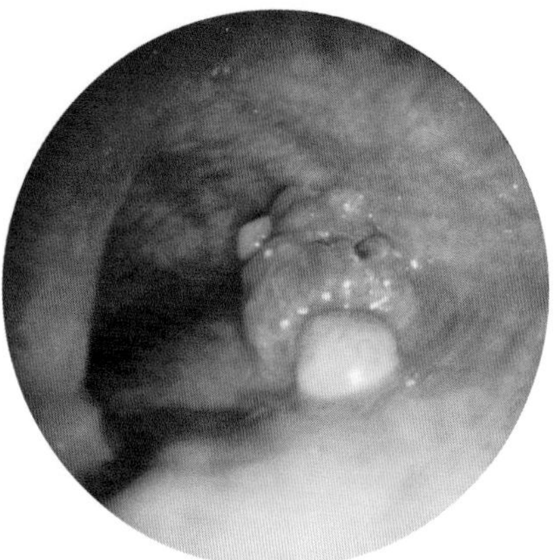

FIG. 172. Esophageal carcinoma with metastasis involving left main bronchus **(left)** and a close-up view of the lesion. Next to posterior wall of trachea, proximal left main bronchus is the airway that is closest to the esophagus. Direct extension and formation of tracheoesophageal fistula can be expected in these locations, and sometimes more distally.

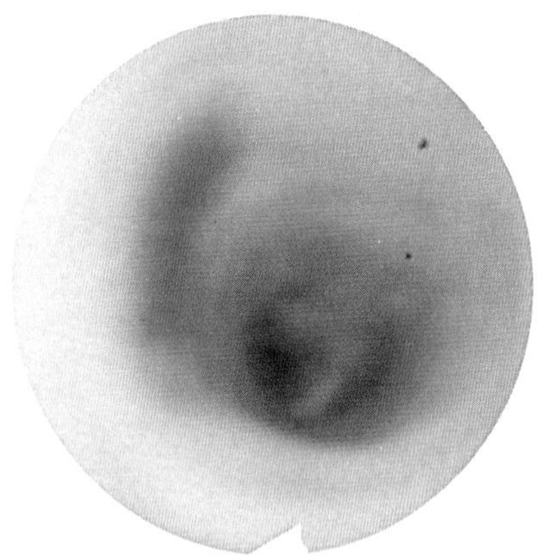

FIG. 173. Kaposi's sarcoma involving the trachea in a patient with AIDS. The lesion is violaceous in color and produces negligible airway obstruction. Nearly 50% of patients with cutaneous Kaposi's sarcoma demonstrate endobronchial involvement (103). Larger lesions can cause lobar atelectasis (104).

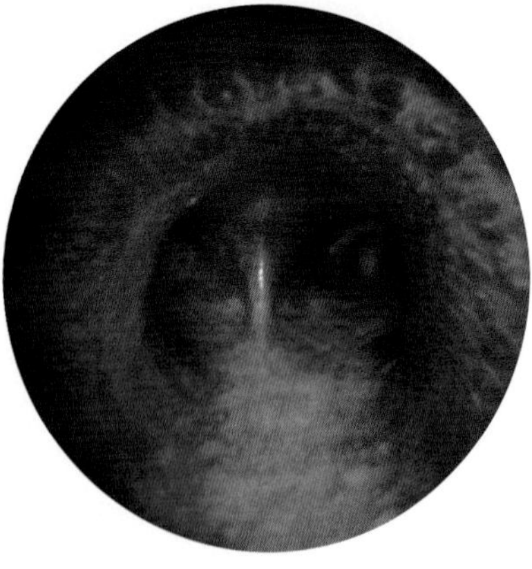

FIG. 174. Kaposi's sarcoma of distal trachea in a patient with AIDS. Multiple dark red mucosal lesions are seen studded throughout.

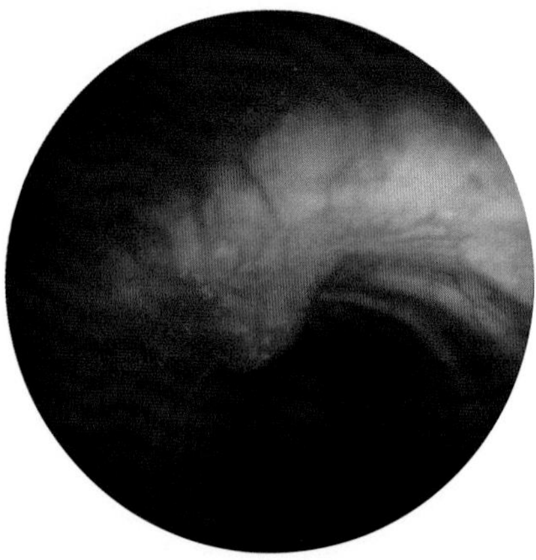

FIG. 175. Kaposi's sarcoma of midtrachea in a patient with renal transplant. Occurrence of endobronchial Kaposi's sarcoma in recipients of renal transplant is rare, although a case has been described (105).

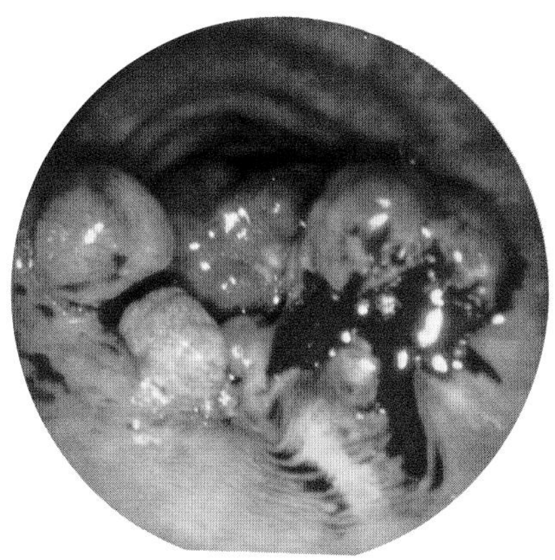

FIG. 176. Melanoma with extensive tracheal metastases. Melanoma is reported to be among the common nonpulmonary tumors to metastasize to lungs (97).

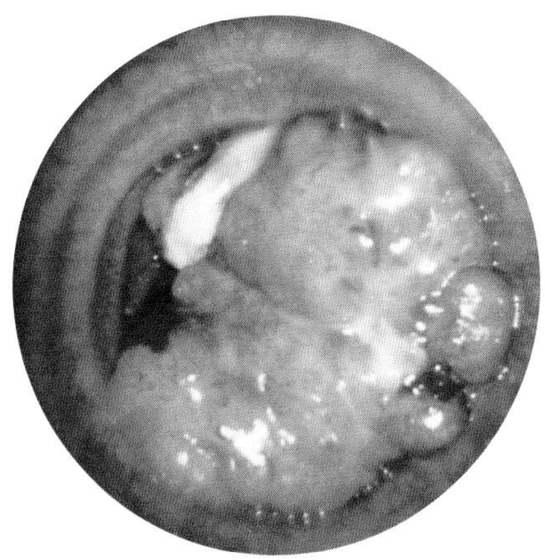

FIG. 177. Melanoma with tracheal metastasis. Nd:YAG laser therapy and mechanical debulking via the rigid bronchoscope resulted in excellent initial response. Recurrences in the same location required eight additional treatments. Patient succumbed 15 months after the first treatment.

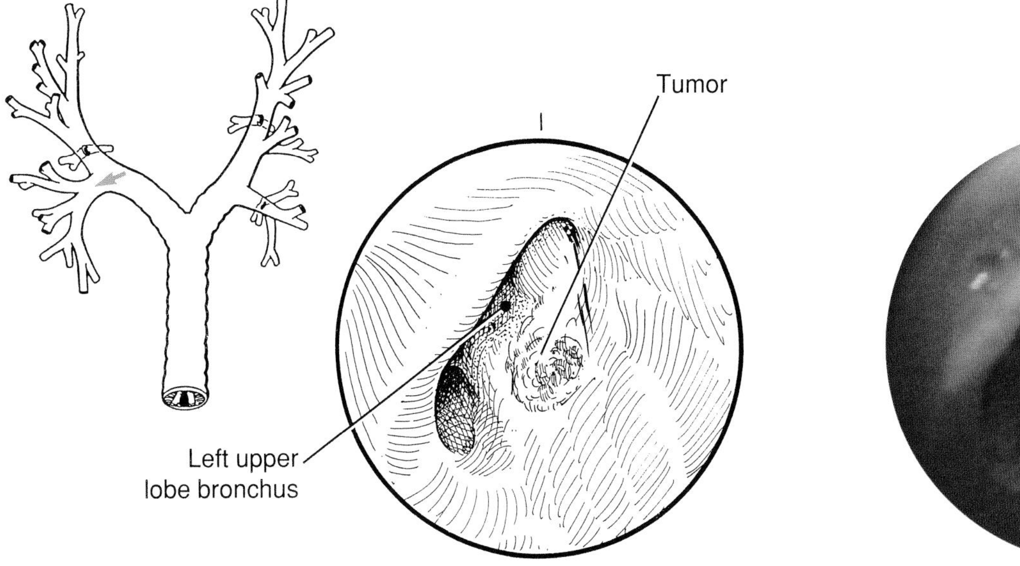

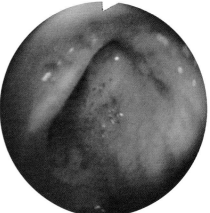

FIG. 178. Osteogenic sarcoma of right distal femur with endobronchial metastasis. Flexible bronchoscopic biopsy was impossible because of the hardness of the lesion but a good biopsy was possible with rigid bronchoscopic forceps. Eventually the patient developed obstruction to the left upper lobe. Nd:YAG laser therapy was not effective because of the inability to treat the bony portion of the metastatic lesion.

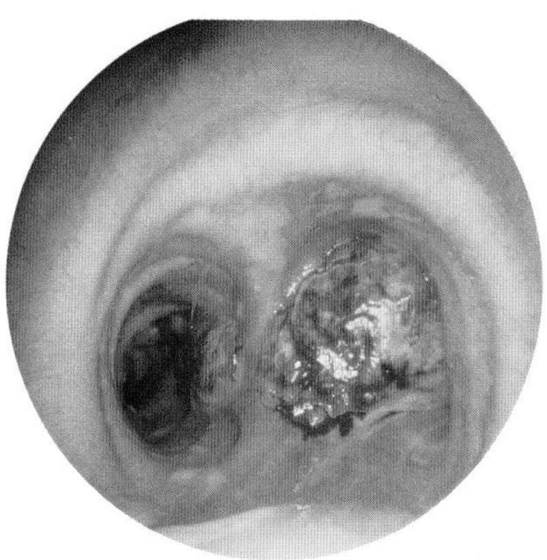

FIG. 179. Ovarian cancer with metastasis primarily to right main bronchus. Endobronchial metastases from ovarian cancer are rare, with only four cases reported in a literature review (106).

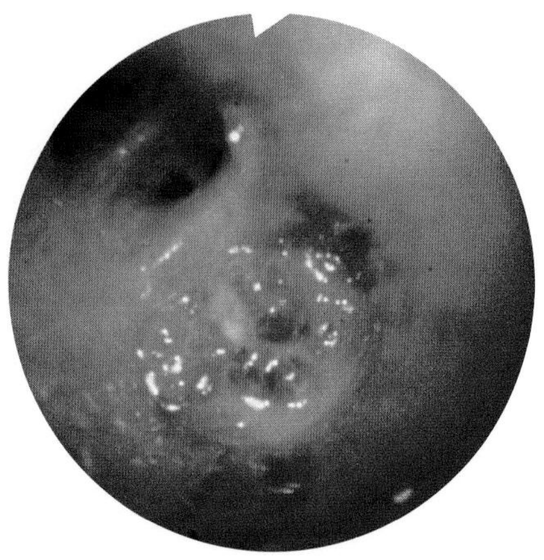

FIG. 180. Ovarian carcinosarcoma with metastasis to left lower lobe bronchus.

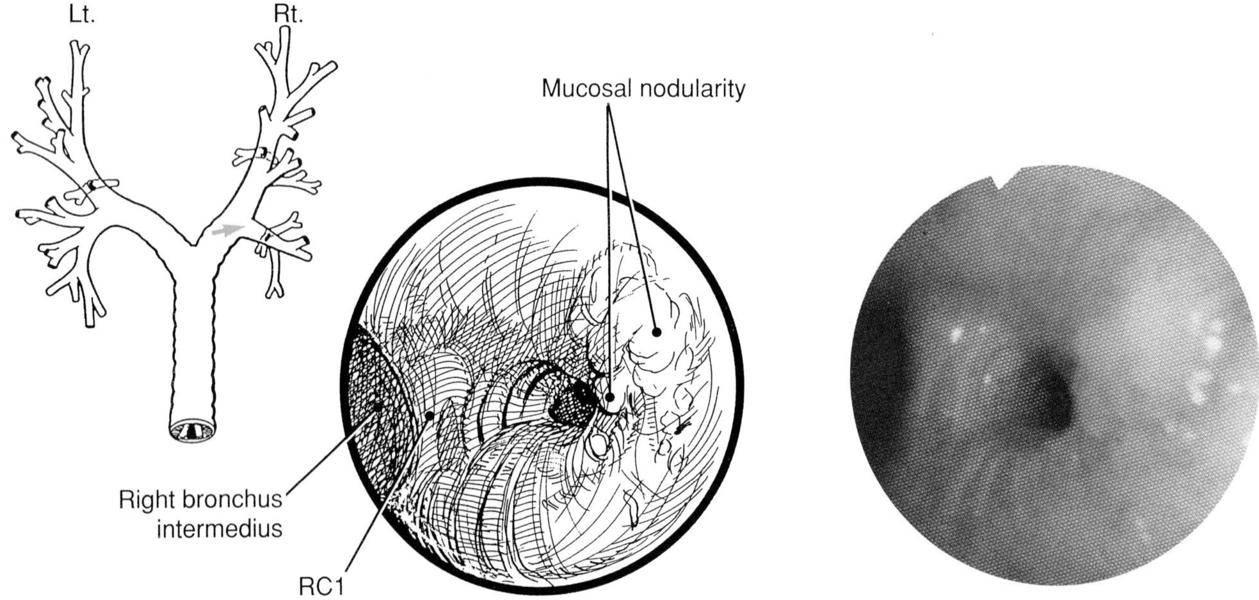

FIG. 181. Prostate carcinoma with endobronchial metastasis. Among elderly men, prostate is one of the common malignant tumors to produce endobronchial metastasis (107,108).

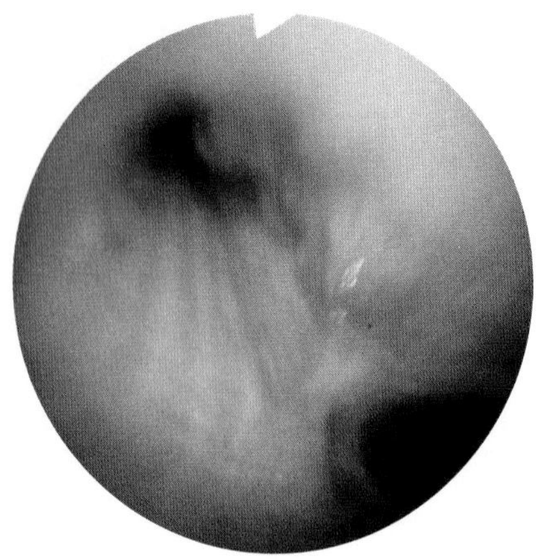

FIG. 182. Prostate carcinoma with endobronchial metastasis involving LC-2 and left upper lobe bronchus. Lobar collapse due to endobronchial metastasis from primary prostate cancer has been described (108).

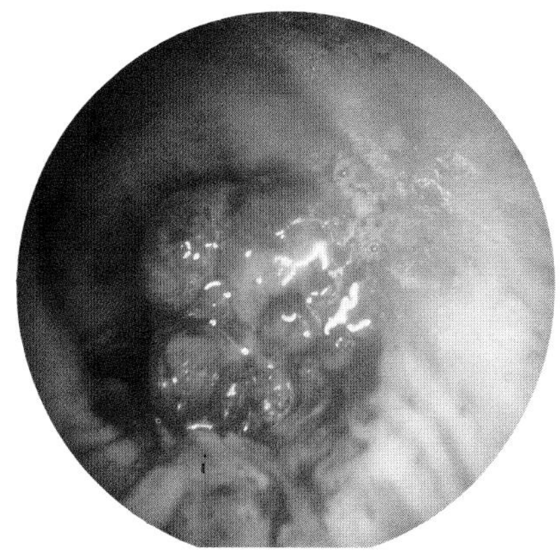

FIG. 183. Renal carcinoma (hypernephroma) with metastasis involving medial wall of left main bronchus. Endobronchial metastases from hypernephroma are relatively common (97,109,110). Generally, the endobronchial tumors are vascular, grow rapidly, and cause hemoptysis. Occasionally, patients expectorate necrotic tumor fragments.

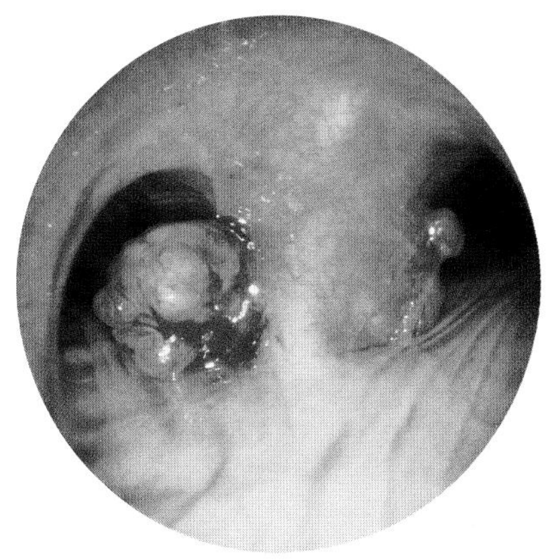

FIG. 184. Renal carcinoma with polypoid metastases to both main bronchi. Metastases limited to the bronchi are amenable to laser therapy. Twenty-two patients, treated at intervals of 6 months, have had 2–5 year survival (s.c.).

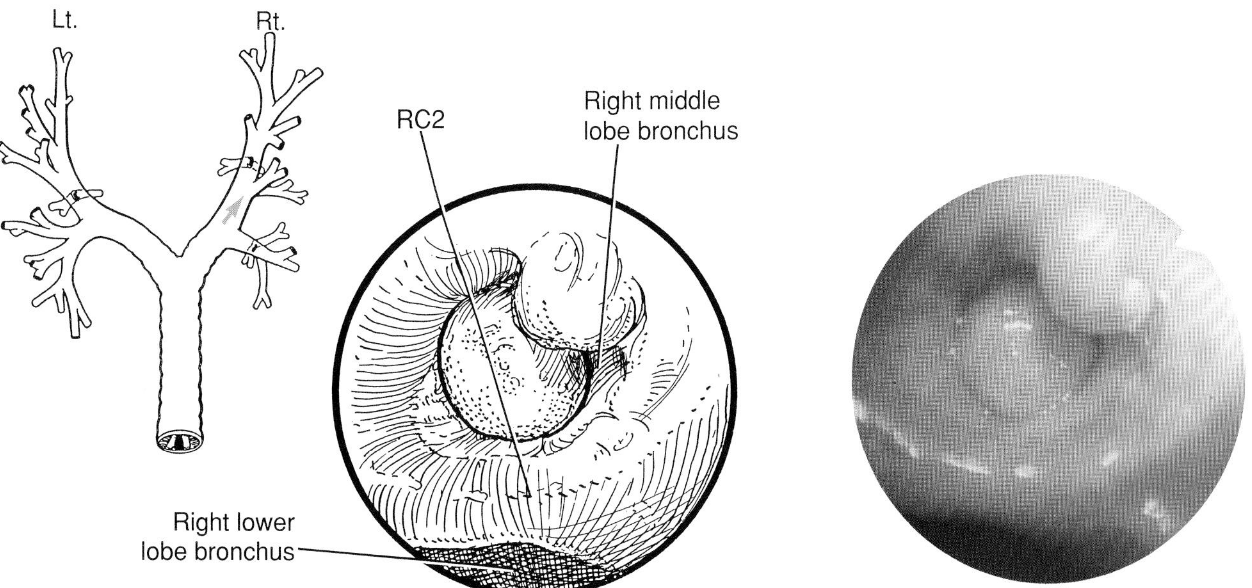

FIG. 185. Renal carcinoma with multiple nodular metastases. Histological analysis revealed clear cell carcinoma identical to the morphology of renal tumor resected 18 months earlier.

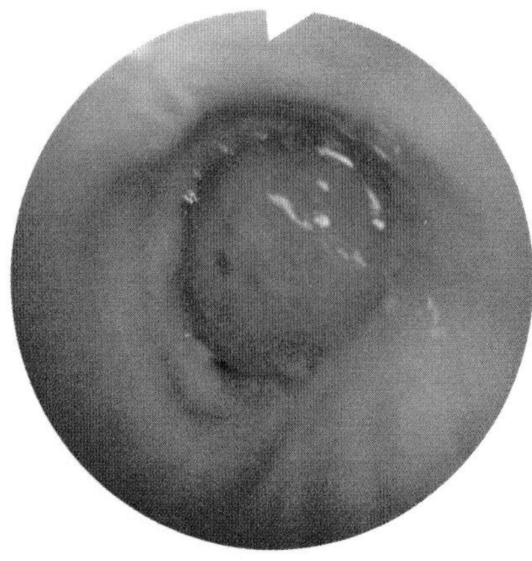

FIG. 186. Renal carcinoma with metastatic mass obstructing right distal main bronchus.

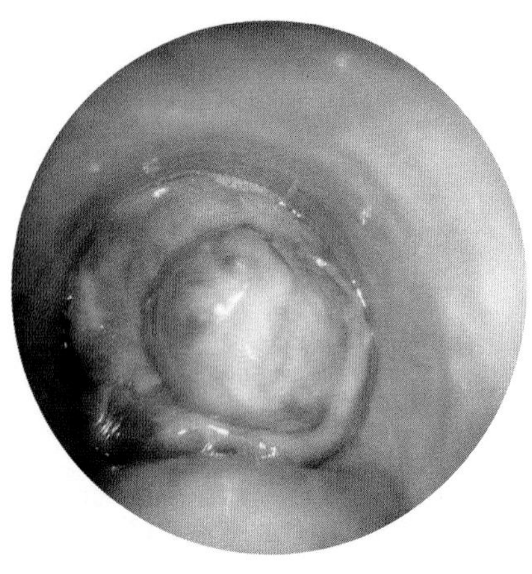

FIG. 187. Seminoma metastatic to trachea and right main bronchus. This association has been described (111).

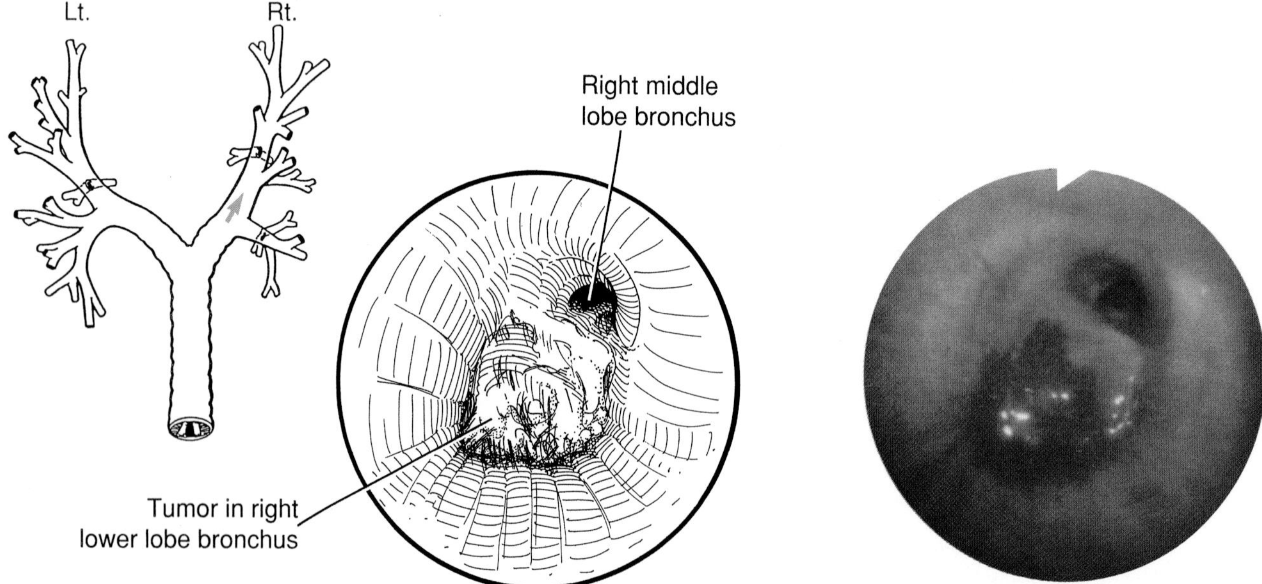

FIG. 188. Thymoma (malignant) with local extension and endobronchial metastasis. Tracheobronchial involvement is usually due to direct extension or extrinsic compression (112). Endobronchial polypoid lesions from thymoma are also described (113).

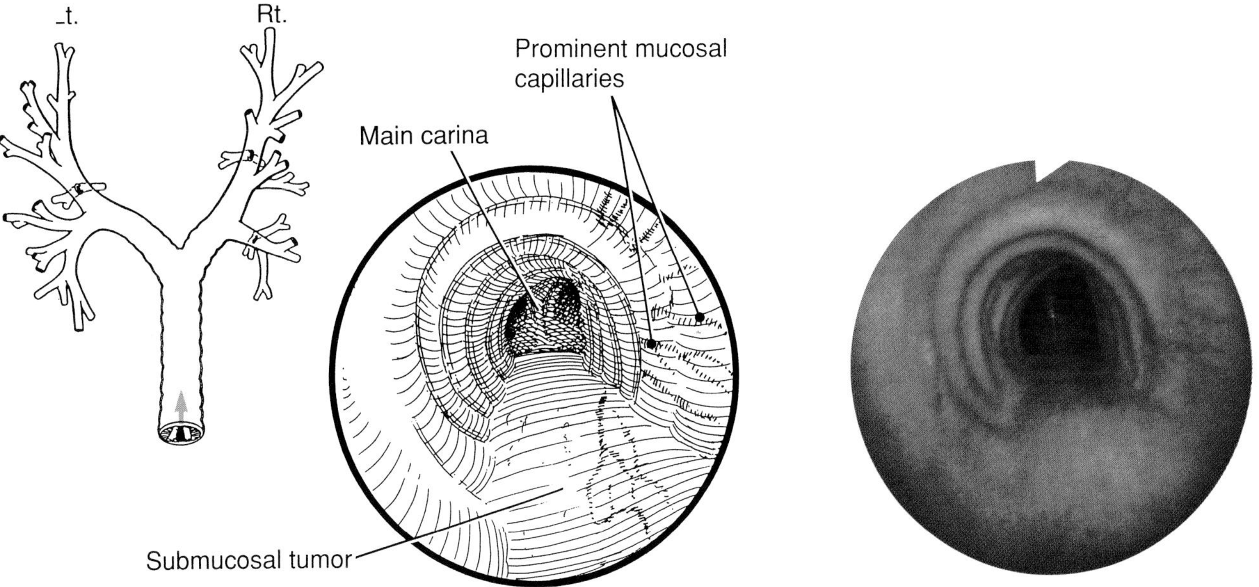

FIG. 189. Thyroid carcinoma with submucosal infiltration of right lateral and posterior walls of upper and midtrachea. Direct invasion of tracheal lumen leads to hemoptysis and symptoms of airway obstruction (114,115).

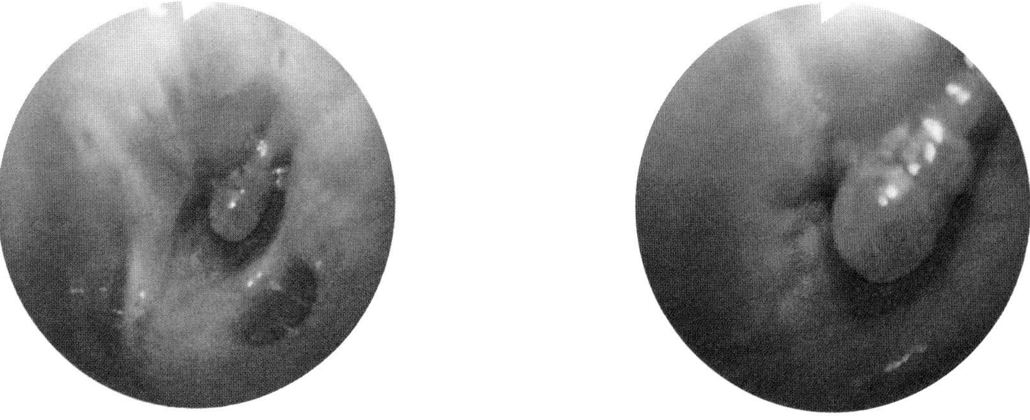

FIG. 190. Thyroid carcinoma (Hurthle cell type) with endobronchial metastasis **(left)**, and a close-up view of the lesion **(right)**. Endobronchial metastasis from Hurthle cell thyroid carcinoma has been described (116).

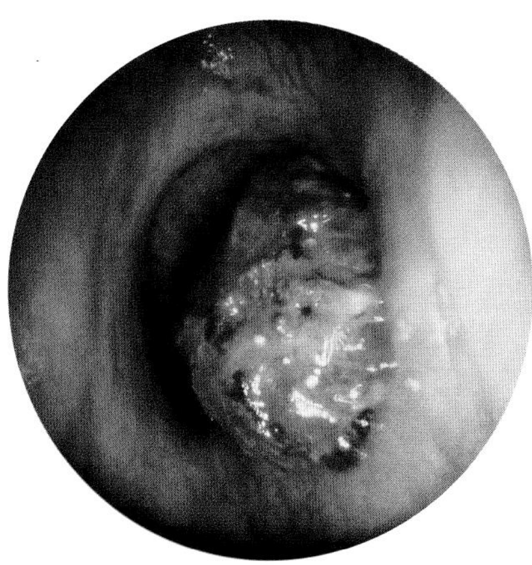

FIG. 191. Thyroid carcinoma with tracheal metastasis.

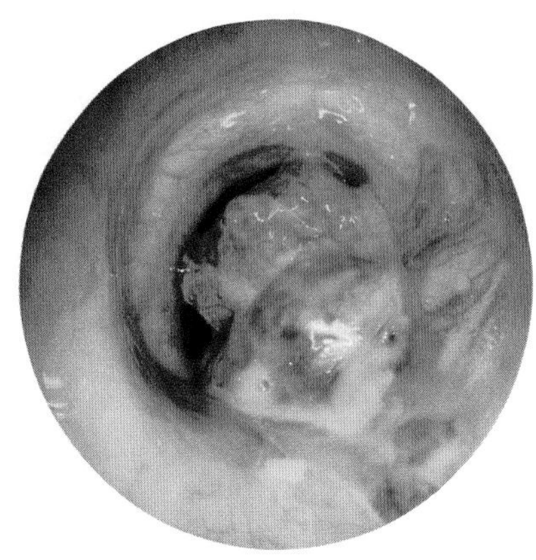

FIG. 192. Thyroid carcinoma with a large metastatic lesion in the trachea. This lesion may require urgent Nd:YAG laser therapy to relieve respiratory distress.

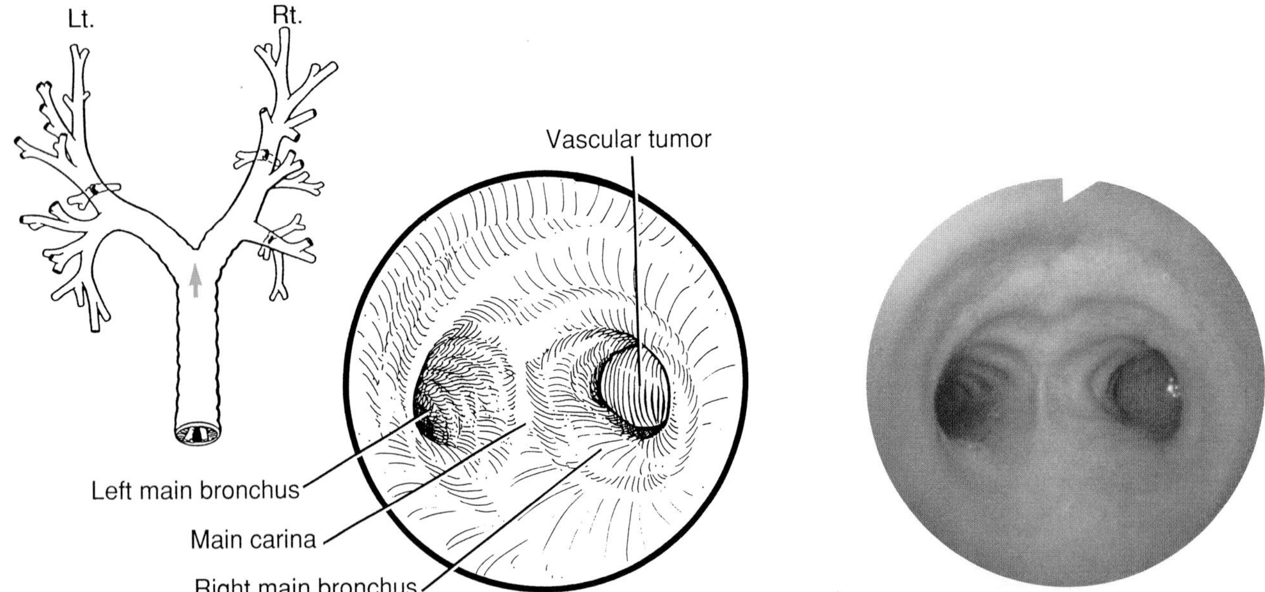

FIG. 193. Uterine leiomyosarcoma with metastasis to right main bronchus. Nd:YAG laser therapy resulted in reexpansion of totally atelectatic right lung. Patient survived for 18 months. Endobronchial metastases from uterine cervical squamous cell carcinoma and leiomyosarcoma have been described (117–119).

RELAPSING POLYCHONDRITIS (Figs. 194–195)

Relapsing polychondritis is an uncommon disease of possibly an autoimmune etiology characterized by recurrent episodes of cartilaginous inflammation, fever, anemia, scleritis, iritis, cataracts, and elevated sedimentation rate. A review of the literature observed 62 patients with serious airway compromise; there were 47 females and 17 males, with an average age of 40.3 years. Major symptoms included hoarseness, dyspnea, cough, stridor, wheezes, and tenderness over laryngotracheal cartilages. Death occurred in 13 patients despite tracheostomy or corticosteroid therapy, or both (120).

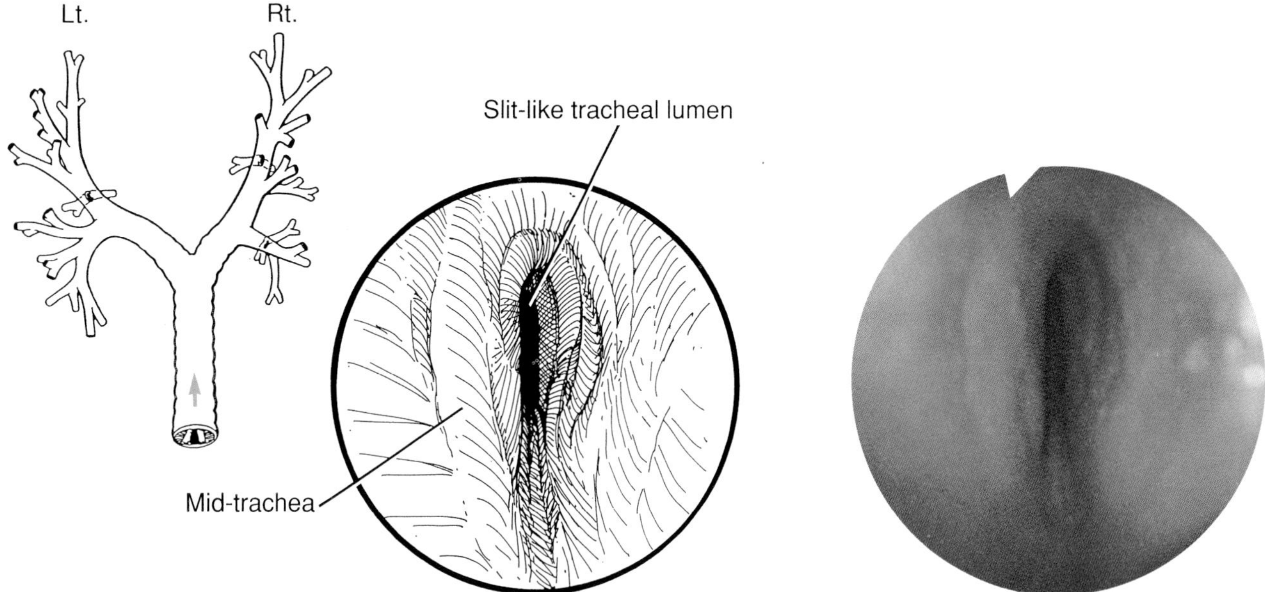

FIG. 194. Relapsing polychondritis. A slit-like tracheal lumen is seen. Patient required long-term tracheostomy. The bronchoscopic appearance is that of "saber sheath" or "scabbard" trachea.

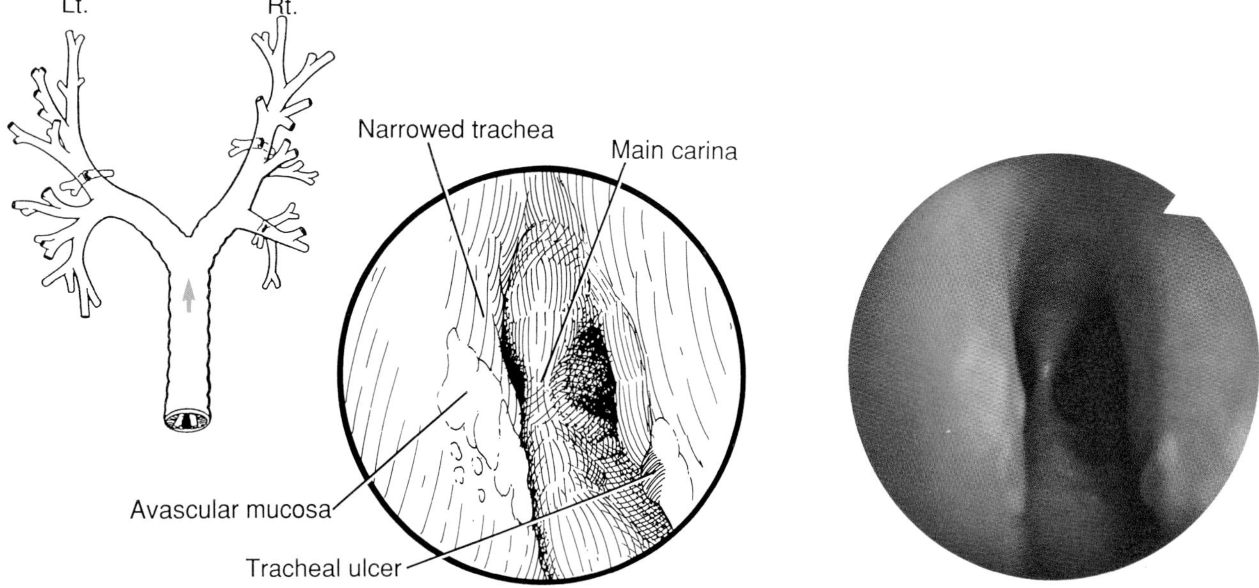

FIG. 195. Relapsing polychondritis with tracheal ulcerations caused by repeated apposition of lateral tracheal walls during coughing.

SARCOIDOSIS (Figs. 196–199)

Sarcoidosis is a relatively common disease in Western countries. It is a multisystem disorder of unknown etiology characterized by defective T-lymphocyte function, proliferation of B lymphocytes, and formation of noncaseous granulomata in various parts of the body. The most common intrathoracic manifestation is the presence of bilateral hilar and paratracheal lymphadenopathy. Endobronchial involvement is seen in 8–10% of patients with all stages of sarcoidosis. The bronchoscopic findings may include nonspecific bronchitis changes, mucosal granularity, islands of raised waxy lesions in the tracheobronchial mucosa, or bronchial stenosis in chronic cases (121–124).

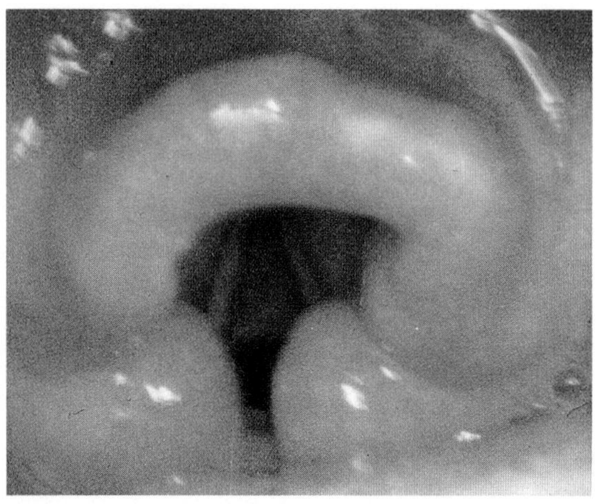

FIG. 196. Sarcoidosis involving epiglottis, and laryngeal structures. Sarcoidosis of upper airways is uncommon, noted in only 6 percent of 818 patients with multisystem sarcoidosis (125). Courtesy of Thomas J. McDonald, M.D.

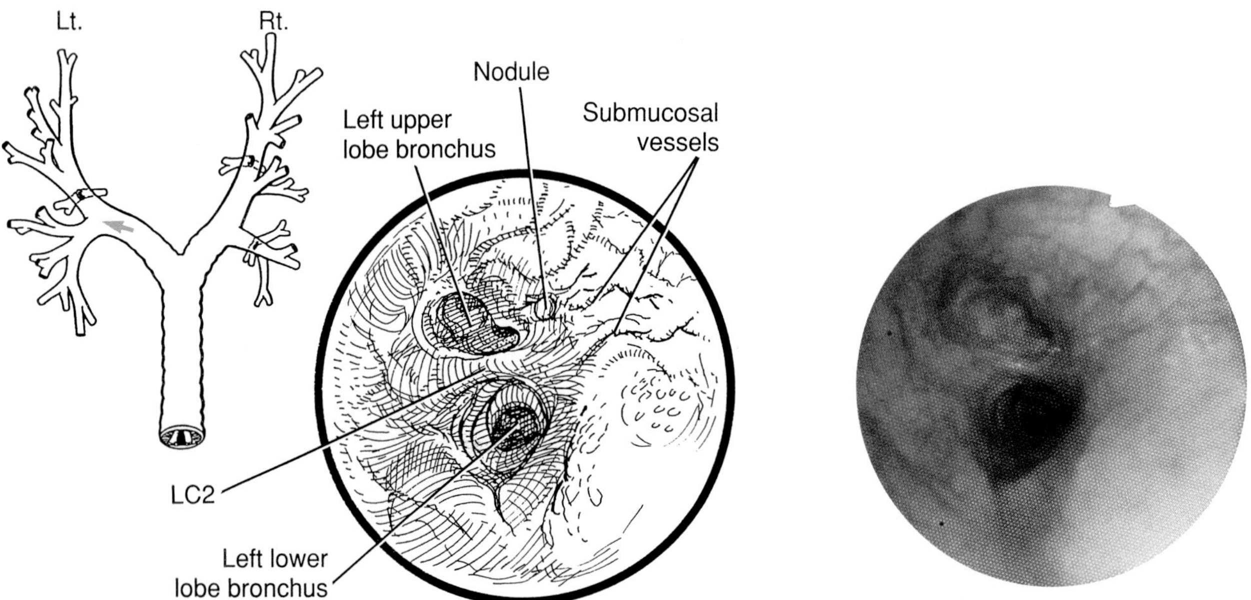

FIG. 197. Sarcoidosis with chronic mucosal changes and mild bronchial narrowing. Mucosal biopsy revealed noncaseous granulomas.

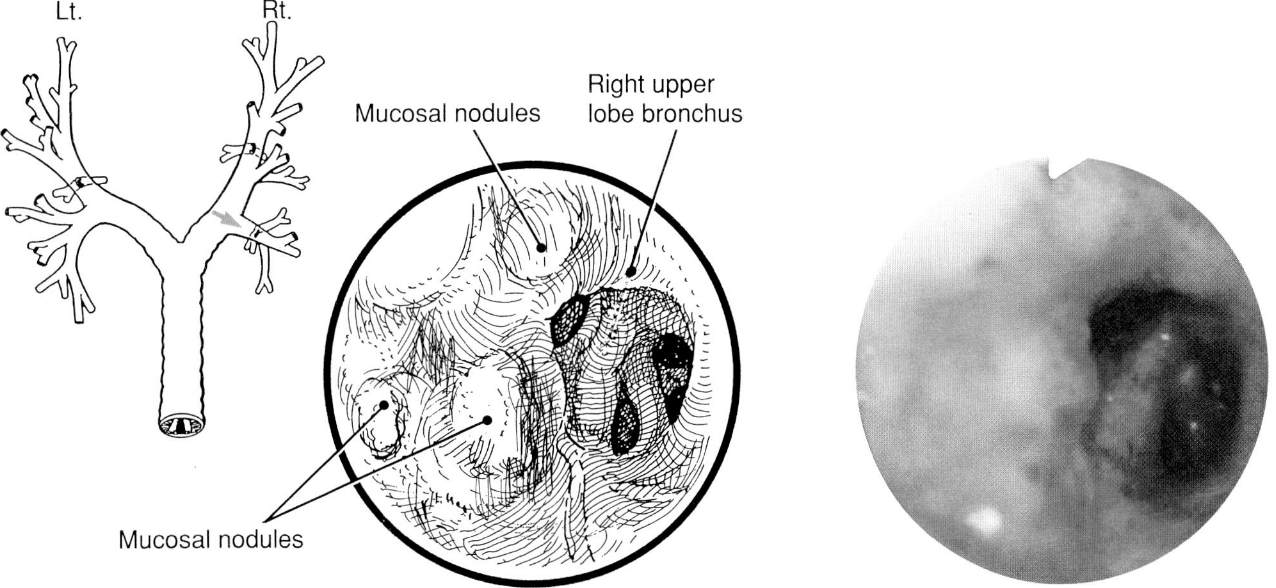

FIG. 198. Sarcoidosis with endobronchial nodules. These nodules are different from the yellowish tinged, waxy-appearing distinct mucosal nodules seen in some patients with sarcoidosis.

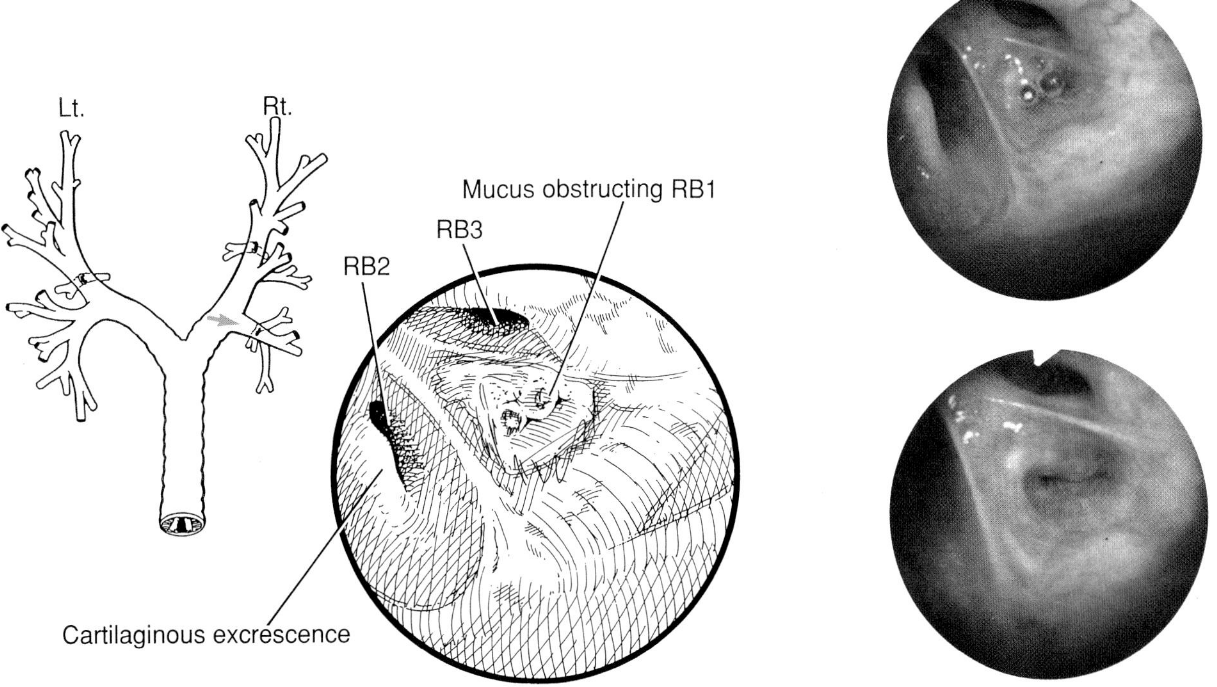

FIG. 199. Sarcoidosis with chronic bronchial stenosis. A small amount of mucus covers the bronchial orifice **(top)**. After removal of mucus **(bottom)**.

STENOSIS/STRICTURE (Figs. 200–209)

Pathogenetic etiologies of tracheobronchial stenosis or stricture can be broadly classified into extrinsic, intrinsic (in the wall of the airways), or intraluminal. The basic mechanisms involved in the formation of tracheobronchial stenosis are discussed in Chapter 21. Nonmalignant tracheobronchial stenoses are difficult to manage and often recur because the results of Nd:YAG laser treatment depend mainly on how much of the tracheobronchial wall is involved. It is well known that inflammatory processes frequently lead to ulceration of the wall with cartilage involvement. However, immediate results are almost always good in all types of stenosis. On the contrary, long term results are not as good and recurrence occurs in about 50% of the cases. Therefore lasertherapy is extremely useful for restoring ventilation, particularly in emergencies. Several of the etiologies are depicted under other headings in this section. The accompanying bronchoscopic portraits show some of the nonmalignant disorders that cause the stenosis.

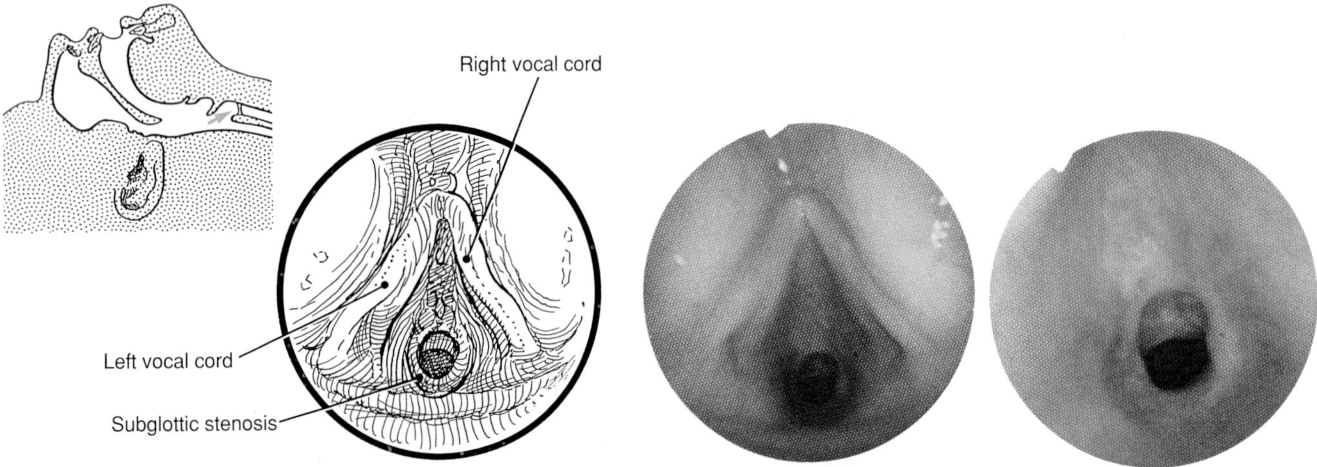

FIG. 200. Benign subglottic tracheal stenosis following endotracheal intubation **(left)**, and a close-up view of the lesion **(right)**.

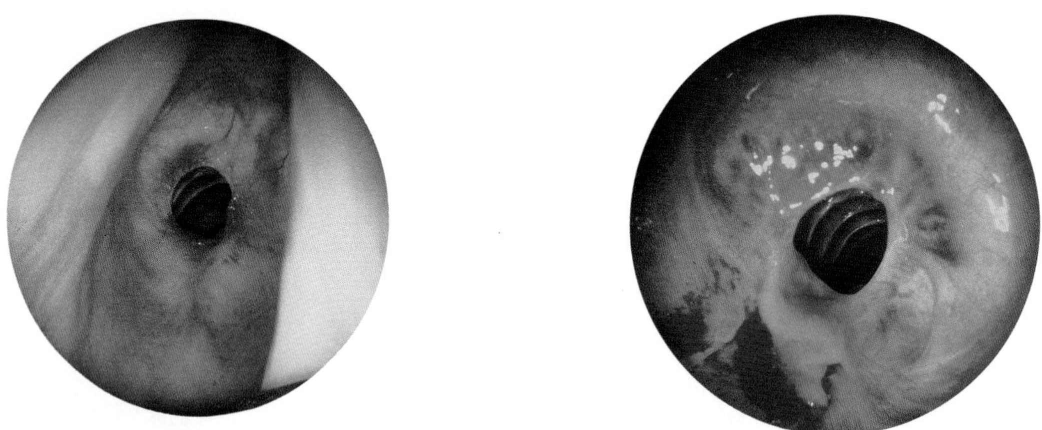

FIG. 201. Benign subglottic tracheal stenosis following endotracheal intubation **(left)**, and a close-up view of the lesion **(right)**.

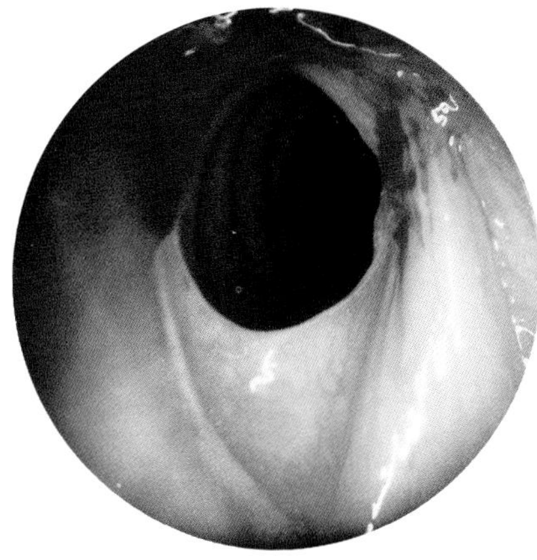

FIG. 202. Benign subglottic tracheal stenosis following endotracheal intubation. Note the thin, web-like stenosis.

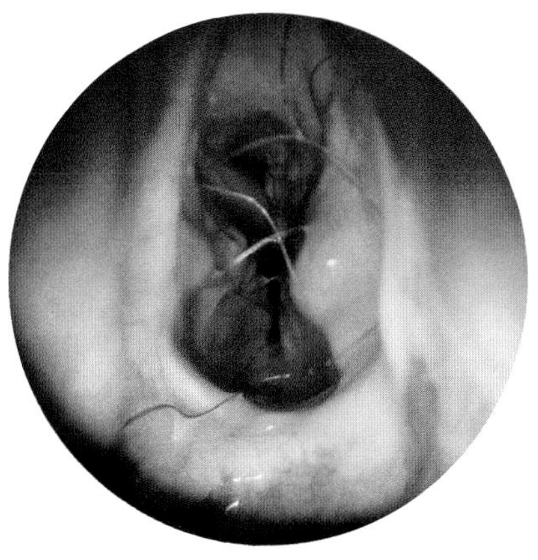

FIG. 203. Benign tracheal stenosis following tracheal trauma. Note intraluminal hair growth presumably caused by involution of skin into the tracheal lumen.

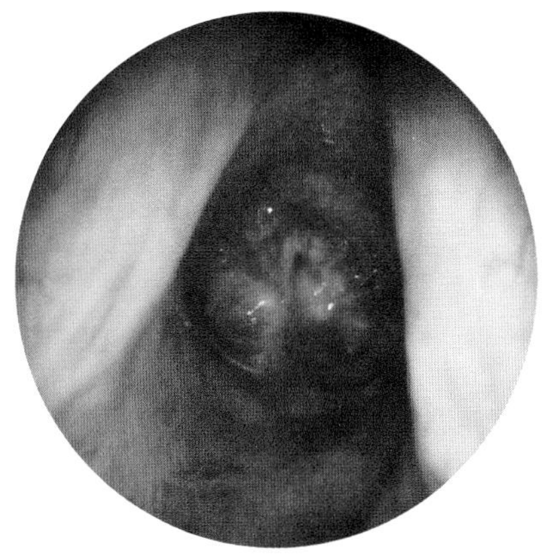

FIG. 204. Benign subglottic stenosis with complete obliteration of tracheal lumen in a patient with tracheostomy in place. Significant posttracheostomy tracheal stenosis occurs in 8% of patients (126).

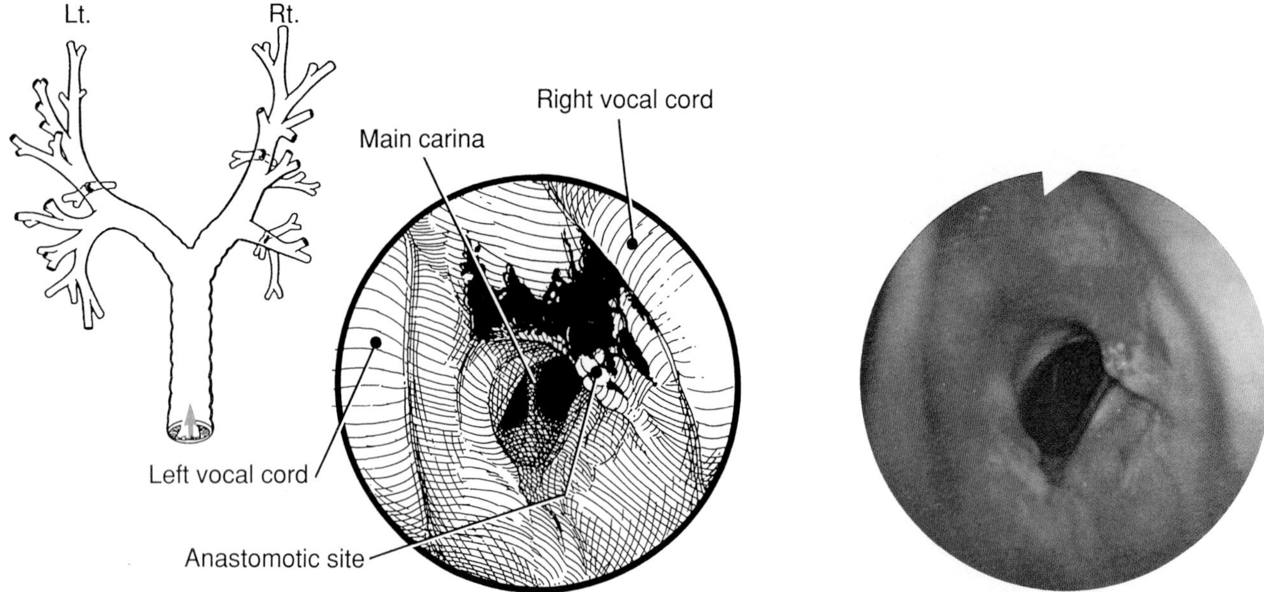

FIG. 205. Postanastomotic stricture of upper trachea in a patient who underwent tracheal resection and reanastomosis for treatment of benign stenosis.

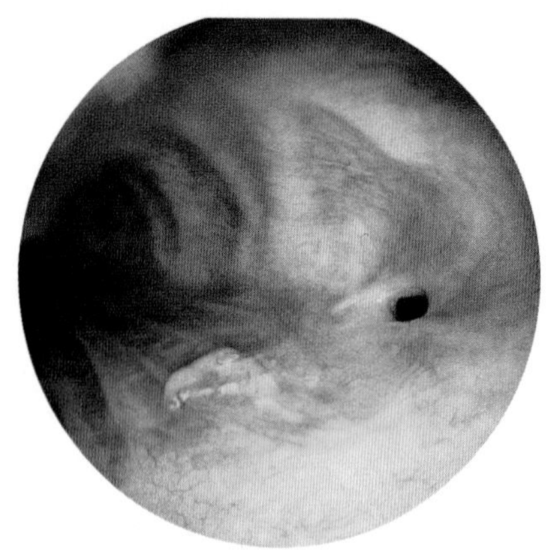

FIG. 206. Severe stenosis of right main bronchus secondary to tuberculosis.

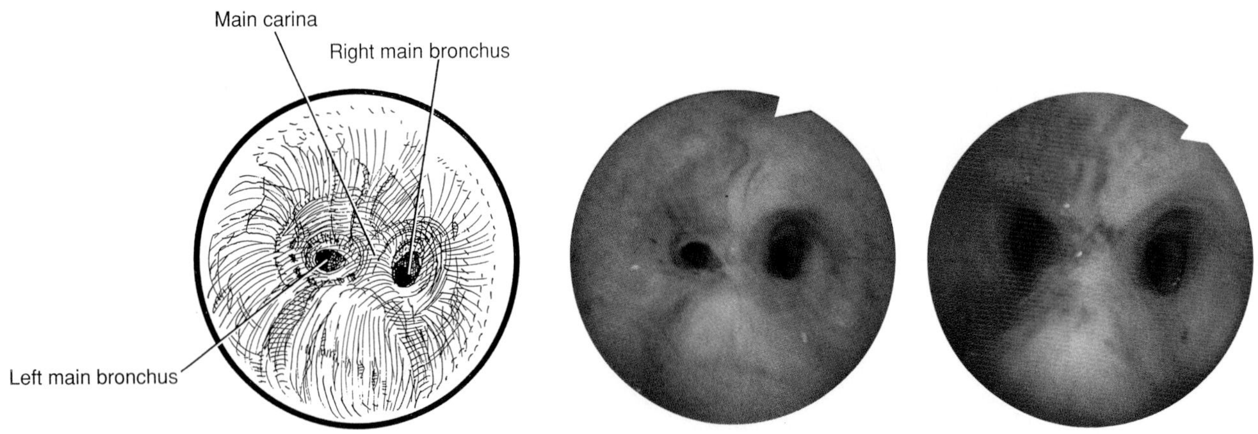

FIG. 207. Severe stenosis of left main bronchus and moderate stenosis of right main bronchus in a patient with mediastinal fibrosis before bronchoscopic balloon dilatation **(left)** and after **(right)**.

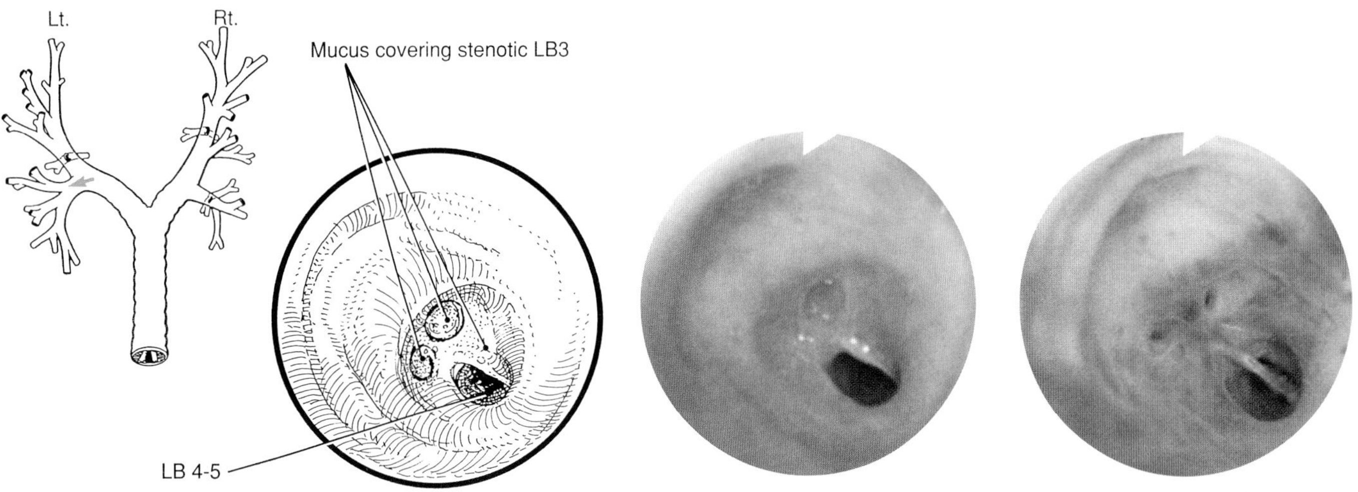

FIG. 208. Severe bronchial stenosis secondary to histoplasmosis. Before suctioning of mucus **(left)** and after bronchoscopic suction **(right)**.

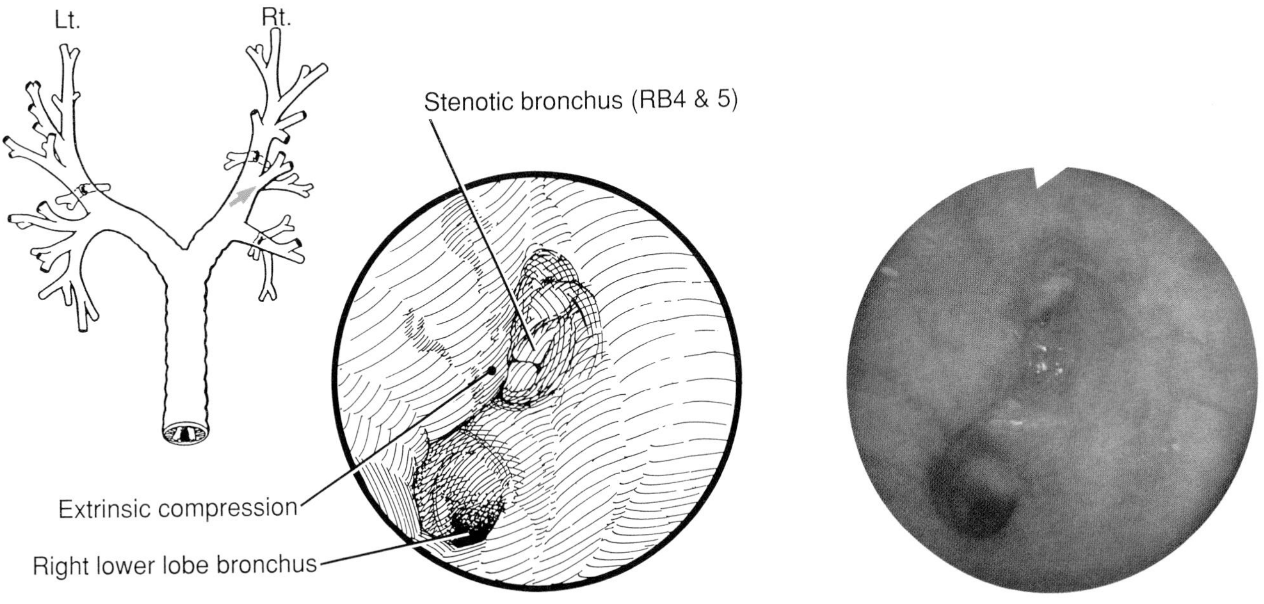

FIG. 209. Stenosis of right middle lobe bronchus caused by chronic atelectasis and peribronchial calcific lymphadenopathy secondary to tuberculosis. Clinically the patient had right middle lobe syndrome.

TRACHEOBRONCHOPATHIA OSTEOCHONDROPLASTICA (Figs. 210–213)

Also known by its shorter name, tracheopathia osteoplastica, this is a rare disease of obscure etiology characterized by cartilaginous or bony outgrowths into the lumen of the tracheobronchial tree. This disorder is neither the end result of nor in any way associated with amyloidosis. The nodular excrescences represent exostoses or ecchondroses from the cartilaginous trachea, which often ossifies. The posterior membranous trachea is always spared from the development of bony/cartilaginous ecchondroses. Histologically, the overlying mucosa is normal. The nodular changes are most pronounced in the trachea. Clinical manifestations include cough, wheeze, and occasional hemoptysis. Bronchoscopy is diagnostic (127–129).

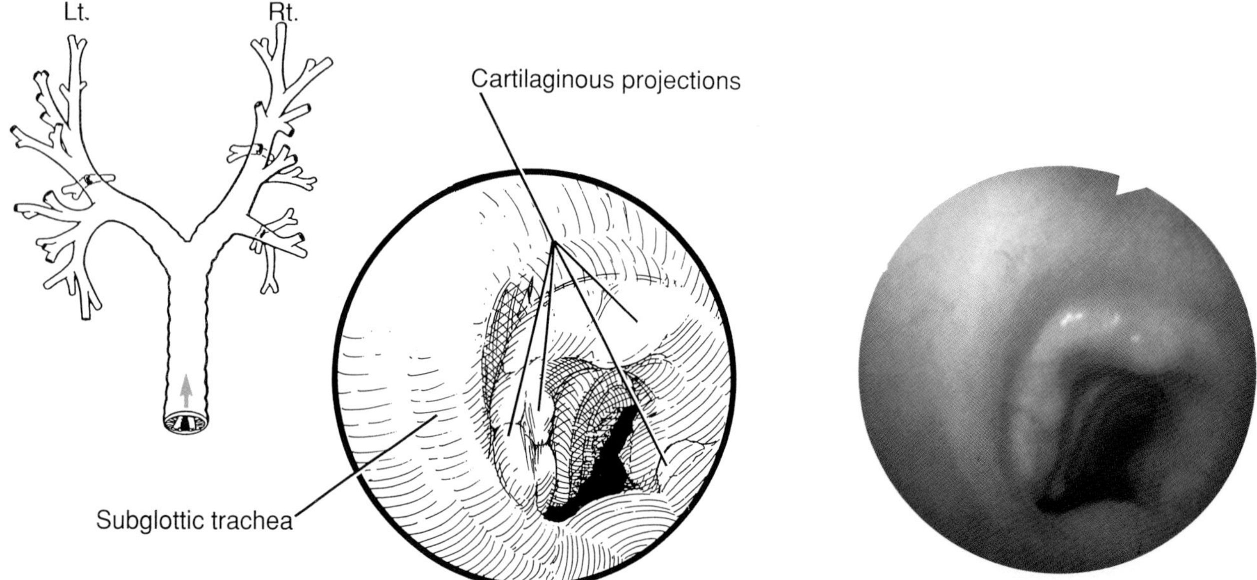

FIG. 210. Tracheopathia osteoplastica of upper tracheal cartilaginous rings. Tracheal luminal deformity and narrowing can be seen.

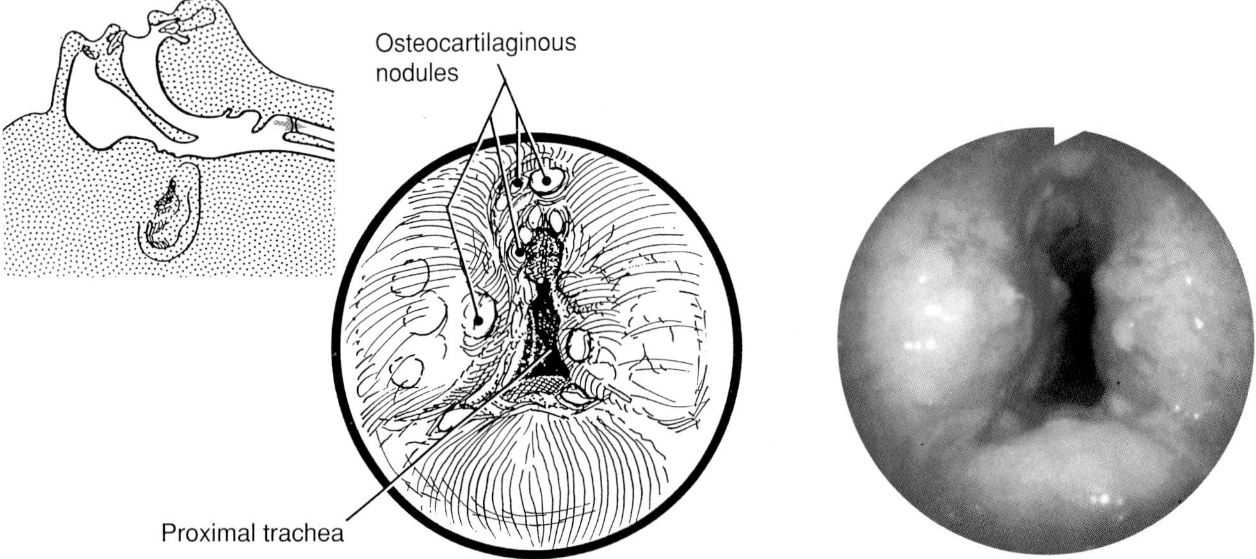

FIG. 211. Tracheopathia osteoplastica causing narrowing of the lateral dimensions of trachea. Multiple nodular excrescences can be seen.

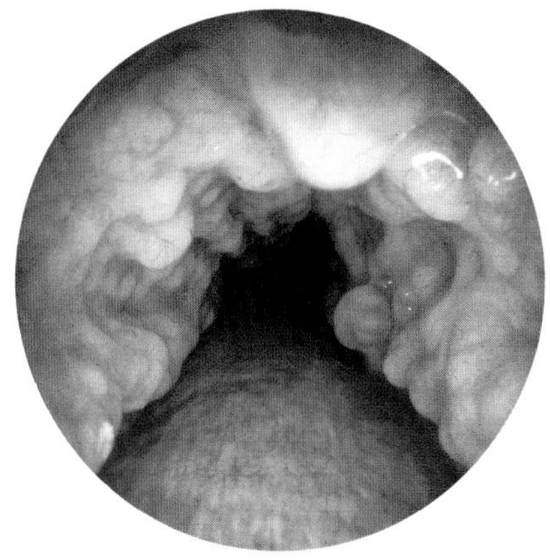

FIG. 212. Tracheopathia osteoplastica producing extensive involvement of the trachea. Sparing of posterior membranous portion is a characteristic finding.

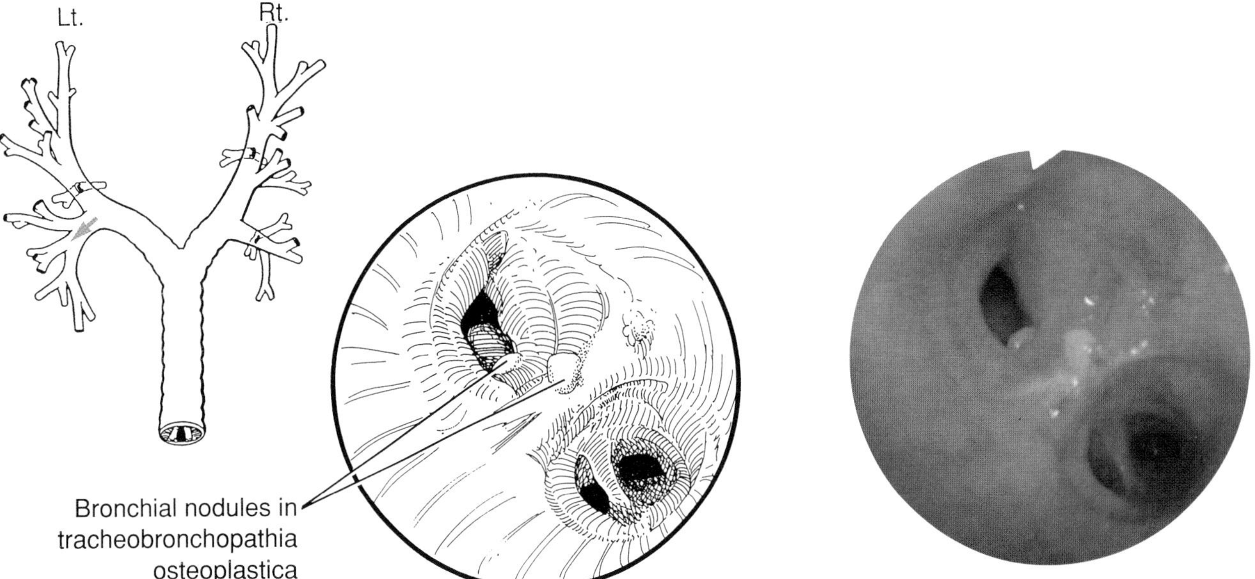

FIG. 213. Tracheopathia osteoplastica involving segmental bronchi. These nodules are generally difficult to biopsy with a flexible bronchoscopic forceps.

TRACHEOMEGALY (Figs. 214–215)

Tracheobronchomegaly is occasionally encountered during bronchoscopy for unrelated reasons. Pathological states associated with tracheobronchomegaly include Mounier–Kuhn syndrome, Ehlers–Danlos syndrome, cutis laxa, and acromegaly. However, many cases of asymptomatic tracheobronchomegaly are idiopathic in nature (130,131).

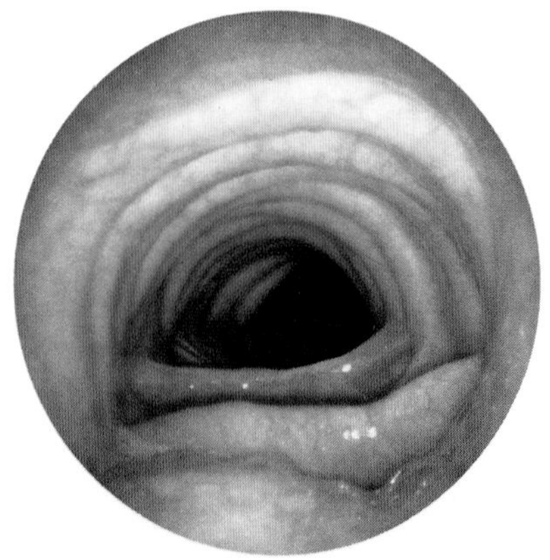

FIG. 214. Tracheomegaly. Note redundant mucosal folds in the posterior membranous portion.

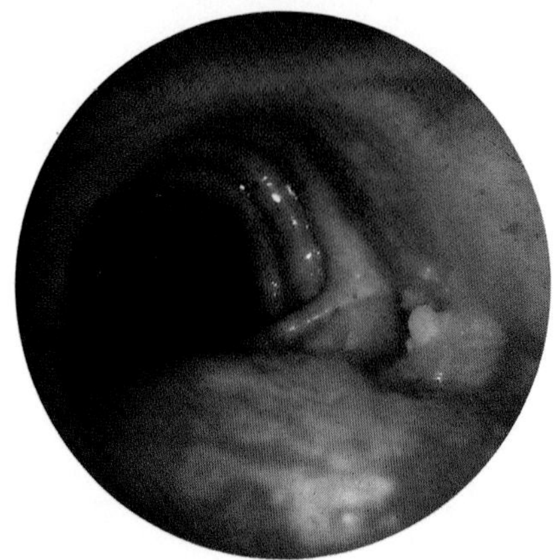

FIG. 215. Tracheomegaly. Diverticular changes can be seen.

VASCULAR LESIONS (Figs. 216–223)

Extrinsic compression of the tracheobronchial tree by major vascular anomalies was discussed above. Bronchoscopically visible vascular lesions are usually submucosal in location and are easily seen during bronchoscopy. The abnormalities include mucosal and submucosal varicosities, telangiectasia, and capillary proliferation caused by various diseases.

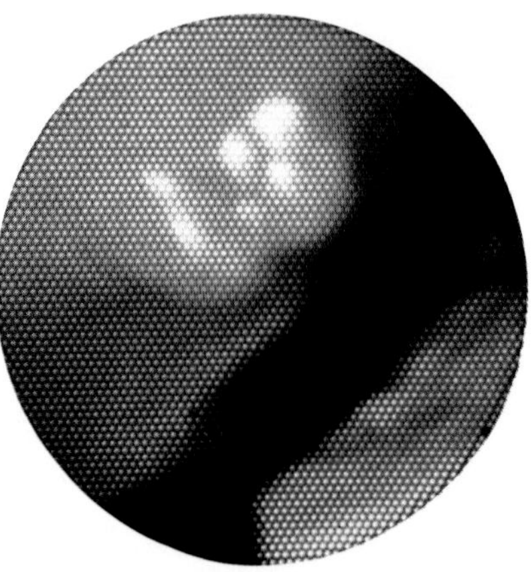

FIG. 216. Arteriovenous malformation of the nasal septum of a patient with hereditary hemorrhagic telangiectasia (Osler–Rendu–Weber syndrome). This lesion was treated with Nd:YAG laser therapy using a flexible bronchoscope (132). From ref. 12, with permission.

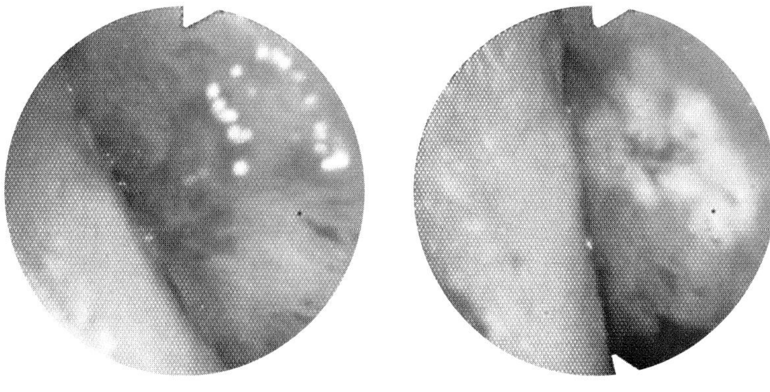

FIG. 217. Arteriovenous malformation of the bronchial mucosa in a patient with hereditary hemorrhagic telangiectasia (Osler–Rendu–Weber syndrome). Before laser therapy **(left)** and after laser coagulation **(right)**. Isolated bronchial telangiectasia has been described in patients with hereditary hemorrhagic telangiectasia (133,134). Courtesy of Atul C. Mehta, M.D.

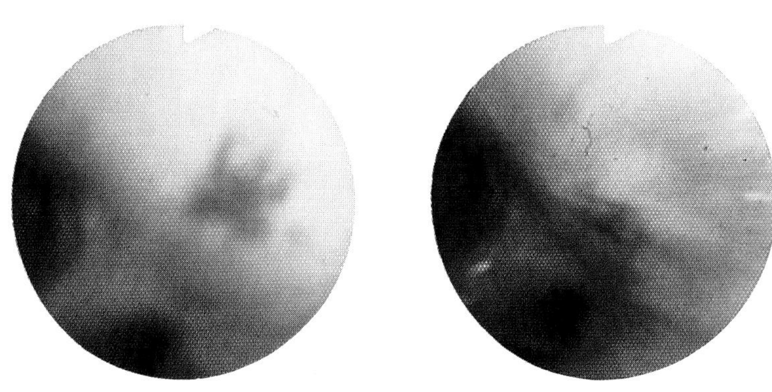

FIG. 218. Arteriovenous malformation of the bronchial mucosa in a patient with hereditary hemorrhagic telangiectasia (Osler–Rendu–Weber syndrome). Before laser therapy **(left)** and after laser coagulation **(right)**. Courtesy of Atul C. Mehta, M.D.

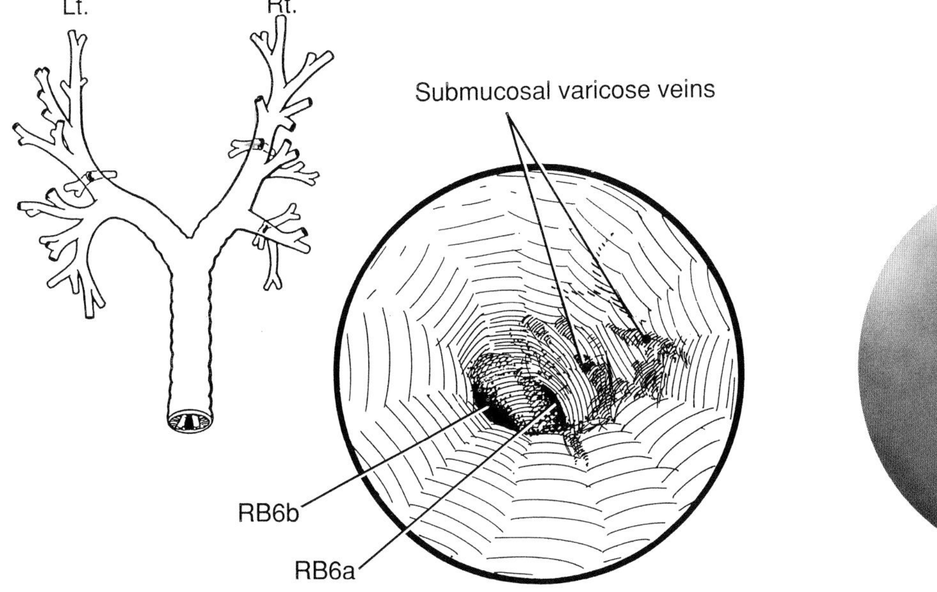

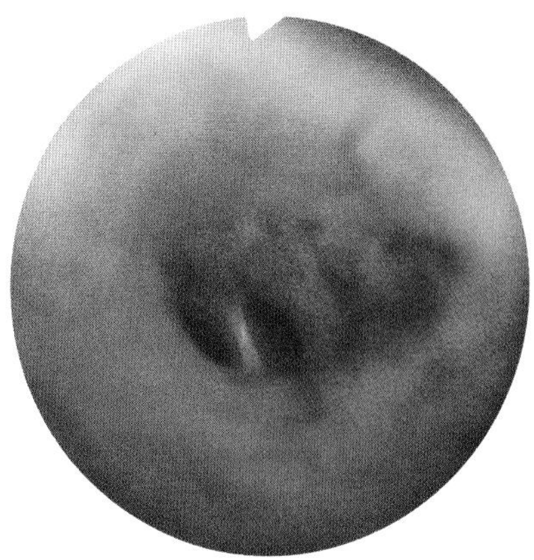

FIG. 219. Venous varicosities in the submucosa. This patient presented with recurrent hemoptysis. Flexible bronchoscopic needle injection of sclerosing agent (tetradecyl sulfate) produced sclerosis and hemoptysis subsided.

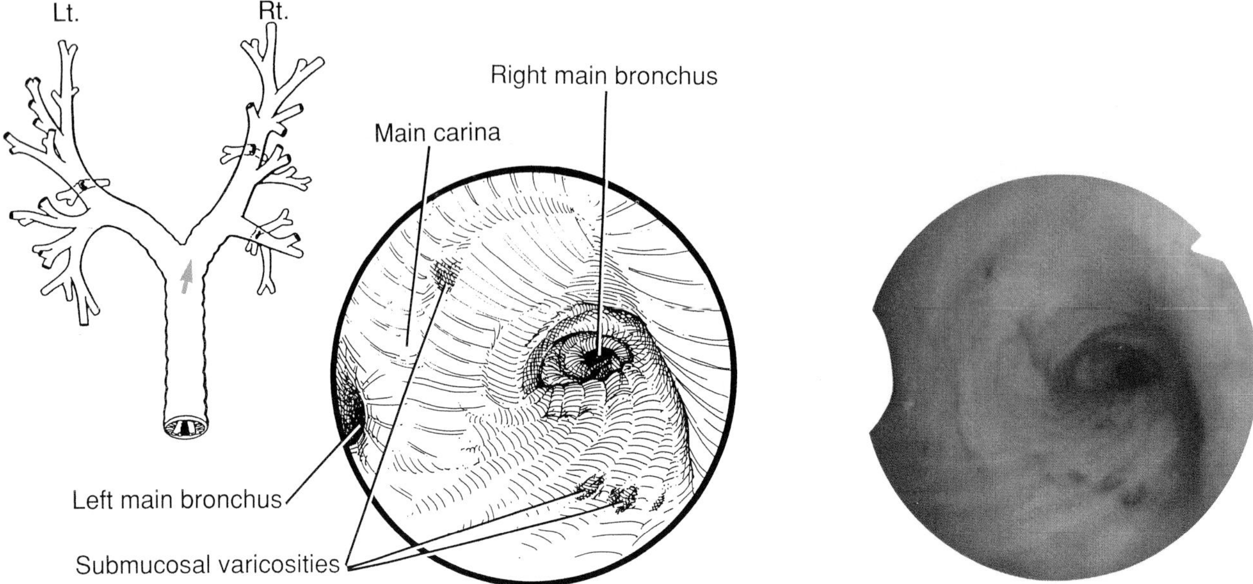

FIG. 220. Venous varicosities in the submucosa. Same patient as in Fig. 219. These mucosal changes were misdiagnosed as anthracotic pigment depositions. Submucosal varicosities and venous lakes are not uncommon in elderly patients. These lesions rarely produce clinical problems.

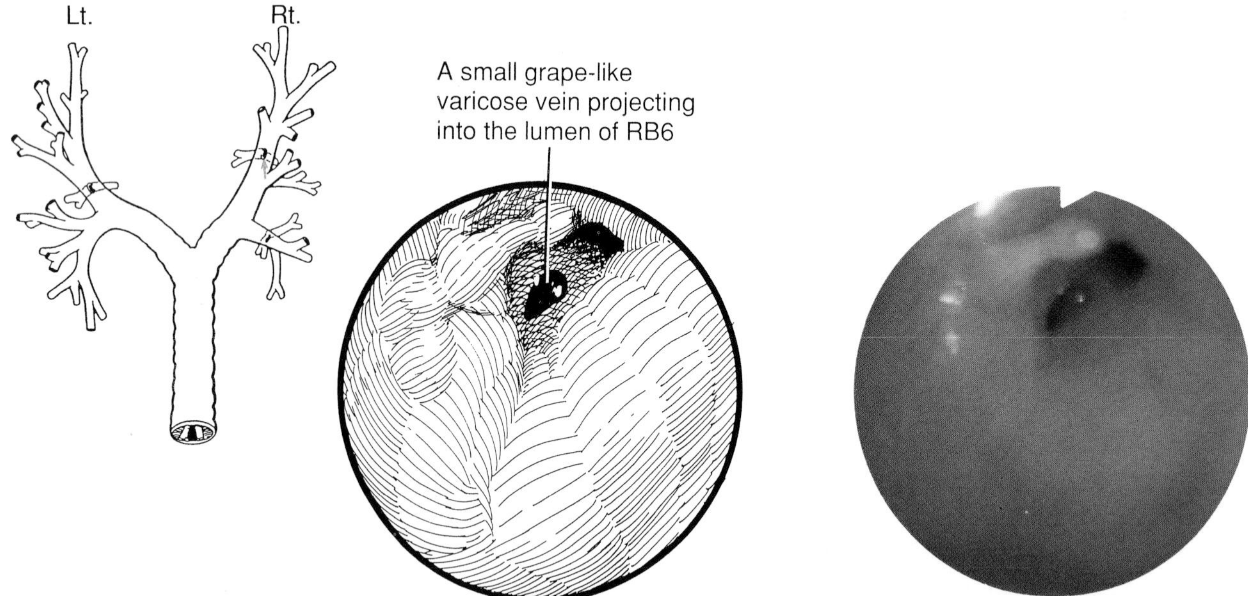

FIG. 221. Varicose vein bulging into the lumen of a bronchus. Same patient as in Fig. 219. This lesion was also treated with sclerosing agent.

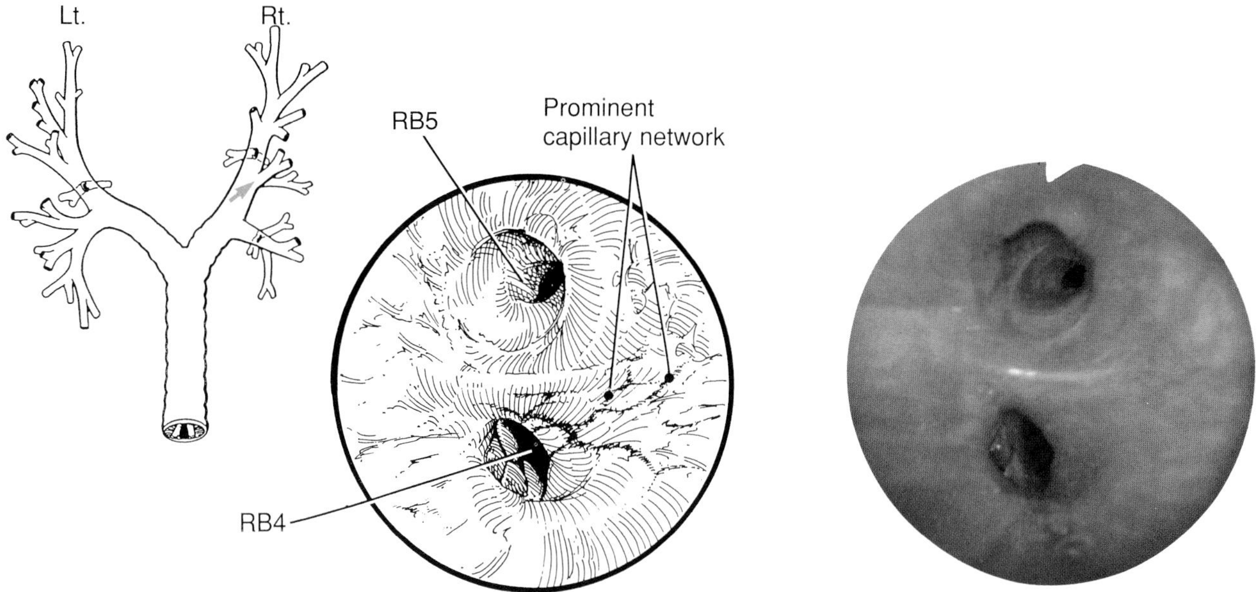

FIG. 222. Submucosal capillary proliferation in a patient with mitral stenosis and hemoptysis.

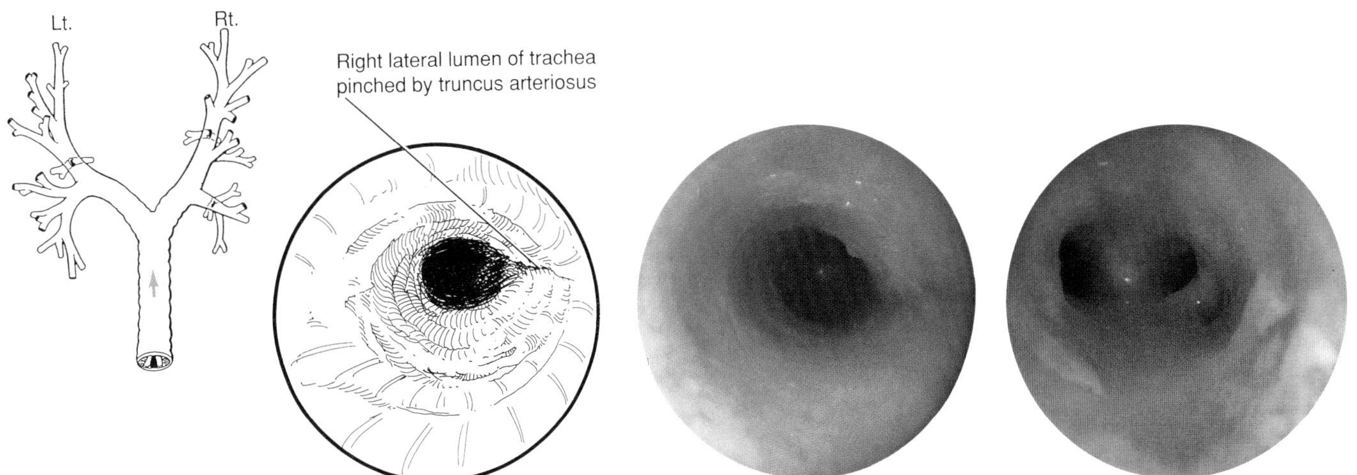

FIG. 223. Mucosal hyperemia and hemoptysis secondary to severe extrinsic compression of trachea by congenital aortic deformity. Before surgical correction of aortic abnormality **(left)** and after surgical correction **(right)**. An accessory tracheal bronchus was identified only after surgical correction of the aorta.

WEGENER'S GRANULOMATOSIS (Figs. 224–229)

Among the various respiratory vasculitides, Wegener's granulomatosis deserves special consideration in bronchoscopy for a number of reasons. First, hemoptysis is a common symptom in Wegener's granulomatosis and therefore many patients undergo bronchoscopy for the evaluation of this symptom. Second, tracheobronchial mucosal ulcerations and stenoses are not uncommon in this disorder (135–138). Third, bronchoscopy and bronchoalveolar lavage is frequently indicated in patients with Wegener's granulomatosis who are immunosuppressed and develop diffuse pulmonary infiltrates.

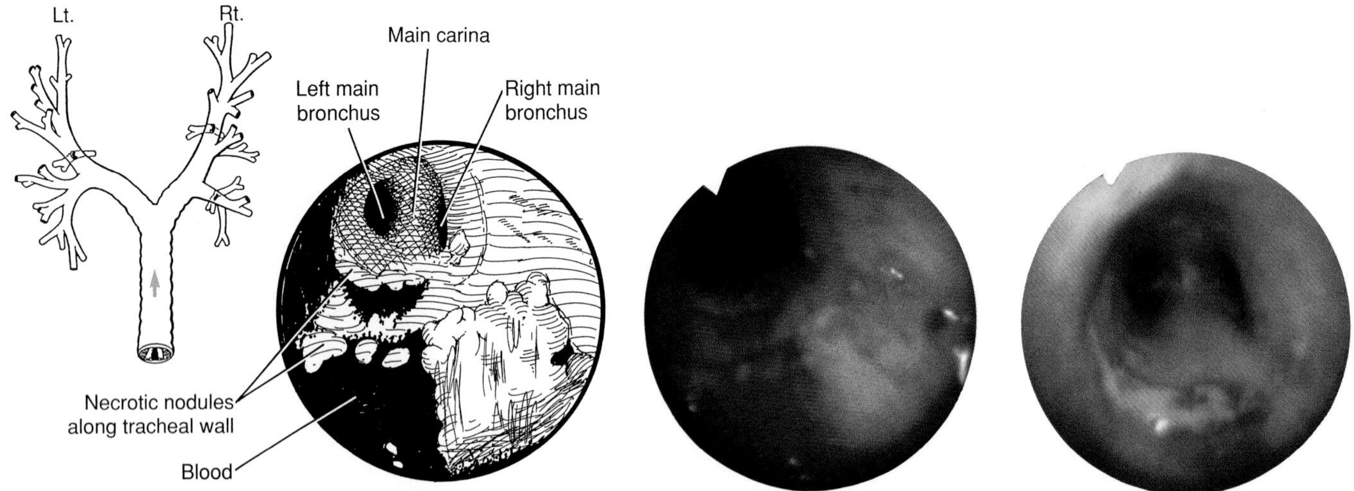

FIG. 224. Wegener's granulomatosis with tracheal mucosal ridges and ulcerations **(left)**, and a close-up view of the lesion **(right)**.

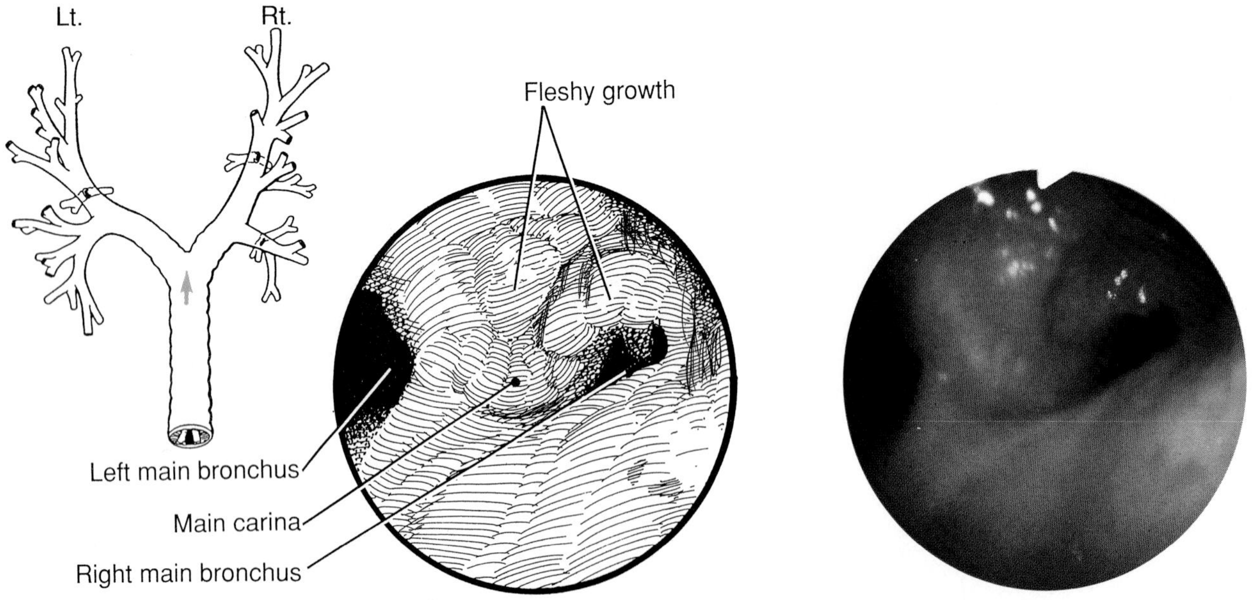

FIG. 225. Wegener's granulomatosis involving proximal right main bronchus. Biopsy revealed changes typical of Wegener's granulomatosis.

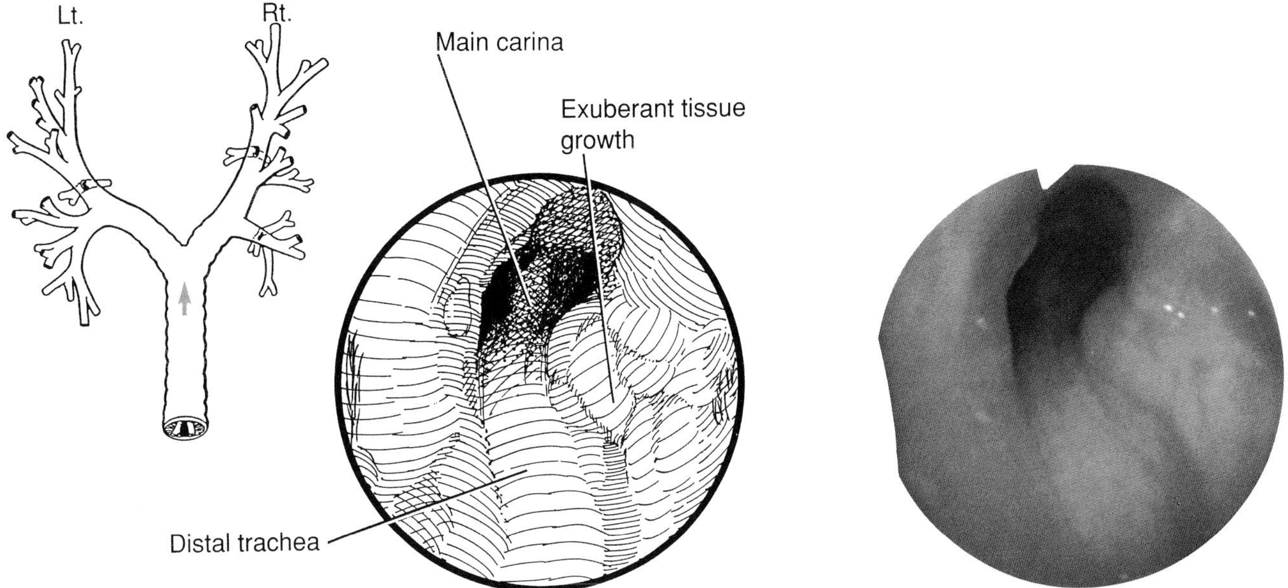

FIG. 226. Wegener's granulomatosis presenting with distal tracheal mass, hemoptysis, and respiratory distress. Despite appropriate medical therapy, the patient required tracheal stent for airway management. This is an unusual presentation of Wegener's granulomatosis.

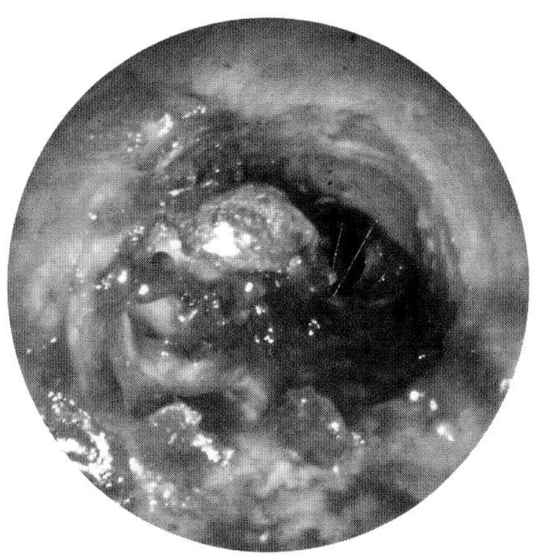

FIG. 227. Wegener's granulomatosis with extensive involvement of distal trachea and main bronchi.

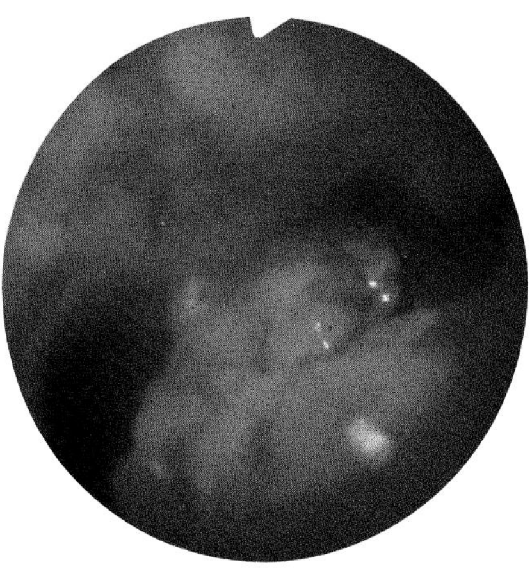

FIG. 228. Wegener's granulomatosis with pseudopolyp formation of RC-1.

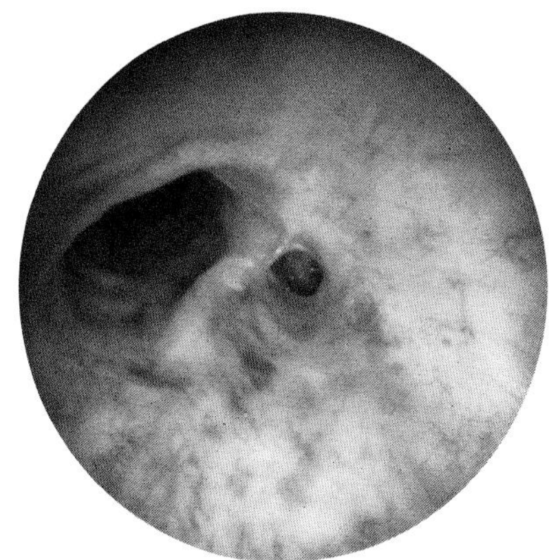

FIG. 229. Wegener's granulomatosis with stenosis of right main bronchus. Lobar atelectasis caused by endobronchial Wegener's granulomatosis has been described (135). Repeated bronchoscopic dilatations have been used to dilate chronic stenotic lesions (136).

MISCELLANEOUS (Figs. 230–235)

Mucosal and submucosal changes caused by nonmalignant lesions may be subtle or obvious. These abnormalities include edema, erythema, irregularity, or discolorations. Submucosal discoloration may be secondary to radiation-induced mucositis, deposition of anthracotic pigment, submucous venous varicosities or venous lakes, submucous capillary proliferation, or ochronosis. Occasionally, submucosal spread of metastatic melanoma may give rise to black discoloration of the airways. Physical and chemical trauma to tracheobronchial mucosa can produce acute or chronic changes.

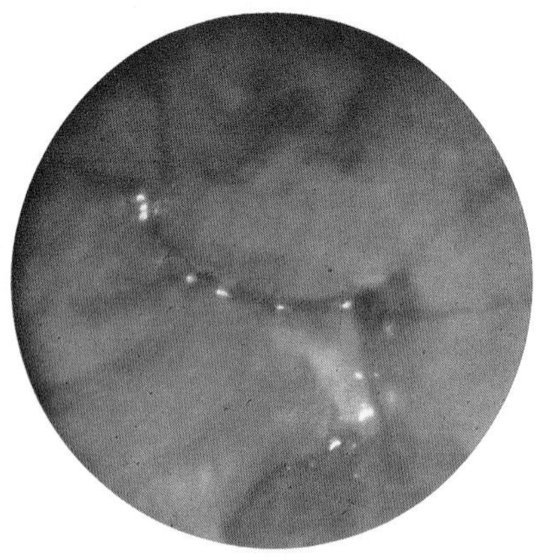

FIG. 230. Chemical burn of proximal trachea caused by ingestion and aspiration of a caustic (lye). Severe mucosal edema, hyperemia, and hemorrhage was eventually followed by tracheal stricture.

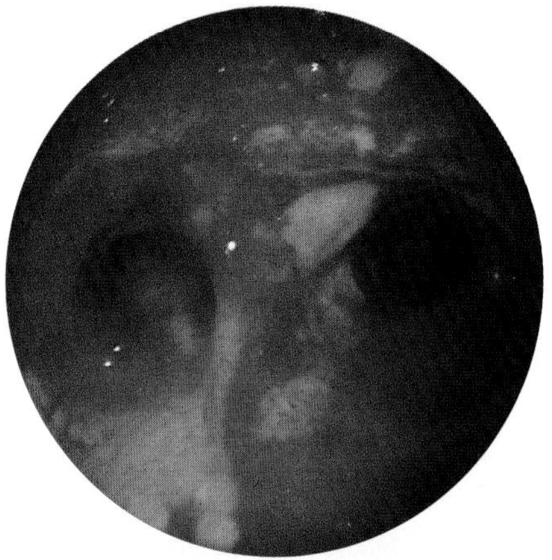

FIG. 231. Chronic hemorrhagic bronchitis caused by mustard gas inhalation. Chemical burns produce hemorrhagic bronchitis, bronchiectasis, and tracheobronchial strictures (139,140). Courtesy of Lutz Freitag, M.D.

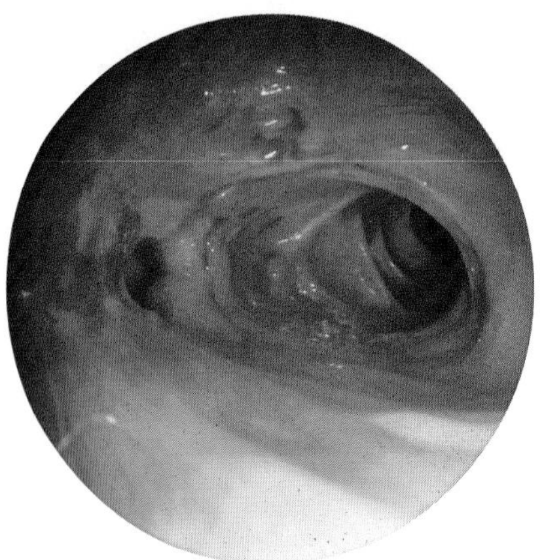

FIG. 232. Stenosis of left main bronchus caused by exposure to mustard gas inhalation. Courtesy of Lutz Freitag, M.D.

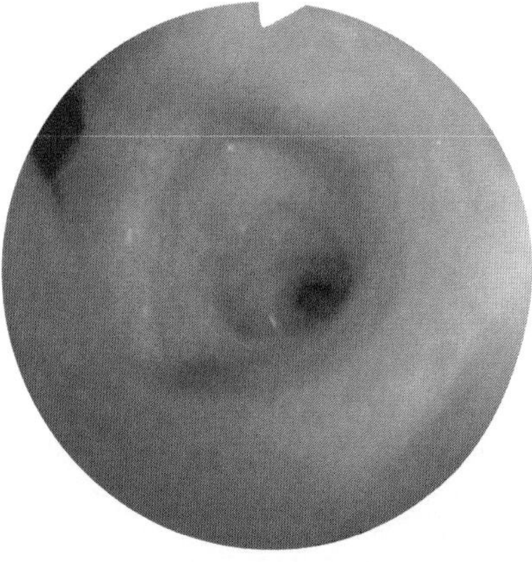

FIG. 233. Anthracotic pigment deposition in bronchial submucosa. It is a common finding and generally does not produce symptoms. Bronchoscopic appearance can be identical to that in submucosal varicosities.

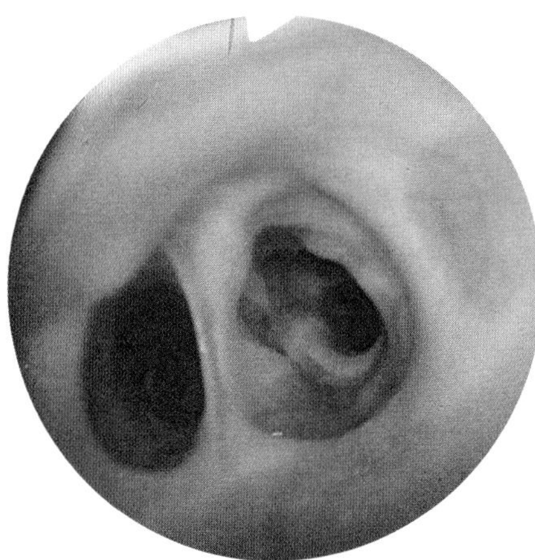

FIG. 234. Ochronosis with hyperpigmentation of tracheal cartilages.

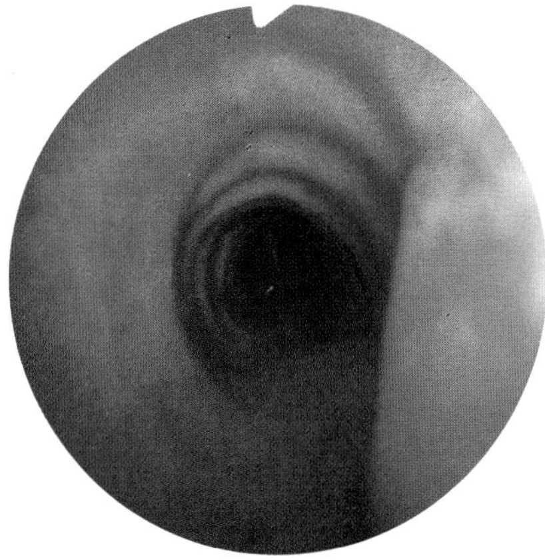

FIG. 235. Physical trauma to upper trachea caused by an automobile accident and complicated by tracheal submucosal hematoma formation. Bronchoscopy is an important tool in the diagnosis and management of physical trauma to the thoracic cage (141).

ACKNOWLEDGMENT

Figs. 33, 35, 54–56, 86, 116, 119, 125, 140, 177, and 187 are reproduced with permission from: Atlas of Therapeutic Bronchoscopy. Cavaliere S and Beamis JF, eds. Tipolitografia F. Apollonio and Co, Brescia, Italy, 1991.

REFERENCES

1. Cordier JF, Loire R, Brune J. Amyloidosis of the lower respiratory tract. Clinical and pathologic features in a series of 21 patients. *Chest* 1986;90:827.
2. Chen KT. Amyloidosis presenting in the respiratory tract. *Pathol Annu* 1989;73:1989.
3. Russchen GH, Wouters B, Meinesz AF, Janssen S, Postmus PE. Amyloid tumour resected by laser therapy. *Eur Resp J* 1990;3:932.
4. Fukumura M, Mieno T, Suzuki T, Murata Y. Primary diffuse tracheobronchial amyloidosis treated by bronchoscopic Nd YAG laser irradiation. *J Med* 1990;29:620.
5. Hoskins MC, Evans RA, King SJ, Gishen P. "Sabre sheath" trachea with mediastinal lipomatosis mimicking a mediastinal tumour. *Clin Radiol* 1991;44:417.
6. Callan E, Karandy EJ, Hilsinger RL Jr. "Saber-sheath" trachea. *Ann Otol Rhinol Laryngol* 1988;97:512.
7. Barat M, Konrad HR. Tracheal bronchus. *Am J Otolaryngol* 1987;8:118.
8. Jackson GD, Littleton JT. Simultaneous occurrence of anomalous cardiac and tracheal bronchi: a case study. *J Thorac Imaging* 1988;3:59.
9. Pounder DJ, Pieterse AS. Tracheopathia osteoplastica: a study of the minimal lesion. *J Pathol* 1982;138:235.
10. Stradling P, Stradling JR. *Diagnostic bronchoscopy. A teaching manual.* Edinburgh: Churchill Livingstone; 1991:75.
11. Anderson WM. Mucoid impaction of upper lobe bronchi in the absence of proximal bronchiectasis. *Chest* 1990;98:1023.
12. Cairns-Bazarian AM, Conway EE Jr, Yankelowitz S. Plastic bronchitis: an unusual cause of respiratory distress in children. *Pediatr Emerg Care* 1992;8:335.
13. Jett JR, Tazelaar HD, Keim LW, Ingrassia TS III. Plastic bronchitis: an old disease revisited. *Mayo Clin Proc* 1991;66:305.
14. Muller W, von-der-Hardt H, Rieger CH. Idiopathic and symptomatic plastic bronchitis in childhood. A report of three cases and review of the literature. *Respiration* 1987;52:214.
15. Trastek VF, Pairolero PC, Ceithaml EL, Piehler JM, Payne WS, Bernatz PE. Surgical management of broncholithiasis. *J Thorac Cardiovasc Surg* 1985;90:842.
16. Cole FH, Cole FH Jr, Khandekar A, Watson DC. Management of broncholithiasis: is thoracotomy necessary? *Ann Thorac Surg* 1986;42:255.
17. Friese KK, Dulce MC, Higgins CB. Airway obstruction by right aortic arch with right-sided patent ductus arteriosus: demonstration by MRI. *J Comput Assist Tomogr* 1992;16:888.
18. Bose S, Hurst TS, Cockcroft DW. Right-sided aortic arch presenting as refractory intraoperative and postoperative wheezing. *Chest* 1991;99:1308.
19. Gikonyo BM, Jue KL, Edwards JE. Pulmonary vascular sling: report of seven cases and review of the literature. *Pediatr Cardiol* 1989;10:81.
20. Fesmire FM, Pesce RR. Tracheal obstruction presenting as new-onset wheezing. *Am J Emerg Med* 1989;7:173.
21. Yamaguchi M, Ohashi H, Hosokawa Y, Oshima Y, Tsugawa C, Kimura K. Surgical treatment of airway obstruction associated with congenital heart disease in infants and small children. *Eur J Cardiothorac Surg* 1991;5:479.
22. Horvath P, Hucin B, Hruda J, et al. Intermediate to late results of surgical relief of vascular tracheobronchial compression. *Eur J Cardiothorac Surg* 1992;6:366.
23. Hawkins JA, Bailey WW, Clark SM. Innominate artery compression of the trachea. Treatment by reimplantation of the innominate artery. *J Thorac Cardiovasc Surg* 1992;103:678.
24. Schuster T, Hecker WC, Ring-Mrozik E, Mantel K, Vogl T. Tracheal stenosis by innominate artery compression in infants: surgical treatment in 35 cases. *Prog Pediatr Surg* 1991;27:231.
25. Filston HC, Ferguson TB Jr, Oldham HN. Airway obstruction by vascular anomalies. Importance of telescopic bronchoscopy. *Ann Surg* 1987;205:541.
26. Prakash UBS, Abel MD, Hubmayr RD. Mediastinal mass and tracheal obstruction during general anesthesia. *Mayo Clin Proc* 1988;63:1004.
27. Sairanen H, Leijala M, Louhimo I. Primary mediastinal tumors in children. *Eur J Cardiothorac Surg* 1987;1:148.
28. Mogilner JG, Fonseca J, Davies MR. Life-threatening respiratory distress caused by a mediastinal teratoma in a newborn. *J Pediatr Surg* 1992;27:1519.
29. Azoulay D, Regnard JF, Magdeleinat P, Diamond T, Rojas-Miranda A, Levasseur P. Congenital respiratory-esophageal fistula in the adult. Report of nine cases and review of the literature. *J Thorac Cardiovasc Surg* 1992;104:381.
30. Schmittenbecher PP, Mantel K, Hofmann U, Berlien HP. Treatment of congenital tracheoesophageal fistula by endoscopic laser coagulation: preliminary report of three cases. *J Pediatr Surg* 1992;27:26.
31. Antonelli M, Cicconetti F, Vivino G, Gasparetto A. Closure of a tracheoesophageal fistula by bronchoscopic application of fibrin glue and decontamination of the oral cavity. *Chest* 1991; 100:578.
32. Nicholas JM, Dulchavsky SA. Successful use of autologous fibrin gel in traumatic bronchopleural fistula: case report. *J Trauma* 1992;32:87.
33. York EL, Lewall DB, Hirji M, Gelfand ET, Modry DL. Endo-

scopic diagnosis and treatment of postoperative bronchopleural fistula. *Chest* 1990;97:1390.
34. Borro JM, Ramos F, Vicente R, Sanchis F, Morales P, Caffarena JM. Bronchial fistula to the mediastinum in a heart-lung transplant patient. *Eur J Cardiothorac Surg* 1992;6:674.
35. Limper AH, Prakash UBS. Tracheobronchial foreign bodies in adults. *Ann Intern Med* 1990;112:604.
36. Cordasco EM Jr, Mehta AC, Ahmad M. Bronchoscopically induced bleeding. A summary of nine years' Cleveland clinic experience and review of the literature. *Chest* 1991;100:1141.
37. Shure D. Endobronchial suture. A foreign body causing chronic cough. *Chest* 1991;100:1193.
38. Keller C, Frost A. Fiberoptic bronchoplasty. Description of a simple adjunct technique for the management of bronchial stenosis following lung transplantation. *Chest* 1992;102:995.
39. Colt HG, Janssen JP, Dumon JF, Noirclerc MJ. Endoscopic management of bronchial stenosis after double lung transplantation. *Chest* 1992;102:10.
40. Ono R, Ikeda S, Suemasu K. Hematoporphyrin derivative photodynamic therapy in roentgenographically occult carcinoma of the tracheobronchial tree. *Cancer* 1992;69:1696.
41. McCaughan JS Jr, Hawley PC, Brown DG, Kakos GS, Williams TE Jr. Effect of light dose on the photodynamic destruction of endobronchial tumors. *Ann Thorac Surg* 1992;54:705.
42. Miller KL, Harrell JH II. Obstructing endobronchial bands complicating radiation therapy for lung carcinoma. *Chest* 1992; 101:1714.
43. Takayama S, Miura H, Kimula Y. A case of "bronchial string"—a rare anomaly of the bronchus. *Respiration* 1991; 58:115.
44. Cunningham MJ. The old and new of acute laryngotracheal infections. *Clin Pediatr* 1992;31:56.
45. St-John RC, Pacht ER. Tracheal stenosis and failure to wean from mechanical ventilation due to herpetic tracheitis. *Chest* 1990;98:1520.
46. Sherry MK, Klainer AS, Wolff M, Gerhard H. Herpetic tracheobronchitis. *Ann Intern Med* 1988;109:229.
47. Harris JB, Lusk R, Wagener JS, Andersen RD. Acute viral laryngotracheitis complicated by herpes simplex virus infection. *Otolaryngol Head Neck Surg* 1987;96:190.
48. Kasian GF, Bingham WT, Steinberg J, et al. Bacterial tracheitis in children. *Can Med Assoc J* 1989;140:46.
49. Kurasawa T, Kuze F, Kawai M, et al. Diagnosis and management of endobronchial tuberculosis. *Intern Med* 1992;31:593.
50. Nakamura K, Terada N, Ohi M, Matsushita T, Kato N, Nakagawa T. Tuberculous bronchial stenosis: treatment with balloon bronchoplasty. *Am J Roentgenol* 1991;157:1187.
51. Van-den-Brande P, Lambrechts M, Tack J, Demedts M. Endobronchial tuberculosis mimicking lung cancer in elderly patients. *Resp Med* 1991;85:107.
52. Choe KO, Jeong HJ, Sohn HY. Tuberculous bronchial stenosis: CT findings in 28 cases. *Am J Roentgenol* 1990;155:971.
53. Wasser LS, Shaw GW, Talavera W. Endobronchial tuberculosis in the acquired immunodeficiency syndrome. *Chest* 1988; 94:1240.
54. Maguire GP, Delorenzo LJ, Brown RB, Davidian MM. Endobronchial tuberculosis simulating bronchogenic carcinoma in a patient with the acquired immunodeficiency syndrome. *Am J Med Sci* 1987;294:42.
55. Mehle ME, Adamo JP, Mehta AC, Wiedemann HP, Keys T, Longworth DL. Endobronchial *Mycobacterium avium-intracellulare* infection in a patient with AIDS. *Chest* 1989;96:199.
56. Mathisen DJ, Grillo HC. Clinical manifestation of mediastinal fibrosis and histoplasmosis. *Ann Thorac Surg* 1992;54:1053.
57. Prechter GC, Prakash UBS. Bronchoscopy in the diagnosis of pulmonary histoplasmosis. *Chest* 1989;95:1033.
58. Hall J, Heimann P, Costas C. Airway obstruction caused by *Aspergillus* tracheobronchitis in an immunocompromised patient. *Crit Care Med* 1990;18:575.
59. Berlinger NT, Freeman TJ. Acute airway obstruction due to necrotizing tracheobronchial aspergillosis in immunocompromised patients: a new clinical entity. *Ann Otol Rhinol Laryngol* 1989;98:718.
60. Pervez NK, Kleinerman J, Kattan M, et al. Pseudomembranous necrotizing bronchial aspergillosis. A variant of invasive aspergillosis in a patient with hemophilia and acquired immune deficiency syndrome. *Am Rev Resp Dis* 1985;131: 961.
61. Edmonds LC, Prakash UBS. Lymphoma, neutropenia, and wheezing in a 70-year-old man. *Chest* 1993;103:585.
62. Spear RK, Walker PD, Lampton LM. Tracheal obstruction associated with a fungus ball. A case of primary tracheal candidiasis. *Chest* 1976;70:662.
63. al-Majed S, al-Kassimi F, Ashour M, Mekki MO, Sadiq S. Removal of endobronchial mucormycosis lesion through a rigid bronchoscope. *Thorax* 1992;47:203.
64. Brown RB, Johnson JH, Kessinger JM, Sealy WC. Bronchovascular mucormycosis in the diabetic: an urgent surgical problem. *Ann Thorac Surg* 1992;53:854.
65. Watts WJ. Bronchopleural fistula followed by massive fatal hemoptysis in a patient with pulmonary mucormycosis. A case report. *Arch Intern Med* 1983;143:1029.
66. Hansen LA, Prakash UBS, Colby TV. Pulmonary complications in diabetes mellitus. *Mayo Clin Proc* 1989;64:791–9.
67. Edmonds LC, Stubbs SE, Ryu JH. Syphilis: a disease to exclude in diagnosing sarcoidosis. *Mayo Clin Proc* 1992;67:37.
68. Kawaida M, Kohno N, Kawasaki Y, Fukuda H. Surgical treatment of large epiglottic cysts with a side-opened direct laryngoscope and snare. *Auris Nasus Larynx* 1992;19:45.
69. Ramesar K, Albizzati C. Laryngeal cysts: clinical relevance of a modified working classification. *J Laryngol Otol* 1988; 102:923.
70. Brin MF, Fahn S, Moskowitz C, et al. Localized injections of botulinum toxin for the treatment of focal dystonia and hemifacial spasm. *Mov Disord* 1987;2:237.
71. Dedo HH, Behlau MS. Recurrent laryngeal nerve section for spastic dysphonia: 5- to 14-year preliminary results in the first 300 patients. *Ann Otol Rhinol Laryngol* 1991;100:274.
72. Blitzer A, Brin MF. Laryngeal dystonia: a series with botulinum toxin therapy. *Ann Otol Rhinol Laryngol* 1991;100:85.
73. Cordier JF, Chailleux E, Lauque D, et al. Primary pulmonary lymphomas. A clinical study of 70 cases in nonimmunocompromised patients. *Chest* 1993;103:201.
74. Ieki R, Goto H, Kouzai Y, et al. Endobronchial non-Hodgkin's lymphoma. *Resp Med* 1989;83:87.
75. Kavuru MS, Mehta AC, Eliachar I. Effect of photodynamic therapy and external beam radiation therapy on juvenile laryngotracheobronchial papillomatosis. *Am Rev Resp Dis* 1990; 141:509.
76. Hunt JM, Pierce RJ. Tracheal papillomatosis treated with Nd-Yag laser resection. *Aust N Z J Med* 1988;18:781.
77. Douzinas M, Sheppard MN, Lennox SC. Leiomyoma of the trachea—an unusual tumour. *Thorac Cardiovasc Surg* 1989; 37:285.
78. Yamada H, Katoh O, Yamaguchi T, Natsuaki M, Itoh T. Intrabronchial leiomyoma treated by localized resection via bronchotomy and bronchoplasty. *Chest* 1987;91:283.
79. Bouros D, Gazis A, Blatsios V, Melissinos C. Leiomyoma of the trachea. *Eur J Resp Dis* 1987;71:206.
80. Uyama T, Monden Y, Harada K, Sumitomo M, Kimura S. Pulmonary leiomyomatosis showing endobronchial extension and giant cyst formation. *Chest* 1988;94:644.
81. Lossos IS, Breuer R, Lafair JS. Endotracheal neurofibroma in a patient with von Recklinghausen's disease. *Eur Resp J* 1988; 1:464.
82. Neis PR, McMahon MF, Norris CW. Cartilaginous tumors of the trachea and larynx. *Ann Otol Rhinol Laryngol* 1989;98:31.
83. Robin J, Wilson AC. Polypoid neurilemmoma of the trachea: an unusual cause of major airway obstruction. *Aust N Z J Surg* 1988;58:912.
84. Frank JL, Schwartz BR, Price LM, Neifeld JP. Benign cartilaginous tumours of the upper airway. *J Surg Oncol* 1991;48:69.
85. Hurt R. Benign tumours of the bronchus and trachea, 1951–1981. *Ann R Coll Surg Engl* 1984;66:22.
86. Chen TF, Braidley PC, Shneerson JM, Wells FC. Obstructing tracheal lipoma: management of a rare tumor. *Ann Thorac Surg* 1990;49:137.
87. Grillo HC, Mathisen DJ, Wain JC. Management of tumors of the trachea. *Oncology* 1992;6:61.
88. Harpole DH Jr, Feldman JM, Buchanan S, Young WG, Wolfe WG. Bronchial carcinoid tumors: a retrospective analysis of 126 patients. *Ann Thorac Surg* 1992;54:50.

89. Toledo J, Roca R, Anton JA, Martin-de-Nicolas JL, Varela G, Yuste P. Conservative and bronchoplastic resection for bronchial carcinoid tumours. *Eur J Cardiothorac Surg* 1989;3: 288.
90. Satomi F, Mori H, Ogasawara H, Kumoi T, Uematsu K. Subglottic plasma cell granuloma: report of a case. *Auris Nasus Larynx* 1991;18:391.
91. Barker AP, Carter MJ, Matz LR, Armstrong JA. Plasma-cell granuloma of the trachea. *Med J Aust* 1987;146:443.
92. Muthuswamy PP, Alrenga DP, Marks P, Barker WL. Granular cell myoblastoma: rare localization in the trachea. Report of a case and review of the literature. *Am J Med* 1986;80:714.
93. Cunningham L, Wendell G, Berkowitz L, Schulman ES, Promisloff R. Treatment of tracheobronchial granular cell myoblastomas with endoscopic bipolar cautery. *Chest* 1989; 96:427.
94. Garcia-Prats MD, Sotelo-Rodriguez MT, Ballestin C, Martinez-Gonzalez MA, Roca R, Alfaro J, De-Miguel E. Glomus tumour of the trachea: report of a case with microscopic, ultrastructural and immunohistochemical examination and review of the literature. *Histopathology* 1991;19:459.
95. Shin DH, Park SS, Lee JH, Park MH, Lee JD. Oncocytic glomus tumor of the trachea. *Chest* 1990;98:1021.
96. Shapshay SM, Strong MS. Tracheobronchial obstruction from metastatic distant malignancies. *Ann Otol Rhinol Laryngol* 1982;91:648.
97. Rovirosa-Casino A, Bellmunt J, Salud A, et al. Endobronchial metastases in colorectal adenocarcinoma. *Tumori* 1992;78:270.
98. Poe RH, Ortiz C, Israel RH, et al. Sensitivity, specificity, and predictive values of bronchoscopy in neoplasm metastatic to lung. *Chest* 1985;88:84.
99. Ettensohn DB, Bennett JM, Hyde RW. Endobronchial metastases from carcinoma of the breast. *Med Pediatr Oncol* 1985; 13:9.
100. Kreisman H, Wolkove N, Finkelstein HS, Cohen C, Margolese R, Frank H. Breast cancer and thoracic metastases: review of 119 patients. *Thorax* 1983;38:175.
101. Albertini RE, Ekberg NL. Endobronchial metastasis in breast cancer. *Thorax* 1980;35:435.
102. Carlin BW, Harrell JH II, Olson LK, Moser KM. Endobronchial metastases due to colorectal carcinoma. *Chest* 1989; 96:1110.
103. Mitchell DM, McCarty M, Fleming J, Moss FM. Bronchopulmonary Kaposi's sarcoma in patients with AIDS. *Thorax* 1992; 47:726.
104. Nathan S, Vaghaiwalla R, Mohsenifar Z. Use of Nd:YAG laser in endobronchial Kaposi's sarcoma. *Chest* 1990;98:1299.
105. Chanez P, Mourad G, Aubas P, et al. Kaposi's sarcoma of the bronchial tree in a renal transplant recipient. *Respiration* 1988; 53:259.
106. Mateo F, Serur E, Smith PR. Bronchial metastases from ovarian carcinoma. Report of a case and review of the literature. *Gynecol Oncol* 1992;46:235.
107. Lee DW, Ro JY, Sahin AA, Lee JS, Ayala AG. Mucinous adenocarcinoma of the prostate with endobronchial metastasis. *Am J Clin Pathol* 1990;94:641.
108. Taylor H, Braude S. Lobar collapse due to endobronchial metastatic prostatic carcinoma: re-expansion with antiandrogen treatment. *Thorax* 1990;45:66.
109. Merine D, Fishman EK. Mediastinal adenopathy and endobronchial involvement in metastatic renal cell carcinoma. *J Comput Tomogr* 1988;12:216.
110. Noy S, Michowitz M, Lazebnik N, Baratz M. Endobronchial metastasis of renal cell carcinoma. *J Surg Oncol* 1986;31:268.
111. Varma VA, Lipper S, Kahn SB. Endobronchial metastasis from testicular seminoma. *Arch Pathol Lab Med* 1981;105:680.
112. Honma K, Mishina M, Watanabe Y. Polypoid endobronchial extension from invasive thymoma. *Virchows Arch Pathol Anat Histopathol.* 1988;413:469.
113. Asamura H, Morinaga S, Shimosato Y, Ono R, Naruke T. Thymoma dispalying endobronchial polypoid growth. *Chest* 1988; 94:647.
114. Harada T, Katagiri M. Hemostasis of the thyroid carcinoma invading the skin and trachea. Conservative treatment. *Thyroidol Clin Exp* 1990;2:29.
115. Britto E, Shah S, Parikh DM, Rao RS. Laryngotracheal invasion by well-differentiated thyroid cancer: diagnosis and management. *J Surg Oncol* 1990;44:25.
116. Lossos IS, Breuer R. Endobronchial metastasis from Hurthle cell thyroid carçinoma. *Chest* 1990;97:768.
117. Coaker LA, Sobonya RE, Davis JR. Endobronchial metastases from uterine cervical squamous carcinoma. *Arch Pathol Lab Med* 1984;108:269.
118. Giudice JC, Komansky H, Gordon R. Endobronchial metastasis of uterine leiomyosarcoma *JAMA* 1979;241:1684.
119. Flynn KJ, Kim HS. Endobronchial metastasis of uterine leiomyosarcoma. *JAMA* 1978;240:2080.
120. Eng J, Sabanathan S. Airway complications in relapsing polychondritis. *Ann Thorac Surg* 1991;51:686.
121. Udwadia ZF, Pilling JR, Jenkins PF, Harrison BD. Bronchoscopic and bronchographic findings in 12 patients with sarcoidosis and severe or progressive airways obstruction. *Thorax* 1990;45:272.
122. Abramowicz MJ, Ninane V, Depierreux M, de-Francquen P, Yernault JC. Tumour-like presentation of pulmonary sarcoidosis. *Eur Resp J* 1992;5:1286.
123. Murray ME, Stokes TC. Endobronchial sarcoidosis presenting as severe upper airways narrowing with normal chest radiograph. *Resp Med* 1991;85:425.
124. Armstrong JR, Radke JR, Kvale PA, Eichenhorn MS, Popovich J Jr. Endoscopic findings in sarcoidosis. Characteristics and correlations with radiographic staging and bronchial mucosal biopsy yield. *Ann Otol Rhinol Laryngol* 1981;90:339.
125. James DG, Barter S, Jash D, MacKinnon DM, Carstairs LS. Sarcoidosis of the upper respiratory tract. *J Laryngol Otol* 1982;96:711.
126. Wood DE, Mathisen DJ. Late complications of tracheotomy. *Clin Chest Med* 1991;12:597.
127. Prakash UBS, McCullough AE, Edell ES, Nienhuis DM. Tracheopathia osteoplastica: familial occurrence. *Mayo Clin Proc* 1989;64:1091.
128. Molloy AR, McMahon JN. Rapid progression of tracheal stenosis associated with tracheopathia osteo-chondroplastica. *Intensive Care Med* 1988;15:60.
129. Nienhuis DM, Prakash UBS, Edell ES. Tracheobronchopathia osteochondroplastica. *Ann Otol Rhinol Laryngol* 1990;99:689.
130. Van-Schoor J, Joos G, Pauwels R. Tracheobronchomegaly—the Mounier—Kuhn syndrome: report of two cases and review of the literature. *Eur Resp J* 1991;4:1303.
131. Woodring JH, Barrett PA, Rehm SR, Nurenberg P. Acquired tracheomegaly in adults as a complication of diffuse pulmonary fibrosis. *Am J Roentgenol* 1989;152:743.
132. Mehta AC, Livingston DR, Levine HL. Fiberoptic bronchoscope and Nd-YAG laser in treatment of severe epistaxis from nasal hereditary hemorrhagic telangectasia and hemangioma. *Chest* 1987;91:791.
133. Masson RP, Altose MD, Mayock RL. Isolated bronchial telangiectasia. *Chest* 1974;65:450.
134. Lincoln MJ, Shigeoka JW. Pulmonary telangiectasia without hypoxemia. *Chest* 1988;93:1097.
135. Amin R. Endobronchial involvement in Wegener's granulomatosis. *Postgrad Med J* 1983;59:452.
136. Eagleton LE, Rosher RB, Hawe A, Bilinsky RT. Radiation therapy and mechanical dilation of endobronchial obstruction secondary to Wegener's granulomatosis. *Chest* 1979;76:609.
137. Flye MW, Mundinger GH Jr, Fauci AS. Diagnostic and therapeutic aspects of the surgical approach to Wegener's granulomatosis. *J Thorac Cardiovasc Surg* 1979;77:331.
138. Lebovics RS, Hoffman GS, Leavitt RY, et al. The management of subglottic stenosis in patients with Wegener's granulomatosis. *Laryngoscope* 1992;102:1341.
139. Freitag L, Firusian N, Stamatis G, Greschuchna D. The role of bronchoscopy in pulmonary complications due to mustard gas inhalation. *Chest* 1991;100:1436.
140. Prakash UBS. Chemical warfare and bronchoscopy. *Chest* 1991;100:1486.
141. Hara KS, Prakash UBS. Fiberoptic bronchoscopy in the evaluation of acute chest and upper airway trauma. *Chest* 1989; 96:627.

Subject Index

G

H

M